Free Radicals in Biology and Medicine

FOURTH EDITION

Barry Halliwell

B.A. (OXON), D.PHIL. (OXON), D.SC (LOND)

and

John M.C. Gutteridge

PHD (LOND), D.SC (LOND)

Do not follow where the path may lead. Go instead where there is no path and leave a trail.

Muriel Strode

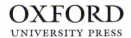

OXFORD
UNIVERSITY PRESS

OXFORD

UNIVERSITY PRESS

Great Clarendon Street, Oxford OX2 6DP

Oxford University Press is a department of the University of Oxford.
It furthers the University's objective of excellence in research, scholarship,
and education by publishing worldwide in

Oxford New York

Auckland Cape Town Dar es Salaam Hong Kong Karachi
Kuala Lumpur Madrid Melbourne Mexico City Nairobi
New Delhi Shanghai Taipei Toronto

With offices in

Argentina Austria Brazil Chile Czech Republic France Greece
Guatemala Hungary Italy Japan Poland Portugal Singapore
South Korea Switzerland Thailand Turkey Ukraine Vietnam

Oxford is a registered trade mark of Oxford University Press
in the UK and in certain other countries

Published in the United States
by Oxford University Press Inc., New York

First edition published 1985
Second edition published 1989
Third edition published 1999
This edition published 2007

Reprinted 2008, 2010, 2012

British Library Cataloguing in Publication Data
Data available

Library of Congress Cataloging in Publication Data
Data available

Typeset by Newgen Imaging Systems (P) Ltd., Chennai, India
Printed in Great Britain
on acid-free paper by
CPI Group (UK) Ltd, Croydon, CR04YY

ISBN 978–0–19–856868–1   978–0–19–856869–8 (Pbk.)

10 9 8 7 6 5

Dedication

We dedicate this edition to two pioneers in the field who died recently, Professors Dan Gilbert and Bernard Babior.

The same thing that makes you live can kill you in the end.

Neil Young

Preface to the fourth edition

When the first edition of *Free Radicals in Biology and Medicine* appeared in 1985, free radicals were mainly studied by radiation chemists and those involved in industrial processes and research relating to rubber, plastics, oils, paint and food (Table below). Two major scientific advances changed all this; the discovery of CuZnSOD by McCord and Fridovich in 1968, and the report by Bernie Babior in 1973 that activated neutrophils produce superoxide for microbicidal purposes. At this time, most of our indirect methodology for measuring the damage caused by free radicals came from the food industry, where the thiobarbituric acid (TBA) assay was widely used to detect and measure lipid rancidity. In hindsight, this distorted our interpretations by focusing attention on lipid peroxidation as a major causative event in disease processes. It also triggered a corresponding rush to find antioxidants that would protect against it. The explosive growth of interest that followed necessitated the writing of a second edition 4 years later (1989). The third edition (1999) reflected an enormous expansion in new methodologies to detect and measure oxidative damage to proteins, carbohydrates, DNA and lipids. These changes quickly led to the realization that free radicals and other reactive species are consequential to most (fortunately not all) disease processes, and by implication antioxidants would in general terms be limited and selective in their efficacy. A new free radical, nitric oxide ($NO^\bullet$), gained prominence, some of the discoverers of its biological role being awarded a Nobel Prize. Nitric oxide research reinforced the increasingly recognized concept that free radicals and other 'reactive species' have purposeful and beneficial roles to play in biology, with cell and molecular biology techniques making a significant contribution to this development. Some remain sceptical about the whole concept of free radicals

and antioxidants in biological processes. We remain convinced that they permeate the whole of biology and knowledge of them is essential to understand how aerobic life works. For sceptics we can always replace the free radical/ reactive species/ antioxidant terminology with phrases such as 'biological electron transfers', 'vitamins' and 'trace nutrients'. The signalling and messenger functions of reactive species are major areas expanded in the fourth edition. Superoxide, $NO^\bullet$ and hydrogen peroxide are poorly reactive (see editions 1, 2 and 3) and better suited to signalling functions than to overwhelmingly destructive chemical reactions. Nevertheless, their potential for selective cytotoxicity is clear. Precise molecular characterisation of oxidative damage is gradually replacing TBA and carbonyl assays, and revealing a wealth of new information about molecular processes in ageing and disease.

We hope that the fourth edition becomes the 'Fourth bridge' (edition 3) to span the gap between experts and novices. Will we need a fifth edition, and when? We think so, but as Norman Krinsky once said 'It is hard to make predictions, particularly about the future'.

B.H.

Deputy President (Research and Technology)
Executive Director, Graduate School for
 Integrative Sciences and Engineering
National University of Singapore, Singapore

J.M.C.G

Visiting Scientist
Royal Brompton and Harefield National Health
 Service Trust
National Heart and Lung Institute
Imperial College School of Medicine,
 London, UK

Milestones in free radical research

Discovery	Year
Demonstration of oxygen toxicity	1785 (Joseph Priestley)
Discovery of selenium	1817
First attempts to study oil oxidation by O_2 uptake	1820
Oxygen causes rancidification of natural oils	1822
Fenton reaction first described	1876
First report of a free radical (triphenylmethyl)	1900, by Gomberg
Discovery of vitamin E	1922
Isolation of vitamin C	1928
Postulation of the Haber–Weiss reaction	1934
Basic mechanism of lipid peroxidation elucidated	1940s
Sperm discovered to be susceptible to oxidative damage	1943
Development of electron spin resonance	1945
Proposal that free radicals account for damage by ionizing radiation	1954
Identification of retinopathy of prematurity as an O_2 toxicity	1954
Proposal that free radicals cause ageing	1956
Discovery of glutathione peroxidase	1957
Synergy between ascorbate and α-tocopherol suggested	1968
Spin traps first developed	1968
Discovery of the SOD activity of CuZnSOD	1968–69
First identification of $O_2^{\bullet-}$ production by an enzyme	1969
First description of phagocyte $O_2^{\bullet-}$ production*	1973
Aromatic hydroxylation introduced as an assay for $OH^{\bullet}$	1975
First description of the effects of ROS on the vascular system	1981
FIRST EDITION OF THIS BOOK	1985
Term 'oxidative stress' introduced	1985
Identification of nitric oxide as the endothelium-derived relaxing factor	1987
SECOND EDITION OF THIS BOOK	1989
Discovery of OxyR and SoxR	1990
Introduction of the isoprostanes as an assay for lipid peroxidation	1991
ROS activate the transcription factor NF-κB in some systems	1991
Detailed characterization of peroxiredoxins	1994 onwards
THIRD EDITION OF THIS BOOK	1999

* By Bernie Babior, one of the pioneers to whom this book is dedicated.

Preface to the third edition

When we first sat down (in January 1996) to write a third edition, we optimistically assumed that it could be finished by June. We underestimated the pace of advance in this subject: almost every section has needed extensive updating. Sometimes our job was easier: new data have often clarified the previously obscure, especially data obtained using the techniques of modern molecular, cellular, and structural biology. More often, however, new data have transformed the way in which scientists think about a particular topic, requiring complete rewriting. We have tried to maintain the essential simplicity of our approach and readability of the text, and hope that we have succeeded. Several reviewers of the second edition requested specific referencing in the text. This is more difficult than it seems because many of the statements made are distilled from several published papers and interpreted through the scientific experiences (or prejudices) of the authors. Citing every relevant paper would generate a book three times the length, out-of-date within six months and too expensive for most people to buy. As a compromise each major statement in the text is now provided with at least one reference, either cited as a superscript in the text or placed in the legend of an adjacent figure or table. References quoted are not always the seminal ones, as we have tried to choose references (often reviews or recent papers) that should make it easy for the reader to access further literature. We hope that experts will forgive us if they find their pet paper uncited.

During the rewriting of the second edition, we felt like painters of the Forth Bridge. Having completed the third edition, we feel like early retirement.

London
September 1998

B.H.
J.M.C.G.

Preface to the second edition

The explosive growth of interest in free radicals, and the enormous amount of research work undertaken since 1984, has necessitated the writing of a second edition of this book after only three years. During the extensive rewriting necessary, we have sometimes felt like painters of the Forth Bridge. Production of the revised edition has been helped by information and critical comments provided by the following scientists, to whom we are very grateful. Any remaining errors are the entire responsibility of the authors, however.

B.N. Ames	T. Connors	D.J. Hockley	Philips Analytical
B. Anderton	F. Corongiu	R.L. Hoult	E.A. Porta
B.M. Babior	J.T. Curnutte	V. Kagan	W.A. Pryor
D.R. Blake	C. Dahlgren	D. Leake	C. Rice-Evans
J.M. Braughler	A.T. Diplock	T. Lindahl	G. Rotilio
L. Breimer	E.A. Dratz	M. Matsuo	L.L. Smith
G. Burton	H. Esterbauer	M.J. Mitchinson	T.F. Slater
R. Cammack	I. Fridovich	D.P.R. Muller	Y. Sugiura
C.J. Chesterton	E. Getzoff	H.J. Okamoto	S.P. Wolff
			R.L. Willson

London
October 1988

B.H.
J.M.C.G.

Preface to the first edition

The importance of radical reactions in radiation damage, food preservation, combustion, and in the rubber and paint industry, has been known for many years to people in the respective fields, but it has rarely been appreciated by biologists and clinicians. The interest in radicals shown by the latter groups has been raised recently by the discovery of the importance of radical reactions in normal body chemistry and in the mode of action of many toxins. The discoveries of hypoxic cell sensitizers that potentiate radiation-induced radical damage to cancerous tumours, of the enzyme superoxide dismutase, and of the mechanism of action of such toxins as paraquat and carbon tetrachloride provide major examples of this importance.

Any expanding field attracts the charlatans, such as those who make money out of proposing that consuming radical scavengers will make you live for ever or that taking tablets containing superoxide dismutase will enhance your health and sex life. In evaluating these and other less obviously silly claims, it is useful to understand the basic chemistry of radical reactions.

This book is aimed mainly at biologists and clinicians. It assumes virtually no knowledge of chemistry and attempts to lead the reader as painlessly as possible into an understanding of what free radicals are, how they are generated, and how they can react. Having established this basis, the role of radical reactions in several biological systems is critically evaluated in the hope that the careful techniques needed to prove their importance will become more widely used. We believe that free-radical chemists should also find these latter chapters useful.

London

B.H.
J.M.C.G.

Acknowledgements

Production of the fourth edition was aided by advice and/or permission to reproduce their published material from the following experts, acknowledged in alphabetical order of surname. We are most grateful for their help, but the responsibility for any errors in the text is solely ours.

Jeffrey Armstrong (Singapore)
Brian Backsai, Charlestown (USA)
James Barber, London (UK)
Shannon Bailey, Birmingham (USA)
Karim Bensaad, Glasgow (UK)
Ranjita Betarbet, Atlanta (USA)
Michael Betenbaugh, Baltimore (USA)
Guy Brown, Cambridge (UK)
Urs Boelsterli (Singapore)
John Butler, Salford (UK)
Ioav Cabantchik, Jerusalem (Israel)
Robin Carrell, Cambridge (UK)
Vincent Castranova, Morgantown (USA)
Pierre-Etienne Chabrier, Les Ulis (France)
Colin Chignell, Bethesda (USA)
Marie Clement (Singapore)
Marcus Cooke, Leicester (UK)
Peter Crack, Melbourne (Australia)
James Crapo, Denver (USA)
Carroll Cross, Davis (USA)
Jeffrey Cummings, Los Angeles (USA)
Brain Day, Denver (USA)
Miral Dizdaroglu, Gaithersburg (USA)
Mark Evans, Leicester (UK)
Gerald Evans, San Francisco (USA)
Christine Foyer, Rothamsted (UK)
Irwin Fridovich, Durham (USA)
Erroll Friedberg, Dallas (USA)
Jurgen Fuchs, Frankfurt (Germany)
Helen Galley, Aberdeen (UK)
David Gems, London (UK)
Elizabeth Getzoff, La Jolla (USA)
Boon Cher Goh (Singapore)

Timothy Greenamyre, Pittsburgh (USA)
Jan Gruber (Singapore)
Fred Guengerich, Nashville (USA)
Jeremiah Harnett, Les Ulis (France)
Ralph Hückelhoven, Giesen (Germany)
Peter Jenner, London (UK)
Balyanaraman Kalyanaraman, Milwaukee (USA)
Frank Kelly, London (UK)
Ronan Kelly (Singapore)
Michael Kemeny (Singapore)
Vuokko Kinnula, Helsinki (Finland)
Nick Lane, Oxford (UK)
Peter Libby, Boston (USA)
Valter Longo, Los Angeles (USA)
Jamie Macdonald, Aberdeen (UK)
Gerassimos Makrigiorgos, Boston (USA)
Jason Marrow, Nashville (USA)
Ronald Mason, Research Triangle Park (USA)
Joshua McElwee, London (UK)
Marilyn Merker, Milwaukee (USA)
Giorgio Minotti, Chieti (Italy)
Vincent Monnier, Cleveland (USA)
Philip Moore (Singapore)
Martin Mueller, Würzburg (Germany)
Robert Murphy, Denver (USA)
Tetsuo Nagano, Tokyo (Japan)
Etsuo Niki, Tokyo (Japan)
Peter O'Brien, Toronto (Canada)
Takashi Okamoto, Nagoya (Japan)
Lester Packer, Berkeley (USA)
Mario Podda, Sassari (Italy)
Alfonso Pompella, Siena (Italy)

Franklyn Prendergast, Rochester (USA)
Gregory Quinlan, London (UK)
Sue Goo Rhee, Bethesda (USA)
Robert Ridley, Geneva (Switzerland)
Ivonne Rietjens, Wageningen (Netherlands)
Jackson Roberts II, Nashville (USA)
Dirk Roos, Philadelphia (USA)
Pauline Rudd, Oxford (UK)
Aziz Sancar, Chapel Hill (USA)
Kim Ping Sit (Singapore)
Roland Stocker, Sydney (Australia)
John Tainer, La Jolla (USA)
Toshifumi Tetsuka, Nagoya (Japan)
Shane Thomas, Sydney (Australia)
Michael Toledano, Gif-sur-Yvette (France)

Paul Tordo, Marseilles (France)
Shinya Toyokuni, Kyoto (Japan)
Maret Traber, Corvallis (USA)
Gabriel Travis, Los Angeles (USA)
Julio Turrens, Mobile (USA)
Karen Vousden, Glasgow (USA)
Nigel Webster, Aberdeen (UK)
Matthew Whiteman (Singapore)
Christine Winterbourn, Christchurch
 (New Zealand)
Karel Wirtz, Utrecht (Netherlands)
Boon Seng Wong (Singapore)
John Eu Li Wong (Singapore)
Moussa Youdim, Rehovot (Israel)
Ben-Zhan Zhu, Corvallis (USA)

Contents

Abbreviations

Where the same abbreviation is used for more than one item, the one listed first is that most commonly used in this book.

AA	Arachidonic acid
A2E	N-retinylidene-N-retinylethanolamine
A2PE-H$_2$	Dihydro-N-retinylidene-N-retinyl-phosphatidylethanolamine
AAPH	2,2′-Azobis(2-amidinopropane) dihydrochloride
Aβ	Beta-amyloid peptides
ABAD	Amyloid β-binding alcohol dehydrogenase
ABTS	2,2′-Azinobis (3-ethylbenzothiazoline-6-sulphonate)
ACE	Angiotensin converting enzyme
AD	Alzheimer's disease
AdhE	Alcohol dehydrogenase E (*E. coli*)
ADMA	Asymmetrical dimethylarginine
AEOL	Aeolus (pharmaceuticals)
AGE	Advanced glycation end-product
AHPR	Alkyl hydroperoxide reductase
AHR	Aryl hydrocarbon receptor
AHSP	α-Haemoglobin stabilizing protein
AIDS	Acquired immunodeficiency syndrome
AIPH	2,2′-Azobis[2-(3-imidazolin-2-yl) propane dihydrochloride]
δ-ALA	δ-Aminolaevulinic acid
ALS	Amyotrophic lateral sclerosis
AMPA	α-Amino-3-hydroxy-5-methyl-4-isoxazole-4-propionate
AMPK	AMP-activated protein kinase
AMVN	2,2′-Azobis(2,4-dimethylvaleronitrile)
AOC	Allene oxide cyclase
AOS	Allene oxide synthase
AP	Apurinic/apyrimidinic (site) *or* alternative pathway
α_1-AP	α_1-Antiproteinase
AP-1	Activator protein 1
APAF-1	Apoptotic proteinase activating factor 1
APE1	Apurinic/apyrimidinic endonuclease 1
APF	2-[6-(4′-Amino) phenoxy-3H-xanthen-3-on-9-yl] benzoic acid
apoA1	Apolipoprotein A-1
apoA2	Apolipoprotein A-2
apoB	Apolipoprotein B
apoE	Apolipoprotein E
APP	Amyloid precursor protein
ARDS	Acute respiratory distress syndrome
ARE	Antioxidant response element
AREDS	Age-related eye disease study
ARP	Aldehyde-reactive probe
ASAP	Antioxidant supplementation in atherosclerosis prevention (trial)
ASK	Apoptosis signal-regulating kinase
At	*Arabidopsis thaliana*
ATBC	α-Tocopherol β-carotene cancer prevention study
ATM	Ataxia telangiectasia mutated
AVED	Ataxia with isolated vitamin E deficiency
AZN	Azulenylnitrone
AZT	Azidodeoxythymidine
BAL	British anti-lewisite
BAT	Brown adipose tissue

BB	Biobreeding (rat)
BCI	Bleomycin-chelatable iron
BCNU	*N,N*-bis(2-chloroethyl)-*N*-nitrosourea
BDNF	Brain-derived neurotrophic factor
BER	Base excision repair
BHA	Butylated hydroxyanisole
BHF	British Heart Foundation
BHT	Butylated hydroxytoluene
BLM	Bleomycin
BNB	*tert*-Butylnitrosobenzene
BPD	Bronchopulmonary dysplasia
BPDS	Bathophenanthroline disulphonate
BrdU	5-Bromo-2′-deoxyuridine
BSD	Bypass SOD deficiency (gene)
BSE	Bovine spongiform encephalopathy
BSO	Buthionine sulphoximine
C11-BODIPY$^{581/591}$	
	4,4-Difluoro-5-(4-phenyl-1,3-butadienyl)-4-bora-3a,4a-diaza-*s*-indacene-3-undecanoic acid
CAD	Caspase-activated deoxyribonuclease
CAL	Calcein
CALPAIN	Calcium-activated non-lysosomal proteinase
CARET	*β*-Carotene and retinol efficiency trial
CASPASE	Cysteine-aspartyl-specific protease
CCA	Coumarin-3-carboxylic acid
CCP	Cytochrome *c* peroxidase
CCS	Copper chaperone for SOD
CD	Cluster of differentiation
CdK	Cyclin-dependent protein kinase
CDNB	1-Chloro-2,4-dinitrobenzene
α-CEHC	2,5,7,8-Tetramethyl-2-(2′-carboxyethyl)-6-hydroxychroman
γ-CEHC	2,7,8-Trimethyl-2-(2′carboxyethyl)-6-hydroxychroman
CF	Cystic fibrosis
CFTR	Cystic fibrosis transmembrane conductance regulator
CGD	Chronic granulomatous disease

CHAOS	Cambridge heart antioxidant study
CHD	Coronary heart disease
CHO	Chinese hamster ovary
CJD	Creutzfeldt–Jakob disease
vCJD	Variant Creutzfeldt–Jakob disease
CK	Creatine kinase
CLA	Conjugated linoleic acid
Clk-1	Clock-1 (gene)
CNS	Central nervous system
CNTF	Ciliary neurotrophic factor
COMT	Catechol-*O*-methyltransferase
COPD	Chronic obstructive pulmonary disease
COPs	Cholesterol oxidation products
CoQ	Coenzyme Q (ubiquinone)
CoQH$_2$	Reduced coenzyme Q (ubiquinol)
COX	Cyclooxygenase
CP	Classical pathway
CR	Caloric restriction
CRP	C-reactive protein
11cRAL	11-*cis*-Retinal
11cROL	11-*cis*-Retinol
CS	Cockayne's syndrome *or* cigarette smoke
CSF	Cerebrospinal fluid *or* Colony-stimulating factor
CuZnSOD	Copper-and-zinc-containing superoxide dismutase
CUPRAC	Cupric reducing antioxidant capacity
CyclodA	8,5′-Cyclo-2′-deoxyadenosine
CyclodG	8,5′-Cyclo-2′-deoxyguanosine
CYP	Cytochrome P450
DAB	Diaminobenzidine
DABCO	1,4-Diazabicyclooctane
DAF-2DA	4,5-Diaminofluorescein diacetate
DAG	Diacylglycerol
DBNBS	3,5-Dibromo-4-nitroso-benzene-sulphonic acid
DCF	2′,7′-Dichlorofluorescein
DCFH	2′,7′-Dichlorodihydrofluorescein
DCFDA	Dichloroflorescin (2′,7′-dichlorodihydrofluorescein) diacetate
ddC	Dideoxycytidine
ddI	Dideoxyinosine
DDTC	Diethyldithiocarbamate

DED	Death effector domain	EGF	Epidermal growth factor
DEPMPO	5-Diethoxyphosphoryl-5-methyl-1-pyrroline-*N*-oxide	EGFR	Epidermal growth factor receptor
		EL	Ethyl linoleate
DETAPAC	Diethylenetriaminepenta-acetic acid	EMPO	5-Ethoxycarbonyl-5-methyl-1-pyrroline-*N*-oxide
DFO	Desferrioxamine	EPA	Eicosapentaenoic acid
DHA	Dehydroascorbate *or* docosahexaenoic acid	EPO	Eosinophil peroxidase
		EPR	Electron paramagnetic resonance
2,3-DHB	2,3-Dihydroxybenzoate	ER	Endoplasmic reticulum
2,5-DHB	2,5-Dihydroxybenzoate	ERK	Extracellular signal related kinase
DHE	Dihydroethidium	Ero	Endoplasmic reticulum oxidoreductase
DHF	Dihydroxyfumarate		
DHLA	Dihydrolipoate	ESR	Electron spin resonance
DHR	Dihydrorhodamine 123	ETS	Environmental tobacco smoke
DIABLO	Direct inhibition of apoptosis protein binding with low ρI	ETYA	5,8,11,14-Eicosatetraynoic acid
		EUK	Eukarion (company)
DISC	Death-induced signalling complex	EURAMIC	European Community multicentre study on antioxidants, myocardial infarction and breast cancer
DMEM	Dulbecco's Modified Eagle's Medium		
DMF	Dimethylformamide	FA	Freidreich's ataxia *or* Fanconi's anaemia
DMPO	5,5-Dimethylpyrroline-*N*-oxide		
DMSO	Dimethylsulphoxide	Fas	Fibroblast-associated cell surface
DMT1	Divalent metal transporter-1	FAD	Flavin adenine dinucleotide
DMTU	Dimethylthiourea	$FADH_2$	Reduced flavin adenine dinucleotide
DNPH	2,4–Dinitrophenylhydrazine		
DOD-8C	(*N*-[4-dodecyloxy-2-(7'-carboxy-hept-1'-yloxy)benzylidene]-*N-tert*- butylamine *N*-oxide)	FAK	Focal adhesion kinase
		FALS	Familial amyotrophic lateral sclerosis
DOPA	L-Dihydroxyphenylalanine	FAPyG	2,6-Diamino-4-hydroxy-5-formamidopyrimidine
DOPAC	3,4-Dihydroxyphenylacetic acid		
DPI	Diphenylene iodonium	FGF	Fibroblast growth factor
DPPD	N,N'-Diphenyl-*p*-phenylenediamine	FMN	Flavin mononucleotide
		$FMNH_2$	Reduced flavin mononucleotide
DPPH	1,1-Diphenyl-2-picrylhydrazyl	FOXO	Forkhead transcription factor, class O
Dpr	Dps-like peroxide resistance protein		
		Fur	Ferric uptake regulator
Dps	DNA binding protein during stationary phase		
		GABA	γ-Aminobutyrate
DS	Down's syndrome	γGCS	γ-Glutamylcysteine synthetase
DTNB	5,5'-Dithiobis(2-nitrobenzoic acid)	γGGT	γ-Glutamyl transpeptidase
DUOX	Dual oxidase	G3PDH	Glyceraldehyde-3-phosphate dehydrogenase
EBV	Epstein–Barr virus	G6PDH	Glucose-6-phosphate dehydrogenase
EC-SOD	Extracellular superoxide dismutase		
		GA	Glucuronic acid
EDRF	Endothelium-derived relaxing factor	GABA	γ-Aminobutyrate
EDTA	Ethylenediamine tetraacetic acid	GADD	Growth arrest on DNA damage

GC	Gas chromatography	HPII	Hydroperoxidase II
GFP	Green fluorescent protein	HPD	Haematoporphyin derivative
GHz	Gigahertz	12-HPETE	12-Hydroperoxy-5,8,11,14-eicosatetraenoic acid
GI-GPx	Gastrointestinal glutathione peroxidase (see GPx2)	HPF	2-[6-(4′-Hydroxyl)phenoxyl-3H-xanthen-3-on-9-yl] benzoic acid
GI tract	Gastrointestinal tract	HPLC	High-performance liquid chromatography
GM-CSF	Granulocyte-macrophage colony stimulating factor	HPO	High-pressure oxygen
GO	Galactose oxidase	HRP	Horseradish peroxidase
GOT	Glutamate-oxaloacetate transaminase	HSF	Heat-shock transcription factor
GPx	Glutathione peroxidase	HSP	Heat-shock protein
GPx2	Intestinal glutathione peroxidase (see GI-GPx)	5-HT	5-Hydroxytryptamine
GPx3	Extracellular glutathione peroxidase	HTGL	Hepatic triglyceride lipase
		HTLV	Human T-cell leukaemia virus
GPx4	Phospholipid hydroperoxide glutathione peroxidase	HX	Hypoxanthine
GPT	Glutamate-pyruvate transaminase	IAP	Inhibition of apoptosis protein
GR	Glutathione reductase	IBD	Inflammatory bowel disease
GSH	Reduced glutathione	ICAD	Inhibitor of caspase-activated deoxyribonuclease
GSSG	Oxidized glutathione		
GST	Glutathione-S-transferase	ICAM	Intercellular adhesion molecule
Gy	Gray (radiation dose)	ICE	Interleukin-1β converting enzyme
		IDO	Indoleamine dioxygenase
HBED	N,N-*bis*(2-hydroxybenzyl) ethylenediamine-N,N-diacetic acid	IgA	Immunoglobulin A
		IgE	Immunoglobulin E
HBO	Hyperbaric oxygen	IGF-1	Insulin-like growth factor 1
HBV	Hepatitis B virus	IgG	Immunoglobulin G
HCS	Hypoxic cell sensitizer	IgM	Immunoglobulin M
HD	Huntington's disease	IL-1	Interleukin-1
HDC	6-Hydroxy-1,4-dimethylcarbazole	ILBD	Incidental Lewy body disease
HDL	High-density lipoproteins	IP	Isoprostane
12-HETE	12-Hydroxy-5,8,11,14-eicosatetraenoic acid	IP-10	Inducible protein 10
		IP$_3$	Inositol triphosphate
HGF	Hepatocyte growth factor	IRE	Iron responsive element
HHE	*Trans*-4-Hydroxy-2-hexenal	IRP	Iron regulatory protein
HHT	12-Hydroxy-5,8,10-heptadecatrienoic acid	I-TAC	Interferon-inducible T-cell α-chemoattractant
HIF	Hypoxia inducible factor		
HIV	Human immunodeficiency virus	JNK	c-Jun N-terminal kinase
HL	Hydroperoxide lyase		
HMGB1	High mobility group 1 protein	KA	Kainic acid
HNE	4-Hydroxy-2-*trans*-nonenal	Keap-1	Kelch-like (erythroid cell-derived protein with CNC homology)-associated protein-1
HNF-1α	Hepatic nuclear factor 1α		
HO	Haem oxygenase		
HOPE	Heart outcomes prevention evaluation (study)	αKGDH	α-Ketoglutarate dehydrogenase
		KGF	Keratinocyte growth factor
HPI	Hydroperoxidase I	kJ	Kilojoule

LA	Lipoic acid
LCAT	Lecithin-cholesterol acyltransferase
LDH	Lactate dehydrogenase
LDL	Low-density lipoproteins
LEC	Long–Evans Cinnamon (rat)
LFA	Lymphocyte function antigen
LGD_2	Levuglandin D_2
LGE_2	Levuglandin E_2
LHON	Leber's hereditary optic neuropathy
LIP	Labile iron pool
LOX	Lipoxygenase
LOX-1	Lipoxygenase-1 *or* Lectin-like oxidised low density lipoprotein receptor-1
LP	Lectin pathway
LPL	Lipoprotein lipase
LPO	Lactoperoxidase
LPS	Lipopolysaccharide (endotoxin)
LRAT	Lecithin retinol acyltransferase
LTA_4	Leukotriene A_4
LTB_4	Leukotriene B_4
LTC_4	Leukotriene C_4
LTD_4	Leukotriene D_4
LTE_4	Leukotriene E_4
M	Molar
μM	Micromolar
mM	Millimolar
nM	Nanomolar
pM	Picomolar
M_1G	Pyrimido [1,2α] purine 10(3H)-one
MAC	Membrane attack complex
MAO-A	Monoamine oxidase A
MAO-B	Monoamine oxidase B
MAP	Mitogen activated protein (kinase)
MAT	Methionine adenosyltransferase
MBL	Mannose binding lectin
MCI	Mild cognitive impairment
MCLA	2-Methyl-6-(4-methoxyphenyl)-3,7-dihydroimidazo[1,2-α] pyrazin-3-one
MCP-1	Monocyte chemoattractant protein 1
MCSF	Macrophage colony-stimulating factor

MDA	Malondialdehyde *or* 3,4-Methylenedioxyamphetamine
MDMA	3,4-Methylenedioxymethylamphetamine
MDT	Marine-derived tocopherol
MEG	Mercaptoethylguanidine
MELAS	Mitochondrial encephalomyopathy, lactic acidosis and stroke-like episodes
MEOS	Microsomal ethanol-oxidizing system
fMet–leu–phe	*N*-formylmethionylleucylphenylalanine
Mig	Monokine induced by interferon-γ
MIP	Monocyte inflammatory protein
MMP	Matrix metalloproteinase
MnSOD	Manganese-containing superoxide dismutase
MODS	Multiple organ dysfunction syndrome
MODY	Maturity onset diabetes of the young
MOG	Myelin oligodendrocyte glycoprotein
MOX	Mitogenic oxidase
MPB	3-(*N*-maleimidylpropionyl) biocytin
$MPDP^+$	1-Methyl-4-phenyl-2,3-dihydropyridine ion
MPG	Mercaptopropionylglycine
MPO	Myeloperoxidase
MPP^+	1-Methyl-4-phenylpyridinium ion
MPT	Mitochondrial permeability transition
MPTP	1-Methyl-4-phenyl-1,2,3,6-tetrahydropyridine
MR	Methaemoglobin reductase
MRC	Medical Research Council (UK)
MRI	Magnetic resonance imaging
MS	Multiple sclerosis
MSR	Methionine sulphoxide reductase
MT	Metallothionein
MTH1	Mut T homologue one
MTT	3-(4,5 Dimethylthiazol-2-yl)-2,5-diphenyl-2-H tetrazolium bromide
MYA	Million years ago
hMYH	Human mut Y analogue

NAAQS	National ambient air quality standard (USA)		NSAID	Non-steroidal anti-inflammatory drug
NAc	*N*-acetylcysteine		Nt	*Nicotiana tabacum*
NAD$^+$	Nicotinamide adenine dinucleotide		NTA	Nitrilotriacetate
NADH	Reduced nicotinamide adenine dinucleotide		NTBI	Non-transferrin-bound iron
NADP$^+$	Nicotinamide adenine dinucleotide phosphate		ODS	Osteogenic disorder Shionogi (rat)
			6-OHDA	6-Hydroxydopamine
NADPH	Reduced nicotinamide adenine dinucleotide phosphate		8OHdG	8-Hydroxy-2′-deoxyguanosine
			8OHG	8-Hydroxyguanine
NAG	*N*-Acetylglucosamine		ORAC	Oxygen radical absorbance capacity
NBT	Nitroblue tetrazolium		OTC	L-2-Oxothiazolidine-4-carboxylate
NCL	Neuronal ceroid lipofuscinoses		Ox-LDL	Oxidized low-density lipoprotein
NDGA	Nordihydroguaiaretic acid		8oxodG	8-Oxo-7-hydro-2′-deoxyguanosine
NER	Nucleotide excision repair			
8-NG	8-Nitroguanine		OxPAPC	Oxidized 1-palmitoyl-2-arachidonoyl-*sn*-glycero-3-phosphorylcholine
NGF	Nerve growth factor			
NHANES	National Health and Nutrition Examination Survey			
NHPA	3-Nitro-4-hydroxyphenylacetate		PAF	Platelet-activating factor
NIA	National Institute of Aging (USA)		PAL	Present atmospheric level
NiSOD	Nickel-containing superoxide dismutase		PAPC	Palmitoyl-2-arachidonoyl-*sn*-glycero-3-phosphorylcholine
NIST	National Institute of Standards and Technology (USA)		PARP	Poly(ADP-ribose) polymerase
			PBG	Porphobilinogen
NK	Natural killer (cell)		PBN	α-Phenyl-*tert*-butylnitrone
NMDA	*N*-Methyl-D-aspartate		PC	Plastocyanin *or* phosphatidylcholine
NMMA	N^G-Monomethyl-L-arginine			
NMP	3-Nitratomethyl-PROXYL		PCC	Phenanthroline-chelatable copper
NNK	4-(Methylnitrosamine)-1-(3-pyridyl)-1-butanone		PCD	Programmed cell death
			PCP	Pentachlorophenol
NNO	Nitronylnitroxide		PCR	Polymerase chain reaction
NOD	Non-obese diabetic (mouse)		PD	Parkinson's disease
NOS	Nitric oxide synthase		PDGF	Platelet-derived growth factor
eNOS	Endothelial nitric oxide synthase		PDH	Pyruvate dehydrogenase
iNOS	Inducible nitric oxide synthase		PDI	Protein disulphide isomerase
nNOS	Neuronal nitric oxide synthase		PDK	Phosphoinositide-dependent kinase
NP	Neuroprostane			
Nramp1	Natural murine resistance associated macrophage protein-1		PE	Phosphatidylethanolamine
			PECAM	Platelet-endothelial cell adhesion molecule
N-ret-PE	*N*-Retinylidene-phosphatidylethanolamine			
			PEG	Polyethylene glycol
NRF1	Nuclear respiratory factor 1		PFL	Pyruvate–formate lyase
Nrf2	Nuclear factor erythroid 2 p4–5-related factor 2		PFOR	Pyruvate–ferredoxin oxidoreductase
NRF2	Nuclear respiratory factor 2		PG	Prostaglandin

pGPx	Plasma glutathione peroxidase (*also see* GPx3)	RBS	Reactive bromine species
PHGPx	Phospholipid hydroperoxide glutathione peroxidase (also see GPx4)	RCS	Reactive chlorine species
		RDA	Recommended dietary allowance
		atRE	all-*trans*-Retinyl esters
Phox	Phagocyte oxidase	Ref-1	Redox effector factor 1
PI	Propidium iodide	RNR	Ribonucleotide reductase
PIH	Pyridoxal isonicotinoyl hydrazone	RNS	Reactive nitrogen species
		atRAL	all-*trans*-Retinal
PKA	Protein kinase A	atROL	all-*trans*-Retinol
PKB	Protein kinase B	ROS	Reactive oxygen species
PKC	Protein kinase C	ROP	Retinopathy of prematurity
PLC	Phospholipase C	RPE	Retinal pigment epithelium
PLD	Phospholipase D	RS	Reactive species
PMA	Phorbol myristate acetate	RSS	Reactive sulphur species
4-POBN	α-(4-Pyridyl-1-oxide)-*N-tert*-butylnitrone	RSV	Respiratory syncytial virus
Pol γ	DNA polymerase γ	SAM	*S*-Adenosyl methionine
PON-1	Paraoxonase-1	SAR	Systemic acquired resistance
PPAR	Peroxisome proliferator activated receptor	SCA	Senescent cell antigen
		SCID	Severe combined immunodeficient
PPP	Pentose phosphate pathway	SDA	Semidehydroascorbate
PQ	Plastoquinone	SDS	Sodium dodecyl sulphate
PR	Promethazine	SERPIN	Serine proteinase inhibitor
Prx	Peroxiredoxin	SF	Synovial fluid
PS	Phosphatidylserine	SFRR	Society for Free Radical Research
PSI	Photosystem I	SHEEP	Stockholm heart epidemiology programme
PSII	Photosystem II		
PTEN	Phosphatase and tensin homologue	SHR	Spontaneously hypertensive rat
		SIH	Salicylaldehyde isonicotinoylhydrazone
PUFA	Polyunsaturated fatty acid		
PUVA	Psoralen ultraviolet A (therapy)	Sir	Silent information regulator
		SIRS	Systemic inflammatory response syndrome
QR	Quinone reductase		
		SIRT	Sirtuin
RA	Rheumatoid arthritis	Sirtuin	Silent information regulator-like protein
RAGE	Receptor for advanced glycation end-products		
		SMAC	Second mitochondria-derived activator of caspases
atRAL	all-*trans*-Retinal		
RANK	Receptor for activator of NF-κB	SLE	Systemic lupus erythematosus
RANKL	Receptor for activator of NF-κB, ligand	SN	Substantia nigra
		SNAP	*S*-nitroso-*N*-acetyl-DL-penicillamine
RANTES	Regulation upon activation, normal T-cell expressed and secreted.		
		SNP	Sodium nitroprusside
		SOD	Superoxide dismutase
RBOH	Respiratory burst oxidase homologue	SOR	Superoxide reductase
		SOTS	Di(4-carboxybenzyl) hyponitrite

SRA	Scavenger receptors A		TRAIL	Tumour necrosis factor related apoptosis inducing ligand
SREBP	Sterol regulatory element binding protein		TRBP	Telomere repeat binding protein
STAZN	Stilbazulenyl nitrone		TRPM	Transient receptor potential melastatin-related (ion channels)
SUVIMAX	Supplementation en vitamins et mineraux antioxidant		Trx	Thioredoxin
SVCT	Sodium-vitamin C transporter		α-TTP	α-Tocopherol transfer protein
			TUNEL	TdT-mediated X-dUTP nick end-labelling
TAC	Total antioxidant capacity		TX	Thromboxane
Tat	Transactivator of transcription			
TBA	Thiobarbituric acid		UCHL1	Ubiquitin carboxy-terminal hydrolase L1
TBARS	Thiobarbituric acid-reactive substances		UV	Ultraviolet
TBHQ	*tert*-Butylhydroquinone			
TCBQ	Tetrachlorobenzoquinone		VA	Veratryl alcohol
TCDD	2,3,7,8-Tetrachlorodibenzo-*p*-dioxin		VAP	Vascular adhesion protein
TCHQ	Tetrachlorohydroquinone		VCAM	Vascular cell adhesion molecule
TCR	Transcription-coupled repair		VDAC	Voltage-dependent anion-selective channel
TDO	Tryptophan 2,3-dioxygenase			
TDS	Translesional DNA synthesis		VEAPS	Vitamin E atherosclerosis prevention study
TdT	Terminal deoxynucleotidyl transferase		VEGF	Vascular endothelial growth factor
TEAC	Trolox equivalent antioxidant capacity		VHL	von Hippel–Lindau
TGF-β	Transforming growth factor β		VLDL	Very low-density lipoproteins
THF	Tetrahydrofolate		Vtc	
THOX	Thyroid oxidase		mutant	Vitamin C mutant (in *Arabidopsis*)
TIBS	*Trends in Biochemical Sciences*			
TIMP	Tissue inhibitor of metalloproteinases		WAVE	Women's angiographic vitamin and oestrogen (trial)
TiP	Thioredoxin interacting protein		WR	Walter Reed (army hospital, USA)
TMINO	1,1,3-Trimethyl-isoindole *N*-oxide			
tNB (NtB)	*tert*-Nitrosobutane (nitroso-*tert*-butane)		XDH	Xanthine dehydrogenase
			XIAP	X-linked inhibitor of apoptosis
TNB	Thionitrobenzoate		XO	Xanthine oxidase
TNF	Tumour necrosis factor		XOR	Xanthine oxidoreductase
TPP	Thiamine pyrophosphate *or* triphenylphosphonium		XP	Xeroderma pigmentosum
TRADD	Tumour necrosis factor receptor-associated death domain		XTT	2,3-*bis*(2-Methoxy-4-nitro-5-sulphophenyl)-2-tetrazolium 5-carboxyanilide
TRAP	Total (peroxyl) radical trapping antioxidant parameter		ZDF	Zucker diabetic fat (rat)

CHAPTER 1

Oxygen is a toxic gas—an introduction to oxygen toxicity and reactive species

Oxygen has been a trouble-maker since the very beginning.

Doris Aberlo

1.1 The history of oxygen: an essential air pollutant[1,2]

The element oxygen (chemical symbol O) surrounds us as a diatomic molecule, O_2. Over 99% of the O_2 in the atmosphere is the isotope oxygen-16 but there are traces of oxygen-17 and oxygen-18 (see the Appendix for further details). Except for some anaerobic and aerotolerant species, all organisms require O_2 for efficient production of energy by the use of electron transport chains that ultimately donate electrons to O_2, such as those in the mitochondria of eukaryotic cells and the cell membranes of many bacteria. This need for O_2 obscures the fact that it is a toxic, mutagenic gas and a serious fire risk; aerobes survive only because they have evolved antioxidant defences.

Oxygen appeared in significant amounts in the Earth's atmosphere over 2.2 billion years ago (Figs 1.1 and 1.2), almost entirely due to the evolution of photosynthesis by cyanobacteria.[a] They evolved to use energy from the Sun to split water. Thereby, they gained reducing power (hydrogen atoms) to drive their metabolism, but the by-product, tonnes of O_2, was discarded into the atmosphere. Initially, most of this O_2 was consumed by the formation of

[a] Cyanobacteria (previously called blue–green algae) are prokaryotes that combine plant—type photosynthesis and cytochrome oxidase-based respiration in the same cell.

the oxide deposits that exist in rocks and ores today (Fig. 1.1). Only when this was largely complete did O_2 build up in the atmosphere. The inexorable rise in atmospheric O_2 concentration was advantageous in at least two ways; it led to formation of the ozone (O_3) layer in the stratosphere and it removed ferrous (Fe^{2+}) iron from aqueous environments, helping to prevent Fenton chemistry (Section 2.4.4). Iron is the fourth most abundant element on the Earth, and by forming insoluble, unreactive ferric complexes, most Fe^{2+} was precipitated from solution, leaving sea water today containing only trace amounts of soluble iron. The ability of O_3 and O_2 to filter out much of the intense solar ultraviolet (UV-C) radiation bombarding the Earth helped living organisms to leave the sea and colonize land, but the increasing O_2 levels must have placed a severe stress on the organisms present.

When living organisms first appeared on Earth, they did so under an atmosphere containing much N_2 and CO_2 but very little O_2, that is they were anaerobes. Anaerobic microorganisms still exist today, but usually their growth is inhibited and often they are killed by exposure to 21% O_2, the current atmospheric level. As the O_2 content of the atmosphere rose, many primitive species must have died out. Present-day anaerobes are presumably the descendants of

1

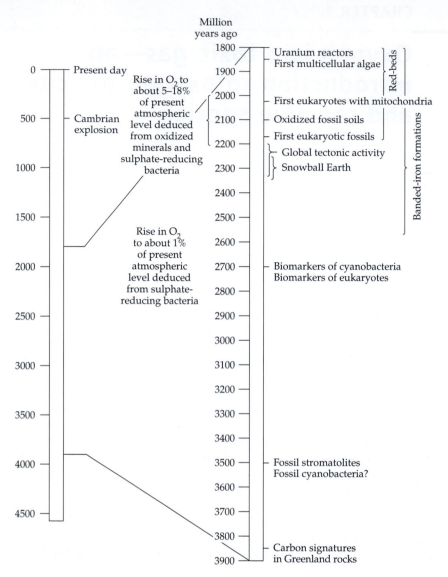

Figure 1.1 Geological timeline expanding the mid-Precambrian period (Archaean and early Proterozoic). Note the burst of evolutionary activity in the period 2.3 to 2 billion years ago, as oxygen levels rose to about 5–18% of present atmospheric levels. Oxygen may have eliminated many anaerobes but it also provided the means for multicellular organisms to evolve. 'Snowball Earth' refers to an ice age. From[2] by courtesy of Dr Nick Lane and Oxford University Press.

organisms that followed the evolutionary path of 'adapting' to rising atmospheric O_2 levels by restricting themselves to environments into which the O_2 did not penetrate (Fig 1.3). Other organisms instead began to evolve antioxidant defence systems (producing new ones and realigning ancient molecules to new functions) to protect against O_2 toxicity. In retrospect, this was a fruitful path to follow. Organisms that tolerated O_2 could also evolve to use it for metabolic transformations catalysed by oxidase, oxygenase and hydroxylase enzymes, such as tyrosine hydroxylase, cytochromes P450 and the proline and lysine hydroxylases needed for collagen

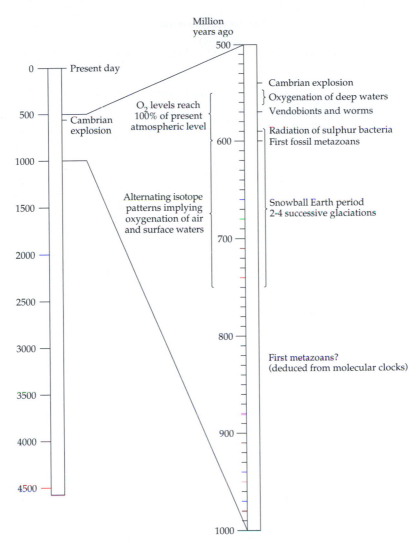

Figure 1.2 Geological timeline expanding the late Precambrian period and Cambrian explosion. From[2] by courtesy of Dr Nick Lane and Oxford University Press.

biosynthesis. Best of all, O_2 could facilitate efficient energy production, employing electron transport chains with O_2 as the terminal electron acceptor. This switch to aerobic metabolism increased the yield of ATP that could be made from food molecules, such as glucose, by over 15-fold. Mitochondria make 80% or more of the ATP needed by almost all animal cells, and the lethal effects of inhibiting this, for example by cyanide, show how important mitochondria now are.

Evolution of efficient energy production allowed the development of complex multicellular organisms, which then also needed systems to ensure that O_2 could be distributed throughout the organism (Fig. 1.3). A further advantage of evolving such systems is that delivery of O_2 can be controlled: for example most cells in the human body are never exposed to the full force of atmospheric O_2 (Fig. 1.4). There must then be mechanisms for monitoring O_2 levels in the body and altering

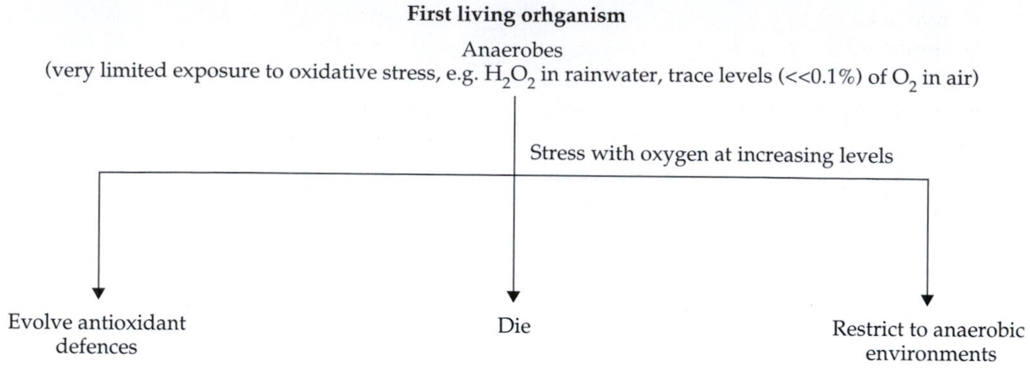

First living orhganism

Anaerobes
(very limited exposure to oxidative stress, e.g. H_2O_2 in rainwater, trace levels (<<0.1%) of O_2 in air)

Stress with oxygen at increasing levels

Evolve antioxidant defences   Die   Restrict to anaerobic environments

Figure 1.3 Evolutionary adaptations to the appearance of O_2. Development of antioxidant defences allowed evolution of O_2-using enzymes and electron-transport chains, enabling oxidation of food material more efficiently. Aerobic respiration produces much more energy per unit mass of food, allowing the development of complex multicellular organisms. The bigger organisms then have to develop mechanisms for delivering O_2 at the right level to their cells, so that many cells are shielded from the full brunt of 21% O_2, perhaps itself a driving force for the evolution of multicellularity.

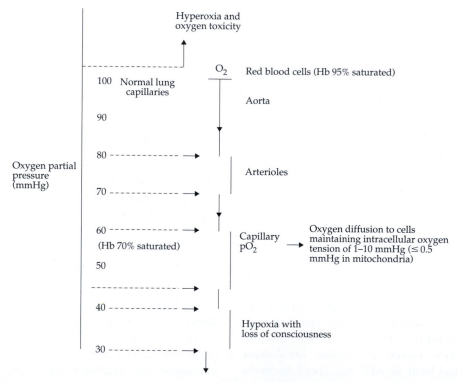

Figure 1.4 Approximate O_2 concentrations in the human body. Most cells are exposed only to fairly low O_2 concentrations: this may be regarded as an antioxidant defence mechanism, although it also renders aerobic cells vulnerable to interruptions of the O_2 transport mechanism. The cornea and respiratory tract are obvious exceptions, but the skin is somewhat shielded by its outer layer of dead cells (Section 6.12). Electron spin resonance (ESR) can be used to measure cellular O_2 concentrations (Section 5.2.2). Cells circulating in the blood (except erythrocytes) and cells in the vessel walls (especially vascular endothelium which has a high metabolic activity) will consume some of the O_2 unloaded from haemoglobin (Hb) before it diffuses into the tissues.

respiration rate and blood flow to control O_2 supply. As multicellular organisms got bigger, they needed structural support; skeletons and connective tissue. Hence collagen biosynthesis (an O_2-requiring process) came into its own, since collagen is a major protein in connective tissue and bone.

1.1.1 The paradox of photosynthesis

Since O_2 is poisonous and photosynthetic organisms expose themselves to high O_2 levels, how was it possible for cyanobacteria to evolve photosynthesis in a 'preantioxidant' world? Even in present-day plants, much of the protein synthesis in illuminated chloroplasts is used to repair the oxidative damage being done (Section 6.8). Were some of the antioxidants in place already? It has been speculated that the part of the photosynthetic system that splits water, photosystem II (Section 6.8.3), could have evolved from a manganese-containing form of the enzyme catalase.[2,3] If true, it follows that catalase-like enzymes must have been present *prior* to a rise in atmospheric O_2 levels. How can this be? Catalase is specific for H_2O_2; was H_2O_2 present to drive its evolution?

Under an atmosphere mainly composed of N_2 and CO_2 with no O_3 screen, UV radiation must have bombarded the face of the Earth. Even at the low O_2 levels present 3.5 billion years ago ($<0.1\%$), there could have been substantial H_2O_2 levels in rainwater generated by photochemical reactions with traces of O_2.[2] Iron was freely available then in a soluble form, Fe^{2+}. Hence Fenton chemistry (Section 2.4.4) was a threat, so H_2O_2 must be eliminated. One suggestion is that the evolutionary precursors of photosystem II used H_2O_2 as a *substrate*,[3] and only later evolved the increased chemical ferocity needed to split water. Decomposition of H_2O_2 by catalase, of course, generates traces of O_2.

1.1.2 Hyperoxia in history?

Oxygen is now the commonest element in the Earth's crust (atomic abundance 53.8%) and 21% of the atmosphere. The barometric pressure of dry air at sea level is 760 mm mercury,[b] giving an O_2 partial pressure of about 159 mmHg.

Oxygen levels may have been even higher at periods in the Earth's history. In the mid-to-late Devonian period, O_2 increased from about 18% to 20%, but then rose sharply to 35% by the late Carboniferous as plant life flourished, CO_2 levels fell drastically and huge deposits of coal and oil formed (Fig. 1.5). This increased O_2 concentration may have permitted insects (whose O_2 distribution system depends largely on diffusion) to become larger. For example the giant Carboniferous dragonfly *Meganeura monyi* had a wingspan of up to 75 cm and a thoracic diameter of about 2.8 cm, compared with about 10 cm and 1 cm, respectively, for present-day dragonflies.[2] Most of the insects that attained exceptionally large body sizes during the Carboniferous did not persist after the Permian, when O_2 concentrations fell again. The plants and animals existing in Carboniferous times must presumably have had enhanced antioxidant defences, which would be fascinating to study if they could be resurrected.

1.1.3 Oxygen in solution

Oxygen is also found dissolved in seas, lakes, rivers and other bodies of water. The solubility of O_2 in sea water exposed to air at 10 °C is about 0.284 millimolar (mM), and decreases at higher temperatures (e.g. 0.212 mM at 25 °C). Oxygen is more soluble in fresh water, for example in distilled water solubility is 0.258 mM at 25 °C and 0.355 mM at 10 °C. The O_2 concentration experienced by cells within a multicellular organism will depend on how far the O_2 has to move to reach them as well as on how quickly they and other cells around them consume it. Mitochondrial respiration can function well at low O_2, so one way of diminishing O_2 toxicity has been to decrease the concentration to which cells within the body are exposed (Fig. 1.4). For example, the O_2 level in human venous blood

---

[b] 1 atmosphere = 760 mmHg = 0.1013 megapascals (approved SI unit).

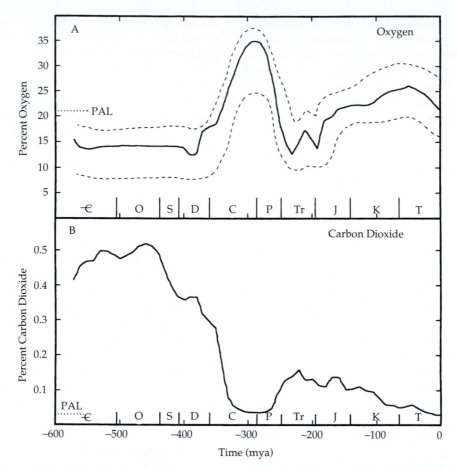

Figure 1.5 Changes in O_2 and CO_2 during the Earth's history. (a) Calculated palaeoatmospheric O_2 concentration showing the estimate (solid line) and its range (dashed lines). Between the mid-to-late Devonian (380–360 million years ago (mya)), O_2 increased from ~18 to 20%, and then rose sharply to ~35% by late Carboniferous (286 mya). The present atmospheric level (PAL) of 21% is indicated. Oxygen steadily declined throughout the Permian (286–250 mya) and dropped to about 15% by the end of the Palaeozoic (250 mya), causing many species 'adapted' to high O_2 to die out (*Science* **308**, 398, 2005). (b) Palaeozoic atmospheric CO_2 model. This gas was present in relatively large amounts in the Ordovician–Silurian, fell precipitously during the Devonian–Carboniferous, and increased in the late Permian. The minimum value shown for the late Carboniferous and early Permian approximates present CO_2 levels (about 0.036%; dotted line). Data from *Nature* **375**, 118, 1995 by courtesy of Dr J.B. Graham and his colleagues and the publishers.

is only around 40 mmHg (53 micromolar O_2). Within most or all eukaryotic cells, there is an O_2 gradient, decreasing in concentration from the cell membrane to the O_2-consuming mitochondria (Fig. 1.4).

However, O_2 is five to eight times more soluble in organic solvents than in water, a point worth bearing in mind when considering oxidative damage to the hydrophobic interior of biological membranes (Section 4.11). One practical consequence of this is the inability of some

plastic culture vessels to maintain anoxia in laboratory experiments; O_2 is soluble in plastic and passes through many types of it readily.[4]

1.2 Oxygen and anaerobes

As O_2 levels rose in the atmosphere, living organisms began to experience O_2 toxicity: oxidations in the cell harmful to the organism and in some cases lethal. This created pressure to evolve protective mechanisms, or to retreat to anoxic environments (Fig. 1.3). Studies of O_2 toxicity in present-day anaerobes may help us understand what happened to the primitive species that failed to adapt and were lost during evolution.

The term 'anaerobic organism' covers a wide range of biological variation.[5–8] There are 'strict' anaerobes such as the bacterium *Treponema denticola* and several *Clostridium* spp. that will grow in the laboratory only if O_2 is absent (or at least as absent as it can ever be). Indeed, the treatment of gangrene due to *Clostridium* infections by exposing patients to pure O_2 at pressures higher than atmospheric (**hyperbaric oxygen therapy**) is in part based on the sensitivity of *Clostridium* spp. to O_2. Hyperbaric treatment is not without problems, however (Section 1.5.2 below). The so-called 'strict anaerobe' *Bacteroides fragilis* even seems to benefit from nanomolar (10^{-9} M) levels of O_2, and has been called a **nanaerobe**.[8] The great difficulty in maintaining zero O_2 levels in the laboratory suggests that much early work on the O_2-tolerance of bacteria needs re-evaluation.

'Moderate' anaerobes can grow under atmospheres containing up to about 10% O_2 (e.g. *Bacteroides fragilis* or *Clostridium novyi* Type A), whereas **microaerophiles**, such as *Campylobacter jejuni* (a major cause of diarrhoea in humans) and *Treponema pallidum* (the causative agent of syphilis), require some O_2 for growth but cannot tolerate 21%. Even so-called 'strict anaerobes' display a spectrum of O_2 tolerance. Some are killed by a brief exposure to O_2 whereas for others O_2 inhibits growth but does not kill, for example *Methanobacterium* AZ ceases growth at 0.01 p.p.m. O_2 but survives exposure for several days to 7 p.p.m. dissolved O_2. Sometimes the induction of antioxidant defence systems (Section 3.4.4) is involved in such tolerance.

Many terrestrial and aquatic environments develop a low enough O_2 concentration to harbour anaerobes. For example, in the human mouth, anaerobes can be cultured from pockets in the gums, from decaying teeth, and from the deeper layers of dental plaque (e.g. *T. denticola*); whereas less strict anaerobes and microaerophiles can be found in the more superficial layers of plaque.[6] The human colon (over 90% of faecal bacteria are anaerobes), rotting material, polluted waters, the deep layers of soil and gangrenous wounds all provide niches for anaerobes to thrive.

1.2.1 Why does oxygen injure anaerobes?

The damaging effects of O_2 on anaerobes are, in essence, due to oxidation of essential cellular components.[7,9] The contents of anaerobic cells are highly reduced, and by oxidizing such essential biomolecules as thiols, iron–sulphur proteins, and reduced pteridines, O_2 can halt metabolism. These oxidations often simultaneously reduce O_2 to oxygen free radicals and other toxic 'reactive oxygen species, ROS' (Table 2.2). Some enzymes in anaerobes are inhibited directly by O_2, although more often enzyme inactivation is due to ROS. Because O_2 is itself a radical, it reacts rapidly with other radicals (Section 1.8 below). Certain enzymes essential to anaerobic metabolism (such as pyruvate-formate lyase and ribonucleotide reductase type III; Sections 7.2.3 and 7.3) use glycyl radicals as catalytic intermediates, and these are rapidly destroyed by O_2. The nitrogen-fixing enzyme **nitrogenase** of *Clostridium pasteurianum* is inactivated by oxidation of essential components at its active site. Nitrogenase catalyses reduction of atmospheric N_2 to ammonia (NH_3), and is essential for growth in environments poor in nitrogen compounds.

Indeed, most[c] known nitrogenase enzymes are inactivated by O_2 to some extent.[10,11] Surprisingly, perhaps, not all N_2-fixing species are strict anaerobes, and they use a variety of ways to cope with this problem. *C. pasteurianum* simply avoids O_2. Several aerotolerant N_2-fixing bacteria surround themselves with a thick capsule to restrict the entry of O_2; this strategy of 'antioxidant defence' is also used by certain streptococci.[13] Some photosynthetic N_2-fixing organisms locate their nitrogenase in specialized, thick-walled, O_2-resistant cells known as **heterocysts**. The photosynthetic organism *Gloeocapsa* contains both nitrogenase and an O_2-evolving photosynthetic apparatus within the same cell, but organizes its metabolism such that

[c] One exception is the O_2-insensitive nitrogenase of *Streptomyces thermoautotrophicus*.[12]

nitrogenase is only highly active when the rate of photosynthesis is low.[10]

In *Azotobacter*, an electron transport system in the plasma membrane is thought to scavenge O_2 and keep the cytoplasm anoxic; if it is overwhelmed by O_2, the nitrogenase is converted into an inactive but O_2-tolerant complex by binding with a protective protein.[11] In the root nodules of leguminous plants that are symbiotic with N_2-fixing bacteria, an O_2-binding protein, (**leghaemoglobin**) is present. It apparently functions to control the O_2 concentration and protect the N_2-fixing system of the bacteria in the nodule (further discussed in Section 6.8.11). A molecule resembling haemoglobin is found in the perienteric fluid of the parasitic nematode *Ascaris lumbricoides*; it has been proposed to protect the parasite against O_2, although here by eliminating O_2 in a complex series of reactions involving nitric oxide, rather than simply binding it.[14]

Anaerobes can teach us a lot about the evolution of antioxidant defences, and we will return to them in Chapter 3.

1.3 Oxygen and aerobes

1.3.1 Oxygen transport in mammals

Complex multicellular organisms such as mammals have evolved mechanisms to ensure that O_2 is delivered to all the cells that need it. Some O_2 travels dissolved in blood plasma, but the solubility of O_2 in water at body temperature is limited (Section 1.1.3). Most O_2 in the blood is carried by **haemoglobin**. This protein has four subunits, two α-chains and two β-chains. Each carries a **haem** group (Fig. 1.6) with iron in the Fe^{2+} state. The O_2 reversibly attaches to haem, binding at high O_2 concentrations as blood flows through the lungs and dissociating again at the lower O_2 levels in tissues (Fig. 1.4).

$$Fe^{2+} + O_2 \rightleftharpoons Fe^{2+} - O_2$$

Only the ferrous form (Fe^{2+}) of haemoglobin can bind O_2. Haemoglobin also helps to control pH in body fluids.

Heart and many other muscles (the so-called 'red muscles') contain **myoglobin**. This contains a single polypeptide chain (bearing one haem), whose structure resembles that of the haemoglobin subunits. Myoglobin appears to act as a store of O_2 in tissues: it binds O_2 more tightly than haemoglobin and only releases it if O_2 levels falls abnormally low; lack of myoglobin impairs heart function in mice.[15] A monomeric **neuroglobin** found in the brain is thought by some to help regulate intracellular pO_2 in neurons (Section 9.16.6.1).

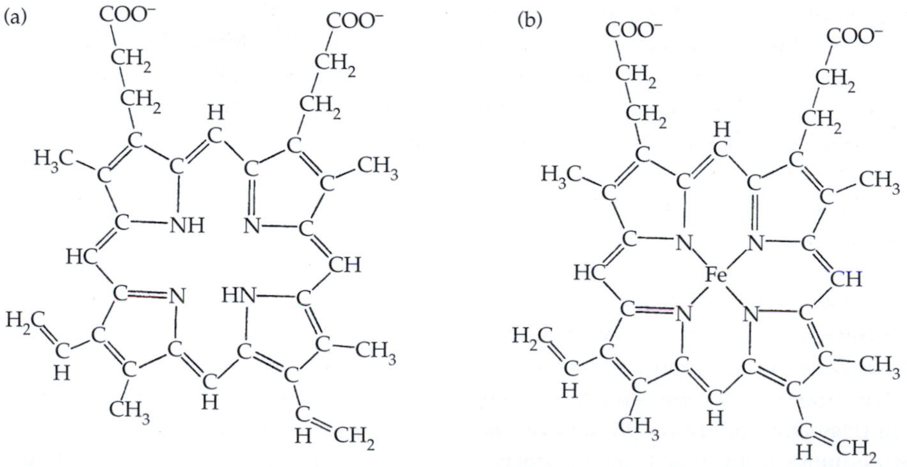

Figure 1.6 The structures of protoporphyrin IX (a) and of iron-protoporphyrin IX or haem (b). The porphyrin ring contains four pyrrole units linked by methene ($-CH=$) bridges. The haem ring gives haemoglobin and myoglobin their distinctive reddish-brown colour. In haemoglobin and myoglobin the Fe^{2+} is co-ordinated to the four nitrogens in the protoporphyrin IX ring. It also ligands to a histidine residue from the protein, and O_2 forms the sixth ligand in the oxy-proteins.

Haem is made not only by animals but also by many bacteria, including some anaerobes. Two steps in the haem biosynthetic pathway, catalysed by the enzymes **coproporphyrinogen oxidase** and **protoporphyrinogen oxidase**, use O_2 in eukaryotes, but other electron acceptors in anaerobic bacteria.[16] The anaerobic bacterium *Porphyromonas gingivalis*, involved in the development of periodontal disease in humans, uses haem in a different way. It requires haem for growth, converting it to a dark pigment that appears able to bind O_2 and act as an 'oxidant buffer', protecting the organism buried deep in the gingival pockets against transient rises in O_2. The pigment can also catalyse H_2O_2 degradation.[17]

1.3.2 Oxygen sensing[18]

Animals need O_2 and must act quickly at the whole organism (e.g. increasing respiration rates) and cellular levels if the supply is compromised. The **carotid bodies** that sense O_2 in the arterial circulation, and the neuroepithelial bodies that detect O_2 in the respiratory tract, play key roles in regulating breathing and heart rate. The O_2 sensor in the carotid body is generally thought to involve the enzyme haem oxygenase (Section 3.17) although roles for ROS have also been proposed, whereas that in the neuroepithelial cell system may involve an NADPH oxidase that produces ROS (Section 7.10.5). Activation of the carotid bodies sends nerve impulses to the brain respiratory centre to increase breathing. In hypoxia cells shift their metabolism, breaking down glycogen (if present) or taking in more glucose, and thus accelerating glycolysis (Fig. 1.7). Energy is temporarily reallocated, RNA and protein synthesis being largely shut down to spare ATP to maintain ion gradients.

If hypoxia persists the cells must adapt, and the **hypoxia inducible factor**s (**HIFs**), especially **HIF-1**, play a key role. The HIFs are transcription factors that promote expression of genes encoding proteins that help cells to respond to low O_2. These proteins include glucose transporters to allow more glucose into the cells, vascular endothelial growth factor (VEGF) to promote **angiogenesis** (the growth of new blood vessels), and **erythropoietin**, a protein hormone required for **erythropoiesis**, the formation of

new red blood cells. Others include transferrin, transferrin receptors and caeruloplasmin, proteins involved in iron delivery to cells (Section 3.15).

The HIFs are heterodimers of α and β subunits. Cells maintain approximately constant levels of HIF-1β. Although HIF-1α subunits are produced, they are degraded rapidly under normoxic conditions. Degradation is promoted by the hydroxylation of proline residues in HIF-1α by prolyl hydroxylase enzymes resembling those involved in collagen biosynthesis. When O_2 is limited the enzymes cannot work, the prolines remain unmolested and the HIF-1α is not degraded, allowing complete HIF-1 to assemble, and bind to DNA. As usual in life it's a bit more complicated; various growth factors and cytokines also act to stabilize HIF-1α, and phosphorylation is involved in the ultimate activation of HIF-1 to a functional transcription factor. Also, transcription of the HIF-1α gene increases in hypoxia. An O_2-dependent **asparagine hydroxylase** enzyme provides a second 'O_2-checking' step: if the enzyme is active, hydroxylation of asparagine residues prevents HIF-1α from working. The HIFs are important in cancer (Section 9.13.4.4).

1.3.3 Mitochondrial electron transport

Mitochondria are the major source of ATP in animals, non-photosynthetic plant tissues and leaves in the dark and they use about 80% of the O_2 we breathe in.[19-21] Metabolic energy production is simple in essence (but not in detail!); food materials are oxidized, losing electrons that are captured by electron carriers. The most important carriers are **nicotinamide adenine dinucleotide** (NAD$^+$) and flavins (**flavin mononucleotide**, FMN, and **flavin adenine dinucleotide**, FAD). The resulting reduced nicotinamide adenine dinucleotide (NADH) and reduced flavins (FMNH$_2$ and FADH$_2$) (Fig. 1.7) are reoxidized by O_2 in mitochondria, producing large amounts of ATP. Oxidation is catalysed in several steps to release the energy gradually. This is achieved by the **electron transport chain** in the inner mitochondrial membrane (Fig. 1.8). Electrons pass from NADH to non-haem iron proteins, which accept the electrons by converting their iron from Fe(III) to Fe^{2+}. They pass on the electrons by reoxidizing to Fe(III). Later in the chain, the

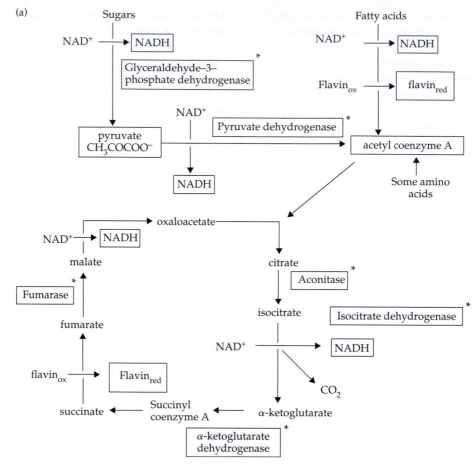

Figure 1.7 The essence of aerobic metabolism in plants and animals: the Krebs cycle and its inputs. Enzymes that are potential targets of damage by reactive oxygen species are highlighted by *. Amino acids often generate various intermediates of the Krebs cycle instead of, or in addition to, acetyl coenzyme A. **Glyceraldehyde-3-phosphate dehydrogenase** (G3PDH) is an essential enzyme in **glycolysis**, the pathway converting glucose to pyruvic acid. Glycolysis generates two ATP molecules per glucose and is upregulated by HIFs (Section 1.3.2). NAD^+ accepts two electrons.

$$NAD^+ + H^+ + 2e^- \rightleftharpoons NADH$$

Cells contain 'pools' of NAD^+ and NADH; the ratio of their concentrations is one factor regulating the activity of NAD^+-using enzymes. The active part of NAD^+ is derived from the B-vitamin **nicotinamide**. **Flavoproteins** contain derivatives of the vitamin **riboflavin**, either FMN or FAD. They also accept two electrons.

$$FMN + 2e^- + 2H^+ \rightleftharpoons FMNH_2$$
$$(FAD) \qquad\qquad\qquad (FADH_2)$$

FMN or FAD are usually attached to the active sites of the enzymes that use them, not free as a pool. Most enzymes in the Krebs cycle use NAD^+ as an electron acceptor but one enzyme in fatty acid metabolism and the Krebs cycle enzyme **succinate dehydrogenase** are flavoproteins.

$$succinate + FAD \rightleftharpoons fumarate + FADH_2$$

If O_2 is absent, glycolysis stops at pyruvate, which is reduced to **lactate** to regenerate NAD^+, by **lactate dehydrogenase (LDH)**.

$$CH_3COCOO^- + NADH + H^+ \rightleftharpoons CH_3CHOHCOO^- + NAD^+$$

and only two ATP can be made per glucose. When O_2 is restored, LDH catalyses the reverse reaction and normal metabolism resumes. Lactic acid accumulation causes **acidosis**, abnormally-low pH.

cytochromes work in the same way, except that their iron ions are present in haem (Fig. 1.8, legend).

The segment of the electron transport chain that uses O_2 is the terminal oxidase enzyme, **cytochrome oxidase**. It removes one electron from each of four reduced (Fe^{2+}–haem) cytochrome c molecules, oxidizing them to ferric cytochrome c. It adds the four electrons on to O_2; the overall reaction is

$$O_2 + 4H^+ + 4e^- \rightleftharpoons 2H_2O$$

(CoQ$_{10}$, shown in the figure) but it is nine (CoQ$_9$) in rats and the worm *C. elegans* and eight (CoQ$_8$) in *E. coli* (Section 10.3.1). The NADH-coenzyme Q complex contains flavoproteins (FMN at active site) and **non-haem-iron proteins** (iron ions are present but not in haem). Coenzyme Q can accept one electron to form a semiquinone (free radical) or two to form a fully reduced (**ubiquinol**) form. Coenzyme Q also accepts electrons from reduced flavoproteins generated by the Krebs cycle (succinate dehydrogenase) and β-oxidation of fatty acids. The enzyme **dihydroorotic acid dehydrogenase**, which catalyses a step in pyrimidine synthesis, also feeds electrons into the electron transport chain at several points in the region of CoQ. The assembly of proteins transferring electrons from succinate to CoQ is called **complex II**. From Q the electrons pass through another multiprotein complex (**coenzyme Q-cytochrome *c* reductase** or **complex III**, which contains an iron-sulphur protein plus cytochromes *b* and *c$_1$*) and on to cytochrome *c*. Cytochromes are haem proteins which accept electrons by allowing Fe(III) at the centre of the haem ring to be reduced to Fe^{2+}, that is they accept or donate single electrons.

$$\text{cytochrome} - \text{Fe(III)} + e^- \rightleftharpoons \text{cytochrome} - \text{Fe}^{2+}$$

Different cytochromes, designated by small letters, contain different proteins and different haem groups. Finally, reduced cytochrome *c* is reoxidized by a multienzyme complex, **cytochrome *c* oxidase** (**complex IV**) which contains cytochrome *a*, cytochrome *a$_3$* and copper ions. For every four electrons taken in by this complex, one oxygen molecule is fully reduced to two molecules of water. The electron transport chain is a gradient of reduction potential (Section 2.3.1.2); as electron travel through the electron transport chain, protons are taken from the mitochondrial matrix and delivered to the intermembrane space, creating a pH difference plus a charge difference (an **electrochemical gradient**) across the inner mitochondrial membrane. The energy of this gradient is used by an **ATP synthase** enzyme (**complex V**) to generate ATP. ATP is transferred across the inner membrane in exchange for ADP by an **adenine nucleotide translocase** and thus made available to the rest of the cell. Like certain Krebs cycle enzymes (Fig. 1.7) this translocator can be a target of oxidative damage (Section 10.4)

The outer mitochondrial membrane is much more permeable to metabolites than the inner membrane, which has very restricted permeability due to the need to maintain the electrochemical gradient. However, it is not totally impermeable to protons (Fig. 1.9, legend); there is a **proton leak**.

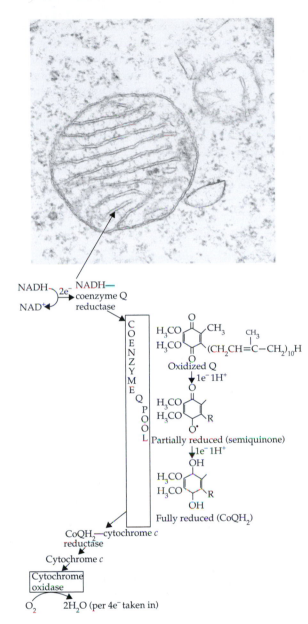

Figure 1.8 The electron transport chain of animal mitochondria (photograph shows HL60 cell mitochondria, courtesy of Dr Jeffrey Armstrong). Mitochondria have an outer membrane and an infolded inner membrane which contains the electron transport chain. The central space of mitochondria (the **matrix**) contains many enzymes, including those of the Krebs cycle (Fig. 1.7), and those that break down fatty acids to acetyl coenzyme A. During the operation of the electron transport chain, NADH is oxidized to NAD^+ by a multienzyme complex known as **NADH-coenzyme Q reductase** (sometimes called **NADH dehydrogenase** or **complex I**) and the two electrons released are eventually passed on to **coenzyme Q** (**ubiquinone**). The number of 'repeats' in the coenzyme Q side chain is variable; it is most often ten in the human

However, it is impossible to add four electrons to O_2 at once—it must be done in stages (Section 2.3). Cytochrome oxidase is a large and complex multiprotein assembly, in part because it catalyses multiple reduction steps.[21] Another reason for complexity is that partially reduced oxygen species are damaging and so cytochrome oxidase must keep them safely bound until they can be fully reduced to water. The haem iron and the copper ions in cytochrome oxidase play key roles in both O_2 reduction and safe binding. Mammalian cytochrome oxidase has a high affinity for O_2: it still works at O_2 levels of less than 1 mmHg.[21,23] Hence ATP production by

mitochondria can continue at low O_2. This ability is very important—oxygenated blood leaving the lungs has an O_2 level of some 100 mmHg, but this falls rapidly in the tissues as oxyhaemoglobin unloads O_2. Cells deep within a tissue may experience levels of only 5 to 15 mmHg, and O_2 still has to cross the cell to reach mitochondria (Fig. 1.4). The sequestration of partially reduced species by cytochrome oxidase and the operation of cells at low intracellular pO_2 can be interpreted as attempts to minimize damage by O_2, that is as antioxidant defences. Mitochondria are also a major source of heat, helping to maintain body temperature (Fig. 1.9).

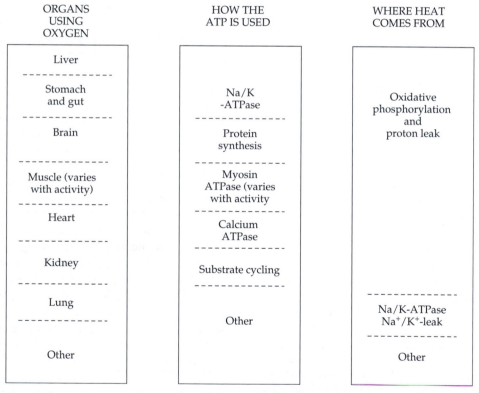

Figure 1.9 Energy utilization in resting adult humans. Indicated within each column are the approximate relative contributions to (from left to right): O_2 utilization by various organs; the contribution of various cellular processes to ATP utilization; the processes contributing to heat production. The inner mitochondrial membrane is not completely impermeable to protons, so that some leak back. This is a major contributor to the body's heat production. **Uncoupling proteins** (Section 1.10.6) play an important part in this proton leak. If mitochondria are subjected to severe stress, the inner membrane becomes suddenly permeable to protons and ATP production ceases: this so-called **mitochondrial permeability transition (MPT)** can be blocked by the drug **cyclosporine**. The transition usually involves a rearrangement of proteins in the mitochondria (including the adenine nucleotide translocator, the **cyclophilin D** protein, and the **voltage-dependent anion transporter (VDAC)** in the outer membrane) to create a non-specific 'pore' across the membranes, although MPT can still occur in mice lacking the translocator. Activation of MPT often plays a key role in cell death induced by O_2 deprivation (also see Section 4.3.2.3)[20,22] and in apoptosis (Section 4.4.1). Adapted from *The Biochemist*, April 2000 issue by courtesy of Dr Guy Brown and the UK Biochemical Society.

1.3.4 The evolution of mitochondria

It is still widely believed (although dissent is rising!) that mitochondria evolved following the engulfment of bacteria by primitive eukaryotic cells (also see Section 3.2.2.2).[24] The bacterial cell wall was eventually lost, and exchange transporter systems (such as the adenine nucleotide translocator, legend of Fig. 1.8) evolved to swap metabolites, so that the cell could deliver oxidizable substrates to the bacteria and collect the ATP they produced. There was a transfer of genes, so that now the great majority of mitochondrial proteins are encoded in the nuclear genome rather than in mitochondrial DNA, and the mitochondria are permanently enslaved. Hence mitochondrial protein import mechanisms also had to evolve. What was the advantage to the eukaryotic cells of the engulfment, prior to the evolution of transport systems? It has been suggested[2] that the capacity of these early bacteria to consume O_2 and reduce it to water constituted an early antioxidant defence mechanism for primitive eukaryotic cells.

1.3.5 Bacterial electron transport chains

Many bacteria, such as *Salmonella typhimurium* and *Escherichia coli*, can grow under both aerobic and anaerobic conditions. *E. coli* can adapt its respiratory chain to work with different terminal electron acceptors.[9,16] In the presence of O_2, substrates such as glucose are oxidized by metabolic pathways including the Krebs cycle (Fig. 1.7) and electrons fed into an electron transport chain containing quinones, *b*-type cytochromes and a cytochrome oxidase, either **cytochrome *bo* oxidase** or **cytochrome *bd* oxidase**. The former (unlike mammalian cytochrome oxidase) has a low affinity for O_2 but a high maximum velocity; it could serve to consume O_2 rapidly when O_2 is abundant (another antioxidant defence perhaps?). At lower O_2 levels cytochrome *bd* oxidase, with a 100-fold greater affinity for O_2, is used. Oxygen level regulates both the function and the amount of these two cytochrome oxidases. When O_2 is absent, for example, levels of cytochrome *bo* fall whereas those of *bd* rise. Anaerobic *E. coli* cells can use at least five different terminal electron acceptors, depending on what is available in its environment.

For example **fumarate reductase** donates electrons to fumarate to give succinate, **nitrate reductases** reduce nitrate (NO_3^-) to nitrite (NO_2^-) and **sulphoxide reductases** work on sulphoxides, such as dimethyl-sulphoxide. If no electron acceptor is available, *E. coli* switches to fermentation as a (much less efficient) source of energy.

1.4 Oxidases and oxygenases in aerobes

The O_2 taken up by aerobic eukaryotes that is not used in mitochondria is mostly consumed by oxidase and oxygenase enzymes. For example, D-**amino acid oxidase** uses O_2 to oxidize unwanted D-amino acids, and **xanthine oxidase** oxidizes xanthine and hypoxanthine into uric acid. During collagen synthesis, proline and lysine hydroxylases use O_2 to add $-OH$ groups onto proline and lysine residues. Like the proline hydroxylase acting on HIF-1α (section 1.3.2), collagen proline and lysine hydroxylases require ascorbate and α-ketoglutarate as cofactors. Synthesis of the hormones **epinephrine (adrenalin)** and **norepinephrine (noradrenalin)** begins with addition of an $-OH$ group to the amino acid tyrosine by an O_2-requiring **tyrosine hydroxylase** enzyme. In general, oxidases and oxygenases have lower affinity for O_2 than cytochrome oxidase. Hence they are often O_2-limited in their action at normal cellular O_2 concentrations and their activities can increase if O_2 levels rise.[25]

1.4.1 Cytochromes P450[26,27]

The endoplasmic reticulum (ER), and often other organelles, of many animal and plant tissues contain cytochromes known collectively as cytochromes P450. Over 500 genes encoding the **cytochrome P450** (often abbreviated to **CYP**) **superfamily** have been described in various species. Cytochromes P450 are involved in the metabolism of drugs and other xenobiotics, arachidonic acid, eicosanoids, cholesterol, vitamin D_3 and retinoic acid (Table 1.1). The name P450 was given because the reduced forms of CYPs bind carbon monoxide, generating an adduct that absorbs light strongly at 450 nm.

The CYPs catalyse oxidation of substrates by O_2. One oxygen atom enters the substrate and the other forms water, such a reaction being known as **mono-oxygenase** or **mixed function-oxidase** reaction. A reducing agent (RH_2) is needed, and the overall reaction catalysed can usually be represented by the equation below, where SH is the substrate (Fig. 1.10)

$$SH + O_2 + RH_2 \rightarrow SOH + R + H_2O$$

The CYPs are haem proteins containing a single polypeptide chain: four ligands to the iron are provided by the haem and a fifth as a thiolate

Table 1.1 A few of the many forms of cytochrome P450 found in humans

Family	Examples of subfamilies	Examples of isoenzymes	Examples of inducers	Representative substrates
CYP1 (polycyclic aromatic hydrocarbon-inducible)	CYP1A	CYP1A1 (aryl hydrocarbon hydroxylase)	3-methylcholanthrene, TCDD (Section 8.3.2)	7-ethoxyresorufin, benzpyrene, benzanthracene
CYP2 (phenobarbital family)	CYP2B	CYP2B1	phenobarbital, aroclor	olefins, acetylenes, dimethylbenzanthrene, benzphetamine
	CYP2E	CYP2B2 CYP2E1	phenobarbital ethanol, ether, acetone, dimethylsulphoxide	dimethylbenzanthracene ethanol, other alcohols, toluene, xylenes, chlorzoxazone (a muscle relaxant)
CYP3 (steroid-inductible)	CYP3A	CYP3A4	rifampicin	methadone, oestradiol, testosterone
CYP4	CYP4A		clofibrate and some other peroxisome proliferators (Section 9.14.2.1)	prostaglandins, fatty acids

Other families include CYP11 (mitochondrial proteins; steroid metabolism), CYP17 (steroid 17α-hydroxylase), CYP21 (steroid 21-hydroxylase), CYP19 (aromatase) and CYP46, involved in brain cholesterol metabolism (Section 9.20.1). The types of P450 present vary between different organisms, tissues and cells and can be affected by changes in gene expression induced by CYP substrates. CYP3A4 in human liver and intestine can be up to 50% of total P450 there. Each P450 family (identified based on amino acid sequence similarities and denoted by a number) is divided into subfamilies (denoted by a capital letter) and the members of each subfamily are identified by numbers. Members of a family are at least 40% identical in sequence; those with 55% or more homology belong to the same subfamily.

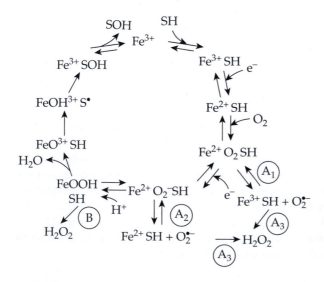

Figure 1.10 A generalized P450 cycle including 'abortive' oxygen reduction. The substrate (SH) binds to the Fe(III) state of a CYP. One electron reduction (e.g. by NADPH-cytP450 reductase in liver) converts the iron to Fe^{2+}, and O_2 binds. This species can occasionally 'leak' $O_2^{\bullet-}$ and regenerate P450 (pathways, A_1, A_2). More usually, a second reduction step generates a bound peroxide which protonates to Fe^{2+}–OOH. This can sometimes break down to release H_2O_2 (pathway B), also produced by dismutation of $O_2^{\bullet-}$ (pathways A_2, A_3). Loss of water from FeOOH generates an oxo-haem species, variously written as FeO^{3+}, Fe(V) = O, or $[Fe(IV) = O]^{\bullet+}$. It may be an Fe(IV) oxoporphyrin radical cation, resembling that in peroxidase compound I (Section 3.13.4). For the majority of substrates, this powerfully oxidizing species abstracts hydrogen from SH, generating a substrate radical which immediately recombines in an **oxygen rebound** with the haem-bound reactive oxygen species. The oxidized substrate (SOH) is released and the cycle repeats. Adapted from [27] by courtesy of Prof FP Guengerich and the American Chemical Society.

anion (S^-) from a cysteine residue. In the 'resting' enzymes, the sixth ligand is water. Figure 1.10 shows a commonly accepted mechanism for substrate hydroxylation by CYPs, but the exact chemical nature of the hydroxylating species at the active site is still debated.

Liver ER is especially rich in CYPs, and feeding substrates of these enzymes to animals often increases synthesis of one or more CYPs. One such inducer is the barbiturate **phenobarbital**, hydroxylation of which increases its solubility and aids its excretion from the body. Excessive intake of ethanol by mammals increases synthesis of **CYP2E1**, the **ethanol-inducible cytochrome P450** (Section 8.8.1.1). Other substrates for CYPs (Table 1.1) include insecticides such as heptachlor and aldrin, hydrocarbons such as benzpyrene and drugs such as amphetamine and paracetamol. Usually CYPs oxidize xenobiotics into products that are less toxic and more readily metabolized to forms that can be excreted, but this is not always the case (Sections 8.9, 8.10 and 9.14).

In liver, the electrons required by CYPs come from NADPH, via the enzyme **NADPH–cytochrome P450 reductase**, which contains FMN and FAD. By contrast, adrenal cortex mitochondria contain a CYP involved in the hydroxylation of cholesterol to give the adrenal steroid hormones (e.g. aldosterone, hydrocortisone and corticosterone); this enzyme receives electrons from a non-haem-iron protein, **adrenodoxin**. A flavoprotein enzyme transfers electrons from NADH to adrenodoxin.

Cytochromes P450 are found in some bacteria, for example in *Pseudomonas putida* a CYP serves to hydroxylate camphor. Electrons are supplied to it by the non-haem-iron protein **putidaredoxin**, which is kept reduced at the expense of NADPH by a flavoprotein enzyme. Hydroxylated camphor is metabolized by the cells to provide energy.

1.5 Oxygen toxicity in aerobes

1.5.1 Bacteria and plants[19,28,29]

Despite its many advantages, even 21% O_2 damages aerobes. Scientists realized this only when they began to measure oxidative damage in aerobes under ambient O_2, and found significant levels

(Chapters 4 and 5). More usually, O_2 toxicity has been studied as the effects of exposing organisms to elevated O_2. Oxygen at levels above 21% has been known for decades to be toxic to plants, animals and bacteria. Indeed, studies of bacterial chemotaxis to O_2 (**aerotaxis**) show that several strains swim away from regions of high O_2 concentration and tend to settle in regions of optimal 'redox state' for their growth. The nematode *C. elegans*, much used in research into ageing (Section 10.3.1) and apoptosis (Section 4.4.1), lives in soil, where O_2 levels can vary sharply. It avoids O_2 levels outside the range of 5 to 12%. At higher levels, the worms cluster and feed together, at optimal O_2 levels they are loners. Maybe the cluster consumes O_2 faster, protecting the worms in the middle.[30]

Plots of the logarithm of survival time against the logarithm of O_2 pressure have shown inverse, approximately linear relationships, for protozoa, mice, rats, rabbits, fish and insects.[28] Plants are damaged at elevated O_2—there is inhibition of chloroplast development, decrease in seed viability and root growth, membrane damage, shrivelling and shedding of leaves.[19] Photosynthetic plant tissues have a particular problem, since they produce O_2 during photosynthesis (Section 6.8). One study revealed that raising the O_2 level from 21 to 35% decreased the growth rate of all plants examined, but the 'evolutionarily older' groups of plants that evolved during the Carboniferous period (e.g. ferns, gingko and cycads) fared better than those that evolved more recently.[2,31] Is this because they are better protected, having evolved during an era of elevated O_2 (Section 1.1.2)?

Figure 1.11 shows a bacterial example of O_2 toxicity: exposure of *E. coli* to high pressure O_2 causes rapid growth inhibition. This is temporarily reversed by adding certain amino acids (e.g. valine) to the culture medium, indicating that one deleterious effect of excess O_2 is to block their synthesis. However, growth soon ceases again due to interference with other metabolic pathways. For example, **quinolinate synthetase**,[32] an enzyme involved in the biosynthesis of NAD^+ and $NADP^+$, is inactivated.

Another effect of O_2 is to enhance the damaging effects of ionizing radiation to bacterial, plant and animal cells (Fig. 1.12).

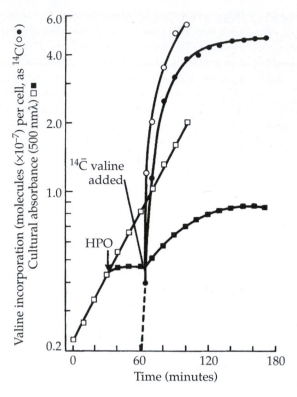

Figure 1.11 Inhibition of the growth of *E. coli* by exposure to high-pressure O_2. The growth medium was mineral salts, glucose and amino acids (no valine) at 37 °C. At the point marked HPO, the atmosphere was changed from air to 80% O_2 at 5 atm total pressure. When valine was added, growth was restored. Closed symbols: HPO experiment; open symbols: normal air control. Growth soon ceases again, however, because of damage to other enzymes, for example those involved in the biosynthesis of NAD(P)$^+$. From Brown and Yein *Biochem. Biophys. Res. Commun.* (1978) **85**, 1219, by courtesy of the authors and Academic Press.

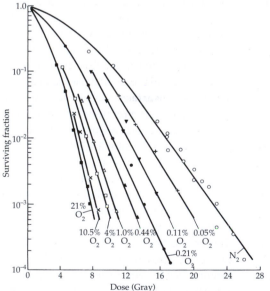

Figure 1.12 The 'oxygen effect': O_2 potentiates damage by ionizing radiation, illustrated here using cultured Chinese hamster ovary cells (CHO) exposed to X-rays. Figure by courtesy of Dr H.B. Michaels.

1.5.2 Oxygen toxicity in animals[33–36]

The toxicity of O_2 to humans is important in relation to diving, underwater swimming, the care of premature babies, design of the gas supply in spacecraft and submarines, and in the use of hyperbaric O_2 (HBO) in the treatment of some cancers (combined with radiation), infections by anaerobes and multiple sclerosis

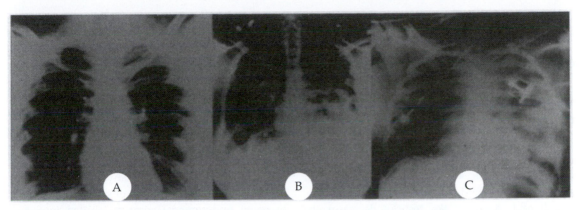

Figure 1.13 Oxygen toxicity in humans. (**A**) Initial chest X-ray of a patient with mild respiratory discomfort after administration of pure O_2 for a non-pulmonary condition. No significant abnormalities visible. (**B**) Further exposure causing X-ray-visible damage with diffuse, irregular pulmonary densities of various sizes in both lungs. (**C**) Late radiological manifestations of pulmonary O_2 toxicity with extension and joining up of lesions. Radiological manifestations are due to fluid accumulation (oedema), **atelectasis** (incomplete expansion or collapse of alveoli) and accumulation of cellular debris in alveolar spaces and in the terminal airways. There is laboured, gasping breathing often accompanied by frothy, bloody sputum. The damaged lungs cannot absorb sufficient O_2 for the body, resulting in **cyanosis** (a blue colour of the skin caused by lack of O_2). From Huber, GL and Drath, DB Chapter 14 in[33], by courtesy of the authors and the publisher.

(treatment of multiple sclerosis in this way is now going out of fashion). Rises in the O_2 partial pressure to which an organism is subjected can result from an increase in the percentage of O_2 in the air and/or from an increase in the total pressure, as in diving at depth, and also in recompression treatment for divers who have surfaced too rapidly. Rapid surfacing causes bubbles of gas, mostly N_2, to form and hinder the blood circulation. High-pressure O_2 forces the gases back into solution and replaces N_2 by O_2; the pressure is then gradually decreased.

High-pressure O_2 can cause acute central nervous system toxicity in animals (including humans), producing convulsions. Oxygen at 1 atm does not do this, but inspired O_2 levels of 360 mmHg or more gradually damage the lungs. For example adult rats show severe lung damage within 72 h of exposure to pure O_2 and often die within 4 to 7 days.[28] Even 28% O_2 for 1 h increases lipid peroxidation in the respiratory tract (Section 6.3). Exposure of humans to pure O_2 at 1 atm for as little as 6 h leads in some subjects to chest soreness, cough and a sore throat; 24 h exposure usually damages the aveoli. Lung injury is first manifested as oedema, mainly due to damage to the capillary/interstitial barrier, allowing proteins to leak from the blood plasma into the interstitial space. This occurs because endothelial cells lining the capillaries are injured by elevated O_2. Further O_2 exposure causes the death of alveolar epithelial cells, and the penetration of protein-rich fluid into the alveoli, interfering with gas exchange.

The lung is a primary target of O_2 toxicity because it is exposed to higher O_2 levels than other body tissues (Fig. 1.4). The epithelium lining the alveoli is a monolayer containing thin so-called **type I cells** and the more cuboidal **type II cells**. The latter secrete **surfactant**, an agent that lowers surface tension and permits the alveoli to function. Type I cells are specialized to aid diffusion of gas from alveoli to the blood capillaries surrounding them: their surface area is large and type I cells cover most of the alveolar surface. Type I cells are more easily damaged/killed by excess O_2 (and many other toxins) than type II cells; after reversible injury, type II cells usually proliferate and differentiate into type 1 cells. However, type II cells can also be injured by excess O_2, for example surfactant production can be inhibited. Lung damage can eventually result in the laying down of inelastic fibrous material in the lung (**fibrosis**), permanently impairing gas exchange. Reactive oxygen species may be involved in fibrosis (Section 4.2.1). Figure 1.13 shows the gradual development of pulmonary O_2 toxicity as seen on chest X-rays.

Oxygen may also worsen lung damage caused by other means even at concentrations thought to be 'safe', that is if the lungs are already injured, elevated O_2 can aggravate the injury.

1.5.3 Retinopathy of prematurity and brain damage

Tissues other than lung are also damaged by hyperoxia. High O_2 levels can cause a general 'stress reaction' in animals, which stimulates the action of some endocrine glands.[28,35] Removal of, for example, the thyroid gland or the testicles decreases the pulmonary and other toxic effects of O_2 in some animals, whereas administration of thyroxine, cortisone or adrenalin can worsen O_2 toxicity.[28,37] Exposure of pregnant animals to elevated O_2 has been reported to increase the risk of foetal abnormalities.[28]

The condition originally called **retrolental fibroplasia** (from the Latin for 'formation of fibrous tissue behind the lens'), but now more usually called **retinopathy of prematurity** (ROP), appeared in the early 1940s among human infants born prematurely, and quickly became widespread. Premature babies have not yet completed development of their antioxidant defence systems, and so are unprepared to tolerate even 21% O_2, let alone higher levels (Section 6.11.8). Not until 1954 was it realized that ROP is associated with the use of high O_2 in incubators for premature babies, and careful control of O_2 use (continuous monitoring, with supplemental O_2 given only when needed to maintain blood O_2) has decreased the severity of ROP. Sadly, the problem has not vanished, since the most premature babies (birth weights of 1000 g or less) need high O_2 levels in order to survive.[38] Administration of α-tocopherol has been reported to ameliorate the severity of ROP in some studies, but the extent of the benefit is not clear.[38]

What goes wrong in ROP? A similar syndrome is observed in newborn rats, rabbits and kittens exposed to elevated O_2. The excess O_2 appears to inhibit the growth of retinal blood vessels. On return to air, the resulting hypoxia induces retinal cells to secrete angiogenic agents (especially VEGF) that cause excessive regrowth of blood capillaries, which sometimes occurs to an extent that causes detachment of the retina and subsequent blindness.

The new vessels lack structural integrity and often bleed. Hyperoxia can also damage the brains of premature babies, potentially leading to cognitive, behavioural and motor defects (Section 6.11.8.2).

1.5.4 Resuscitation of newborns

Resuscitation of non-breathing newborn babies is often done using pure O_2. However, this has been questioned: use of room air may be equally effective and cause less oxidative stress.[38,39] Along similar lines, administration of supplemental O_2 to women undergoing Caesarean section improved the oxygenation of the foetus somewhat, but also raised levels of markers of oxidative damage in both the maternal circulation and the cord blood.[40]

1.5.5 Factors affecting oxygen toxicity

The damaging effects of O_2 on aerobes vary with the species used, age, physiological state and diet.[28,41] Different tissues and different cells within tissues (e.g. type I versus type II cells in the lung) can be affected differently. For example buoyancy in many fish is regulated by the **swim bladder**, which is filled mainly with O_2 plus some N_2 and CO_2. With increasing pressure at higher depths, many fish keep the swim bladder volume constant by increasing its O_2 content, often up to 90% of the total gas. The O_2 partial pressure in the swim bladder of deep-sea fish can be hundreds of times greater than ambient, yet the bladder remains undamaged.[42] The fish as a whole cannot tolerate such O_2 levels, and so its swim bladder (and the **gas gland** responsible for filling it with O_2) must be specially protected (Section 6.1). Cold-blooded animals, such as turtles and crocodiles, are fairly resistant to O_2 toxicity at low environmental temperatures, but become more sensitive at higher temperatures.[28] Newborn rats appear more resistant to O_2 than adult rats, but begin to lose this advantage when about 30 days old.

What about diet? The amounts of vitamins A, E and C, zinc, iron, copper, synthetic antioxidants (now added to many animal and human foods), and polyunsaturated fatty acids can all make a difference. For example adult female Sprague–Dawley rats fed on a fat-free base diet supplemented with cod liver oil tolerated pure O_2 better than when coconut oil was added.[41] In recent years, increased amounts of antioxidants such as α-tocopherol have been added to the diets of laboratory animals, sometimes making it difficult to repeat observations in the older literature.[43]

1.6 What causes the toxic effects of oxygen?

The earliest suggestion was that O_2 directly inhibits essential enzymes.[28,44] Indeed it can, as we saw in Sections 1.2.1 and 1.5.1. Another example comes from plants, where O_2 inhibits the first enzyme in the metabolic pathway that fixes CO_2 (Section 6.8.4). Hence at elevated O_2 there is less CO_2 fixation and less plant growth.[18]

However, most enzymes in aerobes are unaffected by O_2, and for those that are the rates of direct inactivation by O_2 are often too slow to account for O_2 toxicity. In a seminal paper in 1954, Rebecca Gershman and Daniel L. Gilbert (one of the pioneers to whom this book is dedicated) drew a parallel between the effects of O_2 and those of ionizing radiation and proposed that most of the damaging effects of O_2 are due to **oxygen radicals**.[33] For example valine synthesis in *E. coli* exposed to hyperbaric O_2 (Fig. 1.11) is impaired because the enzyme **dihydroxyacid dehydratase**, required for valine production, is inactivated. The enzyme is not directly inhibited by O_2, but rather by oxygen radicals such as superoxide,[9] $O_2^{\bullet-}$. Other enzymes inactivated by $O_2^{\bullet-}$ in *E. coli* exposed to high-pressure O_2 include the Krebs cycle enzymes aconitase and fumarase (Fig. 1.7). *E. coli* contains three fumarases: fumarases A and B are inactivated by $O_2^{\bullet-}$ whereas fumarase C is not. Levels of fumarase C increase when *E. coli* is exposed to oxidizing conditions, perhaps as a 'replacement' for the $O_2^{\bullet-}$-sensitive fumarases A and B.[45] Aconitase is an important target of damage by $O_2^{\bullet-}$ in mammalian tissues exposed to hyperoxia.[46]

The neurological effects of HBO may also involve oxygen radical formation, as measured by free radical trapping[47] or increased levels of oxidative damage. The free radical nitric oxide (Section 2.5.6) also seems to be involved, since inhibition of its formation delays the onset of convulsions in animals.

Nitric oxide may react with $O_2^{\bullet-}$ to generate the cytotoxic species peroxynitrite (Section 2.6.1).[48] Similarly, mice lacking endothelial nitric oxide synthase (Section 2.5.6.6) were less sensitive to ROP and a role for peroxynitrite in causing retinal damage has been proposed.[49] Upregulation of $O_2^{\bullet-}$-producing NADPH oxidase enzymes may also be involved, for example, in the excess VEGF production (Section 7.10). The lung damage caused by exposure of animals to elevated O_2 also involves free radicals, both generated in the lung itself and produced by white blood cells that are recruited to the site of injury.[50] Increased oxidative DNA damage in white blood cells has been observed in humans subjected to HBO, although this damage is quickly repaired.[36]

1.7 So free radicals cause most oxygen toxicity? What then are free radicals?

To understand this section, the reader must know what is meant by such terms as 'covalent bond', 'Pauli principle', 'atomic orbital', 'antibonding molecular orbital', 'spin quantum number' and 'Hund's rule'. We have provided an appendix if help is needed. Although we focus this section on oxygen free radicals, Chapter 2 will reveal that there are many other types of free radical in biology and chemistry.

There are several definitions of 'free radical', as well as debates about whether the word 'free' is superfluous. We adopt a simple definition: **a free radical is any species capable of independent existence** (hence the term 'free') **that contains one or more unpaired electrons**. An unpaired electron is one that occupies an atomic or molecular orbital by itself. A superscript dot after the chemical formula is used to denote a free radical. The simplest free radical is atomic hydrogen, $H^{\bullet}$, since a hydrogen atom has only one electron, which must therefore be unpaired.

The presence of one or more unpaired electrons usually causes free radicals to be attracted slightly to a magnetic field (i.e. to be **paramagnetic**), and sometimes makes them highly reactive, although the chemical reactivity of radicals varies widely. Many free radicals exist in living systems, although most molecules *in vivo* are non-radicals. Radicals can be formed by losing a single electron from a non-radical

$$X - e^- \rightarrow X^{\bullet+} \text{ (radical cation)}$$

or by gaining one

$$Y + e^- \rightarrow Y^{\bullet-} \text{ (radical anion)}$$

Radicals can also be formed when a covalent bond is broken if one electron from the bonding pair remains on each atom, a process known as **homolytic fission**.[51] The energy required to dissociate covalent bonds can be provided by heat, ultraviolet light, or ionizing radiation, for example. Many covalent bonds only dissociate at high temperatures, for example 450 to 600 °C is often required to rupture C–C, C–H or C–O bonds. Hence many studies of free-radical chemistry have been carried out in the gas phase at high temperatures; combustion is well known as a free radical process. Other covalent bonds fragment more easily: merely cutting your fingernails can cleave disulphide bonds to generate sulphur radicals (Section 2.5.5.1).[52] The fracture and grinding of bone can generate free radicals by mechanical damage to covalent bonds, mostly in the collagen present.[52] The process of freeze-drying (**lyophilization**) can generate radicals capable of damaging many biomolecules, a problem in the manufacture of proteins and peptides for clinical or laboratory use. The protein can be directly damaged by radicals, and/or by products generated from radical attack upon molecules (usually carbohydrates) added during the lyophilization procedure.[53]

If A and B are two covalently-bonded atoms (: representing the electron pair), homolytic fission can be written as:

$$A : B \rightarrow A^{\bullet} + B^{\bullet}$$

For example, homolytic fission of one of the O–H covalent bonds in water will yield a hydrogen radical (H[•]) and a hydroxyl radical (usually written as OH[•]; although some authors write it as [•]OH, presumably to emphasize the location of the unpaired electron on the oxygen). The opposite of homolytic fission is **heterolytic fission**, in which one atom receives both electrons when a covalent bond breaks, that is

$$A : B \rightarrow A^- + B^+$$

A receives both electrons. This gives A a negative charge, B is left with a positive charge, and neither species is a free radical. Heterolytic fission of water gives the hydrogen ion H^+ and the hydroxyl (sometimes called hydroxide) ion OH^-. Pure water is slightly ionized in this way and contains 10^{-7} M each of H^+ and OH^- ions at 25 °C, giving a pH of 7. **Hydroxyl radical** and **hydroxyl ion** are sometimes confused in the biomedical literature: Fig. 1.14 clarifies the differences between them.

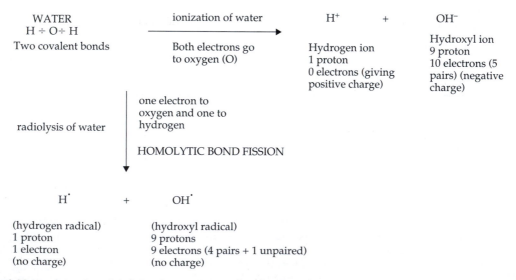

Figure 1.14 Homolytic or heterolytic fission of water. Water can be split into ions (with all electrons paired in OH^- and no electrons in H^+) or free radicals (with unpaired electrons). Molecules can, of course, be both radicals and ions; they are then called radical cations or radical anions.

Let us now examine O_2 and its derivatives to see which are and are not free radicals. Over 60% of the animal body is water, fortunately not a free radical.

1.8 Oxygen and its radicals

Figure 1.15 reveals that the diatomic oxygen molecule qualifies as a free radical: it has two unpaired electrons, each located in a different $\pi*$ antibonding orbital. We should thus write it as $O_2^{\bullet}$, but nobody ever does so we won't either. The two electrons in O_2 have the same spin quantum number (or, as is often written, they have **parallel spins**). This is the most stable state, or **ground state**, of O_2 and is the form it takes in the air around us. Oxygen can act as an oxidizing agent (for definitions see Table 1.2). However, if O_2 attempts to oxidize another atom or molecule by accepting a pair of electrons from it, both electrons must have the same spin in order to fit into the vacant spaces in the $\pi*$ orbitals (Fig. 1.15). A pair of electrons in an atomic or molecular orbital cannot meet this criterion, since they would have opposite spins, in accordance with Pauli's Principle. This **spin**

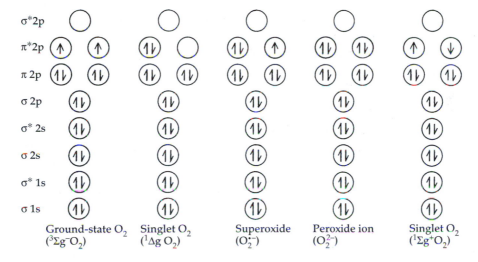

Figure 1.15 A simplified version of bonding in the diatomic oxygen molecule and its derivatives. The oxygen atom has eight electrons, O_2 16 electrons.

Table 1.2 Definitions of oxidation and reduction

Term	Definitions	Example
Oxidation	gain in oxygen or loss of electrons	$C + O_2 \rightarrow CO_2$ (carbon is oxidized to carbon dioxide) $Na \rightarrow Na^+ + e^-$ (a sodium atom is oxidized to a sodium ion) $O_2^{\bullet-} \rightarrow O_2 + e^-$ (a superoxide radical is oxidized to oxygen)
Reduction	loss of oxygen or gain in hydrogen or gain of electrons	$CO_2 + C \rightarrow 2CO$ (CO_2 is reduced to carbon monoxide; C is oxidized to CO) $C + 2H_2 \rightarrow CH_4$ (carbon is reduced to methane) $Cl^{\bullet} + e^- \rightarrow Cl^-$ (a chlorine atom is reduced to a chloride ion) $O_2 + e^- \rightarrow O_2^{\bullet-}$ (oxygen is reduced to superoxide radical)
Oxidizing agent	oxidizes another chemical by taking electrons from it, or by taking hydrogen, or by adding oxygen	
Reducing agent	reduces another chemical by supplying electrons to it, by supplying hydrogen or by removing oxygen	

restriction makes O_2 prefer to accept its electrons one at a time, and contributes to explaining why O_2 reacts sluggishly with most non-radicals.[33] According to basic thermodynamics, the complex organic compounds of the human body should immediately combust in the O_2 of the air (Section 2.3). Fortunately, the spin restriction and other factors slow our oxidation rate. Oxygen *can* react fast with other radicals, but by single electron transfers. Fortunately again, most molecules in the human body are non-radicals.

1.8.1 Singlet oxygen

More reactive forms of O_2, the **singlet oxygens**, can be generated by an input of energy (Section 2.6.4). The $^1\Delta gO_2$ state (Fig. 1.15) has an energy 93.6 kJ (22.4 kcal)[d] above the ground state. The $^1\Sigma g^+ O_2$ state is even more reactive, 157 kJ (37.5 kcal) above the ground state. Singlet O_2 $^1\Delta g$ is not a radical; there are no unpaired electrons (Fig. 1.15). In both forms of singlet O_2 the spin restriction is removed and so the oxidizing ability of the O_2 is greatly increased.

1.8.2 Superoxide radical

If one electron is added to the ground-state O_2 molecule, it enters one of the $\pi*$ antibonding orbitals (Fig. 1.15). The product is **superoxide radical**, $O_2^{\bullet-}$. With only one unpaired electron, superoxide is less 'radical' than O_2, despite its 'super' name.

Addition of another electron to $O_2^{\bullet-}$ will give O_2^{2-}, the **peroxide ion**, a non-radical. Since the extra electrons in $O_2^{\bullet-}$ and O_2^{2-} are located in antibonding orbitals, the strength of the oxygen–oxygen bond drops. In ground-state O_2 the atoms are effectively bonded by two covalent bonds, but in $O_2^{\bullet-}$ only by one-and-a-half bonds (there is an extra electron in an antibonding orbital), and in O_2^{2-} by one bond only. Hence the oxygen–oxygen bond in O_2^{2-} is weaker than in O_2. Addition of two more electrons to O_2^{2-} eliminates the bond entirely since they go into the $\sigma*2p$ orbitals, giving two O^{2-} (**oxide ions**). Usually in

biology the two electron reduction product of O_2 is hydrogen peroxide (H_2O_2), and the four-electron product, water.

$$O_2 \xrightarrow[\text{reduction (plus } 2H^+)]{\text{two-electron}} H_2O_2 \text{ (protonated form of } O_2^{2-})$$

$$O_2 \xrightarrow[\text{reduction (plus } 4H^+)]{\text{four-electron}} 2H_2O \text{ (protonated form of } O^{2-})$$

1.9 Saying it correctly: oxygen radicals, oxygen-derived species, reactive oxygen species or oxidants?

Reactive oxygen species (ROS) is a collective term that includes not only the oxygen radicals but also some non-radical derivatives of O_2 (Table 1.3), such as H_2O_2, hypochlorous acid (HOCl), and ozone (O_3). *Hence all oxygen radicals are ROS, but not all ROS are oxygen radicals.* 'Reactive' is a relative term; $O_2^{\bullet-}$ and H_2O_2 are highly selective in their reactions with biological molecules, leaving most of them unscathed, whereas $OH^\bullet$ attacks everything around it. Hence some authors prefer the term **oxygen-derived species** to ROS. Strictly, however, water is classifiable as an O_2-derived species but it is not much of a threat to us unless we drown in it. Another popular collective term is **oxidants**. However, since $O_2^{\bullet-}$, H_2O_2 and some other ROS can act as both oxidizing and reducing agents in different systems, we do not recommend that term. The term reactive species has been expanded to include **reactive nitrogen, chlorine, bromine** and **sulphur species** (Section 2.1).

1.10 Sources of superoxide in aerobes

A popular theory to explain O_2 toxicity is the **superoxide theory of O_2 toxicity**,[54] which proposes that excess O_2 causes over-production of $O_2^{\bullet-}$, leading to damage to metabolically important enzymes and other biomolecules. We evaluate this theory in Chapter 3 after reviewing the chemistry of $O_2^{\bullet-}$ in Chapter 2, but it is

---

[d] Energies should by convention be expressed in kilojoules (kJ) but the use of kilocalories is still widespread. 1 kcal is 4.18 kJ.

Table 1.3 Reactive oxygen species

Radicals	Non-radicals
Superoxide, $O_2^{\bullet-}$	Hydrogen peroxide, H_2O_2
Hydroperoxyl, $HO_2^{\bullet}$	Peroxynitrite, $ONOO^{-a}$
Hydroxyl, $OH^{\bullet}$	Peroxynitrous acid, $ONOOH^a$
Peroxyl, $RO_2^{\bullet}$	Nitrosoperoxycarbonate, $ONOOCO_2^-$
Alkoxyl, $RO^{\bullet}$	Hypochlorous acid, $HOCl^b$
Carbonate $CO_3^{\bullet-}$	Hypobromous acid, $HOBr^c$
Carbon dioxide $CO_2^{\bullet-}$	Ozone, O_3
Singlet $O_2^{1}\Sigma g^+$	Singlet oxygen $^1\Delta g$

[a] Could equally well be called a 'reactive nitrogen species' (Section 2.6.1).
[b] Could equally well be called a 'reactive chlorine species' (Section 2.6.3).
[c] Could equally well be called a 'reactive bromine species' (Section 2.6.3).

convenient here to review how $O_2^{\bullet-}$ may be produced *in vivo*.

1.10.1 Enzymes

Some $O_2^{\bullet-}$ is produced 'deliberately' *in vivo*, for example by NADPH oxidase enzymes in phagocytic cells and elsewhere (Sections 7.7 to 7.10). Several other enzymes reduce O_2 to $O_2^{\bullet-}$ (Table 1.4), one of the most studied being **xanthine oxidase (XO)** (Fig. 1.16). However, most of the xanthine/ hypoxanthine oxidation *in vivo* is catalysed by a **xanthine dehydrogenase (XDH)** enzyme, which transfers electrons from the substrates to NAD^+ rather than to O_2, and so does not produce $O_2^{\bullet-}$. The term **xanthine oxidoreductase (XOR)** is sometimes used to refer to both XO and XDH. The enzymes have molybdenum, FAD and iron–sulphur centres essential for catalytic activity. Xanthine dehydrogenase can be converted to XO by proteolytic enzymes or by oxidation of thiol (−SH) groups.[55] Conversion can occur *in vivo* when tissues are injured, and leads to $O_2^{\bullet-}$ production (Section 9.5.2). Xanthine dehydrogenase and XO may also catalyse O_2-dependent oxidation of NADH, generating $O_2^{\bullet-}$. In the presence of NADH or (hypo)xanthine, they can reduce nitrate to nitrite and nitrite to $NO^{\bullet}$ under hypoxic conditions. Xanthine oxidoreductase may play a

role in defending the gastrointestinal tract against pathogens.[56]

1.10.2 Auto-oxidation reactions

Many biologically important molecules are oxidized by O_2 to yield $O_2^{\bullet-}$; they include glyceraldehyde, $FMNH_2$, $FADH_2$, adrenalin, noradrenalin, L-DOPA (dihydroxyphenylalanine), dopamine, tetrahydrobiopterin and other tetrahydropteridines and thiol compounds such as cysteine.[57–59] In general, the oxidations start slowly but once some $O_2^{\bullet-}$ is produced it further oxidizes the compound, setting up a chain reaction and generating more $O_2^{\bullet-}$. Tetrahydropteridines are cofactors for several oxygenase enzymes, including nitric oxide synthase (Table 1.4), phenylalanine hydroxylase and tyrosine hydroxylase.

Since O_2 is poorly reactive, how can these 'auto-oxidations' begin? Their rates are greatly accelerated by adding transition metal ions, especially manganese, iron and copper ions. Since it is impossible to free laboratory solutions from contaminating metal ions, it is possible that all 'auto-oxidations' are catalysed by metal ions.

1.10.3 Haem proteins

The iron in the haem of haemoglobin and myoglobin is in the Fe^{2+} state, and mostly remains so when O_2 binds, although some electron delocalization takes place

$$\text{haem–}Fe^{2+}\text{–}O_2 \rightleftharpoons \text{haem–}Fe(\text{iii}) - O_2^{\bullet-}$$

The bonding is intermediate between Fe^{2+} bonded to O_2, and $Fe(\text{iii})$ bonded to $O_2^{\bullet-}$. Occasionally, $O_2^{\bullet-}$ is released.[60]

$$\text{haem–}Fe^{2+} - O_2 \rightarrow O_2^{\bullet-} + \text{haem–}Fe(\text{iii})$$

The $Fe(\text{iii})$ product (**methaemoglobin**, or **metmyoglobin**) cannot bind O_2. It has been estimated that about 3% of the haemoglobin present in human erythrocytes undergoes oxidation every day,[60] and so these cells are exposed to a constant flux of $O_2^{\bullet-}$. Section 6.4 explores how they cope.

Haemoglobin and myoglobin oxidation is accelerated by nitrite (NO_2^-) or by certain transition

Table 1.4 Some enzymes that generate superoxide radical[9,25,54]

Enzyme	Location	Comments/representative references
Cytochromes P450	–	Fig. 1.10.
Peroxidases	Plants and bacteria, some animal tissues (e.g. phagocyte myeloperoxidase, thyroid peroxidase)	$O_2^{\bullet-}$ produced during the oxidase reactions (Sections 3.13 and 7.7 to 7.10)
Cellobiose oxidase	White-rot fungus (*Sporotrichum pulverulentum*)	Contains FAD and a *b*-type cytochrome. Oxidizes a range of disaccharides, $O_2^{\bullet-}$ produced (Section 7.5.4)
Nitropropane dioxygenase	*Hansenula mrakii* (a yeast), *Neurospora crassa* (a fungus)	Catalyses oxidation of propyl−2−nitronate formed from 2−nitropropane into acetone. Superoxide produced and involved in the catalytic mechanism. Superoxide dismutase inhibits the oxidation (*J. Biol. Chem.* **253**, 226, 1978; *Arch. Biochem. Biophys.* **433**, 157, 2005)
Nitric oxide synthases (NOS)	Most mammalian cells	Generate nitric oxide from the amino acid L-arginine. Reported to release $O_2^{\bullet-}$ when tetrahydrobiopterin and arginine levels are low (*J. Biol. Chem.* **273**, 22635, 1998 and **279**, 32243, 2004; *Free Radic. Res.* **37**, 121, 2003). Production of $O_2^{\bullet-}$ from tetrahydrobiopterin oxidation may sometimes contribute to vascular dysfunction (Section 9.3)
Indoleamine 2,3-dioxygenase	Most animal tissues, especially small intestine, not liver	Section 7.4.2.
Tryptophan dioxygenase	Liver	Same reaction as above but specific for tryptophan
Aldehyde oxidase	Liver	Contains molybdenum, iron. Broad substrate specificity; oxidizes a range of aldehydes and other compounds, produces $O_2^{\bullet-}$ (*Q. Rev. Biophys.* **21**, 299, 1988)

metal ions, especially copper.[61–63] The presence of excessive nitrate in the water supply of some rural areas, due to over use of inorganic fertilizers, has caused problems in bottle-fed babies: NO_3^- in the water used to make up feeds is reduced by gut bacteria to NO_2^-, which is then absorbed and causes sufficient methaemoglobin formation to interfere with tissue oxygenation (the 'blue baby' syndrome[e]).[64] This is facilitated by the poor ability of newborns to convert methaemoglobin back to haemoglobin (Section 6.11.8.1). Several abnormal haemoglobins resulting from gene mutations oxidize faster than normal, as do the isolated α- or β-chains that accumulate in **thalassaemia**; Section 3.15.5.3).[62] Oxyleghaemoglobin (Section 1.2.1) can also release $O_2^{\bullet-}$.

[e] The 'blue' refers to cyanosis (Section 6.4.2).

Several bacteria and yeasts contain haemoglobin- or myoglobin-like proteins, often dimeric haem-containing proteins or monomeric haem flavoproteins. For example the flavohaemoglobin **Hmp** found in *E. coli*, contains haem and FAD, and readily reduces O_2 to $O_2^{\bullet-}$ *in vitro*.[65] Bacterial flavohaemoglobins may play several metabolic roles, including protection of the bacteria against nitric oxide.[66] Similarly, both haemoglobin (Section 2.5.6) and myoglobin[15] participate in metabolism of $NO^\bullet$ in animals.

1.10.4 Mitochondrial electron transport

The most important source of $O_2^{\bullet-}$ *in vivo* in many (perhaps all) aerobic animal cells is usually said to be the mitochondrial electron transport chain (we discuss chloroplasts in Section 6.8). The drastic

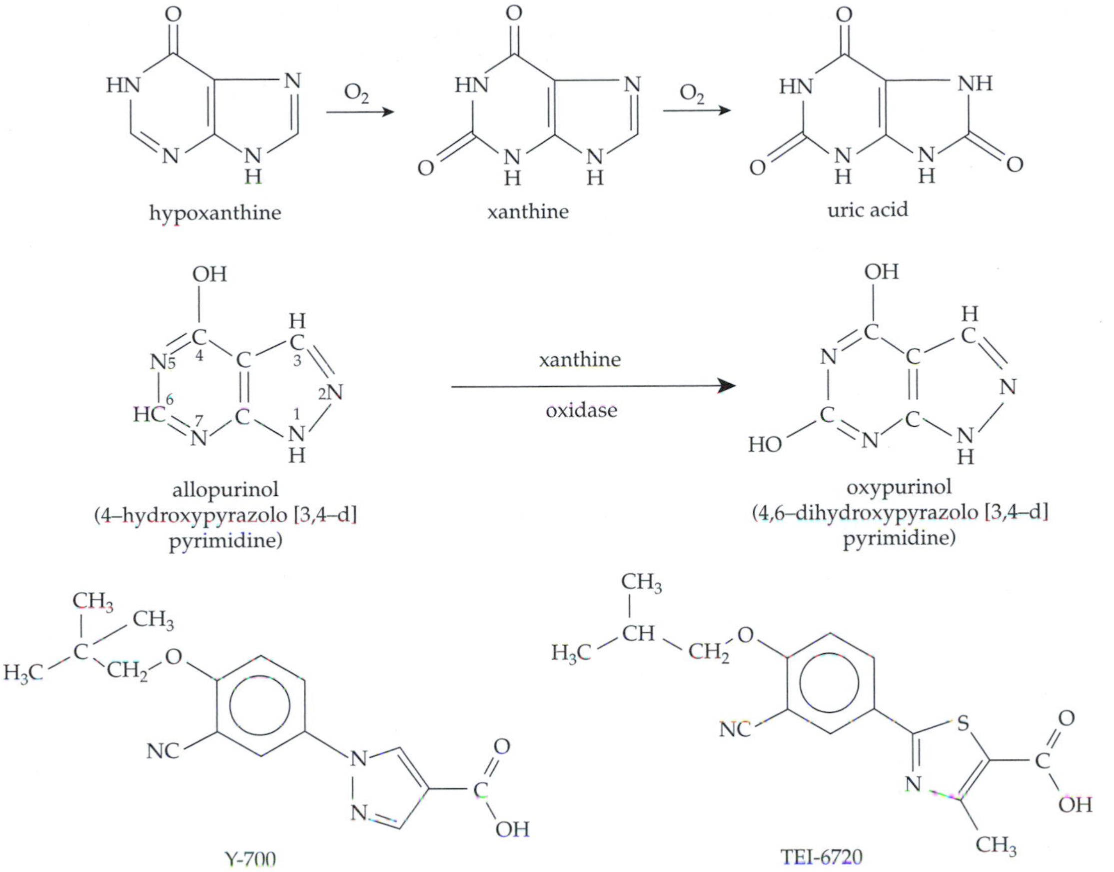

Figure 1.16 Xanthine oxidase (XO) catalyses oxidation of hypoxanthine to xanthine and on to uric acid whilst reducing O_2 to both $O_2^{\bullet-}$ and H_2O_2. It also acts on many other substrates, including acetaldehyde (ethanal, CH_3CHO). **Allopurinol** structurally resembles xanthine and is a powerful inhibitor. It is oxidized by XO to **oxypurinol**, which binds tightly to the active site and causes the inhibition. Indeed, oxypurinol is the major metabolite of allopurinol in humans. Hence allopurinol has been called a 'suicide substrate' of XO. Allopurinol is widely used in clinical medicine to inhibit uric acid accumulation, in gout. More powerful inhibitors of XO are **Y-700** (*J. Pharm. Exp. Ther.* **311**, 519, 2004) and **TEI-6720**, (2-(3-cyano-4-isobutoxyphenyl)-4-methyl-5-thiazolecarboxylic acid (*J. Biol. Chem.* **278**, 1848, 2003). The last is used clinically as **febuxostat** (*N. Engl. J. Med.* **353**, 2450, 2005). Others that have been described are **Iodoxamide, amflutizole** and **B1OZU**, an analogue of oxypurinol in which the oxygen at position 6 is replaced by sulphur. Commercial XO is often used as a laboratory source of $O_2^{\bullet-}$, for example in assays of SOD. The commercial enzyme is often obtained from cream, and the purification process employed by some manufacturers involves the use of proteolytic enzymes to free the oxidase from the milk fat globule membranes. Sometimes these proteases are still present in the final preparation and can cause biological effects mistakenly attributed to $O_2^{\bullet-}$ (e.g. *Circ. Res.* **78**, 1016, 1996; *Arch. Biochem. Biophys.* **426**, 11, 2004). Phospholipases may also contaminate commercial XO preparations, and chelating agents such as EDTA are often present. If contaminating iron is present in the reaction mixture (as it usually is), Fe-EDTA can convert $O_2^{\bullet-}$ and H_2O_2 to $OH^{\bullet}$. Mice lacking XDH die soon after birth, mostly of kidney damage (*Circ. Res.* **95**, 1118, 2004).

consequences of eliminating mitochondrial SOD activity in transgenic animals (Section 3.4.2) are consistent with this, as is the observation that yeast cells without mitochondrial electron transport can survive deletions of the genes encoding SODs (Section 3.4.1) better than normal yeast. Mitochondrial ROS production can be a bad thing, but it might also serve useful purposes in redox regulation (Section 4.5.7).

Whereas cytochrome oxidase releases no ROS, some earlier components of the mitochondrial electron transport chain can leak electrons directly to O_2, although passing the bulk of them on to the next component in the chain.[23,67] This leakage generates $O_2^{\bullet-}$. Whereas mammalian cytochrome oxidase is saturated at low O_2 tensions, the rate of electron leakage (and hence $O_2^{\bullet-}$ production) by mitochondria is, in general, increased by raising O_2 levels (although its not quite so simple; leakage is also favoured by high levels of reduced carriers, which can decrease when O_2 is high). For example, in slices of rat lung exposed to air, about 9% of O_2 uptake led to $O_2^{\bullet-}$ formation, but under 85% O_2, $O_2^{\bullet-}$ formation accounted for 18% of total O_2 uptake.[68]

It has often been suggested that about 1 to 3% of the O_2 reduced in mitochondria may form $O_2^{\bullet-}$. The true rate could be lower, since many experiments are done exposing mitochondria to room air, which is grossly hyperoxic for them.[69] The leakage rate *in vivo* is kept low by at least three factors. First, low intramitochondrial O_2 concentration. Second, the arrangement of electron carriers into complexes (Fig. 1.8) facilitates electron movement to the next component of the chain rather than escape to O_2. Third is the uncoupling proteins (Section 1.10.6 below). It follows that damage to mitochondrial organization can favour leakage and increase $O_2^{\bullet-}$ production. Freeze–thawing of yeast increases mitochondrial $O_2^{\bullet-}$ generation, for example.[70] An intramitochondrial $O_2^{\bullet-}$ concentration of 10^{-11} to 10^{-12} M during normal respiration has been estimated.[71] Inhibitors of electron transport such as **rotenone** (acts on complex I), **antimycin A** (targets cytochrome *bc*) and **cyanide** (inhibits cytochrome oxidase) can increase mitochondrial $O_2^{\bullet-}$ production, presumably by increasing the levels of reduced carriers and facilitating electron transfer to O_2.[72] By contrast, **uncoupling agents** (such as **2,4-dinitrophenol**), which decrease the proton gradient and accelerate electron transport, usually decrease $O_2^{\bullet-}$ production.[73] However, uncoupling by the MPT (Fig. 1.9) can, under certain circumstances, increase $O_2^{\bullet-}$ production by distorting the arrangement of electron carriers in complex I.[74]

There is a wide variation in rates of ROS production by mitochondria from different species and tissues and even from apparently similar mitochondrial preparations in different laboratories.[67,69,73,74] For example, isolated rat heart mitochondria produce more H_2O_2 (presumably derived from $O_2^{\bullet-}$) than isolated rat liver mitochondria, and avian mitochondria produce less ROS than rat ones.[75] Leakage of electrons to O_2 to form $O_2^{\bullet-}$ can take place from components of complexes I and III and, under certain circumstances, from complex II and the coenzyme Q (CoQ) pool.[67,73] Most $O_2^{\bullet-}$ is released into the matrix, but some of that from complex III into the intermembrane space.[73] Superoxide's major fate is probably dismutation to H_2O_2 by SODs present in both compartments (Section 3.2), but cytochrome *c* can also intercept some $O_2^{\bullet-}$. The relative role of each complex in forming $O_2^{\bullet-}$ depends on the source of the mitochondria (e.g. complex I is a major source in brain) and the redox state of the electron transport chain. Mitochondria have several enzymes that remove H_2O_2 (Section 3.12.1). Artefacts to consider in determining mitochondrial $O_2^{\bullet-}/H_2O_2$ production include the presence of contaminating catalase, and of fragmented mitochondria (which produce more ROS) in the mitochondrial preparation,[76] interference with the assays by endogenous molecules such as ascorbate (Sections 5.4 and 5.8), and rapid depletions of O_2 in the reaction mixtures due to fast respiration; as O_2 falls less ROS may be made.

1.10.5 Mitochondrial DNA (mtDNA)

ROS production by mitochondria could contribute to damage to mitochondrial proteins, lipids and DNA. However, at least some claims that the level of oxidative DNA damage in mtDNA is higher than that in nuclear DNA, based on measurements of 8-hydroxydeoxyguanosine, do not rest on a firm experimental foundation (Section 4.8.3).[77] A mitochondrion contains up to 11 double-stranded, circular DNA molecules, each containing about 16 500 base pairs. Mitochondrial DNA encodes only 13 of the mitochondrial proteins (seven of the 26 subunits in complex I, one in complex III, three in complex IV, two in complex V), 22 transfer RNAs and two ribosomal RNAs. Most mitochondrial proteins are encoded in nuclear DNA, synthesized on ribosomes in the cytoplasm, which then have to be imported. Unlike nuclear DNA, mtDNA is not coated with histone proteins and so may be more susceptible to damage. Indeed, mutations in mtDNA (especially deletions of base sequences and substitutions) accumulate in old tissues.[77] This may contribute to ageing and is frequently (but possibly erroneously; Section 10.4) attributed to oxidative DNA damage. Mitochondrial mutations cause several human diseases, including **Leber's hereditary optic neuropathy, LHON** (degeneration of the optic nerve) and **MELAS** (mitochondrial encephalomyopathy, lactic acidosis and stroke-like episodes). The former is caused by mutations in genes encoding constituents of complex I, and the latter by mutations in genes encoding a transfer RNA carrying the amino acid leucine. Optic nerve degeneration in LHON has been suggested to involve increased ROS production,[78] as indeed may the defects in some or all of the other mitochondrial disorders.[79]

There are other sources of ROS in mitochondria, including monoamine oxidase (which generates H_2O_2) in the outer mitochondrial membrane (Section 9.16.5). The Krebs cycle enzyme α-ketoglutarate dehydrogenase (Fig. 1.7) is not only a target of damage by ROS, but may also be able to generate $O_2^{\bullet-}$ from its flavoprotein constituents if substrate is present but NAD^+ levels are very low, so that electrons cannot be passed on.[80]

1.10.6 Uncoupling proteins as antioxidants?[81]

Mitochondria in brown adipose tissue (BAT) contain an **uncoupling protein (UCP1)** in their inner membrane, which allows the passage of protons and so collapses the proton gradient. As a result, all the energy released by electron transport appears as heat rather than ATP, explaining the specialized role of BAT in heat production. Homologues of UCP1 (**UCP2** and **UCP3**) have been detected in mitochondria of other tissues, at lower abundances. It has been proposed that these proteins acts as antioxidants, both by allowing some proton leak and preventing a 'back up' of electrons to escape to O_2, and perhaps by other mechanisms (e.g. acting as a 'channel' to transport mitochondrial ROS out of this organelle).[82] Indeed, knockout of UCP3 in mice led to increased oxidative damage in skeletal muscle,

where this protein is normally expressed. Formation within mitochondria of $O_2^{\bullet-}$ or of hydroxynonenal, an end product of lipid peroxidation (Section 4.12.5.3), seems to lead to activation of UCPs, which should then decrease the membrane potential and hence limit formation of more $O_2^{\bullet-}$.

1.10.7 Bacterial superoxide production

Studies in E. coli[9] suggest that, although some cytosolic enzymes can generate $O_2^{\bullet-}$, most comes from electron transport chains, for example NAD(P)H dehydrogenases, sulphite reductase, succinate dehydrogenase and fumarate reductase, the last being especially active in $O_2^{\bullet-}$ production. Most $O_2^{\bullet-}$ arises by oxidation of partially reduced, solvent-exposed flavins in these enzyme complexes.[9] However, most of these studies are based on work with isolated complexes, and electron leakage may be slower in vivo.[83] The rate of $O_2^{\bullet-}$ production in E. coli was estimated as $5\,\mu M/s$, which, given bacterial levels of SOD, translates[9] to a very approximate steady-state concentration of less than $10^{-10}\,M$ (Section 3.4.1). For comparison, in E. coli grown on glucose-containing medium, levels of intracellular H_2O_2 were estimated as about $10^{-8}\,M$.[9,83]

1.10.8 Endoplasmic reticulum

Isolated subcellular fractions containing ER (**microsomal fractions**) produce $O_2^{\bullet-}$ and H_2O_2 rapidly when incubated with NADPH, and even more so at elevated O_2 concentrations. These ROS largely arise from the CYP in two ways.[27,84] First, the catalytic cycle can short circuit to release $O_2^{\bullet-}$ and H_2O_2 (Fig. 1.10). Phenobarbital-inducible (CYP2B) and ethanol-inducible (CYP2E1) CYPs show especially high rates of O_2 reduction. Some substrates can facilitate such leakage, for example 1,1,1-trichloroethane binds to P450 and starts the reaction cycle but is a poor substrate for oxygenation, facilitating ROS release. For P. putida CYP (Section 1.4.1), little $O_2^{\bullet-}$ or H_2O_2 is released with camphor as substrate. However, the smaller substrate norcamphor fits loosely in the active site, and only about 12% of the electrons fed into the CYP are used in substrate hydroxylation, the rest forming $O_2^{\bullet-}$ and H_2O_2.[84] Second, electrons can escape to O_2 from the flavins in the NADPH-P450 reductase enzyme or other CYP-reducing systems.

In addition, liver ER contains an enzyme system, **desaturase**, that introduces carbon–carbon double bonds into fatty acids and is related to methaemoglobin reductase (Section 6.4.2). The system requires O_2, NADH or NADPH, and a b-type cytochrome, cytochrome b_5. Electrons from NAD(P)H are transferred to cytochrome b_5 by a flavoprotein enzyme, and reduced cytochrome b_5 then donates electrons to the desaturase. Both cytochrome b_5 and the flavoprotein can leak electrons to O_2 to make $O_2^{\bullet-}$, and this might be an additional source of $O_2^{\bullet-}$ *in vivo*. The mechanism that cells use for folding proteins in the ER may also contribute to ROS generation (Section 3.11).

1.10.9 Other cell membranes

The nuclear membrane has been reported to contain an electron transport chain, that can 'leak' electrons to give $O_2^{\bullet-}$ at a rate increasing with O_2 concentration, in the presence of NADH or NADPH.[85,86] Little work has been reported on this system recently and its physiological role is unknown, but it could be important *in vivo* because any ROS it might generate would be close to nuclear DNA. Plasma membranes contain redox systems that transfer electrons from NADH to external electron acceptors, such as ascorbate (Section 7.10.8), dichlorophenol–indophenol and ferricyanide. These systems can be a source of $O_2^{\bullet-}$ in the presence of certain phenolic compounds such as capsaicin.[87] In most cases the physiological role of plasma membrane redox systems is unknown, but sometimes it is, one example being the reduction of iron ions to facilitate their uptake.

1.10.10 Quantification

Production of $O_2^{\bullet-}$ is thought to occur within all aerobic cells, to an extent dependent on O_2 concentration. About 0.5% of electrons from respiratory substrates in *E. coli* have been estimated to form $O_2^{\bullet-}$. In mitochondria, 1 to 3% of electrons are often to said to form $O_2^{\bullet-}$. These numbers do not seem large, but please remember that aerobes can consume a lot of O_2 during respiration. Hence ROS can be made in large amounts (Box 1.1).

1.11 Artefacts in cell culture

Bacteria are often grown in the laboratory in culture media containing autoxidizable molecules, such as thiols. This can confuse studies of O_2 toxicity: on exposure of the cultures to O_2, media constituents can be oxidized to generate *extracellular* $O_2^{\bullet-}$ and other ROS that could damage the bacteria.[57,88] Artefacts can also affect the interpretation of eukaryotic cell culture studies.[89] Culture media are often deficient in antioxidants (e.g. vitamins C and E) and antioxidant precursors (e.g. selenium) and contain 'free' metal ions, present as contaminants or even added deliberately (e.g. iron(III) salts are added to Dulbecco's modified Eagle's medium). Given that most animal cells are cultured as a monolayer under 95% air/5% CO_2 (about 152 mmHg O_2), they are also in a hyperoxic environment, which is likely to increase their rates of ROS formation.[25,89] Thus in one study the intracellular pO_2 of cultured lung endothelial cells was measured as about 140 mmHg,[90] way above physiological levels (Fig. 1.4). It is essential to be cautious when interpreting effects of antioxidants and autoxidizable compounds on cells in culture, first examining the potential reactions of such

---

Box 1.1 How much superoxide is made in the human body?

An adult at rest utilizes approximately 3.5 ml/kg/min O_2 or 352.81 per day (assuming 70 kg body mass) or 14.7 mol per day. If 1% makes $O_2^{\bullet-}$ this is 0.147 mol per day or 53.66 mol per year or about 1.7 kg per year (of $O_2^{\bullet-}$). This calculation is taken from *Nutr. Rev.* 52, 255, 1994.

compounds with the culture medium. For example many studies of telomeres and cellular senescence are affected by artefacts (Section 10.3.5.1). Other problems with cell culture include the use of proteinases such as trypsin in subculturing, and the fact that cells are no longer exposed to growth factors, hormones and the influence of surrounding cells. For example, neurons in culture are often delicate, but in the brain glia help to protect them (Section 9.16).

CHAPTER 2

The chemistry of free radicals and related 'reactive species'

A radical is a man with both feet firmly planted in the air.

Franklin D. Roosevelt

2.1 Introduction

Although Chapter 1 focused on oxygen radicals and other reactive oxygen species (ROS), many types of free radical can be made in living systems (Table 2.1). For example, **carbon-centred** radicals are intermediates in lipid peroxidation. **Transition-metal ions** qualify as free radicals under our broad definition. Some **oxides of nitrogen** ($NO^{\bullet}$, $NO_2^{\bullet}$) are free radicals: indeed, just as the term ROS has been introduced into biology, so have the terms **reactive nitrogen species** (RNS), **reactive chlorine species** (RCS), **reactive bromine species** (RBS) and **reactive sulphur species** (Table 2.2).[1]

2.2 How do radicals react?

If two free radicals meet, they can join their unpaired electrons to form a covalent bond. Thus, atomic hydrogen forms diatomic hydrogen:

$$H^{\bullet} + H^{\bullet} \rightarrow H_2$$

A more biologically relevant example is the fast reaction of nitric oxide ($NO^{\bullet}$) and $O_2^{\bullet-}$ to form a non-radical product, **peroxynitrite**:[2]

$$NO^{\bullet} + O_2^{\bullet-} \rightarrow ONOO^- (peroxynitrite)$$

However, most biological molecules are non-radicals. When a free radical reacts with a non-radical, a new radical results, and **chain reactions** may occur:

1. A radical ($X^{\bullet}$) may add on to another molecule. The adduct must still have an unpaired electron.

$$X^{\bullet} + Y \rightarrow [X-Y]^{\bullet}$$

Example: $OH^{\bullet}$ adds to position 8 in the ring structure of guanine in DNA; the initial product is an 8-hydroxyguanine radical (Section 4.8.2).

2. A radical may be a reducing agent, donating a single electron to a non-radical. The recipient then has an unpaired electron.

$$X^{\bullet} + Y \rightarrow X^+ + Y^{\bullet-}$$

Example: carbon dioxide radical, $CO_2^{\bullet-}$, reduces Cu^+ to Cu

$$CO_2^{\bullet-} + Cu^+ \rightarrow CO_2 + Cu$$

3. A radical may be an oxidizing agent, taking a single electron from a non-radical. The non-radical must then have an unpaired electron left behind.

Example: hydroxyl radical oxidizes the sedative drug promethazine (PR) to a radical cation

$$PR + OH^{\bullet} \rightarrow PR^{\bullet+} + OH^-$$

4. A radical may abstract a hydrogen atom from a C–H bond. As $H^{\bullet}$ has only one electron, an unpaired electron must be left on the carbon.

Example: hydroxyl radical abstracts $H^{\bullet}$ from a hydrocarbon side-chain of a fatty acid residue.

A chain reaction may then occur, since carbon-centred radicals can react with O_2 to make peroxyl radicals (Table 2.1)

Table 2.1 Different types of free radical

Name	Formula	Comments/examples
Hydrogen atom	$H^\bullet$	The simplest free radical.
Trichloromethyl	$CCl_3^\bullet$	A carbon-centred radical (i.e. the unpaired electron resides on carbon). Formed during metabolism of CCl_4 in the liver and contributes to its toxic effects (Section 8.2). Carbon radicals usually react rapidly with O_2 to make peroxyl radicals, e.g. $CCl_3^\bullet + O_2 \rightarrow CCl_3O_2^\bullet$
Superoxide	$O_2^{\bullet-}$	An oxygen-centred radical (Section 2.5.3).
Hydroxyl	$OH^\bullet$	A highly reactive oxygen-centred radical (Section 2.5.1).
Thiyl/perthiyl	$RS^\bullet/RSS^\bullet$	Radicals with unpaired electrons residing on sulphur (Section 2.5.5).
Peroxyl, alkoxyl	$RO_2^\bullet$, $RO^\bullet$	Oxygen-centred radicals formed (among other routes) during the breakdown of organic peroxides (Section 2.5.4). **Peroxychloroformyl radical** $Cl-\overset{\overset{O}{\|}}{C}-OO^\bullet$ has been detected in the atmosphere of Venus (*Proc. Natl. Acad. Sci. USA* **101**, 14007, 2004).
Nitrogen-centred radicals	$C_6H_5N = N^\bullet$	The example shown is phenyldiazine radical formed during oxidation of phenylhydrazine (Section 6.5). Nitrogen-centred radicals are often used to measure total antioxidant capacity (Section 5.17).
Chlorine radical	$Cl^\bullet$	Produced by homolytic fission of chlorine, e.g. by UV light.

which propagate the chain reaction of **lipid peroxidation** (Section 4.11).

2.3 Radical chemistry: thermodynamics versus kinetics

Classical **thermodynamics** deals with the possibility of chemical reactions occurring: are they possible or impossible? A reaction is thermodynamically possible if its **free energy change**, ΔG, is negative. For example, thermodynamic calculations have been used to predict the reactions of peroxynitrite (Section 2.6.1 below). If a reaction is possible, how fast does it occur? This is the area of chemical **kinetics**; a thermodynamically-possible reaction may be very slow, or not occur at all. Catalysts such as enzymes can only speed up thermodynamically possible reactions.

Application of thermodynamics to living organisms is fraught with difficulty, however, since numerical values of thermodynamic parameters such as ΔG in the chemical literature often refer to reaction conditions inappropriate to living organisms. In addition, biochemical reactions are closely inter-linked; for example, an 'impossible' reaction can be coupled to a possible one so that the combination is feasible.

2.3.1 Oxidation and reduction

A frequently used parameter in understanding the chemistry of reactive species (RS) is **reduction potential**, a thermodynamic quantity which determines the feasibility and direction of oxidation and reduction reactions. For example, a compound is said to be **autoxidizable** if its reduced form can be oxidized by O_2. Reduction potentials can predict which compounds should or should not be autoxidizable. Even when autoxidation is thermodynamically possible, its rate is usually slow or zero in the absence of transition-metal ion catalysts (Section 1.10.2).

The reference standard for reduction potentials is the **standard hydrogen electrode**, a platinum electrode dipped in a 1 M solution of H^+ ions and exposed to pure hydrogen (H_2) gas at one atmosphere pressure at 25°C. A reversible reaction occurs:

$$\tfrac{1}{2} H_2 \rightleftharpoons H^+ + e^-$$

Table 2.2 Nomenclature of reactive species

Free radicals	Non-radicals
Reactive oxygen species (ROS)	**Reactive oxygen species (ROS)**
Superoxide, $O_2^{\bullet-}$	Hydrogen peroxide, H_2O_2
Hydroxyl, $OH^{\bullet}$	Hypobromous acid, HOBr[a]
Hydroperoxyl, $HO_2^{\bullet}$	Hypochlorous acid, HOCl[b]
Carbonate, $CO_3^{\bullet-}$	Ozone, O_3
Peroxyl, $RO_2^{\bullet}$	Singlet oxygen, $O_2\,^1\Delta g$
Alkoxyl, $RO^{\bullet}$	Organic peroxides, ROOH
Carbon dioxide, $CO_2^{\bullet-}$	Peroxynitrite, $ONOO^{-}$[c]
Singlet $O_2\,^1\Sigma g^+$	Peroxynitrate, O_2NOO^{-}
	Peroxynitrous acid, ONOOH[c]
	Nitrosoperoxycarbonate, $ONOOCO_2^{-}$
	Peroxomonocarbonate, $HOOCO_2^{-}$
Reactive chlorine species (RCS)	**Reactive chlorine species (RCS)**
Atomic chlorine, $Cl^{\bullet}$	Hypochlorous acid, HOCl[b]
	Nitryl chloride, NO_2Cl[d]
	Chloramines
	Chlorine gas, Cl_2
	Bromine chloride, BrCl[a]
	Chlorine dioxide, ClO_2
Reactive bromine species (RBS)	**Reactive bromine species (RBS)**
Atomic bromine, $Br^{\bullet}$	Hypobromous acid, HOBr[b]
	Bromine gas, Br_2
	Bromine chloride, BrCl
Reactive nitrogen species (RNS)	**Reactive nitrogen species (RNS)**
Nitric oxide, $NO^{\bullet}$	Nitrous acid, HNO_2
Nitrogen dioxide, $NO_2^{\bullet}$	Nitrosyl cation, NO^+
Nitrate, $NO_3^{\bullet}$	Nitroxyl anion, NO^-
	Dinitrogen tetroxide, N_2O_4
	Dinitrogen trioxide, N_2O_3
	Peroxynitrite, $ONOO^{-}$[c]
	Peroxynitrate, O_2NOO^{-}
	Peroxynitrous acid, ONOOH[c]
	Nitronium (nitryl) cation, NO_2^+
	Alkyl peroxynitrites, ROONO
	Alkyl peroxynitrates, RO_2ONO
	Nitryl chloride, NO_2Cl
	Peroxyacetyl nitrate, $CH_3C(O)OONO_2$[e]

'Reactive oxygen species' is a collective term that includes both oxygen radicals and certain non-radicals that are oxidizing agents and/or are easily converted into radicals (HOCl, HOBr, O_3, $ONOO^{-}$, $^1O_2$, H_2O_2). **All oxygen radicals are ROS, but not all ROS are oxygen radicals.** Peroxynitrite and H_2O_2 are frequently erroneously described as free radicals, for example. 'Reactive nitrogen species' is a similar collective term that includes $NO^{\bullet}$ and $NO_2^{\bullet}$ as well as non-radicals such as HNO_2 and N_2O_4. 'Reactive' is not always an appropriate term: H_2O_2, $NO^{\bullet}$, and $O_2^{\bullet-}$ react fast with few molecules, whereas $OH^{\bullet}$ reacts fast with almost everything. Species such as $RO_2^{\bullet}$, $NO_3^{\bullet}$, $RO^{\bullet}$, HOCl, HOBr, $CO_3^{\bullet-}$, $CO_2^{\bullet-}$, $NO_2^{\bullet}$, $ONOO^{-}$, NO_2^+ and O_3 have intermediate reactivities.

[a] HOBr and BrCl could also be regarded as RBS.

[b] HOCl and HOBr are often included as ROS.

[c] $ONOO^{-}$ and ONOOH are often included as ROS.

[d] NO_2Cl can also be regarded as a RNS.

[e] An oxidizing species formed in polluted air.

If this electrode system is connected to a system containing a zinc rod in a 1 M solution of Zn^{2+} ions, electrons flow from the Zn/Zn^{2+} half-cell into the hydrogen electrode, thus the overall reaction is

$$Zn \rightarrow Zn^{2+} + 2e^- \text{ (zinc is oxidized)}$$

$$2H^+ + 2e^- \rightarrow H_2 \text{ (H}^+ \text{ is reduced)}$$

Net: $Zn + 2H^+ \rightarrow Zn^{2+} + H_2$

The measured voltage is given a negative value. If a copper rod/1 M Cu^{2+} solution is connected to the hydrogen electrode, electrons flow the other way, that is

$$Cu^{2+} + 2e^- \rightarrow Cu \, (Cu^{2+} \text{ is reduced)}$$

$$H_2 \rightarrow 2H^+ + 2e^- \, (H_2 \text{ is oxidized)}$$

Net: $Cu^{2+} + H_2 \rightarrow Cu + 2H^+$

The measured voltage is given a positive value. These voltages are called **standard reduction potentials**, symbolized by E°. A system with a negative E° should reduce (i.e. donate electrons to) one that has a positive one. Thus if we connect the Cu/Cu^{2+} half-cell to the Zn/Zn^{2+} half-cell, the latter should reduce the former, that is the predicted reaction is

$$Zn \rightarrow Zn^{2+} + 2e^- (\text{zinc is oxidized})$$

$$Cu^{2+} + 2e^- \rightarrow Cu \, (Cu^{2+} \text{ is reduced)}$$

Net: $Zn + Cu^{2+} \rightarrow Zn^{2+} + Cu$

In living systems, redox-active biomolecules are not separated by electric wires and salt bridges into half-cells. Nevertheless, the same principle applies: a system with a negative E° should reduce a system with a less negative, zero or positive E°. To illustrate this,[3] consider Table 2.3, a list of values for some biologically relevant species in ascending order (the numbers are corrected for pH so as to be the value at pH 7.0, often written as $E^{\circ\prime}$). Top of the list is the hydrated electron $\left(e_{aq}^-\right)$, formed by radiolysis of water (Section 2.3.3.1 below). This should reduce

everything else below it. For example hydrated electrons are thermodynamically capable of reducing paraquat to paraquat radical, ferric EDTA to ferrous EDTA and oxygen to $O_2^{\bullet-}$. Bottom of the list is hydroxyl radical. This is thermodynamically capable of oxidizing everything else on the list, that is everything else should donate electrons to $OH^\bullet$.

Table 2.3 can be used to predict the directions of reactions away from these extremes. Thus the ascorbate/ascorbyl radical system should be able to reduce tocopheryl radical to α-tocopherol. Ubiquinol should do the same. Some reactions are, by contrast, thermodynamically impossible ('unlikely' is a more realistic term—see the caveats below). Thus $O_2^{\bullet-}$ is unlikely[4] to reduce ferric transferrin to ferrous transferrin ($E^{\circ\prime} = -0.4\,V$), but it should be able to reduce ferric iron in ferritin to Fe^{2+} ($E^{\circ\prime} = -0.19\,V$).

2.3.1.1 Caveats

Do not get too excited by the predictive value of E°, $E^{\circ\prime}$ or other thermodynamic parameters, for two reasons. First, reaction conditions make a big difference. Consider the half-cell Zn/Zn^{2+}: the E° refers to a solution with 1 M Zn^{2+} ions. At lower Zn^{2+} concentrations, the electron donating capacity will rise, as the equilibrium

$$Zn \rightleftharpoons Zn^{2+} + 2e^-$$

shifts to the right. At higher Zn^{2+} concentrations, the electron-donating capacity falls. If protons are involved in a reaction, pH is obviously important. Although the values in Table 2.3 are corrected to pH 7, pH in living organisms can vary widely, from <2 in the gastric juice to 8 in the stroma of illuminated chloroplasts (Fig. 6.16). Thus 'real' reduction potentials *in vivo* can differ enormously from standard values. Temperature is often different from 25°C. To correct E° values for the effects of concentration and temperature (T) the **Nernst equation** is used

'effective' reduction potential
$$= E^\circ + \frac{RT}{nF} \log_{10} \frac{[oxidized]}{[reduced]}$$

The second caveat is that E° values predict what is feasible, but not what necessarily occurs. An

Table 2.3 Some biologically relevant standard reduction potentials

	Couple	Standard reduction potential (V)
Highly reducing	H_2O/hydrated electron (e^-_{aq})	−2.84
	$CO_2/CO_2^{\bullet -}$	−1.80
	O_2, $H^+/HO_2^{\bullet}$	−0.46
	Paraquat/paraquat$^{\bullet -}$	−0.45
	Fe(III)-transferrin/Fe^{2+}-transferrin	−0.40 (pH 7.3)
	$O_2/O_2^{\bullet -}$	−0.33
	NAD^+, $H^+/NADH$	−0.32
	Fe(III)-ferritin/ferritin, Fe^{2+}	−0.19
	FAD, $2H^+/FADH_2$	−0.18
	Dehydroascorbate/ascorbate$^{\bullet -}$	−0.17
	Fe(III)-EDTA/Fe^{2+}-EDTA	−0.12
	Ubiquinone, H^+/ubisemiquinone	−0.04
	Fe(III)-ADP/Fe^{2+}-ADP	∼0.10
	Fe(III)-citrate/Fe^{2+}-citrate	∼0.10
	Ubisemiquinone, H^+/ubiquinol	0.20
	Ferricytochrome c/ferrocytochrome c	0.26
	ascorbate$^{\bullet -}$, H^+/ascorbate$^-$	0.28
	H_2O_2, H^+/H_2O, $OH^{\bullet}$	0.32
	$\alpha T^{\bullet}$, $H^+/\alpha TH$ (α-tocopherol)	0.50
	$HU^{\bullet -}$, H^+/UH_2^- (urate)	0.59
	$RO_2^{\bullet}$, $H^+/ROOH$	∼0.77–1.44[a]
	$RS^{\bullet}/RS^-$ (cysteine)	0.92
	$O_2^{\bullet -}$, $2H^+/H_2O_2$	0.94
	$HO_2^{\bullet}$, H^+/H_2O_2	1.06
	$RO^{\bullet}$, H^+/ROH (aliphatic alkoxyl)	∼1.60 (results variable)
	$CO_3^{\bullet -}$, H^+/HCO_3^-	1.78
Highly oxidizing	$OH^{\bullet}$, H^+/H_2O	2.31

Data largely from,[3] and are corrected to pH 7.0 unless otherwise stated, i.e. they are $E^{\circ\prime}$ values rather than E° values. Values quoted in different papers often vary. For each couple the oxidized species is on the left and the reduced species on the right.

[a] For example, the value for $CCl_3OO^{\bullet}$, H^+/CCl_3OOH is 1.19 V.

impossible reaction should never occur, but a feasible one might not either. Rates of reaction depend upon temperature and concentration of reactants, and reacting molecules need to have a certain energy when they collide to break the first bonds and get the reaction going. If this required **activation energy** is high, the reaction can be very slow or may not occur at all.

2.3.1.2 *Thermodynamics of oxygen reduction*

In aqueous solution, O_2 is an excellent oxidizing agent; the $E^{\circ\prime}$ for the 4e$^-$ reduction to water

$$O_2 + 4H^+ + 4e^- \rightarrow 2H_2O$$

is about 0.8 V. Thus thermodynamically, the human body should immediately be oxidized by O_2 in the air. Fortunately, there is a large activation energy for this process! In crematoria, bodies are heated to a sufficiently high temperature to overcome this, and will then burn fiercely. We saw in Section 1.3.5 that *E. coli* can utilize different electron acceptors, and it seems to prefer the one with the highest reduction potential. Thus it 'chooses' O_2 ($E^{\circ\prime} = 0.8$ V) and nitrate ($E^{\circ\prime} = 0.43$ V) over fumarate ($E^{\circ\prime} = 0.03$ V). The mitochondrial electron-transport chain (Fig. 1.8) is a gradient of reduction potential from negative to positive: for example, −0.32 V ($NAD^+/NADH$), −0.18 V ($FAD/FADH_2$), and 0.26 V (oxidized/reduced cytochrome c).

Direct 4e$^-$ oxidations by O_2 probably never happen, whatever thermodynamics says. Reactions of O_2 usually proceed in single electron steps. Conversion of O_2 to $O_2^{\bullet -}$ seems to need quite powerful reducing systems

$$O_2 + e^- \rightarrow O_2^{\bullet -} \quad E^{\circ\prime} = -0.33 \text{ V}$$

However, O_2 concentration is an important variable: this value refers to 1 atm of O_2 (as does the value of +0.8 V for $O_2/2H_2O$).[5] At lower (physiological) O_2 levels, the reduction potential will rise (i.e. become less negative). For a 1 M concentration of O_2, the value rises to −0.16 V, and it will rise further at lower O_2 levels, even becoming positive at the low intracellular O_2 levels *in vivo* (Fig. 1.4). Thus if the level of $O_2^{\bullet -}$ is 10^{-10} M and that of O_2 is 10^{-5} M, the value is +136 mV.

Most of the oxidizing power of O_2 does not become available until the third electron reduction, generating $OH^{\bullet}$. The $E^{\circ\prime}$ values are approximately

$$O_2^{\bullet -} + e^- + H^+ \rightleftharpoons H_2O_2 \quad\quad +0.94 \text{ V}$$

$$H_2O_2 + e^- + H^+ \rightleftharpoons H_2O + OH^{\bullet} \quad +0.32 \text{ V}$$

$$OH^{\bullet} + e^- + H^+ \rightleftharpoons H_2O \quad\quad +2.31 \text{ V}$$

2.3.2 Reaction rates and rate constants: definitions

The rate of a thermodynamically possible reaction depends on temperature, activation energy and concentration of the starting materials (**reactants**). Rates can be measured by following loss of reactants, or formation of products. Reaction rate is the amount of product formed in unit time, or the amount of reactant used up in unit time. Note that these values will only be the same if 1 mole of reactant forms 1 mole of product. Time is usually quoted in seconds (s) and the amount in moles (mol). To take a simple case, suppose 1 mol of compound A in $1 \, dm^3$ of solution is reacting to form another compound, B:

$$A \rightarrow B$$

Suppose further that after one second (s), 0.01 mol of A have been converted into B. The reaction rate (R) can then be expressed either as 0.01 mol of B formed per dm^3 per second, or as 0.01 mol of A used up per $1 \, dm^3$ per second.

The mathematical relationship between reaction rate and reactant concentration is called the **rate law**. In this case it is likely that R is proportional to the concentration of A, expressed in molar (mol/dm^3) terms. This is mathematically equivalent to saying that R is equal to the concentration of A multiplied by a constant, the **rate constant** for the reaction. Thus the rate law is $R = k_1[A]$, where k_1 is the rate constant, and [A] means the molar concentration of A. Once reaction has started, A is used up, [A] falls and so R will fall. Hence rate measurements are often made in the first few seconds of a reaction so that the concentration of reactants has not changed significantly from that originally present (so-called **initial rate measurements**). Rate constants, and hence rates of reactions, increase with temperature, so should be quoted for a specified temperature (Table 2.4), but often are not in the free radical literature, sadly.

In the rate law $R = k_1[A]$, the rate of reaction depends only on the first power of the concentration of A; another way of saying this is that the reaction is **first order with respect to A**. The rate constant k_1 is called a **first-order rate constant** with units of s^{-1}. Now consider another reaction in which there are two different reactants, for example $A + B \rightarrow$ products. This type of equation often represents the reaction of a free radical (A$^\bullet$) or other RS with some other molecule (B) and it usually follows the rate law $R = k_2[A^\bullet][B]$. The reaction is first order with respect to A$^\bullet$, first order with respect to B and second order overall; k_2 is a **second-order rate constant**, with units of $dm^3mol^{-1}s^{-1}$ ($M^{-1}s^{-1}$).

As an example of the information that can be gleaned from rate constants, let us look at the formation of hydroxyl radicals (OH$^\bullet$) from H_2O_2 in the presence of Fe^{2+} or Cu^+ ions.

$$H_2O_2 + Fe^{2+} \rightarrow Fe(\text{III}) + OH^- + OH^\bullet$$
$$k_2 = 76 \, M^{-1}s^{-1}$$

(Fenton reaction)

$$H_2O_2 + Cu^+ \rightarrow Cu^{2+} + OH^- + OH^\bullet$$
$$k_2 = 4.7 \times 10^3 \, M^{-1}s^{-1}$$

If equal concentrations of H_2O_2 are mixed with equal concentrations of Fe^{2+} or Cu^+, the initial rate of OH$^\bullet$ formation with Cu^+ will be greater by a factor of $4.7 \times 10^3/76$, that is 61.8. Values of the rate constant can be applied to see how quickly a reaction might occur *in vivo*. For example, intracellular concentrations of H_2O_2 and Fe^{2+} are usually very low. Let us assume they are in the $10^{-8} \, M$ range for H_2O_2 (Section 2.6.2 below) and the micromolar ($10^{-6} \, M$) range for Fe^{2+} (Sections 3.15 and 4.3.3) and that the Fe^{2+} is chelated to ATP (Table 2.4). If $10^{-8} \, M \, H_2O_2$ comes into contact with $1 \, \mu M \, Fe^{2+}$-ATP, how much OH$^\bullet$ radical will be formed at 37°C? The rate law is:

$$\begin{aligned} R &= k_1[H_2O_2][Fe^{2+} - ATP] \\ &= 1.6 \times 10^4 (10^{-8})(10^{-6}) \\ &= 1.6 \times 10^{-10} \, mol \, dm^{-3}s^{-1} \end{aligned}$$

This seems a tiny figure, but remember that one mole of a substance contains 6.023×10^{23} molecules (**Avogadro's number**). Hence the *number* of hydroxyl radicals formed per dm^3 per second is 9.6×10^{13}—much more impressive! If the cell volume is 10^{-12} to $10^{-11} \, dm^3$ (average volumes

Table 2.4 Rate constants for reactions of physiological iron chelates with various peroxides

Chelate	Peroxide	$k(M^{-1}s^{-1})$	
		25°C	37°C
Fe^{2+}-ATP	H_2O_2	6.7×10^3	1.6×10^4
	t-Butylhydroperoxide	1.3×10^3	2.7×10^3
	Cumene hydroperoxide	3.1×10^3	6.5×10^3
Fe^{2+}-citrate	H_2O_2	4.9×10^3	Not determined
	t-Butylhydroperoxide	1.8×10^3	3.4×10^3
	Cumene hydroperoxide	2.2×10^3	4.2×10^3

Data abstracted from *FEBS Lett.* **275**, 114, 1990.

for a liver cell) this means approximately 100 to 1000 hydroxyl radicals formed per cell every second. Of course, as the reaction proceeds Fe^{2+} and H_2O_2 will be used up and the rate of OH• production will fall unless they are continuously replenished (as indeed they tend to be *in vivo*). Thus, even reactions with low rate constants (such as the Fenton reaction) can be biologically important if they produce highly reactive products. Indeed, substantial OH• production by Fenton chemistry could be detected in *E. coli* even when H_2O_2 concentrations were <1 μM (Section 3.15.4.2).

2.3.3 Reaction rates and rate constants: measurements

Many radical reactions are fast and so special techniques are required to measure their rates. Two techniques are commonly used, **pulse radiolysis** and **stopped flow**.

2.3.3.1 *Pulse radiolysis*[6]
Pulse radiolysis of solutions allows direct observation of reactions of RS and can also be used to determine pK_a values and reduction potentials. The compound (X) to be studied is dissolved (often in water, sometimes in organic solvents) and placed in a reaction cell. Radicals are formed in the cell by a rapid (10^{-6}–10^{-10} s) 'pulse' of high energy electrons, for example from a linear accelerator (Fig. 2.1), and attack X. The resulting X-derived

radicals are monitored over time (typically 10^{-9}–10 s). Since many radicals absorb light or fluoresce at wavelengths different from their parent compound, the progress of the reaction can be followed by changes in the absorbance/fluorescence spectra. Other methods such as electron spin resonance (ESR) (Section 5.2) can also be used.

What radicals can be formed to attack X? During radiolysis of dilute aqueous solutions, most of the energy is absorbed by water to produce ionization and excitation within 10^{-16} s:

$$2H_2O \rightarrow H_2O^+ + e^- + H_2O^*$$

where e^- represents an electron and H_2O^* an excited-state water molecule. H_2O^* undergoes homolytic fission in 10^{-14} to 10^{-13} s:

$$H_2O^* \rightarrow H^\bullet + OH^\bullet$$

Within the same time scale H_2O^+ also reacts to give OH•

$$H_2O^+ + H_2O \rightarrow H_3O^+ + OH^\bullet$$

Electrons become surrounded by clusters of water molecules within 10^{-12} to 10^{-11} s. These **hydrated electrons** are powerful reducing agents (Table 2.3) and are written as e_{aq}^- where 'aq' is an abbreviation for 'aqueous'. Hence three different radicals are produced on 'pulsing' an aqueous solution: H•, OH• and e_{aq}^-. These radicals form initially in clusters called **spurs**, microregions of high radical concentration. Radical recombinations within spurs, which produce H_2O_2 and H_2, are over in

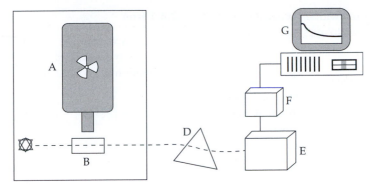

Figure 2.1 Pulse radiolysis. Ionizing radiation from an accelerator (A) in a shielded room is used to irradiate the sample in a cell (B). Light from a lamp (C) passes through the cell, a monochromator (D), photomultiplier (E), digitizer (F) and computer (G) which displays the spectra. Diagram by courtesy of Dr John Butler. Radiolysis of deaerated water at neutral pH generates $OH^•$(0.27), $H^•$(0.06) and e_{aq}^- (0.27). The yields in brackets are expressed as **G-values** in micromolar radicals produced per Gray, where the **Gray** (Gy) is the unit of absorbed radiation dose, equal to one J/kg. Hydrogen gas (H_2, 0.05) and H_2O_2 (0.07) are also generated.

10^{-8} s and afterwards the distribution of radicals is essentially homogeneous in the solution.[6]

Can we select a particular radical to react with X? Yes we can. If the aqueous solution is saturated with nitrous oxide (N_2O) gas before pulsing, e_{aq}^- are removed and converted into $OH^•$.

$$e_{aq}^- + N_2O + H^+ \rightarrow N_2 + OH^•$$

By contrast, if the solution is saturated with O_2 and also contains sodium formate (HCOONa), the following reactions occur

$$e_{aq}^- + O_2 \rightarrow O_2^{•-}$$

$$H^• + HCOO^- \rightarrow H_2 + CO_2^{•-}$$

$$OH^• + HCOO^- \rightarrow H_2O + CO_2^{•-}$$

The carbon dioxide radical is powerfully reducing (Table 2.3) and converts O_2 to more $O_2^{•-}$

$$CO_2^{•-} + O_2 \rightarrow O_2^{•-} + CO_2$$

Thus relatively 'clean' sources of $OH^•$ or $O_2^{•-}$ can be produced, so that they and their reactions with X can be studied.

Pulse radiolysis has been very useful in investigating the rates and mechanisms of reactions of $OH^•$ and $O_2^{•-}$ with biological molecules.[6] As well as direct observations of absorbance, fluorescence or ESR spectra, 'competition methods' may be used to

measure reaction rates. For examples, $OH^•$ reacts with thiocyanate ion (SCN^-) to give a radical anion strongly absorbing around 500 nm, $(SCN)_2^{•-}$

$$OH^• + SCN^- \rightarrow OH^- + SCN^•$$

$$SCN^• + SCN^- \rightleftharpoons (SCN)_2^{•-}$$

If another compound (X) that reacts with $OH^•$ is added, it will intercept some of the $OH^•$, and the absorbance change due to $(SCN)_2^{•-}$ formation will be smaller. Knowing the concentrations of SCN^- and X, and the rate constants for the above reactions, the rate constant for reaction between X and $OH^•$ can be calculated.

Pulse radiolysis can be used to study many types of radical, including those formed by one-electron reduction of quinones, and the ascorbyl radical. For example, ascorbyl radical can be generated in a pulse radiolysis apparatus by reducing dehydroascorbate with e_{aq}^- or by oxidizing ascorbate with $OH^•$:

$$ascorbate^- + OH^• \rightarrow OH^- + ascorbate^•$$

or with another oxidizing radical such as $Br_2^{•-}$, formed by adding bromide (Br^-) ions

$$OH^• + 2Br^- \rightarrow OH^- + Br_2^{•-}$$

Reduction potentials can be determined by pulse radiolysis, for example by studying the changes in concentration when a standard system of known potential $(S/S^{\bullet-})$ is mixed with the unknown $(A/A^{\bullet-})$ and the mixture allowed to approach equilibrium

$$A + S^{\bullet-} \rightleftharpoons A^{\bullet-} + S$$

2.3.3.2 Stopped-flow methods

Stopped-flow methods are sometimes used to study RS, especially when the reaction rates are too slow to be measured conveniently by pulse radiolysis, yet too fast to be measured by standard biochemical techniques (e.g. in the millisecond range). Solutions of the compounds to be reacted are contained in separate syringes, connected to a quartz reaction cell. To start the reaction the plungers are pushed so that the syringe contents are forced simultaneously into the reaction cell, where they mix and react. Absorbance (or other) changes can be measured and recorded and so reaction rates can be calculated. For example, a solution of $O_2^{\bullet-}$ (as its potassium salt, $K^+O_2^{\bullet-}$) in an organic solvent can be placed in one syringe and mixed with a compound in aqueous solution from the other to measure the rate of reaction. Stopped-flow has been used to study reactions of hypochlorous acid,[7] peroxynitrite, and potassium ferrate, an Fe(VI) species (K_2FeO_4).[8]

2.4 Chemistry of transition metals

Most of the metals in the first row of the d-block in the periodic table (see Appendix if more explanation is needed) contain unpaired electrons in their atoms and/or ions and thus qualify as free radicals: one exception is zinc (Table 2.5). Indeed, it is appropriate to classify most transition-metal ions as radicals, since many of their biological effects, whether beneficial (Table 2.5) or deleterious, involve the ability to accept or donate single electrons. The single-electron transfers they promote can overcome the spin restriction on direct reaction of O_2 with non-radicals. The reduction potentials of transition-metal ions depend on the ligands to the metal, and thus can be altered in different enzymes to allow the same metal to catalyse different reactions. The danger is that, unless their availability is carefully controlled, transition metals will catalyse unwanted free-radical reactions such as autoxidations and $OH^{\bullet}$ formation.

2.4.1 Iron

Iron has two common oxidation numbers in which the electron configurations (see the appendix for an explanation if needed) are:

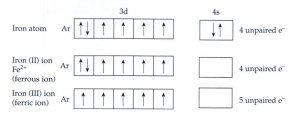

Iron (IV), (V) and (VI) species also exist. For example, **ferryl** (iron (IV)) species are involved in the mechanism of action of catalases, peroxidases, and CYPs (Sections 1.4.1 and 3.13). Potassium ferrate, K_2FeO_4, an Fe(VI) species, is a strong oxidizing agent. One-electron reduction of it (e.g. by $O_2^{\bullet-}$) yields an Fe(V) species, also reactive. For example it oxidizes amino acids.[8]

$$Fe(V) + amino\ acid \rightarrow Fe(III) + NH_3 + \alpha-keto\ acid$$

In solution in the presence of air, iron's most stable oxidation state is Fe(III), whereas Fe^{2+} salts are weakly reducing and ferryl compounds are powerful oxidizing agents. If a solution of an Fe^{2+} salt, for example ferrous sulphate $(FeSO_4)$, is left exposed to air, it slowly oxidizes to the iron (III) state. The Fe^{2+} undergoes one-electron oxidation, and O_2 dissolved in the solution is reduced[9] to $O_2^{\bullet-}$

$$Fe^{2+} + O_2 \rightleftharpoons [Fe^{2+}-O_2 \rightleftharpoons Fe(III)-O_2^{\bullet-}] \rightleftharpoons Fe(III) + O_2^{\bullet-}$$
$$\text{Intermediate complexes}$$

The rate of oxidation of Fe^{2+} is markedly affected by binding ligands to it. In Fe^{2+}, all five 3d orbitals have the same energy and the electron configuration follows Hund's rule. The iron has four unpaired electrons and is said to be in the **high-spin state**. Surrounding the Fe^{2+} with ligands can alter the energy levels of some of the 3d orbitals; if the energy differences between different 3d orbitals are sufficient, the electrons can pair up into the lower-energy orbitals. The Fe^{2+} is then in a **low-spin state**, with no unpaired electrons, and is more difficult to oxidize. This state is present in

Table 2.5 Biological importance of some d-block elements

Metal	Biochemical significance	Selected references
Copper (Cu)	Essential in diet for enzymes such as EC-SOD, CuZnSOD, cytochrome oxidase, lysine oxidase, dopamine-β-hydroxylase and caeruloplasmin. About 80 mg total Cu in adult humans (highest concentrations in liver and brain). Toxic in excess; both excess and deficiency can cause oxidative stress.	Section 2.4.2 and 3.15.2
Zinc (Zn)	Non-transition element, fixed oxidation number of 2(Zn^{2+}); 2–3 g present in adult human body (level second only to iron). Often suggested that Zn can act as an antioxidant by displacing iron ions from their binding sites and inhibiting iron-dependent oxidative damage. Essential in diet; found in RNA polymerase, carbonic anhydrase, CuZnSOD, glyoxalase I, EC-SOD, 'zinc fingers'. Important to the immune system. Toxic in excess, especially to neurons.	*Science* **271**, 1081, 1996 *J. Leuk. Biol.* **64**, 571, 1998 *J. Nutr.* **133**, 2543, 2003; **130**, 1447S, 2000 Section 8.15.12
Vanadium (V)	Essential in animal diet and thought to be so in humans. Suspected to be involved in regulation of glucose metabolism. Accumulated in large amounts in some tunicates. Vanadate inhibits the ATPase enzyme which exchanges Na^+ and K^+ ions across cell membranes and may also affect protein kinase and phosphatase enzymes.	*Mol. Cell Biochem.* **153**, 17, 1995 Section 8.15.9
Chromium (Cr)	Possibly essential in human diet, suggested to be involved in regulation of glucose metabolism. Chromates can damage DNA.	*J. Nutr.* **130**, 715, 2000; Section 8.15.4
Manganese (Mn)	Essential in diet. Needed for MnSOD, arginase, also activates a number of hydrolase and carboxylase enzymes. Toxic in excess; in brain can cause a Parkinsonian-type syndrome (Section 8.6.6). Plays a key role in photosynthesis (Section 6.8.3).	*Fed. Proc.* **45**, 2817, 1986 *FEBS Lett.* **551**, 1, 2003
Iron (Fe)	Essential in diet: deficiency causes anaemia. Most abundant transition metal in human body (about 4–5 g present). Needed for haemoglobin, myoglobin, cyclo-oxygenases, cytochromes, many hydroxylase/oxidase enzymes, ribonucleotide reductase, aconitase, succinate dehydrogenase, catalase and many others. Both iron excess and iron deficiency can cause oxidative stress.	Sections 2.4.1 and 3.15.1
Cobalt (Co)	Essential in vitamin B_{12}. Cobalt compounds can cause DNA damage.	*Nutr. Rev.* **43**, 79, 1985 Sections 7.2 and 8.15.5
Nickel (Ni)	Possibly essential in animals, requirement in humans not established. Carcinogenic in excess. Found in urease in plant cells and bacteria (including *H. pylori*) and in several bacterial enzymes, such as *E. coli* glyoxalase I, and some bacterial hydrogenases and carbon monoxide dehydrogenase. Some nickel-containing SOD enzymes exist (Section 3.2.4).	*Curr. Opin. Chem Biol.* **2**, 208, 1998
Tungsten (W)	No reports of involvement in animal metabolism. Can inhibit xanthine oxidase when administered to animals, by replacing essential molybdenum. Has antidiabetic effects in animals. Tungsten-containing enzymes reported in several anaerobic bacteria, e.g. aldehyde-ferredoxin oxidoreductase in *Pyrococcus furiosus*.	*J. Biol. Inorg. Chem.* **1**, 292, 1996 *J. Biol. Chem.* 278, 47285, 2003
Molybdenum (Mo)	Essential in trace amounts in human diet for some flavin metalloenzymes, e.g. xanthine dehydrogenase, aldehyde oxidase and sulphite oxidase.	*Q. Rev. Biophys.* **21**, 299, 1998

oxyhaemoglobin and oxymyoglobin. By contrast, Fe^{2+} in the deoxy-proteins is in the high-spin state.

2.4.2 Copper

Copper has two common oxidation numbers, copper (I) and copper (II), as shown below. The one-electron difference between Cu^+ and Cu^{2+}, or Cu^{2+} and Cu(III), allows copper to promote radical reactions. Under appropriate conditions, for example, copper ions interact rapidly[10] with $O_2^{\bullet-}$

$$Cu^{2+} + O_2^{\bullet-} \rightarrow Cu^+ + O_2$$
$$k = (5-8) \times 10^9 \, M^{-1}s^{-1}$$

$$H^+ + Cu^+ + HO_2^{\bullet} \rightarrow Cu^{2+} + H_2O_2$$
$$k \approx 10^9 \, M^{-1}s^{-1}$$

$$O_2^{\bullet-} + Cu^+ + H_2O \rightarrow Cu^{2+} + OH^- + HO_2^-$$
$$k \approx 10^{10} \, M^{-1}s^{-1}$$

$$\text{Net: } O_2^{\bullet-} + O_2^{\bullet-} + 2H^+ \rightarrow H_2O_2 + O_2$$

The copper, by changing its oxidation number, is **catalysing** the conversion of two $O_2^{\bullet-}$ radicals and two H^+ ions to H_2O_2 and O_2, that is, it is catalysing the dismutation of $O_2^{\bullet-}$ (Section 2.5.3 below).

2.4.3 Manganese

Manganese is most stable in aqueous solution as Mn^{2+}; oxidizing species such as Mn(III), Mn(IV) and Mn(VII) also exist. Mn^{2+} can interact[10] with $O_2^{\bullet-}$

$$Mn^{2+} + O_2^{\bullet-} \rightarrow Mn(O_2)^+$$

$$Mn(O_2)^+ + O_2^{\bullet-} + 2H^+ \rightarrow Mn^{2+} + H_2O_2 + O_2$$

$$Mn(O_2)^+ + 2H^+ \rightarrow H_2O_2 + Mn(III)$$

Like copper, Mn^{2+} is thus capable of catalysing the dismutation of $O_2^{\bullet-}$ to H_2O_2, to an extent considerably affected by the ligands bound to it. This is physiologically important in some bacteria (Section 3.5.2). In contrast to Fe^{2+} and Cu^+, unchelated Mn^{2+} appears not to react with H_2O_2 to form $OH^{\bullet}$ at a measurable rate.[11] However, it can catalyse the decomposition of H_2O_2 in Tris buffer if both CO_2 and HCO_3^- are present, and in HCO_3^- buffer Mn^{2+} and H_2O_2 can oxidize LDL and amino acids.[12]

2.4.4 The Fenton reaction

Fenton chemistry is a prime example of damaging free-radical reactions catalysed by transition metals.[13] A mixture of H_2O_2 and an Fe^{2+} salt oxidizes many different organic molecules, as Fenton first reported in 1876 using tartaric acid.

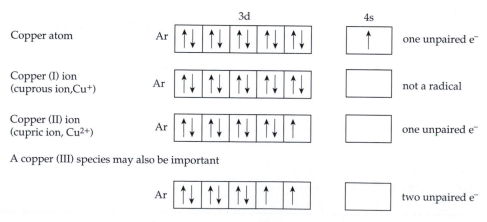

A copper (III) species may also be important

Copper (I) readily undergoes self-reaction if it accumulates

$$Cu^+ + Cu^+ \rightarrow Cu + Cu^{2+}$$

Over 130 years later, we are still debating the mechanism of oxidation. Although the majority of evidence favours $OH^{\bullet}$ as the primary damaging species, other RS may be generated on the pathway to $OH^{\bullet}$ formation.[13–16]

$$Fe^{2+} + H_2O_2 \rightarrow \text{intermediate oxidizing species}$$
$$\rightarrow Fe(III) + OH^{\bullet} + OH^-$$

The Fenton reaction is thermodynamically favoured since $E^{\circ\prime}$ for $H_2O_2/OH^{\bullet}$ is $\sim 0.32\,V$, whereas $E^{\circ\prime}$ for aqueous iron ions at pH 7.0 is $\sim 0.11\,V$, although this value is affected by the ligand to the metal (Table 2.6). The identity of any reactive species other than $OH^{\bullet}$ formed during Fenton chemistry is uncertain; although Fe(IV) species are often suggested, there is no compelling evidence for their existence in Fe^{2+}–H_2O_2 systems (although they do form when haem-iron reacts with H_2O_2). Ferryl might be the intermediate oxidizing species indicated in the equation above.

Iron(III) attached to some ligands can react further with H_2O_2, although this is usually slower than the reaction of H_2O_2 with Fe^{2+} attached to the same ligands. Generation of $OH^{\bullet}$ by mixtures of certain Fe(III) chelates (e.g. ferric EDTA) and H_2O_2

appears to involve $O_2^{\bullet-}$, since it is inhibited by SOD.[17] The reaction is often written as

$$Fe(III) + H_2O_2 \rightarrow \text{intermediate complex(es)}$$
$$\rightarrow Fe^{2+} + O_2^{\bullet-} + 2H^+$$

but no direct evidence for this chemistry has been obtained. By contrast, SOD does not inhibit $OH^{\bullet}$ generation by Fe^{2+}/H_2O_2 mixtures. Many more reactions are possible in Fenton systems,[16] including

$$OH^{\bullet} + Fe^{2+} \rightarrow Fe(III) + OH^-$$

$$OH^{\bullet} + H_2O_2 \rightarrow H_2O + H^+ + O_2^{\bullet-}$$

Which reactions occur depends on the experimental conditions, especially pH and the concentrations of H_2O_2 and Fe^{2+}. If nothing else is added for $OH^{\bullet}$ to attack, it will react with H_2O_2 or oxidize Fe^{2+} to Fe(III) ($k_2 \approx 3.5 \times 10^8\,M^{-1}s^{-1}$). Thus high concentration of Fe^{2+} or H_2O_2 can *decrease* the yield of $OH^{\bullet}$. The overall reaction, unless some other reagent is added, is an iron-catalysed decomposition of H_2O_2

$$2H_2O_2 \xrightarrow[\text{catalyst}]{\text{Fe salt}} O_2 + 2H_2O$$

Added organic molecules are attacked by the $OH^{\bullet}$, generating radicals that can undergo further reactions, often including oxidizing or reducing the iron ions.

Table 2.6 Some standard reduction potentials for iron chelators in relation to interaction with superoxide[3]

Couple	$E^{\circ\prime}$ (V)
$O_2/O_2^{\bullet-}$	−0.33
Likely reductions	
Fe(III)/Fe^{2+} (aq)	+0.11
Fe(III)-(1,10 phenanthroline)$_3$/Fe^{2+}-(1,10 phenanthroline)$_3$	+1.15
Fe(III)-citrate/Fe^{2+}-citrate	+0.1
Fe(III)-ADP/Fe^{2+}-ADP	+0.1
Fe(III)-EDTA/Fe^{2+}-EDTA	+0.12
Fe(III)-DETAPAC/Fe^{2+}-DETAPAC	+0.03
Fe(III)-ferritin/Fe^{2+}-ferritin	−0.19
Fe(III)-cytochrome c/Fe^{2+}-cytochrome c	+0.26
Unlikely reductions	
Fe(III)-transferrin/Fe^{2+}-transferrin	−0.40
Fe(III)-desferrioxamine/Fe^{2+}-desferrioxamine	−0.45

Remember that these are thermodynamic data; reactant concentrations and rates of reaction must be considered. Thus Fe(III)-EDTA is reduced by $O_2^{\bullet-}$ much faster than is Fe(III)-DETAPAC even though both reductions are thermodynamically favourable. DETAPAC, diethylenetriaminepenta-acetic acid. Also, remember that the $E^{\circ\prime}$ for $O_2/O_2^{\bullet-}$ is given for one atmosphere O_2 (Section 2.3.1.2).

2.4.5 Iron chelators and Fenton chemistry: speed it up or slow it down?

The rate constant for reaction of Fe^{2+} with H_2O_2 is $< 10^2\,M^{-1}s^{-1}$, but larger when the iron is attached to certain ligands (Table 2.4) including ATP, citrate, oxalate and pyrophosphate.[15] Ligands can also facilitate the reaction by keeping Fe^{2+} in solution, preventing it from oxidizing to Fe(III) and precipitating. However, ligands can also scavenge $OH^{\bullet}$; the ligand, being at a high local concentration, is an easy target of attack by newly formed $OH^{\bullet}$. For example, iron-EDTA chelates are excellent Fenton reagents, but some EDTA is destroyed during the reaction.[19]

There is much confusion in the literature about chelators as 'inhibitors' or 'promoters' of Fenton chemistry. From simple chemical principles, an iron chelator that affects the observed rate of OH• production from an iron/H_2O_2 system could do so by:

(a) altering the reduction potential of iron to favour (e.g. EDTA) or disfavour (e.g. transferrin) oxidation by H_2O_2 (Table 2.6);
(b) blocking access of H_2O_2 to the iron;
(c) promoting oxidation of Fe^{2+} to Fe(III), which is less reactive with H_2O_2; this will result in a short 'burst' of $O_2^{•-}$ production

$$\text{chelate} - Fe^{2+} \rightarrow \text{chelate} - Fe(III) + O_2^{•-}$$

(d) intercepting OH• before it can escape from the vicinity of the iron chelate, a process that depends on the geometry of the ligand-iron complex and the rate of reaction of the ligand with OH•;
(e) intercepting OH• precursors (such as the putative ferryl intermediate);
(f) if the chelator is in excess over the iron, some of the unbound chelator could scavenge OH• in free solution;
(g) keeping iron ions in solution at higher concentrations than in the absence of the chelator;
(h) any combination of the above actions.

These principles are important in the design of chelators for therapeutic use (Section 10.7).

2.4.6 Reaction of copper ions with H_2O_2

This may also be a significant source of OH• *in vivo*

$$Cu^+ + H_2O_2 \rightarrow Cu^{2+} + OH^• + OH^-$$

Copper binds avidly to many biological molecules, which will 'target' OH• to the binding site, making it difficult to scavenge by any added OH• scavengers. Thus failure of OH• scavengers to inhibit damage by Cu/H_2O_2 systems cannot be used as evidence that the RS formed is not OH•. For example, Cu ions promote H_2O_2-dependent damage to the Na^+, K^+-ATPase ion transporter at the specific sites to which the copper binds.[20] Another suggestion is that Cu^+ reacts with H_2O_2 not to give OH•; but instead an oxo-copper oxidizing species in which the copper is in the Cu(III) state. However, Cu(III) could result from reaction of Cu^{2+} with OH•. Singlet O_2 formation has also been proposed to

occur in Cu/H_2O_2 systems.[21] Currently, the majority of evidence suggests that OH• is a product of Cu/H_2O_2 systems,[22] although probably not the only oxidizing species formed.[21–23]

2.5 Chemistry of other biologically important radicals

2.5.1 Hydroxyl radical[24]

2.5.1.1 *Generation*
Hydroxyl radical can be generated by reaction of metal ions with H_2O_2, or by UV-induced homolytic fission of the O–O bond in H_2O_2

$$H-O-O-H \xrightarrow{\text{UV}} 2OH^•$$

This might even happen in sunlight-exposed skin (Section 6.12). In the laboratory, steady-state generation of OH• from H_2O_2 can be carried out using a low wavelength UV source. Hydroxyl radicals can also be generated from ozone and peroxynitrite (Sections 2.6.1 and 2.6.5 below). Other sources include:

1. *Ionizing radiation.* Since the major constituent of living cells is water, exposure to high-energy radiation such as γ-rays will result in OH• production by homolytic fission of water. Hydroxyl radicals are responsible for much of the damage done to cellular DNA, proteins and lipids by ionizing radiation (Section 8.19).
2. *From hypochlorous acid*[7] reacting with $O_2^{•-}$:

$$HOCl + O_2^{•-} \rightarrow O_2 + Cl^- + OH^•$$
$$k = 7.5 \times 10^6 \, M^{-1}s^{-1} \text{at } 25°C$$

HOCl can also react with Fe^{2+} and certain iron chelates, such as ferrocyanide and Fe^{2+}-citrate, to generate a 'RS' that can hydroxylate aromatic compounds. The simplest explanation would be

$$Fe^{2+}\text{-Chelate} + HOCl \rightarrow Fe(III)\text{-Chelate}$$
$$+ OH^• + Cl^-$$
$$k \sim 1.3 \times 10^4 \, M^{-1}s^{-1} \text{at } 25°C$$

However, the RS produced may be a higher oxidation state of iron[7] instead of OH•.

3. *Ultrasound.*[25] Sonication of aqueous solutions produces OH$^\bullet$. Ultrasound causes formation, growth and collapse of gas bubbles, an event called **acoustic cavitation**. Transient cavitations lead, upon collapse, to 'hot spots' in which temperatures of several thousand degrees and pressures of hundreds of atmospheres coexist, causing homolytic fission of H_2O to H$^\bullet$ and OH$^\bullet$. Unlike radiolysis, hydrated electrons are not normally produced. It seems unlikely that damaging levels of radical production occur during the use of ultrasound in medical diagnostic imaging, although formation of radicals by ultrasonication of human amniotic fluid *in vitro* has been demonstrated.[26] Hydroxyl radical formation during cataract removal by **pharmacoemulsification** (use of an ultrasonic probe to break up the lens within the eye, followed by aspiration) has also been reported, although the use of hyaluronic acid-containing fluids may minimize any biological impact,[27] since hyaluronic acid is a powerful scavenger of OH$^\bullet$.

Kidney stones can be fragmented by **shock wave lithotripsy** techniques, using rapid sonic pulses. Studies in pigs suggest that these techniques cause oxidative damage *in vivo* and revealed a protective effect of allopurinol, presumably by XO inhibition.[28] Sonication of lipids in the preparation of liposomes for studies of lipid peroxidation (Section 4.11.6.1) is also likely to lead to generation of free radicals and lipid oxidation.

4. *Decomposition of* **N-hydroxythiopyridones** has been suggested as a simple laboratory source of OH$^\bullet$, although the reaction also produces a sulphur radical (Fig. 2.2), whose reactivity must be considered. **N-hydroxypyridones** are an alternative, producing OH$^\bullet$ and an alkoxyl radical (Fig. 2.2B). Some of the OH$^\bullet$ will be intercepted by the aromatic ring of the molecule itself.

5. *Production from quinones.* Quinones and semiquinones can generate OH$^\bullet$ from H_2O_2 by redox reactions involving iron ions (Section 8.6.2). Recently it was proposed that tetrachlorobenzoquinone (TCBQ),

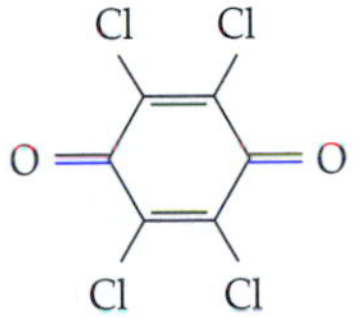

a metabolite of the carcinogenic wood preservative pentachlorophenol (Section 8.3.2), can generate OH$^\bullet$ from H_2O_2 by direct, metal ion-independent reactions.[29] One proposed mechanism was that an intermediate semiquinone radical is formed (exactly how is not clear) which then directly donates an electron to H_2O_2

$$\text{tetrachlorosemiquinone} + H_2O_2$$
$$\rightarrow \text{tetrachloroquinone} + OH^\bullet + OH^-$$

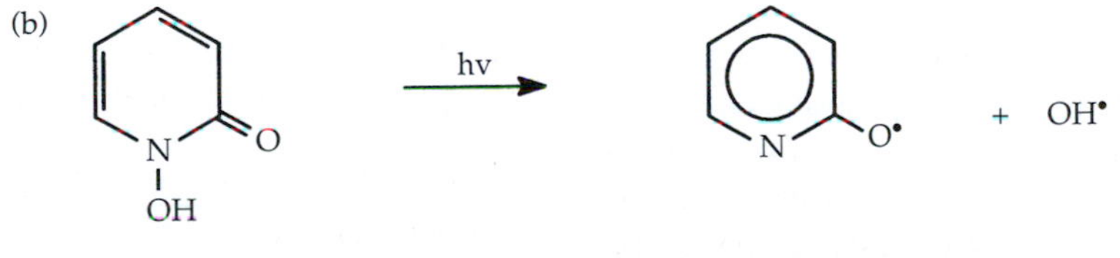

Figure 2.2 Formation of OH$^\bullet$ from (a) *N*-hydroxy-2-thiopyridone and (a) *N*-hydroxy-2-pyridone. Adapted from *Anal. Biochem.* **206**, 309, 1992 by courtesy of Dr T.A. Dix and Academic Press. The compounds release OH$^\bullet$ on exposure to visible light. Note that a thiyl radical is produced, which can sometimes contribute to biological effects. If the —OH group is replaced by —OR, then alkoxyl (RO$^\bullet$) radicals can be generated (*Free Rad. Biol. Med.* **24**, 234, 1998). *N*-hydroxy-4-thiopyridones have also been used. *N*-hydroxy-2-pyridone (*J. Am. Chem. Soc.* **118**, 10124, 1996; *Meth. Enzymol.* **300**, 194, 1999), generates aromatic alkoxyl instead of aromatic thiyl radicals.

Alternatively, TCBQ might combine with H_2O_2 to generate hydroperoxide or hydroperoxide–quinone intermediates, which then decompose by homolytic fission to generate $OH^\bullet$ (Ben-Zhan Zhu, personal communication). This seems intrinsically more likely since 'organic Fenton reactions' of the type shown above, although thermodynamically feasible, have not been convincingly shown to occur at significant rates.

2.5.1.2 *Chemistry*[24]

In the trophosphere, $OH^\bullet$ exists in the gaseous state. It can be formed, among other reactions, by photolysis of atmospheric nitrous acid

$$HNO_2 \rightarrow OH^\bullet + NO^\bullet$$

and readily oxidizes organic compounds in the trophosphere. In aqueous solution, $OH^\bullet$ has a nondescript absorbance spectrum, with a weak absorbance peak at 230 nm. It ionizes at very alkaline, biologically irrelevant, pH values:

$$OH^\bullet \rightleftharpoons O^- + H^+ \qquad pK_a \approx 12$$

If two $OH^\bullet$ radicals meet, they can form H_2O_2:

$$OH^\bullet + OH^\bullet \rightarrow H_2O_2 \qquad k = 5 \times 10^9\,M^{-1}s^{-1}$$

Although this reaction has a high rate constant and occurs in spurs during radiolysis (Section 2.3.3.1), it is unlikely to occur *in vivo* because the steady-state concentration of $OH^\bullet$ is effectively zero. As soon as $OH^\bullet$ is formed, it reacts very fast with molecules in its immediate vicinity (Table 2.7).

Rate constants for $OH^\bullet$ reactions have mainly been determined by pulse radiolysis, although other methods exist, such as the deoxyribose method (Section 5.3.3). The values are almost always very high (Table 2.7); indeed, $OH^\bullet$ is the most reactive oxygen radical known, with a highly positive reduction potential (Table 2.3). For example, it is difficult to demonstrate $OH^\bullet$ reactions *in vitro* in solutions containing Tris, Tricine or HEPES buffers, since $OH^\bullet$ attacks them rapidly and buffer-derived radicals are produced. One end-product of $OH^\bullet$ attack on Tris is formaldehyde.[30]

Reactions of $OH^\bullet$, are of three main types: **hydrogen abstraction**, **addition**, and **electron transfer**. Remember that reaction of a free radical with a non-radical produces a different radical? Let's demonstrate this with $OH^\bullet$. One example of $H^\bullet$ abstraction is the reaction of $OH^\bullet$ with alcohols. The $OH^\bullet$ abstracts $H^\bullet$ and instantly combines with it to form water, leaving behind an unpaired electron on the carbon atom, for example with ethanol:

$$
\begin{array}{c}
\text{H\ \ H} \\
|\ \ \ | \\
\text{H}-\text{C}-\text{C}-\text{O}-\text{H}+\text{OH}^\bullet \\
|\ \ \ | \\
\text{H\ \ H}
\end{array}
\rightarrow
\begin{array}{c}
\text{H} \\
| \\
\text{H}-\text{C}-\text{C}^\bullet-\text{O}-\text{H}+\text{H}_2\text{O} \\
|\ \ \ | \\
\text{H\ \ H}
\end{array}
$$

hydroxyethyl radical

Reactions of the carbon radical can then occur, often with O_2.

$$CH_3\overset{\bullet}{C}HOH + O_2 \rightarrow {}^\bullet O_2CH_3CHOH$$
peroxyl radical

or (if O_2 levels are low), covalent bond formation to form a non-radical:

$$
CH_3\overset{\bullet}{C}HOH + CH_3\overset{\bullet}{C}HOH \rightarrow
\begin{array}{c}
CH_3CHOH \\
| \\
CH_3\overset{}{C}HOH
\end{array}
$$

Reaction of $OH^\bullet$ with aromatic compounds often proceeds by addition. For example, $OH^\bullet$ adds to guanine in DNA to form an **8-hydroxyguanine radical** (Section 4.8.2.1). Similarly, $OH^\bullet$ can add on to double bonds.

$$\ce{>C=C<} + OH^\bullet \rightarrow \ce{>C-\overset{\bullet}{C}<}\ (OH)$$

This happens with thymine; the thymine radical then undergoes further reactions, for example with O_2 to give a thymine peroxyl radical (Section 4.8).

Hydroxyl radicals can take part in electron-transfer reactions, for example with halide ions:

$$Cl^- + OH^\bullet \rightarrow Cl^\bullet + OH^-$$

$$Cl^\bullet + Cl^- \rightarrow Cl_2^{\bullet -}$$

and with nitrite:

$$NO_2^- + OH^\bullet \rightarrow NO_2^\bullet + OH^-$$

Reaction of $OH^\bullet$ with carbonate or bicarbonate is also important.

Table 2.7 Second-order rate constants for reactions of the hydroxyl radical

Compound tested	pH	Rate constant ($M^{-1}s^{-1}$)
Fe^{2+}	2.1	3.5×10^8
H_2O_2	7	4.5×10^7
Adenine	7.4	3.0×10^9
Adenosine	7.7	2.5×10^9
AMP	5.4	1.8×10^9
Arginine	7	2.1×10^9
Ascorbic acid	1	7.2×10^9
Benzene	7	3.2×10^9
Benzoic acid	3	4.3×10^9
Butan-1-ol (n-butanol)	7	2.2×10^9
Butylated hydroxyanisole		6×10^9
Butylated hydroxytoluene		6×10^9
Catalase	–	2.6×10^{11}
Citric acid	1	3.0×10^7
Cysteine	1	7.9×10^9
Cystine	2	2.0×10^9
Cytidine	2	2.0×10^9
Cytosine	7	2.9×10^9
Deoxyguanylic acid	7	4.1×10^9
Deoxyribose	7.4	3.1×10^9
Desferrioxamine		1.3×10^{10}
Dimethylsulphoxide		3.5×10^9
EDTA		2.8×10^9
Ethanol	7	7.2×10^8
Formate		3.5×10^9
Glucose	7	1.0×10^9
Glutamic acid	2	7.9×10^9
Glutathione	1	8.8×10^9
Glycylglycine	2	7.8×10^7
Glycyltyrosine	2	5.6×10^9
Guanine	–	1.0×10^{10}
Haemoglobin	–	3.6×10^{10}
HEPES buffer	–	5.1×10^9
Histidine	6.7	3.0×10^9
Hydroxyproline	2	2.1×10^8
Lactate ion	9	4.8×10^9
Lecithin	–	5.0×10^8
Mannitol	7	2.7×10^9
Methanol	7	4.7×10^8
Methionine	7	5.1×10^9
Nicotinic acid	–	6.3×10^8
Phenol	7	4.2×10^9
Phenylalanine	6	3.5×10^9
Propan-1-ol	7	1.5×10^9
Pyridoxal phosphate	–	1.6×10^9
Ribonuclease	–	1.9×10^{10}
Ribose	7	1.2×10^9
Plasma albumin	–	$> 10^{10}$
Thiourea	7	4.7×10^9
Thymine	7	3.1×10^9
Tris buffer		1.1×10^9
Tricine buffer	–	1.6×10^9
Tryptophan	6	8.5×10^9
Uracil	7	3.1×10^9
Urea	9	$< 7.0 \times 10^5$

Values mostly taken from *Int. J. Appl. Radiat. Isotopes* **18**, 493, 1967; some from *Anal. Biochem.* **165**, 215, 1987. The value for mannitol is from *Free Radic. Res. Commun.* **4**, 259, 1998 and those for HEPES, TRIS and Tricine buffers from *FEBS Lett.* **199**, 92, 1986. Note that $OH^\bullet$ reacts with almost all biomolecules so rapidly that often the reaction is limited only by the rate at which $OH^\bullet$ contacts the molecule in solution (**a diffusion-controlled rate**). Urea is a rare exception: its rate constant is low for a reaction with $OH^\bullet$ but still high when compared with that of many other reactions (e.g. Fenton reactions: Table 2.4). A compendium of rate constants for $OH^\bullet$ and several other RS can be accessed on the NIST database (*kinetics.nist.gov/solution/index.php*)

2.5.2 Carbonate radical[31]

Carbonate radicals are formed when $OH^\bullet$ reacts with carbonate or bicarbonate ions, and it has only recently dawned on most of the free radical community that the CO_2/HCO_3^- content of reaction systems is an important parameter in determining the molecular nature of oxidative damage. The rate constants are lower than for most reactions of $OH^\bullet$. Nevertheless, HCO_3^- levels *in vivo* are high (e.g. $25\,mM$ HCO_3^- in blood plasma) making reaction feasible.

$$CO_3^{2-} + OH^\bullet \rightarrow CO_3^{\bullet -} + OH^-$$
$$k \sim 2 \times 10^8\,M^{-1}s^{-1}$$

$$HCO_3^- + OH^\bullet \rightarrow H_2O + CO_3^{\bullet -}$$
$$k \sim 1 \times 10^7\,M^{-1}s^{-1}$$

Carbonate radical is also produced when $ONOO^-$ reacts with CO_2 (Section 2.6.1) and when Mn^{2+} reacts with H_2O_2 in the presence of HCO_3^- and CO_2.[12] It can be made in the laboratory by the decomposition of cobalt(III) carbonato complex, $[Co(NH_3)_5CO_3]^+$, induced by UV light.[32]

Carbonate radical is a potent one-electron oxidizing agent ($E^{\circ\prime} = 1.78\,V$) and oxidizes a range of biomolecules, including hyaluronic acid. For example, it can abstract $H^\bullet$ from cysteine,

$$\text{cys}-\text{SH} + \text{CO}_3^{\bullet -} \rightarrow \text{HCO}_3^- + \text{cysS}^{\bullet}$$
$$k = 4.6 \times 10^7\,\text{M}^{-1}\text{s}^{-1}$$

or tyrosine

$$\text{Tyr}-\text{OH} + \text{CO}_3^{\bullet -} \rightarrow \text{Tyr}-\text{O}^{\bullet} + \text{HCO}_3^-$$
$$k = 4.5 \times 10^7\,\text{M}^{-1}\text{s}^{-1}$$

or NAD(P)H (Section 2.6.1.1 below) and it can oxidize ascorbate, methionine, and guanine. Carbonate radical is also involved in the 'peroxidase' reactions of CuZnSOD (Section 3.2.1.6). Overall, however, it is less damaging to proteins, lipids and DNA than is OH$^{\bullet}$. More work is needed to ascertain the contribution of $\text{CO}_3^{\bullet -}$ to oxidative damage *in vivo*.

Another species of possible biological interest is **peroxomonocarbonate**, HCO_4^-, reversibly formed[33] when H_2O_2 interacts with HCO_3^- (or CO_2)

$$\text{H}_2\text{O}_2 + \text{HCO}_3^- \rightleftharpoons \text{H}_2\text{O} + \text{HOOCO}_2^-$$

It can be reduced (e.g. by Cu^+) to release $\text{CO}_3^{\bullet -}$

$$\text{HOOCO}_2^- + \text{Cu}^+ \rightarrow \text{Cu}^{2+} + \text{CO}_3^{\bullet -} + \text{OH}^-$$

2.5.3 Superoxide radical[10,24]

Superoxide is far less reactive than OH$^{\bullet}$ and does not react at all with most biological molecules in aqueous solution. It does react quickly, however, with some other radicals, such as NO$^{\bullet}$ (Section 2.5.6 below), iron–sulphur clusters in certain enzymes (Section 3.6) and some **phenoxyl radicals**, for example that formed by abstracting hydrogen from the −OH group of tyrosine.[34] The reaction of tyrosine phenoxyl radical with $\text{O}_2^{\bullet -}$ is quite fast ($k = 1.5 \times 10^9\,\text{M}^{-1}\text{s}^{-1}$) and a **tyrosine hydroperoxide** results, which can then undergo cyclization and loss of the peroxide group. 'Repair' of the tyrosine radical can also occur

$$\text{Tyr}-\text{O}^{\bullet} + \text{O}_2^{\bullet -} + \text{H}^+ \rightarrow \text{Tyr}-\text{OH} + \text{O}_2$$
$$\text{Tyrosine}$$

The reactivity of $\text{O}_2^{\bullet -}$ with non-radicals is influenced by solvent and pH. The pK_a of the reaction

$$\text{HO}_2^{\bullet} \rightleftharpoons \text{H}^+ + \text{O}_2^{\bullet -}$$

is approximately 4.8. Table 2.3 shows that HO$_2^{\bullet}$ radical (**hydroperoxyl**) is a more powerful

reducing agent than $\text{O}_2^{\bullet -}$ ($E^{\circ\prime}$ values of -0.46 and -0.33 V, respectively). Although at the pH of most body tissues the ratio of $[\text{O}_2^{\bullet -}]/[\text{HO}_2^{\bullet}]$ will be large (100/1 at pH 6.8, 1000/1 at pH 7.8), the greater reactivity of HO$_2^{\bullet}$ and its uncharged nature, which might allow it to cross membranes more readily than the charged $\text{O}_2^{\bullet -}$, suggest that it has the potential to cause damage. In general, superoxide does not readily cross membranes, although it can pass through the **anion exchange proteins** present in some cells, for example erythrocytes and lung (Sections 6.3 and 6.4).

2.5.3.1 *Making superoxide in the laboratory*[10,24,36]
Various methods are available:

1. Oxygen may be reduced electrochemically in the presence of an organic solvent such as dimethylsulphoxide or acetonitrile.

2. Tetraalkylammonium superoxides such as tetramethylammonium superoxide ($(\text{CH}_3)_4\text{N}^+\text{O}_2^{\bullet -}$), or trimethylphenylammonium superoxide, ($(\text{CH}_3)_3\text{PhN}^+\text{O}_2^{\bullet -}$), can be dissolved in organic solvents.

3. Potassium metal can be burned in oxygen to form the ionic compound **potassium superoxide**, $\text{K}^+\text{O}_2^{\bullet -}$ (although usually it is far from pure). This salt is slightly soluble in organic solvents and its solubility can be increased by the addition of **crown ethers**, such as **dicyclohexyl-18-crown-6** (Fig. 2.3), cyclic molecules which bind K^+. They are soluble in organic solvents and so 'drag into solution' the central K^+ ion together with its associated $\text{O}_2^{\bullet -}$. The reaction of $\text{O}_2^{\bullet -}$ with another compound added to the organic solvent can be observed, or the KO$_2$-containing organic solvent can be mixed with an aqueous solution of the compound, for example in stopped-flow experiments (Section 2.3.3.2). Superoxide dissolved in organic solvents is stable if water is kept away, but disappears rapidly if moisture from the air is allowed in.

4. Pulse radiolysis (Fig. 2.1) generates $\text{O}_2^{\bullet -}$; it can be detected by its UV-absorbance (maximal absorption around 245 nm; for HO$_2^{\bullet}$ 225 nm) or its ESR spectrum.

5. Enzymes and photochemical reactions are often used to generate $\text{O}_2^{\bullet -}$. Mixtures of xanthine or

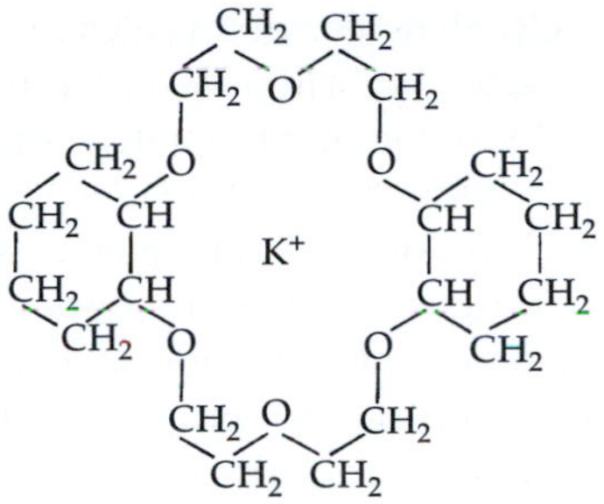
CH2 CH2
CH2 O CH2
CH2 O O CH2
CH2 CH CH CH2
K+
CH2 CH CH CH2
CH2 O O CH2
CH2 O CH2
CH2 CH2

Figure 2.3 Structure of dicyclohexyl-18-crown-6. The K^+ ion fits into the central 'hole'.

hypoxanthine with XO are widely used in biological laboratories, but this enzyme also makes H_2O_2; some points to consider in its use are listed in Fig. 1.16. Xanthine oxidase preparations and laboratory buffers are frequently contaminated with iron, meaning that $OH^\bullet$ radicals can be made.

$$H_2O_2 + Fe^{2+} \rightarrow Fe(\text{III}) + OH^\bullet + OH^-$$

$$Fe(\text{III}) + O_2^{\bullet-} \rightarrow Fe^{2+} + O_2$$

This pair of reactions adds up to

$$H_2O_2 + O_2^{\bullet-} \xrightarrow{\text{Fe catalyst}} OH^\bullet + OH^- + O_2$$

and is often called the **superoxide-assisted (or driven) Fenton reaction**. Some papers have attributed effects of the xanthine/XO system to $O_2^{\bullet-}$ when they are in fact due to H_2O_2 or to $OH^\bullet$. This can be avoided by adding sufficient catalase to remove all H_2O_2 generated.

6. Some azo compounds decompose to generate $O_2^{\bullet-}$

$$X{-}N = N{-}Y \rightarrow X^\bullet + N_2 + Y^\bullet$$

$$X^\bullet(Y^\bullet) + O_2 \rightarrow X^+(Y^+) + O_2^{\bullet-}$$

One example is SOTS, di(4-carboxybenzyl) hyponitrite.

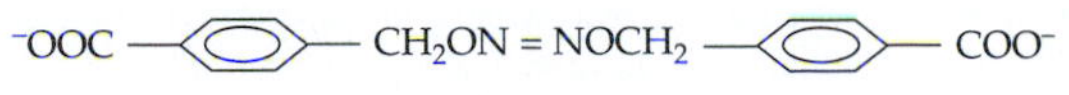
⁻OOC
CH2ON = NOCH2
COO⁻

Its decomposition in water at 37 °C, pH 7 (half-life ~82 min)[35] gives a steady source of $O_2^{\bullet-}$.

2.5.3.2 *Reactions of superoxide*[10]

The rapid disappearance of $O_2^{\bullet-}$ in aqueous solution is due to the **dismutation reaction**. One $O_2^{\bullet-}$ is oxidized (to O_2) and another is reduced (to H_2O_2)—the definition of dismutation is a chemical reaction in which the same species is both oxidized and reduced. The overall reaction is

$$O_2^{\bullet-} + O_2^{\bullet-} + 2H^+ \rightarrow H_2O_2 + O_2$$

However, the rate constant for this reaction as written is close to zero ($<0.3\,M^{-1}s^{-1}$). By contrast, the reaction

$$HO_2^\bullet + O_2^{\bullet-} + H^+ \rightarrow H_2O_2 + O_2$$

has $k_2 = 9.7 \times 10^7\,M^{-1}s^{-1}$, and the reaction

$$HO_2^\bullet + HO_2^\bullet \rightarrow H_2O_2 + O_2$$

has $k_2 = 8.3 \times 10^5\,M^{-1}s^{-1}$. Hence dismutation under physiological conditions usually proceeds by protonation of $O_2^{\bullet-}$ followed by reaction of $HO_2^\bullet$ with $O_2^{\bullet-}$. Dismutation is thus most rapid at the acidic pH values needed to protonate $O_2^{\bullet-}$ and slows down at more alkaline pH values. For example, it may be calculated that in aqueous solution the dismutation reaction has a 'rate constant' of about $10^2\,M^{-1}s^{-1}$at pH 11 and about $5 \times 10^5\,M^{-1}s^{-1}$ at pH 7.0. Any molecule that reacts with $O_2^{\bullet-}$ in aqueous solution will be competing with the dismutation reaction. It also follows that any aqueous system generating $O_2^{\bullet-}$ will produce H_2O_2, unless all the $O_2^{\bullet-}$ is intercepted by some other molecule.

Superoxide in aqueous solution can act as a reducing agent, for example it donates an electron to cytochrome *c*.

$$\text{cyt}\,c\,(Fe(\text{III})) + O_2^{\bullet-} \rightarrow O_2 + \text{cyt}\,c(Fe^{2+})$$

and to the chloroplast copper-containing protein plastocyanin (Section 6.8):

$$\text{plastocyanin}(Cu^{2+}) + O_2^{\bullet-} \rightarrow O_2 + \text{plastocyanin}(Cu^+)$$

It reduces the yellow dye **nitroblue tetrazolium** (NBT^{2+}) to produce the blue product **formazan**, although the reaction mechanism is complex (Fig. 2.4). Reduction of cytochrome *c* and NBT^{2+} by $O_2^{\bullet-}$ are used in assays of SOD (Section 3.2.5).

Superoxide can also act as an oxidizing agent, for example with dopamine and adrenalin (Section 3.2.5) and with ascorbate (AH_2):

$$AH_2 + O_2^{\bullet-} \rightarrow A^{\bullet-} + H_2O_2$$

The rate constant for the above reaction has been quoted as $2.7 \times 10^5 M^{-1}s^{-1}$ at 25 °C and pH 7.4. Superoxide does not oxidize NADPH or NADH at measurable rates, but it can interact with NADH bound to the active site of lactate dehydrogenase (LDH) to form an NAD$^{\bullet}$ radical

$$LDH-NADH + O_2^{\bullet-} + H^+ \\ \rightarrow LDH-NAD^{\bullet} + H_2O_2$$

Unlike $O_2^{\bullet-}$, $HO_2^{\bullet}$ does oxidize NADH directly ($k_2 = 1.8 \times 10^5 M^{-1}s^{-1}$). NADH bound at the active site of the glycolytic enzyme G3PDH (Fig. 1.7) is oxidized faster by $HO_2^{\bullet}$ ($k_2 = 2 \times 10^7 M^{-1}s^{-1}$), although G3PDH does not promote reaction of $O_2^{\bullet-}$ with bound NADH (unlike LDH).

In general, however, $O_2^{\bullet-}$ in aqueous solution at pH 7.4 is not highly reactive. Its rates of reaction with DNA, lipids, amino acids and most other biomolecules are low, or zero. For example, its reaction with GSH proceeds, if at all, with a rate constant[37] $\leq 200 M^{-1}s^{-1}$. Biological damage by $O_2^{\bullet-}$ is highly selective and usually involves its reaction with other radicals, for example NO$^{\bullet}$ or iron ions in iron–sulphur proteins (Section 3.7). It also reacts with HOCl and chloramines (Section 2.6.3 below) and interacts with mitochondrial uncoupling proteins (Section 1.10.6).

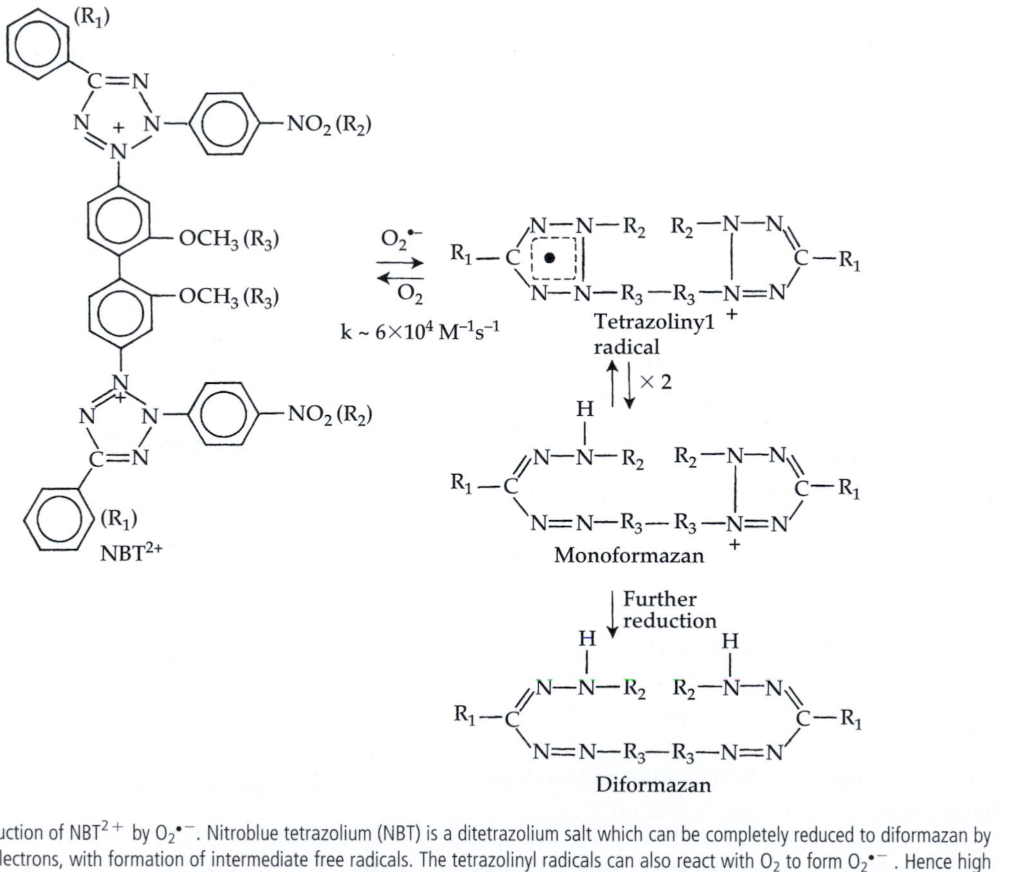

Figure 2.4 Reduction of NBT^{2+} by $O_2^{\bullet-}$. Nitroblue tetrazolium (NBT) is a ditetrazolium salt which can be completely reduced to diformazan by addition of four electrons, with formation of intermediate free radicals. The tetrazolinyl radicals can also react with O_2 to form $O_2^{\bullet-}$. Hence high O_2 concentrations depress formazan production from $O_2^{\bullet-}$ plus NBT^{2+}. NBT^{2+} should not therefore, be used as a specific detector of $O_2^{\bullet-}$ in biological systems, since its reduction to a radical by other mechanisms (e.g. by enzymes such as glucose oxidase or thioredoxin reductase) can lead to $O_2^{\bullet-}$ formation (*J. Phys. Chem.* **84**, 830, 1980; *Arch. Biochem. Biophys.* **318**, 408, 1995; *Free Rad. Biol. Med.* **31**, 1287, 2001). The $CO_2^{\bullet-}$ radical can also generate formazan from NBT^{2+}.

2.5.3.3 *Superoxide–iron interactions*[10,13,16]

Work in Bielski's laboratory established the following rate constants for reaction of $O_2^{\bullet-}$ with aqueous iron salts

$$Fe^{2+} + HO_2^{\bullet} + H^+ \rightarrow Fe(III) + H_2O_2$$
$$1.2 \times 10^6 \, M^{-1}s^{-1}$$

$$Fe^{2+} + O_2^{\bullet-} + H^+ \rightarrow Fe(III) + HO_2^-$$
$$1 \times 10^7 \, M^{-1}s^{-1}$$

$$Fe(III) + O_2^{\bullet-} \rightarrow Fe^{2+} + O_2 \qquad 1.5 \times 10^8 \, M^{-1}s^{-1}$$

$$Fe(III) + HO_2^{\bullet} \rightarrow Fe^{2+} + H^+ + O_2$$
$$<10^3 \, M^{-1}s^{-1}$$

Thus $O_2^{\bullet-}$ can reduce Fe(III), but also oxidize Fe^{2+}. The former reaction may proceed through intermediates, such as **perferryl**

$$Fe(III) + O_2^{\bullet-} \rightleftharpoons [Fe^{2+}-O_2 \leftrightarrow Fe(III)-O_2^{\bullet-}]$$
$$\rightleftharpoons Fe^{2+} + O_2$$

The above rate constants can be changed by binding ligands to the iron. For example, Fe(III) bound to EDTA is still reduced by $O_2^{\bullet-}$:

$$Fe(III) - EDTA + O_2^{\bullet-}$$
$$\rightleftharpoons (intermediate \ complexes)$$
$$\rightleftharpoons Fe^{2+} - EDTA + O_2$$

$$k_2 = 1.3 \times 10^6 \, M^{-1}s^{-1} \ at \ pH \ 7$$

whereas Fe(III) attached to transferrin, lactoferrin or desferrioxamine is not, as predicted by the relative reduction potentials (Tables 2.3 and 2.6). Reduction of Fe(III) chelates of citrate, ADP and DETAPAC by $O_2^{\bullet-}$ is possible (Table 2.6) but the rate constants appear fairly low (e.g. $6 \times 10^3 \, M^{-1}s^{-1}$ for Fe(III)–DETAPAC). Superoxide, produced in sunlit natural waters by photochemical reactions involving dissolved organic matter, helps maintain some dissolved iron as Fe^{2+}, and can also interact with dissolved copper ions.[38]

2.5.3.4 *Reductants and Fenton chemistry*

Superoxide can accelerate OH$^{\bullet}$ production by the Fenton reaction (Section 2.5.3.1). Other reducing agents, such as ascorbate, can do the same: the **Udenfriend system** for hydroxylating aromatic compounds is a mixture of Fe(III)–EDTA, H_2O_2 and ascorbate. Ascorbate stimulates OH$^{\bullet}$ generation by recycling Fe(III) to Fe^{2+}, but too much ascorbate can decrease the yield of OH$^{\bullet}$ by scavenging it (rate constant $>10^9 \, M^{-1}s^{-1}$).

2.5.3.5 *Semiquinones and quinones*

Superoxide can reduce quinones and oxidize diphenols, and often semiquinones reduce O_2 to $O_2^{\bullet-}$ (Fig. 2.5). Essentially these are reversible reactions. However, dismutation of $O_2^{\bullet-}$ in aqueous solution favours reaction of semiquinones with O_2 by removing $O_2^{\bullet-}$. Thus adding SOD can inhibit semiquinone-dependent reactions by causing the equilibrium

$$semiquinone + O_2 \rightleftharpoons quinone + O_2^{\bullet-}$$

to move to the right.

2.5.3.6 *Superoxide in hydrophobic environments*[39]

When $O_2^{\bullet-}$ is dissolved in organic solvents, its abilities to act as a base (H$^+$ acceptor) and a reducing agent are increased. For example, it can reduce dissolved sulphur dioxide (SO$_2$) gas in organic solvents but not in aqueous solution:

$$SO_2 + O_2^{\bullet-} \rightarrow O_2 + SO_2^{\bullet-}$$

Also, if protons are not available, dismutation is prevented and the $O_2^{\bullet-}$ persists longer. Further, it

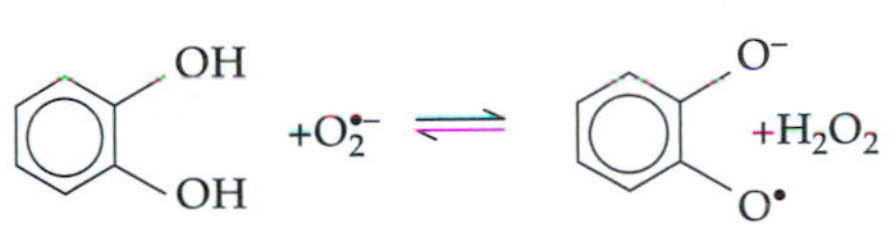

Figure 2.5 Reaction of $O_2^{\bullet-}$ with quinones and diphenols. Some quinones can be reduced to semiquinones by $O_2^{\bullet-}$ and some diphenols oxidized to semiquinones. Reactions are often reversible, i.e. semiquinones can reduce O_2 to $O_2^{\bullet-}$. Above: reduction of benzoquinone (rate constant $\sim10^9 \, M^{-1}s^{-1}$); below: oxidation of catechol (rate constant $\sim10^9 \, M^{-1}s^{-1}$).

acts as a much better **nucleophile**, an agent that attacks the centre of positive charge in another molecule. Consider, for example an ester molecule of general formula:

$$R - \overset{\overset{\textstyle O^{\delta-}}{\|}}{\underset{\delta+}{C}} - O - R'$$

where R and R′ are hydrocarbon groups. Since oxygen is more electronegative than carbon, the carbonyl group is slightly polarized (see the Appendix for explanation if needed). Superoxide will be attracted to the $\delta+$ charge and will attack the molecule, leading to displacement of the alcohol and formation of a carboxylic acid. Indeed, $O_2^{\bullet-}$ in organic media can even nucleophilically displace chloride ion from chlorinated hydrocarbons such as chloroform, tetrachloromethane (CCl_4), hexachlorobenzene (C_6Cl_6), and polychlorobiphenyls, important environmental toxins.[40] For example, in the case of CCl_4 the reaction

$$CCl_4 + O_2^{\bullet-} \rightarrow CCl_3O_2^{\bullet} + Cl^-$$

is followed by further displacements. By contrast, the nucleophilicity of $O_2^{\bullet-}$ in aqueous solution is low, in part because of dismutation and also because hydration of $O_2^{\bullet-}$ decreases its charge density.

Superoxide in organic solvents usually only acts as an oxidizing agent towards compounds that can donate H^+ ions, such as ascorbate, catechol and α-tocopherol. Tocopherol (TocH) is slowly oxidized by $O_2^{\bullet-}$ in organic solvents to give tocopheryl radical (Toc$^{\bullet}$); suggested reactions include:

$$O_2^{\bullet-} + TocH \rightarrow Toc^- + HO_2^{\bullet}$$
(deprotonation by $O_2^{\bullet-}$ giving tocopherol ion)

$$HO_2^{\bullet} + TocH \rightarrow H_2O_2 + Toc^{\bullet}$$
(oxidation of tocopherol by $HO_2^{\bullet}$)

$$O_2 + Toc^- \rightarrow O_2^{\bullet-} + Toc^{\bullet}$$

$$2Toc^{\bullet} \rightarrow \text{dimer and other products}$$

In aqueous solution, however, $O_2^{\bullet-}$ does not react with α-tocopherol at a significant rate, in part because α-tocopherol is poorly soluble in water.

2.5.4 Peroxyl and alkoxyl radicals[24,41]

2.5.4.1 Chemistry

Peroxyl ($RO_2^{\bullet}$) and alkoxyl ($RO^{\bullet}$) radicals are usually good oxidizing agents, having highly positive $E^{\circ\prime}$ values (Table 2.3). Indeed $HO_2^{\bullet}$, protonated $O_2^{\bullet-}$, can be regarded as the simplest peroxyl radical. For example, ($RO_2^{\bullet}$) radicals oxidize ascorbate and NADH, the latter leading to $O_2^{\bullet-}$ formation in the presence of O_2

$$RO_2^{\bullet} + NADH \rightarrow RO_2H + NAD^{\bullet}$$

$$NAD^{\bullet} + O_2 \rightarrow NAD^+ + O_2^{\bullet} \qquad k \sim 10^9\,M^{-1}s^{-1}$$

Alkoxyl and $RO_2^{\bullet}$ radicals can abstract $H^{\bullet}$ from other molecules, a reaction important in lipid peroxidation (Section 4.12). Some $RO_2^{\bullet}$ break down to liberate $O_2^{\bullet-}$, for example α-hydroxylalkyperoxyl radicals. When glucose reacts with $OH^{\bullet}$, six different $RO_2^{\bullet}$ radicals are formed, since $H^{\bullet}$ abstraction by $OH^{\bullet}$ can occur at any of the six carbon atoms. Five of these eliminate $O_2^{\bullet-}$ rapidly, for example

$$R - \overset{\overset{\textstyle R^1}{|}}{\underset{\underset{\textstyle OH}{|}}{C}} - O_2^{\bullet} \rightarrow R - \overset{\overset{\textstyle O}{\|}}{C} - R + H^+ + O_2^{\bullet-}$$

Peroxyl radicals can react with each other, for example by the **Russell mechanism**, to generate singlet O_2 ($^1O_2$):

$$\text{\textbackslash CHOO}^{\bullet} + \text{\textbackslash CHOO}^{\bullet} \longrightarrow \text{\textbackslash CHOH} + \text{\textbackslash C=O} + {}^1O_2$$

A **tetraoxide** intermediate

$$\text{C-O-O-O-O-C}$$

may be involved.

Aromatic alkoxyl and peroxyl radicals tend to be less reactive than aliphatic ones, since electrons are delocalized into the benzene ring. For example, when tyrosine phenoxyl radical (TyrO$^{\bullet}$) is generated in biological systems, it often cross-links to give **bityrosine** (Fig. 2.6), although it can also react with $O_2^{\bullet-}$ (Section 2.5.3). Tyrosyl radicals are very useful in biology, for example in ribonucleotide reductase (Section 7.2), photosynthesis (Section 6.8) and prostaglandin biosynthesis (Section 7.12).

2.5.4.2 *Generation of* $RO_2^{\bullet}/RO^{\bullet}$ *radicals*

Carbon-centred radicals react with O_2 (rate constants often $> 10^9 \, M^{-1} s^{-1}$) to form $RO_2^{\bullet}$ radicals. Decomposition of organic peroxides (ROOH) generates both $RO_2^{\bullet}$ and $RO^{\bullet}$, and the latter can also be produced by substituted *N*-hydroxypyridones (Fig. 2.2). Most peroxides are stable at room temperature, but they can be decomposed by heating, exposure to UV light (in some cases) or by addition of transition metal ions, for example

$$ROOH + Fe(III) \rightarrow RO_2^{\bullet} + Fe^{2+} + H^+$$

$$ROOH + Fe^{2+} \rightarrow RO^{\bullet} + OH^- + Fe(III)$$

These reactions account for much of the stimulation of lipid peroxidation by iron (Section 4.11.6), but protein peroxides are decomposed by metal

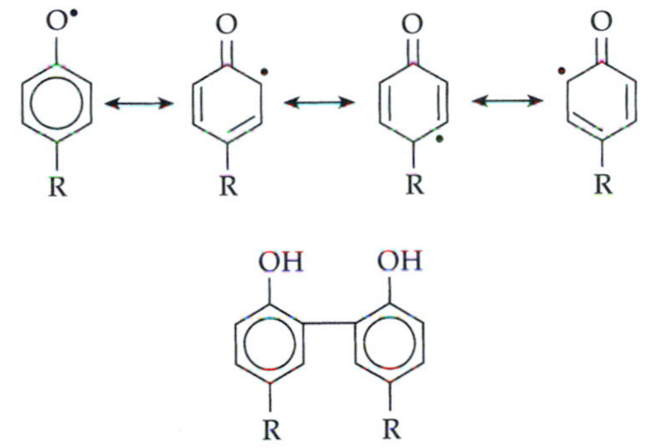

Figure 2.6 Cross-linking of tyrosine residues (see *Amino Acids* **25**, 227, 2003). The tyrosyl (tyrosine phenoxyl) radical has various resonance structures (upper diagram) and can cross-link in different ways, forming several bityrosines. R is the side-chain of the amino acid. The lower diagram shows **3, 3′ — bityrosine**, sometimes called *ortho,ortho-***bityrosine** or **dityrosine** (counting the — OH group on tyrosine as position 4). This compound has an intense fluorescence around 420 nm when excited at 315 nm (alkaline solutions) or 284 nm (acidic solutions). Bityrosine cross-links are found in proteins from the cuticle of *C. elegans* and certain insects, some yeast and fungal cell walls, the fertilization envelope of the sea-urchin (Section 7.5.3) and the thyroid gland (Section 7.5.1). Any radical reactive enough to abstract H$^{\bullet}$ from tyrosine residues in proteins may lead to bityrosine formation. Tyrosyl radical can react with ascorbate, cysteine, GSH and $O_2^{\bullet-}$ (Section 2.5.3), e.g. TyrO$^{\bullet}$ + R–SH $\rightarrow$ TyrOH + R–S$^{\bullet}$.

ions as well (Section 4.13). Lipid peroxides might also react with $HO_2^{\bullet}$ to form $RO_2^{\bullet}$

$$HO_2^{\bullet} + ROOH \rightarrow RO_2^{\bullet} + H_2O_2$$

Azo initiators[42] can be used in the laboratory to generate $RO_2^{\bullet}$ radicals (and $O_2^{\bullet-}$ radicals[35]) (Fig. 2.7). Whereas AAPH is water-soluble, AMVN is hydrophobic and can enter membranes to generate radicals in the lipid phase. The compound AIPH has been used in animals. All three decompose at a temperature-controlled rate to give carbon-centred radicals

$$A - N = N - A \rightarrow N_2 + 2A^{\bullet}$$

which then react rapidly with O_2 to give $RO_2^{\bullet}$ radicals. However, the A$^{\bullet}$ radicals can themselves react with some biological molecules, perhaps including DNA and albumin–SH groups,[43] so it is essential to ensure that sufficient O_2 is present to ensure complete conversion of them to $RO_2^{\bullet}$ The peroxyl radical from AAPH is positively charged, whereas many biologically derived peroxyl radicals are negatively charged (e.g. fatty acid peroxyls) or neutral (phospholipid peroxyls), although some amino acid peroxyls can be positive. Charge influences reactivity: for example in one study AAPH-derived peroxyl radicals could cleave double-stranded plasmid DNA, whereas the negative and neutral peroxyl radicals examined could not.[44] Peroxyl radicals from azo initiators can induce lipid peroxidation and damage proteins, for example they inactivate the enzyme lysozyme.[45] Indeed, they are often used to assess antioxidant activity, for example in the TRAP assay (Section 5.17).

Trichloromethylperoxyl radical[46] is formed from CCl_4 *in vivo* (Section 8.2) and when $O_2^{\bullet-}$ attacks CCl_4 in organic solvents (Section 2.5.3.6). It can be generated in the laboratory by radiolysis of an aqueous mixture of propan-2-ol and tetrachloromethane (CCl_4)

$$e_{aq}^- + CCl_4 \rightarrow CCl_3^{\bullet} + Cl^-$$

$$OH^{\bullet} + CH_3CHOHCH_3 \rightarrow CH_3\overset{\bullet}{C}OHCH_3 + H_2O$$

$$CH_3\overset{\bullet}{C}OHCH_3 + CCl_4 \rightarrow CH_3COCH_3 + H^+ \\ + CCl_3^{\bullet} + Cl^-$$

$$CCl_3^{\bullet} + O_2 \rightarrow CCl_3O_2^{\bullet}$$

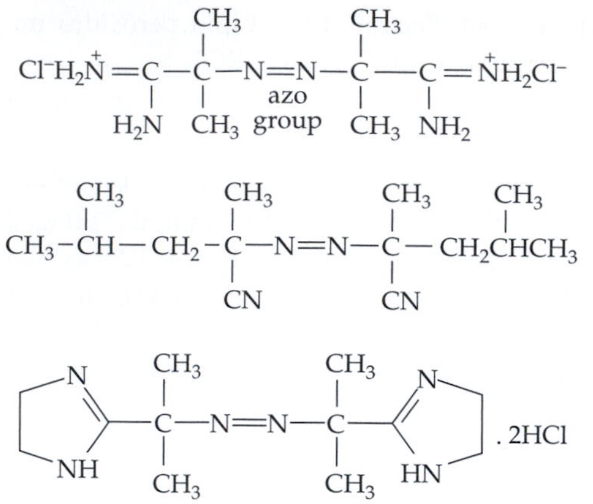

Figure 2.7 Structure of the 'azo initiators' 2,2'-azobis(2-amidino-propane) dihydrochloride (**AAPH**, top), 2,2'-azobis(2,4-dimethylva-leronitrile) (**AMVN**, middle) and 2,2'-azobis[2-(2-imidazolin-2-yl) propane] dihydrochloride (**AIPH**, bottom).

It is very oxidizing ($E^{\circ\prime} = 1.19\,\text{V}$) and reacts rapidly with many antioxidants (Section 8.2.3).

2.5.5 Sulphur radicals[1,47–50]

In vivo, thiols (especially reduced glutathione, GSH) mostly act as antioxidants (Section 3.9). Evidence is emerging that **hydrogen sulphide** (H_2S), essentially hydrogen thiol, H–SH, is a signalling molecule *in vivo*[51] and it has been hypothesized to act as an antioxidant in the brain.[52]

However, thiols can generate free radicals.

2.5.5.1 Formation

Thiyl radicals are formed when thiols react with carbon-centred radicals,

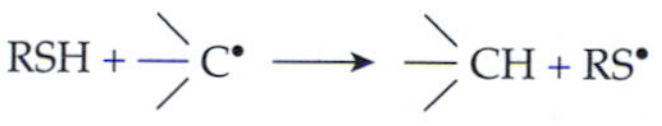

$$RSH + \overset{}{\underset{}{>}}C^{\bullet} \longrightarrow \overset{}{\underset{}{>}}CH + RS^{\bullet}$$

with several oxygen radicals, including $OH^{\bullet}$, $RO^{\bullet}$, $CO_3^{\bullet-}$, $RO_2^{\bullet}$ and (at a much[37] lower rate) $O_2^{\bullet-}$

$$RSH + OH^{\bullet} \rightarrow RS^{\bullet} + H_2O$$

$$RSH + RO_2^{\bullet} \rightarrow RS^{\bullet} + ROOH$$

with transition metal ions

$$RSH + Fe(\text{III}) \rightarrow RS^{\bullet} + Fe^{2+} + H^+$$

$$RSH + Cu^{2+} \rightarrow RS^{\bullet} + Cu^+ + H^+$$

and by the homolytic fission of disulphides, including disulphide bridges in proteins

cysteine–S–S–cysteine
$$\rightarrow \text{cysteine–S}^{\bullet} + {}^{\bullet}\text{S–cysteine}$$

Human fingernails are composed largely of **α-keratin**, a protein rich in disulphide bonds, and sulphur-centred radicals can be produced by cutting fingernails. Indeed, grinding of proteins, especially at low temperatures, is well-known to generate free radicals, and this can be a problem in the food industry, for example in flour milling. Sulphur, carbon and (in the presence of O_2), $RO_2^{\bullet}$ radicals can result.[47] Thiyl radicals also form when thiols react with nitrogen dioxide ($NO_2^{\bullet}$) or peroxynitrite (Section 2.6.1 below) and during the oxidation of thiols by peroxidases (Section 3.13.3). The damaging actions of several toxins on animals may involve thiyl radicals (Section 6.5.2).

2.5.5.2 Reactions

It is often assumed that $RS^{\bullet}$ radicals are essentially inert and disappear by dimerization, for example

$$GS^{\bullet} + GS^{\bullet} \rightarrow GSSG \qquad k = 1.5 \times 10^9\,M^{-1}s^{-1}$$

However, this is unlikely *in vivo* because steady-state levels of $RS^{\bullet}$ would normally be low and thus these radicals would be unlikely to meet. By contrast, GSH levels in cells are in the millimolar range. The pK_a of the GSH thiol group is 9.2

$$GSH \rightleftharpoons GS^- + H^+$$

and so about 1 to 2% is ionized at pH 7.4. Ionized glutathione reacts rapidly with $GS^{\bullet}$

$$GS^{\bullet} + GS^- \rightarrow GSSG^{\bullet-} \qquad k = 8 \times 10^8\,M^{-1}s^{-1}$$

Unlike the oxidizing $GS^{\bullet}$ radical (reduction potential ~0.9 V), $GSSG^{\bullet-}$ is powerfully reducing ($E^{\circ\prime}$ for $GSSG/GSSG^{\bullet-}$ is about $-1.5\,V$). Thus it can reduce metal ions, as well as form $O_2^{\bullet-}$ from O_2

$$GSSG^{\bullet-} + O_2 \rightarrow GSSG + O_2^{\bullet-}$$
$$k = 5 \times 10^8\,M^{-1}s^{-1}$$

Ascorbate also reacts with $RS^{\bullet}$ radicals

$$AH^- + RS^{\bullet} \rightarrow RSH + A^{\bullet-}$$
$$k \approx 5 \times 10^8\,M^{-1}s^{-1}(\text{for } GS^{\bullet})$$

as can NADH and NADPH

$$RS^\bullet + NADH \rightarrow RS^- + NAD^\bullet + H^+$$
$$k = 2.3 \times 10^8 \, M^{-1}s^{-1}$$

which, if O_2 is present, is likely to be followed by

$$NAD^\bullet + O_2 \rightarrow NAD^+ + O_2^{\bullet -}$$
$$k = 1.9 \times 10^9 \, M^{-1}s^{-1}$$

Cysteine thiyl radicals ($CysS^\bullet$) can abstract hydrogen from linoleic, linolenic and arachidonic acids with rate constants of 10^6 to $10^7 \, M^{-1}s^{-1}$, initiating fatty acid peroxidation.[49] Cysteamine thiyl radicals are capable of abstracting hydrogen from the DNA base thymine ($k = 1.2 \times 10^4 \, M^{-1}s^{-1}$)[53] and cysteine thiyl radicals from deoxyribose ($2.7 \times 10^4 \, M^{-1}s^{-1}$).[54]

Alternative fates of thiyl radicals are reaction with $NO^\bullet$ (Section 2.5.6 below) and formation of peroxyl radicals by reaction with O_2, for example

$$GS^\bullet + O_2 \rightleftharpoons GSOO^\bullet \qquad k \approx 3 \times 10^7 \, M^{-1}s^{-1}$$

Thiyl peroxyl radicals are unstable and rapidly form other species. For example, $RSOO^\bullet$ radicals derived from GSH, cysteine or the anti-inflammatory drug **penicillamine** (Section 9.10.6.2) can react with more thiol to produce **sulphinyl radical** ($RSO^\bullet$) or isomerize (in a light-dependent reaction) to **sulphonyl radical** ($RSO_2^\bullet$) which then reacts with O_2 to give $RSO_2OO^\bullet$, **sulphonyl peroxyl**. Thus for cysteine

$$CysS^\bullet + O_2 \longrightarrow CysSOO^\bullet$$
$$CysSOO^\bullet + CysSH \longrightarrow CysSO^\bullet + CysSOH$$
$$CysSOO^\bullet \xrightarrow{h\gamma} CysSO_2^\bullet + (cysS^+ \underset{O^-}{\overset{O^\bullet}{\diagdown}})$$
$$CysSO_2^\bullet + O_2 \longrightarrow Cys\,SO_2OO^\bullet$$

$$\overset{\displaystyle O}{\underset{\displaystyle O}{\overset{\displaystyle \|}{(CysSOO^\bullet)}\underset{\displaystyle \|}{}}}$$

Similarly, end products of GSH oxidation by ROS under aerobic conditions include GSSG, sulphenic acid (GSOH) and sulphonic acid (GSO_3H)

$$GSO^\bullet \xrightarrow[\text{sulphenic acid}]{\text{reduction}} GSOH$$

$$GSO_2OO^\bullet \xrightarrow{\text{reduction}} GSO_2OOH \xrightarrow[\text{sulphonic acid}]{\text{reduction}} GSO_3H + H_2O$$

Hence oxidizing thiols generate a series of potentially-cytotoxic oxygen, sulphur and oxysulphur radicals. Indeed, it was shown decades ago[50] that mixtures of cysteine and copper ions are toxic to mammalian cells, and later work used ESR techniques to identify sulphur radicals in such systems (Section 5.2.7). Thiols may be involved in the oxidation of LDL during atherosclerosis (Sections 9.3 and 10.5.9), and oxysulphur radicals contribute to the toxic effects of SO_2 (Section 8.11.3).

2.5.5.3 Artefacts involving sulphur compounds

Thiols are unstable in commonly used cell culture media,[55] oxidizing to produce radicals and H_2O_2. Some scientists add thiols to cells to study 'redox regulation', without considering reactions in the culture medium. Both copper and iron accelerate cysteine oxidation, copper far more effectively. However, somewhat paradoxically, copper-catalysed oxidation of cysteine is *slowed down* by the simultaneous presence of traces of iron.[56]

[^{35}S]-methionine labelling of cells is commonly used to study protein turnover and protein movement within the cell. However, it can lead to DNA damage, apoptosis and ROS formation.[57]

2.5.6 Nitric oxide

2.5.6.1 Basic chemistry[2,58]

Nitric oxide (officially called **nitrogen monoxide**) is a colourless gas, moderately soluble in water (up to 2 mM at 20 °C, about 1.6 mM at 37 °C) and (like O_2) more soluble in organic solvents. Hence $NO^\bullet$ can cross membranes and diffuse readily between and within cells. Nitric oxide has an unpaired electron in a π^*2p antibonding orbital: thus it is a free radical. If the unpaired electron is removed, **nitrosonium cation**, NO^+, is produced (Table 2.8). One-electron reduction gives **nitroxyl anion**, NO^-, which can also exist as a protonated form, HNO. There has been considerable debate in the literature on the pK_a of HNO, with values ranging from 4.7 to 11.4. However, the higher values seem more likely to be correct,[59] meaning that any NO^- formed *in vivo* should protonate to HNO.

Nitroxyl is a reactive short-lived species, for example it reacts with O_2 to give peroxynitrite

$$NO^- + O_2 \rightarrow ONOO^-$$

Table 2.8 Some reduction potentials of the reactive nitrogen species

Couple	$E^{\circ\prime}$ (V)
$ONOOH^{*}/NO_2^{\bullet}$	2.10
$NO_2^{+}/NO_2^{\bullet}$	1.60
$NO^{+}/NO^{\bullet}$	1.21
$NO_2^{\bullet}/NO_2^{-}$	0.99

Selected from the compilation by Koppenol in Weil *et al.* (eds), *Nitric Oxide and Radicals in the Pulmonary Vasculature*, p 358. Futura Publishing Co., Armonk, NY, 1996. These values apply to pH 7.0 and 1 M gas concentration. Peroxynitrous acid can act as both a one- or two-electron oxidizing agent ($E^{\circ\prime} = 1.4$ V and 0.99 V for ONOOH, H^{+}/NO$_2^{\bullet}$, H$_2$O and ONOOH, H^{+}/NO$_2^{-}$, H$_2$O respectively). The $E^{\circ\prime}$ of the putative activated *trans*-peroxynitrous acid ($ONOOH^{*}$ above) is calculated to be close to that of OH$^{\bullet}$ (2.31 V).

and oxidizes GSH ($k > 10^5\,M^{-1}s^{-1}$).[59] It can also combine with NO$^{\bullet}$ to give **hyponitrite radical**, $ONNO^{\bullet -}$. The physiological significance (if any) of NO^{-}/HNO, is unclear. A frequently used source of HNO is **Angeli's salt**,[59] the sodium salt of trioxodinitrate, $-ON = NO_2^{-}$, which decomposes rapidly at room temperature

$$N_2O_3^{2-} + H^+ \rightarrow HN_2O_3^{-}$$

$$HN_2O_3^{-} \rightarrow HNO + NO_2^{-}$$

On exposure to air, NO$^{\bullet}$ reacts with O$_2$ to form the brown gas **nitrogen dioxide**, a far more reactive free radical (Section 8.11). The overall reaction is

$$2NO^{\bullet} + O_2 \rightarrow 2NO_2^{\bullet}$$

and it follows a **third-order** rate law, that is

$$R = k[NO]^2[O_2] \qquad k \sim 8.4 \times 10^6\,M^{-2}s^{-1} \text{at } 37^{\circ}C$$

Essentially the same rate law applies to NO$^{\bullet}$ and O$_2$ in solution. This law has biological implications, in that the rate of NO$^{\bullet}$ oxidation depends upon the square of NO$^{\bullet}$ concentration. The half-life of 1 μM NO$^{\bullet}$ is several minutes in air-saturated solutions and doubles with each 50% decrease in NO$^{\bullet}$ concentration. Physiological levels of NO$^{\bullet}$ may be in the 1 to 10 nM range and *in vivo* O$_2$ concentrations are also low (Fig. 1.4). Thus if reaction of NO$^{\bullet}$ with O$_2$ to form NO$_2^{\bullet}$ were its only fate *in vivo*, the lifetime of NO$^{\bullet}$ would be hours. The oxidation of

NO$^{\bullet}$ dissolved in aqueous solutions produces mainly nitrite (NO$_2^{-}$); the overall equation is

$$4NO^{\bullet} + O_2 + 2H_2O \rightleftharpoons 4H^+ + 4NO_2^{-}$$

and may be the sum of the equations

$$2NO^{\bullet} + O_2 \rightleftharpoons 2NO_2^{\bullet}$$

$$NO_2^{\bullet} + NO^{\bullet} \rightleftharpoons N_2O_3 (\text{addition of two radicals})$$

$$N_2O_3 + 2OH^- \rightleftharpoons 2NO_2^{-} + H_2O$$

although the role of NO$_2^{\bullet}$ is uncertain. Reaction of NO$^{\bullet}$ with O$_2$ can proceed faster in hydrophobic environments such as the interior of membranes and lipoproteins because both NO$^{\bullet}$ and O$_2$ can concentrate there.[60]

2.5.6.2 *Nitric oxide as a free radical scavenger*[58,61,62]
Nitric oxide is low down on the 'reactivity scale' of free radicals, and reacts slowly, if at all, with most biological molecules, including thiols ($k < 1\,M^{-1}s^{-1}$ at pH 7.4). To generate **thionitrites** (more commonly called **nitrosothiols**) from thiols, NO$^{\bullet}$ must first form ONOO^{-} or a higher oxide of nitrogen such as N$_2$O$_3$ (Table 2.9). By contrast, NO$^{\bullet}$ is highly

Table 2.9 Some terms frequently confused

Nitrosylation	The attachment of an NO (**nitroso**) group to a thiol (**S-nitrosylation**) or a metal. Usually reversible.
Nitration	Attachment of a $-NO_2$ (**nitro**) group to a compound. Usually not easily reversible.

Various reactive nitrogen species (RNS) can oxidize, nitrate, and/or nitrosylate proteins, lipids and DNA (*Free Radic. Res.* **38**, 1, 2004). Nitric oxide rarely reacts directly with $-SH$ groups; usually NO^{+}, N$_2$O$_3$, NO$_2^{\bullet}$ or ONOO^{-} are needed to generate nitrosothiols. For example, exposure of cells to excess NO$^{\bullet}$ can cause covalent modification of $-SH$ groups on G3PDH and damage to iron–sulphur proteins in mitochondria. However, these effects are probably due to NO$^{\bullet}$-derived oxidation products rather than NO$^{\bullet}$ itself. Indeed this may be true of many alleged cellular effects of NO$^{\bullet}$, which is often applied at absurdly high levels in laboratory studies, so that its oxidation to more-reactive NO$_2^{\bullet}$ and N$_2$O$_3$ is rapid. Direct toxic effects of excess NO$^{\bullet}$ include inhibition of ribonucleotide reductase and cytochrome oxidase. Nitrosylation of specific proteins *in vivo* is favoured by (i) their colocalization with NOS enzymes and/or (ii) the presence of highly-reactive cysteine–SH groups on the proteins.

reactive with other free radicals (Table 2.10). Thus NO$^\bullet$ can scavenge OH$^\bullet$

$$NO^\bullet + OH^\bullet \rightarrow HNO_2 \qquad k > 10^{10}\,M^{-1}s^{-1}$$

peroxyl radicals

$$RO_2^\bullet + NO^\bullet \rightarrow ROONO \qquad k > 10^9\,M^{-1}s^{-1}$$

and tyrosyl radicals, the latter probably by a reversible addition reaction. Nitrosothiols can also be formed by addition of NO$^\bullet$ to thiyl radicals

$$RS^\bullet + NO^\bullet \rightarrow RSNO$$

The literature on the free radical reactions of NO$^\bullet$ has largely focused on its reaction with $O_2^{\bullet-}$ to give peroxynitrite (Section 2.6.1 below). Another potentially deleterious effect of NO$^\bullet$ is its ability to reversibly inhibit ribonucleotide reductase by reacting with a tyrosyl radical essential for catalytic function (Table 2.10; Section 7.2.2). However, it may be that the ability of NO$^\bullet$ to react fast with free radicals (Table 2.10) is, overall, beneficial *in vivo*. Thus the ability to scavenge $RO_2^\bullet$ radicals makes NO$^\bullet$ a powerful inhibitor of lipid peroxidation, which may contribute to its antiatherosclerotic effect (Section 9.3.5). Nitric oxide also decreases the pro-oxidant properties of haem proteins in the presence of peroxides (Section 3.15.3), quenching both haem ferryl species and amino acid radicals,[63] and it

Table 2.10 Some rate constants for reaction of nitric oxide with other free radicals[62]

Radical	Rate constant ($M^{-1}s^{-1}$)
Superoxide/HO$_2^\bullet$	$> 10^9$
Peroxyl	$> 10^9$
Tyrosyl	$> 10^9$
Tryptophanyl	$> 10^9$
Hydroxyethyl	$> 10^9$
Hydroxyl (OH$^\bullet$)	$> 10^9$
e$^-$(aq)	$> 10^{10}$
H$^\bullet$	$> 10^{10}$

Nitric oxide can also bind to various Fe^{2+}-chelates (e.g. Fe^{2+}-NTA, Fe^{2+}-citrate) to decrease their reactivity with H_2O_2 in the Fenton reaction (*J. Biol. Inorg. Chem.* **10**, 732, 2005). It may also decrease their reactivity with lipid peroxides.

can bind to Fe^{2+} to decrease its reactivity with H_2O_2 to make OH$^\bullet$ (Table 2.10).

2.5.6.3 *Physiological roles*[64,65]

Nitric oxide has multiple, important physiological roles (Table 2.11). It readily binds to certain transition metal ions, and many of its physiological effects arise from its binding to Fe^{2+}–haem groups in the enzyme **guanylate cyclase**. For example, NO$^\bullet$ synthesized by the **vascular endothelial cells** that line the interior of blood vessels presumably diffuses in all directions, but some of it will reach the underlying smooth muscle, bind to guanylate cyclase and activate it. As a result, more **cyclic GMP** is made, which lowers intracellular free Ca^{2+} and relaxes the muscle, dilating the vessel and lowering the blood pressure.

2.5.6.4 *Removal of NO$^\bullet$ in vivo*[67]

Much of the NO$^\bullet$ generated in the vascular system is eventually removed by interaction with haemoglobin. Nitric oxide forms complexes with Fe^{2+} and ferrous compounds (a process called **nitrosylation**, Table 2.9), including deoxyhaemoglobin.

$$HbFe^{2+} + NO^\bullet \rightleftharpoons HbFe^{2+}NO$$

Nitric oxide also reacts with oxyhaemoglobin, oxidizing it to methaemoglobin (HbFe(III)) and forming nitrate ($k > 10^7\,M^{-1}s^{-1}$). As a result, once NO$^\bullet$ has entered an erythrocyte, its half-life is $<1\,\mu sec$. The rate of entry of NO$^\bullet$ into erythrocytes limits its reaction with oxyhaemoglobin and it has been estimated that the half-life of NO$^\bullet$ in whole blood is about 1.8 msec. Free oxyhaemoglobin scavenges NO$^\bullet$ much faster[67] and as a result can cause problems, for example in the brain (Section 9.17). Nitric oxide can also interact with peroxidases,[68] being oxidized in the presence of H_2O_2 to NO_2^-. Indeed, myeloperoxidase can oxidize NO$^\bullet$ to NO_2^-, and then oxidize NO_2^- further to $NO_2^\bullet$. Nitric oxide can bind to CYPs to inhibit their catalytic activity; indeed, the loss of CYPs observed during incubation of liver cells in culture may involve over-production of NO$^\bullet$ during cell isolation.[69] Nitric oxide is also oxidized by oxymyoglobin, a reaction possibly important in heart and other muscles[70] and it competitively inhibits binding of O_2 to cytochrome oxidase and so can decrease

Table 2.11 Some examples of the physiology and pathology of nitric oxide

Physiological role	Excess implicated in tissue injury in	Effect of 'knock-out' of the relevant gene in mice
Nervous system		
Response to excitatory amino acids (especially glutamate); neurotransmission/ neuromodulation; synaptic plasticity (strengthening of synapses that are most often used; plays a role in long-term memory)	Epilepsy, stroke, excitotoxicity (implicated in multiple neurodegenerative diseases)	nNOS: obstruction of the pylorus (the muscle controlling entry of food into the stomach); less sensitive to brain damage by ischaemia—reperfusion or trauma; inappropriate and excessive sexual and aggressive behaviour
Vascular system		
Control of blood pressure; inhibition of platelet aggregation; killing of foreign organisms (e.g. *Leishmania*, *Trypanosoma*, *Plasmodium*, *Mycobacteria*, *Listeria*, *Toxoplasma* spp.); see *J. Clin. Invest.* **99**, 2818, 1997. Generally antiatherosclerotic (*Circulation* **108**, 2049, 2003)	Septic shock (vasodilation, low blood pressure); chronic inflammation (rheumatoid arthritis, ulcerative colitis); sequelae of infection, including increased cancer risk; transplant rejection. Inhibitors of NOS such as N^G-methylarginine, have been used to treat septic shock but need to be used with caution (*Crit. Care Med.* **27** 855, 1999).	iNOS: increased susceptibility to tuberculosis, *Listeria* and *Leishmania* infection, and lymphoma cell proliferation (e.g. *Proc. Natl. Acad. Sci. USA* **94**, 5243, 1997); resistance to endotoxin-induced hypotension and carrageenan-induced inflammation eNOS: deficient vasodilation in response to acetylcholine; hypertension
Other systems		
Penile erection, bladder control, lung vasodilation, gastrointestinal function (e.g. peristalsis), wound healing	Asthma	

NO• has been implicated in multiple physiological processes, some of which are listed above, yet excess production of NO• (often by iNOS) may cause cell injury. In rodent models of disease, phagocytes (especially macrophages) are usually the cells over-producing NO•, but the ability of human phagocytes to make NO• appears more limited. Cell injury by NO• can be direct (e.g. inhibition of ribonucleotide reductase[61] or cytochrome oxidase[66]) or it can involve conversion of NO• into other reactive nitrogen species, e.g. ONOO⁻. The iNOS enzyme is sometimes called **NOS2**; eNOS is sometimes called **NOS3**; and nNOS is sometimes called **NOS1**.

mitochondrial electron transport and ATP production.[66] Prolonged inhibition can increase $O_2^{•-}$ formation from the electron transport chain, allowing ONOO⁻ to form and damage the mitochondria (Section 2.6.1.3). Cytochrome oxidase[71] can also oxidize NO• into NO_2^-.

2.5.6.5 *Nitrate and nitrite: inert end-products or physiologically important?*

Blood plasma NO_3^- levels in humans on a low NO_3^- diet have been reported as about 30 μM, although they rise rapidly after intake of nitrate or nitrite-rich foods.[72] This basal level presumably results from the oxidation of endogenously produced NO•. Nitrate is eventually excreted in urine. Levels

of NO_2^- in plasma are much lower (0.15–1.0 μM) and it has been proposed that they reflect short-term rates of endothelial NO• synthesis.[73] Nitrite can also be absorbed from the diet and is present at high levels in saliva. Whereas oxyhaemoglobin can oxidize NO_2^- to NO_3^-, deoxyhaemoglobin can reduce NO_2^- to NO• (the rate is maximal when about half the haemoglobin exists in the deoxy form)

$$NO_2^- + HbFe^{2+} + H^+ \rightarrow NO^• + HbFe(III) + OH^-$$
$$\text{methaemoglobin}$$

and it has been suggested that this promotes vasodilation when O_2 levels are falling,[67,74] conditions which hinder the O_2-dependent NOS enzymes. Nitrite enters erythrocytes readily, probably through the band 3 channel (Section 6.4). Xanthine dehydrogenase also converts NO_2^- to $NO^\bullet$ (Section 1.10.1). Nitrite is a scavenger of hypochlorous acid, and it is possible that it could protect against damage by this species at sites of inflammation.[75] Hence NO_2^- is not merely an end-product of $NO^\bullet$ oxidation—it has metabolic roles in its own right.

Dietary nitrates are found in vegetables, to an extent depending on such factors as soil composition and fertilizer use. Nitrate is reduced to NO_2^- in the gut, and NO_2^- absorbed. In addition, nitrites and nitrates have been used since ancient times (and still are) as preserving and curing agents for meats; usually bacon, sausages and tinned meats. Nitrites inhibit the growth of many bacteria in foods, particularly the anaerobe, *Clostridium botulinum*, which causes **botulism**, a potentially lethal type of food poisoning. Indeed, this bacterium moves away from NO_2^--treated meat. Another use of NO_2^- is to make meat look better; meat tends to darken in colour because the Fe^{2+}—haem in myoglobin oxidizes to give dull-red metmyoglobin.[76] Nitric oxide binds to myoglobin to give a red (better looking!) complex, slowing oxidation

$$MbFe^{2+}-O_2 + NO^\bullet \rightarrow MbFe^{2+}NO + O_2$$

One concern about the use of nitrites is that during cooking or in the stomach they might react with secondary amines in food to generate **nitrosamines**, potential carcinogens

$$R_2NH + HNO_2 \rightarrow R_2-N-N=O + H_2O$$
$$\text{nitrosamine}$$

The stomach contents are acidic (often as low as pH 2) and dietary NO_2^- will form **nitrous acid** (HNO_2) that decomposes to oxides of nitrogen. In addition, the salivary glands concentrate NO_3^- from plasma and excrete it into saliva, where some of it is reduced to NO_2^- by oral bacteria. Average salivary NO_2^- levels in fasting subjects have been reported as 100 μM. Generation of oxides of nitrogen from HNO_2 is thought to be an antibacterial and gastroprotective mechanism in the stomach.[76] Yet nitrous acid can damage DNA and its potential carcinogenicity has been debated but not clearly established (Section 6.2).[77]

2.5.6.6 Synthesis of nitric oxide[65,78]

Although $NO^\bullet$ can arise from NO_2^-, most $NO^\bullet$ is synthesized *in vivo* in animals by the **nitric oxide synthase** (NOS) enzymes, which convert L-arginine into $NO^\bullet$ and another amino acid, L-citrulline. Plants also make $NO^\bullet$, but how exactly is uncertain (Section 6.7). Animal NOS enzymes require O_2 and contain four cofactors: FAD, FMN, tetrahydrobiopterin and haem, all compounds whose reduced forms can autoxidize to make $O_2^{\bullet-}$ (Section 1.10). The haem centre resembles those of CYPs; like CYPs, NOS enzymes can bind $NO^\bullet$ and this decreases their enzyme activity. The NOS enzymes can even generate $O_2^{\bullet-}$ if L-arginine is present and tetrahydrobiopterin levels are low (Table 1.4) and these reactions may contribute to vascular dysfunction in atherosclerosis.[79] The electrons required by NOS are supplied by NADPH.

The activity of NOS is carefully regulated. There are three types: **neuronal NOS** (nNOS, NOS1) was originally identified in nervous system tissues and is a constitutive enzyme. It is also important in skeletal muscle, where the $NO^\bullet$ it produces helps to regulate contraction. **Endothelial NOS** (eNOS, NOS3) is expressed constitutively in endothelial cells and synthesizes the $NO^\bullet$ needed for regulation of blood pressure (Table 2.11). Nitric oxide from vascular endothelium was originally identified as an **endothelium-derived relaxing factor** (EDRF), a 'factor' that relaxes blood vessels. The eNOS and nNOS enzymes require Ca^{2+} and the calmodulin proteins for their action, so that the low intracellular 'free' Ca^{2+} within cells restricts NOS activity (Section 4.2). At sites of inflammation, an 'extra' NOS is often present, called **inducible NOS** (iNOS, NOS2). This enzyme was first identified in macrophages and liver cells after treatment with endotoxin[a] or certain cytokines (Section 4.7).

---

[a] Endotoxin (sometimes called **lipopolysaccharide**, LPS) is a complex glycolipid found in the cell walls of Gram-negative bacteria.

The iNOS enzymes bind calmodulin tightly and their activity is essentially Ca^{2+}-independent. They catalyse rapid $NO^{\bullet}$ generation, generating much higher localized concentrations than normal, perhaps as high as the micromolar range. Another rate-limiting factor can be O_2 level; K_m values for eNOS, iNOS and nNOS have been quoted as 4, 135 and 400 µM respectively.[80]

The activity of NOS is also affected *in vivo* by the presence of circulating NOS inhibitors; N^G, N^Gdimethyl-L-arginine (sometimes called **asymmetrical dimethylarginine** or **ADMA**) and N^G-monomethyl- L-arginine (**L-NMMA**). The inhibitor L-NMMA was used for years in the laboratory before it was realized that it is present *in vivo* (Figure 2.8). Excess levels of these agents (especially ADMA) can contribute to hypertension and atherosclerosis.[81]

Although eNOS is constitutive, its levels can be increased in vascular endothelium, for example by shear stress.[82] The iNOS enzyme does not always have to be induced; it is present in normal epithelium in respiratory tract and nasal sinuses, perhaps to release $NO^{\bullet}$ as an antibacterial mechanism.[83] Levels of nNOS can also be raised in neurons by certain treatments. Excess $NO^{\bullet}$ production, often

(but not always) involving iNOS, occurs in various diseases (Table 2.11). In rats and mice, phagocytes (especially macrophages) are prolific producers of $NO^{\bullet}$ during inflammation, but human phagocytes are more reluctant to generate $NO^{\bullet}$, at least *in vitro* and may require prolonged exposure to cytokines.[84]

2.5.6.7 Nitric oxide donors

Nitrovasodilators have been used for more than a century as treatment for diseases with abnormal vasoconstriction (e.g. angina pectoris; Section 9.5.6) and sometimes (e.g. **amyl nitrite**) as recreational drugs. They act largely or entirely as $NO^{\bullet}$ donors. These drugs include organic nitrates and nitrites (e.g. **nitroglycerine** and amyl nitrite), inorganic nitroso compounds (e.g. **nitroprusside**), **sydnonimines** such as **linsidomine** (sometimes called **SIN-1**), and nitrosothiols such as SNAP (Table 2.12; Figs 2.9 and 2.10). Many of these compounds are used as $NO^{\bullet}$ donors in laboratory experiments, but in assessing their effects it is important to understand what else they generate, for example cyanide ions in the case of sodium nitroprusside (Table 2.12). A popular agent is **S-nitroso-N-acetylpenicillamine** (SNAP).

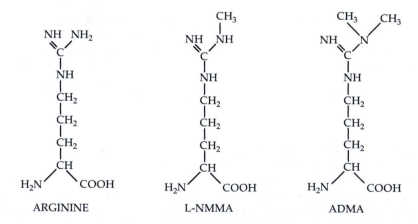

Figure 2.8 Structures of L-arginine and endogenous methylarginines, N^Gmonomethyl-L-arginine (L-NMMA) and $N^G N^G$dimethylarginine (ADMA), both NOS inhibitors.

Table 2.12 Some nitric oxide donors

Type of compound	Examples	Comments
Metal nitrosyl complexes	Sodium nitroprusside (SNP) $Na_2Fe(CN)_5NO$ Ruthenium nitrosylpentachloride, (RNP) $K_2Ru(Cl)_5NO$	Nitric oxide forms one of the ligands to iron. Sodium nitroprusside is widely used in pharmacology but it is not always clear how it makes $NO^\bullet$: this can involve photochemical decomposition or reductive breakdown $[Fe(CN)_5NO]^{2-} \xrightarrow{e^-} [Fe(CN)_5]^{3-} + NO^\bullet$ Similarly, RNP is photolabile and has been used as a source of 'caged $NO^\bullet$'. Nitroprusside breakdown releases toxic cyanide ions and its breakdown products may promote Fenton chemistry (*Free Rad. Biol. Med.* **24**, 1065, 1998).
FK409 (Fungal-derived NO donor) and derivatives		Commonly used in Japan (e.g. *J. Pharm. Exp. Ther.* **252**, 236, 1997). $t_{1/2}$ approx. 40 min at 37°C
S-Nitrosothiols (thionitrites) $R-S-N=O$	Nitrosocysteine (half-life in seconds) GSNO ($t_{1/2} \approx 160\,h$) *S*-Nitroso-*N*-acetyl-DL- penicillamine, SNAP ($t_{1/2} \approx 1\,h$)	Generated by reaction of several RNS (but not $NO^\bullet$ directly) with thiols. Found *in vivo*, e.g. *S*-nitrosoalbumin and GSNO. Decomposition accelerated by light, transition metal ions (especially copper) and reducing agents. $2RSNO \xrightarrow[\text{or light}]{2e^-} RSSR + 2NO^\bullet$ $Cu^+ + RSNO \rightarrow [RSNOCu]^+ \rightarrow RS^- + NO^\bullet + Cu^{2+}$ $Cu^{2+} + RS^- \rightarrow Cu^+ + RS^\bullet$ $RSNO + RS^\bullet \rightarrow RSSR + NO^\bullet$ Note the production of thiyl radicals. Transnitrosation reactions can also occur between thiols, $RSNO + R'S^- \rightleftharpoons RS^- + R'SNO$ including thiols on proteins such as albumin and thioredoxin.
SIN-1	See Fig. 2.10	Decomposition generates both $O_2^{\bullet-}$ and $NO^\bullet$, therefore likely to produce $ONOO^-$. Breakdown accelerated by light. Active metabolite of the antiangina drug **molsidomine**
Organic nitrates/nitrites	Isosorbide dinitrate Nitroglycerine (glycerol trinitrate ester) Amyl nitrite $[(CH_3)_2CH(CH_2)_2-O-N=O]$	Used in medicine and/or as recreational drugs for many years. Reduction (e.g. by mitochondrial aldehyde dehydrogenase in the case of nitroglycerine; *Proc. Natl. Acad. Sci.* **102**, 12159, 2005) releases $NO^\bullet$, producing vasodilation. Some GSH transferases (Section 3.9.5) catalyse reaction of organic nitrites with RSH to give nitrosothiols. Organic nitrates become less effective on prolonged therapy (**nitrate tolerance**), a process which may involve increased vascular $O_2^{\bullet-}$ production (*J. Clin. Invest.* **113**, 352, 2004).

Table 2.12 (*Cont.*)

Type of compound	Examples	Comments
NONOates Contain the [N(O) NO]$^-$ functional group 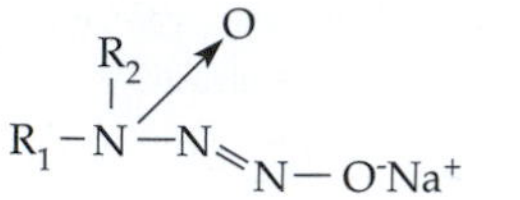	DETA: $R_1 = R_2 = H_2NCH_2\ CH_2$, $t_{1/2} \approx 20\,h$ at 37°C. Spermine: $R_1 = H_2N(CH_2)_3\overset{+}{N}H_2(CH_2)_4$, $R_2 = H_2N$ $(CH_2)_3$, $t_{1/2} = 39\,min$. PAPA: $R_1 = CH_3CH_2CH_2$, $R_2 = H_3N(CH_2)_3$, $t_{1/2} = 15\,min$. MAHMA: $R_1 = CH_3NH_2(CH_2)_6$ $R_2 = CH_3$, $t_{1/2} = 1–2\,min$	Generate NO$^\bullet$ at variable rates depending on the structure. $t_{1/2}$ values vary according to reaction conditions: the values given are only illustrative. Commonly used ones to give slow steady fluxes of NO$^\bullet$ include NOC-5 ($t_{1/2} \approx 93\,min$, $R_1 = CH$ $(CH_3)_2$; $R_2 = (CH_2)_3(NH_2)$ and NOC-18 (DETA NONOate).
NO-releasing polymers	Various NO-releasing agents (e.g. NONOates) embedded in a matrix, e.g. of silicone rubber, PVC or polyurethanes, or PEG–nitrosoalbumin.	*Free Rad. Biol. Med.* **37**, 926, 2004 *J. Pharm. Exp. Ther.* **314**, 1117, 2005

For details, see Packer, L. (ed.) *Meth. Enzymol*, volume 268, 1996 and *Expert Opin. Invest. Drugs* 11, 587, 2002. Many compounds have been used to generate NO$^\bullet$ for chemical or pharmacological studies; some are used as NO$^\bullet$ donors *in vivo*. Often the mechanism of NO$^\bullet$ generation is unclear and is influenced by reaction conditions. One must be aware of what else can be generated (e.g. CN$^-$ or RS$^\bullet$) by some NO$^\bullet$ donors. Several drugs in which NO— or NO$_2$— groups are linked to other pharmacological agents have been designed, such as **nitro-aspirin (NCX-4016), nitrosocaptopril, NO–ferulic acid** (*J. Neurochem.* **89**, 484, 2004) and NO-histamine receptor antagonists.

How do nitrosothiol species generate NO$^\bullet$? Homolytic fission would yield thiyl radical

$$RSNO \rightarrow RS^\bullet + NO^\bullet$$

but, in fact, decomposition of many RSNO is catalysed by transition-metal ions, especially copper, or is light-dependent (Table 2.12) and a variety of end products results. **Never assume that a cellular effect of an NO$^\bullet$ donor is a direct effect of NO$^\bullet$.**

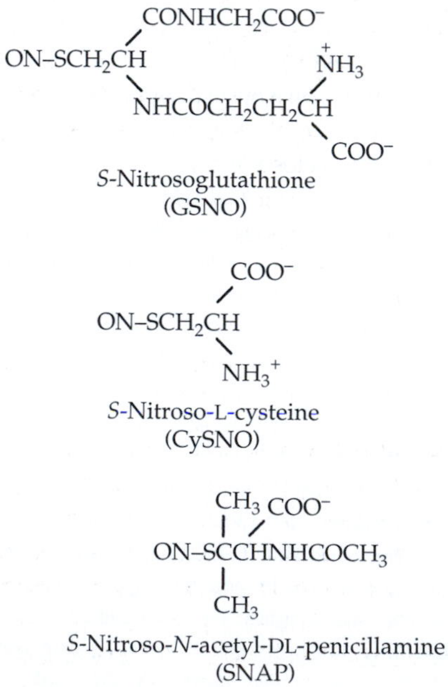

Superoxide can be generated in cell culture media by a variety of mechanisms (Section 1.11). If this occurs, then the availability of NO$^\bullet$ from added NO donors can be diminished, and ONOO$^-$ also formed.[85]

2.6 Chemistry of biologically important non-radicals

2.6.1 Peroxynitrite[2,86]

Since we have just examined NO$^\bullet$, it seems logical to look at peroxynitrite next. We must first point out that NO$^\bullet$ and its oxidation products can interact with ROS in several ways. For example, mixtures of HOCl and NO$_2^-$ can form **nitryl chloride**, NO$_2$Cl.[87] This is a reactive oxidizing, nitrating and chlorinating agent *in vitro*, although its importance *in vivo* is unclear. Hydrogen peroxide and NO$^\bullet$ exert synergistic effects in some systems, although the chemistry of their interaction is uncertain. For example, H$_2$O$_2$ enhances the inhibitory effect of NO$^\bullet$ on platelet aggregation[88] and H$_2$O$_2$ and NO$^\bullet$ can increase or decrease each other's cytotoxicity to cultured cells,[89] depending on the cell type, the NO$^\bullet$ donor used, reagent concentrations and whether cells were pre-exposed

CONHCH$_2$COO$^-$
ON–SCH$_2$CH
$\overset{+}{N}H_3$
NHCOCH$_2$CH$_2$CH
COO$^-$
S-Nitrosoglutathione
(GSNO)

COO$^-$
ON–SCH$_2$CH
NH$_3^+$
S-Nitroso-L-cysteine
(CySNO)

CH$_3$ COO$^-$
ON–SCCHNHCOCH$_3$
CH$_3$
S-Nitroso-*N*-acetyl-DL-penicillamine
(SNAP)

Figure 2.9 Some nitrosothiols. Low levels of nitrosothiols, including nitrosoalbumin, are found in the bloodstream.

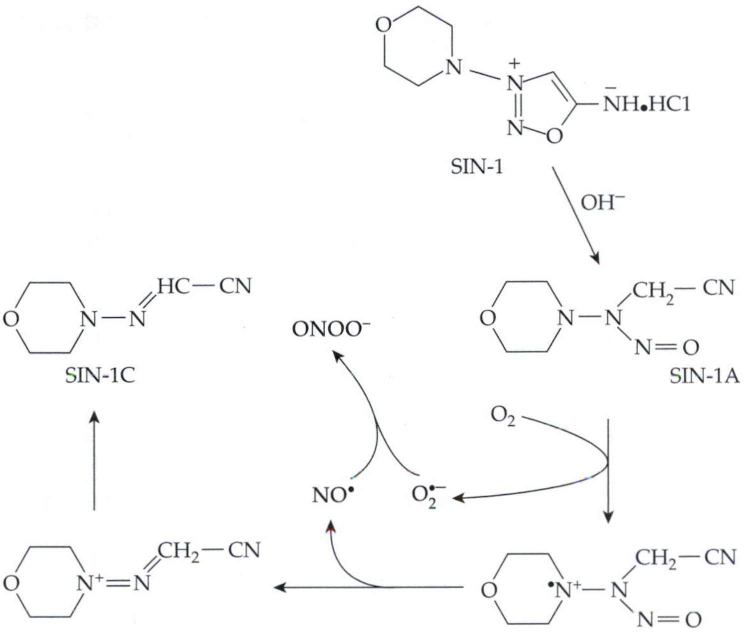

Figure 2.10 The structure of SIN-1. SIN-1 generates $O_2^{\bullet-}$ and $NO^{\bullet}$, leading to $ONOO^-$ generation. SIN-1C can react with ONOOH, giving a range of products that have biological effects in some systems. Hence never assume that an effect of SIN-1 is necessarily an effect of $ONOO^-$ (*Free Rad. Biol. Med.* **35**, 662, 2003). Some biological oxidizing agents can promote the formation of $NO^{\bullet}$ rather than $ONOO^-$ from SIN-1 by catalysing direct oxidation of SIN-1A (*Arch. Biochem. Biophys.* **361**, 331, 1999).

to $NO^{\bullet}$. To take an example, induction of apoptosis by H_2O_2 in bovine aortic endothelial cells requires uptake of iron from the medium and subsequent Fenton chemistry. Nitric oxide decreased the toxicity by blocking iron uptake through the transferrin receptor.[90]

Nevertheless, most attention has been given to **peroxynitrite** (officially called **oxoperoxonitrate** (1-)), which can be formed from NO^- and O_2 (Section 2.5.6) or, more commonly, by the combination of $NO^{\bullet}$ and $O_2^{\bullet-}$

$$NO^{\bullet} + O_2^{\bullet-} \rightarrow ONOO^- \qquad k > 6 \times 10^9 \, M^{-1} s^{-1}$$

The above reaction has a greater rate constant than reaction of $NO^{\bullet}$ with haem compounds ($k < 10^8 \, M^{-1} s^{-1}$) or even reaction of $O_2^{\bullet-}$ with SOD (Section 3.2). Combination of $NO^{\bullet}$ and $O_2^{\bullet-}$ is important, for at least two reasons. First, it means that $NO^{\bullet}$ and $O_2^{\bullet-}$ antagonize each other's biological actions. It has been known for decades that $NO^{\bullet}$-mediated effects can be enhanced by adding SOD.[64] This was first demonstrated in

bioassays of EDRF: adding SOD slowed the rate of loss of the relaxing factor. The system must have been producing $O_2^{\bullet-}$, which combined with some of the $NO^{\bullet}$. Adding SOD removed $O_2^{\bullet-}$ and so raised the $NO^{\bullet}$ level. *In vivo*, excess $O_2^{\bullet-}$ production in or close to vascular endothelium can cause vasoconstriction, and excess $O_2^{\bullet-}$ is involved in hypertension (Section 7.10.3). Similarly, if an injury system is $O_2^{\bullet-}$-dependent, $NO^{\bullet}$ can protect by removing $O_2^{\bullet-}$.

The second reason is that $ONOO^-$ is formed. Addition of $ONOO^-$ to cells, tissues or body fluids leads to its rapid protonation (Fig. 2.11), followed by depletion of $-SH$ groups and other antioxidants, oxidation and nitration of lipids, DNA strand breakage, nitration and deamination of DNA bases (especially guanine; Section 4.8.2.10), nitration of aromatic amino acid residues in proteins as well as oxidation of cysteine, methionine (to methionine sulphoxide) and other residues. The most studied reaction in proteins has been conversion of tyrosine to **3-nitrotyrosine**,[2,91] but tryptophan and phenylalanine can also be nitrated.

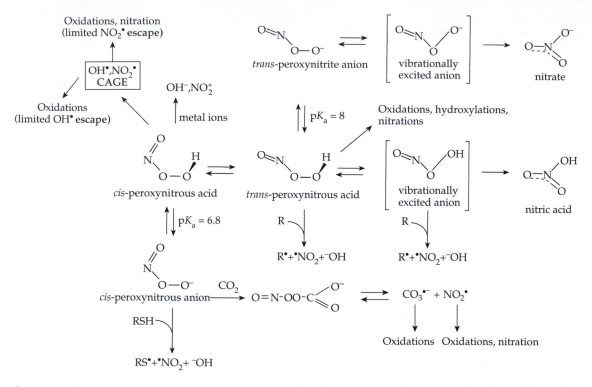

Figure 2.11 The complexities of peroxynitrite. Homolytic fission of ONOOH to OH$^\bullet$ and NO$_2$ may occur, but the caged radicals easily recombine and only limited amounts escape. Certain metal complexes cause heterolytic fission to NO$_2^+$ and OH$^-$. At pH 7.4 about 20% of ONOO$^-$ will exist as ONOOH (p$K_a = 6.8$), which rapidly decomposes. Species able to cause damaging oxidations include OH$^\bullet$, NO$_2^\bullet$, cis-ONOO$^-$ and cis-ONOOH (limited reactivity, but can oxidize, for example −SH compounds), the trans isomers and the excited states of those trans isomers, especially of ONOOH. Activated trans-ONOOH has a reduction potential close to that of OH$^\bullet$ (Table 2.8) and so is potentially highly oxidizing. Some added biomolecules (including thiols) may be oxidized by these various species to radicals, generating NO$_2^\bullet$ also, e.g. trans-ONOOH + R →R$^\bullet$ + NO$_2^\bullet$ + OH$^-$. Diagram adapted from Augusto, O and Radi, R (1996) In: *Biothiols in Health and Disease* (eds Packer, L and Cadenas, E), p. 89, by courtesy of Drs Radi and Augusto and the publishers. Reactions of CO$_2$ with ONOO$^-$ generates O = NOOCO$_2^-$, which can fragment into NO$_2^\bullet$ and CO$_3^{\bullet-}$ radicals.

Haemoglobin is rapidly oxidized to methaemoglobin[67] by ONOO$^-$.

Nitration of tyrosine residues (*not* nitrosylation as is often written in the literature; see Table 2.9) is widely used as a biomarker of ONOO$^-$ generation *in vivo* and has been observed in a vast range of human diseases, although it is not necessarily a specific biomarker for ONOO$^-$ (Section 5.6.1). In some animals, levels of nitrotyrosine in tissues rise with age (Section 10.4.5). Nitration often (but not always) leads to enzyme inactivation (e.g. tyrosine nitration by ONOO$^-$ decreases the activities of MnSOD[92]) and to interference with signal transduction, in part because nitration decreases the pK_a of the tyrosine −OH group from about 10 to 7.5, causing considerable ionization at pH 7.4. Nitration of tyrosines might block phosphorylation by certain tyrosine kinases, yet can facilitate translocation and activation of others, for example protein kinase C, isoform ε.[2,86,91,93–95] Other protein targets attackable upon ONOO$^-$ addition include xenobiotic-metabolizing enzymes such as N-acetyltransferases,[96] CYP2B1[97] and glutathione transferases,[98] structural proteins such as actin and neurofilament L[99], cyclooxygenases,[100] prostacylin synthase,[101] mitochondrial carnitine palmitoyltransferase 1,[102] iNOS,[103] and caeruloplasmin, which releases copper ions when attacked by ONOOH.[104] Addition of ONOO$^-$ to rat neurons caused toxicity due to intracellular Zn^{2+} release, probably from metallothionein (Section 8.15.12). Nitrated **fibrinogen**, a protein important in blood-clotting, is present in the plasma of patients with heart disease and appears to promote clot formation more readily than normal.[105]

Tyrosine nitration is not always the cause of enzyme inactivation by ONOO$^-$ (indeed, sometimes it can activate enzymes!),[98] since ONOO$^-$ addition modifies many other amino acid residues. For example, inactivations of *N*-acetyltransferases,[96] tyrosine hydroxylase, and isocitrate dehydrogenase are caused by oxidation of cysteine residues.[106,107] Inactivation of the latter enzyme decreases cellular NADPH generation, an important component of antioxidant defence (Section 3.9.3).

2.6.1.1 *How does peroxynitrite cause damage?*[2,86,91,103]

The ONOO$^-$ anion is fairly unreactive (although it can oxidize a few molecules, such as thiols and methionine) and solutions of it in alkali are stable for weeks if kept frozen. Peroxynitrite is usually synthesized in the laboratory by reacting nitrite with H_2O_2 at low pH (Table 2.13)

$$NO_2^- + H^+ \rightarrow HONO \text{ (nitrous acid)}$$

$$HONO + H_2O_2 \rightarrow HOONO + H_2O$$

and immediately stabilizing the ONOO$^-$ by adding excess sodium hydroxide. These solutions can be standardized by using the absorbance of ONOO$^-$ at 302 nm in alkali ($\varepsilon = 16770\,M^{-1}cm^{-1}$). However, be aware that the 'ONOO$^-$' obtained is contaminated with NO_2^-, NO_3^- and H_2O_2 as well as excess alkali, causing large pH rises if added to poorly buffered solutions and tissue irritation if injected into animals. A popular control experiment is to compare the effect of the ONOO$^-$ preparation with 'decomposed ONOO$^-$' (Table 2.13). However, the possibility that two agents could be involved in causing damage must not be forgotten (e.g. a cytotoxic effect could involve both H_2O_2 and

ONOO$^-$). Problems also exist with other laboratory methods of making ONOO$^-$ (Table 2.13).

Carbon dioxide reacts with ONOO$^-$ ($k_2 = 4.6 \times 10^4\,M^{-1}s^{-1}$) to form an adduct, **nitrosoperoxycarbonate**, $O=NOOCO_2^-$, which probably mediates many of the reactions attributed to ONOOH (Fig. 2.11), such as nitration of tyrosine and guanine. Animal body fluids and intracellular compartments have high concentrations of CO_2/HCO_3^- (e.g. approximately 1 mM CO_2 and 25 mM HCO_3^- in human blood plasma), making reaction with CO_2 a likely fate of ONOO$^-$ *in vivo*. Nitrosoperoxycarbonate may split harmlessly to NO_3^- and CO_2 or undergo homolytic fission to generate $NO_2^\bullet$ and carbonate radicals. For example, $CO_3^{\bullet-}$ plays a role in the oxidation of NAD(p)H induced by ONOO$^-$, resulting in $O_2^{\bullet-}$ formation[108]

$$CO_3^{\bullet-} + NADH \rightarrow NAD^\bullet + HCO_3^-$$
$$k = 1.4 \times 10^9\,M^{-1}s^{-1}$$

$$NAD^\bullet + O_2 \rightarrow NAD^+ + O_2^{\bullet-}$$
$$k = 1.9 \times 10^9\,M^{-1}s^{-1}$$

Nitrosoperoxycarbonate is less bactericidal than ONOO$^-$; indeed, inhibition of CO_2 production by the enzyme urease in *Helicobacter pylori* aggravated the toxicity of ONOO$^-$ to this organism (Section 9.12.2).

At physiological pH, any ONOO$^-$ that does not react with CO_2 or other molecules rapidly protonates to peroxynitrous acid (HO–O–N=O) and rearranges, forming nitrate as the major end-product, plus some NO_2^-. Addition of ONOO$^-$ to aromatic compounds leads to both hydroxylation and nitration.[2,109] Initially, it was suggested that ONOOH undergoes homolytic fission to generate OH$^\bullet$ and $NO_2^\bullet$. Some thermodynamic arguments suggested that this reaction is disfavoured, whereas others proposed it as a preferred reaction pathway.[110] Experimental data were equally confused. Some groups detected OH$^\bullet$ from decomposing ONOO$^-$ at physiological pH, but assays can be confounded because ONOO$^-$ interferes with the method. For example spin-trapping of OH$^\bullet$ with DMPO is affected by direct reaction of ONOOH with the spin adduct, and products of aromatic

Table 2.13 Some methods for laboratory preparation of peroxynitrite

Method	Basis of method	Comments
Simultaneous generation of $O_2^{\bullet-}$ and $NO^\bullet$	Generate fluxes of $O_2^{\bullet-}$ and $NO^\bullet$ that combine to effect a steady rate of $ONOO^-$ production. This may be a better model for biological $ONOO^-$ generation than bolus addition of $ONOO^-$, although the complexity of the generation systems must be considered.	SIN-1 (Fig. 2.10) is often used. Alternatively, mix spermine NONOate (Table 2.12) and the $O_2^{\bullet-}$ generator SOTS (Section 2.5.3), which generate $NO^\bullet$ and $O_2^{\bullet-}$ respectively with equal rate constants at 37°C (*Chem. Res. Toxicol.* **13**, 1287, 2000). $NO^\bullet$ donors have been mixed with xanthine/xanthine oxidase, but urate produced by the enzyme scavenges ONOOH. Stopped-flow mixing of KO_2 dissolved in DMSO and spermine NONOate has also been used (*J. Biol. Chem* **275**, 32460, 2000). **GEA3162**, used as a $NO^\bullet$ donor may also make $ONOO^-$ (*Br. J. Pharmacol.* **143** 179, 2004). Use of Hepes and other Good's buffers should be avoided as $ONOO^-$ reacts with them (*J. Biol. Chem.* **273**, 12716, 1998).
Reaction of H_2O_2 with HNO_2, made from $NaNO_2$ and HCl	Section 2.6.1.1. HOONO has a $t_{1/2}$ of $\sim$1 s but can be stabilized by rapidly adding excess NaOH.	Currently the most popular method. Product contaminated with Cl^-, NO_2^-, NaOH and H_2O_2. 'Decomposed control' often made by adding solution to phosphate (or other) buffer at pH 7.4; $ONOO^-$ protonates to ONOOH and decomposes within seconds whereas other products remain. Alternatively, H_2O_2 may be removed using manganese dioxide (MnO_2), although with loss of some $ONOO^-$ and contamination by metal ions.
Hydroxylamine method	NH_2OH in alkali plus EDTA or DETAPAC is bubbled with O_2 and oxidized to NO^-, which reacts with O_2 to give $ONOO^-$ $NH_2OH + OH^- + O_2 \rightarrow H_2O_2 + NO^- + H_2O$	H_2O_2 also produced. Some NO_2^-, alkali and NH_2OH remain as contaminants.
Irradiation of NO_3^-	Exposure of $NaNO_3$ or KNO_3 to short-wavelength UV light causes some isomerization to peroxynitrite, mainly the cis form (*J. Am. Chem. Soc* **125**, 15571, 2003).	Poor yield ($\sim$0.3%), some NO_2^- also formed. High NO_3^- levels remain. Formation of peroxynitrite from NO_3^- in Martian soil may have caused false-positive results in tests for 'life' carried out by the *Viking* lander probe.
Ozone/azide system	$N_3^- + 2O_3 \rightarrow ONOO^- + N_2O + O_2$ Solution of sodium azide bubbled with O3 at 0–4°C in weakly alkaline solution.	Solutions are less alkaline than the above methods and contain little, if any H_2O_2, but presence of unreacted azide can be a problem since it inhibits many enzymes.
Reaction of H_2O_2 with alkyl nitrites	H_2O_2 in alkali reacts with RONO (e.g. isoamyl nitrite) $H_2O_2 + OH^- + RONO \rightarrow ONOO^- + ROH + H_2O$	An alcohol (ROH) contaminates the reaction mixture. One approach to avoid this is to mix alkaline H_2O_2 with a water-soluble (e.g. isoamyl) nitrite; $ONOO^-$ stays in the aqueous phase whereas isoamyl alcohol remains in the organic phase and can be separated. Low contamination by NO_2^- and H_2O_2 if H_2O_2 and alkyl nitrite are used in equimolar amounts.

Table 2.13 (*Cont.*)

Method	Basis of method	Comments
Reaction of $NO^\bullet$ with potassium super-oxide	Gaseous $NO^\bullet$ is passed over solid KO_2 $KO_2 + NO^\bullet \rightarrow K^+ONOO^-$	Product can be extracted into alkaline solution, but dismutation of unreacted KO_2 can generate some H_2O_2
Reaction of $O_2^{\bullet-}$ with nitrosothiols	$RSNO + O_2^{\bullet-} \rightarrow RSH + NO^\bullet + O_2$ $O_2^{\bullet-} + NO^\bullet \rightarrow ONOO^-$	Superoxide decomposes RSNO to $NO^\bullet$ (which is a slow reaction, *J. Biol. Chem.* **277**, 2430, 2002). The $NO^\bullet$ then reacts with another $O_2^{\bullet-}$. See *J. Biol. Chem.* **273**, 7828, 1998.

For references see *Meth. Enzymol.* **233**, 299, 1994 and **269,** 285, 1996 and *Prog. Inorg. Chem.* **41**, 599, 1994.

hydroxylation can be oxidized by $ONOO^-$.[109] Even when these problems were overcome, the amount of $OH^\bullet$ detected was usually small. Probably, the radicals produced by homolytic fission are in close proximity (**caged**), rapidly recombine and only small amounts escape to cause damage or be detected by '$OH^\bullet$ traps' (Fig. 2.11).

Addition of certain metal chelates, such as Fe(III)-EDTA or even CuZnSOD, increases the yield of aromatic nitration products from $ONOO^-$, probably by promoting heterolytic fission of ONOOH to **nitronium ion** (NO_2^+), a good nitrating species

$$ONOOH \rightarrow NO_2^+ + OH^-$$

For example, bovine CuZnSOD can be nitrated on tyr108 by $ONOO^-$ addition, and can promote the nitration of adjacent proteins.[99,103] By contrast, human CuZnSOD lacks this tyrosine residue and is not a substrate for nitration, although it can be nitrated (and oxidized) on its single tryptophan residue.[111] Why does adding CO_2 enhance tyrosine nitration? Carbonate radical oxidizes tyrosine readily to its radical, which reacts fast with $NO_2^\bullet$; both species are formed from $ONOOCO_2^-$.

An additional proposal (Fig. 2.11)[2] is that an 'activated transition state form' of peroxynitrous acid on the pathway to NO_3^- is the major reactive oxidizing/hydroxylating/nitrating species. It has been suggested that ONOOH exists in *cis* and *trans* forms with different pK_a values (6.8 and 8.0) and that an excited state of the *trans* isomer is the active species. The more stable *cis* form predominates at high pH, but protonation removes repulsion of the negative char-

ges and allows formation of more *trans* form, which has the higher pK_a and so can reionize. The *trans* forms of ONOOH and $ONOO^-$ can undergo transition to a vibrationally excited state, which involves bending of the N–O–O bond and lengthening of the O–O bond. These activated intermediates can cause damage and/or rearrange to nitrate.

2.6.1.2 *Toxicity of nitrotyrosine and nitrated proteins?*[103,112,113]

Nitrotyrosine added to certain cells at high levels can be toxic, for example by undergoing redox cycling (Section 8.18.1), by interfering with signal transduction or by becoming incorporated into the microtubule protein **tubulin** and distorting the cytoskeleton. Nitrated proteins might also trigger an immune response, a possible contribution to autoimmunity,[114] and they are abundant in pollen (Section 8.18.1). Not much is known about the fate of nitrated proteins *in vivo*; they may be degraded by the proteasome system (Section 4.14.2) and possibly by **denitrase** enzyme systems,[115] whose biochemistry remains to be elucidated.

2.6.1.3 *Nitric oxide, superoxide and peroxynitrite: a balance*

Just as $O_2^{\bullet-}$ reacts fast with $NO^\bullet$, it can react with $NO_2^\bullet$, giving **peroxynitrate,**

$$O_2^{\bullet-} + NO_2^\bullet \rightarrow O_2NOO^-$$

a species to which little attention has been paid but may well be injurious (Section 8.11.2). Nevertheless, $NO^\bullet$ can be beneficial in many ways; for example it deters phagocyte adherence to vascular endothelium, and platelet aggregation. The presence of excess NO• can sometimes inhibit damage by ONOO⁻. For example, whereas equal fluxes of $O_2^{•-}$ and NO• can form ONOO⁻ and stimulate lipid peroxidation, a high ratio of NO• to $O_2^{•-}$ can decrease peroxidation because of the ability of NO• to scavenge peroxyl and alkoxyl radicals (Section 2.5.6.2). Such reactions yield nitro, nitroso and nitrated lipid adducts, whose biological significance remains to be elucidated, although some might activate the PPARγ receptor (described in Section 9.3.4) and can decompose to regenerate NO• and form lipid radicals, the former causing vasodilation. Nitrated linoleic acid has been detected in human plasma (79±35 nM free and 550±275 nM esterified) and red blood cell membranes and has been shown to suppress human neutrophil $O_2^{•-}$ formation *in vitro*, so that it might be anti-inflammatory. Nitrated derivatives of oleic, linolenic and arachidonic acid have also been detected in human body fluids.[116,117]

In normal blood vessels, the NO•/$O_2^{•-}$ ratio experienced by the vascular endothelial cells is probably high. Lowering that ratio might favour pro-oxidant (via ONOO⁻) rather than antioxidant effects of NO•. Nevertheless, addition of ONOO⁻ to thiols or urate leads to reactions[118] that regenerate some NO•. In other words, under certain circumstances ONOO⁻ formation could be a mechanism of removing excess $O_2^{•-}$ by NO•, provided that the damaging ONOO⁻ is swiftly removed by antioxidants, which return some of it as NO•.

By contrast, exposure of mitochondria to excess NO• inhibits cytochrome oxidase, and the back-up of electrons in the electron transport chain can result in more $O_2^{•-}$. Peroxynitrite can form, and damage the mitochondria. Complex I[119] and mitochondrial creatine kinase[120] are potential targets. Peroxynitrite has been reported to damage eNOS, promoting 'uncoupling' of the enzyme to decrease NO• synthesis and increase $O_2^{•-}$ formation.[94]

2.6.1.4 *Experimental artefacts*

In aqueous solution, ONOOH is powerfully oxidizing and nitrating. It can react directly with spin traps (Section 2.6.1.1) and 'probes' for OH• such as thiourea.[121] In one study, an inhibitor of caspase-1 blocked the toxicity of SIN-1 to rat neurons in culture. However, the cell death was not apoptotic;

the inhibitor simply scavenged the toxic ONOO⁻-derived species.[122] Some PARP inhibitors, for example 3-aminobenzamide (Section 4.2.4), can exert the same non-specific effects, and probably many other compounds do so as well. Watch out for direct scavenging of RS by so-called 'selective' inhibitors of various cell injury pathways.

2.6.2 Hydrogen peroxide

Hydrogen peroxide (H_2O_2) is a pale-blue, covalent, viscous liquid, boiling point 150°C. Its structure is shown in Fig. 2.12. It is toxic to many cells at levels in the 10 to 100 μM range, causing senescence or apoptosis, but at lower levels it can promote proliferation of certain cell types, and at higher levels it suppresses apoptosis and promotes necrotic cell death (Section 4.4.1). Indeed, production of high levels of H_2O_2 by L-amino acid oxidases contributes to the toxicity of certain snake venoms[123] and to the antibacterial action of the mucus of the giant snail *Achatina Fulica Férussac*.[124] The weak antiseptic activity of honey, used in wound treatment since ancient times, is partly due to the formation of H_2O_2.[125] Honey also contains other antimicrobial agents, such as **propolis**, a resin collected from trees (Section 3.22.4).[126]

Hydrogen peroxide mixes readily with water and can diffuse within and between cells *in vivo*. Physiologists recognized years ago that water crosses cell membranes much faster than can be explained by simple diffusion of such a polar molecule. Although some water does appear to diffuse across the lipid bilayer, much appears to pass through membrane water channels, the **aquaporins**. Hydrogen peroxide can also traverse

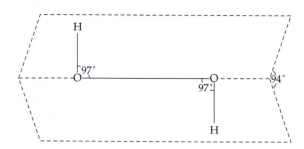

Figure 2.12 The structure of hydrogen peroxide.

these channels,[127] but this may not be the only mechanism by which it crosses membranes. For example, adaptation of yeast to H_2O_2 seemed to involve changes in plasma membrane lipid composition to slow H_2O_2 entry.[128]

2.6.2.1 *Production of H_2O_2*

Several enzymes generate H_2O_2, including xanthine, urate, coproporphyrinogen III, glucose, lysyl, monoamine and D-amino acid oxidases, as well as SOD. Ascorbate and some flavonoids oxidize in commonly used cell culture media to generate H_2O_2, an artefact that has led to some misinterpretations about their effects on cells.[129] Superoxide and H_2O_2 can also be produced in media by photochemical reactions, usually involving riboflavin.[130]

Hydrogen peroxide is continually produced in many, if not all, tissues *in vivo* and studies on perfused rat liver suggest steady-state concentrations of 10^{-7} to 10^{-8} M (Fig. 5.10). Mitochondria may be significant contributors to cellular H_2O_2 generation, both by monoamine oxidases (in brain) and by dismutation of $O_2^{\bullet-}$ from the electron transport chain, although mitochondria can also consume H_2O_2 (Section 3.11.1). H_2O_2 has been estimated to reach a steady-state concentration of about 5 nM in the matrix,[131] although there may be a wide variation in levels between mitochondria from different tissues. Hydrogen peroxide can be detected in exhaled air (Section 5.14.8) and in urine (urinary levels are very variable—usually $<10\,\mu M$ but sometimes $>100\,\mu M$).[132] Drinking coffee raises urinary H_2O_2 levels; the compound **hydroxyhydroquinone** (Section 3.22.3) is absorbed from the coffee, re-excreted and rapidly oxidizes in the urine to produce $O_2^{\bullet-}$ and H_2O_2.[132] *E. coli* growing exponentially on glucose has been estimated to generate about 14 μM H_2O_2 every second (also see Sections 1.10.7 and 3.4.1).[133]

2.6.2.2 *A ROS that is not very reactive*

Perhaps fortunately, given its widespread presence *in vivo*, H_2O_2 is only a weak oxidizing or reducing agent and is generally poorly reactive. Indeed, this probably allows it to play a role in signal transduction (Section 4.5). For example, no oxidation occurs when DNA, lipids or most proteins are incubated with H_2O_2, even at mM levels. However, H_2O_2 is capable of inactivating a few enzymes directly, usually by oxidation of hyper-reactive —SH groups essential for catalysis. These include the glycolytic enzyme G3PDH[134] (Fig. 1.7), chloroplast fructose bisphosphatase (Section 6.8.4), some protein phosphatases (Section 4.5.5) and the caspases involved in apoptosis (Section 4.4.1). Hydrogen peroxide can also oxidize certain keto-acids such as pyruvate (CH_3COCOO^-) and 2-oxoglutarate (Section 3.18.2).

Despite its poor reactivity, H_2O_2 can be cytotoxic and at high concentrations is often used as a disinfectant. Some bacterial strains are especially sensitive to H_2O_2, as is the worm *C. elegans*.[135] Many animal cells in culture are injured or killed if H_2O_2 is added to the medium at concentrations at or above the 10 to 100 μM range. For example, H_2O_2 produced by the pathogen *Mycoplasma pneumoniae* can attack epithelial cells in the trachea.[136] Coinfection of human lymphocytes with the HIV-1 virus and a mycoplasma leads to cell damage involving H_2O_2 generation.[137]

Although some cellular damage by H_2O_2 is direct, for example G3PDH inactivation, addition of H_2O_2 frequently leads to lipid, DNA and protein oxidation that cannot be mediated by H_2O_2 alone. It crosses cell membranes and reacts with iron, and possibly copper, ions to form more damaging species such as $OH^\bullet$. Indeed, $OH^\bullet$ accounts for most or all of the damage done to DNA in H_2O_2-treated cells.[138] Hydrogen peroxide also interacts with haem proteins to cause oxidative damage (Section 3.15.3). Sometimes, exposing cells to H_2O_2 can increase $O_2^{\bullet-}$ production, by activating NADPH oxidases (section 7.10)[138A].

2.6.2.3 *The Russell effect*[139]

In 1896, Becquerel found that uranium compounds could affect a photographic plate wrapped in light-proof paper. This early description of radioactivity excited much curiosity amongst scientists, one of whom was William Russell. During his experiments, Russell made a mask of perforated zinc sheet and placed it between the uranium salts and the photographic plate, intending to produce a shadow of the zinc sheet on the film. To his surprise, he found that the zinc sheet affected the plate more than the uranium. This **Russell effect** is shown by many freshly abraded metals, notably magnesium, cadmium, nickel, aluminum and lead. Wood, leaves, oils, and paper can all give images, particularly if they have been previously exposed to light or, in the case of wood, if it has been recently charred. Russell discovered that the effect is due to H_2O_2 or organic peroxides produced in minute amounts from the material tested, and it illustrates the ubiquitous nature of peroxides.

Most modern photographic films are much less sensitive to H_2O_2, but they can be used to show the Russell effect if specially pretreated. The detection of room temperature degradation of materials of antiquity is important for development of new conservation methods. In cases where autoxidation contributes, the Russell effect is one sensitive method to detect it.

2.6.3 Hypochlorous acid[140–142]

Hypochlorous acid is produced by the enzyme **myeloperoxidase** (MPO) (Section 7.7.3)

$$H_2O_2 + Cl^- \xrightarrow{MPO} HOCl + OH^-$$

It is a weak acid, pK_a approximately 7.5. Hence HOCl is about 50% ionized at pH 7.4

$$HOCl \rightleftharpoons H^+ + OCl^-$$

Hypochlorite (OCl^-) absorbs light at 292 nm (molar extinction coefficient $\varepsilon = 350\,dm^3\,mol^{-1}cm^{-1}$) and so concentrations of HOCl can easily be determined by adding alkali and reading the absorbance, or by adding acid and reading the absorbance of HOCl at 235 nm ($\varepsilon = 100\,dm^3\,mol^{-1}cm^{-1}$). Studies with HOCl are facilitated by the ease with which it can be made in the laboratory, by simple acidification of solutions of sodium hypochlorite (Na^+OCl^-), a constituent of many bleaches. Hypochlorous acid readily decomposes to liberate chlorine (Cl_2) gas, a reaction favoured at low pH

$$HOCl + H^+ + Cl^- \rightleftharpoons Cl_2 + H_2O$$

Although its importance in bacterial killing by phagocytes is uncertain (Section 7.7.3), HOCl has attracted attention because of its high reactivity

(Table 2.14) and ability to damage biomolecules, both directly and by decomposing to form chlorine. It is a powerful two-electron oxidizing agent. For example, addition of HOCl to bacteria such as *E. coli* inhibits ATP synthesis by damaging electron transport chain components and the ATP synthase.[143] Part of the toxicity of HOCl to *E. coli* involves other ROS, although the exact mechanism has not been elucidated.[144] In animal systems, HOCl can attack many targets. It can inactivate α_1-**antiproteinase** within seconds at pH 7.4. α_1-Antiproteinase, formerly called α_1-**antitrypsin**, is produced in the liver and released into extracellular fluids, where it serves to inhibit several proteolytic enzymes, including elastase. Elastase hydrolyses elastin and if uncontrolled can do severe damage, especially in the lung. An inborn deficiency in α_1-antiproteinase in humans can cause the disease **emphysema**, in which the elastic fibres in the lung are destroyed and gas exchange impaired because the lung cannot expand and contract properly. Hypochlorous acid attacks a methionine residue on the α_1-antiproteinase, forming **methionine sulphoxide**. Peroxynitrite inactivates α_1-antiproteinase by the same mechan-

Table 2.14 Some rate constants for reactions of hypochlorous acid

Compound	pH	k(M^{-1}s^{-1})
Monochlorodimedon[a]	5.0	7×10^6
NADH	7.0	$> 2 \times 10^5$
Taurine	7.0	4.8×10^5
GSH[b]	7.4	$> 10^7$
Ascorbate	7.4	$\sim 6 \times 10^6$
Ferrocyanide, Fe(CN)$_6^{4-}$	7.0	~ 220
Fe^{2+}	~ 4	1.7×10^4
Fe(II)-citrate	5.0	1.3×10^4
Superoxide	5.0	7.5×10^6

Data from [7] and values are for 25°C. HOCl is a powerful two-electron oxidizing agent; $E^{\circ\prime}$ for the couple HOCl/H$_2$O, Cl$^-$ about 1.1 V. Oxidations/chlorinations caused by HOCl addition are not necessarily achieved by this molecule; it may decompose to give such species as Cl$^\bullet$, Cl$_2$, etc.
[a] This compound, full name **1, 1-dimethyl-4-chloro-3,5-cyclohexane-dione**, is chlorinated by HOCl; the resulting rise in absorbance at 290 nm is often used to assay HOCl production by myeloperoxidase.
[b] Reaction of GSH with HOCl gives a mixture of products, including GSSG, GSO$_2$SG (glutathione thiosulphonate), and a glutathione sulphonamide (*Biochem. J.* **326**, 87, 1997).

ism.[145] **Thrombomodulin**,[146] a glycoprotein in endothelial cells that regulates the blood coagulation pathway by modifying the action of thrombin, is also inactivated by HOCl, again by attack on methionine. Of course, whether α_1-antiproteinase and thrombomodulin are major targets of attack by HOCl *in vivo* depends on what else is around them, since HOCl react with many biomolecules.

Indeed, HOCl oxidizes thiols, ascorbate, NAD(P)H and DNA. It also chlorinates DNA bases (especially pyrimidines)[147] and tyrosine residues in proteins (generating **3-chlorotyrosine** and **3,5-dichlorotyrosine**). It causes side-chain damage, fragmentation and aggregation of proteins by multiple reactions, not only oxidation of cysteine and methionine residues but also reaction with side-chain $-NH_2$ groups to give chloramines (Section 2.6.3.1 below).[148] Metal ions held in proteins by thiolate (S^-) ligands can be released after HOCl treatment, for example Zn^{2+} is lost from metallothionein.[149] Hypochlorous acid might also participate in formation of singlet O_2 (Section 2.6.4 below) and nitryl chloride (Section 2.6.1), and it can oxidize[75] NO_2^- to NO_3^-. In addition, HOCl oxidizes thiocyanate to **hypothiocyanite**,[150] $OSCN^-$

$$HOCl + SCN^- \rightarrow Cl^- + OSCN^- + H^+$$

HOCl can cross membranes, causing damage to membrane proteins and lipids on its passage and, if any survives to enter the cytoplasm, to intracellular constituents. Yet despite all this, HOCl held at the active sites is used by chloroperoxidase enzymes (Section 3.13.6) to bring about chlorination reactions.[151]

2.6.3.1 Chlorhydrins, chloramines and hydroxyl radical from HOCl[141,148,152]

How does HOCl attack lipids? It can add across double bonds in unsaturated fatty acid residues in phospholipids or esterified to cholesterol

to give **chlorohydrins**. Similar products (**bromohydrins**) are formed when **hypobromous acid** (HOBr), produced by certain phagocytes (Section 7.8), is added to lipids. Hypochlorous acid and HOBr readily oxidize plasmalogens (Section 4.12.8).

Reaction of HOCl with $O_2^{\bullet-}$ or Fe^{2+} generates $OH^\bullet$ or species with comparable reactivity (section 2.5.1); a long time ago Fenton reported that the H_2O_2 in his $Fe^{2+}/H_2O_2/$ tartaric acid system could be replaced by 'chlorine water'. Indeed, *E. coli* mutants with elevated intracellular iron are hypersensitive to HOCl (Section 3.6.2.2).[152]

Taurine (2-aminoethanesulphonic acid) is present at high levels in many mammalian tissues as an end-product of the metabolism of sulphur-containing amino acids (Fig. 7.16). It reacts with HOCl to generate **taurine chloramines**

$$R-NH_2 + HOCl \rightarrow RNHCl + H_2O$$

which can also inactivate α_1-antiproteinase. Chloramines were initially identified as 'long-lived oxidants' generated by reaction of HOCl with body fluids.[142] Similar products are formed by HOCl from amino groups on proteins, lipids, DNA and amino sugars found in proteoglycans (to many of which MPO binds avidly). Hypobromous acid can similarly form **bromamines**, RNHBr. Both HOCl and chloramines have been reported to interfere with DNA repair processes in cells. Chloramines can react with $O_2^{\bullet-}$ to produce nitrogen-centred radicals

$$RNHCl + O_2^{\bullet-} \rightarrow RNH^\bullet + Cl^- + O_2$$

and the presence of $O_2^{\bullet-}$ increases damage to proteins and proteoglycans by HOCl.[148] Chloramines can oxidize thiols, ascorbate and methionine, but much more slowly than does HOCl (rate constants $<10^3 M^{-1}s^{-1}$).[150]

2.6.4 Singlet oxygen[153]

Two singlet states of O_2 exist (Fig. 1.15). In both, the spin restriction that slows reaction of O_2 with non-radicals is removed, so that singlet oxygens are much more oxidizing than ground-state O_2. The $^1\Sigma g^+$ state rapidly decays to the $^1\Delta g$ state, so only the latter is usually considered in biological systems. Hence references to 'singlet O_2' in this book refer to the $^1\Delta g$ state. Note that $^1\Delta g$ O_2 is not a free radical.

Singlet O_2 in solution can transfer its excitation energy to the solvent, so its lifetime is affected by the solvent used. Thus in water its lifetime is about 4 µs, in deuterium oxide (D_2O) 62 µs and in hexane 31 µs.

2.6.4.1 *Singlet O_2 from photosensitization*

Singlet O_2 is often generated by **photosensitization reactions**. If certain molecules are illuminated with light of the correct wavelength, they absorb it and the energy raises the molecule into an **excited state**. The excitation energy can then transfer onto an adjacent O_2 molecule, converting it to a singlet state whilst the photosensitizer returns to its ground state. Popular sensitizers of $^1O_2$ formation in the laboratory include the dyes **acridine orange**, **methylene blue, rose Bengal** and **toluidine blue**, but many biomolecules are sensitizers, including vitamin B_2 (riboflavin) and its derivatives FMN and FAD, **hypocrellins A and B**, chlorophylls *a* and *b* (Section 6.8), the bile pigment **bilirubin,** and various porphyrins, both free and bound to proteins (Figs 2.13 and 2.14).

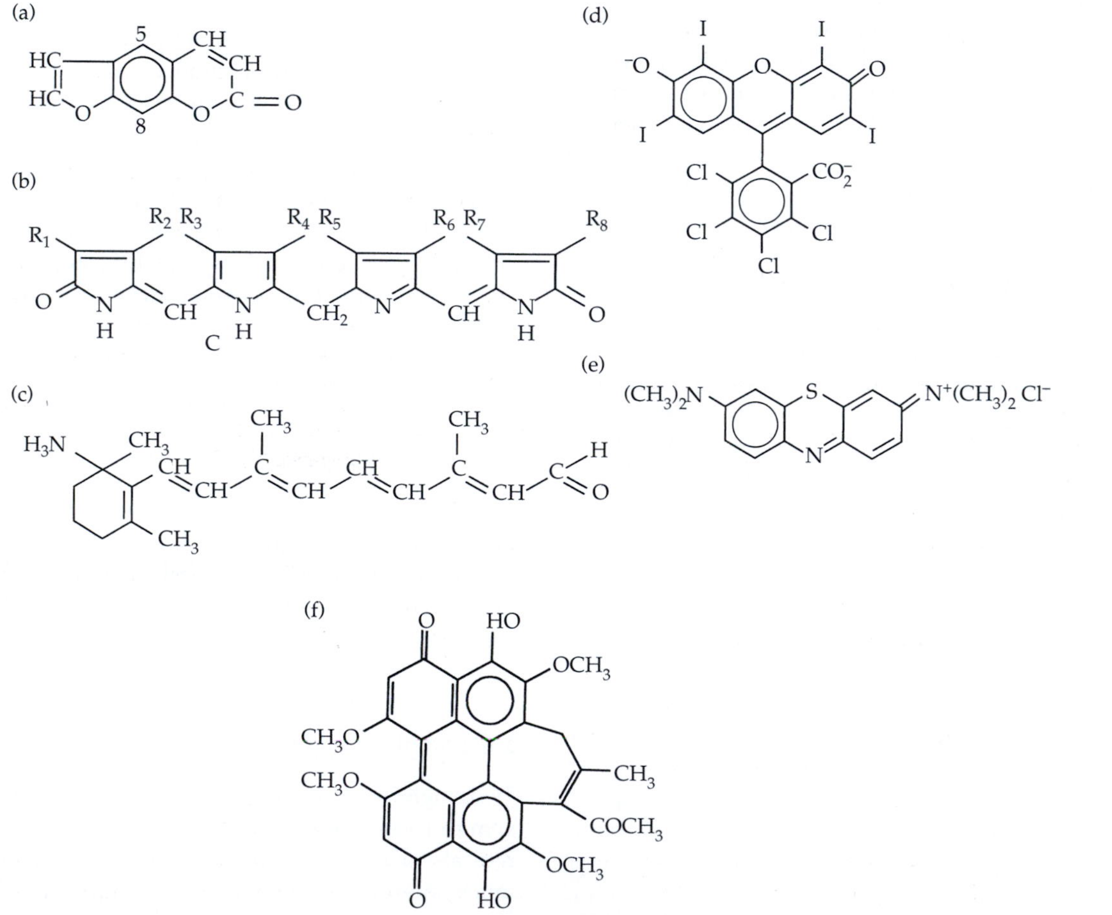

Figure 2.13 Some compounds that sensitize formation of $^1O_2$ when illuminated with light of the correct wavelength. (a) Psoralen, (b) bilirubin, (c) all-*trans* retinal, a compound important in vision (Section 6.10), (d) rose Bengal, (e) methylene blue, chloride salt, (f) hypocrellin B. Hypocrellins are produced by a parasitic fungus found in China, *Hypocrella bambuase*. Other plant-derived photosensitizers are shown in Fig. 6.14.

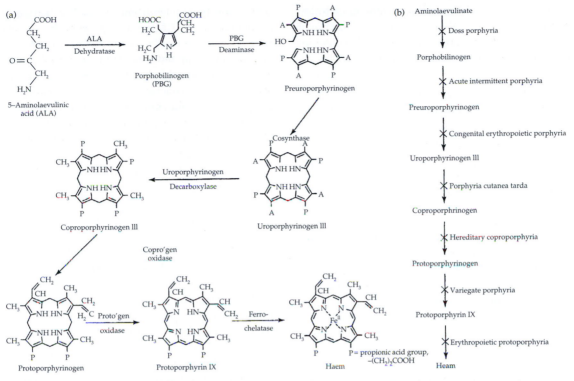

Figure 2.14 Biosynthesis of haem. Eight steps are involved (including the synthesis of ALA); the first four happen in the cytosol and the last four in mitochondria (*Blood* **105**, 1867, 2005). Different porphyrias result from inborn errors in different enzymes. For example, hereditary copro-porphyria and variegate porphyria are frequently associated with skin lesions (coproporphyrin accumulates in the former, protoporphyrinogen in the latter). In **porphyria cutanea tarda**, uroporphyrinogen decarboxylase is decreased and skin lesions are common. This disease is not always inherited: it can result from exposure to certain toxins (Section 8.3.2). Loss of ferrochelatase activity also leads to skin damage, due to protoporphyrin IX accumulation. From *Trends Biochem. Sci.* **21**, 231, 1996, by courtesy of Dr Martin Warren and his colleagues and Elsevier. **5-Aminolaevulinic acid** (ALA), which accumulates in acute intermittent porphyria and also in lead poisoning (Section 8.15.8) is an autoxidizable molecule; rats chronically treated with it showed increased levels of 8OHdG in liver DNA (*Carcinogenesis* **15**, 2241, 1994).

The $^1O_2$ produced on illumination of photo-sensitizers can not only react with any other molecules present but also attack the photo-sensitizer itself. Hence illuminated solutions of flavins lose their orange colour and chlorophylls their green colour as they are attacked (**photo-bleaching**). Reactions of this type cause the dyes in clothes and curtains and the paint on cars to fade when exposed to sunlight. Indeed, exposure of cells in culture to high-intensity visible light leads to damage, especially to the mitochondria, which are rich in haem proteins and flavoproteins. Haem-containing enzymes such as catalase are also inactivated. Cell culture media frequently contain riboflavin, which aggravates these effects,

since the intensity of lighting in many laboratories is sufficient to allow flavin-sensitized $^1O_2$ formation.[130]

2.6.4.2 *Type I and II reactions*

Not all photosensitization damage need involve $^1O_2$, since the excited state of the photosensitizer can sometimes itself cause damage (said to occur by a **type I mechanism**, whereas that caused by $^1O_2$ is described as a **type II mechanism**). Both mechanisms may operate simultaneously and their relative importance depends on the target molecule, the efficiency of energy transfer from the sensitizer to O_2, and the O_2 concentration. In addition, illumination of several photosensitizers, including porphyrins and acridine dyes, in aqueous solution produces $OH^\bullet$ and $O_2^{\bullet-}$ in addition to $^1O_2$. Thus it must never be assumed that $^1O_2$ is the species responsible for any damage observed.[154]

2.6.4.3 *Biological damage by photosensitization*[153,155]

Photosensitization reactions, usually mediated by $^1O_2$, are important *in vivo*, especially in skin (Section 6.12.1.1), chloroplasts (Section 6.8.1) and the eye (Section 6.10). Illumination of milk or milk products can cause development of 'off-flavours' as the riboflavin present photosensitizes the degradation of milk proteins and lipids.[156]

Several diseases can lead to excessive singlet O_2 formation. For example, the **porphyrias** (a term derived from *porphuros*, Greek for purple) are caused by defects in the biosynthesis of haem (Fig. 2.14). In some (the **cutaneous porphyrias**), porphyrins accumulate in the skin, exposure of which to light causes eruptions, scarring and thickening (Fig 2.15). The severity of the damage depends upon which porphyrin is accumulated and thus differs in different types of porphyria. Oral β-carotene, a singlet O_2 quencher, can offer some protection (Section 3.21). The British King George III (1738–1820) is believed to have suffered from an

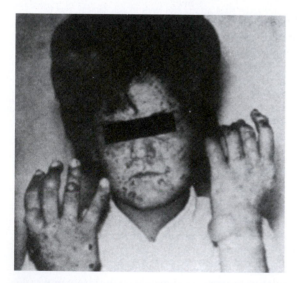

Figure 2.15 Skin and tissue damage in a porphyria patient. Note the blistering and swelling. From *Angew-Chem. Int. Ed.* **21**, 343, 1982, with permission.

acute porphyria syndrome (possibly variegate porphyria; Fig. 2.14) causing periodic severe attacks of abdominal pain, vomiting, psychiatric disturbances and reddish-brown or purple urine, perhaps aggravated by arsenic in the drugs he was given by his physicians.[157] The discoloration of urine is due to autoxidation of excreted porphyrin precursors. Even healthy skin can be exposed to $^1O_2$ from small amounts of porphyrins generated by bacteria (Section 6.12.1.1).

Several clinically used drugs are capable of sensitizing $^1O_2$ formation, including some antidepressants, tetracycline and fluoroquinolone antibiotics (Section 8.16), and certain non-steroidal anti-inflammatory drugs, such as **carprofen**. Clinically, most problems appear to arise with the fluoroquinolones.[158] **Benoxaprofen** was introduced as an anti-inflammatory agent but is no longer used, in part due to phototoxicity. Various constituents of sunscreens and perfumes have also been suggested to be photosensitizers (Section 6.12.1.1) and certain herbicides damage plants by increasing $^1O_2$ formation (Section 6.9).

Photosensitization reactions are also important in veterinary medicine.[159] Digestion of chlorophyll in ruminants forms the pigment **phylloerythrin,** which is absorbed from the gut and excreted in the bile. Liver malfunction hinders excretion, allowing phylloerythrin to enter the bloodstream and deposit in the tissues. When the animals are exposed to sunlight the pigment in the skin causes damage that results in reddening and swelling. The fungal product **sporidesmin** achieves a similar effect by inhibiting bile production. **Buckwheat** synthesizes a compound that sensitizes $^1O_2$ formation and is toxic to farm animals. The same is true of **St John's wort**, a plant which produces the sensitizer **hypericin** (Section 6.10.1.1).

2.6.4.4 *Uses of photosensitization*

Sometimes photochemical effects are useful. A well-established case is the treatment of the jaundice often developed by premature infants soon after birth.[160] The yellow colour is due to accumulation of bilirubin (Fig. 2.13) in the skin. It arises from the breakdown of haemoglobin and travels in the blood attached to albumin, which can bind two molecules of bilirubin per molecule of protein. Usually, the liver takes up bilurubin and converts it into a water-soluble product using the enzyme **uridine diphosphoglucuronyl transferase**, which catalyses the reaction:

$$\text{bilirubin} + 2\text{UDP} - \text{glucuronic acid}$$
$$\rightarrow \text{bilirubin diglucuronide} + 2\text{UDP}$$

The soluble diglucuronide is excreted into bile. Premature babies often have insufficient glucuronyl transferase in the liver, so that the lipid-soluble bilirubin accumulates in the blood, and deposits in tissues with a high lipid content, such as the brain, where it can cause irreversible damage. The jaundice can be ameliorated by careful exposure of the babies to blue light from a sunlamp. This causes a light-induced rearrangement (**photoisomerization**) of the structure of bilirubin to give water-soluble products that can be excreted, although $^1O_2$ may also be involved.[160]

Other examples of the medical relevance of photosensitization include the use of **psoralens** (Fig. 2.13), powerful photosensitizers produced by some plants (e.g. celery), for skin diseases such as psoriasis. Treatment consists of the combined application of ultraviolet light and a psoralen, and is often referred to as **PUVA therapy** (psoralen ultraviolet A). This therapy is helpful in psoriasis, but there is debate about its safety, for example whether it increases the risk of skin cancer.

Certain porphyrins are taken up by malignant tumours.[161] After injection of HPD (**haematoporphyrin derivative**, a mixture of porphyrins), porphyrins are accumulated by the tumour, enabling its detection by observing fluorescence. Irradiation with light of the correct wavelength to excite HPD constituents can then damage the tumour. Such methods are under development for cancer treatment, especially for oesophageal and some forms of lung cancer, in which the tumour can be illuminated with light from a flexible fibre-optic tube, as well as for skin cancers. Both $OH^\bullet$ and $^1O_2$ appear to be involved in HPD-mediated tumour damage. The HPD

preparation is a complex mixture and more recently a simpler mixture (**Photofrin II**) enriched in the tumour-localizing fractions has been employed. Hypocrellins (Fig. 2.13) and several other compounds have also been tested. Another approach is to supply ALA or its esters (Fig. 2.14)—this stimulates a transient build-up of protoporphyrin IX which especially affects tumour tissues since their ferrochelatase activities seem lower than normal.[161] Photodynamic therapy is also being tested for the treatment of macular degradation (Section 6.10).

2.6.4.5 *Other sources of singlet* O_2

Peroxyl radicals can form $^1O_2$ by the Russell mechanism (Section 2.5.4), for example during lipid peroxidation (Section 4.11.8.1). Another system used to generate $^1O_2$ in the laboratory is a mixture of H_2O_2 and hypochlorite

$$OCl^- + H_2O_2 \rightarrow Cl^- + H_2O + O_2(\text{singlet})$$

The singlet O_2 arises from the H_2O_2. Hypobromite (OBr^-) reacts similarly. Hypochlorite is formed by MPO (Section 2.6.3) and several groups have measured 'singlet O_2' from activated neutrophils. However, $HOCl/OCl^-$ is itself highly reactive, which can cause problems in attempts to detect singlet O_2 formation. Reaction of ozone with some biomolecules generates $^1O_2$ (Section 2.6.5 below).

A 'clean' method of producing $^1O_2$ without other ROS is the decomposition of aromatic endoperoxides, such as the substituted naphthalene endoperoxides. Depending on the R group, these can be water-soluble or hydrophobic

Generation of $^1O_2$ in this way has been used to assess its effects on antioxidants in human blood plasma.[162] Exposure of plasma to a water-soluble $^1O_2$ generator led to depletion of ascorbate, urate, protein $-SH$ groups and bilirubin, but not of α-tocopherol or β-carotene. Lipid-soluble $^1O_2$ generators led to faster loss of bilirubin, protein thiols, ubiquinol and ascorbate but lower rates of urate degradation.

2.6.4.6 *Reactions of singlet oxygen*[153]

Singlet O_2 interacts with other molecules in essentially two ways: it can react chemically with them, and/or transfer its excitation energy to them, returning to the ground state while the other molecule enters an excited state. The latter

can occur—the $^1O_2$ adds and the double bond changes position:

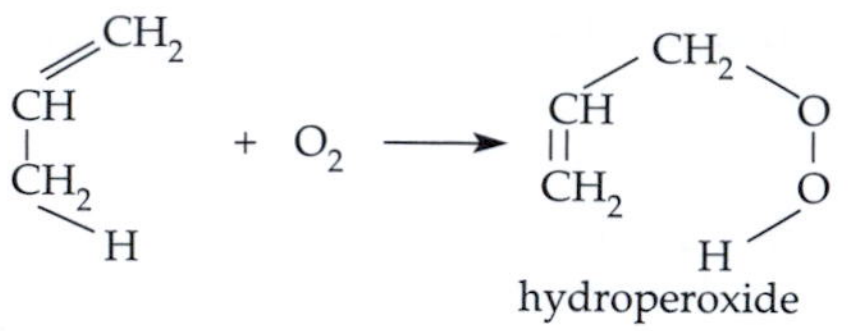

If there is an electron-donating atom, such as N or S, adjacent to the double bond, $^1O_2$ may cause **dioxetane** formation.

Dioxetanes are unstable and decompose to give compounds containing carbonyl groups,

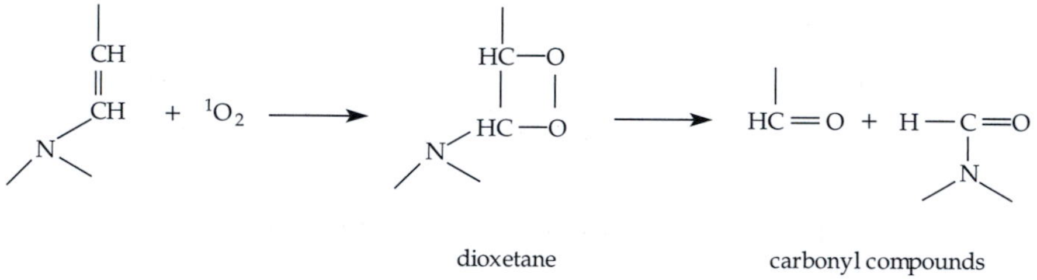

dioxetane   carbonyl compounds

phenomenon is called **quenching** of singlet O_2. Molecules used in the laboratory as 'singlet O_2 quenchers/scavengers' include histidine, DABCO, azide and diphenylisobenzofuran. Sometimes both quenching and chemical reactions occur with the same molecule (Fig. 2.16).

Singlet O_2 reacts rapidly with compounds containing carbon–carbon double bonds. Molecules containing two double bonds separated by a single bond (known as **conjugated double bonds**) often react to give **endoperoxides**.

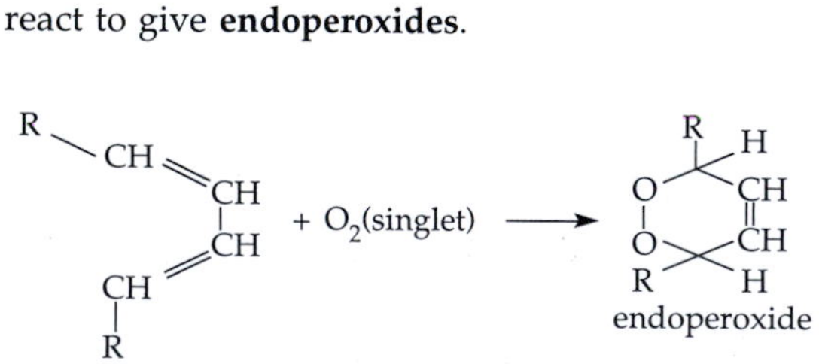

endoperoxide

Diphenylisobenzofuran reacts in this way (Fig. 2.16). If one double bond is present, the **ene-reaction**

Tryptophan is an example (Fig. 2.16).

2.6.5 Ozone[163]

Ozone is an irritating, non-free radical triatomic gas, poorly soluble in water. It has a characteristic pungent smell and its name is derived from the Greek *ozein*, 'to smell'. The two oxygen–oxygen bonds in O_3 are of equal length and intermediate in structure between O–O and $O=O$ bonds. Ozone performs an essential 'antioxidant' function in the higher levels of the atmosphere by screening out UV light. Ozone is produced there by the photodissociation of O_2 into oxygen atoms, which then combine with O_2. Recently there has been concern over the commercial use of fluorinated hydrocarbons because they may deplete the O_3 layer. Free radicals are involved yet again! Homolytic photodissociation of chlorofluorocarbon gases such as CF_2Cl_2 and $CFCl_3$ produces **chorine radicals** (chlorine atoms) in the atmosphere, which react with ozone by such reactions as

$$Cl^{\bullet} + O_3 \rightarrow O_2 + ClO$$

Compound	Structure	Comments
DNA	Guanosine	Forms unstable endoperoxide; opening of the ring can eventually form 8OHdG. $^1O_2$ can then oxidize 8OHdG further (Section 4.8.2.5) 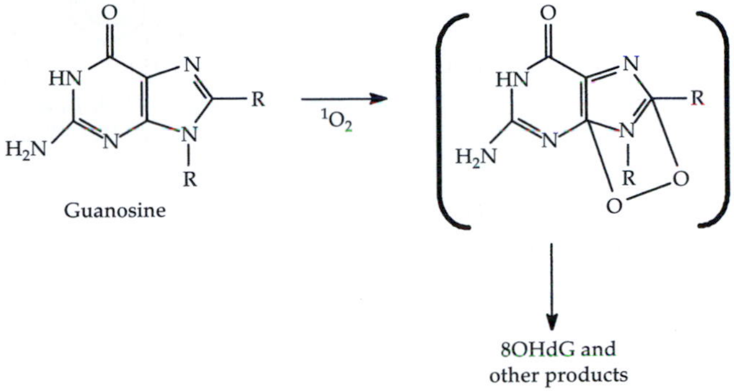 $\xrightarrow{^1O_2}$ 8OHdG and other products
Methionine	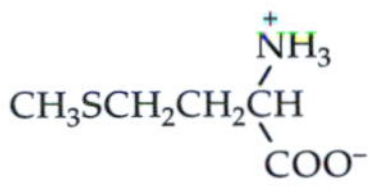 $CH_3SCH_2CH_2\overset{\overset{+}{N}H_3}{\underset{COO^-}{CH}}$	Forms methionine sulphoxide 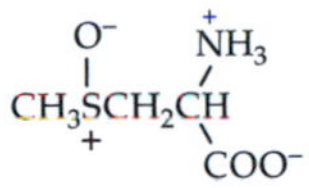 $CH_3\overset{\overset{O^-}{S^+}}{S}CH_2\overset{\overset{+}{N}H_3}{\underset{COO^-}{CH}}$
Cystine	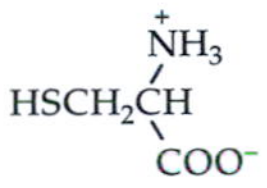 $HSCH_2\overset{\overset{+}{N}H_3}{\underset{COO^-}{CH}}$ (R—SH)	Reactions not fully characterized: both cystine and cysteic acid (RSO_3H) are formed. Cystine can react further with $^1O_2$.
Histidine	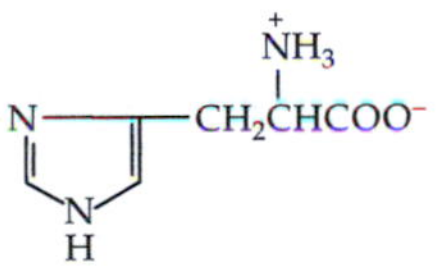 $\overset{}{N}\text{—}CH_2\overset{\overset{+}{N}H_3}{CHCOO^-}$	Probably reacts to give an endoperoxide 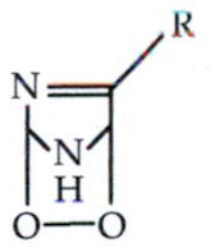 which decomposes to a complex mixture of products
Tryptophan	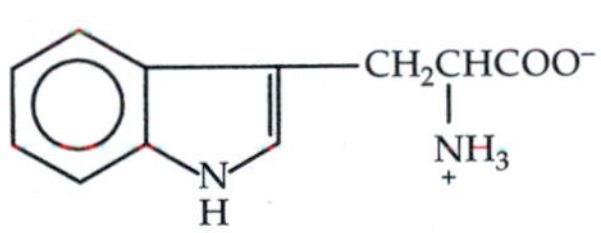 (indole)—$CH_2\underset{\overset{+}{N}H_3}{CHCOO^-}$	Reacts by several mechanisms, including an ene-reaction to give initially 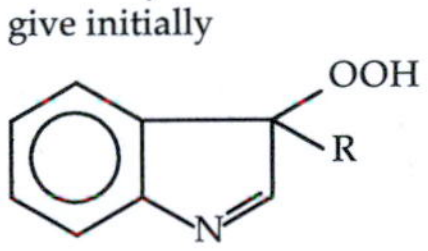 OOH, R (R is the side-chain) and also formation of a dioxetane

Figure 2.16 Reactions of singlet O_2 with various biomolecules, antioxidants and 'singlet quenchers/scavengers'.[153,155] Calculations based on reaction rate constants suggest that most $^1O_2$ generated *in vivo* will react with amino acid residues on proteins. Protein peroxides formed can then decompose into free radicals to propagate damage.

Compound	Structure	Comments

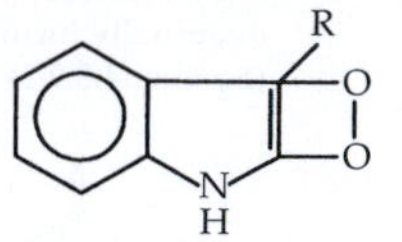

which decomposes to *N*-formylknurenine, itself a photosensitizer of $^1O_2$ formation

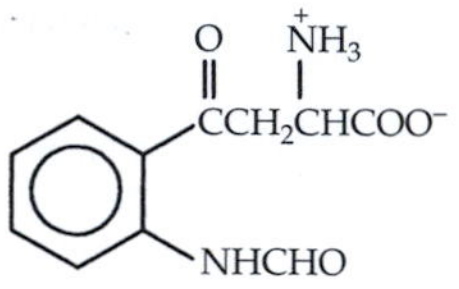

| DABCO (1,4-diazabicyclooctane) | 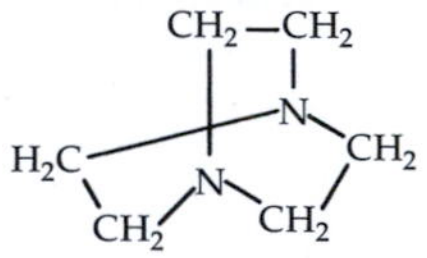 | Quencher |

| Azide ion | N_3^- | Mostly quenching |

| α-Tocopherol | Section 3.20 | Mostly quenching but some chemical reaction to give |

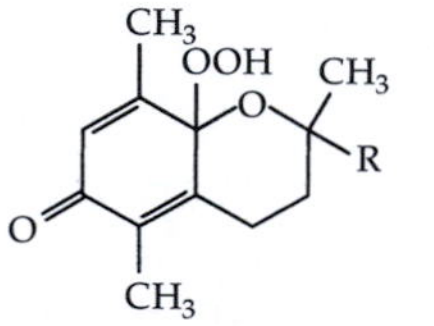

which decomposes to various products including α-tocopherylquinone (R is the side chain)

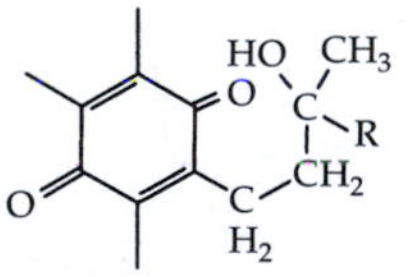

Major product is the 5α-hydroperoxide.

Figure 2.16 (*Cont.*)

Compound	Structure	Comments
Cholesterol	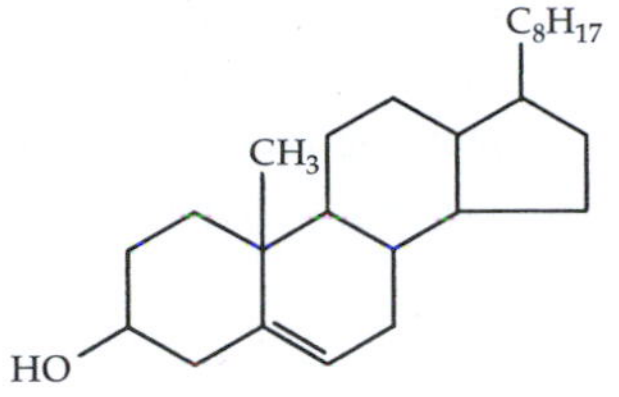	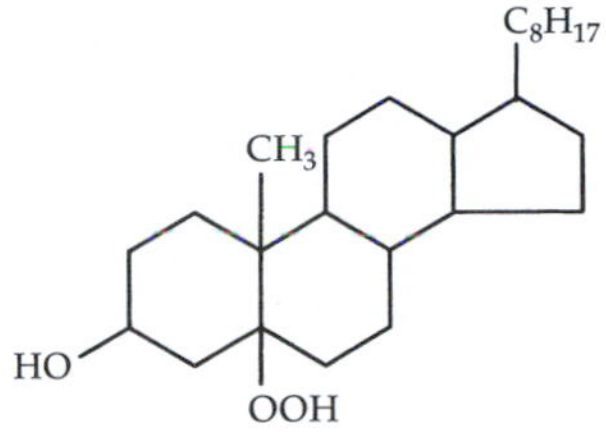 but some 6α and 6β-OOH can form. Cholesterol can be used to detect $^1O_2$.
β-Carotene	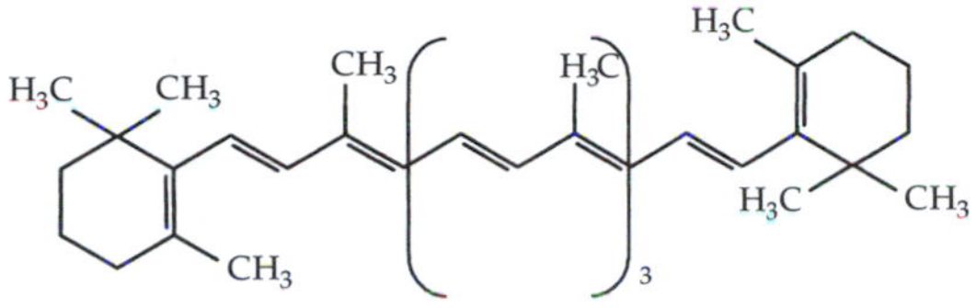	Mostly quenching, some (complex) chemical reactions (Section 3.21).
Ascorbate	Produces unstable hydroperoxides 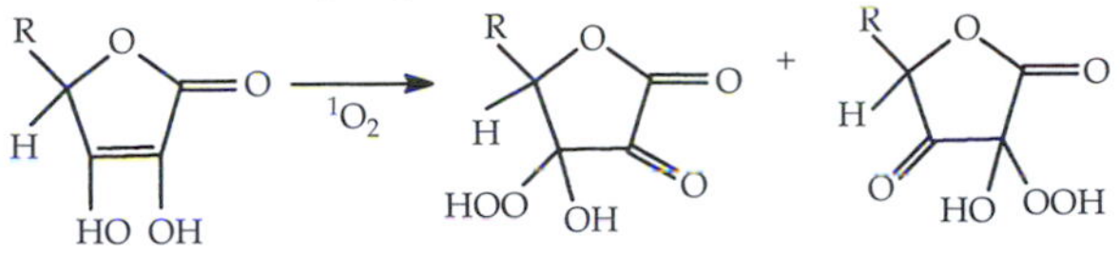	
Diphenylisobenzofuran	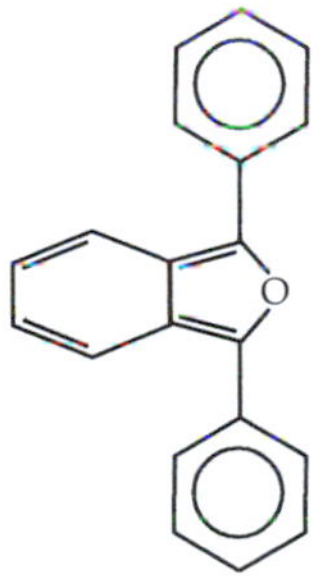	Endoperoxide formation accompanied by loss of absorbance at 415 nm 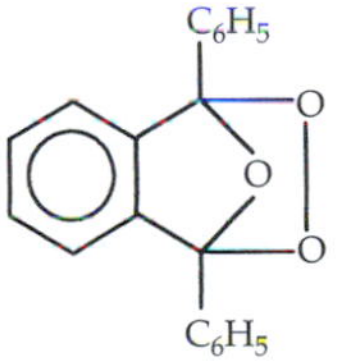

Figure 2.16 (*Cont.*)

However, O_3 is a nuisance if formed in the lower atmosphere. It can arise by photochemical reactions between oxides of nitrogen and hydrocarbons: motor vehicle exhausts are a good source of the necessary gas mixture. Millions of people in the USA and Europe are regularly exposed to O_3 above the recommended levels (Section 8.11.1).

Ozone levels as low as 0.5 p.p.m can cause lung damage (especially loss of ciliated cells and type I alveolar cells) in a few hours. Some photocopying machines have been reported to produce significant amounts of O_3.[164] Ozone induces inflammation, activating pulmonary macrophages and recruiting neutrophils to the lung; RS produced by these cells are an additional source of oxidative stress after O_3 exposure. Damage to lung macrophages can also decrease resistance to infections. Ozone irritates the eyes and can oxidize proteins (e.g. lysozyme) and lipids in tear fluids.[165] Ozone also damages plants and skin (Sections 6.9.3 and 6.12.1.4).

Ozone is a powerful oxidizing agent. It adds directly across double bonds in lipids to generate **ozonides**, which can decompose to cytotoxic aldehydes (Fig. 2.17). Ozone also oxidizes proteins,[163,166] attacking $-SH$, tyrosine, tryptophan, histidine and methionine residues, among others. Both lipids and proteins (e.g. in surfactant) may be targets of direct attack by O_3 in the respiratory tract. In aqueous solution, O_3 decomposes to form some $OH^\bullet$, but this is a slow process at physiological pH (favoured at highly alkaline pH). Nevertheless, aromatic hydroxylation studies (Section 5.3.1) have detected more $OH^\bullet$ in rats or humans breathing ozone.[167] Reaction of O_3 with several biomolecules (NADH, NADPH, cysteine, albumin, methionine, uric acid or GSSG) has been shown[168]

to produce some $^1O_2$, which could then cause further oxidations, as could the H_2O_2 produced when O_3 reacts with lipids (Fig. 2.17). Ozonation has been used as an alternative to chlorination for the sterilization of drinking water in some places since it is highly bactericidal.

2.6.5.1 *Endogenous ozone?*[169]

We usually regard O_3 as an exogenous toxin, but it may be generated *in vivo*. Products consistent with the ozonolysis of cholesterol (Fig. 2.16) have been detected in human atherosclerotic lesions, and O_3 was measurable when the phagocytes in such tissues were stimulated by adding phorbol myristate acetate (Section 7.7.2). It was suggested that antibodies can catalyse the oxidation of H_2O to H_2O_2 by $^1O_2$ via a process involving the trioxygen species H_2O_3, **dihydrogen trioxide**. Ozone might also arise from H_2O_3. These studies may have revealed a series of biologically-relevant **reactive trioxygen species**, although more work on the chemistry and methodology is required.[170]

CHAPTER 3

Antioxidant defences: endogenous and diet derived

Sometimes scientific progress is not based on a discovery or the generation of new data but on a change of viewpoint that allows one to see a set of already existing data in a new light

Michael Reth

3.1 Introduction

Oxygen is poisonous: aerobes survive in its presence only because they have evolved **antioxidant defences**. Antioxidants can be synthesized *in vivo* or taken in from the diet. Defences against reactive nitrogen species (RNS) such as peroxynitrite (Section 2.6.1) and reactive chlorine species such as HOCl (Section 2.6.3) are also needed. In this Chapter we will use **reactive species (RS)** to encompass ROS, RNS and reactive halogen and sulphur species.

3.1.1 The simplest defence: avoid O_2 as much as possible

Some mobile organisms avoid O_2 toxicity by swimming away from regions with high O_2 levels. In several bacteria, including *Salmonella typhimurium* and *E. coli*, there is an intracellular 'redox sensor' which measures the redox state of the respiratory chain and transmits a signal to the flagellae involved in swimming.[1] Other adaptations may have been to pack redox constituents together in electron transport chains in a way that makes 'escape' of electrons to O_2 less likely, and to evolve a cytochrome oxidase that works fast even at low pO_2, and does not release ROS, allowing intramitochondrial pO_2 to be kept low. This need to use the minimum intracorporeal O_2 levels that permit aerobic respiration may have been one force

driving the evolution of multicellularity (Fig. 1.4). Insects, for example, seem to open and shut their spiracles to maintain a low constant internal pO_2, subject to the need to allow CO_2 to escape.[2] Food manufacturers exploit this technique when they seal foods under nitrogen or in vacuum packs, and some stem cells may lurk in hypoxic environments until they are needed (Section 3.1.2 below).

3.1.2 Other antioxidant defences

These can comprise:

(a) agents that catalytically remove RS, such as the superoxide dismutase (SOD), superoxide reductase, catalase and peroxidase enzymes;

(b) agents that decrease RS formation, e.g. mitochondrial uncoupling proteins (Section 1.10.6). Under this category one can include proteins that minimize the availability of pro-oxidants such as iron ions, copper ions or haem. Examples are transferrins, albumin, haptoglobins, haemopexin, haem oxygenases, metallothionein and (possibly) polyamines (Section 4.12.9). This category includes proteins that oxidize Fe^{2+} ions, such as caeruloplasmin;

(c) proteins that protect biomolecules against oxidative damage by other mechanisms, e.g. chaperones;

(d) the physical 'quenching' of RS, e.g. of singlet O_2 by carotenoids;

(e) the replacement of molecules sensitive to oxidative damage by molecules resistant to it; an example is the fumarase C of *E. coli* (Section 1.6); (f) 'sacrificial agents' that are preferentially oxidized by RS to preserve more important biomolecules; examples are GSH, α-tocopherol, bilirubin, ascorbate, urate, albumin (Section 3.16.3.5 below) and plasmalogens (Section 4.12.8).

The levels and composition of antioxidant defences differ from tissue to tissue and cell type to cell type (possibly even from cell to cell of the same type) in a given tissue. For example, several papers suggest that adult and embryonic stem cells are exceptionally rich in antioxidant defences, which decrease as the cells differentiate.[3,4] Haematopoietic stem cells may reside in hypoxic niches in the bone marrow, perhaps ameliorating cumulative damage by ROS over time.[4] Extracellular fluids have different protective mechanisms from the intracellular environment (Section 3.16.3 below). Antioxidant defences are often increased after exposure of organisms to RS and to some cytokines (Section 4.7).

Antioxidant defences are not 100% effective, since oxidative damage to DNA, proteins, lipids and other molecules can be demonstrated in living systems under ambient O_2. Hence even 21% O_2 is toxic (Table 4.1). In part, this may be because several RS are used as messengers (Chapter 4), so the challenge is to evolve antioxidant defences that allow this role whilst minimizing damage. Thus some authors classify the **repair systems** needed to cope with damaged molecules (e.g. to repair DNA, reassemble [Fe–S] clusters in enzymes [Section 3.6.1 below], or to degrade damaged lipids and proteins) as antioxidant defences. Others consider the two as separate, but in any case antioxidant defences and repair processes are intimately linked.

3.1.3 What is an antioxidant? A new definition

Antioxidant, like **oxidative damage** and **oxidative stress**, is a term widely used but surprisingly difficult to define clearly. Food technologists use antioxidants to inhibit lipid peroxidation and consequent rancidity in foods, so they often define an antioxidant as a good inhibitor of lipid peroxidation. Museum curators use 'antioxidants' to preserve their exhibits.[5] Polymer scientists use 'antioxidants' to control polymerization in the manufacture of rubber, plastics and paint and for the protection of clear plastics against ultraviolet light.[6] Combustion is a free-radical process: the oil industry makes extensive use of antioxidants and a knowledge of free-radical mechanisms in the design of better fuels and lubricating oils.[6] All these scientists have their own views on what a good antioxidant should be.

What about living organisms? When RS are generated *in vivo*, many antioxidants come into play. Their relative importance depends upon:

- which RS is generated
- how it is generated
- where it is generated, and
- what target of damage is measured.

For example, when human body fluids are exposed to O_3 or $NO_2^{\bullet}$, urate appears to be a protective antioxidant (Section 8.11). By contrast, urate provides little protection against damage to blood plasma constituents by HOCl. If the oxidative stress is the same but a different damage target is measured, different answers result. For example, exposure of human blood plasma to gas-phase cigarette smoke causes peroxidation of plasma lipids, which is inhibited by ascorbate. By contrast, ascorbate does not protect against damage to plasma proteins by cigarette smoke, as measured by the carbonyl assay (Section 8.12.1).

To encompass these various complexities, the third edition of this book proposed a broad definition of an antioxidant as **any substance that, when present at low concentrations compared with those of an oxidizable substrate, significantly delays or prevents oxidation of that substrate**. The term **oxidizable substrate** includes almost every molecule found *in vivo*. This definition emphasizes the importance of the damage target studied and the source of RS used when antioxidant action is examined. It is also imperfect, like us all. For example, plasma albumin may bind copper and protect low density lipoproteins (LDL) against oxidative damage (Section 3.16.3.5 below), but here the albumin is in considerable molar *excess* over the LDL. The definition does not take into account chaperones, repair systems or inhibitors of RS generation. Thus we now simplify the definition to **any substance that delays, prevents or removes oxidative damage to a target molecule**. There is no universal 'best' antioxidant, as illustrated by the cigarette smoke/plasma experiments mentioned above.

Let us now examine the known antioxidant systems, always bearing in mind two questions; (i) what can they do? and (ii) what evidence exists that what they do is important *in vivo*?

3.2 Antioxidant defence enzymes: superoxide dismutases (SODs)

The discovery of SODs provided much of the basis for our current understanding of antioxidant defence, since it led to the postulation of the superoxide theory of O_2 toxicity and the realization that free radicals are important metabolic products.[7] Hence it is appropriate to consider SODs first.

3.2.1 Copper-zinc SOD[7,8]

In 1938, Mann and Keilin isolated a blue-green protein containing copper (**haemocuprein**) from bovine blood. In 1953, a similar protein was isolated from horse liver and named **hepatocuprein**. Other proteins of this type were later isolated, such as **cerebrocuprein** from brain. In 1970, it was discovered that the erythrocyte protein contains zinc as well as copper. No enzymic function was detected in any of these proteins, so it was often suggested that they served as metal stores. However, in 1969 McCord and Fridovich reported that the erythrocyte protein is able to remove $O_2^{\bullet-}$ catalytically, that is it functions as a copper- and zinc-containing **superoxide dismutase** enzyme (CuZnSOD). Figure 3.1 illustrates this using pulse radiolysis (Section 2.3.3.1).

The SOD enzymes are highly efficient in catalytic removal of $O_2^{\bullet-}$. However, they can promote a few other reactions *in vitro*. For example, nitroxyl anion (NO^-) can reduce Cu^{2+} in the enzyme, and in the presence of $O_2^{\bullet-}$ CuZnSOD can catalyse[9] conversion of NO^- to $NO^{\bullet}$

$$NO^- + O_2^{\bullet-} + 2H^+ \rightleftharpoons NO^{\bullet} + H_2O_2$$

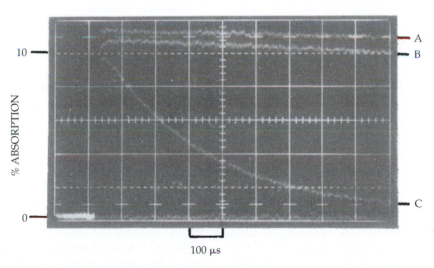

Figure 3.1 The catalytic action of CuZnSOD as demonstrated by pulse radiolysis. The oscilloscope shows the decay at pH 8.8 of $O_2^{\bullet-}$ radical (initial concentration 32 μM) as followed by the loss of its absorbance at 250 nm. Trace A, spontaneous dismutation of $O_2^{\bullet-}$; trace C, plus 2 μM of SOD; trace B, as for trace C but SOD boiled for 5 min to destroy enzyme activity. Data from *Biochim. Biophys. Acta* **268**, 605, 1972 by courtesy of Professor G. Rotilio and Elsevier.

The CuZnSOD enzymes also promote nitration of tyrosine residues by $ONOO^-$ (Section 2.6.1) and can oxidize the ionized form of hydrogen sulphide (H_2S) to **hydrosulphide radical**.[10]

$$E-Cu^{2+} + HS^- \rightarrow E-Cu^+ + HS^\bullet$$

They have also been reported to catalyse oxidation of cysteine and cysteamine (but not GSH), forming H_2O_2 and disulphide.[11]

The CuZnSODs are unusually stable enzymes. In purifying CuZnSOD from erythrocytes, the cells are lysed and haemoglobin removed by treatment with chloroform and ethanol, followed by centrifugation. The enzyme enters the organic phase, from which it can be precipitated by addition of cold acetone and then further purified by ion-exchange chromatography. Not many enzymes will tolerate such procedures. Most CuZnSODs are fairly resistant to heating, attack by proteinases and denaturation by such reagents as guanidinium chloride, sodium dodecyl sulphate (SDS) and urea.

3.2.1.1 *CuZnSOD in eukaryotes and prokaryotes*

The CuZnSODs are present in almost all eukaryotic cells. In animal cells, most CuZnSOD is located in the cytosol, but some appears present in lysosomes, nucleus and the space between inner and outer mitochondrial membranes. Peroxisomes have also been reported to contain CuZnSOD.[7,12]

The CuZnSODs were originally thought to be rare in prokaryotic cells, but examples of their presence have accumulated fast. The first to be discovered was a CuZnSOD in the luminescent bacterium *Photobacterium leiognathi*. This organism exists in a symbiotic relationship with the ponyfish, occupying a special gland and imparting a characteristic luminescence to the fish. It was initially suggested that the bacterium obtained the gene for its CuZnSOD by gene transfer from its host fish, although this is doubtful.[7] Indeed, CuZnSODs occur in many other bacteria, including *Neisseria*, *Caulobacter*, *Legionella*, *Brucella*, *Salmonella* and *Haemophilus* species and in *Mycobacterium tuberculosis*.[13] Often (e.g. in *E. coli*) the CuZnSOD is located in the **periplasmic space** (the space between the bacterial cell wall and cell membrane). It may help to defend against external sources of RS, such as

activated phagocytes, and against any $O_2^{\bullet-}$ generated in the periplasmic space itself.[13,14]

3.2.1.2 *Catalytic ability of CuZnSOD*

The CuZnSOD enzymes from eukaryotes usually have relative molecular masses of about 32 000 and contain two protein subunits, each of which has an active site containing one copper and one zinc ion.[7] A different type of CuZnSOD, extracellular SOD (EC-SOD), sometimes called SOD3, is considered in Section 3.16.3.1 below. Bacterial CuZnSODs are also usually dimers with one Cu per subunit, although a few, including the *E. coli* enzyme, are monomers.[13]

The CuZnSODs function to accelerate the dismutation of $O_2^{\bullet-}$ (Fig. 3.1)

$$O_2^{\bullet-} + O_2^{\bullet-} + 2H^+ \rightarrow H_2O_2 + O_2 \text{ (ground-state)}$$

Whereas the overall rate constant for the uncatalysed dismutation of $O_2^{\bullet-}$ depends on pH (Section 2.5.3) and is about $5 \times 10^5 \, M^{-1}s^{-1}$ at pH 7.0, the reaction catalysed by bovine erythrocyte CuZnSOD is almost independent of pH in the range 5.3 to 9.5, and the rate constant for reaction of $O_2^{\bullet-}$ with the active site is at least $1.5 \times 10^9 \, M^{-1}s^{-1}$, over three orders of magnitude greater. Also, non-enzymic dismutation requires $O_2^{\bullet-}$ and $HO_2^\bullet$ to collide, which is difficult given their low intracellular concentrations (10^{-9}–10^{-10} M). Superoxide is more likely to collide with SOD, present in many cells at $\sim 10^{-5}$ M. The copper ions in CuZnSODs catalyse dismutation by undergoing alternate oxidation and reduction,

$$\text{Enzyme-Cu}^{2+} + O_2^{\bullet-} \rightarrow \text{Enzyme-Cu}^+ + O_2$$

$$\text{Enzyme-Cu}^+ + O_2^{\bullet-} + 2H^+ \rightarrow$$
$$\text{Enzyme-Cu}^+ + H_2O_2$$

Net reaction: $O_2^{\bullet-} + O_2^{\bullet-} + 2H^+ \rightarrow H_2O_2 + O_2$

The Zn^{2+} does not function in the catalytic cycle but helps stabilize the enzyme. Indeed, the *M. tuberculosis* enzyme seems not to contain zinc yet dismutes $O_2^{\bullet-}$ efficiently.[15] In eukaryotic cells, a **metallochaperone** known as **CCS** (**copper chaperone for SOD**), delivers copper to the **apoenzyme** (metal-free enzyme) whilst ensuring correct dis-ulphide bridge formation in the SOD molecule (Section 3.15.2 below).[16] Mammalian CCS has considerable structural similarity to CuZnSOD. Knockout of CCS in yeast or the plant *Arabidopsis thaliana* (Section 6.8.7) abolishes CuZnSOD activity. However, in animals some activity remains; apparently there is a secondary pathway involving Cu delivery by GSH.[17]

Ions of most other transition metals, including iron and manganese, cannot replace the copper of CuZnSOD to yield a functional enzyme, but cobalt, mercury or cadmium ions can replace Zn^{2+} in increasing enzyme stability.[7] If the Cu^{2+} is replaced by cobalt ions (Co^{2+}), however, the enzyme has been claimed to still catalyse $O_2^{\bullet-}$ dismutation,[18] although with a rate constant of only $4.8 \times 10^6\,M^{-1}s^{-1}$.

3.2.1.3 *CuZnSOD structure*

The complete amino acid sequences (and, in some cases, three-dimensional structures) of CuZnSOD from multiple plants and animals have been determined and, in general, are very similar.[7] The first CuZnSOD to have its detailed structure determined was the bovine erythrocyte enzyme. Each of the two subunits is composed primarily of eight antiparallel strands of β-pleated sheet struc-ture that form a flattened cylinder, plus 'loops'. The copper ion is held at the active site by interaction with the nitrogens in the imidazole ring structures (Fig. 3.2) of four histidine residues (numbers 44, 46, 61 and 118 in the amino acid sequence), whereas the zinc ion is bridged to the copper by interaction with the imidazole of His61 and it also interacts with His69 and His78 and the carboxyl group of Asp81. Histidine 61 (his63 in the human enzyme), which interacts with both metals, may be involved in supplying the protons needed for dismutation. Human CuZnSOD shows similar structure: it is a dimeric enzyme with ellipsoidal dimensions of about $30 \times 40 \times 70\,\text{Å}$. Each subunit contains 153 amino acid residues plus one zinc and one copper ion (Fig. 3.3, Plate 1). In dimeric prokaryotic CuZnSODs the structure is broadly similar, but the loop regions (Fig. 3.3, Plate 1) differ and the interactions holding the two subunits together are generally less strong.[13]

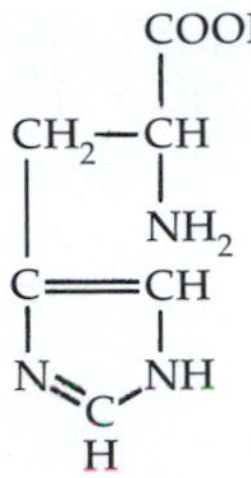

Figure 3.2 Structure of the amino acid histidine. The ring structure is known as the **imidazole ring** and contains two nitrogen atoms. Each has five electrons in its outermost shell, three of which are being used in covalent bonding. The remaining two constitute a **lone pair** and can act as ligands to metal ions.

In CuZnSODs, much of the surface of each subunit is negatively charged, repelling $O_2^{\bullet-}$, except for positively charged 'tracks' that lead into the active site (Fig. 3.4, Plate 2). A similar arrangement prob-ably exists in the manganese and iron SODs (Sections 3.2.2 and 3.2.3 below). Hence, $O_2^{\bullet-}$ approaching the enzyme is 'guided' into the active site. Modification of these positively charged amino acid side-chains decreases enzyme activity, and high ionic strength does the same, both by interfering with this **elec-trostatic facilitation** of $O_2^{\bullet-}$ dismutation. Variants of SOD have been developed in the laboratory that work faster than the wild-type enzyme by enhancing this mechanism (Fig. 3.4d, Plate 2d).

3.2.1.4 *Inhibitors of CuZnSOD*

Cyanide is a powerful, albeit non-specific, inhibitor of CuZnSODs. They are also inactivated on incubation with **diethyldithiocarbamate (DDTC)**

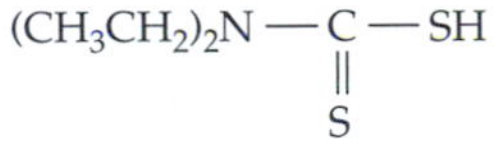

a compound that binds to copper and removes it from the active sites. Diethyldithiocarbamate has been used to inhibit CuZnSOD in cells and whole animals. For example, 3 h after its injection into mice, the SOD activity of blood had decreased by 86%, that of liver by 71% and that of brain by 48%.[19] However, use DDTC with caution, since it inhibits several other copper-containing enzymes and also xanthine oxidase.[20] As a thiol, DDTC can exert direct antioxidant properties, form RS$^\bullet$ radicals, chelate metals and inhibit apoptosis (Section 4.4) in some

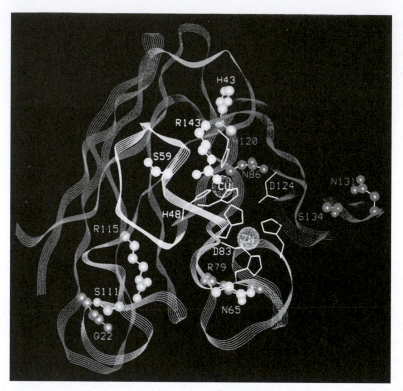

Figure 3.3 (see plate 1) Human CuZnSOD β-structure framework (blue) and loop regions, along with conformationally important side chains. The α-carbon backbone is shown as a ribbon coloured to highlight the various loops. Critical side chains that form multiple side-chain-main-chain hydrogen bonds are shown in ball-and-stick representation, labelled by residue number and the one-letter amino acid code, and colour-coded to match the loops they stabilize: Gln22 for the purple insertion loop II, His43 for the light-blue Greek-key connection (loop III); Ser59 and Arg143 for the yellow disulphide subloop (IV); Asn65 and Arg79 for the gold Zn-ligand subloop (IV); Ser111 and Arg115 for the green Greek-key loop (VI); and Asn86, Asn131 and Ser134 for the red electrostatic loop (VII). Metal ligands His48, His120 and Asp83 also make side-chain to main-chain hydrogen bonds to the loop regions. The copper ligands (**His46, His48, His63 and His210**) form distorted square-planar geometry, while the zinc ligands (**His63, His71, His80 and Asp83**) are tetrahedral. The copper and zinc are linked directly by the **bridging histidine** (His63) and indirectly by the side-chain carboxylate of buried Asp124, which hydrogen bonds to both a copper- and a zinc-ligating histidine. Photograph by courtesy of Drs John Tainer and Elizabeth Getzoff and the American National Academy of Sciences; see *Proc. Natl. Acad. USA* **89**, 6109, 1992.

cells. Hence its effects *in vivo* can be hard to interpret. 2-Methoxyoestradiol has been claimed to inhibit SOD, but probably does not.[21]

3.2.1.5 *Isoenzymes of CuZnSOD*

SOD activity can be visualized by gel electrophoresis (Fig. 3.5), and inhibition by cyanide used to identify CuZnSOD. Electrophoresis of tissue extracts, or even of purified SOD enzymes, often shows the presence of multiple bands. Exercise caution in attributing such multiple bands to SOD isoenzymes since they can arise as a consequence of attack on the SOD protein by proteolytic enzymes present in the extract. Partial loss of metal ions increases the net negative charge and can also cause multiple bands. Some animal CuZnSODs, for example the human and chicken-liver enzymes, contain cysteine–SH groups that can oxidize and aggregate on storage, as well as form mixed disulphides (Section 3.9.6 below) with other thiols, such as GSH.[22]

However, purification of the different enzymes has confirmed the existence of isoenzymes of CuZnSOD in several species, including maize, *Arabidopsis* and *Drosophila*.[23,24] Indeed a variant of human CuZnSOD has been found in Northern Sweden and Finland.[23] Most of the population is homozygous for 'normal' SOD, but there are some heterozygotes with both forms of the enzyme and a few homozygotes for the variant form. The two

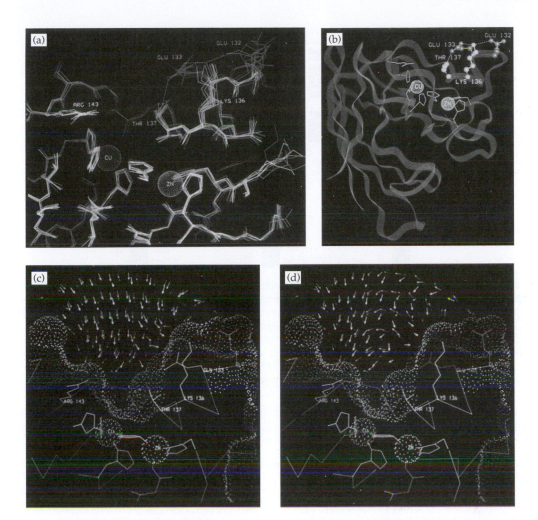

Figure 3.4 (see plate 2) Network of human SOD residues involved in electrostatic recognition of superoxide: Glu132, Glu133, Lys136 and Thr137. The colour-code is: red, most negative; yellow, negative; green, neutral; light blue, positive; blue, most positive. Copper (gold) and zinc (blue) ions are shown as spheres. The SOD enzyme shown, and used as a control for construction of electrostatic mutants, is the double mutant Cys6 → Ala, Cys111 → Ser. This mutant maintains the activity and rate-versus-pH profile of wild-type human SOD but is more stable. (a) Superimposed copies of the SOD active site. Dotted lines (upper right) show hydrogen bonds linking side chains of electrostatically important residues: Thr137 (green, centre) to Glu133 (red, top centre), to Lys136 (blue, upper right), to Glu132 (red, upper right). All other residues are shown colour-coded by subunit, and appear white where superimposed. (b) Overview of mutated residues in the electrostatic loop and their structural relationship to the active site and overall β-barrel protein fold (blue ribbon following polypeptide chain) in one subunit of the SOD homodimer. Electrostatically important side chains Glu132, Glu133, Lys136 and Thr137 (coloured and oriented as in panel a) form a hydrogen-bonding network (ball-and-stick models with dashed hydrogen bonds) on the solvent-edxposed helical turn of the electrostatic loop overhanging the active-site channel (upper right). This helix is orientated so that its C-terminal carbonyl oxygen atoms and helical dipole stabilize and are stabilized by zinc binding. Side chains of copper and zinc ligands and of active-site Arg143 are shown as lines. (c) Cross-section of the active site channel for wild-type human SOD, with colour-coded molecular surface dots and arrows indicating the direction of the electrostatic force on the negative charge of $O_2^{\bullet-}$. (d) Corresponding view for (Glu133 → Gln) mutated SOD. Neutralizing negatively charged Glu by converting it to uncharged glutamine increases the reaction rate by guiding $O_2^{\bullet-}$ more directly downward to the catalytic copper ion. Photographs by courtesy of Drs John Tainer, Elizabeth Getzoff and Nature Publishing Group; see *Nature* **358**, 347, 1992.

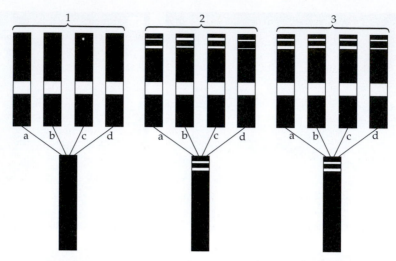

Figure 3.5 Visualization of SOD on polyacrylamide gels. After electrophoresis, the gel is soaked in a solution of nitroblue tetrazolium (NBT) and exposed to an $O_2^{\bullet-}$ generating system. Superoxide reduces NBT to the blue-coloured formazan (Section 2.5.3) and so the gel turns blue except where SOD activity is located. The enzyme removes $O_2^{\bullet-}$, prevents formazan production, and a white 'achromatic zone' is detected (*Anal. Biochem.* **44**, 276, 1971). The figure shows the pattern obtained after electrophoresis of extracts from (a) brain, (b) heart, (c) liver and (d) lung of (1) rat, (2) mouse, (3) chicken. Upper panel, no cyanide added. Lower panel, 2mM CN^- ions present, which inhibit CuZnSODs. Figure from *Biochim. Biophys. Acta* **556**, 32, 1979 by courtesy of the authors and Elsevier, Amsterdam. The activity **tetrazolium oxidase**, extensively studied by geneticists, is actually SOD (*Arch. Biochem. Biophys.* **159**, 798, 1973). Other proteins that react with $O_2^{\bullet-}$, including some copper and iron proteins (e.g. caeruloplasmin, haem peroxidases), can also produce achromatic bands.

forms can be separated by gel electrophoresis at high pH. This mutant SOD is rarely detected in other populations, except in one of the Orkney islands; perhaps the Vikings may have introduced the altered gene on one of their rampages. It has also been found in some Mormons in Utah; between 1850 and 1905, over 30 000 Mormon converts left Scandinavia for the USA.[25] The variant enzyme has a slightly lower specific activity, but homozygotes appear to suffer no ill effects.[23] The term **SOD-2** was originally used to describe this mutant form, but is now more generally employed in the literature as a synonym for MnSOD (Section 3.2.2 below).

3.2.1.6 *Pro-oxidant effects of CuZnSOD?*[26,27]
Superoxide reacts fast with the active site copper of CuZnSOD ($k_2 > 10^9$ $M^{-1}s^{-1}$). The reaction product H_2O_2 can also react with the copper, but much more slowly

$$E-Cu^{2+} + H_2O_2 \rightarrow E-Cu^+ + O_2^{\bullet-} + 2H^+$$

$$E-Cu^+ + H_2O_2 \rightarrow E-Cu^{2+} + OH^\bullet + OH^-$$

Thus CuZnSOD in the presence of mM levels of H_2O_2 can generate $OH^\bullet$, or a species that resembles

it (possibly Cu(III); Section 2.4.6) at its active site. This mixture of SOD and H_2O_2 can catalyse oxidation of several substrates *in vitro*, including azide, urate, nitrite (to $NO_2^\bullet$), ABTS (Section 5.17) and the spin-trap DMPO (Section 5.2.4). Addition of CO_2/HCO_3^- increases the rates of many of these oxidations, possibly by forming carbonate radical ($CO_3^{\bullet-}$) by reaction of CO_2/HCO_3^- with $OH^\bullet$ at the active site,[a] followed by escape of the $CO_3^{\bullet-}$ from the enzyme to oxidize the substrate. Bicarbonate has no effect where the substrate itself can enter the active site, e.g. for NO_2^- oxidation. Another possibility is that HO_2^- reacts with CO_3^{2-} bound to the enzyme to form peroxomonocarbonate (Section 2.5.2).

$$E-Cu^+ - CO_3^{2-} + HO_2^- \rightarrow$$
$$E-Cu^+ - CO_4^{2-} + OH^-$$

$$E-Cu^+ - CO_4^{2-} + 2H^+ \rightarrow E-Cu^{2+} - CO_3^{\bullet-} + H_2O$$

The CuZnSOD protein is damaged during incubation with high H_2O_2 levels, suffering oxidation of

[a] Some papers suggest that HCO_3^- enters the active site, others that CO_2 does so.

amino acid residues (e.g. active-site histidine to 2-oxohistidine, oxidation of tryptophan by $CO_3^{\bullet-}$) and aggregation. Pro-oxidant copper ions can also be released; some of them bind to the SOD protein surface and target further damage there.

Addition of CO_2/HCO_3^- also facilitates oxidation of cysteine[11] by CuZnSOD plus H_2O_2.[28]

3.2.2 Manganese SOD (sometimes called SOD2)

The SOD first isolated from *E. coli* turned out to be entirely unlike CuZnSOD. It was pink rather than blue-green, not inhibited by CN^- or DDTC, had a relative molecular mass of 40 000 rather than 32 000, was destroyed by treatment with chloroform plus ethanol (and hence did not survive the typical purification methods for CuZnSOD) and contained manganese at its active site, as Mn(III) in the 'resting' enzyme. Almost all manganese SODs are more labile to denaturation by heat, organic solvents or detergents than CuZnSODs.

Despite these differences, MnSODs catalyse essentially the same reaction as CuZnSODs. The (simplified) reaction mechanism can be written as

$$Mn(III) + O_2^{\bullet-} \rightleftharpoons [Mn(III)\text{-}O_2^{\bullet\bullet}] \longrightarrow Mn^{2+} + O_2$$

$$Mn^{2+} + O_2^{\bullet-} \rightleftharpoons [Mn^{2+}\text{-}O_2^{\bullet-}] + 2H^+ \longrightarrow Mn(III) + H_2O_2$$

$$\updownarrow$$

$$[Mn\text{-}X\text{-}SOD]$$

The intermediate of the second reaction is in equilibrium with a less-active form of the enzyme, designated as Mn-X-SOD above, in which the $O_2^{\bullet-}$ is attached in a non-productive manner.[29] At pH 7.0 the rates of $O_2^{\bullet-}$ dismutation for CuZnSOD and MnSOD are similar, but, unlike many CuZnSODs, the rates for MnSODs decrease at alkaline pH (e.g. for the *E. coli* enzymes, the rate constant at pH 7.8 is 1.8×10^9, but $0.33 \times 10^9 \, M^{-1}s^{-1}$ at pH 10.2).

3.2.2.1 *Where is MnSOD found?*
The MnSODs are widespread in bacteria, plants and animals (Table 3.1). In most animal tissues and yeast, MnSOD is largely (and usually entirely) located in the mitochondria,[7] although the yeast *Candida albicans* expresses a cytoplasmic MnSOD under certain growth conditions.[30] Other exceptions are

some crustacea that use the copper-containing protein haemocyanin for O_2 transport, for example the blue crab *Callinectes sapidus* contains MnSOD in both mitochondria and cytosol, but no CuZnSOD.[31]

The relative amounts of MnSOD and CuZnSOD in animals depend on the tissue and species; one obvious variable between tissues is the number of mitochondria present. Mammalian erythrocytes (with no mitochondria) contain no MnSOD, but it forms about 10% of total SOD activity in rat liver. For bacteria and fungi (and maybe green plants), growth conditions can make a difference. Thus in a normal growth medium, the fungus *Dactylium dendroides* contains 80% of its SOD activity as CuZnSOD and 20% as MnSOD. However, if its copper supply is restricted, more MnSOD is synthesized to maintain the total cellular SOD activity approximately constant. This 'extra' MnSOD appears in the cytosol.[32] Diet could even have an effect in animals, for example rises in CuZnSOD and falls in MnSOD activity were observed in the livers of chickens fed a Mn-restricted diet.[33]

A polymorphism in the mitochondrial 'targeting sequence' for MnSOD has been described in humans, where position 16 can be either alanine or valine. The frequency of the ala-encoding allele varies from 0.13 to 0.50 depending on population, and individuals can be val/val or ala/ala homozygotes, or ala/val heterozygotes. It has been suggested that this polymorphism affects mitochondrial uptake and activity of MnSOD, but despite several epidemiological studies no clear link to human disease has emerged.[34]

3.2.2.2 *Structure of MnSOD*
The MnSODs from higher organisms usually contain four protein subunits and have 0.5 or 1.0 ions of Mn per subunit (Table 3.1). Figure 3.6 (also Plate 3) shows the subunit structure of human MnSOD as determined by X-ray crystallography. By contrast, most, but not all, of the bacterial enzymes have two subunits (Table 3.1). Removal of Mn from the active site causes loss of catalytic activity; the Mn cannot usually be replaced by iron or any other metal ion to yield a functional enzyme.

The amino acid sequences of MnSODs, whether from animals, plants or bacteria, are similar to each other and unrelated to the CuZnSOD sequences.[7]

Table 3.1 Some organisms from which manganese-containing SODs have been purified

Organism	No. of subunits	Moles of Mn/mol enzyme
Higher organisms		
Maize	4	2
Bovine adrenal cells	4	2
Bovine heart mitochondria	4	2
Pleurotus olearius (a luminous fungus)	4	2
Pea (*Pisum sativum*)	4	1
Chicken liver	4	2
Rat liver	4	4
Human liver	4	4
Saccharomyces cerevisiae	4	4
Bullfrog (*Rana catesbeiana*)	4	4
Blue crab (*Callinectes sapidus*)	2	2
Aspergillus fumigatus	4	4
Bacteria		
Halobacterium halobium	2	1–2
Rhodopseudomonas spheroides	2	1
E. coli	2	1
Bacillus stearothermophilus	2	1
Mycobacterium phlei	4	2
Mycobacterium lepraemurium	2	1
Thermus thermophilus	4	2
Streptococcus faecalis	2	1
Streptococcus mutans	2	1–2
Propionibacterium shermanii	2	3
Bacillus subtilis	2	1
Serratia marcescens	2	1–2
Gluconobacter cerinus	2	1
Acholeplasma laidlawii	2	1
Actinomyces naeslundii	4	2.3
Pseudomonas carboxydohydrogena	–	1

This is consistent with the **endosymbiotic theory** for the origin of mitochondria, which suggests that these organelles evolved (Section 1.3.4) from a symbiosis between a primitive eukaryote (with CuZnSOD) and a prokaryote (with MnSOD). The latter eventually became incorporated into the eukaryote cytoplasm, wrapped in a membrane (which gave rise to the outer mitochondrial membrane).

3.2.3 Iron and cambialistic SODs

Four SOD enzymes can be purified from *E. coli*, including periplasmic CuZnSOD and MnSOD. A third SOD was found to be an iron-containing dimer (**FeSOD**), and similar enzymes were later found in many other bacteria, algae, trypanosomes and higher plants (Table 3.2). The fourth *E. coli* SOD is a hybrid enzyme containing subunits of the manganese and iron enzymes in the same molecule. In *E. coli*, both FeSOD and MnSOD are found in the cell cytoplasm.[7]

Iron-containing SODs usually contain two protein subunits, although some tetrameric enzymes have been described and some dimers associate to form tetramers under certain conditions (Table 3.2). The dimeric enzymes usually contain one or two iron ions per molecule. The iron in 'resting' FeSODs

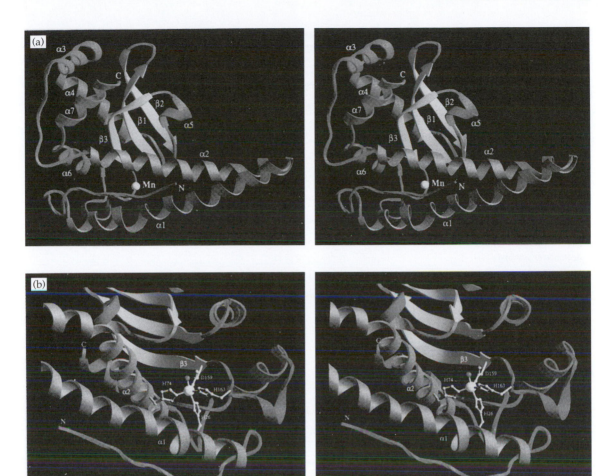

Figure 3.6 (see plate 3) Structure of human MnSOD. Manganese ions are shown as light pink spheres. (a) MnSOD subunit coloured to emphasize secondary structure and organization. The N-terminal domain (bottom) is made up of an N-terminal loop (blue) and two long α-helices (α1 and α2) shown in purple. The C-terminal α/β domain (top) is composed of five α-helices (α3–α7) shown in blue and three β-strands (β1–β3), in yellow. The manganese lies between the two domains. MnSOD subunits have approximate dimensions 40 $\times$ 47 $\times$ 49 Å. (b) Active site geometry of MnSOD. The five manganese ligands are drawn in a ball-and-stick representation. Amino acids from both domains contribute to the active site, His26 in α1 and His74 in α2 from the N-terminal domain and Asp159 in β3 and His163 from the C-terminal domain. The fifth co-ordination site is occupied by a water molecule (blue sphere). The four active sites of the MnSOD tetramer are grouped in pairs across the dimer interfaces, with residues Glu162 and Tyr166 from one subunit contributing to the active site of the neighbouring subunit. Photographs by courtesy of Drs John Tainer and Elizabeth Getzoff, and Cell Press (see *Cell* **71**, 107, 1992).

is Fe(III) and oscillates between the Fe(III) and Fe^{2+} states during catalysis.

$$Fe(III) - enzyme + O_2^{\bullet-} \rightarrow Fe^{2+} - enzyme + O_2$$

$$Fe^{2+} - enzyme + O_2^{\bullet-} + 2H^+ \rightarrow$$
$$Fe(III) - enzyme + H_2O_2$$

Net reaction: $O_2^{\bullet-} + O_2^{\bullet-} + 2H^+ \rightarrow H_2O_2 + O_2$

although this is probably an oversimplification of the mechanism. Like MnSODs, FeSODs show decreased catalytic activity at high pH and are not inhibited by CN$^-$.

The amino acid sequences of FeSODs are similar to those of MnSODs, which explains why a hybrid SOD can occur in *E. coli*. Despite this structural similarity, MnSODs and FeSODs are usually only effective with the correct metal at the active site. However, the SODs from

Table 3.2 Some organisms from which iron-containing SODs have been purified

Organism	No. of subunits	Moles of Fe/mol enzyme
Bacteria		
Acidianus ambivalens	2	1
Streptococcus mutans	2	1–2
E. coli	2	1–1.8
Desulphovibrio desulphuricans	2	1–2
Thiobacillus denitrificans	2	1
Chromatium vinosum	2	2
Photobacterium leiognathi	2	1[a]
Pseudomonas ovalis	2	1–2
Helicobacter pylori	2	–
Methanobacterium bryantii	4	2–3
Azotobacter vinelandii	2	2
Bacillus megaterium	2	1
Mycobacterium tuberculosis	4	4
Propionibacterium shermanii	2	2
Sulpholobus acidocaldarius[b]	2	1
Aquifex pyrophilus	4	~3
Ralstonia metallidurans	2	2
Other organisms		
Tomato (*Lycopersicon esculentum*)	2	1–2
Mustard (*Brassica campestris*)	2	1–2
Water-lily (*Nuphar luteum*)	2	1
Porphyridium cruentum	2	1
Spirulina platensis	2	1
Plectonema boryanum	2	1
Anacystis nidulans	2	1
Euglena gracilis	Not reported	1
Nostoc PCC 7120	2	Not reported
Crithidia fasciculata (trypanosome)	2	2–3
Acanthamoeba castellanii (protozoan)	2	Not reported
Rhodotorula glutinis (a yeast)	Not reported	~1
Gingko biloba	2	1

[a] Plus some 'non-specifically bound' iron.

[b] Enzyme is a dimer at room temperature but forms a tetramer at the elevated temperatures at which this organism lives. It is one of the most thermostable enzymes known, being able to tolerate 24 h at 95 °C. It is also very resistant to denaturing agents (*J. Mol. Biol.* **285**, 689, 1999).

several bacteria, such as *Bacteroides fragilis*, *Chloroflexus aurantiacus*, *Sinorhizobium meliloti*, *Streptococcus mutans* and *Propionibacterium shermanii*, appear to be active with either (or both) metals present and are often called **cambialistic SODs**.[35] Cambialistic SODs have also been isolated from the diatom *Thalassiosira weissflogii*[36] and from seeds of the camphor tree,

Cinnamomum camphora.[37] The tertiary structures of FeSODs and cambialistic SODs from several organisms, including *Pseudomonas ovalis*, *E. coli* and *P. shermanii* have been determined by X-ray crystallography.

A few species have been reported to contain SODs with both Fe and Zn, FeZnSOD. *Streptomyces coelicolor* is one example.[38]

Table 3.3 Representative data for SOD levels in human tissues

Tissue	CuZnSOD[a] (µg/mg protein)	CuZnSOD activity[b] (units/g wet wt)	MnSOD activity[b] (units/g wet wt)
Cerebral grey matter	3.7	ND	ND
Liver	4.71	106 900	2260
Erythrocytes	0.52[c]	–	0
Renal cortex	1.93	24 800	1510
Renal medulla	1.31	(total kidney)	(total kidney)
Thyroid	0.38	10 700	276
Testis	2.16	ND	ND
Cardiac muscle	1.82	ND	ND
Gastric mucosa	0.94	Gut 10 000	358
Pituitary	0.99		
Pancreas	0.39	8630	778
Lung	0.47	7500	86
Thoracic aorta	–	7040	86

[a] An immunological method was used which measures the enzyme protein. Data abstracted from *Clin. Chim. Acta* **36**, 125, 1973.

[b] Enzyme activity determined by the KO_2 method at high pH, which has low sensitivity for MnSOD. Data from *Biochem. J.* **222**, 649, 1984 and *Arterio. Thromb. Vasc. Biol.* **15**, 2032, 1995. Results were obtained from subjects who had died after accidents. Extracellular SOD (EC-SOD) levels in human thoracic aorta were ∼6440 units/g; the mean for other tissues is 63–1260 as compared with a mean of 7500–30 200 for CuZnSOD.

[c] Erythrocyte value per milligram of haemoglobin.

3.2.3.1 *Distribution of* FeSODs

Some bacteria contain either FeSOD or MnSOD, whereas others contain both (e.g. *E. coli*).[7,14] For example, *Bacillus cereus* contains only FeSOD, *B. subtilis* and *Streptococcus sanguis* only MnSOD. *Mycobacterium tuberculosis* and *Photobacterium leiognathi* contain FeSOD in addition to CuZnSOD. One must not be too dogmatic, because growth conditions (e.g. the supply of metals) have a major effect. Growth of *E. coli* under anaerobic conditions for several generations causes loss of MnSOD, but FeSOD remains, apparently to aid survival on reintroduction of O_2 until MnSOD can be synthesized.[7]

No animal tissues have yet been found to contain FeSOD, but some algae, trypanosomes (Section 3.12.1 below), yeasts and higher plants do (Table 3.2). Leaf FeSOD is usually in the chloroplast (Section 6.8.7).

3.2.4 Nickel-containing SODs

Several *Streptomyces* species, and some cyanobacteria, have been reported to contain SODs with nickel at the active site. These are tetrameric or hexameric enzymes that appear structurally different from the other SOD types. The metal oscillates between Ni^{2+} and Ni(III) during catalysis.[39]

3.2.5 Assaying SOD[40,41]

One can measure SOD protein levels and/or enzyme activity. Immunological methods for detecting CuZnSOD and MnSOD have been developed; since these enzymes are structurally different, the antibodies do not cross-react. There is a high level of both MnSOD and CuZnSOD in liver in humans (Table 3.3) and other animals (Table 3.4).

Direct determination of SOD activity can be carried out by pulse radiolysis (Fig. 3.1), which has been useful in studying the mechanism of enzyme action. Similarly, the loss of the ultraviolet absorbance of $O_2^{\bullet-}$ when KO_2 is added to an aqueous solution can be observed, by stopped flow or in a spectrophotometer (Table 3.4). This method can only be used at alkaline pH, when

Table 3.4 Examples of the measurement of SOD activities in animal tissues

Animal	Assay	Tissue	Total SOD activity (units/mg protein)	Reference
Mouse	Disproportionation of KO_2 in alkaline solution (one unit of SOD causes $O_2^{\bullet -}$ to decay at the rate of 0.1/sec in a 3 ml reaction volume)	Pancreatic islets	331	*Biochem. J.* **199**, 393, 1981
		Liver	660	
		Kidney	582	
		Erythrocytes	52	
		Heart	390	
		Brain	408	
		Skeletal muscle	282	
Rat	Riboflavin–light–NBT system (one unit of SOD inhibits NBT reduction by 50%)	Liver	22	*Biochem. J.,* **150**, 31, 1975
		Adrenal	20	
		Kidney	13	
		Erythrocytes	4	
		Spleen	5	
		Heart	9	
		Pancreas (whole)	1.5	
		Brain	3	
		Lung	3	
		Stomach	7	
		Intestine	3	
		Ovary	2	
		Thymus	1	

the rate of non-enzymic $O_2^{\bullet -}$ dismutation is low, and it will underestimate the activity of FeSOD or MnSOD in relation to that of CuZnSOD since FeSOD and MnSOD are less active at high pH (Section 3.2.2). Appropriate correction factors must be used.

However, most laboratories use the **indirect assay methods** for SOD activity, in which $O_2^{\bullet -}$ is generated and reacts with a detector (Fig. 3.7). SOD removes $O_2^{\bullet -}$ and stops its reaction with the detector. In their original work on erythrocyte SOD, McCord and Fridovich used this type of assay; $O_2^{\bullet -}$ was generated by a mixture of xanthine oxidase (XO) and xanthine, and detected by its ability to reduce cytochrome *c*, which causes a rise in absorbance at 550 nm. Adding SOD removes $O_2^{\bullet -}$ and inhibits the absorbance change. One unit

of SOD activity was defined as the amount that inhibits cytochrome *c* reduction by 50% under their assay conditions. Hence units of SOD activity quoted in the literature bear no relation to quoted units for other enzymes (1 enzyme unit is often defined as that amount catalysing transformation of 1 μmol of substrate per minute) and values will be different for each different SOD assay (as Table 3.4 illustrates).

One problem with indirect assays of SOD is that a false SOD activity can be registered by any agent that inhibits $O_2^{\bullet -}$ generation (Fig. 3.7), for example by inhibiting XO. One advantage of using XO is that this artefact can (and should!) be checked for by measuring enzyme activity (e.g. as the production of uric acid). Many tissue extracts contain cytochrome oxidase, which oxidizes reduced

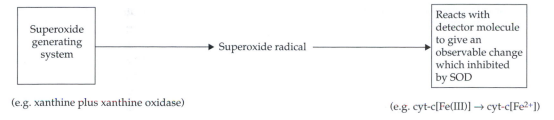

(e.g. xanthine plus xanthine oxidase)   (e.g. cyt-c[Fe(III)] $\rightarrow$ cyt-c[Fe^{2+}])

Figure 3.7 Principles of the indirect assay methods for SOD activity.

cytochrome c and interferes with the assay. Modification of cytochrome c by attachment of acetyl (CH_3CO-) groups to some of its amino acid side chains prevents it from being a substrate for cytochrome oxidase but still allows reaction with $O_2^{\bullet -}$. Hydrogen peroxide produced directly by XO (Section 1.10.1) and by $O_2^{\bullet -}$ dismutation can slowly reoxidize reduced cytochrome c and react with contaminating metal ions to produce OH$^\bullet$. To prevent this, catalase can be added to the reaction mixture. It is essential to ensure that any commercial catalase used is not contaminated with SOD; commercial cytochrome c also often contains traces of SOD.

Detector molecules for $O_2^{\bullet -}$ other than cytochrome c can be used (Table 3.5). For example, NBT is reduced by $O_2^{\bullet -}$ to a deep-blue-coloured formazan, and adrenalin is oxidized by $O_2^{\bullet -}$ to form a pink product, **adrenochrome**. The compound XTT, which forms a water-soluble formazan, has some advantages over NBT (Table 3.5, legend and Fig. 2.4).[42] The ability of $O_2^{\bullet -}$ to oxidize NADH in the presence of lactate dehydrogenase (Section 2.5.3) has also been used. **Luminol** and **luciferin** emit light when exposed to $O_2^{\bullet -}$ and other ROS and have often been used as detector molecules, but the chemistry involved is complex and their validity is suspect (Section 5.11.4). Inhibition of autoxidation reactions has also been used (Table 3.5); one problem is that tissue extracts can contain transition metal ions that accelerate autoxidations.

Each method has its problems and no single assay is suitable for all systems. In some assays, it is difficult to check for artefactual effects of a putative $O_2^{\bullet -}$ scavenger on the rate of $O_2^{\bullet -}$ generation. Our laboratory routinely uses inhibition of NBT or XTT reduction by a xanthine-XO system to assay SOD in

cell or tissue extracts. Although this avoids problems with cytochrome oxidase, it must be remembered that the reaction of NBT with $O_2^{\bullet -}$ is complex (Section 2.5.3).

Whatever assay is used, it should first be calibrated with pure SOD. A known amount of SOD enzyme, added to the extract being examined, should be quantitatively detected on subsequent assay. One should think carefully about possible artefacts interfering with $O_2^{\bullet -}$ generation or $O_2^{\bullet -}$ detection.[41,43] For example, pamoic acid and 2-methoxyoestradiol appeared to inhibit SOD activity in indirect assays, but were in fact interfering with those assays.[21,43] Reducing agents in tissue extracts can react with certain detector molecules: this is a particular problem in autoxidation-based assays (Table 3.5 legend) and with cytochrome c, which is easily reduced by ascorbate and thiols.

3.2.5.1 *Distinguishing between different types of SOD*[7,40]

The CuZnSODs are inhibited by CN$^-$, whereas FeSOD and MnSOD are not. Inhibition by CN$^-$ can thus be used to identify CuZnSOD activity in assays of tissue homogenates or on polyacrylamide gels (e.g. Fig. 3.5). Millimolar levels are required, and one must check for effects on pH (solutions of KCN and NaCN are alkaline) and on cytochrome c, which reacts with CN$^-$. Cyanide does not affect the XTT assay.[44]

Whereas CuZnSOD and FeSOD are inactivated on prolonged exposure to H_2O_2, MnSOD is not. Thus incubating a cell extract with H_2O_2 will inactivate FeSOD but not MnSOD and can be used to distinguish the two. The rate of inactivation of CuZnSOD by H_2O_2 is greater at higher pH values. Another method for distinguishing between different SOD types exploits the fact that FeSODs are

Table 3.5 Some of the indirect methods used to measure SOD activity

Source of superoxide	Detector of superoxide	Reaction measured[a]
Xanthine–xanthine oxidase	Cytochrome *c*	Reduction, ΔA
	Nitroblue tetrazolium, NBT[b]	Reduction, ΔA
	Luminol, luciferin	Light emission
	Adrenalin	Oxidation, ΔA
	NADH + lactate dehydrogenase	Oxidation, ΔA at 340 nm
	Hydroxylamine[c]	Nitrite formation (colorimetric method)
	Spin traps	ESR signal (Section 5.2)
Auto-oxidation reactions[d]	Adrenalin	Oxidation, ΔA
	Sulphite	O_2 uptake
	Pyrogallol	O_2 uptake or ΔA
	6-Hydroxydopamine	Oxidation, ΔA
Directly added $K^+O_2^-$	–	Loss of $O_2^{\bullet-}$, ΔA in UV
	NBT	Reduction, ΔA
	Cytochrome *c*	Reduction, ΔA
	Tetranitromethane	Reduction, ΔA
Illuminated flavins[e]	NBT	Reduction, ΔA; O_2 uptake (SOD accelerates)
	Dianisidine	Oxidation, ΔA ('positive' assay)[f]
NADH + phenazine methosulphate[g]	NBT	Reduction, ΔA

[a] ΔA: reaction results in a measurable absorbance change.

[b] High O_2 concentrations can decrease NBT reduction by $O_2^{\bullet-}$ (Section 2.5.3) and formazan can precipitate in the reaction mixture; tetrazolium salts that generate water-soluble formazans have been described, e.g. sulphonated products such as 2,3-*bis* (2-methoxy-4-nitro-5-sulphophenyl)-2-tetrazolium 5-carboxyanilide (**XTT**); XTT is also not directly reduced by glucose or xanthine oxidases (Section 2.5.3) although some *E. coli* enzymes can reduce it directly (*Anal. Biochem.* **310**, 186, 2002).

[c] Hydroxylamine itself reacts slowly, if at all, with $O_2^{\bullet-}$, and nitrite formation may require $OH^\bullet$. Thus the chemistry of this assay is complex.

[d] These and many other compounds oxidize in solution and produce $O_2^{\bullet-}$. Once formed, $O_2^{\bullet-}$ participates in the oxidation of further molecules, so that addition of SOD slows down the observed rates of oxidation. The rates of these oxidations are usually accelerated by transition-metal ions, and this can cause problems in the assay of crude extracts containing such ions unless metal-ion chelators are added. Even then, some metal chelates are still redox-active (Section 2.4.5). Reducing agents such as ascorbate can interfere by 'recycling' radicals back to the original compound and preventing chromogen formation.

[e] Illumination of a riboflavin solution in the presence of either EDTA or methionine causes reduction of the flavin. It then reoxidizes and simultaneously reduces O_2 to $O_2^{\bullet-}$, which is allowed to react with a detector molecule such as NBT. Adding SOD inhibits formazan production. Flavin photochemistry is complex, however, and $^1O_2$ is also produced. In a variation on this assay, an O_2 electrode is used to measure the rate of O_2 consumption during photochemical generation of $O_2^{\bullet-}$ in the presence of NBT. Reduction of the dye by $O_2^{\bullet-}$ is accompanied by stoichiometric O_2 production, i.e. NBT + $O_2^{\bullet-}$ → NBT radical + O_2. On addition of SOD, two $O_2^{\bullet-}$ molecules are required to make one O_2, and the rate of oxygen uptake increases.

[f] A solution containing riboflavin and the detector molecule *ortho*-dianisidine is illuminated, whereupon the detector is slowly oxidized, accompanied by an absorbance change at 460 nm. Addition of SOD increases the rate of dianisidine oxidation because it removes $O_2^{\bullet-}$, which interacts with an intermediate dianisidine radical and decreases the net rate of oxidation. The assay is called 'positive' because addition of the SOD causes the absorbance change to increase instead of decrease. At alkaline pH values, SOD accelerates the oxidation of **haematoxylin**, a stain used by histologists. This reaction has also been proposed as a positive assay for SOD.

[g] Not recommended; see *J. Am. Chem. Soc.* **104**, 1666, 1982.

generally more sensitive to inhibition by azide. For example, at pH 7.8, 10 mM azide inhibits CuZn, Mn and FeSODs by about 10%, 30% and 70% respectively. There is some variation, however; for example, the *Methanobacterium bryantii* FeSOD is less sensitive to azide than other FeSODs, and CuZnSOD from tomato leaves appears more sensitive to azide than other CuZnSODs.

A third approach has been to remove the metals from SOD proteins in cell extracts, and then to add either Fe^{2+} or Mn^{2+} back to the extract. If a band of enzyme activity observed on electrophoresis before metal removal reappears on addition of, say Fe^{2+} but not Mn^{2+}, then it most likely represented a FeSOD. However, the existence of the cambialistic enzymes means that such results must be interpreted with caution. There is no substitute for purifying the enzyme and characterizing it properly.

3.2.6 Using SOD enzymes as probes for superoxide

The specificity of SOD for $O_2^{\bullet-}$ is often used to establish the involvement of $O_2^{\bullet-}$ in biological processes; if SOD inhibits the process it is assumed that $O_2^{\bullet-}$ is involved. Although SOD under most reaction conditions can be regarded as specific for catalytic removal of $O_2^{\bullet-}$, the SOD proteins (like any other protein) can react directly with some RS, such as $OH^{\bullet}$, $RO_2^{\bullet}$, $RO^{\bullet}$, HOCl, ONOOH (Section 2.6.1) and $^1O_2$. Indeed, CuZnSOD and MnSOD facilitate nitration by $ONOO^-$. For bovine CuZnSOD, one SOD molecule catalyses nitration of a second SOD molecule (or of any other adjacent nitratable protein). Nitration of bovine CuZnSOD occurs at Tyr108, close to the copper ion in the active site.

Thus if a large amount of SOD is added to a system producing the above RS, an artefactual inhibition of damage due to direct scavenging might result. Controls with heat-denatured SOD, other proteins (e.g. albumin) in equimolar amounts or SOD apoenzyme should thus be performed. A similar point applies to the use of other enzymes, such as catalase to implicate H_2O_2 involvement in an observed reaction: any protein at high concentrations can act as a 'general' scavenger of RS.

Inhibitions by SOD must also be interpreted with caution in systems containing quinones and semiquinones. Many semiquinones react reversibly with O_2 (Section 2.5.3.5):

$$semiquinone + O_2 \rightleftharpoons quinone + O_2^{\bullet-}$$

The equilibrium tends to move to the right because of non-enzymic dismutation of $O_2^{\bullet-}$. Addition of SOD, by removing $O_2^{\bullet-}$ faster, decreases the steady-state concentration of semiquinone. Hence a reaction caused by the semiquinone might be mistakenly attributed to $O_2^{\bullet-}$ as a result of the inhibition by added SOD. An example is provided by early studies on vitamin K-dependent carboxylation of glutamic acid residues by enzymes in the ER. Adding SOD inhibits, but by removing semiquinone; $O_2^{\bullet-}$ is not involved in the carboxylation.

A similar artefact can arise using $O_2^{\bullet-}$-generating systems. Frequently, an autoxidizable compound, such as adrenalin, dopamine or **dihydroxyfumarate** (DHF), is added to a cell/tissue and causes damage. Adding SOD inhibits the damage, a result often interpreted to mean that it is caused by $O_2^{\bullet-}$. However, $O_2^{\bullet-}$ is an essential intermediate in dopamine, adrenalin or DHF oxidation, and so SOD inhibits that oxidation. Thus *any product of oxidation*[45] could be causing the damage, not necessarily $O_2^{\bullet-}$.

3.2.7 Superoxide and other metalloproteins[7]

Several copper-containing proteins other than CuZnSOD react with $O_2^{\bullet-}$, as can complexes of Cu^{2+} ions with non-metalloproteins such as immunoglobulin G and albumin (Section 10.6.4). At physiological pH, the rate constant for $O_2^{\bullet-}$ dismutation by each active site of CuZnSOD is at least $1.5 \times 10^9\,M^{-1}s^{-1}$ and the reaction is catalytic (Fig. 3.1). For other copper proteins, the rate constants are lower and the reactions tend not to be catalytic; some representative literature values are $2 \times 10^7\,M^{-1}s^{-1}$ for cytochrome c oxidase, $7 \times 10^5\,M^{-1}s^{-1}$ for caeruloplasmin and $3 \times 10^6\,M^{-1}s^{-1}$ for galactose oxidase. Several haem proteins also interact with $O_2^{\bullet-}$, including catalase, haemoglobin and peroxidases (Sections 3.13.4 and 3.14.1 below).

3.3 Superoxide reductases[46]

Several anaerobic and microaerophilic bacteria, including *Treponema pallidum*, *Desulphoarculus baarsi* and *Pyrococcus furiosus* are able to eliminate $O_2^{\bullet-}$ using **superoxide reductase** (**SOR**) proteins, which reduce $O_2^{\bullet-}$ to H_2O_2

$$O_2^{\bullet-} + e^- + 2H^+ \rightarrow H_2O_2$$

The oxidized SOR proteins are then re-reduced by a cellular electron donor (X). Hence the overall reaction is

$$O_2^{\bullet-} + 2H^+ + X \rightarrow H_2O_2 + X_{(OX)}$$

Unlike SOD, SORs produce no O_2, an obvious advantage for an anaerobe, although the H_2O_2 has to be dealt with, of course. The SORs are non-haem iron-containing proteins of various types, depending on the bacterium. The terminal electron donors for $O_2^{\bullet-}$ reduction by SORs are often NADH or NADPH,[b] via various electron carrier proteins such as **rubredoxin**. Superoxide reductase may even be able to function when introduced into eukaryotic cells (Section 10.6.4).

Genomic studies suggest that SORs may be present in all anaerobic bacteria. Presumably, they allow O_2-intolerant bacteria to survive transient exposure to O_2 and consequent $O_2^{\bullet-}$ production, especially as many anaerobes lack SOD (e.g. *Treponema pallidum* has no SOD, catalase or peroxidase). A few anaerobes contain both SOR and SOD, usually FeSOD. For example *Desulphovibrio vulgaris* contains a cytoplasmic SOR and a periplasmic SOD.[47] In others, for example *Bacteroides fragilis*, SOD appears only if O_2 is present.

In vitro, even SOD can be made to act like a SOR, although this probably has no biological relevance.[48] For example, CuZnSOD can catalyse oxidation of ferrocyanide by $O_2^{\bullet-}$.

$$E-Cu^{2+} + Fe(CN)_6^{4-} \rightarrow E-Cu^+ + Fe(CN)_6^{3-}$$

$$E-Cu^+ + O_2^{\bullet-} + 2H^+ \rightarrow E-Cu^{2+} + H_2O_2$$

or reduction of ferricyanide by $O_2^{\bullet-}$.

$$E-Cu^+ + Fe(CN)_6^{3-} \rightarrow E-Cu^{2+} + Fe(CN)_6^{4-}$$

$$E-Cu^{2+} + O_2^{\bullet-} \rightarrow E-Cu^+ + O_2$$

3.4 Superoxide dismutases; are they important *in vivo*?

The discovery of SOD led to the **superoxide theory of oxygen toxicity**, which proposes that $O_2^{\bullet-}$ is a major factor in O_2 toxicity and that SODs are an important defence against it.[7] The theory is now generally accepted, although several questions remain. Do the available data support this acceptance? Let us see.

3.4.1 Gene knockout in bacteria and yeasts

E. coli has two main SODs, FeSOD and MnSOD (the periplasmic CuZnSOD contributes little to total SOD activity). Touati *et al.*[49] inactivated the genes encoding MnSOD and FeSOD in *E. coli*, generating a bacterium initially thought to have no SOD (we now know that periplasmic CuZnSOD was still present). The resulting mutant would not grow aerobically on a minimal glucose medium. Growth could be restored by removing O_2, restoring SOD to the cells by introducing a gene coding for any SOD (even mammalian CuZnSOD) or enriching the growth medium of the bacteria with amino acids. This is reminiscent of the observation that certain amino acids diminish the growth-inhibiting effects of hyperbaric O_2 on *E. coli* (Fig. 1.11). Even with this supplementation, the SOD-deficient mutant grew slowly; its membranes were leaky to certain ions, it was more sensitive to damage by increased O_2 or by H_2O_2 and it showed elevated mutation rates during aerobic (but not anaerobic) growth on rich media. Addition of DDTC to inhibit periplasmic CuZnSOD inhibited growth even on a rich medium.[50]

The steady-state level of $O_2^{\bullet-}$ in aerobic *E. coli* in the log-phase of growth has been estimated at 20 to 40 picomolar ($1\,pM = 10^{-12}\,M$), rising to about 300 pM in the double mutant.[7] By contrast, intracellular H_2O_2 in wild-type *E. coli* has been estimated as 100 to 200 nanomolar ($1\,nM = 10^{-9}\,M$), over three orders of magnitude greater.[51] Thus an $O_2^{\bullet-}$ concentration of a few hundred picomolar is sufficient to lead to DNA damage and impairment of metabolic activity, and $O_2^{\bullet-}$ must somehow contribute to H_2O_2 toxicity. The reasons are examined in Section 3.6 below.

Similar studies have been carried out on other organisms. *Pseudomonas aeruginosa* lacking Mn- and FeSOD grows poorly aerobically.[52] Inactivating the gene encoding MnSOD in *Saccharomyces cerevisiae* makes it hypersensitive to O_2.[53] Survival of this yeast in stationary phase is decreased, with loss of activity

---

[b] NADPH differs from NADH (Fig. 1.7) by one phosphate group but is oxidized and reduced in the same way.

of aconitase and succinate dehydrogenase in mitochondria.[53] Expression of *E. coli* FeSOD in the yeast mitochondria (but not in yeast cytosol) offered protection.[54] Indeed, MnSOD-deficient yeast in which the electron transport chain was also absent (**Rho°ˢ state**) were more resistant, consistent with the view that electron transport is an important source of $O_2^{\bullet-}$ *in vivo*.[55] Similarly, *S. cerevisiae* lacking CuZnSOD is hypersensitive to O_2 and will not grow aerobically unless supplemented with such amino acids as lysine and methionine. Adding antioxidants, such as ascorbate or GSH, overcame this requirement.[56] When yeast was screened for mutations conferring hypersensitivity to hyperoxia, almost all the mutants found were also sensitive to the $O_2^{\bullet-}$ generator paraquat (Section 8.4), suggesting that $O_2^{\bullet-}$ is a major contributor to hyperoxia damage.[53] Genes required for O_2 tolerance in yeast include not only those encoding CuZnSOD and MnSOD, but also genes for CCS and Cu^{2+} transporters.[53]

3.4.2 Transgenic animals

With transgenic animal technology, it is possible to 'knock out' or overexpress genes. For example, mice expressing the human CuZnSOD gene and containing human CuZnSOD protein in various tissues have been produced. The human CuZnSOD is present in addition to the mouse CuZnSOD, raising total CuZnSOD activity. Such mice show increased resistance to O_2 toxicity and to other ROS-generating toxins, consistent with the superoxide theory of O_2 toxicity, but they are subtly abnormal in some ways[57] (Box 3.1). Mice overexpressing human MnSOD in the lung have been generated (without affecting CuZnSOD, catalase or

Box 3.1 Consequences of overexpressing CuZnSOD in mice (and some comparisons with CuZnSOD knockout mice)

1) Transgenic mice with elevated levels of CuZnSOD:
   a) are more resistant than controls to O_2 toxicity under some but not all experimental conditions;
   b) are more resistant than controls to certain toxins, e.g. ozone, alloxan, MPTP, NMDA receptor agonists (Section 9.16.4), methamphetamine, methylenedioxyamphetamine, methylenedioxymethylamphetamine, 3-nitropropanoic acid, 6-hydroxydopamine (Chapter 8) and to airway changes produced by certain allergens;
   c) suffer more brain infarction after cerebral ischaemia–reperfusion (in young mice), but less in adult mice; adult CuZnSOD-knockout mice suffer greater damage;
   d) still show O_2-induced retinopathy (when exposed to 90% O_2 during the first 5 days of life);
   e) show abnormal neuromuscular junctions in the tongue, altered serotonin metabolism, decreased proteasome activity in the brain cortex, premature involution of the thymus, increased sensitivity to malaria infection and increased angiogenesis in response to growth factors;
   f) may show some of the other neurological defects characteristic of Down's syndrome;
   g) show less colonic inflammation after treatment with dextran sodium sulphate;
   h) show no protection (and possible aggravation of damage) against noise-induced hearing loss, although

CuZnSOD-knockout mice are more susceptible to this, and age-related cochlear hair cell loss is increased in knockout mice;
   i) have eye lenses more susceptible to photochemical damage *in vitro*;
   j) show less damage after traumatic brain injury.
2) Diabetic mice show less renal injury. Pregnant, diabetic animals show less foetal damage by elevated glucose.
3) Peritoneal macrophages show decreased microbicidal capacity and increased ability to produce cytokines and matrix metalloproteinases.
4) Midbrain neurons from transgenic pups survive better in culture.
5) Isolated hearts are less susceptible to ischaemia–reperfusion injury in some model systems, as is intestine *in vivo*. Less rejection observed after hearts from CuZnSOD-overexpressing mice are transplanted.

Data summarized from multiple publications, too numerous to list. Variation in results between laboratories can occur because of the genetic background of the mouse strain used and the extent of the overexpression of CuZnSOD (more is not necessarily more protective). There may also be differences between male and female transgenics (Exp. Neurol. 172, 332, 2001).

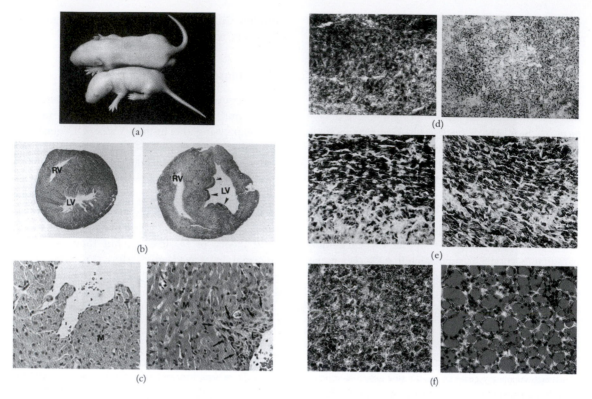

Figure 3.8 (see plate 4) Appearance and histopathology of MnSOD-deficient mice. (a) MnSOD $-/-$ (bottom) and $+/+$ (top) mice, 6 days old. Note the smaller size and yellow tinge of the mutant animal. (b) Transverse section of $+/+$ (left) and $-/-$ (right) hearts showing left (LV) and right ventricles (RV). The left ventricular cavity of $-/-$ mice is enlarged, and the wall is thinner. (c) Haematoxylin and eosin-stained, paraffin-embedded, sections of the ventricles of $+/+$ (left) and $-/-$ (right) mice showing fibrous thickening of the endocardium (arrows) in $-/-$ mice, 100 $\times$. (d) Succinate dehydrogenase (SDH) staining in frozen sections of $+/+$ (left) and $-/-$ (right) hearts showing the lack of functional SDH in the $-/-$ heart, 400 $\times$. (e) Cytochrome c oxidase (COX) staining in frozen sections of $+/+$ (left) and $-/-$ (right) hearts showing comparable levels of COX, 400 $\times$. (f) Oil Red O stain for the detection of lipid deposits in frozen sections of liver from $+/+$ (left) and $-/-$ (right) mice, 400 $\times$. A dramatic increase in the number of lipid vesicles is present in $-/-$ liver. Original magnifications are indicated. Reprinted from *Nature Genet.* **11**, 376, 1995 by courtesy of Prof. C.J. Epstein and Nature Publishers.

glutathione peroxidase activities) and found to be somewhat more resistant to lung damage by hyperoxia than are normal mice.[58] Transgenic strains of the fruit fly *Drosophila* overexpressing bovine CuZnSOD were more resistant to hyperoxia and to paraquat, a $O_2^{\bullet-}$ generator (Section 8.4) than control flies. By contrast, *Drosophilia* lacking CuZn-SOD show decreased lifespan, increased O_2 toxicity and infertility.[59]

More dramatic data come from animals lacking MnSOD. In one study,[60] MnSOD-knockout mice usually died within 10 days after birth, with cardiac abnormalities (Fig. 3.8, Plate 4), fat accumulation in liver and skeletal muscle and metabolic acidosis. Severe mitochondrial damage in heart and, to a

lesser extent, in other tissues is evidenced by decreases in complex I, succinate dehydrogenase and aconitase activities (Fig. 3.8, Plate 4) and rises in oxidative damage to mitochondrial DNA, consistent with an essential role of MnSOD in maintaining normal mitochondrial function.[61] Even SOD2 $(+/-)$ heterozygous mice, which at first seem normal, show increased mitochondrial oxidative damage as they age,[62] as well as increased nuclear oxidative DNA damage and elevated cancer rates (Section 9.13.5.8). Those animals completely lacking MnSOD that manage to survive longer than 10 days soon succumb to a variety of pathologies, including severe anaemia and neurodegeneration.[63] They also show retinal defects (Section 6.10.2.2).

Treatment of MnSOD$^-$ mice with low molecular mass scavengers of $O_2^{\bullet-}$ keeps them alive longer, whereupon they suffer even more retinal damage and brain degeneration, perhaps because the scavengers do not enter the brain.[63] MnSOD knockout mice are also highly susceptible to hyperoxia.[64]

Mice lacking CuZnSOD have also been obtained. When young, they appear normal (although they are more sensitive to paraquat and to ethanol) but as they age, neurological damage, muscle wasting, hearing loss and cancers (especially liver cancer) can develop at an accelerated rate. They have reproductive problems and show impaired vascular reactivity.[65–69] From as early as 3 months of age, their livers showed increased 8OHdG[c] and F_2-isoprostanes;[c] protein carbonyl[c] levels increased only in older animals, carbonic anhydrase III (Section 10.4.5.1) becoming especially oxidized.

3.4.2.1 *A caveat about transgenic animals*

One must be circumspect in interpreting data from transgenic animal experiments. Knockout or over-expression of any gene is likely to lead to a host of compensatory changes. For example, CuZnSOD$^-$ mice show increased metallothionein (Section 3.16.1 below) gene expression in the liver.[70] Also, knockout mice are kept in a laboratory under warm, protected, well-fed conditions. A knockout lethal in the wild might have a relatively mild (or no) apparent phenotype under these conditions. Thus it would be a mistake to interpret the mild phenotype of CuZnSOD$^-$ mice early in life as meaning a limited importance for this enzyme. Yet, even laboratory-bred mice cannot adapt to a lack of MnSOD.

3.4.3 RNA interference

Some laboratories have used antisense oligonucleotides or RNA interference to examine the role of SOD. For example, decrease of CuZnSOD levels by antisense lowered progesterone production by rat luteal cells.[71] RNA interference-mediated silencing of MnSOD expression in *Drosophila* shortened lifespan and caused loss of mitochondrial aconitase and succinate dehydrogenase activities,[72] whereas RNA

[c] For a discussion of these biomarkers of oxidative damage please see Chapter 5.

interference against CuZnSOD promoted senescence in cultured human fibroblasts (Section 10.3.5.1).

3.4.4 Induction experiments

Much evidence other than that from molecular genetic approaches supports the important role of SODs. Exposure of organisms to elevated O_2 should, according to the superoxide theory of O_2 toxicity, cause them to form more $O_2^{\bullet-}$ *in vivo* and this might lead to synthesis of more SOD if there is not enough to cope with the extra $O_2^{\bullet-}$. Data support this.[7] For example, exposing *E. coli* to elevated O_2 increases its MnSOD activity. *E. coli* grown under pure O_2 are more resistant to the toxic effects of high-pressure O_2 than are cells grown under air. Similarly, one can increase the MnSOD activity of *E. coli* (up to about 7% of total cell protein!) by incubating it with compounds that increase intracellular $O_2^{\bullet-}$ generation, such as streptonigrin, paraquat, juglone, menadione and pyocyanin (Section 8.4). Strains of *E. coli* with elevated SOD activity are resistant both to the toxic effects of these compounds, and to O_2 toxicity. Elevated O_2 and many $O_2^{\bullet-}$ generating compounds often also induce H_2O_2-degrading enzymes as well.

Similar experiments correlating SOD activity with O_2 exposure have been carried out in plants, animals and other bacteria. For example, the O_2 produced by the photosynthetic activity of symbiotic algae increases SOD activity in their animal host, the sea anemone *Anthopleura elegantissima*. Anemones that contain symbiotic algae have more SOD and catalase than anemones which do not. Hence the food provided to the anemone by the photosynthetic 'guest' has to be balanced against the cost of increasing antioxidant defences in the host.[73] A similar phenomenon occurs in coral reefs (Section 6.9.5).

3.4.5 SOD and oxygen toxicity in animals[7,64,74–76]

Adult rats placed in pure O_2 rapidly develop lung damage and often die after 60 to 72 h. However, if rats are exposed to somewhat lower O_2 concentrations (e.g. 85% for 7 days) they can adapt to survive for longer when subsequently exposed to 100% O_2. This adaptation is correlated with increased SOD activity in lung homogenates. Transgenic studies also support a protective role for SOD, since mice overexpressing MnSOD or CuZnSOD show increased O_2 tolerance under certain experimental conditions (Section 3.4.3), whereas MnSOD$^-$ mice are more sensitive to hyperoxia. However, a co-ordinated increase in several antioxidant defences (including GSH, catalase, glutathione peroxidase and reductase, HO-1, peroxiredoxins, and chaperones) is essential to obtain maximum protection. Indeed, injection of liposomes containing SOD into rats has limited protective effects against O_2 toxicity, but including catalase gives more protection.[77]

Newborn rats, mice and rabbits appear more resistant to O_2 toxicity than adults, apparently because the SOD and other antioxidant activities of their lungs is increased and maintained more effectively under high O_2 than it is in adults (another possibility is that neonatal cells make less $O_2^{\bullet-}$ than adult cells). By contrast, newborn hamsters and guinea pigs are no better than adults at increasing defences, and they are equally susceptible to hyperoxia. If induction of antioxidant defence enzymes is prevented (e.g. by injection of protein synthesis inhibitors), newborn rats become highly sensitive to hyperoxia. Newborn rats kept in pathogen-free environments have lower SOD activities in lung than normal, and they are more sensitive to O_2 toxicity. Treatment of adult rats with low levels of endotoxin (Section 2.5.6.6) enhances their resistance to O_2, associated with increased lung antioxidant defences. Endotoxin also lowers levels of certain CYPs, a source of $O_2^{\bullet-}$ *in vivo*.[76] Be careful—commercial SOD and catalase can be contaminated with endotoxin. This has caused erroneous results to appear in the literature (Section 10.6.3).

3.4.6 SOD and hibernation

Hibernating animals show decreased O_2 consumption and body temperature. Yet activities of SOD and other antioxidant defences in certain tissues are higher than normal. We have proposed that this is in preparation for the intense metabolic activity (presumably accompanied by rapid ROS production) that occurs during awakening.[78] A similar phenomenon may occur in land snails: they respond to aridity by going into a dormant state, but actually increase their SOD and H_2O_2-removing enzyme activities.[79]

3.5 The superoxide theory of oxygen toxicity: variations and anomalies

3.5.1 Anaerobes with SOD and aerobes without SOD

Some anaerobes contain SOD and many have SOR (Section 3.3), presumably to help them survive transient O_2 exposure. More interesting in relation to the superoxide theory of O_2 toxicity are aerobic bacteria that appear to lack SOD. *Mycoplasma pneumoniae*[80] contains $O_2^{\bullet-}$ generating systems, but neither SOD, nor catalase, activities. A few *Leptospira* strains[81] have been found to be SOD-negative although original reports that the gonococcus (*Neisseria gonorrhoeae*) is SOD-negative have not been confirmed.[82] Gonococci are also exceptionally rich in catalase and peroxidase enzymes and in methionine sulphoxide reductase (Section 4.14.1).[82] *N. gonorrhoeae* colonizes human mucous membranes and provokes a strong neutrophil response, although neutrophils are not good at killing it.[82] Exposure of *N. gonorrhoeae* to H_2O_2 or neutrophils produces a further rise in catalase.[83]

If iron-catalysed OH$^\bullet$ formation is a major contributor to the toxicity of $O_2^{\bullet-}$ in bacteria (Section 3.6 below), it follows that protection could be achieved by the efficient removal of either $O_2^{\bullet-}$ or H_2O_2, or by iron sequestration in non-redox-active forms. All are not necessarily required. This is one possible explanation of the rare 'aerobes without SOD'. There are others, however. Let us look at one.

3.5.2 Manganese can replace SOD

Several aerotolerant strains of Lactobacillaceae contain SOD, but some do not, for example *Lactobacillus plantarum*. It accumulates manganese ions from its growth medium to an internal concentration of 25 mM or more.[84] If this is prevented by removing external manganese, *L. plantarum* will not grow in the presence of O_2. Since chelates of Mn^{2+} with some biomolecules (e.g. polyphosphates) can react with $O_2^{\bullet-}$ (Section 2.4.3) it has been suggested that these chelates catalyse $O_2^{\bullet-}$ removal *in vivo*. *L. plantarum* also possesses a manganese-containing, H_2O_2-degrading enzyme (Section 3.7.7 below).

Manganese might help other organisms as well; thus *E. coli* SOD^- mutants grow better if the medium is enriched with manganese,[85] and such a medium also enhances the resistance of *N. gonorrhoeae* to oxidative stress.[82] Mutants of *S. cerevisiae* lacking CuZnSOD can be 'rescued' by mutations in other genes, such as the *BSD* (**bypass SOD deficiency**)[86] genes. One of these encodes a transport protein, mutation of which allows the cells to accumulate manganese. If extracellular Mn^{2+} is removed, the 'rescue' is inoperative, again suggesting an $O_2^{\bullet-}$ scavenging role for manganese ions.

One feature presumably making it possible to use manganese to remove $O_2^{\bullet-}$ is that Mn^{2+} ions do not catalyse $OH^\bullet$ formation from H_2O_2 (Section 2.4.3).

3.6 Why is superoxide cytotoxic?

3.6.1 Direct damage by superoxide: not very super but super enough?

The evidence reviewed above shows that SOD is important *in vivo*. Since SOD uses only $O_2^{\bullet-}$ as a substrate most or all of the time, it follows that $O_2^{\bullet-}$ is damaging *in vivo*. However, despite its 'super' name, $O_2^{\bullet-}$ seems relatively unreactive in aqueous solution (Section 2.5.3), unlike the indiscriminately reactive $OH^\bullet$. So why is it a problem?

Superoxide can decrease the activity of other antioxidant defence enzymes, such as catalase (Section 3.7 below). Any $O_2^{\bullet-}$ produced in the hydrophobic membrane interior could be very damaging, since $O_2^{\bullet-}$ is highly reactive in organic solvents (Section 2.5.3). The protonated form of $O_2^{\bullet-}$, $HO_2^\bullet$, is more reactive than $O_2^{\bullet-}$, and (unlike $O_2^{\bullet-}$) can initiate peroxidation of fatty acids (Section 2.5.3). Traces of $HO_2^\bullet$ exist in equilibrium with $O_2^{\bullet-}$ at physiological pH, and the pH close to a membrane surface may be more acidic, possibly favouring $HO_2^\bullet$ formation. For example, the pH beneath activated macrophages adhering to a surface was reported[87] to be ≤ 5, and so a considerable amount of any $O_2^{\bullet-}$ that they generate will exist as $HO_2^\bullet$. The uncharged $HO_2^\bullet$ should more readily cross membranes than $O_2^{\bullet-}$. Much $O_2^{\bullet-}$ generated within cells comes from membrane-bound systems (e.g. the electron transport chains of mitochondria and ER), and so $HO_2^\bullet$ formed close to the membrane (or $O_2^{\bullet-}$ within it) might cause damage. However, despite all these suppositions, it simply has not been demonstrated that $O_2^{\bullet-}$ or $HO_2^\bullet$ mediate direct membrane lipid damage *in vivo*.

What about proteins? Here the picture is brighter: the highly-selective reactivity of $O_2^{\bullet-}$ does include the ability to damage some important proteins. In *E. coli*, several enzymes can be attacked: examples are 6-phosphogluconate dehydratase, aconitase, fumarase and dihydroxyacid dehydratase.[88] Dihydroxyacid dehydratase, which catalyses the third step in the biosynthesis of branched-chain amino acids, contains a $[4Fe-4S]^{2+}$ iron–sulphur cluster at its active site, which falls apart upon exposure to $O_2^{\bullet-}$ (or, much more slowly, to O_2). *E. coli* aconitase, fumarase A and fumarase B enzymes, contain similar clusters and are also inactivated by O_2 and $O_2^{\bullet-}$; second-order rate constants for reactions of these enzymes with $O_2^{\bullet-}$ are 10^6 to $10^7\,M^{-1}s^{-1}$ whereas with O_2 they are 10^2 to $10^3\,M^{-1}s^{-1}$. Thus amino acid biosynthesis and energy metabolism in the Krebs cycle are major targets of damage by $O_2^{\bullet-}$. Inactivation is caused by oxidation of the cluster, leading to release of iron, which can then promote Fenton chemistry (Section 3.6.2.2 below).

$$[4Fe-4S]^{2+} + O_2^{\bullet-} + 2H^+ \rightarrow [4Fe-4S]^{3+} + H_2O_2$$

$$[4Fe-4S]^{3+} + O_2^{\bullet-} \rightarrow [3Fe-4S] + Fe^{2+} + O_2$$

$$Fe^{2+} + H_2O_2 \rightarrow Fe(III) + OH^\bullet + OH^-$$

The oxidized enzymes can be 'repaired' *in vivo* by reassembling the iron clusters. Indeed, even the low basal levels of $O_2^{\bullet-}$ in *E. coli* (Section 3.4.1) damage these enzymes, and activity is maintained by constantly repairing them. If $O_2^{\bullet-}$ levels rise, inactivation rates accelerate, repair cannot keep up and metabolic pathways are inhibited.[88] Similar damage to Fe–S clusters may occur in *S. cerevisiae* deficient in CuZnSOD.[89] Mammalian aconitase[90] has a similar cluster and can be inactivated by $O_2^{\bullet-}$. It was also reported that $O_2^{\bullet-}$ can inactivate NADH dehydrogenase in bovine heart submitochondrial particles.[91]

Thus, as in *E. coli*, energy metabolism may be a target of direct damage by $O_2^{\bullet-}$ in animals, a view supported by the loss of enzyme activities in MnSOD-knockout mice (Fig. 3.8). If NADH levels are high, as in diabetes (Section 9.4), the ability of LDH to catalyse a $O_2^{\bullet-}$-dependent oxidation of NADH (Section 2.5.3) could become significant. Superoxide can also interfere with *E. coli* **transketolase**, a key enzyme in the pentose phosphate pathway (Section 3.8.3 below). It oxidizes the dihydroxyethyl reaction intermediate at the active site, inhibiting the enzyme and damaging it.[92] Another possible target is ribonucleotide reductase, essential to provide the precursors of DNA (Section 7.2). This enzyme is inactivated by free radicals that quench its active-site tyrosine radical. Nitric oxide is one example (Section 2.5.6) and $O_2^{\bullet-}$ may be another.[93]

Some mammalian creatine kinases have been reported[94] to be inactivated by $O_2^{\bullet-}$, as has **calcineurin**, a protein involved in signal transduction (Section 4.5.5.3).

3.6.2 Cytotoxicity of superoxide-derived species

3.6.2.1 *Hydrogen peroxide and peroxynitrite*
As well as causing direct damage, $O_2^{\bullet-}$ could be cytotoxic by generating other RS. Dismutation of $O_2^{\bullet-}$ generates H_2O_2, but H_2O_2 is poorly reactive at physiological levels, although it can attack some enzymes directly (Section 2.6.2). A more cytotoxic species is peroxynitrite, which generates a range of noxious species under physiological conditions (Section 2.6.1). For example, addition of $ONOO^-$ inactivates creatine kinase more efficiently[94] than does $O_2^{\bullet-}$.

3.6.2.2 *Hydroxyl radical*
Many studies showing the ability of $O_2^{\bullet-}$-generating systems to kill cells and damage biomolecules found that protection was achieved not only by adding SOD, but also by catalase and 'OH$^\bullet$ scavengers' (such as mannitol, formate, thiourea and dimethylsulphoxide (DMSO)).[95] At first, it was suggested that $O_2^{\bullet-}$ and H_2O_2 react directly to form OH$^\bullet$

$$H_2O_2 + O_2^{\bullet-} \rightarrow O_2 + OH^\bullet + OH^-$$

Indeed, formation of OH$^\bullet$ in a range of $O_2^{\bullet-}$-generating systems has been detected by many methods (Section 5.3). The above reaction was postulated by F. Haber and J. Weiss in 1934 and has become known as the **Haber–Weiss reaction**. However, the rate constant for it in aqueous solution is at or close to zero. Nevertheless, OH$^\bullet$ formation can be accounted for if the Haber–Weiss reaction is catalysed by transition metals, as first suggested by Weiss in 1935.

$$\text{oxidized metal complex} + O_2^{\bullet-} \rightarrow$$
$$\text{reduced metal complex} + O_2$$

$$\text{reduced metal complex} + H_2O_2 \rightarrow$$
$$OH^\bullet + OH^- + \text{oxidized metal complex}$$

$$\text{Net: } O_2^{\bullet-} + H_2O_2 \xrightarrow[\text{catalyst}]{\text{metal}} O_2 + OH^\bullet + OH^-$$

Transition-metal ions, especially iron ions, contaminate most biochemical reagents. Chromium (Cr^{2+}), nickel (Ni^{2+}), cobalt (Co^{2+}), titanium (Ti^{3+}) and vanadium (vanadyl) can participate in OH$^\bullet$ formation *in vitro* and OH$^\bullet$ may be involved in their toxicity (Section 8.15). However, most attention has focused on iron and copper as potential mediators of OH$^\bullet$ generation *in vivo*, and in the 1980s we proposed[96] that iron-dependent OH$^\bullet$ generation occurs *in vivo* and is an important mediator of oxidative damage. However, although the reactions

$$Fe(\textsc{iii}) + O_2^{\bullet-} \rightarrow Fe^{2+} + O_2$$

$$Fe^{2+} + H_2O_2 \rightarrow OH^\bullet + OH^- + Fe(\textsc{iii})$$

or

$$Cu^{2+} + O_2^{\bullet-} \rightarrow Cu^+ + O_2$$

$$Cu^+ + H_2O_2 \rightarrow Cu^{2+} + OH^\bullet + OH^-$$

$$\text{Net: } O_2^{\bullet -} + H_2O_2 \xrightarrow[\text{catalyst}]{\text{metal}} O_2 + OH^{\bullet} + OH^{\bullet}$$

readily occur *in vitro*, is $O_2^{\bullet -}$ likely to be the reductant of the metals *in vivo*? Probably not, since its concentration is low. Other possible reductants present at higher levels include ascorbate, quinones and semiquinones, cysteine, reduced flavins/flavoproteins (such as lipoyl dehydrogenase)[97] and NAD(P)H.[88,98–100] Indeed, the role for $O_2^{\bullet -}$ may be more that of *providing the necessary iron*, for example by releasing it from Fe–S clusters. Iron can then catalyse more $O_2^{\bullet -}$ generation, for example from NAD(P)H and thiols.[98] Superoxide releases iron not only from Fe–S clusters but also from ferritin (Section 3.15.4.2 below), and can also liberate metal ions indirectly, *via* $ONOO^-$. Peroxynitrite displaces iron from Fe–S proteins and degrades caeruloplasmin to release copper (Section 2.6.1).

Manipulations of the intracellular iron content of bacteria reveal its importance in causing damage. Studies on *Staphylococcus aureus* many years ago showed that more intracellular iron increased susceptibility to killing by H_2O_2, and cell-permeable $OH^{\bullet}$ scavengers offered some protection.[101] *E. coli* has a high-affinity iron uptake system, encoded by about 30 genes whose transcription is increased if cell iron content is low.[102] Iron can be taken up as Fe(III) bound to **siderophores** (bacterially produced iron-chelating agents), or directly as Fe^{2+}. Uptake is regulated by the *fur* (**ferric uptake regulator**) gene. The protein encoded by *fur* chelates Fe^{2+} and then binds to a DNA base sequence (the **iron box**) found in the promoter regions of many genes regulated by iron, blocking their transcription. Genes with iron boxes include not only the iron uptake system but also those encoding MnSOD and hydroperoxidases I and II (Section 3.7 below). Indeed, some iron-chelating agents, such as **nalidixic acid** or **bipyridyl**, render fur protein inactive and increase synthesis of MnSOD, even causing it to appear in *E. coli* grown under anaerobic conditions.

E. coli fur mutants accumulate excess iron and become hypersensitive to H_2O_2, especially if MnSOD and FeSOD are also absent. Hydroxyl radical generation and oxidative DNA damage occur.[103] A double mutant, defective in both *fur* and DNA repair, is not viable under aerobic conditions. It can be 'rescued' by addition of an iron chelator (ferrozine), further mutations interfering with iron uptake, overexpression of a bacterial ferritin, increasing SOD activity, or by adding the $OH^{\bullet}$ scavengers DMSO or thiourea. *Fur* mutants are also hypersensitive to hypochlorous acid, suggesting that reaction of this species with iron (Section 2.6.3) might sometimes be significant *in vivo*.[102] However, in *E. coli* stressed by excess $O_2^{\bullet -}$ generation, Fe is not totally bad; some 'labile Fe' is essential to allow reassembly of the Fe–S clusters and recovery of metabolic activity.[104]

Evidence also supports a role of $OH^{\bullet}$ and $O_2^{\bullet -}$ in the toxicity of H_2O_2 to mammalian cells; indeed, nitric oxide can ameliorate damage by H_2O_2 in some cells by decreasing their iron content (Section 2.6.1). Fluorescent probes for 'free' iron[105] have shown its increased availability in mammalian cells subjected to oxidative stress (Section 3.15.1.3 below). The iron content of the cell culture medium is an important variable; it can be transferrin-bound, present as contamination in inorganic form and/or added deliberately, for example Fe(III) as ferric nitrate added to Dulbecco's modified Eagle's medium (Section 1.11). Cells can take up not only transferrin-bound iron but also 'free' iron ions, by a mechanism involving plasma membrane redox systems and Fe^{2+} transporters.[105] For example, in cardiac myocytes some Ca^{2+} channels can also transport iron.[106] Inorganic iron present in the medium can decompose added peroxides, leading to *extracellular* Fenton chemistry, which has confused some experimental results.

Externally added SOD does not usually protect mammalian cells against the toxicity of H_2O_2, but it can do so if allowed to enter the cells, or is overexpressed in them, suggesting that $O_2^{\bullet -}$ plays some role.[107] Permeant iron chelators, such as *o*-phenanthroline, frequently also protect. Hydrogen peroxide added to animal cells causes oxidative damage to DNA, yet neither $O_2^{\bullet -}$ nor H_2O_2 damages

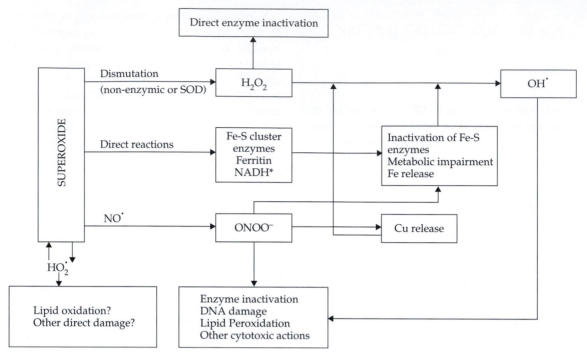

Figure 3.9 Mechanisms of superoxide-dependent damage to biomolecules: a summary. * Catalysed by LDH.

DNA. Analysis of the pattern of damage to DNA bases reveals that OH$^{\bullet}$ is the culprit.[108] Presumably H_2O_2 crosses the plasma membrane (Section 2.6.2), penetrates the nucleus and interacts with transition metal ions bound to DNA to form OH$^{\bullet}$. These metals might always be bound to DNA, and/or metals released from metalloproteins by $O_2^{\bullet-}$ or H_2O_2 could attach to DNA, making it a target of damage.

Hydroxyl radicals, once generated, react with DNA or whatever else is in their immediate vicinity. The lower reactivity of $O_2^{\bullet-}$ and H_2O_2 means that they can diffuse away from their sites of formation, leading to iron ion release and OH$^{\bullet}$ generation in any part of the cell where a sensitive metalloprotein is located.[95] Hence the precise biomolecular damage done by $O_2^{\bullet-}$ or H_2O_2 is influenced by the availability and distribution of metal ions, whether released by $O_2^{\bullet-}$ or available from other sources. The binding of metal ions to biomolecules such as DNA makes such molecules a ready target of oxidative damage by **site specific OH$^{\bullet}$ generation**, that is OH$^{\bullet}$ is generated at the metal-binding site and causes localized destruction.[95]

3.6.2.3 *Singlet oxygen*

Singlet O_2 has been suggested to contribute to the toxicity of $O_2^{\bullet-}$, but claims that it is produced in significant amounts in the non-enzymic dismutation of $O_2^{\bullet-}$ or the Haber–Weiss reaction are not supported by experiment.[109]

Addition of water to suspensions of potassium superoxide ($K^+O_2^{\bullet-}$) in chlorinated hydrocarbon solvents[110] has been shown to produce $^1\Delta g\ O_2$. However, $O_2^{\bullet-}$ reacts with chlorinated hydrocarbons (Section 2.5.3.6). Generation of peroxyl radicals followed by their self-reaction (Section 2.5.4.1) might account for $^1O_2$ production

$$O_2^{\bullet-} + CCl_4 \rightarrow CCl_3O_2^{\bullet} + Cl^-$$

$$CCl_3O_2^{\bullet} + CCl_3O_2^{\bullet} \rightarrow 2\,^1O_2 + CCl_3CCl_3$$

$$O_2^{\bullet-} + CCl_3O_2^{\bullet} \rightleftharpoons CCl_3O_2^- + \,^1O_2$$

Figure 3.9 summarizes various mechanisms of $O_2^{\bullet-}$ toxicity.

Table 3.6 Catalase and glutathione peroxidase (GPx) activities in human tissues

Tissue	Individual	Catalase activity (units per mg protein)	Glutathione peroxidase activity (units per mg protein)
Liver	A	1300	190
	B	1500	120
Erythrocytes	A	990	19
	B	1300	19
Kidney cortex	A	430	140
	B	110	87
Adrenal gland	B	300	120
Kidney medulla	A	700	90
	B	220	73
Spleen	A	56	50
Lymph node	A	120	160
Pancreas	A	100	43
	B	120	110
Lung	A	210	53
	B	180	54
Heart	A	54	69
Skeletal muscle	A	36	38
	B	25	22
Brain (grey matter)	A	11	71
	B	3	66
Brain (white matter)	A	20	76
Adipose tissue	A	270	77
	B	560	89

Data from *Cancer Res.* **42**, 1955, 1982. Glutathione peroxidase was assayed with an organic substrate (see text). Results are expressed as enzyme activity/mg protein. Two individuals, denoted A and B, were used as sources of tissue samples. This is *total* GPx activity: there are different enzymes with different tissue distributions (Section 3.8.1).

3.7 Antioxidant defence enzymes: catalases[111]

Dismutation of $O_2^{\bullet-}$ generates H_2O_2, as do several oxidase enzymes (Section 2.6.2). Hydrogen peroxide can be removed by two types of enzyme. The **catalases** catalyse direct decomposition of H_2O_2 to ground-state O_2

$$2H_2O_2 \rightarrow 2H_2O + O_2$$

Peroxidase enzymes remove H_2O_2 by using it to oxidize another substrate (written SH_2 below)

$$SH_2 + H_2O_2 \rightarrow S + 2H_2O$$

Most aerobes contain catalase, although a few do not, such as *Bacillus popilliae*, *Mycoplasma pneumoniae*,[80] the green alga *Euglena*, several parasitic helminths (e.g. the liver fluke) and *Gloeocapsa*. Some anaerobic bacteria, such as *Propionibacterium shermanii*, contain catalase, but many do not. In animals catalase is present in all organs, but especially concentrated in liver (Table 3.6). Catalase in erythrocytes helps protect them against H_2O_2 generated by dismutation of $O_2^{\bullet-}$ from haemoglobin autoxidation (Section 6.4). Since H_2O_2 crosses membranes, erythrocytes can also protect other tissues against extracellular H_2O_2 by 'absorbing' and destroying it.[112] Brain, heart and skeletal muscle have lower levels of catalase (Table 3.6), although the activity varies between cell types. Several plants, for example maize, appear to have multiple catalases, encoded by several genes, although it has been suggested that in the fungus *Neurospora crassa*, some electrophoretically-separable catalases arise from photochemical modification of the enzyme *in vivo* by singlet O_2.[113]

3.7.1 Catalase structure

Animal catalases contain four subunits, each of which has Fe(III)-haem at its active site.[114] Each subunit of bovine liver catalase consists of a large antiparallel β-pleated sheet domain with helical insertions, followed by a smaller domain containing four α-helices. The haem group is buried at least 20 Å below the molecular surface, only accessible by a channel lined with hydrophobic residues. Ligands to the haem iron are provided by Tyr357 (358 in human catalase), His74 and Asp147. Burying the haems in non-polar pockets, connected to the surface by narrow channels, prevents most molecules other than H_2O_2 from gaining access (Fig. 3.10, Plate 5 shows this for human catalase). Each subunit usually has one molecule of NADPH bound to it. Dissociation of catalase into its subunits, which easily occurs on storage, freeze-drying or exposure of the enzyme

to acid or alkali, causes loss of activity.[115] Commercial catalase preparations can be contaminated with these partial denaturation products, as well as with SOD, antioxidant 'stabilizers' such as thymol (Section 3.22 below) and even with endotoxin. This should be borne in mind when using commercial catalase as a 'probe' for the involvement of H_2O_2 in a reaction, especially in whole animals.[116] Contamination of commercial catalase with arginase has also been reported.[117]

E. coli has two catalases,[118] one of which (known as **hydroperoxidase II**, HPII) is a tetramer with one haem per subunit (but without bound NADPH).[118] It is encoded by the *kat*E gene. By contrast, **hydroperoxidase I** (HPI), encoded by the *kat*G gene, is a tetramer which shows both catalase and peroxidase activities, that is, it is a **bifunctional catalase–peroxidase**. The HPI enzyme is present under both aerobic and anaerobic conditions and levels increase if H_2O_2 is added, whereas H_2O_2 does not induce HPII in *E. coli*. Similar enzymes are present in many other bacteria, including *M. tuberculosis*. By contrast, *Pseudomonas aeruginosa* has three different catalases (**Kat A, Kat B, Kat E**), but no catalase–peroxidase.[119]

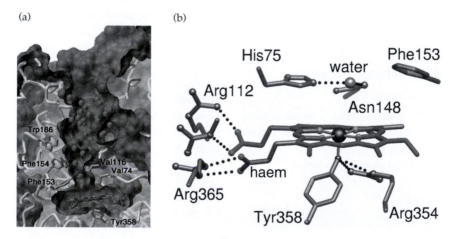

(a)   (b)

Figure 3.10 (see plate 5) Active site of human catalase. (a) A ~25 Å tunnel leads from the enzyme surface to the haem in the active site and forms an hydrophobic constriction 2–3 Å wide, which is critical for the selective utilization of H_2O_2, immediately above the active site. Side-chains making up the hydrophobic channel and the Tyr358 ligand are displayed in green. Backbone shown in white. (b) Stereo view of the human catalase active site. The pentaco-ordinate iron-haem (red) is accessible at the distal side to peroxides and small molecules at the bottom of a long channel filled with a network of water molecules that ends with a water molecule bound by the protein side-chains (green), His75 and Asn148. The reactivity of the haem iron is tuned by electron donation by the Tyr358 ligand, and neutralization of the carboxylate charge by Arg72, Arg112 and Arg365. Adapted from *J. Mol. Biol.* **296**, 295, 2000 by courtesy of Dr John Tainer and Elsevier.

3.7.2 The reaction mechanism of catalase[111,120]

Catalase, like SOD, catalyses a dismutation reaction; one H_2O_2 is reduced to H_2O and the other oxidized to O_2

$$\text{catalase-Fe(III)} + H_2O_2 \xrightarrow{k_1} \text{compound I} + H_2O$$

$$\text{compound I} + H_2O_2 \xrightarrow{k_2} \text{catalase-Fe(III)} + H_2O + O_2$$

Net $2H_2O_2 \rightarrow 2H_2O + O_2$

For rat liver catalase, the rate constants, k_1 and k_2, are $1.7 \times 10^7 \, M^{-1}s^{-1}$ and $2.6 \times 10^7 \, M^{-1}s^{-1}$, respectively. Formation of compound I leads to changes in the absorbance spectrum of catalase (Fig. 3.11), which have been used to assess rates of H_2O_2 production in perfused organs (Section 5.8). In compound I, the iron has been oxidized from Fe(III) to a nominal valency of Fe(V). In fact, an Fe(IV) oxoporphyrin-cation radical, $(\text{haem}^{\bullet+})$ Fe(IV)O, is formed, that is the iron is Fe(IV) and the extra oxidizing capacity is 'parked' by one-electron oxidation of the haem. A similar intermediate is formed in the bacterial catalase-peroxidases. Compound I receives two electrons from H_2O_2 to reform ferric catalase.

Catalase **compound II** can be produced by one electron reduction of compound I and is an inactive Fe(IV) species, catalase-(haem)Fe(IV)O, without the porphyrin radical. Electron transfer can occur within compound I itself, generating a tyrosine radical on the protein, or from an external electron donor such as ferricyanide or $O_2^{\bullet-}$. One role of the bound NADPH may be to help maintain enzyme activity by acting as a preferred electron donor to complex I if H_2O_2 supply is limited, so hindering formation of amino acid radicals. NADPH may also reconvert compound II to active catalase.[121]

It is difficult to saturate catalase with H_2O_2—its maximum velocity (V_{max}) for the destruction of H_2O_2 is enormous. However, the above equations show that complete removal of H_2O_2 requires the impact of two H_2O_2 molecules upon a single catalase active site, which becomes less likely as H_2O_2 concentrations fall. The amount of compound I present in a mixture of catalase and H_2O_2 depends on their relative concentrations and on k_1 and k_2. Chance *et al.*[111] calculated that at all reasonable

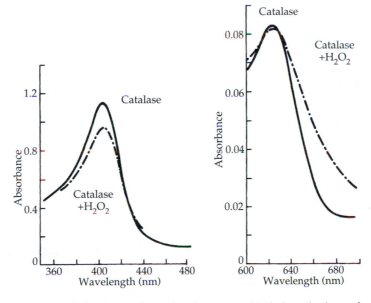

Figure 3.11 Absorbance spectra of purified rat liver catalase and catalase compound I. The large absorbance of catalase around 400 nm is known as the **Soret band**, a feature of most haem proteins.

concentrations, the rate of removal of H_2O_2 is given by the equation:

$$\begin{aligned} \text{Moles } H_2O_2, \\ \text{used}(l^{-1}s^{-1}) &= 2k_2[H_2O_2][\text{compound I}] \\ &= 2k_1[H_2O_2][\text{free catalase}] \end{aligned}$$

Thus if the concentration of H_2O_2 is fixed, the initial rate of its removal will be proportional to the concentration of catalase present and hence will be higher in liver than in, say, brain or heart (Table 3.6). Similarly, for a given concentration of catalase, the initial rate of H_2O_2 removal will be proportional to the H_2O_2 concentration. As a result, the specific activities (μmol H_2O_2 decomposed/min/mg protein) quoted by manufacturers for their catalase preparations are meaningless unless they describe exactly how the assay was done.

3.7.3 Catalase inhibitors

Catalase can be inhibited by azide, cyanide, peroxynitrite, and HOCl, but these are non-specific. A more useful inhibitor[122] is **aminotriazole** (Fig. 3.12), which inhibits catalase *in vivo*. Its inhibitory action is exerted on compound I, so aminotriazole will only inhibit if H_2O_2 is present. It acts by modifying a histidine ligand to the haem (His74 in the bovine enzyme). The observation that aminotriazole inhibits catalase in whole animals or plants confirms that H_2O_2 is produced *in vivo*.

3.7.4 Peroxidatic activity of catalase

Mammalian catalases can also catalyse peroxidase-type reactions,[111] to an extent restricted by accessibility of substrates to the haem (Fig. 3.10). Compound I can oxidize methanol (CH_3OH) and ethanol (CH_3CH_2OH) to their corresponding aldehydes HCHO (formaldehyde or methanal) and CH_3CHO

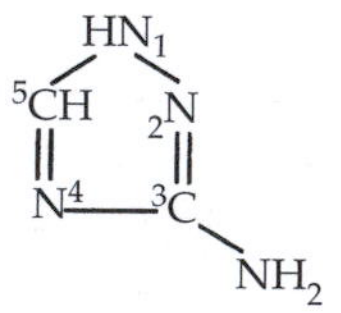

Figure 3.12 Structure of aminotriazole (3-amino-1,2,4-triazole).

(acetaldehyde or ethanal), but propanols or butanols are much poorer substrates. Formic acid (HCOOH) can be oxidized to CO_2 by compound I and nitrite (NO_2^-) to nitrate. Catalase has also been suggested to oxidize elemental mercury (Hg) absorbed into the human body to Hg^{2+} ions.[123]

The presence of peroxidatic substrates for catalase *in vivo* will decrease the concentration of compound I, causing more free catalase to be formed. This is another variable to be considered in assessing how quickly catalase removes H_2O_2 *in vivo*. Separated catalase subunits show little catalase activity, but have peroxidase activity on a wider range of substrates, including NADH, because the haem is more accessible.[115]

The drug **cyanamide** ($H_2NC \equiv N$) is converted *in vivo* into a product (possibly nitroxyl anion; Section 2.5.6) that inhibits aldehyde dehydrogenase (Section 8.8). Consumption of ethanol after taking cyanamide causes ethanal accumulation and unpleasant symptoms, and so cyanamide administration is used to deter alcohol consumption. It has been suggested that catalase is responsible for oxidizing cyanamide to the product that inhibits aldehyde dehydrogenase: during this oxidation, the catalase loses activity.[124]

Nitric oxide reversibly binds to the haems of catalase, causing modest decreases in enzyme activity. Catalase can also use H_2O_2 to slowly oxidize[125] $NO^\bullet$ to NO_2^-, and on to NO_3^-.

3.7.5 Photosensitization by catalase

Exposure of cultured keratinocytes to UVB light causes oxidative stress, and catalase was identified as one of the molecules responsible.[126] Indeed, isolated catalases from a variety of species catalyse light-dependent ROS production. This action is *stimulated* by 3-aminotriazole and azide, but inhibited by CN^-. Catalase, like most proteins, can readily be modified and inactivated by singlet O_2.[113]

3.7.6 Subcellular location of catalase

The catalase activity of animal (except for erythrocytes) and plant cells is largely or completely located in subcellular organelles bounded by a single membrane, the **peroxisomes**.[111] Peroxisomes also contain several enzymes that generate H_2O_2, such as glycollate oxidase, urate oxidase (absent in primates) and the flavoprotein dehydrogenases involved in β-oxidation of fatty acids, a metabolic pathway that operates in both mitochondria and peroxisomes in animals. In mitochondria these flavoproteins donate electrons to the electron transport chain, but in peroxisomes they react with O_2 to give H_2O_2. It seems logical (although logic is sometimes dangerous in the free radical field!) to believe that these H_2O_2-producing enzymes have evolved to colocate in an organelle with high capacity to destroy H_2O_2. This view is supported by mutations affecting the peroxisomal targeting sequence of catalase, so that it stays in the cytoplasm and does not enter peroxisomes. In its absence, H_2O_2 produced in peroxisomes damages them, fatty acids are not properly degraded and severe symptoms result.[127] Some CuZnSOD may also be present in peroxisomes (Section 3.2.1.1).

Mitochondria (at least in skeletal muscle and liver),[111,128] chloroplasts and the ER contain little, if any, catalase. Hence any H_2O_2 produced by these organelles *in vivo* cannot be disposed of by catalase, unless H_2O_2 diffuses out of them to the peroxisomes. Isolated subcellular fractions, especially microsomes and mitochondria, may be heavily *contaminated* with catalase released from peroxisomes, however. Although much of the catalase in homogenates of animal and plant tissues is not organelle-associated, this is generally thought to be due to rupture of peroxisomes, which are fragile organelles, during homogenization. However, some non-peroxisomal catalase may occur in the livers of a few animals, such as guinea pigs.[129] By contrast with other tissues, mitochondria in rat heart do contain some catalase, in the matrix.[128]

S. cerevisiae contains two catalases, one (**catalase A**) in peroxisomes and the other (**catalase T**) in the cytosol, as does the nematode *C. elegans*. Knockout of peroxisomal catalase shortened the lifespan of this worm, but knockout of the cytosolic one did not (Section 10.3.1).

3.7.7 Manganese-containing catalases[130]

Several microorganisms contain Mn-catalases, H_2O_2-degrading enzymes insensitive to inhibition by azide or cyanide and without haem. They are sometimes called **pseudocatalases**. Thus the *Lactobacillus plantarum* Mn-catalase has six subunits, each of which contains a dimanganese active site, the metal being in the Mn(III) state. The dimanganese sites cycle between Mn(III) and Mn^{2+} during catalysis.

3.7.8 Acatalasaemia[131]

The gene encoding catalase in humans is located on chromosome 11, and mutations in it may result in **acatalasaemia**. In the original description of this condition in Japan there was a severe deficiency of catalase activity, but the only observable clinical problem was an increased incidence of gum disease (**Takahara's disease**). Splicing mutations, or a deletion in exon 4 of the catalase gene, have been identified in different Japanese patients. Another series of mutations has been described in Switzerland and results in an active but unstable enzyme, leading to variable decreases in catalase activity in different issues: no clinical effects are apparent. Similarly, transgenic mice lacking catalase grow normally and show no obvious abnormalities,[132] although they are more prone to injury by H_2O_2-generating toxins and possibly more susceptible to ischaemia–reperfusion and to cancer development as they age. *Drosophila* mutants with lowered catalase are also viable, unless activity is decreased to <2% of normal,[133] but *C. elegans* needs its peroxisomal catalase (Section 3.7.6). Studies in Hungary showed no clinical effects of acatalasaemia, but suggested that it is a risk factor for development of diabetes.[131] Changes in the promoter region of the catalase gene may also influence the enzyme activity in humans.[134]

Inactivating catalase genes in bacteria or yeasts has, in general, much less striking effects than deleting SOD genes (one exception is *P. aeruginosa*, where Kat A is required for virulence[119]). This may be due to the presence of other H_2O_2-removing enzymes, or the fact that H_2O_2 can simply diffuse out of the cell to the medium. However, the cells usually become more sensitive to added H_2O_2 or H_2O_2-generating toxins, which could make them hypersensitive to phagocytic killing (Section 7.7). Catalase-deficient plants are considered in Section 6.8.7.

The disease **aniridia** is associated with an increased incidence of mental retardation and of the type of cancer known as **Wilms' tumour**. Aniridia results from a deletion on chromosome 11 and also leads to decreased catalase activity. Whether this contributes to the symptoms of aniridia is unknown.[135]

3.8 Antioxidant defence enzymes: the glutathione peroxidase family[111,136]

Glutathione peroxidases (GPx) remove H_2O_2 by coupling its reduction to H_2O with oxidation of **reduced glutathione**, GSH, a thiol-containing tripeptide (Fig. 3.13)

$$H_2O_2 + 2GSH \rightarrow GSSG + 2H_2O$$

A GPx enzyme was first discovered (in animal tissues) in 1957; GPx are less common in plants or bacteria. However, GSH is present in animals, plants and many aerobic bacteria (e.g. E. coli), at intracellular concentrations frequently in the mM range (Table 3.7), but is found less often in anaerobic bacteria.

The GPx enzymes are widely distributed in animal tissues (Tables 3.6 and 3.7) and are mostly specific for GSH as a hydrogen donor. They can be inhibited by **mercaptosuccinate**.[137] They can also act on peroxides other than H_2O_2. For example they catalyse GSH-dependent reduction of fatty acid hydroperoxides and various synthetic hydroperoxides such as cumene and *t*-butyl hydroperoxides, which are often used as substrates to assay the enzyme *in vitro*. The peroxide group is reduced to an alcohol

$$LOOH + 2GSH \rightarrow GSSG + H_2O + LOH$$

Most GPx enzymes cannot act upon fatty acid peroxides esterified to lipids in lipoproteins or membranes: peroxidized fatty acids must first be released by lipase enzymes.

3.8.1 A family of enzymes[136]

At least four types of GPx exist. One is the 'classical' enzyme, often now called cytosolic GPx, cGPx or **GPx1**. Mammalian plasma contains low levels of a different form, **PGPx** (often called **GPx3**), a glycoprotein. It is also found in other extracellular fluids such as milk, seminal fluid, amniotic fluid, aqueous humor of the eye and lung lining fluid, and

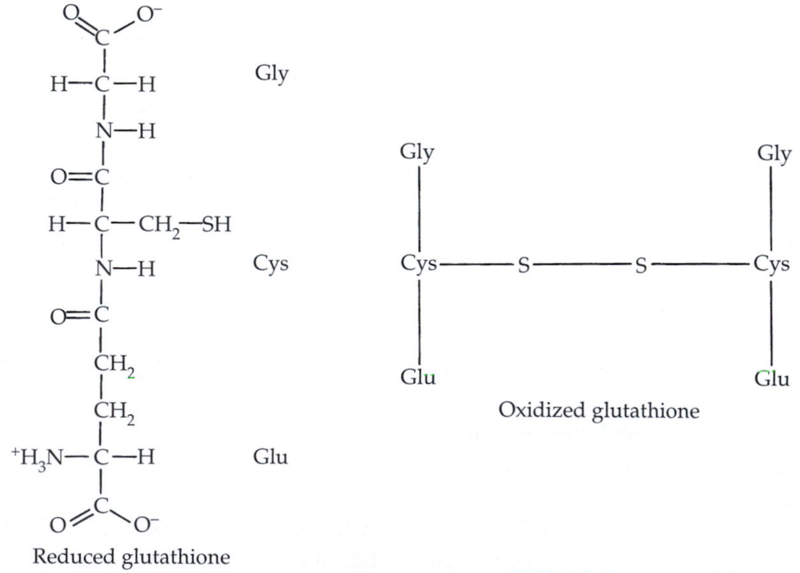

Reduced glutathione

Oxidized glutathione

Figure 3.13 Structures of reduced (GSH) and oxidized (GSSG) glutathione. GSH is a tripeptide (glutamic acid–cysteine–glycine). In GSSG, two GSH molecules join together as the –SH groups of cysteine oxidize to form a disulphide bridge. In **homoglutathione** the glycine residue is replaced by a peptide bond involving the –COOH group of cysteine and the –NH$_2$ group of β-alanine, that is glu–cys–CONHCH$_2$CH$_2$COO$^-$.

Table 3.7 Presence of glutathione and enzymes using it in different organisms—some examples

System studied	GSH[c] concentration	GSH/ GSSG[d] ratio	Glutathione[a] peroxidase (total)	Glutathione[a,b] reductase
Spinach chloroplasts	3.0 mM	>10/1	Absent	High
Rat tissues				
Liver	7–8 mM	>100/1	High	High
Erythrocyte	2 mM	>100/1	Moderate	Moderate
Heart	2 mM	>100/1	Moderate	Moderate
Lung	2 mM	>100/1	Moderate	Moderate
Lens	6–10 mM	>100/1	Moderate	Moderate
Kidney	4 mM	>100/1	Moderate	Moderate
Brain	2 mM	>100/1	Moderate	Moderate
Skeletal muscle	1 mM	>100/1	Low	Low
Blood plasma	20–30 μM	~ 5/1	Low	Traces
Adipose tissue	3.2 mg/10[6] cells	>100/1	Low	Low
Human tissues				
Liver	4 mmol/g wet wt	>100/1	High	High
Kidney	2 μmol/g	>100/1	High	High
Lens	6–10 mM	>100/1	Moderate	Moderate
Erythrocytes	240 μg/ml blood	>100/1	Moderate	Moderate
Whole blood[e]	~ 1 mM	>100/1	High	High
Blood plasma[e]	1–3 μM	varies	Low	Absent
Alveolar lining fluid	40–200 μM	varies (usually >10/1)	Traces[f]	Traces or absent
Neurospora crassa	20 μmol/g dry wt	150/1	Absent	Moderate
E. coli				
Aerobically grown	27 μmol/g[g]	>10/1	Absent	Moderate
Anaerobically grown	7 μmol/g			

Data compiled from a wide range of publications.

[a] The description of enzyme activities is relative rather than absolute. Several forms of GPx exist (Section 3.8.1)

[b] Glutathione reductase is absent from *Drosophila* and *Anopheles* (Section 6.6).

[c] Whenever possible, concentrations are expressed as millimolar but this cannot always be calculated from published data. These GSH values must not be taken too literally, since they (i) may be affected by age, (ii) are different at different times of day in animals, different times of year in humans (*Am. J. Clin. Nutr.* **71**, 1194, 2000) and at different points of the growth cycle in bacteria and fungi, (iii) in animal tissues (especially liver), decrease on starvation, (iv) vary between the different cell types present in tissues, and (v) may depend on the gender of the animal (e.g. *Free Rad. Biol. Med.* **23**, 648, 1997; *Biochem. J.* **112**, 109, 1969).

[d] GSH: GSSG ratios vary in different subcellular compartments: ratios of 3:1 have been estimated for the interior of the ER, where protein folding and disulphide bond formation take place (*Science* **257**, 1496, 1993).

[e] Concentrations of cysteine and cystine in plasma are significantly higher (7–8 μM and 80–90 μM, respectively in humans). Virtually all GSH in whole blood is in the cells, especially erythrocytes.

[f] Mostly the pGPx. Levels reported to rise in asthmatic patients (*FASEB J.* **15**, 70, 2001).

[g] 3.5 mM in log growth: 6.6 mM in stationary phase.

originates mainly from the kidney. Whether it functions as a GPx in plasma is uncertain because of the low levels of GSH: plasma GSH levels are μM (Table 3.7) but the K_m of the enzyme for GSH is in the mM range. It may work better in alveolar lining fluid where GSH levels are higher (Table 3.7). The GPx3 enzymes can also use thioredoxin as a substrate, but there is not a lot of this in plasma either.

Another type of GPx is found in the cells lining the gastrointestinal tract. Intestinal glutathione peroxidase (**GI-GPx**, sometimes called **GPx2**) may serve to metabolize peroxides in ingested food lipids as well as any generated during lipid peroxidation in the intestine itself (Section 6.2.2). Human liver also contains GPx2, as well as GPx1 and GPx4 (see below).

The fourth member of the family is **phospholipid hydroperoxide glutathione peroxidase (PHGPx** or **GPx4)**, with the unique ability to reduce not only H_2O_2 and synthetic organic peroxides but also fatty acid and cholesterol hydroperoxides that are still esterified. By contrast, GPx1 and GPx2 do not act on cholesterol peroxides, and GPx3 hydrolyses them only slowly. In other words, GPx4 can act upon peroxidized fatty acid residues within membranes and lipoproteins, reducing them to alcohols. It is less specific for GSH as a reductant than the other GPx enzymes and can also reduce thymine hydroperoxide,[138] a product of free radical attack on thymine in DNA (Section 4.8). In general GPx4 activity in tissues is lower than that of GPx1. Testis is an exception, with high GPx4; this enzyme plays a key role in sperm maturation by catalysing oxidation of protein thiol groups in the sperm head. The GPx4 ends up incorporated into the sperm capsule in an inactive form.[139]

3.8.2 The role of selenium[136]

The GPx1, 2 and 3 enzymes contain four protein subunits, each of which bears an atom of **selenium** (Se) at its active site. However, GPx4 is an exception, being a monomer of relative molecular mass 19 000, with one Se. Selenium (discovered in 1817 by Jöns Jacob Berzelius and named after the Greek goddess of the moon *Selene*) is an element in group VI of the periodic table, and resembles sulphur in its chemistry, although the Earth's crust contains about 10^3-fold less selenium than it does sulphur. Selenium is present at the active sites as **selenocysteine**, cysteine in which the sulphur atom (R-SH) is replaced by selenium (R-SeH). The presence of Se lowers the pK_a (~8.3 for –SH, 5.2 for –SeH) and so favours ionization to Se$^-$. Selenocysteine is encoded in the GPx genes as TGA (UGA in mRNA), also a stop codon. To prevent reading as 'stop', a selenocysteine insertion sequence must be present downstream of the UGA.

Selenocysteine transfer RNA is first loaded with serine, which is then converted into selenocysteine, the selenium being donated by selenophosphate. Rodent epididymis has been reported to contain a Se-independent GPx (**GPx5**) with cysteine at the active site, but this may not be present in humans.[140]

During catalysis by GPx, the **selenol** (enzyme-Se$^-$) reacts with peroxide to give a **selenenic acid** (enzyme-SeOH)

$$Enzyme\text{-}Se^- + ROOH + H^+ \rightarrow$$
$$ROH + Enzyme\text{-}SeOH$$

Glutathione then binds, followed by

$$Enzyme\text{-}SeOH\text{-}GSH \rightarrow H_2O + Enzyme\text{-}Se\text{-}SG$$

The second GSH binds, followed by

$$Enzyme\text{-}Se\text{-}SG\text{-}GSH \rightarrow Enzyme\text{-}SeH\text{-}GSSG \rightarrow$$
$$Enzyme\text{-}Se^- + H^+ + GSSG$$

Traces of selenium are essential in the diet of animals, one important role being to provide selenocysteine for the GPx family. When rodents are selenium-deprived, GPx activity falls, GPx1 most rapidly whereas GPx2 and 4 activities are preserved for longer, suggesting that they are more important *in vivo*. The role of GPx4 in sperm maturation helps to explain why selenium deficiency impairs reproduction in rats.[139]

However, selenium plays many other metabolic roles. For example, in thyroid hormone biosynthesis it is an essential component of **iodothyronine-5′-deiodinase** enzymes, which convert thyroxine (T_4) to the more biologically active hormone 3,5,3′-triiodothyronine (T_3). Several other selenoproteins are present *in vivo*. For example most selenium in the plasma of humans and other animals is on **selenoprotein P**, a glycoselenoprotein (ten selenocysteines per molecule). It may act as a carrier of Se to tissues such as the testis and brain[141] and has been suggested to have antioxidant properties, possibly by reducing phospholipid hydroperoxides in a GPx-like manner with thioredoxin as the electron donor.[142] **Selenoprotein W**, an intracellular protein found in many tissues, also has antioxidant properties.[143] Selenium is also a component of thioredoxin reductase (Section 3.11 below) and methionine sulphoxide reductase (Section 4.14.1). When animals are Se-deprived, the brain is one of the last tissues to be depleted, suggestive of the importance of this element to brain function (Section 9.16.6.2).

3.8.3 Glutathione reductase

The ratios of reduced to oxidized glutathione in normal cells are high (Table 3.7); conversion of GSSG back to GSH is achieved by **glutathione reductase** enzymes, which catalyse the reaction:

$$GSSG + NADPH + H^+ \rightarrow 2GSH + NADP^+$$

Glutathione reductases contain two subunits,[144] each with FAD at its active site. NADPH reduces the FAD, which then passes its electrons onto a disulphide bridge in the active site. The two –SH groups so formed then interact with GSSG and reduce it to 2GSH, reforming the protein disulphide. Glutathione reductase can be inhibited *in vitro* and *in vivo* by **BCNU, *N,N*-bis(2-chloroethyl)-*N*-nitrosourea**, although this reactive compound is unlikely to be a specific inhibitor.[145]

3.8.3.1 *Sources of NADPH*

NADPH in animal tissues is provided by several mechanisms, a major one being the **pentose phosphate pathway** (PPP).[111] The first enzyme is **glucose-6-phosphate dehydrogenase** (G6PDH)

$$Glucose\ 6\text{-}phosphate + NADP^+ \rightarrow$$
$$6\text{-}phosphogluconate + NADPH + H^+$$

Followed by 6-phosphogluconate dehydrogenase,

$$6\text{-}phosphogluconate + NADP^+ \rightarrow$$
$$CO_2 + NADPH + H^+ + ribulose\ 5\text{-}phosphate$$

The rate of the PPP is controlled by the supply of $NADP^+$; as the action of glutathione reductase lowers the $NADPH/NADP^+$ ratio, the pathway speeds up to replace NADPH. Fibroblasts deficient in G6PDH show premature senescence in culture, accompanied by increased oxidative damage[146] and deficiency of this enzyme has clinical consequences in humans (Section 6.4.5). Indeed, mice

with abnormally low levels of G6PDH in heart show aggravated injury after ischaemia–reperfusion (Section 9.5.4). In several cell types, treatment with GSH-depleting drugs increases synthesis of G6PDH.[147] Of course, NADPH can also make ROS, as a substrate of the NOX enzymes (Section 7.10).

Another source of NADPH, especially in mitochondria (Fig. 1.7), but also in cytosol to some extent, is the enzyme **$NADP^+$-dependent isocitrate dehydrogenase**, a target of damage by RS[148].

3.8.4 Watching GPx in action

A common approach is to measure the PPP activity by supplying 1-^{14}C-labelled glucose and measuring the release of $^{14}CO_2$ in the 6-phosphogluconate dehydrogenase reaction (Section 3.8.3.1). Increased pathway activity is observed upon exposing many cells and tissues to elevated O_2, presumably as more NADPH is used by glutathione reductase as it deals with more GSSG. NADPH is also needed to maintain catalase activity (Section 3.7) but this probably consumes only small amounts.

An alternative approach has been to measure GSSG release: if cells are treated with reagents that oxidize internal GSH to GSSG, such as **diamide**,[149] $(CH_3)_2NCON=NCON(CH_3)_2$, they eject GSSG into the surrounding medium. In intact liver, GSSG is released into bile.[150] The release of GSSG from perfused organs has been used as an approximate measure of GPx activity if glucose is omitted from the perfusing medium, so that NADPH cannot be produced by the PPP (there are other ways to make NADPH however; Section 3.8.3). Exposure of isolated perfused organs (e.g. liver and lung) to elevated O_2 causes increased GSSG release.

Figure 3.14 shows GSSG release when H_2O_2 at increasing concentrations is infused into a perfused rat liver: the 'saturation' of GSSG release is probably related to the increased action of catalase in removing H_2O_2 at higher concentrations. Inclusion of physiological concentrations of glycollate in the perfusing medium causes little increase in GSSG release, suggesting that H_2O_2 generated by glycollate oxidase is largely disposed of by catalase in peroxisomes. As expected, if catalase is inhibited by aminotriazole, glycollate does increase GSSG

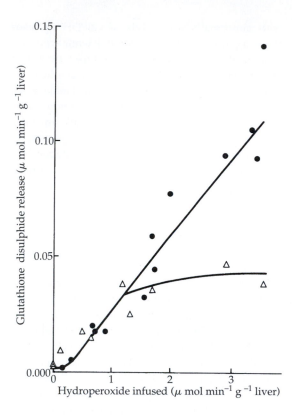

Figure 3.14 Release of GSSG from an isolated perfused liver during infusion of H_2O_2, included in the perfusion medium at the concentration stated (open triangles). The closed circles show the results when an organic hydroperoxide was infused instead. Diagram by courtesy of Professor Helmut Sies (see *Eur. J. Biochem.* **89**, 113, 1978).

release. The undestroyed H_2O_2 presumably diffuses across the peroxisomal membrane and at least some is then dealt with by GPx.

3.9 Glutathione in metabolism and cellular redox state

3.9.1 Cofactor and redox agent

In addition to being a cofactor for the GPx enzymes, GSH is involved in many other metabolic processes, including ascorbate metabolism (Section 3.20.1.2 below), maintaining communication between cells through gap junctions,[151] and generally preventing protein-SH groups from oxidizing and cross-linking. Because high levels are present, the GSSG/2GSH couple is a major contributor to the 'redox state' of the cell. If we assume 10 mM total glutathione in the cytosol with 99% GSH and 1% GSSG, the reduction potential is approximately -250 mV.[152] The value depends both on the GSH/GSSG ratio and on the total concentration of glutathione. For example if this is 1 mM with 1% as GSSG the potential rises to

about -220 mV. It is about -180 mV in the ER, where GSH/GSSG ratios are lower (Table 3.7, legend) and different again in the mitochondrial matrix, because pH is higher than in the cytoplasm due to the proton gradient. Of course, there are many other redox couples in the cell; examples include $NAD^+/NADH$, ascorbate/dehydroascorbate, and $NADP^+/NADPH$.

Reduced glutathione is a radioprotective agent (Section 8.19), may sometimes be involved in supplying copper to CuZnSOD (Section 3.2.1.2) and is a cofactor for several enzymes in different metabolic pathways, including glyoxalases[153] and enzymes involved in leukotriene synthesis (Fig. 7.23). **Methylglyoxal** (CH_3COCHO) reacts with GSH and the complex is oxidized by the **glyoxalase I** enzyme into *S*-lactoylglutathione ($CH_3CHOHCOSG$). This is hydrolysed by **glyoxalase II** into lactate, regenerating GSH. Methylglyoxal is produced from glyceraldehyde 3-phosphate and dihydroxyacetone phosphate (intermediates of glycolysis), from acetone by CYP2E1, and during lipid peroxidation. Rapid removal is essential because of its high reactivity with DNA and proteins, for example covalent binding to cysteine, arginine and lysine residues.[153] **Glyoxal** (CHOCHO), additionally formed from glycolytic intermediates and during lipid peroxidation and equally damaging, is also removed by glyoxalases I and II. Glutathione additionally assists in removal of the toxic aldehyde formaldehyde, converted to *S*-formyl-glutathione by formaldehyde dehydrogenase.

Glutathione plays a role in protein folding (Section 3.10 below) and the degradation of proteins with disulphide bonds, such as insulin (the first step in insulin breakdown is cleavage of disulphide bridges linking the two peptide chains). A special role of GSH is seen in the freshwater coelenterate *Hydra*, which recognizes wounded prey by the release of GSH from damaged cells. The GSH binds to specific receptors, leading to tentacle contractions and mouth opening in the hungry predator.[154]

3.9.2 GSH as an antioxidant

In vitro, GSH can react with $OH^\bullet$, HOCl, $ONOO^-$, $RO^\bullet$, $RO_2^\bullet$, $CO_3^{\bullet-}$, $NO_2^\bullet$, carbon-centred radicals and $^1O_2$, but not $O_2^{\bullet-}$ (or at least, not very fast with $O_2^{\bullet-}$). Since GSH is present at mM intracellular concentrations (Table 3.7) scavenging of these RS is feasible *in vivo*. Reaction with RS can often generate thiyl ($GS^\bullet$) radicals, and in turn $O_2^{\bullet-}$ (Section 2.5.5).

$$GS^\bullet \xrightarrow{GS^-} GSSG^{\bullet-} \xrightarrow{O_2} GSSG + O_2^{\bullet-}$$

The $O_2^{\bullet-}$ can be removed by SOD, and the GSSG reconverted to GSH by glutathione reductase, consuming NADPH. Reaction of GSH with $ONOO^-$ leads to formation of some nitrosothiol (GSNO), which can decompose to regenerate $NO^\bullet$.[155] Hence GSH can, to some extent, 'recycle' $ONOO^-$ to $NO^\bullet$. It also chelates copper ions and can diminish[156] their ability to generate $OH^\bullet$ from H_2O_2.

3.9.3 Glutathione biosynthesis and degradation

Glutathione is synthesized in the cytoplasm of all animal cells, the liver being the most active organ.

Mitochondria contain about 10 to 20% of total cellular GSH yet cannot make it and must acquire GSH from the cytoplasm through transporters in the inner membrane.[157]

Glutamate–cysteine ligase (often called **γ-glutamylcysteine synthetase**, γGCS) catalyses the first, and rate-limiting step, in GSH synthesis

$$\text{L-glutamate} + \text{L-cysteine} + \text{ATP} \rightarrow$$
$$\text{L} - \gamma - \text{glutamyl- L-cysteine} + \text{ADP} + P_i$$

and the dipeptide product is converted to GSH by **glutathione synthetase**

$$\text{L-}\gamma\text{-glutamyl-L-cysteine} + \text{glycine} + \text{ATP} \rightarrow$$
$$\text{GSH} + \text{ADP} + P_i$$

Cells can make the necessary cysteine from methionine (Fig. 10.7), or they can take it up from the surrounding fluids. Some take up cysteine as such, others the disulphide form (**cystine**), which they reduce to cysteine inside the cell. Cysteine and cystine use different transporters, but the latter also transports glutamate. Hence abnormally high extracellular glutamate levels can decrease GSH in some cell types by slowing entry of cystine.[158] In patients with severe burns, metabolic disturbances may decrease glycine availability to an extent that limits GSH synthesis.[158] Glutathione is present in many foods, but only small amounts are absorbed intact by the gut; most is hydrolysed to amino acids, which are then absorbed. γ-Glutamylcysteine synthetase is feedback inhibited by GSH (competitively with glutamate) and does not appear substrate-saturated at normal cellular cysteine levels, so that increased cysteine often promotes GSH synthesis. Variations in cysteine levels might account for the effects of starvation and refeeding on GSH levels (Table 3.7).

Glutamylcysteine synthetase can be inhibited by **buthionine sulphoximine** (BSO), widely used in experiments to deplete cellular GSH. It has the structure

$$\text{CH}_3\text{CH}_2\text{CH}_2\text{CH}_2\overset{\overset{\displaystyle O}{\|}}{\underset{\underset{\displaystyle NH}{\|}}{S}}\text{CH}_2\text{CH}_2\overset{\displaystyle NH_2}{\underset{\displaystyle COOH}{\text{CH}}}$$

Treating isolated cells or whole organisms with BSO is not usually lethal, but substantial falls in

GSH levels make them highly sensitive to ionizing radiation and to toxins that are metabolized by reactions involving GSH. Sprague–Dawley rats treated with BSO suffer vascular oxidative stress and hypertension.[159] It is much more difficult to deplete mitochondrial GSH by using BSO than cytosolic GSH. Very severe GSH depletion, affecting the mitochondrial pool, leads to mitochondrial damage, and is lethal in newborn animals because of multiple organ damage (e.g. to kidney, liver, lung, brain and eye).[160] Tissue injury is ameliorated by replacing GSH, for example with GSH ethyl or methyl esters (Section 10.6.9.1).

Reduced glutathione is in a constant state of turnover; its half-life has been estimated as 4 days in human erythrocytes and 3 h in rat liver. Turnover in red blood cells can involve export of GSSG into plasma by an ATP-dependent transport system similar to the one in liver that excretes GSSG into bile. Liver constantly secretes GSH into plasma, to provide substrates for GSH synthesis in other tissues; it is the main source of plasma GSH and export occurs through several different transporters.[161] However, mammalian cells are inefficient at taking up GSH; in cells other than erythrocytes, **γ-glutamyltranspeptidase** (sometimes called **γ-glutamyltransferase**, γGGT) breaks it down. The enzyme is located on the plasma membrane with its active site facing outwards, and acts on extracellular GSH to transfer the glutamate residue onto other amino acids such as cystine, methionine and glutamine

$$GSH + amino\ acid \rightarrow \gamma\text{-glutamylamino acid} + cysteinyl\text{-glycine}$$

The cys-gly dipeptide can then be hydrolysed by dipeptidases on the plasma membrane, and the cysteine and/or glycine taken up. The γ-glutamylamino acids are also taken up and converted to 5-oxoproline and then to glutamate (Fig. 3.15) or, in the case of Glu-Cys, directly recycled to GSH. K_m values of the transpeptidase for GSH are in the μM range, similar to GSH levels in plasma (Table 3.7). **Acivicin**

is an experimentally used, powerful (but sadly not specific) inhibitor of γGGT, first isolated as a fermentation product of *Streptomyces sviceus*. γ-Glutamyltransferase is also involved in metabolism of glutathione–xenobiotic conjugates (Section 3.9.5 below) and in leukotriene biosynthesis (Fig. 7.23).

In summary, plasma GSH turns over rapidly (half time is a few minutes): it originates largely from the liver and is metabolized by γGGT in other tissues. Kidney is especially rich in γGGT, but lung and intestine also have high levels (Fig. 7.23).

3.9.4 Defects in GSH metabolism: humans and transgenic animals[158,160,162]

Humans with inborn deficiencies of γ-GCS (very rare), GSH synthetase (less rare), glutathione reductase, γGGT, GPx1 and 5-oxoprolinase have been reported. Such individuals often exhibit a tendency to haemolysis and neurological defects. Usually, however, there is some residual enzyme activity; a knockout of γ-GCS in mice, leading to very low GSH levels, was embryonic lethal. Some patients with glutathione reductase deficiency exhibit early cataract formation; cataracts are also observed in newborn mice treated with buthionine sulphoximine. In patients with severe GSH synthetase deficiency (**5-oxoprolinuria**) affecting several tissues, there is decreased feedback inhibition of γ-GCS and thus increased synthesis of γ-glutamylcysteine. Since the latter is a good substrate of γ-glutamyl cyclotransferase (Fig. 3.15), 5-oxoproline is overproduced, leading to life-threatening acidosis. Patients also suffer brain damage. In a milder form of GSH synthetase deficiency, apparently affecting only the erythrocytes, the genetic defect leads to synthesis of an unstable enzyme. Turnover of this active but unstable enzyme compensates for the defect in most cells, but not in the erythrocyte (which does not synthesize protein). Several other diseases have been associated with changes in GSH levels, but the contributions made by this to the disease pathology are uncertain (Table 3.8).

Mice lacking GPx1 develop and survive normally, but are more susceptible to certain toxins such as paraquat, O_3, and the anthracyclines, and to 'insults' such as myocardial or cerebral ischaemia–reperfusion.[163] They may also develop more severe

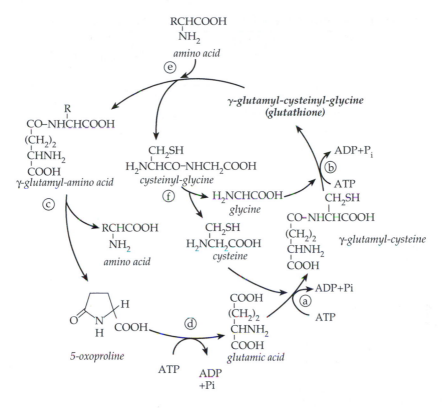

Figure 3.15 Glutathione synthesis and metabolism: (a) Glutamylcysteine synthetase; (b) glutathione synthetase; (c) γ-glutamyl cyclotransferase; (d) oxoprolinase; (e) γ-glutamyltranspeptidase; (f) dipeptidases (including leucine aminopeptidase). Diagram by courtesy of the late Professor Alton Meister and the American Society for Biochemistry and Molecular Biology.

cataracts with age than do control mice (Section 6.10.2.2). Since three other types of GPx exist *in vivo* as well as other peroxide-removing systems such as the peroxiredoxins (Section 3.11 below), this limited phenotype is perhaps predictable. In addition, ability to survive in the warm, well-fed laboratory environment is not necessarily to be interpreted as ability to survive in the stresses of the wild. Indeed, knockout of *both* GPx1 and GPx2 predisposed mice to intestinal inflammation and cancer,[164] and knockout of PHPGPx (GPx4) was reported to be embryonic lethal.[165] Knockout mice lacking γGGT showed elevated plasma and urinary GSH but decreased tissue levels. They suffered growth retardation, developed cataracts, and most died between 10 to 18 weeks of age, illustrating the importance of this enzyme in maintaining tissue GSH levels in mice. Mitochondrial GSH levels were subnormal and mitochondria damaged. Mice

are not men, however; patients with γGGT deficiency show normal cellular GSH levels, although plasma GSH is elevated, and seem to suffer few ill effects.

Mutant bacteria lacking enzymes involved in GSH synthesis are generally viable but often (not always) more sensitive to damage by radiation, peroxides and some other chemicals. Many bacteria, including *E. coli*, have transporters that enable them to take up GSH from the medium.[166] However, GSH-deficient *E. coli* have membranes leaky for K^+ and cannot grow in low-potassium media.[167] Glutathione deficiency may also impair reassembly of the [Fe–S] clusters in enzymes after inactivation by $O_2^{\bullet-}$ (Section 3.6.1). Several yeasts require GSH; knockout of γ-GCS has been reported in some, but not all yeasts, to produce organisms unable to grow unless GSH or its precursors are added to the medium.[168]

Table 3.8 Some human diseases with reported decreases in GSH

Disease	Tissue/body fluid	GSH (% of normal)	Further discussion in Section
AIDS	Variable reports		9.23.1
ARDS	Alveolar lining fluid	<10	9.7
Alcoholic liver disease	Liver	38–66	8.8
	Blood	64	
Non-alcoholic liver disease	Liver	63	8.8
	Blood	51–66	
Alcoholics	Lung lining fluid	14	8.8
Cigarette smokers	Red blood cells	126	8.12
Hereditary tyrosinaemia	Blood	34	–
	Liver	57	–
Idiopathic pulmonary fibrosis	Lung lining fluid	23	–
Kwashiorkor	Blood[a]	50	4.1
Anorexia nervosa	Blood[a]	~70	–
Parkinson's disease	Substantia nigra	60–72	9.19
Wilson's disease	Liver	13	3.15.5.5

Changes of GSH with age have also been reported (Section 10.4.4). ARDS, acute respiratory distress syndrome; ND, not determined. Adapted from *Life Sci,* **51**. 1083, 1992 by courtesy of Prof. A. Wendel and the publishers.

[a] Probably due to insufficient cysteine because of lack of dietary protein (*Am. J. Clin. Nutr.* **76**, 646, 2002; *Eur. J. Clin. Nutr.* **58**, 238, 2004)

3.9.5 The glutathione S-transferase superfamily[169]

Glutathione is also involved in the metabolism of **xenobiotics** ('foreign compounds') (Section 8.1). Many of them are metabolized by conjugation with GSH, catalysed by **glutathione S-transferase (GST)** enzymes

$$RX + GSH \rightarrow RSG + HX$$

For example, maize leaves contain an enzyme which detoxifies the herbicide **atrazine** by combining it with GSH. Some of the **herbicide safeners**, compounds that protect crops from injury by certain herbicides, act in part by raising GSH levels.[170]

Usually, conjugation with GSH is the first step in detoxifying a xenobiotic. Sometimes, however, the resulting products are also damaging. For example GSH conjugates of several halogenated hydrocarbons, including dibromo- and dichloroethane, cause kidney damage. Liver is especially rich in GST enzymes and the glutathione conjugates are often excreted into bile using ATP-dependent 'efflux pumps', some of which are also involved in

export of GSSG from liver.[150] Adducts can additionally be degraded by γGGT to remove glutamate and glycine; the cysteine conjugate is then acetylated to form a *N*-acetylcysteine conjugate (**mercapturic acid**) which can be excreted in the urine. Compounds metabolized by GST enzymes in animals include chloroform, adriamycin, BCNU, organic nitrates, bromobenzene, aflatoxin, DDT, naphthalene and paracetamol (Section 8.10). The presence of large amounts of such xenobiotics can decrease hepatic GSH concentrations, impairing the antioxidant defence capacity of the liver.

The most widely used substrate to assay GST activity is **1-chloro-2,4-dinitrobenzene** (CDNB), which is conjugated with GSH to give *S*-(2,4-dinitrophenyl)–glutathione, whose formation is assayed spectrophotometrically.

3.9.5.1 *Subclasses of GST*

All eukaryotes have multiple cytosolic and membrane-bound (e.g. in mitochondria and the ER) GST isoenzymes, with distinct substrate specificities. As well as their catalytic functions, many GSTs appear to serve as intracellular carrier proteins for haem,

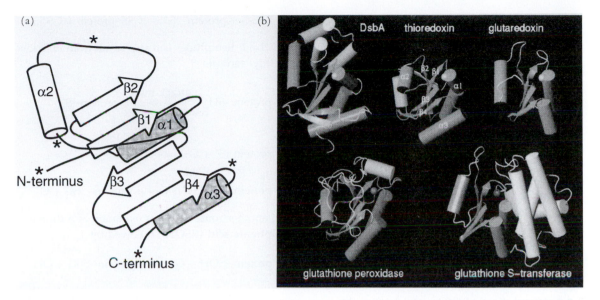

Figure 3.16 (see plate 6) The thioredoxin superfamily. (a) The thioredoxin 'fold' contains about 80 residues and involves β-sheets (β1−4) and α-helices (α1−3). An N-terminal β1α1β2 motif is linked to a C-terminal β3β4α3 motif by a loop of residues also containing a helix (α2). (b) Structural comparison of five proteins to show the presence of thioredoxin folds (in green). The protein **DsbA** is present in the periplasmic space of *E. coli* and involved in the folding of proteins exported from the cytoplasm. The atoms that interact with the cysteine residues of a substrate are shown as coloured balls; yellow is a sulphur atom of the more N-terminal cysteine in thioredoxin, DsbA and glutaredoxin, pink is the selenocysteine residue of bovine erythrocyte GPx and red the tyrosine hydroxyl of rat liver mu class GST. Adapted from *Structure* **3**, 245, 1995 by courtesy of Dr J. L. Martin and the publishers.

bilirubin, bile pigments, thyroid hormones and steroids, which bind non-enzymically to GSTs. The photosensitizer hypericin (Section 2.6.4.3) binds to some GSTs, attenuating its photochemical activity.[171] Cytosolic GSTs are dimers of subunits encoded by multiple gene families, at least seven in animals (alpha, zeta, mu, pi, omega, sigma, and theta). The two subunits can be identical, for example a dimer of type 1 mu subunits is written as GST M1-1. Subunits in the dimer can be different, but always come from the same family, for example a heterodimer of type 1 and 2 alpha subunits is A1-2. Similarly, P denotes pi, K kappa and T theta. For example, human liver contains GSTs A1-1, A1-2 and A2-2, among many others.

The alpha, mu and pi class enzymes are most abundant in mammals, and levels are often increased by exposure of the animal to xenobiotics via 'antioxidant response elements' (Section 4.5.10). Human gene polymorphisms that decrease the activity of certain GSTs (especially the **GSTM1 null genotype**, which abolishes GSTM1 activity) have been claimed to be associated with increased risk of cardiovascular disease and some forms of cancer, and to make humans more susceptible to ozone (Section 8.11.1). These polymorphisms may affect the response of patients to cancer chemotherapy.

In alpha, mu, pi and sigma GSTs, a tyrosine residue is important in GSH binding (e.g. Fig. 3.16, Plate 6) and $ONOO^-$ can inactivate the proteins by tyrosine nitration (Section 2.6.1).

3.9.5.2 *GSTs and lipid peroxidation*[169]

Some GSTs show a GPx-like activity with organic hydroperoxides, which was formerly called **non-selenium glutathione peroxidase**. They catalyse reaction of organic peroxides (but *not* of H_2O_2) with GSH to form GSSG and alcohols. Perfused livers from rats fed a selenium-deficient diet release no GSSG when H_2O_2 is infused, but do so when *tert*-butylhydroperoxide is infused, indicating that the GSTs can function in whole organs (Fig. 3.14). The significance of most GSTs as peroxide-metabolizing systems *in vivo* is uncertain. They can, however, cause confusion if synthetic organic hydroperoxides are used to assay 'GPx' in biological material. For example, cumene hydroperoxide will detect both 'real' GPx and some of the transferases. Thus it is better to use H_2O_2 as a substrate to assay GPx.

However, a few GSTs may be important protectors against lipid peroxidation. Some show PHGPx-like activity on membrane-associated lipid peroxides as well as on isolated fatty acid hydroperoxides, for example GST A1-1 and A1-2. Some can metabolize toxic end-products of lipid peroxidation, such as 4-hydroxynonenal (Section 4.12.5.3) and A_2/J_2 isoprostanes (Section 4.12.3). Thus knockout mice lacking GSTA4 had increased levels of HNE in the liver. In general, knockout of various GSTs produces a mild or null phenotype, probably because the activities of other GSTs often increase.

3.9.6 Mixed disulphides involving glutathione: pathological or protective?

Intracellular free glutathione is almost entirely present as GSH (Table 3.7), but some glutathione may exist as 'mixed disulphides' with other compounds that contain –SH groups. These can include cysteine, coenzyme A and –SH residues of several proteins, sometimes including human CuZnSOD (Section 3.2.1.5). If R–SH is used to represent the other thiols, then the mixed disulphides have the general formula:

$$\begin{array}{ccc} \text{Glu} & \text{Cys} & \text{Gly} \\ & | & \\ & \text{S---S---R} & \end{array}$$

Some may have biological effects, for example a coenzyme A-glutathione adduct was reported to be a powerful vasoconstrictor[172] and a cysteine–glutathione disulphide is a mating signal in the polychaete *Nereis succinea*.[173]

Thiol groups are often essential for protein function and the total level of protein–SH in cells may approach or exceed that of GSH. Similarly, plasma albumin contributes 300 to 500 µM –SH groups and is the major component of 'total –SH groups' in plasma. Protein thiol groups can react with GSSG to form mixed disulphides (a process that has been called **protein-S-glutathionylation**). Reaction with protein thiolate ions occurs much more readily than with unionized –SH groups

$$GSSG + protein –S^- \rightarrow GSS\text{-protein} + GS^-$$

Mixed disulphides can also result from reactions of thiyl radicals

$$protein–SH \xrightarrow[\text{reactive species}]{\text{attack by}} protein–S^\bullet$$

$$protein–S^\bullet + GSH \longrightarrow protein–S–S^{\bullet-}G$$

$$protein–S–S^{\bullet-}G + O_2 \longrightarrow protein–SSG + O_2^{\bullet-}$$

Yet another route involves oxidation of a thiol to a **sulphenic acid** (RSOH), followed by

$$protein–SOH + GS^- \longrightarrow protein–SSG + OH^-$$

The GSS–protein can remain as such, or react with another thiolate group (on the same or a different protein) to give inter- or intraprotein disulphides. Indeed, incubation of several enzymes and other proteins with GSSG *in vitro* causes inactivation, by forming mixed disulphides.[174,175] Examples include adenylate cyclase, isocitrate dehydrogenase, G3PDH, enolase and phosphofructokinase. Formation of GSSG in mitochondria can glutathionylate components of complex I and increase $O_2^{\bullet-}$ formation.[176] GSSG can inhibit protein synthesis in animal cells, and accumulation of GSSG was suggested to account for this inhibition in water-deprived mosses.[177] However, in a few cases glutathionylation activates an enzyme, carbonic anhydrase III (Section 10.4.5.1) being one.

Mixed disulphides of glutathione with proteins and other thiols accumulate in tissues subjected to oxidative stress, in both mitochondria and cytosol. For example, stimulation of the respiratory burst of human monocytes (Section 7.9.3) caused S-thiolation of several intracellular proteins,[178] including G3PDH. This and several other proteins are S-thiolated[174] when cells are treated with H_2O_2 or TNFα. These apparently damaging actions of GSSG may explain why cells keep intracellular GSSG levels low (Table 3.7) under normal conditions, and why some cells export GSSG when under oxidative stress. However, is glutathionylation as bad as it looks? Maybe not; it can also be regarded as protective. S-Thiolation is readily reversible; it may protect protein –SH groups from further oxidations (e.g. conversion of RS$^\bullet$ or RSOH species to **sulphinic** and **sulphonic acids**, RSO_2H and RSO_3H, which are harder to repair) when the cell is under oxidative stress, allowing later regeneration of them using GSH when normal redox balance has been restored. Reversible glutathionylation may even participate in cellular redox modulation. For example it has been suggested to regulate actin polymerization in A431 cells exposed to growth factors.[179]

Deglutathionylation is accelerated by the **glutaredoxin** proteins.[175,176] Glutaredoxin, sometimes called **thioltransferase**, was originally discovered as a cofactor of ribonucleotide reductase in *E. coli* (Section 7.2) but later found to be present in many organisms, including animals. Glutaredoxins are found in both mitochondria and cytosol and can be reduced directly by GSH. They are involved in catalysing thiol-disulphide interchange and the repair of glutathionylated proteins. Hence when cells have suffered excess protein glutathionylation due to oxidative stress, glutaredoxin can step in to help restore things to normal. Glutaredoxins also have **dehydroascorbate reductase** activity[180]

$$2GSH + \text{dehydroascorbate} \rightleftharpoons GSSG + \text{ascorbate}$$

Selenite (SeO_3^{2-}) can react with GSH to form the selenium equivalent of a mixed disulphide[181]

$$2H^+ + 4GSH + SeO_3^{2-} \rightarrow GSSG + GSSeSG + 3H_2O \quad \text{selenodiglutathione}$$

which is a metabolite of selenium in mammalian tissues. Further reduction of GSSeSG leads to **selenide**, Se^{2-}.

3.10 Protein-disulphide isomerase[182]

During folding of newly synthesized proteins, the correct –SH residues must join up to form the right disulphide bridges. **Chaperones** are present within cells to assist generally with protein folding (Section 4.6). **Protein-disulphide isomerase** (PDI) enzymes,

located in the lumen of the ER at concentrations close to mM, catalyse the formation of new disulphide bridges and the rearrangements of incorrect ones, by redox exchange with disulphides at the PDI active sites. The PDI is then reoxidized by **Ero proteins** whose reduced form can react with O_2, possibly producing ROS. The term 'ero' is an abbreviation for 'endoplasmic reticulum oxidoreductase'. The GSH/GSSG ratio is lower within the ER than in the rest of the cell, presumably to give optimum redox state for disulphide bridge formation. Glutathione made in the cytosol (Section 3.9.3) is imported into the ER lumen.

PDI enzymes also have dehydroascorbate reductase activity[180] and are involved in the action of **prolyl hydroxylase**, an ascorbate-dependent enzyme that hydroxylates proline residues during collagen synthesis. Prolyl hydroxylase is a tetramer of two α- and two β-subunits, the latter being identical to PDI and involved in interaction with ascorbate.

3.11 Thioredoxin and peroxiredoxins: key players in peroxide metabolism[183,184]

Thioredoxin has appeared in many guises in biology and only recently has its central importance to antioxidant defence and redox regulation in animals been appreciated (by contrast its role in redox regulation in chloroplasts has been known for decades; Section 6.8.10). Thioredoxin stimulates the growth of various cells in culture and several isolated protein 'factors' such as **adult T cell-leukaemia derived factor, T-hybridoma (MP-6)-derived B cell stimulatory factor** and **early pregnancy factor** were later found to be identical with thioredoxin. *In vivo*, thioredoxin acts as a reducing agent for ribonucleotide reductase (Section 7.2) and **methionine sulphoxide reductases**, enzymes that repair oxidative damage to methionine residues in proteins (Section 4.14.1). In *Drosophila*, glutathione reductase appears to be absent and thioredoxin is used to regenerate GSH from GSSG.[185]

Thioredoxins are polypeptides of relative molecular mass about 12 000, found in both prokaryotes and eukaryotes and widely distributed in mammalian cells. Several different thioredoxins have been described, for example the cytosolic **Trx1** and the mitochondrial **Trx2**. Reduced thioredoxins contain two –SH groups that form a disulphide in oxidized thioredoxin. They undergo redox reactions with multiple proteins

$$\text{Thioredoxin} - (SH)_2 + \text{protein} - S_2 \rightleftharpoons$$
$$\text{thioredoxin} - S_2 + \text{protein} - (SH)_2$$

Thioredoxins bind to target proteins and, via intermediate formation of a mixed disulphide, reduce the protein disulphide bridge whilst oxidizing themselves. The $E^{\circ\prime}$ of thioredoxins is about $-0.27\,V$, indicating their high reducing potential. Thioredoxins can also mediate thiol-disulphide exchange between a protein dithiol and another protein disulphide. Features of the thioredoxin structure are seen in several related proteins including glutaredoxin, GPxs, GSTs and PDI, where the thioredoxin-like domains form the active site. All these proteins may have evolved from a common 'thiol-binding protein' ancestor (Fig. 3.16). Selenite and GSSeSG (Section 3.9.6) can bind to –SH groups on thioredoxin and inhibit its function.[181]

Oxidized thioredoxins are reduced *in vivo* in animals by **thioredoxin reductase** enzymes, which contain selenium (as selenocysteine) and FAD and show similarities to glutathione reductases, including use of NADPH (contrast this with glutaredoxin, which is reduced directly by GSH)

$$\text{thioredoxin-}S_2 + NADPH + H^+ \rightarrow$$
$$NADP^+ + \text{thioredoxin-}(SH)_2$$

However, the chloroplast enzyme uses ferredoxin as an electron donor (Section 6.8.10). Thioredoxin reductase can also reduce PDI and thus achieve an NADPH-dependent reduction of the disulphide bridges of such proteins as insulin. Chloro-2,4-dinitrobenzene (CDNB), a substrate of GSTs (Section 3.9.5), is an inhibitor of thioredoxin reductase. The $-NO_2$ group is reduced to form nitro radicals, which then reoxidize to generate $O_2^{\bullet-}$ (Section 8.18). Hence CDNB converts the enzyme to a $O_2^{\bullet-}$-producing NADPH oxidase.[183] Curcumin does the same (Section 3.22.3 below).

Peroxiredoxins are a family of peroxidases that reduce H_2O_2 and organic peroxides (Figure 3.17). They are homodimers and contain no prosthetic groups: the redox reactions are dependent on cysteine at the active sites. There are at least three classes; the **typical 2-cys** (the most common), the **atypical 2-cys** and the **1-cys** peroxiredoxins. In all cases, the peroxide oxidizes an –SH group on the peroxiredoxin to a sulphenic acid, cys–SOH. In the 2-cys enzymes, this sulphenic acid reacts with another –SH on the protein to give a disulphide that is then reduced by thioredoxin (Fig. 3.17). In typical 2-cys enzymes, the second thiol is on the other subunit, in atypical 2-cys on the same subunit. In 1-cys peroxiredoxins, it is not yet clear which cellular reductant regenerates the –SH group; it's not thioredoxin.

The first peroxiredoxin to be identified was found in yeast and originally named **thiol specific antioxidant**, but we now know that peroxiredoxins are widely distributed in animals, plants and bacteria. Thus the **alkyl hydroperoxide reductase** (AHPR) system of bacteria such as *Salmonella*

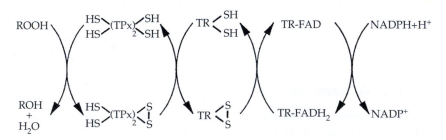

Figure 3.17 Two-cys peroxiredoxins are **thioredoxin-dependent peroxide reductases** (TPx). Trx, thioredoxin; TR, thioredoxin reductase. Adapted from *J. Biol. Chem.* **269**, 27670, 1994 by courtesy of Drs Sue Goo Rhee and Ho Zoon Chae and the American Society for Biochemistry and Molecular Biology.

typhimurium, which uses NAD(P)H to reduce thymine, linoleic acid and cumene hydroperoxides to alcohols, involves a typical 2-cys peroxiredoxin as one of its two subunits (**AhpC**); the other (**AhpF**) is a flavoprotein that mediates the electron supply from NAD(P)H. Peroxiredoxins are even found in the archeae, indicating an ancient evolutionary origin. Several pathogenic bacteria, including *Vibrio cholerae*, contain hybrid proteins with both peroxiredoxin and glutaredoxin domains.[186]

Currently available data indicate that peroxiredoxins are probably more important peroxide-removing systems in animals than catalase or GPx1 and they often constitute 0.1 to 0.8% of the total soluble protein of mammalian cells. At least six different types are known, designated as **prx1**, **prx2** etc. The Prx1 to 4 forms are typical 2-cys peroxiredoxins, prx5 is atypical 2-cys and **prx6** belongs to the 1-cys class. The **Prx3** form occurs only in mitochondria whereas Prx1, -2 and -6 are cytosolic. The **Prx4** form is found in the ER and extracellularly, **prx5** in both mitochondria and peroxisomes.

3.11.1 Catalase, glutathione peroxidases and peroxiredoxins: fitting it all together[184]

These three families of enzymes can remove H_2O_2 *in vivo*, so how do they co-operate and co-ordinate? Low levels of H_2O_2 contribute to redox regulation and signal transduction (Section 4.5), so how does the cell arrange its peroxide-metabolizing enzymes to allow this?

Catalase may be the key enzyme for H_2O_2 removal in peroxisomes (although prx5 might contribute). Mitochondria usually lack catalase; although there is some in rat heart mitochondria, its contribution to H_2O_2 removal appears small.[128] Hydrogen peroxide produced elsewhere in the cell could diffuse into peroxisomes for removal, perhaps the 'ultimate sink'. However, humans and animals can survive without catalase and mice without GPx1. Mitochondria contain GSH, glutaredoxin, thioredoxin, thioredoxin reductase, GPx1 and peroxiredoxins: these organelles generate and release H_2O_2, but they can also catabolize added H_2O_2.[187] Mitochondrial H_2O_2 may sometimes be a redox-signal to the nucleus (Section 4.5.7), yet how

can it be released when so many H_2O_2-catabolizing enzymes are present? We don't know, sorry.

Red blood cells generate H_2O_2 (Section 6.4) and many early papers discussed the relative importance of catalase and GPx in removing it. The general conclusion was that catalase is more important at high fluxes of H_2O_2 (e.g. when H_2O_2 or ROS-producing toxins are added) whereas GPx1 deals with lower 'physiological' levels of H_2O_2 generation. Sadly, however, GPx1-knockout mice do not show haemolysis. By contrast, knockout of prx1 in mice causes shortened lifespan due to early development of both cancers and severe haemolytic anaemia. Anaemia is also seen in pr2– knockouts. Hence peroxiredoxins play a key role in erythrocyte antioxidant defence, at least in older mice. Similarly, knockout of prx6 in mice markedly increased lung damage and decreased survival on exposure to 100% O_2 whereas overexpression of prx6 diminished O_2 toxicity.[188] *S. cerevisiae* lacking peroxiredoxins show an enhanced mutation rate and are more readily damaged by H_2O_2 or $ONOO^-$. They also have increased contents of GSH and glutathione reductase, suggesting an attempt at compensation. Indeed, these yeast were hypersensitive to GSH-depleting agents.[189]

Peroxiredoxins are slower at catalysing H_2O_2 removal than GPx, although the large amounts present and their low K_m for H_2O_2 ($<20\,\mu M$) can compensate for this. They are readily inactivated by H_2O_2, the essential cysteine being oxidized to a sulphinic acid, cys-SO_2H. Indeed, inactivated peroxiredoxins accumulate in cells subjected to such oxidative stresses as treatment with H_2O_2. The eukaryotic enzymes are more susceptible to oxidation than bacterial ones. It has been suggested[184,190] that at low physiological H_2O_2 concentrations, peroxiredoxins dispose of most H_2O_2 generated inside cells. However, when the cell senses extra H_2O_2 (e.g. at a site of inflammation), and a response is required to allow gene expression by redox regulation, the peroxiredoxins are partially inactivated to allow some H_2O_2 to act on transcription factors. Inactivation is both by sulphinic acid formation and by glutathionylation. The cell can then make more peroxiredoxin, and also reactivate the inactive form, so that the extra H_2O_2 can be removed after it has done its job. For the 2-cys peroxiredoxins, reactivation of the sulphinic acid form is achieved by the protein **sulphiredoxin**, which can draw reducing power from either GSH or reduced thioredoxin. Thioredoxin and peroxiredoxins can also form mixed disulphides with glutathione (Section 3.9.6) in some oxidatively stressed cells, perhaps temporarily inactivating them but preventing sulphinic acid generation.

Peroxide metabolism is also influenced by phosphorylation and dephosphorylation, itself subject to cellular redox regulation (Section 4.5.5). The Prx1 and 2 proteins can be phosphorylated by cyclin-dependent kinases (Section 9.13), which decreases peroxiredoxin activity. It is interesting to speculate that this relates to the proproliferative effects of H_2O_2 (Section 4.2.1). By contrast, GPx1 and catalase are phosphorylated by the c-Abl and arg kinases, which activates them (Section 4.5.5).

In *E. coli*, AHPR may be the most important scavenger of metabolically produced H_2O_2, but catalase is important when exogenous levels of H_2O_2 are high, since the activity of AHPR is saturated at low H_2O_2 levels and the supply of NADH may limit its action.[191] *E. coli* also has a periplasmic 'thiol peroxidase' resembling atypical 2-cys-peroxiredoxins, and seemingly important in metabolizing organic peroxides.[192] In *H. pylori* lacking AHPR, organic peroxides accumulated and caused partial inactivation of catalase.[193]

Bacterial peroxiredoxins have also been suggested[194] to play protective roles against $ONOO^-$; a similar role has been suggested for human prx5.[195] In all cases, the reactions are rapid and could conceivably out compete CO_2 or GSH for reaction with $ONOO^-$ *in vivo*.

3.11.2 Selenium deficiency: reinterpretation of an old paradigm

Selenium deficiency in animals produces a variety of diseases similar to those induced by lack of α-tocopherol (Section 3.20.2 below).[196] They include **white muscle disease**, a muscle wasting syndrome (mink, horses, pigs, cattle, sheep), **mulberry heart disease** (pigs) and infertility (many species). The effects of selenium deficiency can often be overcome by giving excess α-tocopherol, and *vice versa*.

Exceptions to this generalization include the observation that selenium cannot protect female rats against foetal reabsorption caused by α-tocopherol lack, nor can α-tocopherol protect rats against the damage to the pancreas that occurs on selenium-deficient diets. Rats fed diets lacking Se and α-tocopherol showed elevated plasma levels of F_2 isoprostanes,[197] a biomarker of lipid peroxidation, and selenium deficiency also causes increased protein oxidation.

In thinking about how selenium relates to antioxidant defence, most emphasis was initially placed on GPx1. We now know that other GPx proteins may be more important (Section 3.8.1), and that Se is required for thioredoxin reductase (Section 3.11) and methionine sulphoxide reductase B (Section 4.14.1). Selenoproteins P and W might also be antioxidants (Section 3.8.2).

3.11.2.1 *Human selenium deficiency*

The importance of selenium in the human diet was appreciated fully after the discovery of a selenium-responsive degenerative heart disease, **Keshan disease**. Symptoms include wasting and enlargement of the heart, heart rhythm disruptions and eventual cardiac arrest in severe cases. The name comes from an episode in 1935 in which 57 out of 286 inhabitants of a village in Keshan country of Heilongjiang province in China died of the disease. Epidemiological studies showed that the incidence of Keshan disease was correlated with that of animal degenerative diseases already known to be related to selenium deficiency. Both Keshan disease and the animal diseases could be prevented by administration of small doses of sodium selenite (Na_2SeO_3). In all affected areas, selenium concentrations in foodstuffs were found to be low. Whole-blood selenium levels in many countries fall into the 1 to 3 μM range but levels in subjects with Keshan disease were much lower (Table 3.9). Measurements of total selenium and GPx activity in whole blood from New Zealanders showed a good correlation between these two parameters at total blood selenium concentrations up to 1.3 μM, but not at higher levels. It seems from this and other data that about 1 μM is the 'threshold figure' at which GPx (at least in blood) reaches maximum activity. This enzyme is the most responsive to Se

Table 3.9 Some illustrative human blood selenium concentrations

	Concentration in whole blood (μM)
Azerbaijan	1.39
Canada	2.31
China, Peoples' Republic of	
High-selenium area with toxicity	40.52
High-selenium area without toxicity	5.57
Moderate selenium area (Beijing)	1.20
Low-selenium area without disease	0.34
Low-selenium area with Keshan disease and/or Kashin–Beck disease	0.15
Egypt	0.86
Finland	0.71
Guatemala	0.29
New Zealand	0.86
Senegal, Velingara	1.11
Sweden	1.52
UK	
1974	4.05
1986	1.52
1991	0.96
Ukraine	5.59
USA	
South Dakota	3.24
Ohio	1.98
Venezuela	
High-selenium area	10.30
Moderate-selenium area	4.50
Zaire	
Karawa schoolchildren	0.39
Karawa cretins	0.29
Businga adults	0.60
Kikwit adults	2.49

Data selected from Diplock, AT (1993) Am. *J. Clin. Nutr. Suppl.* **57**, 256S, by courtesy of Professor AT Diplock. Selenium intakes and blood levels have fallen in the UK due to dietary changes (e.g. less use of flour from selenium-rich wheat imported from the USA).

withdrawal in animal experiments (Section 3.8.2), suggesting it may be a good marker of Se status in the above range.

An abnormally low selenium intake appears to be the major factor leading to Keshan disease, but not the sole cause. For example, Keshan disease was not endemic in all low-selenium areas of China and seasonal variations in disease incidence did not seem to be caused by changes in selenium (or α-tocopherol) intake. One factor predisposing to cardiomyopathy may be infection with **Coxsackie viruses**.

Feeding mice a selenium-deficient diet (or knocking out GPx1) favoured selection and replication of a damaging viral subtype in the heart after inoculation of the animals with a normally-benign strain.[198]

Selenium deficiency has also been implicated in **Kashin–Beck disease** (named after the Russian scientists who first described it), a disabling joint disease seen in children in Northern China, North Korea and East Siberia. Administration of sodium selenite and α-tocopherol during the early stages of the disease has beneficial effects. The geographical distribution of Kashin–Beck disease resembles (but is not identical with) that of Keshan disease, and iodine deficiency may also play a role; both iodine and Se are involved in thyroid hormone metabolism.[199] Another factor may be the level of mycotoxins in food.

A study of blood selenium levels led Chinese scientists to conclude that a minimum adequate dietary intake for humans is about 30 μg. Normal daily intakes in advanced countries are in the range 30 to 200 μg/day and recommended dietary allowances are usually 50 to 70 μg. Larger amounts (>500 μg/day) can produce toxic effects: an early sign of excess selenium intake is deformation and loss of fingernails, toenails and sometimes hair, and a 'garlic breath' smell due to **dimethylselenide**, $(CH_3)_2Se$. Selenium-accumulating plants such as *Astragalus* (**milk vetch**) species can poison cattle (leading to **blind staggers** and **alkali disease**) and are a particular nuisance to farmers in certain parts of the world.[200] Indeed, in 1295 the explorer Marco Polo described a disease of horses that sounds exactly like selenium toxicity. Selenium poisoning has been reported in patients who consumed Se–containing supplements to great excess. The toxicity of selenite (SeO_3^{2-}) to *E. coli* appears to involve[201] production of excess $O_2^{\bullet-}$.

Selenium deficiency has sometimes been claimed to accompany protein–calorie malnutrition or prolonged intravenous feeding, but reports are often inconclusive. Residents of low-selenium areas in Finland or New Zealand appear to suffer no obvious ill-effects, although they may well eat, of course, food that was grown in areas of higher selenium. Nevertheless, suggestions remain that low blood selenium might predispose to cardiovascular disease, cancer or complications of pregnancy. The Finnish government began supplementing fertilizers with selenium in 1984 for this reason. Selenium can be detected in rat and human urine as selenosugars including **1β-methylseleno-N-acetyl-D-galactosamine**.[202]

3.12 Other sulphur-containing compounds involved in antioxidant defence

Reduced glutathione plays key metabolic roles in animals, plants and some bacteria. However, many organisms, especially prokaryotes (some of which do not produce any GSH) and plants, contain other sulphur-containing compounds that could fulfil similar roles. For example. γ-glutamylcysteine is a major thiol in halobacteria,[203] and **homoglutathione** (γ-glutamylcysteinylalanine; Fig. 3.13) accumulates in certain higher plants.[204] Some mycobacteria (including *M. tuberculosis*) and *Streptomycetes* produce a cysteine derivative, **2-(N-acetylcysteinyl)amido-2-deoxyα-D-glucopyranosyl-*myo*-inositol (mycothiol)**,[205] apparently as an alternative to GSH (Fig. 3.18). Sea-urchin eggs contain **ovothiol C**, apparently to scavenge H_2O_2 (Fig. 7.6). The pathogenic amoeba *Entamoeba*

histolytica, which causes the unpleasant intestinal disease amoebiasis in humans, lacks GSH and accumulates cysteine instead.[206] By contrast, *Streptococcus agalactiae* makes GSH, but is unusual in that its γ-GCS and glutathione synthetase activities are not separate enzymes, but part of the same protein.[207]

3.12.1 Trypanothione: an antioxidant defence in some parasites[206,208]

Some parasitic protozoa, such as *Crithidia fasciculata* or *Trypanosoma brucei*, lack GSH but contain **trypanothione**, two glutathione molecules covalently linked to the polyamine **spermidine** (Fig. 3.18). Trypanothione forms part of a system for removing H_2O_2 and organic peroxides that may be especially important to these parasites, since they often lack catalase or GPx, yet contain SODs (usually FeSOD). The system has four components. A peroxiredoxin-like **tryparedoxin peroxidase** removes peroxides by oxidizing the protein **tryparedoxin**. This is re-reduced by trypanothione, the oxidized form of which is regenerated at the expense of NADPH by a

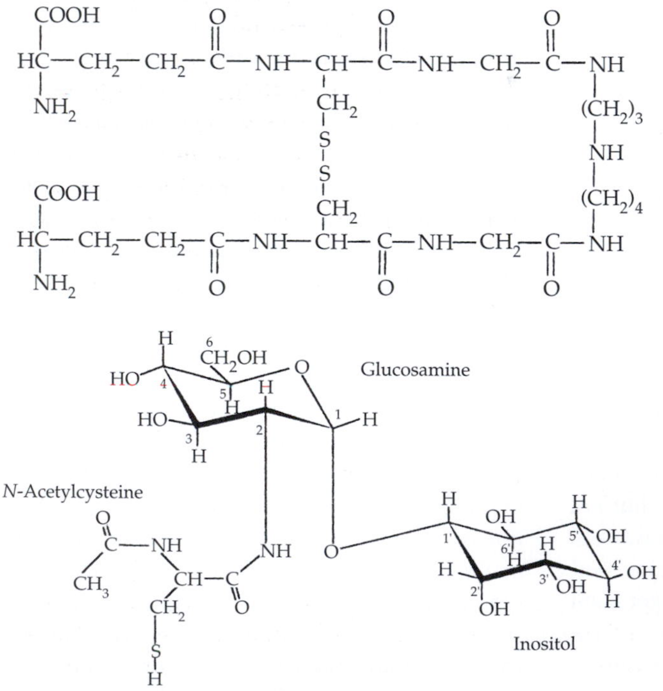

Figure 3.18 Structures of trypanothione disulphide (top) and mycothiol (bottom). Bottom diagram from *Biochem. J.* **325**, 623, 1997 by courtesy of Dr D.J. Steenkamp and the Biochemical Society. Several bacteria replace GSH by other thiols, e.g. *Borrelia burgdorferi* (the causative agent of Lyme disease) accumulates coenzyme A instead (*Mol. Microbiol.* **59**, 475, 2006).

flavoprotein **trypanothione reductase** that resembles glutathione reductase. Many parasites contain additional peroxiredoxins,[209] and sometimes ovothiol A (Fig. 7.6) as well as ascorbate peroxidases (Section 3.13.7 below), the dehydroascorbate being reduced by trypanothione back to ascorbate. Tryparedoxin peroxidase might also help to remove $ONOO^-$.

Compounds that interfere with these systems might be useful in treating diseases caused by parasites, for example African sleeping sickness (*T. brucei*), Chagas' disease (*T. cruzi*) and leishmaniasis. Trivalent **arsenicals** (R-As$=$O) and trivalent **antimonials** (Sb(III)) inhibit trypanothione reductase, and some quinones and nitrocompounds interact with this enzyme to generate ROS and exert cytotoxic effects (Section 8.18).

3.12.2 Ergothioneine[210,211]

Ergothioneine, which exists in equilibrium between thiol and thione forms (Fig. 3.19), was first discovered in *Claviceps purpurea* (the ergot fungus). Early work also detected it in rat erythrocytes and liver and suggested that it arose from dietary plant material, although the distribution of ergothioneine in plants and animals has not been fully investigated. Its presence in human, rat and other animal tissues has been confirmed by HPLC and nuclear magnetic resonance techniques and the genes encoding membrane transporters for it are highly expressed in some cells, for example monocytes, intestine, kidney and trachea.

The function of ergothioneine is unknown. *In vitro*, it forms stable complexes with iron and copper ions, and reacts with HOCl, $ONOO^-$, $OH^\bullet$, $RO^\bullet$, $RO_2^\bullet$ and haem ferryl species. The one-electron oxidation product of ergothioneine can be re-reduced by ascorbate ($k = 6.3 \times 10^8 M^{-1}s^{-1}$).[212] More work is needed to establish the levels, and origin, of ergothioneine in animal tissues and to investigate its putative antioxidant role.

3.13 Antioxidant defence enzymes: other peroxidases

Peroxidases are enzymes that uses a peroxide to oxidize another substrate. Some are specific for a single substrate (such as GP$\times$1 for GSH), but most have a broader specificity.

3.13.1 Cytochrome *c* peroxidase: another specific peroxidase[111,213]

The haem-containing enzyme **cytochrome *c* peroxidase** (CCP) is found in some bacteria (e.g. *N. gonorrhoeae*), fungi (e.g. *Cryptococcus neoformans*), and between the inner and outer membranes of *S. cerevisiae* mitochondria, which contain no catalase (an enzyme mostly present in cytosol and peroxisomes in this yeast).

The CCP enzyme reacts rapidly with H_2O_2 to form a stable enzyme–substrate complex with an absorbance maximum at 419 nm, whereas that of the free enzyme is at 407 nm. Hydrogen peroxide performs two-electron oxidation; the haem Fe(III) is oxidized to a Fe(IV) state and there is one-electron oxidation of a tryptophan residue (Trp191) in the active site to a radical. Two molecules of reduced cytochrome *c* (Fe^{2+}) are then oxidized to the Fe(III) form and the enzyme returns to its resting state. An

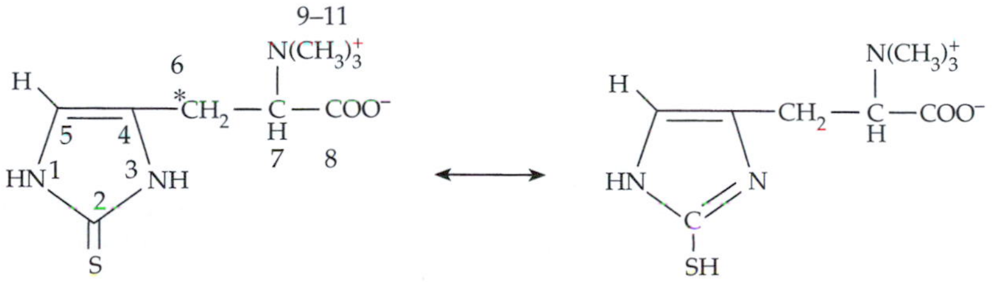

Figure 3.19 Structure of the thiol (right) and thione (left) forms of ergothioneine. The thione predominates at pH 7.4. * A hydroxylated ergothioneine with an extra −OH at position 6 has been isolated from the mushroom *Lyophyllum connatum* (*Biosci. Biotechnol. Biochem.* **69**, 357, 2005).

electron from the first cytochrome c neutralizes the tryptophan radical, leaving compound II (still a ferryl haem species) and the second electron reforms the Fe(III) enzyme. Under some experimental conditions the reverse can happen; the ferryl is reduced first. Spectrophotometric measurement of the CCP enzyme–substrate complex has been used to assay H_2O_2 (Section 5.8).

3.13.2 NADH oxidase

Many bacteria contain enzymes that oxidize NADH and reduce O_2 to H_2O, or sometimes to H_2O_2 (e.g. in *Enterococcus faecium*).[214] It is often suggested that the H_2O-producing enzymes act in anaerobes as 'O_2-scavenging' systems, removing O_2 and preventing O_2 toxicity at the expense of cellular reducing equivalents.[215] However, one must bear in mind that NADH oxidase activities assayed in crude extracts could belong to a variety of enzyme systems. Thus the flavoprotein NADH oxidases reported from *Amphibacillus xylanus* and many other bacteria are probably part of an AHPR system, and serve to *consume* H_2O_2 when the peroxiredoxin-like component (Section 3.11) is added.[216]

13.3.3 'Non-specific' peroxidases

Plants and bacteria often harbour haem-containing peroxidases capable of using H_2O_2 to oxidize a range of substrates, for example *E. coli* HP-I is a bifunctional catalase-peroxidase (Section 3.7.1). 'Non-specific' peroxidases are usually assayed in cell extracts using artificial substrates, which are oxidized in the presence of H_2O_2 to give coloured or fluorescent products. Often the true substrates of these peroxidases *in vivo* have not been identified. Such artificial substrates include **guaiacol** (a phenol produced by certain millipedes, possibly as a defence system; structure shown in Fig. 3.33 below),[217] **benzidine** (Fig. 9.20) and *o*-**dianisidine**.

'Non-specific' peroxidases are also present in animals. **Myeloperoxidase** (MPO) is found in phagocytic cells (Section 7.7.3) and **thyroid peroxidase** helps make the thyroid hormones (Section 7.5.1). **Lactoperoxidase** (LPO) is found in milk, respiratory tract mucus (e.g. in sheep) and

saliva.[218,219] It may have an antibacterial role, since (among many other substrates), LPO can oxidize thiocyanate (SCN^-) ions, found in both milk and saliva, into **hypothiocyanite** ($OSCN^-$). This is toxic to several bacteria, including *E. coli*, streptococci and *Salmonella typhimurium*. It is also produced when HOCl or MPO oxidize SCN^- (Section 2.6.3). Lactoperoxidase may be one of the factors in milk that protect babies against infections of the gastrointestinal tract. The H_2O_2 that it needs to oxidize SCN^- can arise from certain other bacteria (e.g. *Streptococcus sanguis*), which excrete H_2O_2 into their surroundings, and from NADPH oxidases on mucosal surfaces (Section 7.10).[219] Hydrogen peroxide is also often present in beverages (Section 2.6.2).

3.13.4 Horseradish peroxidase[220]

One of the most-studied non-specific peroxidases is **horseradish peroxidase** (HRP), obtained from the roots of the horseradish plant (*Armoracia rusticana*). Several different forms exist, each containing bound carbohydrate and calcium ions, but all have broad substrate specificity. For example, HRPs will oxidize guaiacol, pyrogallol, CN^-, I^-, Br^-, NADH, thiol compounds and phenols. Oxidations by HRP, and probably by most other non-specific peroxidases, usually occur by the following reactions, in which SH_2 is the substrate:

$$\text{peroxidase} + H_2O_2 \rightarrow \text{compound I}$$

$$\text{compound I} + SH_2 \rightarrow SH^{\bullet} + \text{compound II} + H^+$$

$$\text{compound II} + SH_2 \rightarrow SH^{\bullet} + \text{peroxidase} + H^+$$

The haem iron in 'resting' peroxidase is Fe(III). Hydrogen peroxide removes two electrons to give compound I, which contains iron in the Fe(IV) oxidation state (perhaps as Fe(IV)=O), the extra oxidizing capacity being accommodated by one-electron oxidation of the haem to a radical cation (haem$^{\bullet+}$). The two electrons are replaced in two one-electron steps, in each of which a substrate molecule forms a radical, $SH^{\bullet}$. Hence peroxidase–H_2O_2 mixtures have been used to generate free radicals in the laboratory from almost every compound under the sun. Compound II is the intermediate state; the haem iron is still ferryl but the haem$^{\bullet+}$ radical has been neutralized by one-electron addition. In LPO the cation radical can sometimes be reduced by the protein, giving a tyrosine radical plus a haem ferryl species.[221]

The substrate-derived radicals have several fates. They might undergo disproportionation, one reducing the other to SH$_2$ whilst oxidizing itself to S

$$SH^\bullet + SH^\bullet \rightarrow S + SH_2$$

They might link together; for example, tyrosine phenoxyl radicals can produce bityrosine (Fig. 2.6). They could also interact with O$_2$

$$SH^\bullet + O_2 \rightarrow S + O_2^{\bullet-} + H^+$$

Superoxide can give H$_2$O$_2$ by dismutation

$$O_2^{\bullet-} + O_2^{\bullet-} + 2H^+ \rightarrow H_2O_2 + O_2$$

Thus, when HRP is oxidizing a substrate whose radical reduces O$_2$ to O$_2^{\bullet-}$, only trace amounts of H$_2$O$_2$ are needed. For example, oxidation of NADH by HRP occurs without addition of H$_2$O$_2$, since traces of H$_2$O$_2$ are present in NADH solutions due to autoxidation.[222] The HRP-mediated NADH oxidation generates NAD$^\bullet$ radical and O$_2^{\bullet-}$.

$$peroxidase + H_2O_2 \rightarrow compound\ I$$

$$compound\ I + NADH \rightarrow compound\ II + NAD^\bullet \\ + H_2O$$

$$compound\ II + NADH \rightarrow peroxidase + NAD^\bullet \\ + H_2O$$

$$2NAD^\bullet + 2O_2 \rightarrow 2NAD^+ + 2O_2^{\bullet-}$$

$$2O_2^{\bullet-} + 2H^+ \rightarrow H_2O_2 + O_2\ (dismutation)$$

---

overall reaction: $2NADH + O_2 + 2H^+$
$+ 2NAD^+ + 2H_2O$

NAD$^\bullet$ radicals can also form a dimer:

$$NAD^\bullet + NAD^\bullet \rightarrow (NAD)_2$$

but this reaction has a lower rate constant $(3 \times 10^7 M^{-1}s^{-1})$ than the reaction of NAD$^\bullet$ with

O$_2$ $(k_2 = 1.0 \times 10^9 M^{-1}s^{-1})$. NADH oxidation is an example of the **oxidase reactions of peroxidase**, as compared with its 'normal' reactions in which equal amounts of SH$_2$ and H$_2$O$_2$ are used up and no O$_2$ is consumed.

Superoxide can react[223] with HRP to generate **oxyperoxidase**, or **compound III**:

$$enzyme\text{-}Fe(\text{III}) + O_2^{\bullet-} \rightarrow enzyme\ (Fe^{2+} - O_2)$$

Oxyperoxidase oxidizes NADH only slowly, and its accumulation during the reaction slows down the rate of NADH oxidation.[222] Compound III decays spontaneously, but slowly, to release O$_2^{\bullet-}$.

Several non-specific peroxidases (including HRP) can oxidize thiols into thiyl radicals[224] in the presence of H$_2$O$_2$. For example

$$H_2O_2 + 2GSH \rightarrow 2H_2O + 2GS^\bullet$$

These radicals can then participate in several reactions that result in O$_2$ uptake, for example for GS$^\bullet$

$$GS^\bullet + GS^- \rightarrow GSSG^{\bullet-}$$
(ionized form of GSH)

$$GSSG^{\bullet-} + O_2 \rightarrow GSSG + O_2^{\bullet-}$$

$$GS^\bullet + O_2 \rightarrow GSO_2^\bullet$$

Another oxidase reaction of peroxidase is its action on **2-nitropropane** (CH$_3$CH(NO$_2$)CH$_3$),[225] a compound used as a solvent (e.g. in inks, paints and varnishes) and also found in cigarette smoke; a 'standard' US filterless cigarette generates smoke containing about 1 µg of 2-nitropropane. Peroxidases use traces of H$_2$O$_2$ to initiate nitropropane oxidation, generating intermediate radicals that reduce O$_2$ to O$_2^{\bullet-}$. Superoxide then participates in continued oxidation.

3.13.5 Why do plants have so much peroxidase?[220]

Deposition of lignin in plant cell walls involves the polymerization of phenols derived from phenylalanine (Section 7.5.4.1). Peroxidases bound to the cell walls oxidize the phenols into **phenoxyl**

radicals, which polymerize to form lignin. One source of the required H_2O_2 appears to be the simultaneous oxidation by peroxidase of NADH generated by a malate dehydrogenase enzyme, also bound to the cell walls.[226] Lignin destruction by fungi also involves peroxidases (Section 7.5.4.2).

Peroxidases are additionally involved in fruit ripening, defence reactions against pathogens (Section 7.11) and in degradation of the plant growth hormone, **indoleacetic acid** (**auxin**). This reaction is more complex than most peroxidase-catalysed reactions and involves several radicals (Fig. 3.20).

3.13.6 Chloroperoxidase and bromoperoxidase[227]

Chloroperoxidase was first isolated from the fungus *Caldariomyces fumago*. It contains haem and catalyses the usual 'non-specific' peroxidase reactions, and can show catalase activity under certain conditions. In addition, it adds halogen atoms to a range of substrates in the presence of H_2O_2 and chloride, bromide or iodide. If SH is the substrate and X^- the halide, the reaction is

$$\text{substrate-H} + X^- + H_2O_2 + H^+ \rightarrow$$
$$\text{substrate-X} + 2H_2O$$

For example, tyrosine can be converted to chloro-bromo- or iodotyrosine depending on the halide ion added. For chlorination, HOCl is involved in the reaction mechanism.

Many marine organisms are rich in halogenated compounds (possibly produced as antimicrobial agents) and contain similar enzymes. In some cases only one halide is a substrate, for example a bromoperoxidase has been isolated from several marine organisms. Bromoperoxidases from a few fungi, several marine algae (e.g. the brown alga *Ascophyllum nodosum*) and the lichen *Xanthoria parietina* contain vanadium (as vanadate) at the active site instead of haem, as does the chloroperoxidase from the fungus *Curvularia inaequalis*, which again uses HOCl as a reaction intermediate.[227] A vanadium-dependent iodoperoxidase was found in the brown alga *Laminaria digitata*.[228]

3.13.7 Ascorbate peroxidase[229]

Chloroplasts (Section 6.8.7), green algae and cyanobacteria contain **ascorbate peroxidase** enzymes, which catalyse the overall reaction

$$\text{ascorbate} + H_2O_2 \rightarrow 2H_2O + \text{dehydroascorbate}$$

They are haem proteins with some structural resemblance to CCP (Section 3.13.1) but operate by 'classical' peroxidase mechanisms, that is they form ascorbyl radical, which then disproportionates into ascorbate and dehydroascorbate (DHA). They can also oxidize other substrates such as pyrogallol or guaiacol. Compound I is a Fe(IV)-haem cation radical.

When incubated with H_2O_2 in the absence of ascorbate, ascorbate peroxidase is inactivated, apparently by reaction of compound I with H_2O_2 to cause destruction of the haem ring.[230]

3.13.8 Peroxidase 'mimics'

Myoglobin, haemoglobin and complexes of haemoglobin with haptoglobins (Section 3.16.3 below) display some peroxidase activities *in vitro* using H_2O_2 and a suitable electron donor. The peroxidase properties of haemoglobin form the basis of a diagnostic test for gastrointestinal bleeding (**faecal occult blood test**).[231]

3.14 Antioxidant defence enzymes: co-operation

3.14.1 The need for co-operation

Antioxidant defences must operate as a balanced and co-ordinated system. Section 3.11.1 considered how different H_2O_2-removing systems might co-operate, but they must in turn co-operate with other defence systems such as the SODs. As we saw in Section 3.4.5, liposomes containing both catalase and SOD protect rats against O_2 toxicity better than liposomes containing either enzyme alone.[77] Exposure of rats to pure O_2 at high

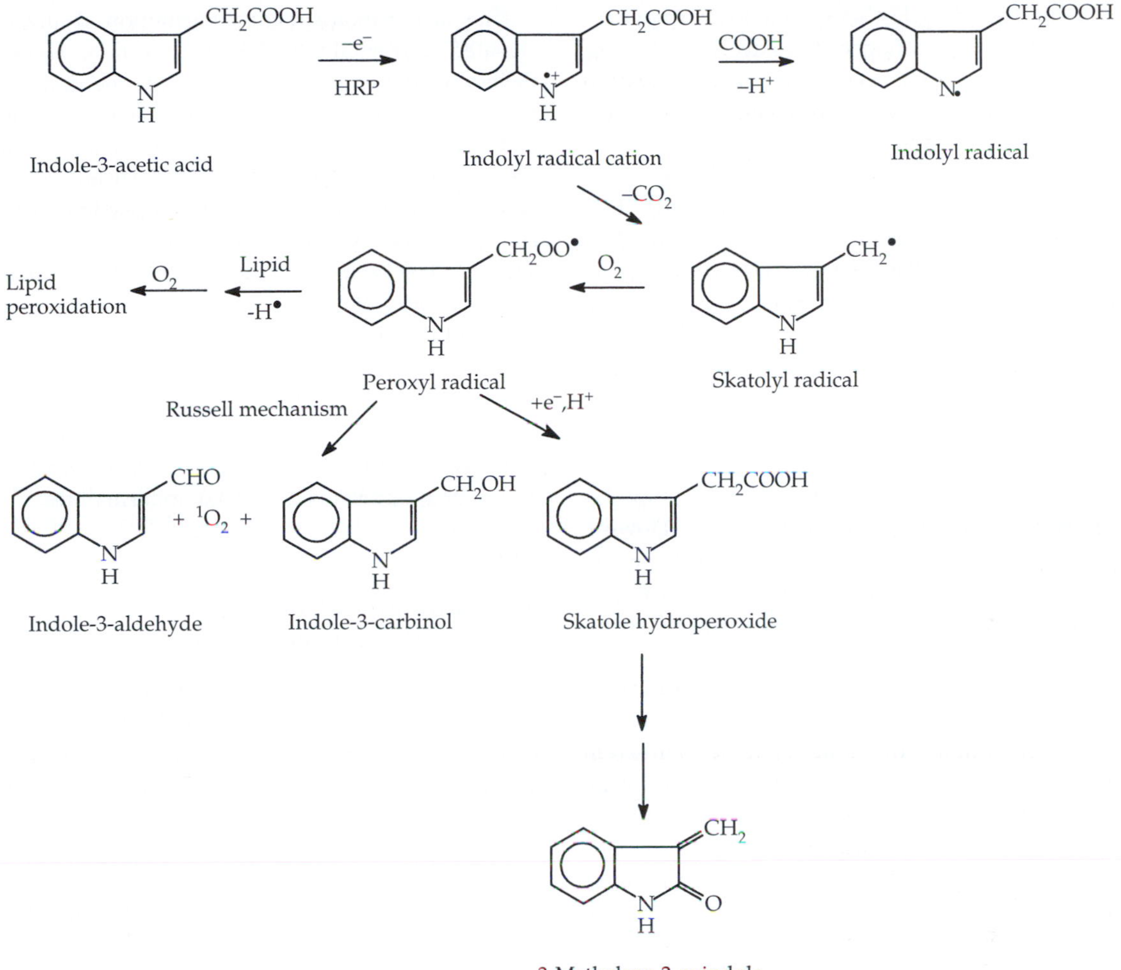

Figure 3.20 Mechanisms of auxin oxidation by horseradish peroxidase. From *Chem. Res. Toxicol.* **17**, 1350, 2004 by courtesy of Dr P.J. O'Brien and the American Chemical Society. Methyleneoxindole and some of the radicals are cytotoxic and IAA/peroxidase conjugated to an antibody delivery system has been evaluated as an antitumour agent (*Biochem. Pharmacol.* **61**, 129, 2001).

pressure causes convulsions (Section 1.5.2); pre-injection of liposomes containing both enzymes delayed the time to onset of convulsions by approximately three-fold. Again, liposomes with SOD alone or catalase alone were less protective.[232] Further evidence[233] for co-operation is provided by transfection experiments. Transfection of a gene encoding CuZnSOD into mouse epidermal cells raised CuZnSOD levels and sensitized them to damage upon incubation with a mixture of xanthine and XO, whereas subsequent transfection with genes encoding catalase or GPx1 rendered the cells equally or more resistant to damage.[233]

The need for co-operation may in part be driven by the fact that RS can damage individual antioxidant enzymes. For example, if not removed by SODs, $O_2^{\bullet-}$ can partially inhibit catalase; the reaction[120]

$$\text{enzyme} - \text{Fe(III)} + O_2^{\bullet-} \rightleftharpoons \text{enzyme} - \text{Fe}^{2+} - O_2$$

generates a **ferroxycatalase** that does not rapidly decompose H_2O_2. In addition, $O_2^{\bullet-}$ can reduce catalase compound I to compound II, again poorly active in degrading H_2O_2 (Section 3.7.2). *Mycoplasma pneumoniae*, a pathogen that infects the human respiratory tract, may decrease the catalase activity of respiratory tract cells by producing $O_2^{\bullet-}$, promoting damage by H_2O_2.[80]

Superoxide dismutases diminish $ONOO^-$ formation and some peroxiredoxins scavenge this species; $ONOO^-$ nitrates and inactivates MnSOD and some CuZnSODs, but can also oxidize and inactivate catalase and GPx. Similarly, if H_2O_2 is not quickly removed, it can inactivate CuZnSOD and FeSOD.

3.14.2 Down's syndrome

An imbalance of antioxidant defences may be important in **trisomy 21**, often called **Down's syndrome (DS)** after the physician John Langdon Down, who described it in 1866. The syndrome is characterized by variable degrees of mental retardation, morphological abnormalities and an increased risk of developing Alzheimer's disease (AD). Down's syndrome is the most common chromosomal abnormality, affecting one in about every 1000 babies. It results from the presence of an extra copy of all or part of chromosome 21, which leads to increased production of many of the proteins encoded by genes on this chromosome. One is CuZnSOD; 1.5 times the normal CuZnSOD activity is found in cells from trisomy 21 patients. Indeed, cells from DS patients are less readily damaged by *M. pneumoniae* (Section 3.14.1).[80]

Is DS related to the rise in CuZnSOD? This question has been examined using transgenic mice (Box 3.1). Animals have been obtained with 1.6- to 6-fold more SOD activity, especially in the brain. Rises in brain catalase activity (but not in GPx) were also observed. The mice appear morphologically normal and are more resistant to several toxins (Box 3.1). However, abnormal neuromuscular junctions were reported in the tongue, apparently similar to those found in tongue muscles of trisomy 21 patients. The mice also showed abnormalities in serotonin metabolism comparable to those reported in patients. However, they did not show the changes in dorsal root ganglia that are found in patients; hence only some of the neurological changes in trisomy 21 occur in the mice.

Thus at the moment the contribution, if any, of elevated CuZnSOD to DS is uncertain. Nevertheless, evidence for increased oxidative damage, for example elevated F_2–isoprostanes, 8OHdG and allantoin levels, has been reported in DS patients.[234–236] Cerebral cortex from young adult DS patients was found at autopsy to contain elevated levels of oxidized RNA and nitrated proteins.[237] The gene encoding amyloid precursor protein is present on chromosome 21 and increased $A\beta$ production (Section 9.20) could contribute to brain oxidative damage and the increased risk of AD in DS patients. Another gene of interest on chromosome 21, *ets-2*, encodes a transcription factor whose presence in excess seems to promote neuronal apoptosis and skeletal abnormalities.[238]

3.15 Antioxidant defence: sequestration of metal ions

Iron and copper are essential in almost all aerobes for the synthesis of proteins involved in respiration, O_2 transport, $NO^{\bullet}$ formation and antioxidant defence. Yet these metals are potentially dangerous pro-oxidants (Table 3.10). It is not only 'free' metal ions that can promote oxidative damage; haem and certain haem proteins can do so as well (Section 3.15.3 below). Hence organisms must be careful in handling metals.

3.15.1 Iron metabolism[239]

The average adult human male contains about 4.5 g of iron, the majority of which is in haemoglobin. Liver (~1 g, mostly in ferritin), skeletal muscle (~300 mg, most in myoglobin) and macrophages (~600 mg in total) are also important iron depots. He absorbs 1 to 2 mg of iron per day from the diet and expels the same amount when in iron balance. Premenopausal women often have less body iron, partly because of menstruation.

Since total plasma iron turnover is some 35 mg/day, efficient mechanisms to regulate body iron content must exist. Even slight disturbances of iron metabolism will lead to either deficiency or overload, both with deleterious consequences (e.g. iron deficiency in growing children can impair mental

Table 3.10 Role of transition-metal ions in converting less reactive to more reactive species[95,96]

Starting agent	More-reactive species produced on addition of metal ions	Metal involved	Comment
H_2O_2 ($\pm O_2^{\bullet-}$)	OH$^{\bullet}$ (and possibly reactive oxo-metal species)	Fe/Cu/Co/Ni/Cr (not Mn)	Iron-dependent and copper-dependent conversion of H_2O_2 to OH$^{\bullet}$ and other oxidizing species
HOCl	OH$^{\bullet}$	Fe	Fe^{2+} reacts with HOCl to form OH$^{\bullet}$ or similar species (Section 2.5.1.1)
Lipid peroxides	Peroxyl radicals, alkoxyl radicals, cytotoxic aldehydes	Fe/Cu	Sections 4.11.6 and 4.12.5
Thiols (R-SH)	$O_2^{\bullet-}$, H_2O_2, RS$^{\bullet}$, OH$^{\bullet}$	Fe/Cu	Oxidation of thiols produces thiyl, oxysulphur and oxygen radicals (Section 2.5.5)
NAD(P)H	NAD(P)$^{\bullet}$, $O_2^{\bullet-}$, OH$^{\bullet}$	Fe/Cu	NAD(P)$^{\bullet}$ radicals reduce O_2 to give $O_2^{\bullet-}$; copper is especially good at promoting NAD(P)H oxidation.
Ascorbic acid	OH$^{\bullet}$, possibly $O_2^{\bullet-}$, semidehydroascorbate radical	Fe, especially Cu	Oxidation of ascorbate produces cytotoxic species (Section 3.20.1.3 below)
Alloxan, adrenalin, DOPA, dopamine, dihydroxyfumarate, tetrahydrofolates, 6-hydroxydopamine, other 'autoxidizable' compounds (including some plant polyphenols)	OH$^{\bullet}$, $O_2^{\bullet-}$, carbon-centred or other radicals derived from the toxin	Fe, Cu, Mn, often other metals	'Autoxidations' depend on the presence of transition-metal ions Section 3.22.3 below
Peroxynitrite (ONOO^{-})	NO_2^{+}	Fe/Cu	Transition-metal ions and some metalloproteins (including SOD) accelerate nitration of aromatic compounds, by facilitating conversion of ONOO^{-} to NO_2^{+} (Section 2.6.1)

development).[240] It has been estimated that more than 500 million people in the world are iron-deficient (although be cautious in equating low blood iron to dietary iron deficiency; chronic infection/inflammation can also cause it; Section 4.7) and several million are iron-overloaded. Iron is lost from the body in sweat, faeces (by loss of unabsorbed iron, and of iron in cells shed from the lining of the gut), urine and blood (especially menstrual bleeding in women), and possibly small amounts are excreted by the lung into mucus (Section 6.3.1) and will be lost if the mucus is expectorated. Body iron stores have a negative

regulatory effect on the efficiency of iron absorption: normally only 10 to 15% of non-haem iron is absorbed but this increases in iron-deficiency anaemia. Foods such as wheat flour and breakfast cereals are fortified with iron in many countries; sometimes infant formulas and some weaning foods are also. It has been estimated that fortification contributes about 10% of adult iron intake in the UK and more than double this for preschool children.

Most inorganic iron in food is in the Fe(III) state, the most stable oxidation state for iron. Agents that solubilize and reduce Fe(III), such as the ascorbate and hydrochloric acid present in the gastric juice, facilitate iron absorption. Gastric juice has higher ascorbate levels than plasma. Many dietary components influence iron uptake. For example, **phytates**, present in cereals, nuts and legumes, chelate iron and slow its absorption. Haem iron is absorbed by a different pathway: haem released by proteolysis of haemoproteins in the gut lumen is taken up and the iron removed from it in the mucosal cells by the action of **haem oxygenase**[241] (Section 3.17 below). A greater percentage of dietary haem iron tends to be absorbed than for non-haem iron, and haem iron uptake is not affected by dietary iron-binding agents such as phytates. Excess intake of meats rich in haem, so that unabsorbed haem enters the faeces, has been suggested to contribute to the development of colon cancer.[242]

The main site of iron uptake is the duodenum, and dietary iron is presented to it in three forms; Fe(III), Fe^{2+} (reduction of some iron by ascorbate in the stomach) and haem. Ferrous iron is taken up by a divalent metal ion transporter called **Nramp2** (also known as **DCT1** or **DMT1**). It can additionally transport manganese, zinc, copper, cobalt and (less desirably) lead, cadmium and nickel. The duodenal mucosa handles Fe(III) using a ferric reductase system, involving a b-type cytochrome (**duodenal cytochrome b; DcytB**), on the cell surface. This system is probably supplied with electrons by intracellular ascorbate. Iron(III) is thus converted to Fe^{2+} for uptake by Nramp2. Reductase activity is increased in hypoxia or iron deficiency, both of which increase iron uptake; duodenal ascorbate also rises.[243]

Iron must then be released from the gut cells to the blood, although some will be stored as ferritin (Section 3.15.1.4 below) within the mucosal cells. Serosal release of iron involves the protein **ferroportin**, encoded by the *IREG1* (**iron-regulated transporter-1**) gene. Ferroportin also plays a role in iron export from macrophages and several other cell types (including lung cells; Section 6.3). Exit of iron from the gut to the plasma is facilitated by **hephaestin**, a copper-containing protein resembling caeruloplasmin (Section 3.15.2.1 below); it has been known for decades that copper deficiency impairs iron uptake. Hephaestin promotes oxidation of Fe^{2+} to Fe(III) for loading onto transferrin, without forming ROS; O_2 is completely reduced to H_2O. Its name is derived from *Hephaestus*, the Greek god of fire and metal workers.

3.15.1.1 *Transferrin*[244]

Some of the iron absorbed from haem or inorganic iron in the diet is retained in the gut mucosal cells within ferritin and other proteins and is lost in the faeces when these cells are shed. The rest enters the circulation bound to **transferrin**. Transferrin also accepts iron released by the destruction of aged red blood cells (estimated as 20–25 mg/day) and it supplies the same amount to the bone marrow to make about 200 billion new red blood cells per day. Circulating transferrin only accounts for about 3 mg of body iron, but it's a busy protein, turning over its iron about 10 times daily. Transferrin is a glycoprotein (relative molecular mass 79 000), mostly synthesized in the liver. It has N-terminal and C-terminal domains, each of which tightly binds one Fe(III) at pH 7.4. Two monoferric forms of transferrin can therefore exist, with iron bound to the N-terminal or the C-terminal domain. Tight binding of iron to either domain requires the presence of carbonate (CO_3^{2-}) anion. In healthy people, transferrin is usually no more than 20 to 30% loaded with iron. Hence human and other animal blood plasmas have considerable iron-binding capacity and their content of 'free' iron ions is essentially zero. The affinity of transferrin for iron at pH 7.4 is high (stability constant $\sim 10^{22}$), slightly more so for the C-terminal domain than for the N-terminal. The strength of binding decreases at lower pH.

Transferrin can bind several metal ions other than Fe(III), although with lower affinity, including aluminium (Al(III), stability constant $\sim 10^{12}$).

3.15.1.2 *Other iron-binding proteins*[245]

A protein similar to transferrin, **lactoferrin**, is found in saliva, vaginal mucus, seminal fluid, tears, bile, nasal secretions, milk (more in human milk than cow's milk) and other secretory fluids and is released by neutrophils during inflammation (Section 7.7.2.6). Lactoferrin also binds two Fe(III) per molecule, but holds it more tightly at low pH than does transferrin. Lactoferrin may have several roles *in vivo*: it binds to DNA and may influence gene transcription, has various effects on cells of the immune system and may be an antibacterial factor (Section 7.7.2).

Many similar iron-binding proteins are known. Egg-white contains **ovotransferrin** (sometimes called **conalbumin**). Melanoma cells can express a **melanotransferrin. Uteroferrin** is a purple protein, synthesized in large amounts by the uterus of pigs after treatment with the hormone progesterone. The colour arises from an active site where iron is co-ordinated with tyrosine. Uteroferrin can also act as a phosphatase enzyme, belonging to the type 5 (tartrate-resistant) acid phosphatase class. In humans, this type of enzyme is found in osteoclasts (cells that destroy the matrix of bone and cartilage: Section 9.10.2) and serum levels increase in diseases where bone resorption is enhanced.[246]

3.15.1.3 *Iron within cells*[105,244,247]

Cells needing iron express **transferrin receptors** on their surface: the more iron they want, the more receptors they make. Receptors bind diferric plasma transferrin, and the complex is internalized by endocytosis and enters the cytoplasm in a vacuole. The liver and many cells in culture can also take up 'low molecular mass' iron chelates, such as Fe–citrate, although this is probably only of much relevance *in vivo* in iron overload. The contents of the vacuole are acidified to about pH 5.5 by the action of an H^+-pumping ATPase; this low pH weakens iron binding to transferrin. The iron is then removed and reduced (possibly by an NADPH-dependent ferrireductase system) and transported out of the vacuole by Nramp2 to form the **labile iron pool, LIP** (see below). The iron-free transferrin (**apotransferrin**) is ejected from the cell for reuse. At pH 7.4, the transferrin receptor has a much higher affinity for iron-loaded transferrin than for the apoprotein, enabling it to collect the iron-bearing protein from the plasma. This order of affinities is reversed at acidic pH, so keeping the apotransferrin on the receptor for ejection from the cell. Two different transferrin receptors exist, **TfR1** and **TfR2**. TfR1-mediated endocytosis is the usual pathway of iron uptake by body cells *in vivo*; TfR2 may be involved in supporting growth in a few cell types, but its exact role is unclear as yet.

The LIP is a transit pool that receives iron from transferrin and supplies it for the synthesis of ferroproteins. The location and chemical nature of the LIP in cells and organelles is unclear, but fluorescent iron chelators such as **calcein** (Fig. 3.21) have demonstrated its presence. It may exist bound to ligands such as proteins, citrate, ATP, GTP, inositol phosphates and other phosphate esters, possibly including phospholipid head groups and the DNA backbone (Section 4.8.2). Using calcein, an average LIP of $0.35\,\mu M$ in human erythroleukaemia cells was calculated. Addition of Fe^{2+} to the cells raised this value, but it returned to normal within 30 to 60 min. Addition of H_2O_2 or *tert*-butyl hydroperoxide also raised the level, and it took longer (60–90 min) to return to normal.[105] Pools in other cells seem to be in the 0.1 to $2\,\mu M$ range. Of course, calcein measures 'calcein-chelatable' iron: it can only bind iron that it comes into contact with (e.g. it may not enter lysosomes) and it is possible that it cannot remove iron from some carriers involved in the transit pool. Laser scanning microscopy using **Phen green** (Fig 3.21) identified 'labile iron' in nucleus, cytosol, mitochondria and the lysosomal–endosome system, the nucleus having the highest level.[248] Mitochondria have been reported to take up iron salts rapidly, and need them to make haem and Fe–S proteins; the synthesis of haem is finalized in the mitochondria (Fig. 2.14) and some of it must then be exported to supply the rest of the cell. ATP-dependent uptake systems for iron-citrate and iron-ATP have been reported in microsomes and nuclei. 'Labile iron' can also be generated in lysosomes by continual degradation of iron-containing proteins during autophagy (Section 4.14).[249]

3.15.1.4 *Ferritin*[250]

Most intracellular iron is stored in **ferritin**. Mammalian ferritins consist of a hollow protein shell, 12 to 13 nm outside diameter (7–8 nm inside diameter), composed of 24 subunits, each with a relative molecular mass of about 20 000. The shell surrounds an iron core that can hold up to 4500 iron ions, but usually has fewer. Traces of other metals can be present, including copper.[251] Most ferritin is intracellular, part in mitochondria but the majority in cytosol. Some is present in blood, and plasma ferritin level is often used clinically as

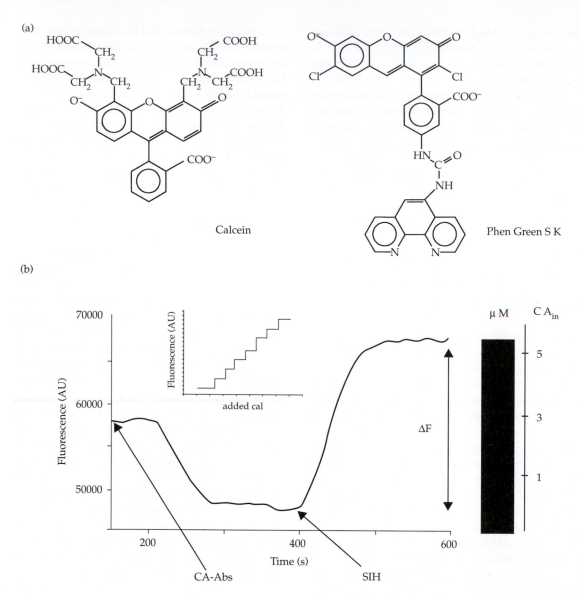

Figure 3.21 Probes for the detection of 'labile' iron. (a) Structures of calcein (CAL) and phen green S K. (b) The CAL method for measuring the labile iron pool (LIP). Cells are loaded with the acetomethoxy derivative of CAL (CAL-AM), which is non-fluorescent and membrane permeable. Upon entry to cells, CAL-AM is hydrolysed to give the fluorescent CAL, which is quenched upon binding of iron. Anti-CAL antibodies are added to ensure that fluorescence is intracellular. The compound SIH, a permeant iron chelator (Table 10.14) restores fluorescence (ΔF) by taking iron away from CAL. The figure shows a representative experiment. CAL-bound iron concentration is given by $[CAL\text{-}Fe] = [CAL]_{tot} * \Delta F$, where $[CAL]$ is obtained from a calibration curve (inset). Knowing the K_d of iron binding to CAL, it is possible to compute the concentration of CAL-detectable free iron. $[CAL\text{-}Fe]$ and $[Fe]_{free}$ together constitute the LIP. Adapted from *Free Rad. Biol. Med.* **33**, 1037, 2002 by courtesy of Professor Z.I. Cabantchik and Elsevier.

an approximate index of body iron stores (e.g. Section 10.5.10).

Mammalian ferritins contain two subunit types (**H-** and **L-chains**), of similar size and about 50% amino acid sequence identity. Ferritins vary widely in H/L ratios and ratios often change in various diseases. In general, ferritins in liver and spleen are richer in L-subunits than those in heart and brain. By contrast, plant and bacterial ferritins are usually homo-polymers of H-type subunits. *E. coli* produces three ferritin-like proteins; bacterial ferritin (24 subunits), **bacterioferritin** (24 subunits, but also contains 12 haem rings) and **Dps** (12 subunits). Levels of Dps (*D*NA binding *p*rotein during *s*tationary phase) increase under stress conditions. These 12-subunit bacterial proteins, sometimes called **miniferritins**, serve to protect DNA against damage by H_2O_2 in several bacteria, including *E. coli* and *Streptococcus suis*. Such proteins may have had an early evolutionary origin, since Fenton chemistry may have been common in the 'preoxygen' world (Section 1.1).[252]

Iron enters animal ferritins as Fe^{2+}, which is oxidized to Fe(III) and deposited in the core as an insoluble hydrated ferric oxide. The chemistry of the oxidation is incompletely understood; the H−chains have a metal-binding site and can oxidize Fe^{2+} to Fe(III) whereas the L-subunits facilitate iron nucleation and storage. The first step is formation of a diferric peroxide,

$$2Fe^{2+} + O_2 \rightarrow Fe(III)-O-O-Fe(III)$$

At low fluxes of iron into ferritin H_2O_2 is produced on the H-chains

$$Fe(III)-O-O-Fe(III) + H_2O \rightarrow$$
$$Fe(III)-O-Fe(III) + H_2O_2$$

whereas at high fluxes Fe^{2+} oxidation occurs on the surface of the growing core, minimizing H_2O_2 production. Tyrosyl radicals and OH• have been detected from ferritin during iron loading but are (fortunately) not stoichiometrically produced as Fe^{2+} is oxidized. Cellular ferritin levels affect the LIP, for example overexpression of ferritin in cells decreases the amount of calcein-detectable iron (Fig. 3.21), and decreasing ferritin raises LIP size.[105]

How cells release iron from ferritin is uncertain; *in vitro*, it can be released (as Fe^{2+}) by several reducing agents, including ascorbate, thiols, urate, $O_2^{\bullet-}$, and reduced flavins. Iron enters and leaves through channels; it can also be released when ferritin is taken up into lysosomes and degraded. Ferritin can be converted in lysosomes into an insoluble product, **haemosiderin**, probably by proteolytic attack.

3.15.1.5 *Regulation of cellular iron balance*[244,247]
Regulation of the synthesis of transferrin receptors and ferritin subunits is synchronized in mammalian

cells. This involves cytoplasmic **iron-regulatory proteins** (**IRPs**) which bind to **iron-responsive** (or **regulatory**) **elements** (**IREs**), special base sequences in the mRNAs for ferritin subunits and transferrin receptors. When cellular iron levels are too low, IRPs bind to IREs. This stabilizes transferrin receptor mRNA, so that more protein is made. By contrast, it prevents translation of ferritin mRNA. When there is enough cellular iron, mRNA for the transferrin receptor is rapidly degraded.

The **IRP-1** protein is identical with a cytosolic form of the enzyme **aconitase** (aconitase also occurs in mitochondria, in the Krebs cycle, Fig. 1.7). It has aconitase activity when its [4Fe−4S] cluster is present, but is an IRP when iron is low and the cluster is absent; switching between these forms depends on cellular iron status. Mutations inactivating the IRE in mRNA encoding ferritin L-subunits are associated with elevated plasma ferritin levels and cataract in humans; the latter may be due to deposition of ferritin aggregates in the lens.[253] Another IRP, **IRP-2**, without aconitase activity, is found in mammalian cells: the presence of iron facilitates binding of haem to IRP-2, leading to ROS production, oxidation at cysteine residues and degradation of oxidized IRP-2 by the proteasome (Section 4.14.2.1).[254] Alternatively, IRP-2 may be degraded after hydroxylation by a 2-oxoglutarate-dependent dioxygenase.[255] Knockout of the IRP-2 gene in mice produced anaemia, iron accumulation in brain, and neurodegeneration.[256]

Iron−sulphur clusters are sensitive to oxidizing agents and so it is not surprising that several ROS, RCS and RNS can influence IRP action and hence cellular iron metabolism.[257] Iron status can also affect the iNOS gene, high iron levels decreasing its transcription in response to cytokines, especially in macrophages.[244] Cytokines such as 1L-2 and TNFα increase ferritin synthesis in several cell types, by encouraging transcription of the gene encoding the H-subunits. The IRPs also affect the synthesis of several other iron-containing proteins, including mitochondrial aconitase and δ-aminolaevulinate synthetase (Fig. 2.12). Binding of IRPs blocks translation of the mRNA encoding the latter enzyme and thus decreases haem production.

The cellular iron level must find a balance between supplying enough iron for metabolic requirements and the risk of accelerated oxidative damage. Too little iron can decrease the activity of essential proteins such as ribonucleotide reductase and mitochondrial Fe–S proteins. Indeed, incubation of cells with iron chelators for long periods can lead to apoptosis. Not only iron overload but also iron deficiency can cause oxidative stress, probably both involving increased mitochondrial ROS production. Thus iron deficiency impairs electron transport, promoting electron leakage.[258]

3.15.2 Copper metabolism[259,260]

Copper ions are powerful catalysts of oxidative damage (Table 3.10), more effective than iron in causing oxidative DNA damage and stimulating peroxidation of LDL (Section 9.3.8), and so organisms must handle them carefully. Essential Cu-containing proteins include SOD1, EC-SOD (Section 3.16.3.1 below) and cytochrome oxidase. Not only too much copper but also copper deprivation can increase oxidative stress, the latter by decreasing SOD and cytochrome oxidase activities and increasing mitochondrial ROS production.[261] Copper may play a role in angiogenesis, and experiments with copper chelators as putative anticancer agents are underway in several laboratories.[260]

An average adult human contains about 80 mg copper and absorbs about 1 mg/day, both from dietary copper and from 'recycled' copper, that released by the liver into bile. Copper is absorbed in the duodenum as chelates with amino acids (such as histidine) or small peptides. Not all the copper entering gut mucosal cells enters the blood: some is stored in these cells and lost from the body when they are shed. The rest enters the blood bound to **transcuprein** and to albumin; each albumin molecule has one high affinity binding site for copper plus a number of weaker binding sites.

3.15.2.1 *Caeruloplasmin and copper chaperones*[259]
Copper is taken up by the liver through the **Ctr1** transporter and enters the cell in the Cu^+ form (it is not clear how it is reduced). The liver incorporates some of the copper into the protein **caeruloplasmin**, relative molecular mass about 132 000. Caeruloplasmin is secreted into plasma, and unwanted copper into the bile. Caeruloplasmin contains six tightly bound copper ions and often a seventh, less well bound. A membrane-bound form of caeruloplasmin attached to glycosylphosphatidylinositol is present in certain tissues, including brain (Section 9.16.6).

Caeruloplasmin is often thought to donate copper to copper-requiring cells, but knockout mice show no impairment in this, suggesting that other mechanisms of copper uptake must exist. Within the cell, copper delivered by Ctr1 binds to transport proteins, the **copper chaperones**, one of which (CCS, Section 3.2.1.2) delivers copper to CuZnSOD, another to the Golgi apparatus for insertion into exported proteins (e.g. caeruloplasmin) and yet another takes copper to mitochondria for incorporation into cytochrome oxidase. Some intracellular copper may exist bound to GSH, providing an additional source of Cu to CuZnSOD (Section 3.2.1.2). Metallothioneins plays a role in copper sequestration (Section 3.16.1 below), and APP (Section 9.20) may be involved in brain. It is essential to keep Cu^+ tightly protein-bound to help suppress its pro-oxidant potential.

3.15.2.2 *A phantom copper pool?*
Human blood plasma normally contains 200 to 400 mg/dm^3 of caeruloplasmin, accounting for 90% or more of total plasma copper. The rest is bound to albumin and transcuprein. In addition, a 'low molecular mass' pool bound to histidine or small peptides is often claimed to exist. *In vitro*, copper can be removed from its amino acid chelates by the metal-binding agent **o-phenanthroline** (Section 4.3.4).[262] However, if mammalian plasma is incubated with phenanthroline, no chelatable copper is detected, which implies that amounts of these non-caeruloplasmin copper chelates in plasma are small.[262,263] Chromatography, dialysis or low-temperature storage of plasma or serum lead to release of copper from caeruloplasmin, which may account for reports of 'non-caeruloplasmin copper' in earlier studies.[262] Copper release in 'aged' plasma appears to occur by the action of a plasma metalloproteinase on caeruloplasmin.[264] Caeruloplasmin has structural similarities to two proteins involved in blood coagulation, **factors V** and **VIII**. These factors are activated by proteolytic cleavage, and the similarity of caeruloplasmin to them may help explain

its sensitivity to proteolysis. Adding $ONOO^-$ to caeruloplasmin also releases copper (Section 2.6.1).

3.15.2.3 Caeruloplasmin as an oxidase[264,265]

In vitro, caeruloplasmin can catalyse oxidation of several polyamines and polyphenols, including catecholamines, but these activities have acidic pH optima and their biological significance is uncertain. Caeruloplasmin also has **ferroxidase** activity; it oxidizes Fe^{2+} to Fe(III) and can facilitate iron loading on to transferrin and possibly ferritin. The physiological importance of caeruloplasmin is illustrated by patients with **acaeruloplasminae-mia**,[266] who carry mutations in the gene encoding it. They show low plasma iron, elevated serum ferritin and elevated iron deposition in the brain (accompanied by increased lipid peroxidation), liver and other tissues. Pathological consequences include diabetes, retinal degeneration and neurological abnormalities. Low plasma iron is due to a slowed *export* of iron from the liver and reticuloendothelial system, which appear to require ferroxidase activity to ensure export as Fe(III) and loading onto transferrin. Indeed, injection of caeruloplasmin raises plasma iron. Copper uptake through the gut and into the liver, and biliary excretion of copper, are normal in knockout mice lacking caeruloplasmin, suggesting that caeruloplasmin is not essential for these roles.[259] Similarly, dietary copper deficiency in animals produces an anaemia that does not respond to iron administration but can be corrected by injection of caeruloplasmin.

Ferrous salts spontaneously oxidize at physiological pH to produce ROS:

$$Fe^{2+} + O_2 \rightarrow Fe(III) + O_2^{\bullet-}$$

$$2O_2^{\bullet-} + 2H^+ \rightarrow H_2O_2 + O_2$$

$$Fe^{2+} + H_2O_2 \rightarrow Fe(III) + OH^{\bullet-} + OH^-$$

By contrast, caeruloplasmin-catalysed Fe^{2+} oxidation does not: four Fe^{2+} are oxidized and one O_2 reduced to $2H_2O$. The same may be true of hephaestin (Section 3.15.1). However, the loosely bound seventh copper of caeruloplasmin has been suggested to catalyse oxidation of LDL and contribute to atherosclerosis (Section 9.3.5).[264]

The ferroxidase activity of caeruloplasmin is inhibited by azide and is often called **ferroxidase I**, to distinguish it from other ferroxidases. In humans, caeruloplasmin accounts for almost all plasma ferroxidase activity, whereas in certain other animals, for example rabbits, plasma additionally contains an azide-resistant ferroxidase, **ferroxidase II**.[263,265] Decreases in plasma ferroxidase activity in the face of unchanged or raised caeruloplasmin protein levels have been observed in several human diseases, including ARDS and rheumatoid arthritis, but their physiological significance is uncertain.

3.15.2.4 Caeruloplasmin as a peroxidase[267]

Caeruloplasmin can remove H_2O_2 and lipid peroxides *in vitro* in the presence of GSH; this could be important in lung lining fluids where GSH levels are high (Table 3.7), but is unlikely to occur at the low plasma GSH levels. Indeed, lung synthesizes some caeruloplasmin and secretes it into the lining fluid.

Caeruloplasmin can also bind to MPO, inhibiting HOCl formation without blocking its own ferroxidase activity.[268]

3.15.3 Haem proteins: potential pro-oxidants

Haemoglobin and myoglobin are normally intracellular proteins in red cells and muscles respectively. Both undergo slow oxidation to form $O_2^{\bullet-}$ and Fe(III) protein, and both can cause damage when mixed with H_2O_2, which readily penetrates to the haem centres. Such damage can occur *in vivo* and during meat processing, the latter causing lipid oxidation and 'off-flavours'.[269] By contrast, neuroglobin (Section 1.3.1) seems not to promote such damage.[270]

When haemoglobin or myoglobin are exposed to excess ($\geq 10:1$ molar ratio) H_2O_2 or lipid peroxides they are degraded, releasing both haem and iron ions (from haem ring breakdown).[271,272] Haem and iron so released can stimulate lipid peroxidation, and iron ions can form $OH^\bullet$ from H_2O_2. At lower H_2O_2 : protein ratios (e.g. $1:1$), haemoglobin and myoglobin are converted to haem ferryl species. Amino acid radicals are also generated; tyrosine and tryptophan peroxyl radicals (Trp/TyrOO$^{\bullet}$) and histidinyl radicals have been identified.[273]

$$\text{haem Fe(III)protein} + H_2O_2 \rightarrow$$
$$\text{haem [Fe(IV) = O]protein}^{\bullet} + H_2O$$

Cross-links between haem and tyrosine can form. Both ferryl and amino acid radicals can stimulate peroxidation of lipids[274] and oxidize other molecules,[275] including thiols, urate and certain proteins, to form secondary radicals, for example urate radical and RS$^{\bullet}$. When added to lipids (including lipoproteins), haem proteins in the *absence* of added H_2O_2 can stimulate peroxidation, probably by promoting the decomposition of pre-existing traces of lipid peroxides in the lipids to alkoxyl and peroxyl radicals (Section 4.11.6.1). Myoglobin can oxidize the anticancer drug doxorubicin in the heart (Section 9.15.2.1).

Hence haem, haemoglobin and myoglobin outside their normal location (e.g. when haemoglobin is released in the brain; Section 9.17.3) are potentially damaging molecules. This pro-oxidant potential, together with the rapid scavenging of NO$^{\bullet}$ by haemoglobin, poses problems in the design of haemoglobin-based blood substitutes.[276] Myoglobin released as a result of severe muscle injury can lead to kidney failure, involving oxidative damage caused by myoglobin with haem–tyrosine crosslinks, haem itself and released iron.[276] Cytochrome *c* plus H_2O_2 also generates free radicals[277] and can oxidize various molecules.[278] It can again be degraded by excess H_2O_2, as can cytochromes P450. For example, kidney damage induced by *cis*-platin administration to rats appeared to involve iron release from CYPs.[279]

Too little haem is also bad; cellular haem deficiency, like iron or copper deficiency, can lead to oxidative stress by increasing mitochondrial ROS production.[280]

3.15.4 Metal ion sequestration: why do it?

3.15.4.1 *Keeping bacteria at bay*[281]
Why do organisms take such care in the handling of iron, copper and other transition metal ions? Almost all bacteria need these metals for growth, although a few (e.g. *Borrelia burgdorferi*, the

causative agent of Lyme disease) have evolved to do without iron.[282] Restricting metal availability in body fluids is thus an antibacterial mechanism. Indeed, some bacteria have evolved mechanisms to circumvent this. They synthesize powerful iron chelators (**siderophores**), able to take iron from transferrin. Others cleave transferrin, for example *Pseudomonas aeruginosa* in cystic fibrosis patients (Sections 8.7 and 9.8). Iron-overloaded subjects are more prone to infection by a range of organisms, including *Vibrio vulnificus* and *Listeria monocytogenes*.

Mammals have evolved to fight back; **lipocalin 2** is secreted by neutrophils and endothelial cells and binds siderophores, helping to internalize them and liberating the iron they carry for host use.[283]

3.15.4.2 *Diminishing free-radical reactions*[95,284]
Another reason for sequestering metal ions is to diminish their pro-oxidant ability (Table 3.10). Manipulations of the iron content of *S. aureus*, *E. coli* and mammalian cells that illustrate this point were discussed in Section 3.6.2.2. Multiple other studies have shown that the toxicity of H_2O_2 or organic peroxides to bacterial, animal, and plant cells is increased by raising their iron content, and decreased by the presence of chelating agents such as phenanthroline, or sometimes desferrioxamine. For example, in *E. coli* lacking H_2O_2-metabolizing enzymes, (AHPR, Kat G, Kat E) intracellular OH$^{\bullet}$ formation was detectable even with <1 μM H_2O_2. Iron chelators eliminated the poor growth and increased DNA damage of these mutants under aerobic conditions.[285] The size of the LIP of animal cells correlates with cellular sensitivity to damage by peroxides.[105,247] Injection of ferric salts bound to the chelating agent **nitrilotriacetate** (**NTA**) into animals causes severe tissue injury, increases oxidative damage to lipids, proteins, and DNA and induces renal cancer (Fig. 5.17),[286] at least in part because ferric–NTA is highly effective at generating OH$^{\bullet}$ from H_2O_2. This chelator has been used in detergents (to prevent mineral build up) and is used in the laboratory to prepare iron-loaded transferrin.

But *are* protein-bound metal ions less effective pro-oxidants than 'unchelated' metals or chelates of iron with such molecules as citrate and ADP? In general yes, with a few caveats.

1. Iron correctly bound within the two iron-binding sites of lactoferrin or transferrin will not stimulate autoxidations, react with $O_2^{\bullet-}$ or H_2O_2 or decompose lipid peroxides at pH 7.4.[284,287]

2. Iron in the ferritin cores is insoluble and not pro-oxidant. However, it can be mobilized by reducing agents, including $O_2^{\bullet-}$. Nevertheless, the amount of $O_2^{\bullet-}$-mobilizable iron in ferritin is a low percentage of the total iron content; whether $O_2^{\bullet-}$ releases iron from the core or merely liberates iron still within the channels or loosely bound to the protein surface, is uncertain.[95,287] Commercial ferritin preparations are often partially degraded and thus easier to mobilize iron from, which has led to some artefactual results in the literature.

3. Haemosiderin iron is less available than that in ferritin, essentially because haemosiderin is insoluble.[288] A comparable strategy is used by the malarial parasite, which packs haem into insoluble haemozoin (Section 6.6).

4. Superoxide releases iron from iron-sulphur clusters, e.g. from aconitases. This is important as a source of oxidative damage in bacteria, and probably also in animals.

5. The six 'tightly bound' caeruloplasmin copper ions do not catalyse oxidative damage; the seventh might.[264]

6. Copper ions attached to albumin can still react with H_2O_2. However, the $OH^{\bullet}$ (or other RS) produced is absorbed by the protein. Albumin binds copper and prevents it from associating with lipoproteins and membranes. If $O_2^{\bullet-}$ or H_2O_2 were produced in plasma (e.g. from activated phagocytic cells) they might still react with copper, but this would damage the albumin. Since plasma albumin levels are high and its turnover rapid, this is unlikely to matter much. Albumin has thus been called a **sacrificial antioxidant**.[284]

7. Haem proteins can promote oxidative damage, so are kept in intracellular environments surrounded by antioxidant enzymes to keep peroxides away from them as far as possible.

8. Iron in uteroferrin and other purple acid phosphatases has been reported to generate $OH^{\bullet}$ from H_2O_2.[246] However, in performing such experiments it essential to check that the proteins remain intact. For example, early reports that haemoglobin converts H_2O_2 to $OH^{\bullet}$ were due to degradation of the protein and iron release in the reaction mixture.

3.15.5 Metal ion sequestration: when it goes wrong

The importance of metal ion sequestration is amply illustrated by the pathology of **iron overload** and **copper overload** diseases. For example, a mouse strain that synthesizes transferrin at less than 1% of the normal rate has been described. Gastrointestinal iron absorption is increased, low molecular mass iron chelates are present in plasma, and iron accumulates in many tissues. The mice die soon after birth unless transferrin is injected.[289] **Atransferrinaemia**, a rare hereditary disorder, produces similar effects in humans and is treated by plasma infusions.[290]

3.15.5.1 *Iron overload: diet-derived*

The body iron content is determined by how much crosses the gastrointestinal tract. Once it has entered the blood, there appears to be no dedicated physiological mechanism for disposing of iron, unless one counts menstrual bleeding. This inability to dispose of excess iron is illustrated in iron overload. Transient iron overload occurs in several diseases (Section 4.3.3). Acute severe iron overload can be caused by ingestion of large quantities of iron salts, usually by children who eat 'iron tablets' (containing ferrous salts) prescribed for their parents. There is vomiting, gastrointestinal bleeding and severe shock, requiring urgent treatment with desferrioxamine. Excess iron salts, particularly as Fe^{2+}, generate $OH^{\bullet}$, degrade the protective layer of gastrointestinal mucus[291] and damage the cells underneath. Some zoo animals, including mynah birds, pandas and the black rhinoceros (*Diceros bicornis*) are sensitive to diet-induced iron overload.[292,293] These species may have efficient uptake systems for iron, because their dietary iron content in the wild is low, whereas zoo feed may have too much iron.[292] Luckily, most humans do not develop overload at high dietary iron intakes because of the efficiency of the regulatory mechanisms that decrease iron uptake from the gut when the body is replete.

3.15.5.2 *Iron overload: genetic*

A more slowly developing iron overload of dietary origin has been described in several parts of Africa and is related both to drinking acidic beer out of iron pots and to a genetic predisposition to iron overload.[294] However, perhaps the best-studied iron-overload conditions are the inherited diseases collectively known as **haemochromatosis**.[295] In these conditions, the normal down-regulation of gut iron uptake when the body has enough does not happen. Indeed, iron uptake is accelerated, so that too much dietary iron is absorbed (absorption of cobalt, lead, manganese and zinc may also be increased). The time taken for clinically significant iron overload to develop in most cases of haemochromatosis is often 40 or more years and depends to some extent on diet and gender, men being more prone than women. In many subjects iron overload may never develop to an extent that causes symptoms.[296]

When overload occurs, the iron-binding capacity of plasma transferrin can be exceeded, so that 'labile iron', often in these conditions called **non-transferrin-bound iron** (NTBI), is present. At least some, and perhaps all, of this iron is bound to plasma citrate,[297] although other organic acids and albumin may also bind some iron. The liver takes up NTBI rapidly, eventually becoming iron-overloaded. The pathology resulting from iron overload can be devastating. It includes liver fibrosis and cirrhosis, an elevated risk of liver cancer, weakness, malaise, weight loss, damage to the gonads, skin pigmentation, diabetes (pancreatic β-cells are damaged), cardiac malfunctions and a chronic joint inflammation resembling rheumatoid arthritis. Haemochromatosis is not rare: the prevalence of the homozygous state in Australian, American and several European populations has been estimated as 0.3 to 0.5%. The heterozygote frequency is about 10%, making this the commonest genetic disorder among Caucasians. Incidence is lower in Asian, African or Hispanic populations.[295]

Type 1 haemochromatosis, the commonest form, results from mutations in the *HFE* (**human gene for haemochromatosis**) gene on chromosome 6. The most frequent mutation changes a cysteine residue at position 282 to tyrosine in the HFE protein, and may have originated by chance in a single Viking (or Celtic) ancestor in Northern Europe some 2000 years ago.[295] **Juvenile haemochromatosis** (onset of iron overload before age 30; sometimes called **type 2 haemochromatosis**) and **neonatal haemochromatosis** also exist, but are rarer and due to different mutations. In the latter, children are born with hepatic iron overload and liver damage, and require transplantation to survive. Mutations in the gene encoding TfR2 are also a rare cause (**type 3 haemochromatosis**); clinically they resemble the type 1 form.

Mice mutated in *HFE* show increased transferrin saturation and liver iron overload. A key player in these events is **hepcidin**,[295] a peptide secreted into blood by the liver. Hepcidin binds to ferroportin and promotes its degradation. Thus low hepcidin raises ferroportin levels and promote increased iron uptake in the duodenum and iron release from macrophages; high levels decrease ferroportin and have the opposite effects, blocking iron uptake from the gut and keeping iron within macrophages. Hepcidin levels are normally decreased by anaemia or hypoxia but increased by iron overload and inflammation. Mice lacking hepcidin show iron overload; indeed iron-overloaded haemochromatosis patients show abnormally low hepcidin levels. Thus the deficit in HFE somehow (we don't yet know the details) blocks the normal response (increased hepcidin production) to elevated body iron. Mutations in the *TfR2* gene may do the same. Mutations in the hepcidin gene cause a few cases of severe juvenile haemochromatosis, although most are due to other mutations, for example in the **haemojuvelin gene (*HFE2*)**. What this gene encodes is uncertain, but its product is probably required for hepcidin production. Finally, haemochromatosis can occur from mutations in the gene encoding ferroportin (**type 4 haemochromatosis**), rendering it resistant to regulation by hepcidin.

3.15.5.3 *Thalassaemias*[281]

Iron overload can result from medical treatment of other diseases. For example, the **thalassaemias** (named from a Greek word meaning 'the sea') are inborn conditions in which the rate of synthesis of a haemoglobin chain is diminished, the prefix α- or β-thalassaemia being used to identity the chain synthesized abnormally slowly. Thalassaemias often arise from splicing mutations. **Thalassaemia major** (sometimes called **Cooley's anaemia**) and **thalassaemia minor** refer to the homozygous and heterozygous states, respectively.

Untreated patients with thalassaemia major die young, but can be kept alive by regular blood transfusions. Since each unit of blood contains about 200 mg of iron, the patients become iron-overloaded, leading to saturation of transferrin and often the appearance of NTBI in the blood. Impaired erythropoiesis also 'sends a signal' to the gut to increase iron uptake. For both these reasons, iron accumulates in tissues, especially in the liver and spleen, with some in the heart. Sadly, heart is sensitive to iron, so that many thalassaemic patients suffer cardiac malfunctions. Ferric haem also circulates in the plasma and can exert pro-oxidant effects, for example to LDL[298] and pro-longed iron overload may impair the microbicidal functions of phagocytes, predisposing (as does the iron overload itself) to infections.[299] Similar problems arise in the treatment of other chronic anaemias by transfusion.

Treatment of iron overload resulting from hae-mochromatosis is usually by blood-letting (**phle-botomy**, sometimes called **venesection**), whereas desferrioxamine is administered to transfused thalassaemic patients in an effort to slow or prevent the accumulation of iron in the body. Desferriox-amine and its iron chelate ferrioxamine are rapidly excreted, in both urine and bile, so removing iron from the body. Desferrioxamine cannot be given by mouth (requiring subcutaneous or intravenous infusion) and it penetrates only slowly into cells. Hence there is interest in developing better chelators (Section 10.7).

3.15.5.4 Non-transferrin-bound iron: is it pro-oxidant?[95]

The NTBI found in the plasma of iron-overloaded haemochromatosis or thalassaemia patients will stimulate lipid peroxidation, and $OH^{\bullet}$ formation from H_2O_2, *in vitro*, which suggests that the pathology of iron overload might be related to increased oxidative damage. The sensitivity of the heart to even modest iron loading might be explained by its relatively poor protection against ROS: cardiac catalase activity is low and activities of SOD and GPx are only moderate (Tables 3.4 and 3.6). Other examples of the sensitivity of the heart to oxidative damage include the cardiomyopathy induced by doxorubicin (Section 9.15.2) and the heart lesions in Keshan disease (Section 3.11.2). L-type Ca^{2+} channels in cardiac muscle may be one route of entry for NTBI.[106] The pancreatic β-cells, often damaged in haemochromatosis, are also sensitive to free radical attack (Section 8.5).

Some evidence consistent with this 'radical hypothesis' of damage induced by iron overload has been obtained. For example, iron-overloaded patients show elevated levels of lipid peroxidation, protein carbonyls, and etheno-DNA adducts (Section 4.12.5) and subnormal levels of coenzyme Q, α-tocopherol, and vitamin C.[300–302] An additional mechanism of damage is the labilization of lysosomal membranes caused by excessive cata-bolism of ferritin within them: this lysosomal damage might be a consequence of iron-stimulated lipid peroxidation. However, present evidence, although suggestive, is not sufficient to prove that free-radical reactions cause the pathology of iron overload.

Methods for the measurement of plasma NTBI are considered in Section 4.3.3.1.

3.15.5.5 Copper overload

The toxicity of excess copper is illustrated by **Wilson's disease**,[260] an inherited recessive disorder often characterized by low concentrations of caeruloplasmin, but not due to defects in the gene encoding this protein. Wilson's disease occurs worldwide with a prevalence of up to 1 in 30 000. Copper is deposited in the liver, kidney, cornea and brain, the last causing damage that leads to lack of co-ordination, tremors and progressive mental retardation.

It seems likely (but is not proven) that copper-stimulated free-radical reactions are involved in the pathology of Wilson's disease. Plasma levels of ascorbate, α-tocopherol and urate are subnormal and increased levels of products of uric acid oxidation (Section 5.12), DNA damage, and lipid peroxidation have been detected in patients.[300,303,304] Treatment involves a copper-restricted diet and use of chelating agents, such as **penicillamine**, that promote copper excretion. Oral administration of zinc salts may also help, by interfering with the intestinal absorption of copper and by raising levels of metallothionein (Section 3.16.1 below), which can store copper. Zinc ions (Zn^{2+}) might also compete with copper for binding to target sites that could be damaged by RS.

The defective gene in Wilson's disease is on chromosome 13 and encodes a **Cu^{2+}-transporting ATPase** enzyme, **ATP7B**; the gene is strongly expressed in liver but also in brain, cornea, spleen and kidney. The **Long–Evans Cinnamon (LEC)** rat has a similar mutation and accumulates copper in the liver, spontaneously developing hepatitis. This is accompanied by increased levels of etheno-DNA adducts[300,305] and elevated OH• formation.[306] The ATP7B transporter helps to deliver copper to newly synthesized proteins in the Golgi apparatus; the low plasma caeruloplasmin often seen in Wilson's disease is secondary to a defect in this delivery. The activity of EC-SOD (Section 3.16.3.1 below) may also be affected, and copper export from liver into bile is impaired.

A related disorder encoded by a gene on the X chromosome, **Menke's disease**, involves a defect in a similar ATPase (**ATP7A**) involved in export of copper from the intestine. Normally, it seems to facilitate copper movement from the cytosol to secretory pathways. When it is defective, copper enters the intestinal cells but is not transported further, resulting in severe copper deficiency in most other body tissues. Patients show a wide range of problems including skeletal defects, aneurysms and degeneration of the nervous system, related to decreased levels of essential copper-containing enzymes such as lysyl oxidase, dopamine-β-hydroxylase, and possibly EC-SOD (Section 3.16.3.1).

3.16 Metal ions and antioxidant defence: intracellular and extracellular strategies[284]

Within cells, iron is in constant transit between the LIP, ferritin and other iron-containing proteins. Oxidative stress can lead to more iron (and possibly copper) release. This may explain why cells rely heavily on enzymes that remove $O_2^{\bullet-}$

(SODs) and peroxides (catalases, peroxiredoxins, the GPx family) for their antioxidant defence; it is important to minimize levels of $O_2^{\bullet-}$ and H_2O_2 before they come into contact with transition metal ions and generate more damaging species (Table 3.10). The use of low levels of peroxides in signal transduction (Section 4.5) means that some oxidative damage is probably inevitable and is dealt with by repair systems.

3.16.1 Metallothioneins[307–310]

Metallothioneins, low molecular mass (about 6500) proteins encoded by genes on chromosome 16 in humans, also contribute to safe segregation of metal ions. They are found in the cytosol and nucleus of eukaryotic cells, especially in liver, kidney and gut. Two isoforms, **MT-I** and **MT-II**, are found in all animal tissues, and a third isoform, **MT-III**, in brain and, to a lesser extent, kidney. A fourth, **MT-IV**, may exist.

Metallothioneins are rich in sulphur (23–33% of the amino acids are cysteine). They therefore are significant contributors to total cellular protein thiol. Each MT molecule can bind five to seven ions of such metals as zinc (Zn^{2+}), silver (Ag^+), copper (Cu^+), cadmium (Cd^{2+}) and mercury (Hg^{2+}). Binding is achieved by association of cysteine–SH groups with the metal ion; for example, Cd^{2+} and Zn^{2+} are linked to four cysteine thiolate ligands (Cys-S$^-$) in a tetrahedral arrangement. Binding of Cu^+ is tighter than that of Cu^{2+} and appears to involve three thiolate ligands. The MT content of tissues can be increased by injection or oral administration of Cd, Cu or Zn salts, and synthesis of MTs is also increased by several hormones, including glucocorticoids, glucagon and adrenalin, and by IL-1 produced during inflammation (Section 4.7). Proposed functions of MTs include storage of heavy metals in a non-toxic form, regulation of cellular copper[307] and zinc metabolism, and control of the absorption of these metals by the gut. For example, cultured mammalian cells that cannot make MTs are sensitive to injury by Cd^{2+} ions, whereas cells overproducing these proteins are resistant to Cd^{2+}.

Metallothioneins might also be antioxidants. Sequestration of copper will diminish RS generation promoted by this metal, and the high content of −SH groups in MTs makes them excellent scavengers of $ONOO^-$, HOCl, singlet O_2 and $OH^\bullet$ radicals, although the fate of the resulting sulphur-centred radicals must be considered. For example, reaction of $OH^\bullet$ with MT can generate a thiyl radical that reacts with an adjacent thiolate on the protein

$$RS^\bullet + RS^- \xrightarrow{O_2} RSSR^{\bullet -} \rightarrow RSSR + O_2^{\bullet -}$$

or combines with O_2 to give a thiyl peroxyl radical

$$RS^\bullet + O_2 \rightarrow RSOO^\bullet$$

Metallothionein-enriched cells are generally more resistant to damage by RS, consistent with an antioxidant role.[308] However, knockout mice defective in MT-I and -II appeared normal, including unaltered levels of oxidative damage,[309] but cells from them were more sensitive to damage by Cd^{2+}, *tert*-butylhydroperoxide, or paraquat (Section 8.4). Hence the 'antioxidant' role of MT-I and -II may be limited in normal animals, but could be important in oxidative stress. Metallothionein levels rise in brain in response to cold injury, and MT-I and -II knockout mice showed an aggravated inflammatory response to such injury. Surprisingly perhaps, mice lacking the brain MT-III were not more susceptible, although overexpression of this protein in the brain has been shown to be protective in some other neuronal injury models.[310]

3.16.2 Phytochelatins

Several plants contain small, cysteine-rich proteins involved in the accumulation and detoxification of cadmium, zinc, copper and other metals. They consist of repetitive γ-glutamylcysteine units and are synthesized from GSH. These **phytochelatins** may function like metallothioneins, some of which also occur in plants.[311]

3.16.3 Extracellular antioxidant defence[284]

Antioxidants in the extracellular fluids of multicellular organisms help to protect the following

against damage by RS:

- the surfaces of the cells with which they are in contact, e.g. seminal plasma helps protect spermatozoa against ROS generated by phagocytes in semen (Section 6.11);
- constituents of the aqueous phase of the fluids (e.g. surfactant in lung lining fluids);
- constituents of the lipid phase of the fluids, e.g. plasma lipoproteins.

In animals, one difference from the intracellular environment is that extracellular fluids such as blood plasma, seminal fluid, respiratory tract lining fluids, cerebrospinal fluid (CSF) and synovial fluid, generally contain little or no catalase activity. The traces of catalase sometimes detected may have leaked from cells; for example slight haemolysis is common during centrifugation of blood for preparation of plasma. There is at least one exception; catalase is present in human and other animal oviductal fluids and may help protect the sperm transiently residing there.[312] The mucus lining the respiratory and gastrointestinal tracts may contain catalases, peroxiredoxins and other peroxidases contributed by lysis of shed cells;[313] indeed damage to underlying cells may 'automatically' increase the antioxidant defence of extracellular fluids by releasing GSH, ascorbate, SODs, GPx, thioredoxin and peroxiredoxins.

Levels of GSH, SOD and GPx are also generally low in extracellular fluids, except that the fluid lining the lower part of the respiratory tract has high GSH levels (Table 3.7). Although there is a plasma GPx, its putative substrates (GSH and thioredoxin; Section 3.8.1) are present only at low levels and it is hard to see how it could function under normal conditions.

3.16.3.1 *Extracellular superoxide dismutase (sometimes called SOD3)*[314]

Of the limited SOD activity present in extracellular fluids, some is CuZnSOD and some MnSOD, both of which might arise, at least in part, by leakage of enzymes from damaged cells. However, most is a different type of CuZnSOD called **extracellular SOD (EC-SOD)**. Plasma EC-SOD activity shows a large interspecies variation, for example rabbits, rats, mice and guinea pigs have levels one or two orders of magnitude greater than pigs, dogs and humans.

Extracellular SOD has a higher relative molecular mass (about 135 000) than CuZnSOD and is a tetrameric glycoprotein, each subunit containing one Cu and one Zn. Like SOD1, EC-SOD can be inactivated by excess H_2O_2. There are several isoforms of EC-SOD (A, B and C); B and C bind to heparin, C more tightly than B. In A, the heparin-binding domains at the C terminal regions of all four subunits are removed by intracellular proteolysis before secretion of the enzyme, in B from only some of the subunits and in C from none of them. It seems likely that *in vivo* most EC-SOD is bound to cell surfaces, largely by association with cell surface carbohydrates, especially in the lung, kidney, uterus and blood vessel walls. For example, human thoracic aorta has fairly low SOD1 activity, but a comparable level of EC-SOD. This is unlike most tissues, where CuZnSOD is the major contributor to total SOD (its in a different place of course!) (Table 3.3). In cartilage, there is a lot of EC-SOD in the matrix (Section 9.10.1). Injection of heparin into animals produces a rise in plasma EC-SOD, by displacing the enzymes from cell surfaces. The heparin-binding domain additionally allows EC-SOD to bind to collagen[315], and the protein **fibulin 5** (which is closely associated with elastin) also helps to bind EC-SOD to blood vessels.[316]

Extracellular SOD may serve to minimize interaction of $O_2^{\bullet-}$ and $NO^{\bullet}$ to form $ONOO^-$, especially in situations such as hypertension when vascular $O_2^{\bullet-}$ production is increased (Section 7.10.3).[317] Indeed, $NO^{\bullet}$ in excess may increase EC-SOD biosynthesis. Transgenic mice lacking EC-SOD appear normal and show no compensatory changes in other antioxidant defence enzymes, but they developed more lung damage and died faster when exposed to pure O_2, showed an exaggerated lung inflammation when exposed to 1.5 ppm ozone[318] and had aggravated joint inflammation in collagen-induced arthritis (Section 7.9.4). There was also an impaired response of erythropoietin synthesis to hypoxia (Section 7.10.5). As always, there must be a balance; mice over-expressing EC-SOD were *more* sensitive to 6 atm hyperbaric O_2, an effect reversed by the SOD inhibitor DDTC (Section 3.2.1.4). This may be because removal of more $O_2^{\bullet-}$ raises the level of $NO^{\bullet}$ and increases cerebral blood flow, preventing the normal vasoconstriction of blood vessels that occurs in hyperbaric hyperoxia and so delivering excess O_2 to the brain (Section 9.16.6). Extracellular SOD knockout mice also display mildly-impaired learning and memory functions under certain experimental situations, and more brain damage after cerebral ischaemia.[314] Nevertheless, a human polymorphism (2–6% of adults) is known in which a single base substitution causes an arg → gly transition in EC-SOD, affects heparin binding and elevates plasma EC-SOD level, presumably also decreasing cell surface levels. There are no obvious physiological consequences, although an increased risk of ischaemic heart disease has been suggested.[319]

Extracellular SOD subunits closely resemble those of SOD1 and it seems likely that the EC-SOD gene evolved by a duplication of the SOD1 gene, followed by later structural modifications.

3.16.3.2 *Other extracellular SODs*

Several parasites, for example *Taenia*, *Trichinella*, *Schistosoma* and *Ascaris* species,[7] secrete SOD1 (and sometimes other antioxidant proteins such as FeSOD and peroxiredoxins)[209] on their surfaces, presumably to protect them against damage by host phagocytes.

3.16.3.3 *Metal-ion sequestration*

In general in extracellular fluids, activities of antioxidant defence enzymes are low (Section 3.16.3). The lipoproteins present contain α-tocopherol and other lipid-soluble antioxidants (Section 9.3.4) whereas vitamin C and urate help defend the aqueous phase (Sections 3.18.6 and 3.20.1 below) against RS produced by enzymes (e.g. plasma XO), autoxidizing compounds and activated phagocytes. Sometimes these RS act as useful signals, for example low levels of H_2O_2 may facilitate cell proliferation, the aggregation of platelets and adherence of phagocytes to vascular endothelium. In whole blood, excess $O_2^{\bullet-}$ and H_2O_2 might (like $NO^{\bullet}$) diffuse into erythrocytes for metabolism (Section 6.4.2). Indeed, H_2O_2 can diffuse into and out of any cell. However, for these things to happen, it is important that $O_2^{\bullet-}$ and H_2O_2 be stopped from forming $OH^{\bullet}$.

Transferrin is present at high levels in plasma and binds iron ions in a form that will not stimulate free-radical reactions. In healthy people, it is only

20 to 30% loaded with iron, so that the content of NTBI in plasma is effectively nil. Hence if enough animal plasma is added to iron-dependent OH•-generating systems or to lipids undergoing iron-dependent peroxidation, the reactions are inhibited. Lactoferrin acts as an antioxidant in the same way and it may be secreted by neutrophils at sites of inflammation to aid in iron sequestration (Section 7.7.2.6). Any Fe^{2+} ions released into plasma will be assisted in binding to transferrin by the ferroxidase activity of caeruloplasmin.

Metal-binding antioxidant defence may be weaker in some other extracellular fluids. Thus human CSF contains little transferrin, albumin or caeruloplasmin and its transferrin is at or close to iron saturation (Section 9.16.5). Synovial fluid has lower concentrations of albumin, transferrin and caeruloplasmin than plasma. The fluids that line the respiratory tract[320] have a low protein content (mainly albumin, but some transferrin) but can contain 'free' iron (Section 6.3).

3.16.3.4 *Haem binding*[284]

Haem and haem proteins can be pro-oxidants (Section 3.15.3), but are often released from damaged cells, for example lysed erythrocytes. Indeed, injected haem or erythrocyte lysate are proinflammatory in animals.[321] Luckily, plasma contains the haemoglobin-binding **haptoglobins**, as well as a haem-binding protein (**haemopexin**). Binding of haemoglobin to haptoglobins, or of haem to haemopexin, decreases their effectiveness in stimulating lipid peroxidation (Fig. 3.22). The haemoglobin–haptoglobin or haem–haemopexin complexes are then removed from the circulation. Macrophages in liver and elsewhere play a key role in uptake and degradation of the haemoglobin–haptoglobin complex.[322] The haem–haemopexin complex is taken up by the liver and then dissociated, the haemopexin being returned to the circulation. Haptoglobin is an acute phase protein (Section 4.7.3), mainly synthesized in the liver but also in the lung and adipocytes.

Haptoglobin- or haemopexin-knockout mice seem normal, but suffer worse renal damage and oxidative stress during haemolysis than do controls.[323] After acute haemolysis, haemopexin levels increased in haptoglobin-null mice, and haptoglobin increased in haemopexin-lacking mice. Double knockouts again appeared normal, but developed

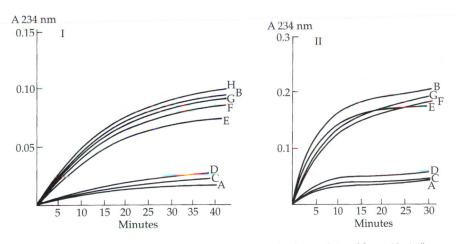

Figure 3.22 Antioxidant effects of haemopexin and haptoglobin. (I) Haemin-stimulated peroxidation of fatty-acid micelles measured as diene conjugation at 234 nm (Section 5.14.4.2). Micelles were incubated at pH 7.4 and 25°C alone (curve A), with haemin (curve B), or with haemin and (C) the lipid-soluble chain-breaking antioxidant BHT, (D) apohaemopexin, a powerful inhibitor, (E) albumin, a weak inhibitor, (F) mixed haptoglobins (little effect). (G) desferrioxamine (little effect), or (H) apotransferrin (no effect). (II) Haemoglobin stimulated lipid peroxidation. Micelles were incubated at pH 6.4 and 25°C alone (curve A), with desferrioxamine and methaemoglobin (curve B), or with desferrioxamine and methaemoglobin plus (C) mixed haptoglobins, a powerful inhibitor, (D) BHT, (E) apohaemopexin (no effect), (F) apotransferrin (no effect) or (G) albumin (no effect). Data abstracted from *Biochem. J.* **256**, 861, 1988. Haemopexin can also protect LDL against oxidation by haem or haemoglobin—presumably released haem is involved in the latter case (*Biochemistry* **35**, 13112, 1996). Mixed haptoglobins refers to a mixture of the 1–1, 1–2 and 2–2 isoforms.

spleen enlargement, liver inflammation and fibrosis after a haemolytic event.[324] Albumin can bind haem, but does not prevent its pro-oxidant effects as well as haemopexin (Fig. 3.22).

The human haptoglobin gene on chromosome 16 is polymorphic, with two alleles, denoted 1 and 2. There are thus three haptoglobin phenotypes, 1–1, 1–2 and 2–2, whose distribution varies in different races. Under certain conditions, the 1–1 form is a better inhibitor of haemoglobin-induced lipid peroxidation than the 2–2 form, and haemoglobin bound to the 1–1 form is more rapidly cleared from the circulation.[325] There are several suggestions that the 2–2 phenotype increases the risk of atherosclerosis, for example in diabetes. Why diabetes? It seems that this haptoglobin is less good at blocking the pro-oxidant activity of glycated haemoglobins (Section 9.4.4).[325]

3.16.3.5 *Albumin*[284]

Albumin has multiple roles, for example it maintains osmotic pressure and transports drugs, bilirubin (Section 3.18.1 below), hormones and fatty acids in the blood. However, it could also be an important extracellular antioxidant. It binds haem and copper ions, protecting more important targets (e.g. LDL) against damage (Section 3.15.4.2). Albumin contains an exposed cysteine —SH group (position 34 in the human protein), contributing up to $500\,\mu M$ to 'total plasma thiols'. Albumin–SH reacts quickly with $ONOO^-$, $NO_2^\bullet$, $CO_3^{\bullet -}$, HOCl, $RO_2^\bullet$, and $RO^\bullet$ and slowly with H_2O_2.

Rats unable to synthesize albumin show increased levels of plasma cholesterol ester hydroperoxides and decreased levels of ascorbate and ubiquinol. In dialysis patients, plasma albumin was reported to show elevated levels of protein carbonyls[327] (a biomarker of oxidative protein damage; Section 5.15.3) and in septic patients there is considerable oxidation of albumin–SH groups.[328] All three observations are consistent with a scavenger role, although there are also suggestions that oxidized albumin may be toxic to vascular endothelium and could provoke phagocyte RS production.[329] Oxidized albumin is probably removed by phagocytes and endothelial cells using scavenger receptors (Section 9.3).[330] A few cases of human **analbuminaemia** (less than one

per million births) have been reported; as in the rat, it is not life-threatening but parameters of oxidative damage have not been studied. Levels of several other plasma proteins are elevated in this condition.

3.16.3.6 *Artefacts with albumin*

Studies of antioxidant (or toxic) effects of albumin in cell culture or *in vivo* must consider the fact that commercial albumin preparations are often partially oxidized at Cys34 and contaminated with endotoxin and metals such as iron, copper and vanadium (Table 4.4).[331] Sometimes transferrin contamination is present.[332] Despite this, infusions of albumin have been used for over 50 years for maintaining plasma volume and to treat hypoalbuminaemia and hyperbilirubinaemia. The clinical benefit of albumin infusion in sepsis or acute respiratory distress syndrome (ARDS) patients (Section 9.7) continues to be debated,[328] especially if oxidized albumin really is toxic.[329]

Table 3.11 summarizes plasma antioxidant defences.

3.17 Haem oxygenase

Haem oxygenase (HO), an enzyme found in the ER, catalyses the breakdown of haem to biliverdin, releasing iron ions and carbon monoxide (Fig. 3.23). Biliverdin is converted to **bilirubin** by the enzyme **biliverdin reductase** in the cytosol. Three isoforms of HO have been characterized; one is a constitutive isoform (**HO-2**) present normally in several tissues. In the carotid body (Section 1.3.2), HO-2 is involved in O_2 sensing; it degrades haem and forms CO that keeps K^+ channels open. In hypoxia, CO formation slows, K^+ channels close and trigger an alarm signal for the body that increases respiration rates.[333]

Another form of HO is a 'stress-inducible' isoform (**HO-1**), identical to the heat shock protein, **hsp32** (Section 4.6). This form is present at high levels in the Kupffer cells of the liver and in the spleen, to destroy haem from the processing of worn-out red blood cells. The third form, **HO-3**, has low activity and may function as a haem-binding protein rather than an HO. Humans, or knockout mice, lacking HO-1 show anaemia and tissue iron accumulation, as well as low plasma bilirubin, indicative of the key role of HO-1 in iron metabolism.[334] Carbon monoxide plays some roles as a signalling molecule, not only in the carotid body but also in liver and brain.[335]

Haem oxygenase enzymes remove a pro-oxidant (haem) whilst generating a putative antioxidant (bilirubin) and another pro-oxidant (iron), so we are not quite sure whether to classify them as antioxidants. For example, mice lacking HO-1 are more susceptible to inflammation and hypoxia (which induces HO-1 in normal animals) but paradoxically they suffered *less* lung damage when exposed to pure O_2.[336] Studies on endothelial and skin cells show that induction of HO-1 by exposing them to haem is accompanied by a rise in ferritin; if this is prevented, exposure of the cells to haem *sensitizes* them to H_2O_2. Hence HO must co-operate with iron sequestration systems to achieve cell protection. Normally, the released iron acts through the IRPs (Section 3.15.1) to increase ferritin synthesis. Studies on transplanted hearts and blood vessel grafts showed that increased levels of HO-1 improve outcome, but the protection could be mimicked by brief exposure to CO, apparently because CO suppresses phagocyte infiltration/

activation and fibroblast proliferation.[337] In some systems, bilirubin and/or biliverdin might contribute to protection.[338]

Haem oxygenases can be inhibited by **tin protoporphyrin**, widely used to study the role of HO. For example, pretreatment of rats with haemoglobin to induce HO-1 decreased the lethality of subsequent endotoxin treatment, but tin protoporphyrin prevented this.[339] However, it may not be specific: tin protoporphyrin can decrease caspase activities and inhibit apoptosis (Section 4.4.1).

3.18 Antioxidant protection by low-molecular-mass agents: compounds synthesized *in vivo*

Several small molecules are thought to be important antioxidants. Some are made *in vivo*, others obtained from the diet. Let us consider some of the former first. Antioxidant effects of GSH and other thiols were considered in Sections 3.9 and 3.12. Other compounds of interest discussed elsewhere are taurine and hypotaurine (Section 7.7.3), polyamines (Section 4.12.9) plasmalogens (Section

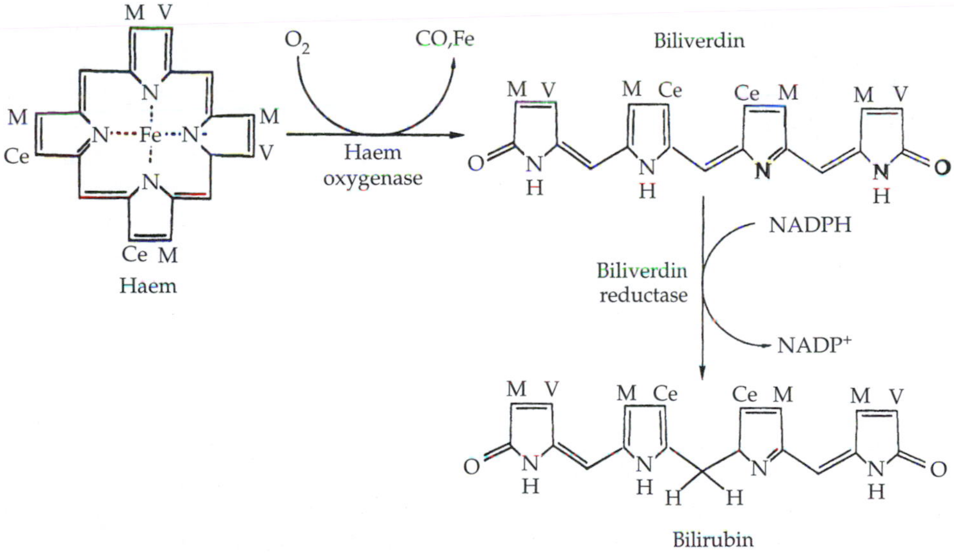

Figure 3.23 Haem degradation by haem oxygenases. Adapted from *Am. J. Respir. Cell. Mol. Biol.* **15**, 9, 1996 by courtesy of Dr Augustine Choi and the publishers. Haem oxygenase enzymes are unusual in that they use haem as both substrate and prosthetic group. NADPH-cytochrome P450 reductase reduces the active site-haem to Fe^{2+}, which then binds O_2. The Fe^{2+}–O_2 complex then generates the oxidizing species, possibly a ferric peroxide (*Acc. Chem. Res.* **31**, 543, 1998). V, vinyl group; M, methyl group; Ce, propionyl group.

Table 3.11 Extracellular antioxidant defences in blood plasma[294]

Defence	Mode of action	Comments
Transferrin, lactoferrin	Bind iron and stop its pro-oxidant activity.	These proteins are not easily damaged by H_2O_2, HOCl, ONOO⁻ or lipid peroxides; only release iron ions at acidic pH
Caeruloplasmin	Catalytically oxidizes Fe^{2+} to Fe(III) *without release* of oxygen radical intermediates. Reacts stoichiometrically with $O_2^{\bullet-}$; reports of greater $O_2^{\bullet-}$–scavenging activity may be due to contamination with EC-SOD; see *Free Rad. Biol. Med.* **2**, 255, 1988). Binds to and inactivates myeloperoxidase. Plays a key role in iron metabolism Speculation that one of its copper ions could be pro-oxidant.	Acute-phase protein, levels go up in disease
Erythrocytes	Can take up $O_2^{\bullet-}$ and H_2O_2 for metabolism by SOD/catalase/GPx1/peroxiredoxins and NO• for oxidation by haemoglobin. Can also convert NO_2^- to NO• when O_2 levels are low.	H_2O_2 could diffuse also into platelets, phagocytes, endothelial cells, etc. for metabolism
Albumins	Bind copper tightly and iron weakly. Present at high concentrations. Possible sacrificial antioxidants; rapidly scavenge HOCl and ONOOH. Provide high –SH level in plasma. Bind haem, can help protect lipoproteins against haem-dependent oxidation. Carry bilirubin.	Liver synthesis and plasma concentration drop during illness, sometimes called 'a negative acute-phase response'

Haptoglobin/haemopexin	Bind free haemoglobin/haem and decrease their pro-oxidant ability (Fig. 3.22). Haptoglobin also suggest to have chaperone activity, possibly protecting other extracellular proteins against damage (*Biochemistry* **44**, 10904, 2005)	Acute-phase proteins
Urate	Inhibits lipid peroxidation and scavenges RS.	Can also bind iron and copper ions. Urate radical can be damaging, but can be removed by ascorbate. Reaction with $ONOO^-$ produces some $NO^•$.
α-Tocopherol	Lipid-soluble antioxidant: chain-breaking by trapping peroxyl radicals.	Major, lipid-soluble, chain-breaking antioxidant in human plasma; important in protecting lipoproteins against oxidation. Coenzyme Q also present, in smaller amounts.
Glucose	Scavenger of $OH^•$ radical; rate constant comparable to that of mannitol. Can exert pro-oxidant effects by glycation of proteins.	Normal plasma concentration around 4.5 mM, greater immediately after carbohydrate-containing meals.
Bilirubin	Postulated antioxidant.	A sensitizer of $^1O_2$ production, and its oxidation products may be vasoactive. Neuroprotective at low levels, too much is neurotoxic.

Extracellular SOD, GPx, thioredoxin and catalase are not included here.

4.12.8), coelenterazine and coelenteramine (Section 7.6.1) and tryptophan-derived products (Section 7.4.2).

3.18.1 Bilirubin

Since we have just studied HO, let us consider its product bilirubin (Fig. 3.22). Its precursor biliverdin is blue-green, whereas bilirubin is bright yellow. Hence the colour of a bruise changes from reddish brown (extravascular haemoglobin), through greenish to yellow as it heals. Biliverdin reductase is not present in birds, reptiles and amphibians, so they excrete biliverdin instead. About 80% of the bilirubin produced in mammals arises from HO-dependent catabolism of haemoglobin from senescent red blood cells, by reticuloendothelial cells in the spleen, liver and bone marrow.[241] The rest comes from other haem proteins such as myoglobin, catalase and cytochromes. Over 270 mg of bilirubin is produced daily in the average adult human.

Bilirubin is insoluble in water at physiological pH and binds tightly to albumin in a 1:1 stoichiometry. This binding prevents uptake by extrahepatic tissues, particularly lipid-rich organs such as the brain, and directs bilirubin to the liver. There the albumin–bilirubin complex dissociates, bilirubin enters the hepatocyte through a carrier protein and binds to cytosolic proteins, mainly GSTs. Bilirubin undergoes conjugation in the ER with glucuronic acid (Section 2.6.4.4), forming mono- and diglucuronides which are water-soluble and excreted in the bile. Impaired conjugation leads to jaundice in premature babies (Section 6.11.8).

In vitro, bilirubin can scavenge ONOOH, $RO_2^\bullet$, $RO^\bullet$ and singlet O_2, actions possibly important in premature babies (Section 6.11.8). Bilirubin is oxidized by some ROS to biliverdin, which can be recycled by biliverdin reductase (Fig. 3.22).[340] Bilirubin bound to albumin can protect the protein itself and albumin-bound fatty acids against free-radical damage. Suggestions that bilirubin is an important antioxidant were initially based largely on experiments showing protective effects in cultured cells, especially neurons, but animal studies are now appearing.[338] For example, bilirubin administration decreased oxidative damage and tissue injury in rats with experimental autoimmune encephalitis.[341] Urinary excretion of bilirubin oxidation products was reported to be elevated in septic patients, consistent with an antioxidant role.[342]

Do not forget, however, that bilirubin can *sensitize* formation of singlet O_2 in the presence of light, and high levels in premature babies are toxic to the brain; the antibiotic minocycline can decrease this neurotoxicity in animals.[343] Oxidative degradation of bilirubin can produce potentially-toxic vasoconstricting compounds, which have been detected in CSF from patients after subarachnoid haemorrhage.[344] Thus the jury is still out as to whether bilirubin is a major, minor, or zero contributor to antioxidant defence *in vivo*.

3.18.2 α-Keto acids[345]

Several keto acids, including pyruvate, glyoxylate and α-ketoglutarate (often called 2-oxoglutarate) react non-enzymically with H_2O_2 and act as 'H_2O_2 scavengers' when they are added at mM levels to cell culture media. Thus pyruvate addition to the reperfusion fluid decreased oxidative injury in pig hearts *in situ*.[346] It is also likely that keto acids can scavenge HOCl and ONOOH. Decarboxylation of 2-oxoglutarate has been used as an assay for H_2O_2 (Table 5.8). Whether such RS scavenging occurs *in vivo* in animals is uncertain, but the non-enzymic conversion of glyoxylate (OHC.COOH) to formate by H_2O_2 may happen in the peroxisomes of illuminated green leaves (Section 6.8.4). Pyruvate is an important metabolic substrate for the early human embryo (Section 6.11) and could also act as an antioxidant to some extent.

3.18.3 Melatonin[347]

Most melatonin is produced by the pineal gland at the base of the brain, but small amounts are made in some other tissues. It also occurs in some foods, for example walnuts. Melatonin regulates circadian rhythms, and has been popularized as a cure for 'jet lag'. It arises by methylation and acetylation of **serotonin** (Fig. 3.24); blood levels of melatonin are low during the day and increase at night as pineal

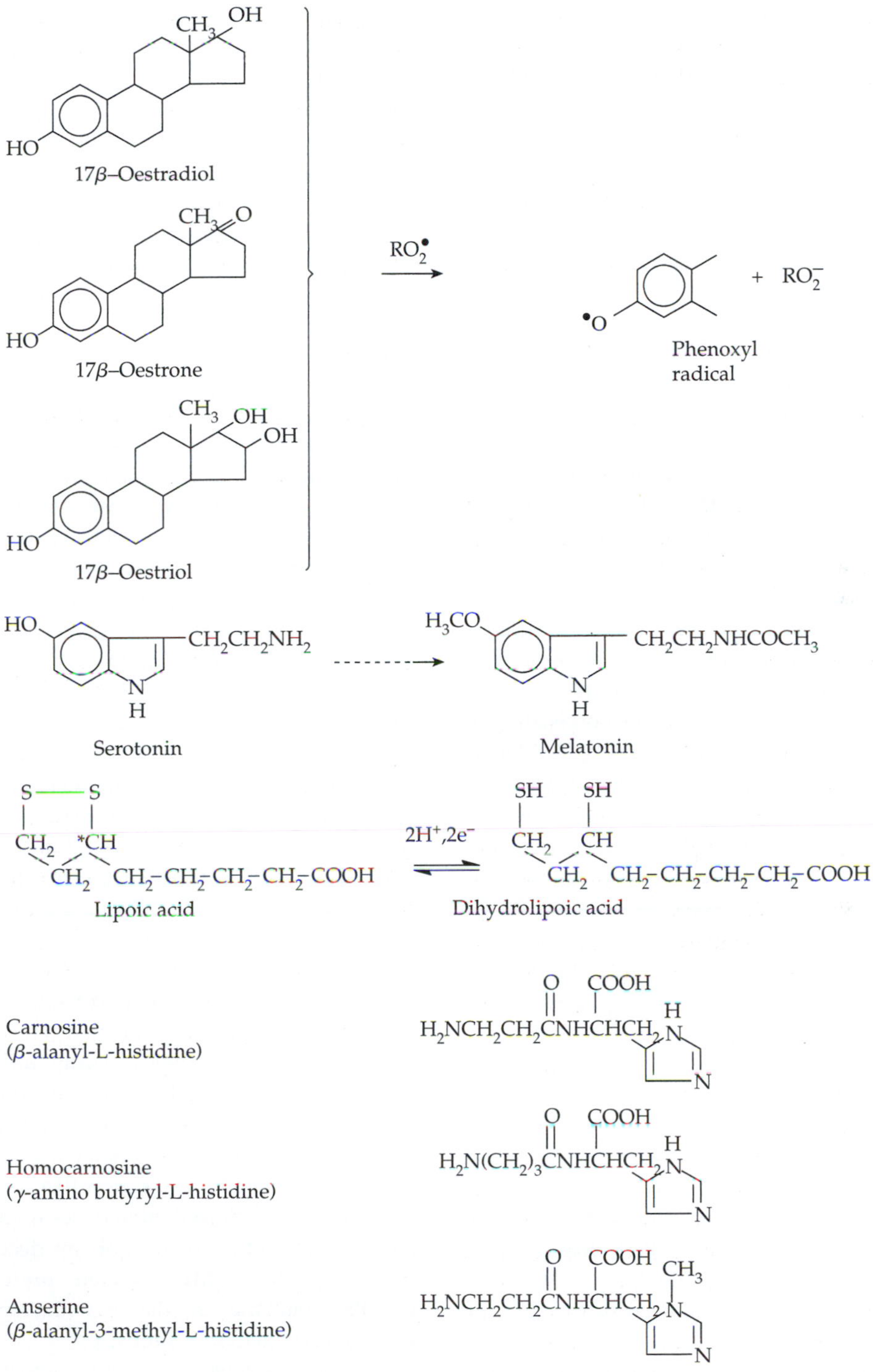

Figure 3.24 (*Cont.*)

Mycosporine–glycine

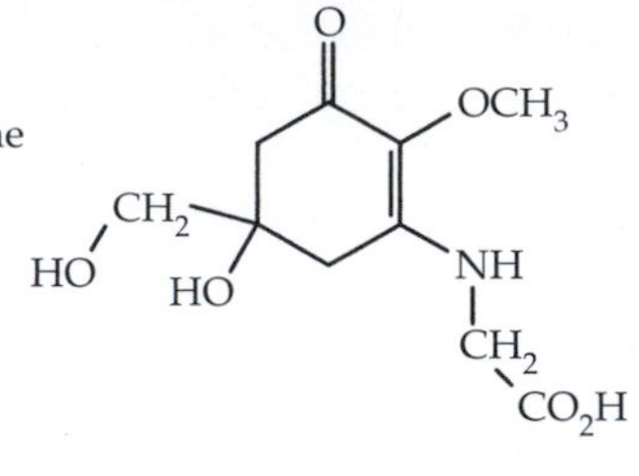

Figure 3.24 Structures of some putative antioxidants. In lipoamide the −COOH group becomes −CONH$_2$. The metabolism of oestrogens is shown in Fig. 9.20.* Represents the chiral centre in lipoic acid.

synthesis accelerates. Melatonin shows modest antioxidant activity *in vitro* (probably by donation of hydrogen by the NH group), but only at concentrations some orders of magnitude higher than those present *in vivo* (which are <1 nM). Its precursor, serotonin, is a better lipid peroxidation inhibitor *in vitro*, as would be expected since it contains a phenolic −OH group which in melatonin is blocked by methylation (Fig. 3.24).[348]

Nevertheless, there are reports of benefits of melatonin administration in oxidative stress situations such as ischaemia–reperfusion and in transgenic mice overexpressing APP (Section 9.20), plus the usual crop of 'no effect' reports.[347,349] Melatonin seems unlikely to exert direct antioxidant effects in animals, and may instead act by increasing the levels of antioxidant defence enzymes, such as GPx and γ-GCS, as well as decreasing production of cytokines and iNOS. By contrast in the dinoflagellate *Gonyaulax polyedra* melatonin levels can be much higher and a direct antioxidant effect is feasible.[350]

3.18.4 Lipoic acid[351]

Lipoic acid, **1,2-dithiolane-3-pentanoic acid** (sometimes called **thioctic acid**), is an essential component (as the *R*-stereoisomer of its amide form, **lipoamide**) of the pyruvate and αKGDH multienzyme complexes (Fig. 1.7). Both the oxidized (disulphide) and reduced (dithiol; Fig. 3.24) forms of lipoic acid show antioxidant properties *in vitro*; they can scavenge RO$_2^\bullet$, HOCl, CO$_3^{\bullet-}$, NO$_2^\bullet$, OH$^\bullet$ and ONOOH and bind iron and copper ions.

With a reduction potential ($E^{0'}$) of −0.32 V, dihydrolipoate (DHLA) is a powerful reducing agent. Thus it can reduce GSSG to GSH,

dehydroascorbate to ascorbate and α-tocopheryl radical to α-tocopherol, the latter both directly and via ascorbate. Indeed, administration of lipoic acid reversed some of the effects produced by α-tocopherol deficiency in mice, and decreased the incidence of cataract in mice treated with buthionine sulphoximine to inhibit GSH synthesis (Section 3.9). *In vivo*, lipoic acid is converted to DHLA by **lipoamide dehydrogenase** enzymes at the expense of NADH or NADPH. Glutathione and thioredoxin reductases may also act on lipoic acid.

Levels of 'free' lipoic acid/DHLA in animal tissues and body fluids are low, so it is unlikely to be an important endogenous antioxidant. However, its range of antioxidant properties and ability to regenerate other naturally-occurring antioxidants have provoked attempts to use it as a therapeutic antioxidant, for example in the treatment of diabetes (Section 9.4). The *R*-stereoisomer of lipoic acid also seems to promote glucose uptake by muscle. Of course, the use of thiols as antioxidants should be undertaken with consideration of the thiyl and oxysulphur radicals that can be produced (Section 2.5.5). Nevertheless, many animal studies have indicated antioxidant effects of lipoic acid in many oxidative stress situations and it has even been speculated to be an 'antiageing' molecule, at least in dilapidated rats (Section 10.4.2). Lipoic acid has other effects as well; high doses in rats lowered food intake and body weight, by decreasing the activity of the **AMP-activated protein kinase (AMPK)** enzyme in the hypothalamus whilst increasing its activity in muscle.[352]

In *Mycobacterium tuberculosis* lipoamide does play a direct role in antioxidant defence by co-operating with a peroxiredoxin, AhpC. This is linked to lipoamide dehydrogenase and lipoamide succinyltransferase proteins through an intermediate 'adaptor protein', **AhpD**, to form a complex that scavenges peroxides and ONOO⁻, helping to defend this pathogen against attack by RS from phagocytes.[353]

3.18.5 Coenzyme Q[354]

Coenzyme Q is essential in mitochondrial electron transport (Fig. 1.8), undergoing oxidation and reduction via a free-radical intermediate, **ubisemiquinone** (CoQH•). It is also found in other cell membranes and in lipoproteins. *In vitro*, ubiquinol (CoQH$_2$) can scavenge RO$_2^•$ radicals and inhibit lipid peroxidation

$$RO_2^• + CoQH_2 \rightarrow RO_2H + CoQH^•$$

For example, the ubiquinol content of LDL affects their resistance to peroxidation (Section 9.3.8). Ubiquinol can regenerate α-tocopherol from its radical in lipoproteins and membranes

$$\alpha\text{-Toc}^• + CoQH_2 \rightarrow CoQH^• + \alpha\text{-TocH}$$

The rate constant for scavenging of RO$_2^•$ by CoQH$_2$ is about one-tenth that of α-tocopherol. It follows that tocopherol recycling is probably more important than direct scavenging of RO$_2^•$ by CoQH$_2$, since the α-tocopherol and coenzyme Q levels in most cell membranes (but not in LDL; Section 9.3.8) are broadly comparable.

The contribution of ubiquinol to antioxidant defence *in vivo* is uncertain. It may be especially important in mitochondria, where the electron transport chain can easily reoxidize/rereduce CoQH•. By contrast, it has been suggested that mitochondrial ubisemiquinone can be a source of O$_2^{•-}$ radicals, although this may not happen without exposure of it to a source of protons, for example by membrane disruption (Section 1.10.4). The enzyme **DT-diaphorase** (Section 8.6.4) can reduce CoQ to CoQH$_2$, as can thioredoxin reductase.[355]

A CoQ-deficient strain of *S. cerevisiae* was abnormally sensitive to damage by oxidation products of PUFAs, consistent with the view that CoQ can exert antioxidant effects in at least some organisms,[356] one of which is *C. elegans* (Section 10.3). Some scientists

have suggested that the ratio of ubiquinol to ubiquinone in human plasma may be an index of oxidative stress.[357] Coenzyme Q administration appears to have some benefit in patients with diabetes[358] and certain neurodegenerative diseases (Section 9.16.6.6), although it is uncertain if this is due to antioxidant or 'mitochondria-protecting' effects, or both.[359]

3.18.6 Uric acid

Uric acid is produced from hypoxanthine and xanthine by XO and XDH enzymes. In most species, the H$_2$O$_2$-producing peroxisomal enzyme **urate oxidase** converts it to allantoin, which is further converted to allantoate and then gloxylate plus urea, all products much more soluble in water than is urate (Fig. 3.25). However, humans and other primates lack a functional urate oxidase gene; a similar DNA sequence is present in the human genome, but a stop codon is present in one of the exons and the defective gene is not transcribed. Urate oxidase activity is thus absent and urate accumulates in blood plasma to high concentrations, usually 0.2 to 0.4 mM. Urate is also present intracellularly and in other human body fluids including milk, respiratory tract lining fluids, saliva, synovial fluid and tear fluid, usually at lower levels than plasma (e.g. 100–200 μM in saliva). Release of urate from dying cells is one of the factors that help provoke an immune response.[360]

At physiological pH almost all uric acid is ionized to urate,[361] bearing a single negative charge, since the pK_a of uric acid is around 5.4. Urate has limited solubility in water: excess production *in vivo* can lead to crystallization from solution. This occurs in **gout**, a disease often treated with allopurinol (Fig. 1.16). The excruciatingly painful character of attacks of gout, caused by joint inflammation triggered by urate crystals, has been recognized since ancient times and afflicted (to name but a few) the Roman emperor Claudius, Henry VIII and Benjamin Franklin. Indeed, urate oxidase 'knockout' mice show elevated plasma urate and develop kidney stones.[362] Several RS, such as OH• and RO$_2^•$, oxidize urate into a free radical, which also bears a single negative charge at pH 7.4, since its pK_a is 3.1. The unpaired electron is

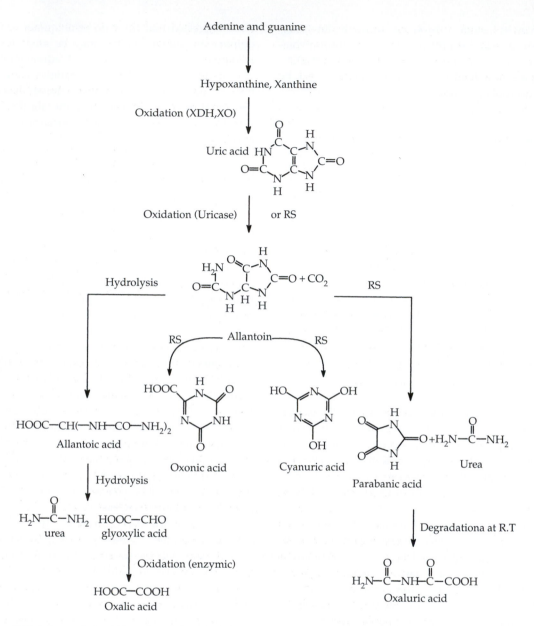

Figure 3.25 Pathways of uric acid formation and degradation, both enzymic and non-enzymic. Urate is formed by enzyme-catalysed breakdown of unwanted purines arising from DNA, RNA, GTP and ATP. Breakdown occurs in the liver, gut and muscles and urate is released into the blood. Some is excreted in urine, but the kidneys reabsorb much urate and return it to the blood. (*Nature* **415**, 393, 2002). Diagram by courtesy of Dr H. Kaur (also see *Chem. Biol. Interac.* **73**, 235, 1990). XDH, xanthine dehydrogenase; XO, xanthine oxidase; RS, reactive species; RT, room temperature.

delocalized over the purine ring, giving a resonance-stabilized radical which does not react rapidly with O_2 to form a peroxyl radical.[361] The reduction potential of the urate/urate radical system at pH 7 is 0.59 V, which is considerably higher than that of ascorbate ($E^{0'} = -0.28$ V). Hence ascorbate would be expected to reduce the urate radical, and this has been demonstrated experimentally (second-order rate constant $\approx 10^6 \, M^{-1} s^{-1}$).

In 1981, Ames *et al.*[363] pointed out that urate is a powerful scavenger of ROS *in vitro*, proposed that it functions as a biological antioxidant and further suggested that loss of urate oxidase was advantageous to primates since it simultaneously removed a source of H_2O_2 (urate oxidase) and allowed a powerful antioxidant to accumulate. This loss must have been accompanied by further adaptations to prevent deleterious effects of the urate.[362] Indeed, urate is a powerful scavenger of O_3 and $NO_2^{\bullet}$ and may help to protect biomolecules against these oxidizing air pollutants in the respiratory tract (Section 8.11). Urate is a substrate for oxidation by haem protein/H_2O_2 systems (Section 3.15.3) and might be able to protect against oxidative damage by being preferentially oxidized. Urate also protects proteins against nitration on addition of $ONOO^-$; its reaction with $ONOO^-$ is complex and produces some nitrosocompounds that decompose to release $NO^{\bullet}$, as well as **triuret**,[364]

$$H_2N - \overset{\overset{\displaystyle O}{\|}}{C} - NH - \overset{\overset{\displaystyle O}{\|}}{C} - NH - CONH_2$$

which might be further oxidized by ONOOH to **aminocarbonyl radical**

$$H_2N - \overset{\overset{\displaystyle O}{\|}}{\underset{\bullet}{C}}$$

Urate can also chelate metal ions: it binds iron and copper ions in forms apparently poorly reactive in catalysing free-radical reactions, although it can also reduce Cu^{2+} to Cu^+ and stimulate LDL oxidation *in vitro* (Section 9.3.8.3).

The high levels of urate *in vivo* make a role in scavenging RS feasible. This is supported by observations that products of urate degradation by RS, especially **allantoin** (Fig. 3.25), increase in concentration in patients subjected to oxidative stress, for example in Wilson's disease, Down's syndrome, haemochromatosis, rheumatoid arthritis, intensive exercise and premature birth (Section 5.12). However, reaction of urate with Cu^{2+}, haem proteins plus H_2O_2, $RO_2^{\bullet}$, $OH^{\bullet}$ or $ONOO^-$ generates urate radical.[361] This is not necessarily innocuous, since it has been shown *in vitro* to lead

to inactivation of some proteins, such as human α_1-antiproteinase.[365] This may not be a significant problem *in vivo* however; inactivation of α_1-antiproteinase can be prevented by the simultaneous presence of ascorbate, presumably because it reduces urate radical.[365] Urate radical can also be reduced by several flavonoids (rate constants $\sim 10^6 \, M^{-1}s^{-1}$) and reacts fast ($k = 8 \times 10^8 \, M^{-1}s^{-1}$) with $O_2^{\bullet -}$, presumably to generate urate and O_2.[366]

There have been suggestions that high plasma levels of urate are risk factors for cardiovascular disease and stroke, but the precise link is uncertain as yet.[367] By contrast, infusion of urate has neuroprotective effects in some animal models, apparently by scavenging[368] $ONOO^-$. Infusion of urate into humans decreased rises in F_2–IPs caused by severe exercise (Section 6.13.1).

3.18.7 Histidine-containing dipeptides[369]

Many mammalian tissues, especially muscle and brain, contain mM concentrations of dipeptides composed of histidine plus another amino acid (Fig. 3.24). They include **carnosine, homocarnosine** and **anserine**. In humans, pigs and turkeys, carnosine is more common than anserine, whereas the reverse is true for chickens and rabbits (don't ask us why; no-one knows!). Carnosine levels in rat and human muscles decline with age (Section 10.4.4). **Carcinine** (β-alanyl-histamine), presumably a decarboxylation product of carnosine, has been detected in several mammalian tissues. It has been suggested that humans can absorb carnosine from meat (the origin of its name) in the diet as well as make it themselves.[370]

In vitro, these dipeptides can exert antioxidant effects;[369,371] for example, the imidazole ring chelates copper ions and prevents copper-dependent oxidative damage. They are weak inhibitors of lipid peroxidation; claims of greater inhibitory effects are often due to the ability[372] of these compounds to interfere with measurement of lipid peroxidation by the TBA test (Section 5.14.9). Contamination of commercial carnosine preparations with **hydrazine**, a powerful reducing agent that reacts fast with aldehydes, may also have led to overestimation of carnosine's antioxidant effects.[373] Nevertheless, the purified dipeptides are able to scavenge $RO_2^\bullet$ and singlet O_2. They also react with cytotoxic end products of lipid peroxidation, such as HNE, converting them to stable adducts, and can be converted to chloramines by HOCl.[373]

Histidine alone *promotes*[374] iron ion-dependent lipid peroxidation *in vitro* and enhances the toxicity of H_2O_2 to mammalian cells in culture.[375] Since the dipeptides do not exert such 'pro-oxidant' effects, they may represent 'safer' ways of accumulating histidine at high levels for use as an intracellular buffer (the histidine imidazole ring has a pK_a of about 6) and, perhaps, copper ion chelator.[372] One exception; both histidine and the dipeptides can *aggravate* $OH^\bullet$ production from H_2O_2 by nickel ions (Section 8.15.3). Another suggestion is that these dipeptides help to protect proteins against glycation, since carnosine is rapidly glycated upon incubation with high levels of glucose (or other sugars) *in vitro*. It also protects proteins against damage by methylglyoxal (Section 3.9.1).[376]

Enzymes (**carnosinases**) that hydrolyse these dipeptides have been described in various muscles and in brain. Some are just 'general dipeptidases' but others may be more specific.[377] It has been hypothesized that genetic variants in these enzymes, helping to raise plasma carnosine levels, may protect against diabetic nephropathy.[378]

3.18.8 Trehalose (α-D-glucopyranosyl-1, 1-α-D-glucopyranoside)[379]

Some bacteria and yeasts (including *S. cerevisiae* and *Candida albicans*) accumulate the trisaccharide **trehalose** on exposure to stress, apparently to protect proteins against damage. In addition, at the very high concentrations that accumulate (up to 500 mM), it may exert radical-scavenging properties. Yeast cells unable to make trehalose are hypersensitive to, oxidative protein damage by H_2O_2.

3.18.9 Melanins: hair, skin, corals, fungi and fish

Melanins (from the Greek word *melanos*, 'dark') are pigments, found throughout the animal kingdom and in some fungi, that are formed by oxidation and polymerization of tyrosine.[380] In humans they are important to the skin and eye (Sections 6.10 and 6.12) and for hair colour. Melanins are made in melanosomes (Fig. 3.26). The first steps are catalysed by **tyrosinases**, copper-containing enzymes that convert tyrosine to L-DOPA and then oxidize L-DOPA to semiquinones and quinones, which polymerize (Fig. 3.26). Assembly of melanin occurs upon a scaffold of the **Pme117** protein, which also sequesters the reactive intermediates from the other parts of the cell (Section 9.20.6). **Tyrosine hydroxylase** enzymes, iron-containing proteins, assist in L-DOPA formation. The end-products of polymerization contain high concentrations of *o*-quinone (oxidizing) and *o*-hydroquinone (reducing) groups as well as semiquinones, and many unpaired electrons. Hence one can regard melanins as large free radicals. The movement of unpaired electrons between different energy levels helps melanins to absorb ultraviolet radiation, especially the brown or black **eumelanins**. Illumination of melanins generates $O_2^{\bullet-}$ within the molecule, but this is usually quickly scavenged; $O_2^{\bullet-}$ can reduce melanin quinones to semiquinones, and oxidize hydroquinones, also to semiquinones (Section 2.5.3.5). Hence, overall, eumelanins are 'radical sinks' for $O_2^{\bullet-}$ and $RO_2^\bullet$.

The red-brown or yellow pigment found in the skin and hair of fair-skinned, red-headed humans is **pheomelanin**, which appears less good as a radical scavenger and could even sensitize skin cells to oxidative damage under certain circumstances.[381] On exposure of pheomelanin to strong light it is degraded, and a net formation of $O_2^{\bullet-}$ can be measured. Pheomelanins contain cysteine, which cross-links with dopaquinone during polymerization to give **cysteinyl DOPAs** (Fig. 3.26). Thus the supply of GSH/cysteine in the melanocyte helps determine whether pheomelanins or eumelanins form. Melanins also bind transition and other metal ions; for example, the binding of iron to neuromelanin is relevant to Parkinson's disease (Section 9.19). Sequestration of metal ions by melanins could conceivably contribute to antioxidant defence, but the metal ions are probably still redox-active and could damage the melanin itself if, for example, H_2O_2 were present. Indeed, the 'pro-oxidant' effect of illuminated pheomelanin *in vitro* seemed to involve iron ions bound to it.[381]

High levels of melanin might contribute to the resistance of some pigmented fungi and of the cancer **melanoma** to ionizing radiation. For example,

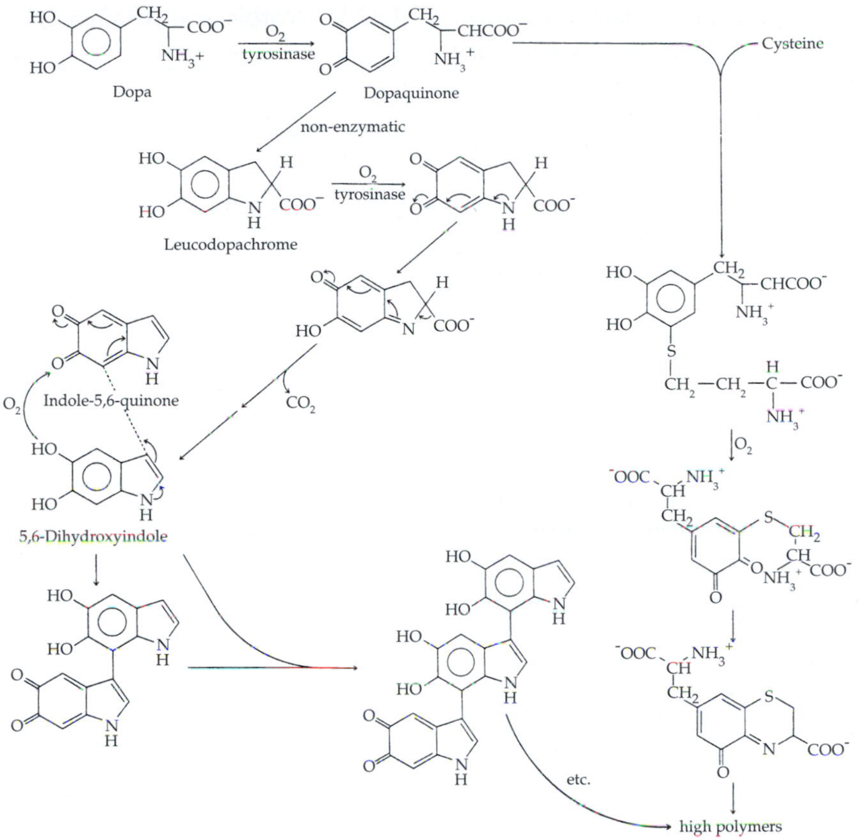

Figure 3.26 Biosynthesis of melanin. The complex reaction pathways involve both enzyme-catalysed and non-enzymic reactions. Melanin is produced by specialized cells called **melanocytes**, formed within them in organelles called **melanosomes**. Melanin can remain there, or be transferred to other cells. Diagram from *Biochemistry, The Chemical Reactions of Living Cells* by courtesy of Dr David E. Metzler and Academic Press. Various mutations can lead to **albinism**; sufferers are prone to photochemical damage to the skin and show impaired eye function. For example, mutations that inactivate tyrosinase produce a complete lack of melanin in skin, eye and hair (*Human Mutation* **13**, 19, 1999).

melanized cells of the pathogenic fungus *Cryptococcus neoformans*, are more resistant to killing by RS than non-melanized cells.[382] Overall, however, the physiological importance of melanins as antioxidants is uncertain. Several marine organisms (including corals and certain fish) appear to protect themselves against UV light by synthesizing UV-absorbing **mycosporine-like amino acids** such as **mycosporine glycine** (Fig. 3.24).[383]

3.19 Gender affects antioxidant defence

In all advanced countries women live longer than men, on average. Many explanations have been advanced (Section 10.5.10), some of which involve antioxidant defences. Thus in certain intervention studies with dietary antioxidants, women showed less benefit than men (Section 10.5.7), suggesting better antioxidant status. Levels of oxidative damage products, 8OHdG and F_2-IPs, are lower in women in some studies.[384,385] Testosterone promotes O_2 toxicity (Section 1.5.2) and castrated males live longer (or does it just feel like longer?); although castration increases free radical production in the prostate gland (Section 7.10) it might decrease it in the body as a whole. Women show lower body iron stores until after the menopause–in one large study, premenopausal women excreted less 8OHdG than men, but postmenopausal females excreted more.[385] Isoprostanes were also lower after brain injury in females.[386]

The female sex hormones oestradiol, oestrone and oestriol can inhibit lipid peroxidation (including LDL peroxidation) *in vitro*, because they possess phenolic–OH groups and can act as chain-breaking antioxidants (Figure 3.24). In general, however, the concentrations of hormones needed to inhibit peroxidation *in vitro* (μM) are larger than physiological (pM range). In addition, the phenoxyl radicals produced during antioxidant activity (Fig. 3.24) are reactive and capable of damaging proteins and DNA[387] (again perhaps unlikely to be relevant at physiological levels, although it could contribute to the cancers induced in rodents by treatment with high levels of these hormones [Section 9.14.1]). The synthetic oestrogen **diethylstilboestrol** is a powerful inhibitor of lipid peroxidation at μM concentrations *in vitro*, although it is carcinogenic in humans.[388]

Oestrogens at physiological levels may act instead by decreasing ROS production and raising antioxidant levels. Thus mitochondrial ROS production appears lower in female than in male rats but is increased by removal of the ovaries (**ovariectomy**), as is vascular iNOS activity. Female rats also show higher levels of some antioxidant defence enzymes, such as MnSOD and GPx1.[389] By contrast, some assays reveal a lower total plasma antioxidant activity in human females, although the physiological importance of this parameter is uncertain (Table 5.17). In ovariectomized animals there is considerable bone loss, apparently related to decreased antioxidant defences and increased ROS, promoting bone reabsorption by osteoclasts (these cells are further discussed in Section 9.10.2). Thus ROS could contribute to **osteoporosis**, the bone-thinning disease that plagues many elderly ladies.[390] Short-term hormone replacement therapy decreased levels of lipid peroxidation, as measured by F_2-IPs, in human volunteers.[391]

3.20 Antioxidant protection by low-molecular-mass agents: compounds derived from the diet

Many dietary constituents have been suggested to act as antioxidants. The health aspects of dietary antioxidants are discussed in Chapter 10; here we examine their basic chemistry.

3.20.1 Ascorbic acid (vitamin C)[392,393]

Ascorbic acid is a white crystalline solid, very soluble in water. It was first isolated from adrenal glands, cabbages, lemons and oranges as an 'acidic carbohydrate' by Szent-Györgyi in 1928. His first paper describing it was rejected by the *Biochemical Journal* because the editor did not like the suggested name *ignose* (from 'I don't know' and –ose for carbohydrate). *Godnose* was also unacceptable, and eventually they agreed on the name *hexuronic acid*. Good dietary sources of vitamin C include citrus fruits, guava, berries, mango, broccoli and peppers.

Ascorbic acid has two ionizable –OH groups (Fig. 3.27). Since pK_{a1} is 4.25 and pK_{a2} is over 11.5, the monoanion is favoured at physiological pH. Hence we use the name **ascorbate** from now on. Plants and most animals can synthesize ascorbate from glucose, but humans, other primates, guinea pigs, some fish and fruit bats lost the enzyme required for the terminal step (**gulonolactone oxidase**) and so need ascorbate in the diet. Gulonolactone oxidase catalyses the reaction:

$$\text{L-gulono-}\gamma\text{-lactone} + O_2 \rightarrow$$
$$\text{L-ascorbate} + H_2O_2$$

Note that H_2O_2 is produced, so that high rates of ascorbate synthesis in animals could, paradoxically, impose oxidative stress.[394] By contrast, the terminal step of ascorbate synthesis in plants does not make H_2O_2 (Section 6.8.8). An extensively mutated and inactive form of the L-gulonolactone oxidase gene is present in human and guinea pig genomes and probably in the other species mentioned above. Inability to make ascorbate (like the lack of urate oxidase) is a universal inborn error of metabolism in humans.

Ascorbate in animals acts as a cofactor for at least eight enzymes, of which the best known are the prolyl and lysyl hydroxylases involved in collagen biosynthesis, and the prolyl and asparaginyl hydroxylases that contribute to O_2 sensing (Section 1.3.2). All contain iron at their active sites. Collagen synthesized in the absence of ascorbate is insufficiently hydroxylated and does not form fibres properly, giving rise to poor wound healing and fragility of blood vessels. For example, impaired collagen synthesis may predispose to premature rupture of the chorioamniotic membranes during pregnancy (Section 6.11.6). Ascorbate is also required by the copper-containing enzyme **dopamine-β-hydroxylase**, which converts dopamine into noradrenalin. Two enzymes in the biosynthesis of **carnitine**, a cofactor important in fat metabolism, require ascorbate. Other ascorbate-requiring enzymes are involved in tyrosine metabolism and in the addition of amide groups to peptide hormones to stabilize them.

Deficiency of ascorbate in the human diet causes **scurvy**. In 1536, the French explorer Jacques Cartier vividly described this disease, which afflicted all but ten of the 110 men aboard his ships wintering in the frozen St Lawrence river: 'The victims' weakened limbs became swollen and discoloured, whilst their putrid gums bled profusely'. Nearly 30 years later, the Dutch physician Ronsseus

advised that sailors consume oranges to prevent scurvy. In 1639, one of England's leading physicians, John Woodall, recommended lemon juice as an antiscorbutic. James Lind, a Scottish naval surgeon, was the first man in medical history to conduct a controlled clinical trial; in May 1747, he tested a variety of reputed remedies on 12 scorbutic sailors. Two of them were restricted to a control diet, but the others were additionally given one of the substances under trial. The two seamen who were provided two oranges and a lemon each day made a speedy recovery. The only others to show any signs of recovery were those who had been given cider (made from apples; apples are a mediocre source of vitamin C and it readily oxidizes in solution). Lind observed no improvement in the condition of those who had been given either oil of vitriol (dilute sulphuric acid), vinegar, sea-water (popular folk-remedies for scurvy at the time) or the control diet.

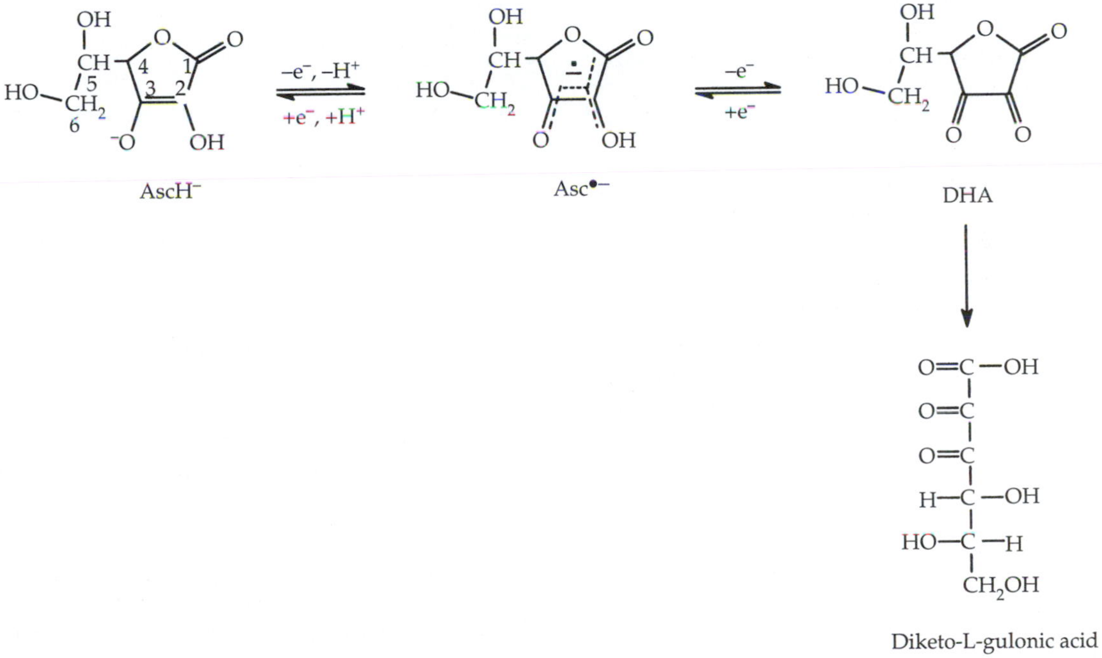

Figure 3.27 Structure of ascorbic acid and its oxidation and degradation products. At physiological pH the acid form is largely ionized (ascorbate) since the pK_{a1} of ascorbic acid is 4.25. Diketogulonate readily spontaneously degrades to a mixture of species, including oxalate, the four-carbon sugar threonate, and 5-carbon sugars,[393] also see *Anal. Biochem.* **265**, 238, 1998. Yeasts (e.g. *S. cerevisiae, C. albicans*) often contain **D-erythroascorbate**, in which the side chain is −CH$_2$OH rather than −CHOHCH$_2$OH. It has very similar biochemical properties to ascorbate; the terminal step in its synthesis also involves an H$_2$O$_2$-producing enzyme, **D-arabinono-1, 4-lactone oxidase** (*Mol. Microbiol.* **30**, 895, 1998).

Box 3.2 Ascorbate as an antioxidant

- Scavenges $O_2^{\bullet-}$ and $HO_2^{\bullet}$ (rate constant $>10^5 M^{-1}s^{-1}$ at pH 7.4)
- Scavenges $OH^{\bullet}$ (rate constant $>10^9 M^{-1}s^{-1}$, although rate constants for reaction of $OH^{\bullet}$ with most other molecules *in vivo* are comparable)
- Scavenges water-soluble peroxyl ($RO_2^{\bullet}$) radicals; lipophilic ascorbate esters have been developed for use in foods and cosmetics and can scavenge lipid-soluble $RO_2^{\bullet}$ radicals
- Scavenges thiyl, and oxysulphur radicals (Section 2.5.5)
- Scavenges ergothioneine-derived radicals (Section 3.12.2)
- A substrate for ascorbate peroxidases, enzymes essential for H_2O_2 removal in chloroplasts and some other organisms
- Prevents damage by radicals arising by attack of $OH^{\bullet}$ or $RO_2^{\bullet}$ upon urate, probably by reacting with urate radicals (Section 3.18.6)
- A powerful scavenger of HOCl, ONOOH (also see *Free Rad. Biol. Med.* **35**, 1529, 2003) and nitrosating agents (Sections 2.6.1 and 2.6.3) although its ability to prevent gastric nitrosation reactions *in vivo* is uncertain
- Inhibits lipid peroxidation induced by haemoglobin–or myoglobin–H_2O_2 mixtures; reduces the haem Fe(IV) species back to the Fe^{2+} state, preventing ferryl-dependent oxidations and haem breakdown (Section 3.15.3)

- A powerful scavenger and quencher of singlet O_2 (Section 2.6.4)
- Co-operates with vitamin E; regenerates α-tocopherol from α-tocopheryl radicals in membranes and lipoproteins (Section 3.20.2)
- Scavenges nitroxide radicals (Section 5.2)
- Infusion or oral administration of gram doses has been shown in some, but not all, studies to improve endothelium-dependent vasodilation in patients with vascular dysfunction, possibly by scavenging ROS and/or by preserving tetrahydrobiopterin for eNOS and thus maintaining $NO^{\bullet}$ levels (*J. Clin. Invest.* **111**, 1201, 2003)
- Protects plasma lipids against peroxidation induced by activated neutrophils and AAPH-derived peroxyl radicals
- Protects membranes and lipoproteins against lipid peroxidation induced by RS in cigarette smoke (Section 8.12)
- A powerful scavenger of O_3 and $NO_2^{\bullet}$ in human body fluids; probably protects lung lining fluids against inhaled oxidizing air pollutants (Section 8.11)
- Inhibits oxidative damage by scavenging radicals generated from certain drugs (e.g. phenylbutazone)
- Protects against phagocyte adhesion to endothelium induced by oxidized LDL

For references see *Free Radic. Res.* **25**, 439, 1996 and *Br. J. Pharmacol.* **142**, 231, 2004.

Lind's conclusions were acted upon by Captain James Cook on his second voyage round the world. Although Cook was at sea for 3 years, not a single member of his crew died from scurvy, thanks to adequate provision of lemon juice, fresh fruit and vegetables. Surprisingly, it was not until 1795 that the British Admiralty agreed to Lind's demands for a regular issue of lemon juice on British ships. The effect was dramatic; in 1780, there had been 1457 cases of scurvy admitted to Haslar naval hospital, but only two admissions took place between 1806 and 1810. Unfortunately, lemon juice was soon replaced by cheaper lime juice in a money-saving exercise rather typical of British governments throughout the ages; hence English sailors were often nicknamed 'limeys'. Scurvy returned and it

took over a century to realize that the lime juice used had only about one-quarter of the antiscorbutic activity of the lemon juice.

3.20.1.1 *Ascorbate as an antioxidant:* in vitro *yes*, in vivo *maybe?*[395-397]

Ascorbate-dependent peroxidases are important H_2O_2-removing systems in plants and some other species (Section 3.13.7 and 6.8.8), and ascorbate may also have direct antioxidant effects. Mammalian cells accumulate ascorbate from body fluids against a concentration gradient, coupled to uptake of Na^+, using two similar transporters **SVCT1** (**sodium-vitamin C transporter 1**) and **SVCT2**, one or both of which is found in most tissues. Mice lacking SVCT2 have decreased levels of ascorbate in many tissues and die quickly after birth, with brain damage (Section 9.16.6.4). Much intestinal uptake of ascorbate is Na^+-dependent, but its oxidation product dehydroascorbate (DHA, Fig. 3.27) can also be absorbed. Hence DHA in foods can act as a source of vitamin C for the body, being reduced within the gut cells to ascorbate for delivery to plasma. In the body, several cell types (especially neutrophils) can take up DHA through some of the glucose transport systems (**GLUT1**, **GLUT3** and **GLUT4**); glucose thus competes with DHA uptake in these cells (but apparently not for DHA uptake from the gut).[398] Little is known about the subcellular distribution and movement of ascorbate, although mitochondria contain ascorbate and appear able to take up and reduce DHA, probably via a glucose transporter in the inner membrane.[399] It is not clear what stops ascorbate from simply reducing cytochrome c, however.

The most striking chemical property of ascorbate is its action as a reducing agent, for example its ability to reduce Fe(III) to Fe^{2+} facilitates iron uptake in the duodenum (Section 3.15.1) and maintains the activity of lysyl, asparaginyl and prolyl hydroxylases; iron at the active site must be Fe^{2+} for hydroxylation to occur. Table 2.3 shows that the reduction potential of ascorbate places it close to the bottom of the 'pecking order' for oxidizing species, that is it will tend to reduce more-reactive species such as $OH^\bullet$, $O_2^{\bullet-}$ and urate radical. Donation of one electron by ascorbate gives the **semidehydroascorbate** (SDA), sometimes called **ascorbyl**, radical (Fig. 3.27), which can be further oxidized to give DHA. Ascorbyl radical is not very reactive, being neither strongly oxidizing nor strongly reducing, nor does it seem to reduce O_2 to $O_2^{\bullet-}$ at a high rate (if at all). The poor reactivity of ascorbyl is the essence of many of ascorbate's antioxidant effects: a RS interacts with ascorbate and a much less reactive (ascorbyl) radical is formed. Indeed, ascorbate has a multiplicity of antioxidant properties *in vitro* (Box 3.2).

Left to itself, ascorbyl undergoes slow disproportionation, regenerating some ascorbate

$$2SDA \rightleftharpoons ascorbate + DHA$$

Dehydroascorbate is unstable and breaks down to a mixture of products (Fig. 3.27). Aqueous solutions of ascorbate are stable at pH 7.4 unless transition metal ions are present, which catalyse its rapid oxidation. Copper salts are excellent catalysts–if you want plenty of vitamin C from vegetables, do not cook them in copper pans! Copper- and iron-induced oxidation of ascorbate produce H_2O_2 and $OH^\bullet$; the multiple literature reports of the ability of ascorbate to degrade DNA and damage various animal cells in culture, including cancer cells, can probably be attributed to the formation of ROS due to the presence of transition metal ions in the reaction solutions or cell culture media.[400] Ascorbate can be stabilized by conversion to sulphate forms (found in some marine organisms), or by phosphorylation: **ascorbate phosphates** and **ascorbate glucosides** have been used as 'non-autoxidizable' delivery vehicles for vitamin C in several cell culture studies.

But is ascorbate an antioxidant *in vivo*? The levels of it present (30–90 μM in human plasma; higher in CSF, aqueous humour of the eye, seminal fluid, gastric juice and lung lining fluid: millimolar intracellular levels in many cell types) are certainly sufficient to exert antioxidant effects. However, direct evidence that ascorbate acts as an antioxidant *in vivo* is limited.[395] A review from the Linus Pauling institute[396] concluded that attempts to demonstrate antioxidant effects *in vivo* in humans using biomarkers of oxidative damage (such as DNA base oxidation products or F_2-IPs) had not given consistent positive effects, and most of the better-designed studies were negative. Suggested vasculoprotective or antihypertensive effects of ascorbate are similarly variable between laboratories and in any case could be due to the preservation of tetrahydrobiopterin for NOS rather than to antioxidant effects (Box 3.2). It may be that ascorbate levels in healthy subjects on a good diet are sufficient to exert maximum antioxidant effects already, so that supplements give no further benefit (Table 10.5). This is illustrated by studies on human sperm; 60 mg ascorbate per day seemed sufficient to normalize the elevations in sperm 8OHdG levels observed in subjects on an ascorbate-poor diet (Section 6.11; Table 6.7). Nevertheless, a significant percentage of the world's population is malnourished, even in advanced countries, and depletions of ascorbate can occur in sick people, for example in the intensive care unit or with kidney failure.[401,402]

There is evidence for rapid oxidation of ascorbate *in vivo* at sites of oxidative stress. It becomes oxidized to DHA in synovial fluid in the knee-joints of patients with active rheumatoid arthritis and in the lungs of patients with ARDS (Section 9.10 and 9.7), presumably as it acts to scavenge RS. Measurement of ascorbyl radical by ESR has been used as an index of oxidative stress in several systems (Section 5.2). Ascorbate levels are lower in cigarette smokers and in diabetics (Sections 8.12 and 9.4).

The effects of ascorbate depletion are often examined in guinea pigs, but can also be studied in a mutant rat strain that cannot make ascorbate.[403] The **ODS rat** was discovered in the laboratories of the Japanese pharmaceutical company Shionogi & Co, as suffering from osteogenic disorders when fed the usual rat chow; hence the name **osteogenic disorder Shionogi** (ODS) rat. Ascorbate intake (in the range 150–900 mg/kg diet) did not alter lipid peroxidation in ODS rats. Again, only when there is a very low ascorbate intake can antioxidant effects of extra dietary ascorbate be convincingly demonstrated.[403]

3.20.1.2 'Recycling' of ascorbate[393,399]

Ascorbate/DHA ratios are high in mammalian body fluids and tissues during health; almost no DHA is present. Oxidation of ascorbate in body fluids usually leads to its depletion, probably by the reactions

$$\text{ascorbate} \xrightarrow{\text{RS attack}} \text{SDA radical}$$

$$2\text{SDA} \xrightarrow{\text{disproportionation}} \text{ascorbate} + \text{DHA}$$

$$\text{DHA} \xrightarrow[\text{breakdown}]{\text{rapid non-enzymic}} \text{multiple products}$$

In addition, erythrocytes, neutrophils and some other cells take up DHA and convert it back to (intracellular) ascorbate. Most tissues possess enzymes that convert ascorbyl radical or DHA back to ascorbate at the expense of GSH or of NADH,

often called **NADH-semidehydroascorbate reductase** or **dehydroascorbate reductase** activities. However, their identity as unique enzymes is uncertain since several proteins involved in thiol–disulphide interchange, including PDI, thioredoxin reductase and glutaredoxin (Sections 3.10 and 3.11) can act as DHA reductases. For example, a 'DHA reductase' purified from human neutrophils was found to be glutaredoxin. In parasites, trypanothione (Section 3.12.1) can reduce dehydroascorbate.

There is evidence that GSH and ascorbate do interact *in vivo*.[160] Severe GSH depletion in newborn rats and guinea pigs is lethal, but death can be prevented by high doses of ascorbate (although not by DHA). The onset of scurvy in guinea pigs fed a diet low in ascorbate is delayed by administering GSH precursors. In isolated hepatocytes, lowering GSH levels increases ascorbate synthesis. In a human study, concentrations of ascorbate and GSH in lymphocytes were correlated, both appearing to decline with age.[404] There was also a seasonal variation in ascorbate concentration, and administration of ascorbate to subjects with the lowest plasma levels of this vitamin raised lymphocyte GSH.[404]

3.20.1.3 Pro-oxidant effects of ascorbate[395,397]

In vitro, vitamin C can also exert pro-oxidant properties. The classic **Udenfriend system** for making OH• in the laboratory consists of ferric-EDTA, H_2O_2 and ascorbate. Ascorbate reduces the iron

$$\text{Fe(III)}-\text{EDTA} + \text{ascorbate} \rightarrow \\ \text{Fe}^{2+}-\text{EDTA} + \text{SDA}$$

$$\text{Fe}^{2+}-\text{EDTA} + H_2O_2 \rightarrow \text{Fe(III)}-\text{EDTA} \\ + \text{OH}^\bullet + \text{OH}^-$$

Ascorbate/Cu^{2+} mixtures inactivate many enzymes, probably by formation of OH• and/or oxo-copper species, and iron salt/ascorbate mixtures have been used for decades *in vitro* to induce lipid peroxidation and other oxidative damage. Instillation of ascorbate plus iron or copper ions into the stomach of animals was reported to lead to OH• generation[405] and the mixture of metal ions and ascorbate in some vitamin pills has been claimed to generate OH[•] as the pills dissolve.[406] Pro-oxidant effects of ascorbate are a problem in the food industry[407] and in the design of fluids for parenteral nutrition (Section 6.11.8.5). Even dissolving ascorbate tablets in tap water can generate OH[•] if, as is often the case, transition metal ions are present.[408]

Are these pro-oxidant effects physiologically relevant? *In vitro* pro-oxidant effects are not unique to ascorbate; they can be demonstrated with several reducing agents in the presence of transition metal ions, including α-tocopherol (Section 3.20.2.5 below), GSH, NAD(P)H, urate, and several plant phenolics (Section 3.22.3 below). Thus if ascorbate's pro-oxidant effects are relevant *in vivo*, pro-oxidant effects of these other reductants might also be expected to occur. One key question is the availability of 'catalytic' transition metal ions. Iron and copper ions in most extracellular fluids are largely sequestered in forms unable to catalyse free-radical reactions (Section 3.16), so that the pro-oxidant properties of ascorbate (and other biological reducing agents) would be limited. In contrast, cells have labile intracellular 'pools' of iron. If these come into contact with ascorbate, pro-oxidant effects could conceivably occur. Whether they do or not is an open question.

Do we learn anything by looking at patients with thalassaemia or haemochromatosis? Plasma ascorbate levels in such patients are often subnormal.[301,409] There are a few published 'case reports' that giving vitamin C to iron-overloaded subjects without administration of desferrioxamine can produce deleterious clinical effects, although some case reports do not find this.[410] The data are inconclusive, although haemochromatosis patients are often cautioned not to take high-dose ascorbate supplements.[409]

Injury to human tissues can liberate transition metal ions (Fig. 9.1). Could the pro-oxidant effects of ascorbate become relevant here? The authors have hypothesized[284] that the decline in ascorbate at sites of tissue injury occurs because: (i) ascorbate scavenges RS and may recycle α-tocopherol; (ii) the resulting DHA is taken up by cells to maintain intracellular ascorbate; and (iii) ascorbate removal from the extracellular environment minimizes its potential pro-oxidant interactions with metal ions released by tissue damage. Thus one can speculate that giving lots of ascorbate to sick people may not be a good thing, an idea supported by some epidemiological studies in diabetes (Section 9.4.6). It's still only speculation, though. Another frequently-asked question is whether ascorbate could favour excess uptake of iron into the body, since Fe(III) reduction to Fe^{2+} by ascorbate facilitates iron uptake in the duodenum. There is little evidence to support this view in healthy subjects; iron uptake is carefully regulated whatever the ascorbate intake. However, the issue needs to be addressed in iron overload.[411]

We conclude that, although the *in vivo* evidence for major antioxidant effects of ascorbate is not compelling, that for metal ion-dependent pro-oxidant effects is even more sparse. However, potentially-damaging effects of ascorbate need not always involve metal ions. Ascorbate can glycate proteins, for example (although metal ions often participate in glycoxidation; Section 9.4).[412] Lee *et al*[413] showed that vitamin C causes lipid peroxide decomposition to cytotoxic aldehydes in the absence of metal ions. However, ascorbate can combine with cytotoxic aldehydes such as HNE (Section 4.12.5.3). Indeed, approximately 1 μM HNE–ascorbate conjugate was detected in the plasma of healthy human subjects, suggesting that this reaction occurs *in vivo*.[414]

3.20.1.4 *Taking ascorbate supplements?*

There is no convincing evidence for toxicity of gram doses of ascorbate in healthy humans (although it can increase urinary oxalate in some subjects and has been hypothesized to increase the risk of kidney stone formation),[415] but no evidence of benefit either. Ascorbate is ultrafiltered and reabsorbed in the kidney, but the active uptake system has limited capacity so that an intake of about 200 mg daily (easily obtainable from a diet with five servings of fruits and vegetables daily) is sufficient to saturate cells and body fluids with ascorbate: any excess is excreted.[416] However, heavy smokers need more vitamin C (Section 8.12). The popular belief that high doses of ascorbate protect against the common cold has been difficult to verify in controlled studies.[417] So take lots of C if you believe in it, it probably does little harm, if not necessarily any good. Be aware that ascorbic acid is quite acidic, whereas the sodium salt will deliver a lot of Na^+ if gram quantities are consumed.

3.20.2 Vitamin E[196,418]

3.20.2.1 *Putting E in its place*

Vitamin E is often said to be the most important (but not the only) inhibitor of lipid peroxidation *in vivo*. However, as with vitamin C, evidence for its antioxidant effect in well-nourished humans is limited. For example, large oral doses over long periods (greater than 2000 mg/day for more than 8 weeks or, in one study, 200 mg/day for one year)[419] are required to decrease lipid peroxidation in humans (ref[420] and J Morrow, personal communication). In any case, the antioxidant action of vitamin E comes at a late stage; lipid peroxidation can be prevented, as an earlier line of defence, by enzymes that scavenge RS and mechanisms that sequester transition metal ions. In addition, vitamin E may have non-antioxidant roles in metabolism.

3.20.2.2 *What is vitamin E?*

'Vitamin E' is not a specific chemical. It is a nutritional term, first used to refer to a fat-soluble 'factor', discovered in 1922 to be essential in the diet of rats to permit normal reproduction. Later work showed that vitamin E is essential in the diets of other animals:[196,421] lack of it causes a variety of symptoms including sterility in male rats, dogs, cocks, rabbits and monkeys, haemolysis in rats and chicks, muscular degeneration in rabbits, guinea pigs, crocodiles, snakes, lizards, elephants, monkeys, ducks, mice and minks, 'white-muscle disease' in lambs, flamingos and calves, yellow fat disease in kittens and degeneration of the cerebellum in chicks. Human muscular dystrophy or multiple sclerosis do not respond to vitamin E administration (Section 9.2).

The dietary intake of vitamin E affects the sensitivity of laboratory animals to certain toxins or to tissue insults such as ischaemia–reperfusion (Sections 9.5 and 9.17). However, short-term absence of vitamin E from the human diet does not cause overt disease.[422] Dietary sources of vitamin E include wheat-germ, vegetable oils and foods containing them (e.g. some margarines), nuts (especially almonds and hazelnuts),[423] grains, and green leafy vegetables.

3.20.2.3 *Chemistry of vitamin E*

Eight naturally-occurring substances have vitamin E activity in the rat reproduction test: **d-α-**, **d-β-**, **d-γ-** and **d-δ-tocopherols**, and **d-α-**, **dβ-**, **d-γ-** and **d-δ-tocotrienols**. Indeed, the name 'tocopherol' comes from the Greek words *tokos* (childbirth) and *phero* (to bring forth). Each tocopherol has three asymmetric carbon atoms, giving eight optical isomers. The most effective form in animals is **RRR–α-tocopherol**, formerly called **d-α-tocopherol** (Fig. 3.28). Plants and their oils often contain a mixture of tocopherols, for example in soy, corn, walnut, and rapeseed oils there is more γ-tocopherol than α-tocopherol. By contrast, almond and sunflower oil have mostly α-tocopherol.[423] Palm oil is rich in tocotrienols (about 75% of their total vitamin E; only about 14% is α-tocopherol).[424]

The terms 'α-tocopherol' and 'vitamin E' tend to be used in the literature interchangeably. This is, strictly speaking, incorrect: 'vitamin E' is a nutritional term and the other tocopherols and tocotrienols do have some vitamin E activity in animal bioassays. For those taking α-tocopherol supplements, *RRR*-α-tocopherol is preferable; synthetic vitamin E supplements (**dl-α-tocopherol**, sometimes called **all-rac-α-tocopherol**) contain about 12.5% of the *RRR*-form, together with seven other isomers that are less biologically active. Supplements of 'mixed tocopherols' $(\alpha,\beta,\gamma,\delta)$ can be purchased.

Tocopherols and tocotrienols inhibit lipid peroxidation because they scavenge lipid peroxyl radicals (LO$_2^{\bullet}$) much faster than these radicals can react with adjacent fatty acid side chains or with membrane proteins. Rate constants for the reaction

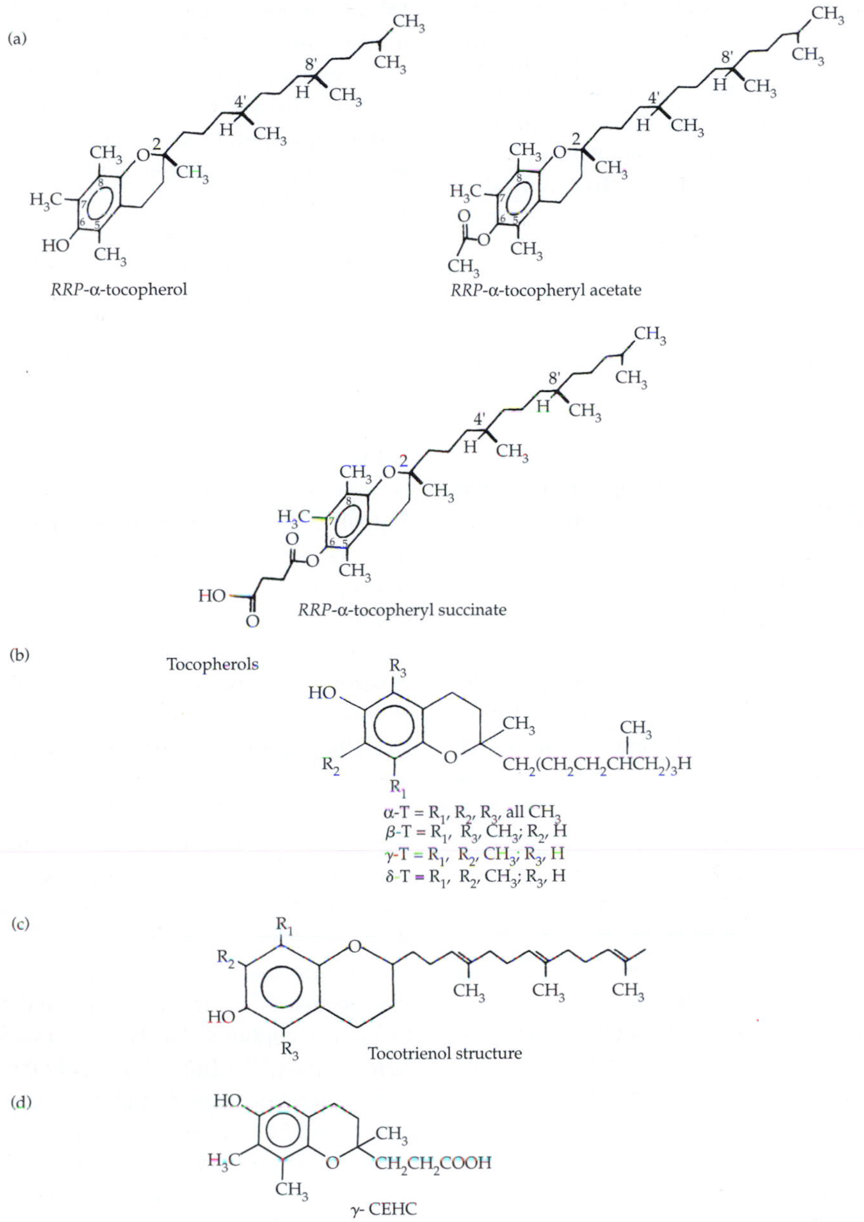

Figure 3.28 Compounds with vitamin E activity. (a) Structures of 'natural vitamin E' (*RRR-α*-tocopherol) and its esters with acetic acid (*RRR-α*-tocopheryl acetate) and succinic acid (*RRR-α*-tocopheryl succinate). The esters are often used in commercial vitamin E preparations because they are more stable on storage, but are rapidly hydrolysed by esterases in the gut. Consumption of the acetate, for example, gives approximately the same plasma levels as unesterified α-tocopherol. (From *Tolerance and Safety of Vitamin E*, by H. Kappus and A.T. Diplock, by courtesy of these authors and the Vitamin E Research and Information Service). Tocopheryl acetate is not common in nature, but may be secreted by the squash beetle, *Epilachna variestis*, during its 'defence response', as a carrier for an irritant chemical (*Experientia* **52**, 616, 1996). **α-Tocopheryl phosphate** has been found at low levels in some animal and plant cells (*Free Rad. Biol. Med.* **39**, 970, 2005). (b) Diagrammatic representation of the structures of α-, β-, γ- and δ-tocopherols. All the tocopherols have a **chromanol** ring structure and a **phytol** side-chain which anchors them in the membrane. (c) Basic structure of the tocotrienols, which have three double bonds in the hydrophobic side chain. Side-chain nomenclature as for the tocopherols. (d) Structure of γ-CEHC, a product of γ–tocopherol degradation. The chromanol ring (and its antioxidant properties) are still intact.

$$\alpha\text{-TocH} + LO_2^{\bullet} \rightarrow \alpha\text{-Toc}^{\bullet} + LO_2H$$

are about $10^6 \, M^{-1}s^{-1}$, some four orders of magnitude faster than those for reaction of $LO_2^{\bullet}$ with lipids.[425] There is little or no difference in antioxidant activity between the different tocopherols and tocotrienols *in vitro*.[426] The α Toc$^{\bullet}$ radical is capable of reacting with another peroxyl radical to give non-radical products

$$LO_2^{\bullet} + \alpha Toc^{\bullet} \rightarrow \alpha TocOOL$$

that is one molecule of α-tocopherol is, in principle, capable of terminating two peroxidation chains. Further products include α-substituted tocopherones and epoxy (hydroperoxy) tocopherones: the former readily hydrolyse to **tocopherylquinone** (Fig. 3.29) and the latter to epoxyquinones.

α-Tocopherol is fat-soluble and therefore concentrates in the interior of membranes and in lipoproteins. For example, mitochondrial membranes contain about one molecule of α-tocopherol per 2100 molecules of phospholipid, but there is more than this in the chloroplast thylakoid membrane (Section 6.8.9) and in the outer segment membranes of the retinal rods (Section 6.10.2.2), both of which are at special risk of peroxidation. Whether α-tocopherol is evenly spread throughout the membrane, or concentrates in certain areas, needs further investigation.[427] Raising the mitochondrial level of α-tocopherol in mice by supplementing the diet lowered the rate of $O_2^{\bullet-}$ generation by subsequently-isolated mitochondria.[428] Whether this is due to scavenging of $HO_2^{\bullet}$ within the mitochondrial membranes by α-tocopherol (Section 2.5.3.6) or an effect on membrane organization to disfavour electron leakage is uncertain. The hydrophobic phytol chain of α-tocopherol anchors the molecule in the membrane, positioning the **chromanol ring** containing the radical-scavenging phenolic $-OH$ group at the hydrocarbon interface. In some cold-water fish such as salmon a **marine-derived tocopherol** (MDT) is present as well as α- tocopherol; MDT has the same structure except for a $=CH_2$ instead of one of the $-CH_3$ groups at the end of the side-chain. This may allow increased mobility within the membrane and thus increased antioxidant efficiency at low temperatures. The MDT may be acquired by the fish from plankton in the diet.[429]

Tocopherols also quench and react with singlet O_2 (Fig. 2.16) and might help to protect chloroplast and retinal membranes against this species. Like most biological molecules, tocopherols do not react readily with $O_2^{\bullet-}$ (Section 2.5.6.3) but do react at diffusion-controlled rates with OH$^{\bullet}$. This is unlikely to be important *in vivo* because everything reacts with OH$^{\bullet}$.

3.20.2.4 *Recycling of α-tocopheryl radicals*

During its action as a chain-breaking antioxidant, α-tocopherol forms a radical. Do mechanisms exist for reducing this radical back to α-tocopherol? Synergy between vitamins E and C was first suggested by Tappel in 1968. Pulse radiolysis studies confirmed that ascorbate reduces α-tocopheryl radical to α-tocopherol with a reasonable rate constant ($\sim 1.5 \times 10^6 \, M^{-1}s^{-1}$) and this reaction has since been shown to occur in isolated membranes, blood plasma (Fig. 5.1), cultured cells and lipoproteins, although it has been difficult to establish conclusively that it occurs *in vivo*. Studies using deuterated α-tocopherol in guinea pigs gave no evidence of recycling by ascorbate,[430] although weanling guinea pigs deficient in both C and E developed progressive paralysis and increased lipid peroxidation in the brain, effects not seen with either deficiency alone.[431] Also consistent with interaction *in vivo* is the observation that feeding guinea pigs, fish, or ODS rats (Section 3.20.1.1) on a C-deficient diet decreases tissue α-tocopherol levels.[403,432] However, in one human study,[419] administration of 200 mg/day of d-α-tocopherol decreased lipid peroxidation (as serum F_2-IPs) by 17%, but adding 500 mg vitamin C had no extra effect, nor did the C itself affect isoprostane levels (maybe the subjects had enough ascorbate already). So the jury is still out on whether C recycles α-tocopherol *in vivo*; it may do so in smokers (Section 8.12.3) but not non-smokers perhaps.

Ubiquinol can also recycle the α-tocopheryl radical in some experimental systems (Section 3.18.5) as can some flavonoids (Section 3.22 below) and GSH. It is generally felt that the ascorbate-dependent recycling system is the most important *in vivo*, although on the basis of an inadequate evidence base.

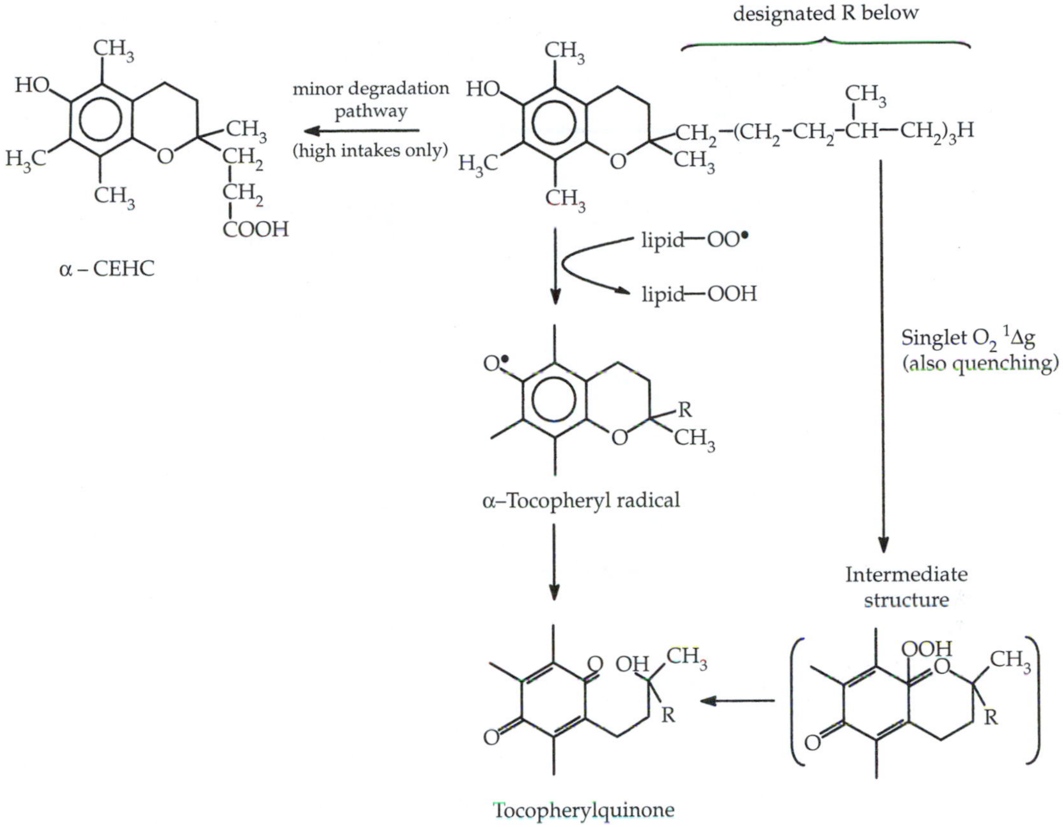

Figure 3.29 Structure of tocopherol and some of its oxidation products. Tocopheryl radical is an aromatic alkoxyl radical (sometimes called **tocopheroxyl radical**). It may be recycled to tocopherol or can undergo further oxidation (e.g. to tocopherylquinone) by a series of mechanisms. Traces of α-tocopherylquinone are found in animal (including human) tissues: it is metabolized by reduction to the hydroquinone (which itself can exert antioxidant properties: *Proc. Natl. Acad. Sci. USA* **94**, 7885, 1997). When high doses of α-tocopherol are consumed some can be degraded by hepatic cytochromes P-450 to **α-CEHC (2,5,7,8-tetramethyl-2-(2'-carboxyethyl)-6-hydroxychroman)**, the ring structure (and antioxidant activity) being retained. Tocopherols are powerful scavengers of $^1O_2$, but can also photosensitize its generation when illuminated at 308 nm (*Free Radic. Res.* **40**, 333, 2006).

3.20.2.5 *Pro-oxidant effects of α-tocopherol?*[407]

Tocopherols can reduce Fe(III) to Fe^{2+} and Cu^{2+} to Cu^+ and can exert pro-oxidant effects *in vitro*. Indeed, this iron-reducing ability is the basis of some colorimetric methods to measure tocopherols. In addition, the α-Toc$^\bullet$ radical is not completely unreactive: it can abstract hydrogen from PUFAs

$$\alpha\text{-Toc}^\bullet + LH \rightarrow L^\bullet + \alpha\text{-TocH}$$

However, the rate constant is about $5 \times 10^{-2} M^{-1}s^{-1}$, four or five orders of magnitude lower than the rate constants for reaction of peroxyl radicals with PUFAs.[425] Nevertheless, if α-Toc$^\bullet$ is generated in a lipid system in the absence of $RO_2^\bullet$ (e.g. if copper ions are added to a tocopherol-containing lipid), it can act as a weak promoter of lipid oxidation. This phenomenon has been observed in the food industry and in studies of the oxidation of LDL (Section 9.3.8). Addition of excess α-tocopherol to lipid emulsions used for intravenous infusion can accelerate peroxidation of the lipids,[433] presumably because no coreductants are present. The poor availability of metals and the recycling of the αToc$^\bullet$ radical by ascorbate and other reducing agents should diminish the likelihood of such occurrences *in vivo*, although

(a)

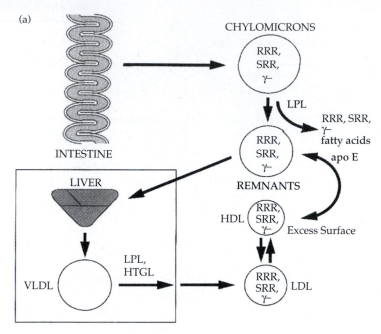

Vitamin E transport during chylomicron catabolism

(b)

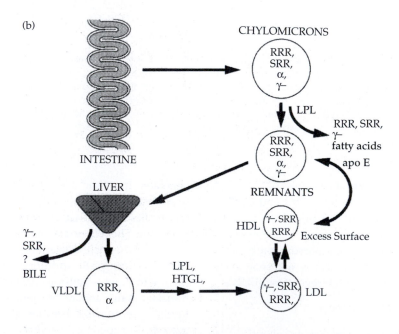

α–Tocopherol transport during VLDL catabolism

dl-α-tocopheryl acetate (400 IU daily) administration *raised* plasma F_2-IPs on smokers on a high-fat diet[434] and increased liver fat content in rats fed a high-fat diet plus ethanol.[435]

High intakes of tocopherols in adults are generally thought to show little toxicity (Section 10.5), although they can affect blood coagulation by interfering with the action of **vitamin K** (further discussed in Fig. 8.6). At least some of this activity is due to the vitamin E metabolite α-**tocopherylquinone** (Fig. 3.29), which is a more powerful anticoagulant.[436] Whether high-dose tocopherol supplements do any good is an open question (Section 10.5).

◀━━━━━━━━━━━━━━━━━━━━

Figure 3.30 Human lipoprotein metabolism in relation to that of vitamin E. Lipoproteins are plasma lipid transport vehicles consisting of a hydrophobic core (with triglyceride and cholesterol ester) and a surface permitting interaction with aqueous environments and usually containing cholesterol, phospholipid and proteins. The four major classes are chylomicrons (CL), very low density lipoproteins (VLDL), low density lipoproteins (LDL) and high density lipoproteins (HDLs). (a) *The transfers of tocopherols during CL catabolism.* The intestine absorbs and processes dietary lipids and secretes CLs that carry various forms of vitamin E (*RRR*- and *SRR*-α-tocopherols, β-, γ- and δ-tocopherols, tocotrienols, etc.) into the lymph, from where they eventually enter the bloodstream. Fat digestion requires bile; defects in bile production impair absorption of fats and fat-soluble vitamins. Chylomicrons are hydrolysed in the circulation by a **lipoprotein lipase** (LPL) enzyme on the surface of capillaries, and fatty acids and tocopherols transfer to tissues. The CL remnants can transfer tocopherols to HDL and can acquire apolipoprotein E (apoE), a protein which directs the CL remnants to the liver. Tocopherols in HDL can transfer to other circulating lipoproteins, such as LDL and VLDL (transfer to circulating VLDL is not shown). (b) *The events following hepatic uptake of CL remnants.* The liver secretes lipids in nascent VLDL. The hepatic α-**tocopherol transfer protein** preferentially transfers *RRR*-α-tocopherol to VLDL. The large typeface indicates that the plasma lipoproteins are enriched in *RRR*-α-tocopherol by this mechanism. Other forms of α-tocopherol (such as *SRR*-α-tocopherol) are passed into bile and so their lifetime *in vivo* is shorter than that of *RRR*-α-tocopherol. Once VLDL is secreted in the circulation, both LPL and hepatic triglyceride lipase (HTGL) participate in its conversion to LDL. Only about half of the VLDL is converted to LDL; the remainder is taken up by the liver (not shown). During triglyceride hydrolysis by LPL and HTGL, tocopherol can be transferred to HDL, in a manner analogous to transfer during CL catabolism (transfer not shown). The secretion of *RRR*-α-tocopherol in nascent VLDL by the liver maintains plasma tocopherol concentrations; the exchange of tocopherols between lipoproteins determines individual lipoprotein concentrations. Plasma levels of α-tocopherol peak at about 11–14 h after consumption. Hyperlipidaemia (*J. Nutr.* **135**, 58, 2005), other dysfunctions of lipid metabolism (Section 3.20.2.8 below) and AVED (Section 3.20.2.6) can impair tocopherol delivery to tissues. Diagram and text by courtesy of Drs Herbert Kayden and Maret G. Traber and the *Journal of Lipid Research*.

Table 3.12 Human blood tocopherol levels in health and disease

Subjects	Total tocopherol (µM)
Healthy adults*	20–35
Children (2–12 years)	28
Term infants	18
Premature infants	9
AVED patients (non-supplemented)	<5
Infants and children with protein–calorie malnutrition	6
Kwashiorkor	7
Gastrointestinal diseases	
cholestatic liver disease	<2
abetalipoproteinaemia	<2
coeliac disease	7
Non-tropical sprue	6
tropical sprue	9
chronic pancreatitis	6
ulcerative colitis	10
Haemolytic anaemias	
β-thalassaemia major	10
thalassaemia intermedia	5
sickle-cell anaemia	4.5–20 (depends on number of transfusions; *Br. J. Haematol.* **114**, 917, 2001)
Glucose 6 phosphate dehydrogenase deficiency	12
Miscellaneous	
Total parenteral nutrition	13
Gaucher's disease	
severe	2
chronic	8

'Normal' values vary among different populations and the data above are only illustrative. Because tocopherol is carried by lipoproteins, the plasma lipid content influences the plasma tocopherol level. Hence plasma α-tocopherol levels are best expressed as a ratio with total plasma lipids or cholesterol (a normal value is 4.5–6.0 µmol α-tocopherol per millimole cholesterol). For example, it has been suggested that some or all of the apparent α-tocopherol depletion in ARDS (Section 9.7) is due to lower plasma lipids. The requirement for vitamin E increases when the intake of PUFAs increases. Attempts have been made to specify a fixed ratio of dietary *RRR*-α-tocopherol to PUFAs, but this has not been completely satisfactory for humans. When the primary PUFA in the diet is linoleic acid, as in most US diets, a ratio of approximately 0.4 mg *RRR*-α-tocopherol to 1 g of PUFA has been suggested as adequate for adult humans. As intakes of vegetable oils increase, vitamin E intake increases as well, because the oils contain it, provided that they have not been over-used, deteriorated or become rancid. Data by courtesy of the Vitamin E Research and Information Service, also see *Nutrition* **13**, 450, 1997.

* For comparison, plasma levels in zoo felines (cheetah, fishing cat, lion, etc.) were also around 20 µM (*J. Nutr.* **133**, 160, 2003).

3.20.2.6 *Processing of dietary vitamin E*[437]

If large oral doses of α-tocopherol are taken, much fails to be absorbed and is excreted in the faeces. Usually 25 to 50% of the α-tocopherol in foods is absorbed, although there are considerable interindividual variations.[438] Being fat-soluble, all forms of vitamin E enter the body in **chylomicrons**. Some dietary fat is thus required for vitamin E uptake, but only a small amount appears sufficient[439] (Fig. 3.30). The gut appears not to discriminate between the different forms of vitamin E for uptake. However, levels of *RRR*-α-tocopherol are higher in plasma because the liver incorporates it selectively into the **very low density lipoproteins** (VLDLs) that it secretes into the blood. Liver secretion of VLDL is an important contributor to maintaining plasma *RRR*-α-tocopherol levels. The VLDLs contain lipids that originated from the diet (by uptake of chylomicron remnant particles by the liver) as well as lipids made by the liver itself.

How does liver achieves this selectivity? A hepatic α-**tocopherol transfer protein** (α-TTP) preferentially picks *RRR*-α-tocopherol to incorporate into VLDL. This protein is important; mutations in the gene encoding it cause the autosomal recessive neurodegenerative disease **ataxia with isolated vitamin E deficiency** (**AVED**). Ataxia means impaired movement due to loss of motor co-ordination. Patients have an impaired ability to incorporate α-tocopherol into VLDL. As a result, their plasma tocopherol levels are very low (Table 3.12) leading eventually to neurodegeneration. After AVED patients consume α-tocopherol, peak blood levels are reached within 6 h (faster than the normal 11–14 h), but drop swiftly, indicative of the importance of the liver α-TTP system in maintaining plasma levels, and the α-tocopherol is rapidly degraded to α-CEHC (Fig. 3.28) which is excreted in urine after sulphation or glucuronidation. Knockout mice lacking α-TTP similarly develop neurological symptoms after about 1 year. They also show retinal degeneration, since α-tocopherol is an important antioxidant in the eye (Section 6.10.2.2). Pregnant α-TTP⁻ mice show severe placental malformations and their embryos die

in utero unless high doses of α-tocopherol are given.

Tissues acquire various tocopherols from chylomicrons, and α-tocopherol from VLDL, LDL and other lipoproteins. During conversion of VLDL to LDL in the circulation (Fig. 3.30), part of the *RRR*-α-tocopherol remains in the LDL, but some is transferred to HDL; LDL and HDL can exchange tocopherol, assisted by the plasma **phospholipid transfer protein** (Fig. 3.30). *RRR*-α-tocopherol taken up by cells from lipoproteins is distributed to organelles (especially the mitochondria) by intracellular transfer proteins. The brain receives more α-tocopherol from VLDL/HDL than from chylomicrons (Fig. 3.30) and so is especially affected in AVED.

The α-TTP recognizes other forms of vitamin E, to a limited extent. Compared to *RRR*-α-tocopherol, its relative affinity for γ-tocopherol is 9%, β- about 38% and α-tocotrienol about 9%. Consuming a lot of α-tocopherol thus decreases plasma levels of other tocopherols, by competition for binding to α-TTP.

3.20.2.7 *The fate of γ-tocopherol*

Steroisomers of α-tocopherol other than the *RRR* form are not efficiently selected by α-TTP and their turnover in plasma is fast, as they are discarded into bile (Fig. 3.30). Gamma tocopherol is degraded by cytochromes P450 (mostly CYPs 4F2 and 3A4) to **2,7,8-trimethyl-2-(2′-carboxyethyl)-6-hydroxychroman** (γ-**CEHC**)(Fig. 3.28) which is excreted in urine after conjugation with glucuronic acid. Tocotrienols and α-tocopherol can be metabolized by a similar route, but the latter only when high doses are given or in AVED (Fig. 3.28); CYP4F2 acts only slowly on α-tocopherol. Because of its rapid metabolism, plasma γ-tocopherol levels rarely exceed 1 to 2 μM even when supplements of it are taken. Tocopherols and tocotrienols bind to the human **pregnane X receptor**, leading to upregulation of CYP3A. α- and γ-Tocotrienols are the most effective *in vitro*.[440] This ability of high intakes of tocopherols to modulate CYP levels could conceivably impact on drug metabolism, for example of antiretroviral drugs (Section 9.23), in patients taking supplements.

In vitro, γ-tocopherol is a better scavenger of RNS such as $ONOO^-$ than α-tocopherol, but it is hard to imagine how it might do this *in vivo* at such a low plasma level, unless it is acting within membranes. Nevertheless, 5-nitro-γ-tocopherol has been detected in human atherosclerotic plaque and plasma, and levels are elevated in patients with heart disease; a contributing factor may be that nitration slows the metabolism of γ-tocopherol to γ-CEHC.[441] Scavenging of RNS might also be important in plants (Section 6.8.9) and in the colon, where higher levels of γ-tocopherol are present.[442] Both γ-tocopherol and γ-CEHC are anti-inflammatory in rats, and effects on COX-2 may be involved.[443]

Epidemiological studies suggest that low plasma levels of γ-tocopherol correlate with a higher incidence of certain diseases, for example cancer and coronary heart disease, although one must be careful in interpreting such data (Section 10.5.3). Also, γ-CEHC can act as a **natriuretic factor**, promoting Na^+ excretion in the urine.[443]

3.20.2.8 α-Tocopherol, a mediocre antioxidant?[418,420]

Supplementing well-nourished humans with α-tocopherol has only modest (if any) effects on lipid peroxidation (Section 3.20.2.1), and more has been learned by examining deficiency states. Many of the signs of α-tocopherol deficiency in animals are partially or completely alleviated by feeding synthetic chain-breaking antioxidants (e.g. ethoxyquin or promethazine) or by raising the selenium content of the diet (Section 3.11.2). It is well-known to veterinary practitioners, zookeepers and farmers that feeding unsaturated fats to animals increases their requirement for α-tocopherol. Thus for every 1% of corn oil fed to young pigs above 4% of the diet, 100 mg extra α-tocopherol is required. Chicks fed on lard, a mainly saturated fat, can remain healthy without α-tocopherol for weeks. Feeding extra α-tocopherol to pigs, chickens and cows has been reported to increase the stability of their meat against rancidity on storage.[444]

Tissue samples from α-tocopherol-deficient animals show evidence of more peroxidation (e.g. as elevated levels of F_2–IPs[197] or, less convincingly, as TBA-reactive material), and tissue homogenates or subcellular fractions from such animals peroxidize faster than normal when incubated *in vitro*. These animals are more sensitive to the toxic effects of pure O_2, exhale more hydrocarbon gases (Section 5.14.8) and accumulate fluorescent pigments in certain tissues more rapidly than normal, especially if they are fed a diet rich in PUFAs. Lack of α-tocopherol in the diets of rodents promotes accumulation of **senescent cell antigen**, a damaged cell-surface protein indicative of 'old' cells (Section 6.4.6). Nevertheless, tocopherol-deficient animals survive. It requires a combined deficiency of both α-tocopherol and vitamin C to produce mortality in weanling guinea pigs, for example.[431] In other animal studies, deficiencies of both selenium and α-tocopherol are required to cause significant morbidity and often (Section 3.11.2) the animals still survive, although perhaps because levels of other antioxidants such as peroxiredoxins and ubiquinol are increased.[445]

Although a short-term lack of α-tocopherol in the human diet does not produce symptoms, it does increase *susceptibility* of membranes to peroxidation, as revealed by an increased rate of haemolysis when erythrocytes are treated with H_2O_2 *in vitro* (**peroxide stress haemolysis test**; Section 6.4.3). Severe depletion of α-tocopherol (Table 3.12) occurs only as a result of impaired fat absorption by the gut, after prolonged intravenous feeding, or as a result of an inborn error in metabolism such as AVED (Section 3.20.2.6). For example, in patients suffering from **abetalipoproteinaemia**, dietary fat is ingested and absorbed, but not transported out of the intestinal mucosal cells. This disease is due to an inherited defect in apoprotein B, an essential component of chylomicrons (Fig. 3.30). Untreated patients with abetalipoproteinaemia have negligible plasma α-tocopherol and eventually develop neuronal damage, retinal degeneration and abnormally shaped erythrocytes (**acanthocytes**). This can be prevented by administering large oral doses of α-tocopherol (sufficient to ensure some uptake by the gut). Patients can also be given *RRR*-α-tocopheryl polyethylene glycol (PEG) succinate, a more hydrophilic molecule in which water-soluble PEG is attached to α-tocopherol succinate.

Neurological and retinal disorders have some-times been observed in patients with cystic fibrosis (Section 9.8) or with congenital defects that impair bile production, both again related to impaired fat absorption.

Newborn babies have low concentrations of plasma α-tocopherol, especially if born prematurely (Table 3.12). Their erythrocytes are more susceptible to lipid peroxidation *in vitro*, although this does not normally cause a clinical problem. Sometimes haemolysis does occur, and this **haemolytic syndrome of prematurity** responds to α-tocopherol therapy (Section 6.11.8). α-Tocopherol might also help protect against retinopathy of prematurity (Section 1.5.3). The occasional haemolysis occurring in patients with thalassaemia (Section 3.15.5.3) or G6PDH deficiency (Section 6.4.5) can be decreased by consumption of extra α-tocopherol, and a similar protective effect has been suggested to occur in sickle cell anaemia. In these diseases there is extra 'oxidative stress' and/or a decrease in other protective mechanisms so that the effects of α-tocopherol are more readily seen.

3.20.2.9 *Vitamin E: an antioxidant or something else?*[418]

γ-Tocopherol and its metabolites may have physiological effects other than antioxidant ones (Section 3.20.2.7). The same might be true for α-tocopherol. Studies on cells in culture reveal that physiological levels of α-tocopherol, but in general not other tocopherols, can inhibit several enzymes including 5-lipoxygenase, protein kinase C and phospholipase A_2. These can lead to inhibitory effects on cell proliferation (e.g. in smooth muscle cells), platelet aggregation and monocyte adhesion/$O_2^{\bullet-}$ production. α-Tocopherol also modulates the expression of several genes, including those encoding tropomyosin, scavenger receptors and matrix metalloproteinase-19. These 'non-antioxidant' effects of α-tocopherol could be[418] more important *in vivo* than its antioxidant effects. One point to consider is that cell culture media often contain little α-tocopherol, so that some cell lines begin with abnormally-low levels.[446] Nevertheless, some (but not all), studies suggest a mild

anti-inflammatory effect of high-dose α-tocopherol in humans.[447]

α-Tocopheryl succinate (Fig. 3.28) has some unusual properties, for example it inhibits proliferation or promotes apoptosis of several tumour cell lines, whereas α-tocopherol does not. Its use to treat cancer is under evaluation. How α-tocopheryl succinate works at the molecular level is uncertain, in that different mechanisms have been proposed in different cell lines.[448] γ-Tocopherol was also reported to induce apoptosis in prostate cancer cells, by interfering with the sphingolipid pathway (Section 4.4.1.2).[449] Tocotrienols have been suggested to inhibit hydroxymethylglutarylcoenzyme A reductase, the first enzyme in cholesterol biosynthesis, but evidence for this effect *in vivo* is limited.[450]

3.21 Carotenoids: bright colours but not sparkling antioxidants?[437,451,452]

Diets rich in fruits, grains and vegetables are protective against several human diseases, especially cardiovascular disease, diabetes and some types of cancer (Section 10.5). It is widely assumed that carotenoids and flavonoids contribute to this protective effect. Is this view justified?

Carotenoids (of which the first to be isolated was from carrots, in 1831) are a group of coloured pigments (usually yellow, red or orange) that are widespread in plant tissues (Figs 3.31 and 3.32). They are also found in some animals (e.g. snails, goldfish, salmon, bird plumage and lobsters) and certain bacteria (e.g. *Staphylococcus aureus*; Section 7.7.2.12) and fungi (e.g. *N. crassa*). Over 700 carotenoids have been described. Carotenoids from the diet are found in human tissues, but many other animals (e.g. rodents, sheep, hares or elephants) do not normally absorb them, although ferrets and gerbils can. In humans, most carotenoids are found in adipose tissue (80–85% of total body amount) and liver (8–12%) but the concentration is highest in the corpus luteum of the ovary and in adrenal gland; testis appears enriched in lutein. Lutein and zeaxanthin are present in the macula (Section 6.10.4). Tissue and plasma

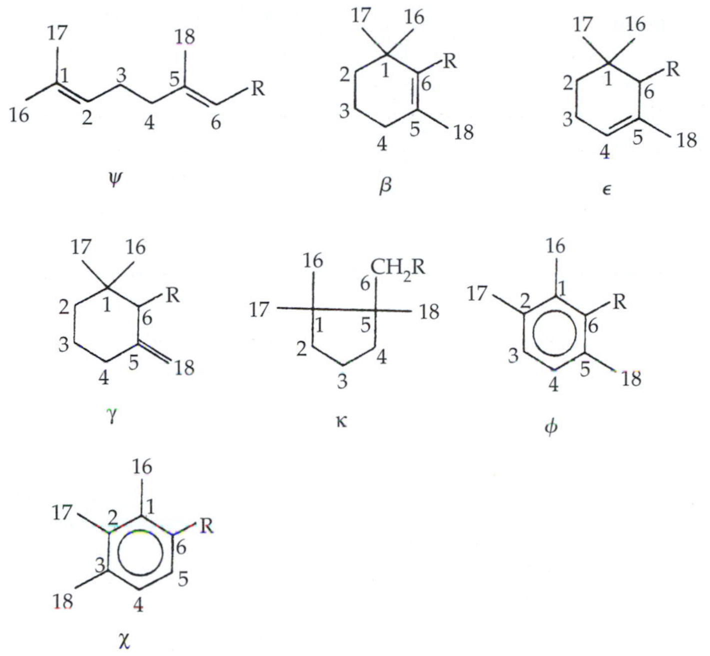

Figure 3.31 The seven different types of end-group found in natural carotenoids. Thus β-carotene has two β-groups, α-carotene has one β- and one ε-group. Diagram from *FASEB J.* **9**, 1551, 1995 by courtesy of Dr George Britton and the publishers.

carotenoid levels vary with diet; human plasma levels are usually in the low micromolar range (e.g. lycopene, 0.5–1.0 µM; β-carotene, 0.2–0.6 µM; α-carotene, 0.05–0.1 µM; lutein, ~0.3 µM).

Absorption of dietary carotenoids in humans is incomplete and depends on what food mixtures are eaten and on how the food is processed. For example, raw tomatoes are rich in lycopene, but little is absorbed. More is taken up from cooked tomatoes or tomato paste, for example on pizzas, although some *trans-cis* isomerization of lycopene occurs during processing. There is also considerable person-to-person variation in absorption. Some dietary fat is required for carotenoid uptake.[439]

3.21.1 Carotenoid chemistry[437,451–453]

Carotenoids have long chains of alternating double and single bonds (Fig. 3.32). This allows extensive electron delocalization, causing carotenoids to absorb in the visible range and generate their beautiful colours. The basic skeleton of carotenoids has 40 carbon atoms and can be modified by cyclization at one or both ends, by reducing certain double bonds, or by addition of oxygen-containing functional groups (Fig. 3.31). Carotenoids that contain one or more oxygens are known as **xanthophylls**, the parent hydrocarbons as **carotenes**.

Carotenoids are usually known by their trivial names, although a semisystematic scheme has been devised based on the stem name *carotene* preceded by two Greek-letter prefixes that indicate the end-groups present (Fig. 3.31). Thus β-carotene should be called β, β-carotene, α-carotene is β, ε-carotene and zeaxanthin is β, β-carotene-3,3'-diol. Some carotenoids have structures with less than 40 carbons; they are called **apocarotenoids** when carbon atoms have been lost from the ends of the molecule or **norcarotenoids** when they are lost from within the chain. In principle, each double bond in a carotenoid could exist as *cis* or *trans* geometric isomers, but *trans* forms are more common in nature, presumably because the most stable form of long polyunsaturated chains is usually a linear, *trans*, extended conformation. *Cis* bonds kink the chain

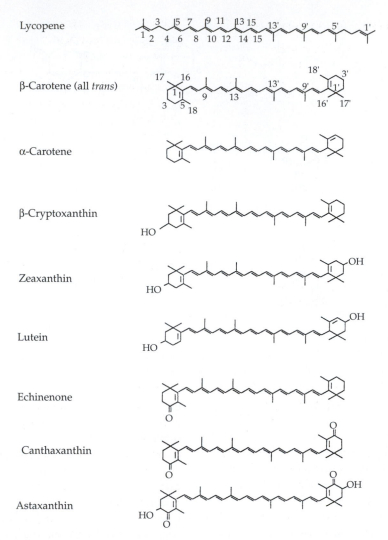

Figure 3.32 Structures of several carotenoids found in plants and animals. The *trans* forms are shown. Structures by courtesy of Professors Catherine Rice-Evans and Norman Krinsky.

and greatly modify the overall molecular shape. Some *cis* isomers do occur, however, including those of lycopene mentioned above, and **9-*cis*-β-carotene**. However, the human gut prefers to absorb all *trans*-β-carotene. Heating of tomatoes isomerizes some of the lycopene from *all-trans* to 9-*cis* and 13-*cis* isomers; both *cis* and *trans* forms can be absorbed.

As would be expected from their structures, carotenoids are very hydrophobic and completely insoluble in water. This causes a problem in cell culture studies—how to deliver them to the cells? Often such organic solvents as tetrahydrofuran are used, but at the levels which cells can tolerate, there is likely to be some carotenoid precipitation in the culture medium. Carotenoids in blood are located in the circulating lipoproteins. In tissues they occur within fat stores, in the hydrophobic interior of membranes and bound to hydrophobic domains of certain proteins.

3.21.2 Metabolic roles of carotenoids[451]

Their best-established role in humans and other animals is as a precursor of the fat-soluble vitamin known as **vitamin A**, sometimes called **retinol**. Cats are an exception; they can absorb β-carotene but cannot make vitamin A from it. Vitamin A is essential for cell growth and differentiation, and in vision (Section 6.10); vitamin A deficiency is the leading cause of childhood blindness in the world. Over 50 carotenoids (not including lycopene) can generate vitamin A, but the most important is β-carotene. Indeed, in individuals eating largely plant-based diets, carotenoids are the major source of vitamin A. A variable percentage of dietary carotenoids is absorbed, mostly in the duodenum. Some are cleaved to retinal by a β-**carotene dioxygenase** enzyme in the duodenal mucosal cells, and the retinal then reduced to retinol. Enzyme levels drop when the body is replete with retinol, so that high doses of β-carotene do not cause excess vitamin A accumulation. Unmolested carotenoids enter the body in chylomicrons (whether specific uptake proteins are also involved is unclear as yet), from where they are distributed to tissues by much the same mechanisms as for tocopherols (Fig. 3.30), that is uptake both from chylomicrons (involving lipoprotein lipase) and from lipoproteins (VLDL, HDL and LDL). The liver (and possibly some other tissues) can also convert β-carotene into retinol.

3.21.3 Carotenoids and vitamin A as antioxidants[451,453]

In plants, carotenoids play a key antioxidant role, helping to quench singlet O_2 and deter its formation during photosynthesis (Section 6.8.5). Indeed, some studies show β-carotene administration to be protective against light-induced skin damage in porphyria patients (Section 2.6.4.3).[454] Sunlight depletes β-carotene in skin, consistent with a protective role even in normal subjects.[455] How important this antisinglet O_2 effect is in skin, eye, and other tissues is uncertain (Section 6.10.4 and 6.12.2), although $^1O_2$ can form during lipid peroxidation (Section 4.11.8.1). Lycopene appears to be the best singlet O_2 quencher *in vitro*, although all the carotenoids are very good.

In vitro studies have shown that β-carotene (albeit at unphysiological levels) inhibits peroxidation of simple lipid systems at low O_2 levels, but not at high O_2 concentration. However, β-carotene does not protect LDL against peroxidation whatever the O_2 concentration.[456] Nevertheless, carotenoids are capable of scavenging some RS. Vitamin A can do the same (as would be expected from its double-bond structure) but no data exist supporting such a role *in vivo*.[457] Indeed, studies (again *in vitro*) have suggested pro-oxidant effects of high levels of retinol, for example it increased levels of oxidative DNA damage in Sertoli cells.[458]

3.21.3.1 *How do carotenoids react with radicals?*

They can interact with oxidizing radicals by electron transfer, for example for nitrogen dioxide reacting with β-carotene (written Car or CarH below) a radical cation results

$$NO_2^{\bullet} + Car \rightarrow Car^{\bullet +} + NO_2^{-} \quad k_2 {\sim} 1 \times 10^8\,M^{-1}s^{-1}$$

Possible fates of $Car^{\bullet +}$ include dismutation

$$2Car^{\bullet +} \rightleftharpoons Car + Car^{2+}$$

and reaction with ascorbate (assuming that $Car^{\bullet +}$ was present near a membrane or lipoprotein surface to interact with ascorbate in the aqueous phase)

$$Car^{\bullet +} + Asc \rightarrow Car + Asc^{\bullet} + H^+$$

Peroxyl radicals can react with carotenoids by electron transfer, for example

$$H^+ + RO_2^{\bullet} + Car \rightarrow Car^{\bullet +} + ROOH$$

by hydrogen abstraction

$$CarH + RO_2^{\bullet} \rightarrow Car^{\bullet} + ROOH$$

or by addition reactions

$$Car + RO_2^{\bullet} \rightarrow [Car-OOR]^{\bullet}$$

Addition products could intercept another radical, or react with O_2 to give a peroxyl radical

$$[\text{Car-OOR}]^\bullet + R^1O_2^\bullet \longrightarrow R^1 - \text{OOCar-OOR}$$
$$\downarrow$$
$$\text{decomposition products}$$

$$[\text{Car-OOR}]^\bullet + O_2 \rightarrow [\text{OO-Car-OOR}]^\bullet$$

Thiyl radicals can add to carotenoids (k_2 for $GS^\bullet$ ~2 $\times 10^8 M^{-1} s^{-1}$)

$$RS^\bullet + \text{Car} \rightarrow [\text{Car-SR}]^\bullet$$

possibly followed by O_2 addition to give a peroxyl radical

$$[\text{Car-SR}]^\bullet + O_2 \rightleftharpoons [\text{RS-Car-OO}]^\bullet$$

Carotenoids also react with $OH^\bullet$ (as does almost everything else)

$$OH^\bullet + \text{CarH} \rightarrow \text{Car}^\bullet + H_2O$$

The carbon-centred ($\text{Car}^\bullet$) radicals formed by the above reactions are stabilized by extensive electron delocalization. Hence reaction with O_2 to give peroxyl radicals

$$\text{Car}^\bullet + O_2 \rightleftharpoons \text{CarO}_2^\bullet$$

is slow. The $\text{Car}^\bullet$ could add to another radical, for example

$$\text{Car}^\bullet + RO_2^\bullet \rightarrow \text{Car-OOR (non-radical product)}$$

Radicals such as $[\text{OO-Car-OOR}]^\bullet$, and $\text{CarO}_2^\bullet$ could propagate lipid peroxidation by abstracting hydrogen. Hence it is easy to see why O_2 concentration affects the antioxidant/pro-oxidant properties of carotenoids. Another factor to be considered is the different solvents in which the above reactions have been studied, which can alter the reaction mechanism.

The rate constants for reaction of carotenoids with these various radicals are high, at first glance perhaps suggesting that carotenoids in membranes and lipoproteins might be capable of reacting with them. Whether or not such reactions would protect the surrounding PUFAs and proteins largely depends on the reactivities of the various

carotenoid-derived radicals that can be formed and on the O_2 level. Animal membranes usually contain more α-tocopherol and ubiquinol than carotenoids, so it is hard to see much contribution of carotenoids as free-radical scavengers. Interactions of α-tocopherol with carotenoids have been suggested to occur, but rather than carotenoids converting α-tocopheryl radical back to α-tocopherol the reverse reaction,

$$\text{Car}^{\bullet+} + \alpha\text{TOH} \rightarrow \text{Car} + \alpha\text{-TO}^\bullet + H^+$$

seems preferred, at least under some reaction conditions.

Overall, the evidence supporting an antioxidant role for carotenoids in animals is weak. However, this does *not* mean they are unimportant; they could exert beneficial effects by other mechanisms, regulating cell–cell communication or gene expression, for example.[459,460] Carotenoids, or sometimes their oxidation products such as **2,7,11-trimethyltetradecehexaene-1,14-dial** from lycopene breakdown),[459] can facilitate cell–cell communication via gap junctions (by stimulating synthesis of the **connexin proteins**). Increased communication decreases growth of transformed cells in culture. Again, however, the relevance of these effects *in vivo* is uncertain.

3.21.3.2 *Stability of carotenoids*
Pure carotenoids, even as solids, are susceptible to oxidation and can break down to a complex mixture of products, as evidenced by loss of the characteristic colour (**bleaching**). Sometimes the oxidation products (particularly epoxides and highly-reactive aldehydes) show cytotoxic effects *in vitro*.[461] It is difficult to stabilize pure carotenoids, especially lycopene, and the possible presence of oxidation products is a factor to be considered by those who wish to consume carotenoid supplements, or to examine the effects of carotenoids on cells in culture.[459,461,462]

3.21.3.3 *The interesting case of lycopene*[463]
Lycopene accumulates in several tissues, including testis and prostate gland. Several epidemiological studies suggest that consumption of tomato products might lower risk of prostate cancer

Table 3.13 Some dietary sources of plant phenols

Compound	Some sources
Flavanols	
Epicatechin	Green teas
Catechin	Red wine
Epigallocatechin	Cocoa, chocolate
Epicatechin gallate	
Epigallocatechin gallate	
Flavanones	
Naringin	Citrus fruits
Taxifolin	
Flavonols	
Kaempferol	Endive, leek, broccoli, radish, grapefruit, black tea
Quercetin	Onion, lettuce, broccoli, cranberry, apple skin, berries, olive, tea, red wine
Myricetin	Cranberry, grapes, red wine
Flavones	
Chrysin	Fruit skin
Apigenin	Celery, parsley
Anthocyanidins	
Malvidin	Red grapes, red wine
Cyanidin	Cherry, raspberry, strawberry, grapes
Apigenidin	Coloured fruits and peels
Pelargonidin	
Hydroxycinnamic acid derivatives	
Caffeic acid	White grapes, white wine, olives, olive oil, spinach, cabbage, asparagus, coffee
p-Coumaric acid	White grapes, white wine, tomatoes, spinach, cabbage, asparagus
Chlorogenic acid	Apples, pears, cherries, plums, peaches, apricots, blueberries, tomatoes, anise, coffee, artichoke, aubergine

Adapted from *Free Rad.Biol. Med.* **20**, 933, 1996 by courtesy of Professor C. Rice-Evans and Elsevier. Chlorogenic acid (5-caffeoylquinic acid) is an ester of caffeic acid with quinic acid. Tea, a beverage that has been prepared from the leaves of the plant *Camellia sinensis* for almost 50 centuries is an important source of dietary phenols to many people. Green tea is rich in catechins, whereas black tea has fewer but additionally contains complex polymers called **theaflavins** and **thearubigins**. These are formed by oxidation of catechins by the enzyme **phenolase** during preparation of the leaves for tea manufacture. In green tea manufacture this enzyme is inactivated by steaming the leaves (*Antiox. Redox. Signal* **3**, 1009, 2001).

(Section 10.5.8) and administration of tomato sauce was reported to decrease levels of oxidative DNA damage both in white cells and in prostate biopsies of human volunteers. In a transgenic mouse model of prostate cancer, administration of a mixture of α-tocopherol, selenium and lycopene slowed cancer development (Section 9.15.4). Remember, however, that lycopene might act by mechanisms other than antioxidant action, for example promoting gap junctional communication or interfering with the proproliferative effects of androgens and growth factors by modulating signal transduction pathways.

Good dietary sources of lycopene include tomato paste/juice, cooked tomatoes, guava, papaya and watermelon. In plants lycopene exists mainly in the *trans* form, but in human plasma about half of it exists as various *cis* isomers. The prostate also contains some *cis* forms. Heating lycopene-containing foods causes some isomerization, but the rest must occur in the gut or after absorption into the body. Its biological significance is unknown.

3.22 Plant phenols[464,465]

A phenol is any compound that contains an —OH group attached to a benzene ring. **Monophenols** have one such aromatic —OH group, **diphenols** two and **polyphenols** more than two. Plants contain a huge range of phenols (Table 3.13), including the tocopherols and tocotrienols (monophenols). Most phenols exert antioxidant effects *in vitro*, inhibiting lipid peroxidation by acting as chain-breaking peroxyl radical scavengers. In addition, phenols often scavenge other RS, such as $OH^{\bullet}$, $NO_2^{\bullet}$, N_2O_3, ONOOH and HOCl. Some can react with $O_2^{\bullet-}$, mostly the di- and polyphenols (Section 2.5.3.5).[466] Phenols with two adjacent —OH groups, or other chelating structures, can bind transition metal ions (especially iron and copper), often in forms poorly active in promoting free-radical reactions; this chelating ability can interfere with uptake of metals from the diet.

Thus, many plant polyphenols are excellent antioxidants *in vitro*. Most attention has been given to the **flavonoids** such as quercetin, found in high levels in onion, wine, teas and many other plant products; Fig. 3.34). The number of phenolic −OH groups and their relative positions are key determinants of antioxidant activity. **Thymol** (Fig. 3.33) is often used as an antiseptic and antioxidant in commercial enzyme suspensions (e.g. of catalase; Section 3.7.1).

3.22.1 Phenols in the diet[465]

The human diet is rich in a variety of phenols. For example, soybean contains tocopherols, isoflavones (e.g. **genistein** and **daidzein**; Fig. 3.33) and caffeic acid. **Taxifolin** (Fig. 3.34) occurs in peanuts. **Resveratrol** is often present at low levels in wine, being produced in the grapes as a defence agent toxic to fungi. **Curcumin** gives the yellow colour to the curry spice **turmeric**, obtained from the roots of *Curcuma longa*. Sesame seed oil contains **sesamol**, esters of caffeic acid (Fig. 3.33) are present in several plants, and green teas are rich in **catechins** (Fig. 3.35) which contribute much of their *in vitro* antioxidant activity (Table 3.33). Catechin, epicatechin and epigallocatechin gallate are significant contributors to the total antioxidant activity of red wine. Cottonseed oil contains a yellow polyphenol, **gossypol** (Fig. 3.33), which has spermicidal effects and has undergone (unsuccessful due to side-effects) clinical trials as a male contraceptive (Section 6.11.4).

Herbs and spices have been used for centuries to preserve foods;[407] in the book of Exodus in the Old Testament it is stated that spices were added to oil to keep it fresh. They are rich sources of antioxidants: extracts of sage, rosemary, red peppers, chilli, tarragon, ginger, thyme and oregano inhibit lipid peroxidation *in vitro*, largely due to the phenols present. These include **carnosic acid** and **rosmaric acid** in rosemary, **dehydrozingerone** in ginger, and phenolic acid amides in black pepper. Oil of cloves contains **eugenol** (Fig. 3.33), sometimes added to dental materials as an analgesic and antiseptic. Wood smoke contains various phenols, such as **guaiacol** (Fig. 3.33), that can inhibit lipid peroxidation in smoked foods. Olives contain **hydroxytyrosol** (Fig. 3.33). Further examples are

given in Table 3.13. Often phenols are present in plants as conjugates with sugars (**glycosides**). For example quercetin can be attached to rhamnose to give **quercitrin** or rutinose (giving **rutin**) or, more usually, to glucose. For example, onion contains **quercetin 4′ glucoside** and **quercetin 3,4′-diglucoside**. Most flavonoids are glycosylated in plants, except for the catechins.

3.22.1.1 Do we absorb them?[465]

Not completely, the amount absorbed varies between species and individuals and depends on the compound. For example, in humans anthocyanins are less well absorbed than quercetin or catechins. Glycosides are usually hydrolysed by intestinal glycosidase enzymes (especially **lactase phloridzin hydrolase**) and the resulting phenols (and *possibly* some intact glycosides) can be absorbed. Unabsorbed phenols enter the colon, where polyphenols are extensively metabolized to monophenols and other products by the gut flora. Those that are absorbed are rapidly metabolized by methylation and glucuronidation of −OH groups, in the gut itself and in the liver. The liver also catalyses sulphation of phenols. For example, when [^{14}C-] quercetin was administered to humans, about 36 to 53% was absorbed; 18 to 27% of the radioactivity appeared in urine, but <5% in faeces. The majority was detected as exhaled $^{14}CO_2$, indicative of extensive degradation.[467] Plama levels of unconjugated polyphenols rarely exceed 1 μM, even in subjects consuming large amounts in the diet, and levels of 'free' quercetin in humans are virtually zero; most is present as glucuronides and some as sulphates.[465] Similarly, plasma levels of resveratrol in wine drinkers are very low (Section 10.3.4). High dietary levels of quercetin and some other flavonoids can decrease intestinal uptake of glucose and ascorbate by binding to their transport proteins.[468]

Dietary flavonoid intake in the USA and Denmark has been estimated as ~20 to 25 mg/day, and total polyphenol intake can be over 100 mg/day in subjects consuming diets rich in fruits and vegetables.[469,470] In Asian countries,

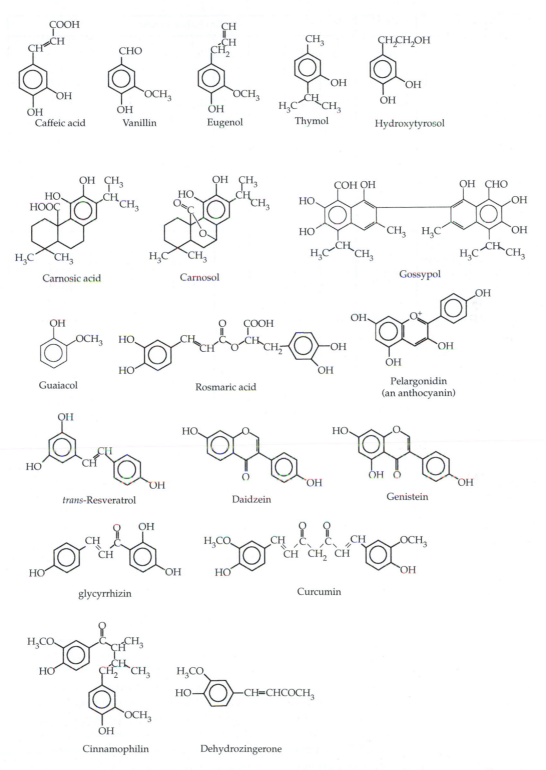

Figure 3.33 Structures of some plant phenols. The isoflavones, such as genistein and daidzein, have a weak antioestrogen-like activity, and contribute to the ability of certain plants (eaten in excess) to interfere with reproduction in farm animals (*Biochem. Pharmacol.* **60**, 1, 2000).

Generic structure	Flavonoid	Hydroxylation pattern								
		2'	3'	4'	5'	3	5	6	7	8
Flavane 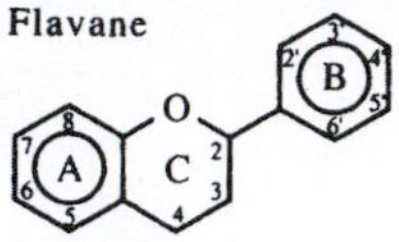	Catechins		•	•		•	•		•	
	Meciadonol		•	•		Methoxy	•		•	
Flavanone 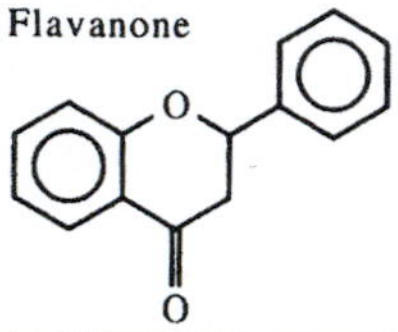	Taxifolin		•	•		•	•		•	
	Naringenin			•			•		•	
	Naringin			•			•		Rhamno-glucoside	
Flavone 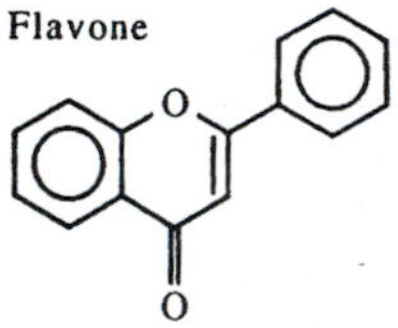	Luteolin		•	•			•		•	
	Apigenin			•			•		•	
Flavonol 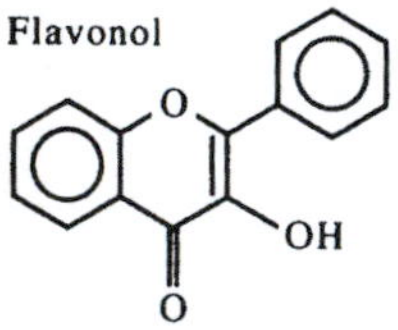	Quercetin		•	•		•	•		•	
	Myricetin		•	•	•	•	•		•	
	Gossypetin		•	•		•	•		•	•
	Fisetin		•	•		•			•	
	Cirsiliol		•	•		H	•		Methoxy	
	Morin	•		•		•	•		•	
	Kaempferol			•		•	•		•	
	Galangin					•	•		•	
	Baicalein					H	•	•	•	
	Rutin		•	•		Rutinose	•		•	
	Quercetrin		•	•		Rhamnose	•		•	
	Gossypin		•	•		•	•		•	Glycoside

Figure 3.34 Structure and hydroxylation pattern of some members of the flavonoid family. Taken from *Food Chem. Toxicol.* **33**, 1061, 1995 by courtesy of Dr Joe Formica and Elsevier. The family members include flavones, 3-hydroxyflavones (flavonols), catechins (flavanols), anthocyanins, isoflavones and flavanones. The flavonoid core structure contains three rings (A, C, B): variations in ring C and type of substituents produce the different members of the flavonoid family.

consumption of soya may deliver up to 20 to 40 mg isoflavones daily. Subjects who drink a lot of coffee may ingest 0.5 to 0.8 g of hydroxycinnamates per day.

3.22.2 Are plant phenols antioxidants *in vivo*?[442,471]

Within plants, some phenols are important biosynthetic precursors (e.g. **caffeic acid** for lignin; Section 7.5.4). Others may be produced to absorb ultraviolet radiation, for example *Arabidopsis* mutants unable to synthesize phenols were more damaged by ultraviolet light.[472] Yet others, especially the red/blue **anthocyanins**, and the yellow **aurones** and **chalcones**, may attract pollinating insects. In some cases, phenols may act as antioxidants in the plant; in the central vacuoles of leaves both phenols and peroxidase may be present. Any H_2O_2 in the leaf that escapes consumption elsewhere can diffuse into the vacuole and be consumed as a cosubstrate in the oxidation of phenols by peroxidase. Ascorbate in the vacuole may recycle the oxidized phenols.[473]

But what about when humans eat phenols? Are they antioxidant *in vivo*? Two observations drew attention to this question. First, phenols in red wine

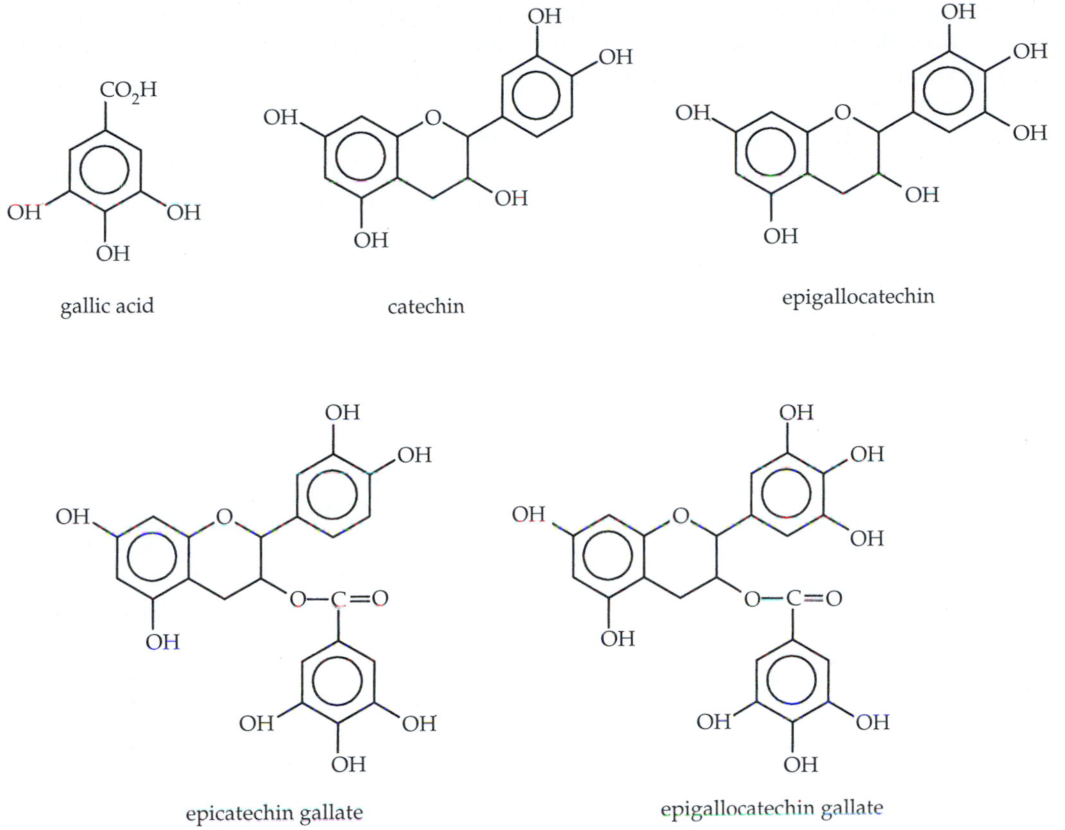

Figure 3.35 Structure of gallic acid and the catechins. Adapted from *Free Rad. Biol. Med.* **20**, 933, 1996 by courtesy of Professor C. Rice-Evans and Elsevier, Amsterdam.

were found to inhibit LDL oxidation *in vitro*, and it was suggested that they could exert cardioprotective effects by limiting LDL oxidation *in vivo*. This was proposed as an explanation of the lower incidence of heart disease in certain areas of France (the **French paradox**) despite the high prevalence there of risk factors, such as smoking and high fat intake.[474] Alcohol alone, however, has cardioprotective effects (at moderate intakes) and the debate continues as to whether wine has any additional benefit due to its flavonoid content (Section 8.8.1). Teetotallers may be pleased to learn that phenols in tea, grape juice, cocoa, dark chocolate and many other foods also inhibit LDL oxidation *in vitro*; wine is not essential.

Second, an epidemiological study in the Netherlands (the **Zutphen study**)[469] suggested an inverse correlation between the incidence of coronary heart disease and stroke and the dietary intake of flavonoids (especially quercetin), which originated mainly from tea, fruits (e.g. apples) and vegetables (e.g. onions) in the population examined. Since then multiple other epidemiological studies have confirmed similar associations, although a few have not. Like the USA and Denmark (Section 3.22.1.1), total daily flavonoid consumption in the Netherlands is estimated as at least 23 mg, of which about 16 mg/day is quercetin, more than the average daily intake of α-tocopherol (7–10 mg).

It was widely assumed that these alleged beneficial effects were due to antioxidant actions of flavonoids. Since then, many studies have used biomarkers of oxidative damage, for example F_2–IPs and 8OHdG, to see if flavonoids exert antioxidant effects *in vivo* in humans. Some positive effects using these biomarkers have been found, for example with several studies involving green tea, soy, chocolate, dealcoholized wine, garlic extracts, and grape juice and with some involving individual phenols, for example hydroxytyrosol. Of course, a protective effect of flavonoid-rich foods or beverages should not necessarily be interpreted as a protective effect of flavonoids. For example, the ability of green or black tea to decrease the incidence of UV-induced skin cancer in hairless mice turned out to be due to the caffeine present.[475] But there are an equal number of negative reports, in which administration of pure phenols or flavonoid-rich foods, or placing subjects on flavonoid-poor diets, has failed to alter parameters of oxidative damage.[442,476] Since plasma levels of unconjugated flavonoids rarely exceed $1\,\mu M$ and the metabolites tend to have lower antioxidant activity because of the blocking of $-OH$ groups by methylation, sulphation or glucuronidation, it seems difficult to imagine a powerful antioxidant effect *in vivo*. However, high levels of phenols exist in the stomach, small intestine and colon and could conceivably exert antioxidant, and other, protective effects there (Section 6.2).[442] Some flavonoids can recycle the α-tocopheryl radical (e.g. in LDL) which could contribute to antioxidant effects *in vivo*.[477]

3.22.2.1 *More than antioxidants?*
Flavonoids are not only antioxidants: they have many other effects *in vitro*. Thus some can inhibit telomerase (Section 10.5), protein glycation, XO, the proteasome, COX-1 and -2 (Section 7.12.3), lipoxygenases (Section 7.12.7) and matrix metalloproteinases, or bind to the aryl hydrocarbon receptor (Section 10.5 and ref [478]). Genistein and daidzein have an antioestrogen action, which is probably more important than their limited antioxidant ability. Flavonoids can modulate signal transduction pathways including MAP kinases, platelet-derived growth factor (PDGF) receptor, AP-1 and NF-κB (Section 4.5).[479] Resveratrol and related compounds can activate the sirtuins (Section 10.3.4). Whether plasma levels of flavonoids are sufficient to exert such effects is unclear, but all these actions are

feasible at the levels present in the gut. For example, ingestion of green tea partially inhibited COX in human rectal mucosa.[480] In apoE-knockout mice, red wine polyphenols slowed atherosclerosis, but did not affect lipid peroxidation (Section 9.3.7), suggestive of action by a different mechanism.

3.22.3 Pro-oxidant effects of phenols?

Phenols do not always chelate transition metal ions in redox-inactive forms; sometimes mixtures of metals and phenols can stimulate oxidative damage to DNA or proteins *in vitro* (but not usually to lipids, since the chain breaking antioxidant effect predominates). As we have already commented for vitamins C and E, the physiological relevance is uncertain. Several studies have shown cytostatic or cytotoxic effects of flavonoids on cells in culture, and a few have demonstrated antitumour effects of administering high levels to animal models of carcinogenesis. Some of the claimed cellular effects could be artefacts: polyphenols rapidly oxidize in commonly-used cell culture media, generating both H_2O_2 and quinines/semiquinones that can injure cells.[481] Phenols also oxidize at high temperatures; for example this produces levels of H_2O_2 in instant coffee $>100\,\mu M$ and in teas $>50\,\mu M$.[482] As a result, these beverages appear mutagenic in some bacterial test systems that are sensitive to H_2O_2. Drinking coffee leads to elevated excretion of H_2O_2 in the urine, since some of the autoxidizable compounds, such as **benzenetriol** (sometimes called **hydroxyhydroquinone**)

are absorbed, re-excreted and continue to generate H_2O_2 in the urine (Section 2.6.2.1). There is no evidence that such levels cause harm: no significant deleterious effects of coffee drinking have been revealed in numerous epidemiological studies and the balance of evidence suggests (but does not

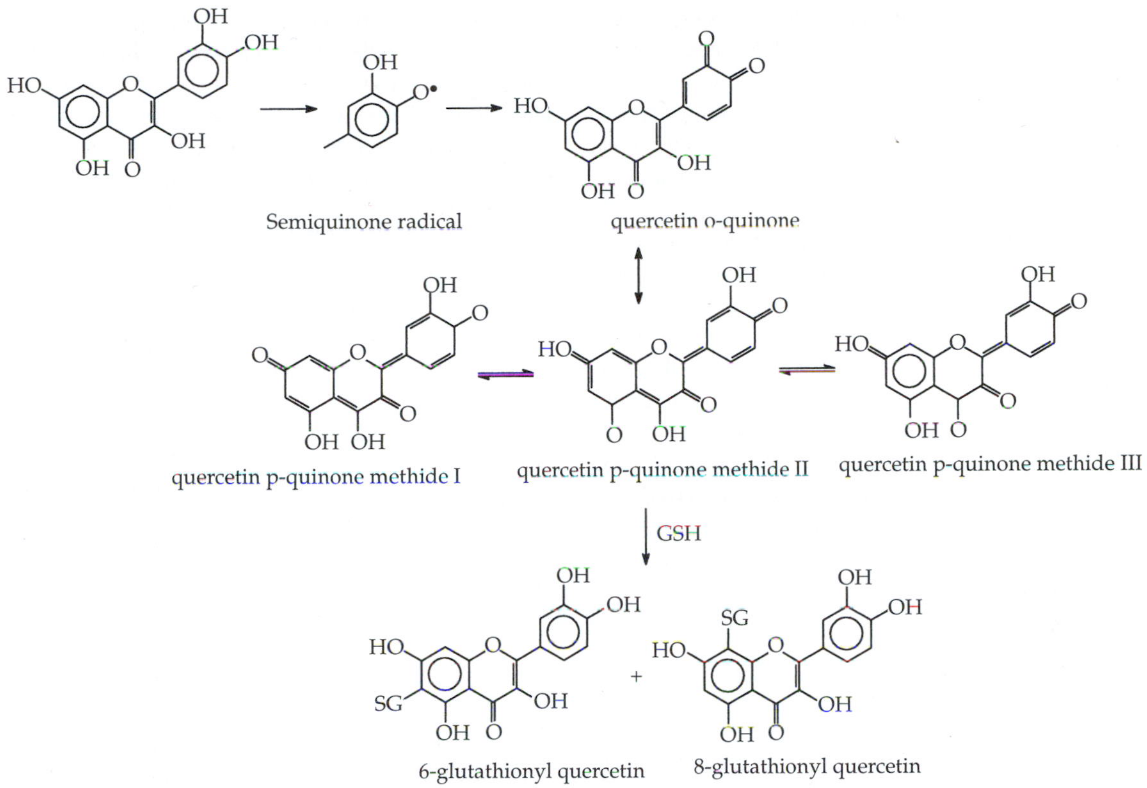

Figure 3.36 Quercetin and some of its oxidation products. Oxidation of the catechol structure in the B ring initially forms a semiquinone radical, which can then form a quinone, which has several isomeric forms. This can react with GSH to give 6- or 8-glutathionyl-quercetins (*FEBS Lett.* **520**, 30, 2002). Adapted from *Free Radic. Res.* **36**, 103S, 2002 by courtesy of Professor Ivonne M.C.M. Rietjens and Taylor and Francis Ltd.

prove) benefit rather than harm from green and black teas. Other phenols that have shown anticancer effects in animal models include resveratrol and curcumin (Fig. 3.33). However, curcumin *increased* lipid peroxidation in the LEC rat (presumably by interaction with copper ions; Section 3.15.5.5)[305] and it inhibits thioredoxin reductase, causing it to become an NADPH-dependent ROS-generating protein (Section 3.11 and ref [483]).

More research is needed to assess the physiological importance of plant phenols as anti- or pro-oxidants *in vivo*. Possible biological effects of any flavonoid-derived radicals generated during antioxidant activity must also be considered, as might be the case for gossypol (Section 6.11.4) and eugenol. Both inhibit lipid peroxidation *in vitro*, but their resulting radicals can damage other molecular targets such as DNA (again *in vitro*). Quercetin oxidation produces quinones that conjugate with

GSH and can deplete GSH levels in cultured cells (Fig. 3.36), although quercetin (and probably other flavonoid-derived) phenoxyl radicals may be reduced back to quercetin by ascorbate *in vivo*.

3.22.4 Herbal medicines[484,485]

There is considerable interest in the development of flavonoids and their derivatives for therapeutic use (Section 10.6.7), for example as anti-inflammatory, anticancer, anti-ischaemic and antithrombotic agents. An extract of the ornamental tree *Ginkgo biloba* has been used 'to improve memory' for thousands of years (Section 9.16.6.7).

Kampo medicines are traditional in Japan; they are extracts of multiple herbs and contain a complex mixture of phenols and other compounds, including **glycyrrhizin** (Fig. 3.33) from roots of the licorice plant, *Glycyrrhiza glabra*. Extracts of

propolis, a resinous substance used by bees in hive construction (Section 2.6.2) have often been used in herbal medicine, and contain many phenolic and other plant-derived compounds, including **caffeic acid phenethyl ester**. Roots of the plant *Polygonum capsidatum*, used extensively in traditional Chinese medicine, are rich in resveratrol.

Never assume that natural products are safe to consume just because they are natural. Examples of noxious agents produced by plants include cyanide and aflatoxin (Section 9.14). Nordihydroguairetic acid (Table 10.15), a powerful inhibitor of lipoxygenase-catalysed and non-enzymic lipid oxidation isolated from the creosote bush *Larrea divaricata*, is no longer used as a food preservative because of adverse toxicological reports. An extract of the plant *Cratoxylum cochinchinense* isolated on the basis of its powerful antioxidant activity turned out to be cytotoxic.[486] Flavonoids increased damage in mouse autoimmune encephalomyelitis, a model for multiple sclerosis.[487] Nevertheless, some clinical studies suggest that *Ginkgo* has a mild antidementia effect (Section 9.16.6.7) and ginger extract seems to help arthritis.[488] Curcumin administration decreased[489] oxidative damage and brain pathology in a transgenic mouse model of Alzheimer's disease and several papers are suggesting neuroprotective effects of flavonoids and flavonoid-rich foods. Don't assume that these are necessarily mediated by antioxidant effects, however (Section 10.6.7).

Cellular responses to oxidative stress: adaptation, damage, repair, senescence and death

Life is pleasant. Death is peaceful. It's the transition that's troublesome.

Isaac Asimov

4.1 Introduction

In healthy aerobes, production of reactive species (RS) is approximately balanced with antioxidant defence systems. The balance is not perfect, however, so that some RS-mediated damage occurs continuously (Table 4.1). In other words, antioxidant defences control levels of RS rather than eliminate them, for example OxyR keeps H_2O_2 levels in *E. coli* at about $0.2\,\mu M$ (Section 4.5.2 below). Why is this? Maintaining excess antioxidant defences would have an energy cost—it could be energetically 'cheaper' to repair or replace damaged biomolecules. Antioxidants may simply be unable to intercept some RS. For example, $OH^{\bullet}$ generated by homolytic fission of water due to our background exposure to ionizing radiation will react with whatever it meets first.

Another factor is that RS play essential roles *in vivo* (some are discussed in Chapter 7). Everyone is familiar with regulation of cellular processes by phosphorylation and dephosphorylation of enzymes and transcription factors, but we have realized in the past decade that regulation by oxidation and reduction (**redox regulation**) is equally important. Not only that, the two systems cross-talk, that is the redox state of the cell influences phosphorylation, and *vice versa* (Section 4.5 below). The antioxidant defence network must minimize the levels of most RS whilst still permitting enough to remain for their essential roles.

4.1.1 Defining oxidative stress and oxidative damage

What happens if this delicate balance is upset, or repair or replacement systems fail? Having too many RS in relation to the available antioxidants is often said to be a state of **oxidative stress**. Although this term is widely used in the free-radical literature it is not clearly defined. Sies, who introduced the term from the title of the book he edited in 1985, *Oxidative Stress*, defined it in 1991 in the introduction to the second edition[2] as *a disturbance in the prooxidant–antioxidant balance in favour of the former, leading to potential damage*. Such damage is often called **oxidative damage**. We[1] have defined this as *the biomolecular damage caused by attack of RS upon the constituents of living organisms*. Not all damage caused by oxidative stress is oxidative damage (Section 4.2 below). Increased oxidative damage can result not only from more oxidative stress, but also from failure of repair or replacement systems.

In principle, oxidative stress can result from:

1. Diminished antioxidants, e.g. mutations decreasing the levels of antioxidant defences, such as GSH or MnSOD. Depletions of dietary antioxidants and other essential dietary constituents (e.g. copper, iron, zinc, magnesium) can also lead to oxidative stress (Table 10.3). Children with the protein deficiency disease **kwashiorkor** suffer

Table 4.1 Evidence that damage by reactive species (RS) occurs *in vivo*

Target of damage	Evidence
DNA (Section 4.8)	Low levels of oxidative base damage products present in DNA isolated from all aerobic cells; levels often increase in animals with cancer or chronic inflammatory diseases or subjected to oxidative stress by toxins, e.g. smoking. Some base damage products are excreted in urine, in part from DNA repair processes.
Protein (Section 4.13)	Attack of RS upon proteins produces carbonyls and other amino acid modifications. Low levels of carbonyls and other products are detected in healthy animal tissues and body fluids. Nitrotyrosines, products of attack on tyrosine by RNS, have been detected in many normal body tissues at low levels, and at higher levels in diseased tissues. Chloro- and bromotyrosine also occur. Bityrosine has been detected in tissues and urine.
Lipid (Section 4.12)	Presence of specific end-products of peroxidation (e.g. isoprostanes, isofurans, HNE-adducts) in tissues and body fluids; levels increase during oxidative stress.
Uric acid (Sections 3.18.6 and 5.12)	Attacked by several RS to generate allantoin, cyanuric acid, parabanic acid, oxonic acid and other products, which are present in human body fluids. Levels increase in several diseases. Only applicable to primates, which accumulate high levels of urate because they lack urate oxidase.

Further details may be found in this chapter, in Chapters 5 and 9, and in ref.[1]

oxidative stress, involving low GSH levels (lack of sulphur-containing amino acids in the diet) and iron overload (inability to make enough transferrin; Table 4.3 below). Whether giving them antioxidants would be of benefit is uncertain.[3]

and/or

2. Increased production of RS, e.g. by exposure to elevated O_2, the presence of toxins that produce RS (Chapter 8), or excessive activation of 'natural' systems producing RS, e.g. inappropriate activation of phagocytic cells in chronic inflammatory diseases (Chapter 9).

4.2 Consequences of oxidative stress: proliferation, adaptation, senescence, damage or death?

Consequences of oxidative stress can include any, or any combination of, the following, to an extent that depends on the cell type and the severity of the oxidative stress (Fig. 4.1).

1. *Increased proliferation.* Many cells respond to mild oxidative stress by proliferating.
2. *Adaptation* of the cell or organism by upregulation of defence systems, which may: (a) completely protect against damage; (b) protect against damage

to some extent but not completely; or (c) 'over-protect'—the cells is then resistant to higher levels of oxidative stress imposed subsequently.
3. *Cell injury.* This involves damage to some or all molecular targets: lipids, DNA, protein, carbohydrate, etc. Such damage can sometimes be the trigger leading to adaptation. *Not all damage caused by oxidative stress is oxidative damage*: secondary damage to biomolecules can result from oxidative stress-related changes in, for example, ion levels (e.g. Ca^{2+} leading to activation of proteinases; Section 4.3.2 below).
4. *Senescence.* The cell survives but can no longer divide (Section 10.3.5).
5. *Cell death.* After injury the cell may: (a) recover from the oxidative damage by repairing it or replacing the damaged molecules; or (b) it may survive with persistent oxidative damage; or (c) oxidative damage, especially to DNA, may trigger death by apoptosis, necrosis, or cell death mechanisms intermediate between these extremes.

Let us elaborate on these events.

4.2.1 Proliferation

Low-level oxidative stress (e.g. by adding small amounts of H_2O_2 or of aldehydes such as

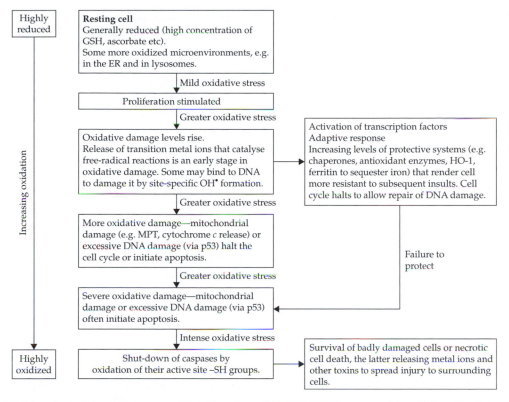

Figure 4.1 How cells respond to oxidative stress. Adapted from *Lancet* **355**, 1179, 2000 by courtesy of the publishers. Stimulation of proliferation by low levels of RS is associated with increased net phosphorylation of multiple proteins (Section 4.5.5 below). The cell is generally a reducing environment, especially the mitochondria ($E°' \sim -0.28$ V) and cytosol (GSH/GSSG >100, $E°' \sim -0.23$ V), but less so in the ER lumen ($E°' \sim -0.18$ V) and probably in endosomes and lysosomes (*Proc. Natl. Acad. Sci. USA* **102**, 17987, 2005). The exact $E°'$ values depend on both the absolute and relative concentrations of GSH and GSSG (Section 3.9.1). An interesting example is stem cells; they seem rich in antioxidant defences which decline as they differentiate. Indeed, low-level ROS may promote differentiation, but too much oxidative stress (e.g. in diabetes) can impair stem cell differentiation (*Antiox. Redox Signal.* **7**, 1409, 2005). Sometimes, cells are injured by 'special' mechanisms, e.g. the HL-60 leukaemia cell line contains myeloperoxidase; H_2O_2-induced apoptosis involves HOCl formation (*Arch. Biochem. Biophys.* **401**, 223, 2002).

4-hydroxynonenal; Section 4.12.5.3 below) stimulates the proliferation of several cell types in culture. Figure 4.2 shows an example. Indeed, the cell culture environment is for many cells a low level oxidative stress, which may be why they grow so well in certain media (Section 1.11). The arrest of growth induced by cell confluence (**contact inhibition**) has been suggested by some to be related to a decrease in intracellular ROS and consequent loss of pro-proliferative stimuli.[4] Pro-proliferative effects of RS may contribute to atherosclerosis (abnormal proliferation of smooth muscle cells; Section 9.5.5), angiogenesis (Section 9.13.5), rheumatoid arthritis (Section 9.10) and to **fibrosis** (abnormal proliferation of fibroblasts) in

several human diseases.[5] Diminishing ROS levels can decrease proliferation (at least in cell culture); for example overexpression of catalase in rat aortic smooth muscle cells lowered H_2O_2 levels and blocked their proliferation,[6] and fibroblasts from mice overexpressing catalase showed decreased growth rates in culture.[7]

4.2.2 Adaptation

Cells usually tolerate mild to moderate oxidative stress, which often results in increased synthesis of antioxidant defences (and/or of other defences such as heat-shock proteins) in an attempt to restore the oxidant/antioxidant balance. For

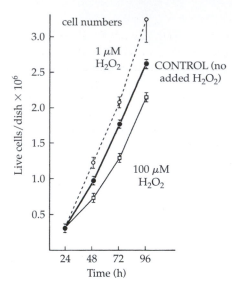

Figure 4.2 The effect of H_2O_2 on the proliferation of baby-hamster kidney fibroblast cells. At 24 h, monolayer cultures were treated with 1 μM H_2O_2, which stimulated cell division, or 100 μM H_2O_2, which inhibited it. Data from *Free Radic. Res.* **29**, 121, 1994, by courtesy of the late Professor Roy Burdon and Harwood Academic Press.

example, if adult rats are gradually acclimatized to elevated O_2 concentrations, they can tolerate pure O_2 for longer than control rats, apparently due to increased synthesis of lung antioxidants (Section 3.4.5). Another example of adaptation is some cases of **ischaemic preconditioning** (Section 9.5.6). A brief period of ischaemia in pig hearts followed by reperfusion led to prolonged depression of contractile function, an effect attenuated by antioxidants.[8] However, repeated brief periods of ischaemia led to quicker return of contractile function on reperfusion, an adaptive response not seen in the antioxidant-treated animals. In other words, ROS produced by ischaemia–reperfusion caused damage leading to depressed contractility, but also led to a response protective against subsequent insult. In some cases, mild oxidative stress can elevate defences sufficiently to protect cells against more severe oxidative stress applied subsequently. Thus exposure of *E. coli* to low levels of H_2O_2 can render it resistant to higher levels (Section 4.5.2 below).

Mechanisms of adaptation need not always involve increased antioxidant defences. For example, by culturing **HeLa cells** (a malignant cell line) at gradually increasing O_2 concentrations over a 21-month period, it was possible to obtain cells capable of growing under 80% O_2, a level lethal to 'normal' HeLa cells.[9] These cells did not show elevated levels of SOD, catalase or GPx and it was proposed that their increased O_2 tolerance is due to an alteration of targets normally vulnerable to oxidative damage. Such a phenomenon occurs with the enzyme fumarase in *E. coli* (Section 1.6). Another possibility is that the mitochondria in these HeLa cells have 'adapted' to produce less ROS.[10]

4.2.3 Cell injury and senescence

'Injury' is a widely used, but vague, term. It can be defined as the result of a chemical or physical stimulus, either in excess or in deficiency, that transiently or permanently alters the homeostasis of the cell.[11] The response to oxidative injury may be reversible; for a variable period the cell is in an altered redox state which does not lead to cell death and it then returns to 'normal'. Events triggered by the altered redox state (e.g. increased expression of genes encoding antioxidant defences or heat-shock proteins, and less expression of some other genes[12]) can persist for a while or even permanently. Moderate levels of oxidative stress tend to halt cell proliferation transiently, by triggering **cell cycle checkpoints** (Section 9.13.1). For example, p53 can be activated when cells are exposed to H_2O_2, leading to cell cycle arrest. Oxidative stress can also affect intercellular communication through gap junctions (Section 3.21.3.1).[13]

Oxidative stress can damage many different biomolecules. Often it is unclear which is the first target, both because injury mechanisms interact widely and because the assays used to measure damage have variable specificities and sensitivities (Chapter 5). For example, measurement of protein carbonyls (Section 5.15.3) would not detect early damage by oxidation of essential −SH groups on membrane ion transporters. The initial target of oxidative stress can vary depending on the cell, the type of stress imposed and its severity. For example, carbon tetrachloride seems to injure cells primarily by lipid peroxidation (Section 8.2). By contrast, DNA is an important early target of damage when H_2O_2 is added to many mammalian cells.

Senescence, a permanent state of non-division (Section 10.3.5) can be induced by high levels of RS. For example, human fibroblasts exposed to 100 to 300 µM H_2O_2 in culture developed a senescent phenotype,[14] showing increased expression of proteins that inhibit the cell cycle. Senescence after prolonged cell culture is in part due to the oxidative stress of the culture process (Section 10.3.5).

4.2.4 Poly(ADP–ribose)polymerase[15,16]

Excessive DNA strand breakage is associated with depletion of cellular ATP and NAD^+ levels. The latter occurs because a chromatin-bound enzyme, **poly(ADP–ribose)polymerase 1 (PARP-1)** binds to damaged DNA, splits the NAD^+ molecule and transfers the ADP–ribose portion onto nuclear proteins, including histones, DNA polymerases, DNA ligases, p53 and PARP-1 itself (**automodification**) (Fig. 4.3). ADP-ribosylation of proteins is important; under conditions of low to moderate DNA damage, it facilitates DNA repair (Section 4.10.3 below) and promotes cell survival. Hence transgenic knockout animals lacking PARP-1 show genomic instability in response to DNA damaging agents such as ionizing radiation.[15] The PARP-1 enzyme also aids removal of oxidized nuclear proteins via the proteasome (Section 4.14.2). After repair is complete, the poly(ADP)–ribose residues are removed by a **poly(ADP)–ribose glycohydrolase** enzyme, which is constitutively active.

However, excessive activation of PARP-1 (i.e. if there are too many DNA strand breaks) can deplete the cellular NAD^+ pool, interfering with ATP synthesis and perhaps even leading to cell death. This cell death has sometimes been called a **suicide response**; since DNA repair is not error-free a cell with extensively damaged DNA may 'commit suicide' in the interests of the organism to avoid the risk of becoming cancerous. Mice lacking PARP-1 show increased resistance to streptozotocin-induced diabetes, which is thought to be an example of 'lethal NAD^+ depletion' (Section 8.5).[16] Treatment of cells with **nicotinamide**, which maintains NAD^+ levels, can often delay or prevent this cell death. Nicotinamide also affects the sirtuin system (Section 10.3.4), so do not assume that a protective effect of nicotinamide always occurs by opposing PARP-1 action.

Several agents inhibit PARP-1, including **theophylline**, **theobromine**, **3-aminobenzamide** and **INO–1001**. They decrease the falls in NAD^+ seen in cells with extensive DNA damage, for example after irradiation or toxin treatment, and often maintain cell viability. Be careful however, in some studies they inhibited $ONOO^-$-induced cell death not by blocking PARP, but simply by reacting directly with $ONOO^-$ (Section 2.6.1.4). PARP-1 is involved in both apoptotic and necrotic cell death (Section 4.4 below).

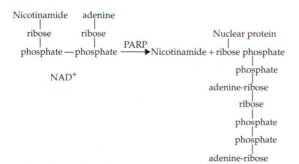

Figure 4.3 The reaction catalysed by poly(ADP–ribose) polymerase-1 (PARP-1). PARPs are sometimes called **poly (ADP–ribose) synthetases** or **poly(ADP–ribose) transferases**. ADP–ribose is usually attached to the side-chain carboxyl groups of glutamate residues on the target proteins, and chains can be more than 200 units long.[15] Several other PARPs have been identified; PARP-1 and PARP-2 are involved in spindle formation during mitosis (Nature **432**, 645, 2004).

4.3 Oxidative stress causes changes in cellular ion metabolism

4.3.1 Basic principles

Reactive species can affect ion movements in several ways,[17] including

1. Redox regulation of genes encoding ion channel proteins.
2. Redox regulation of ion channel proteins themselves, e.g. by oxidizing and reducing essential thiol groups or nitrating tyrosine residues to modulate channel function. Such modifications may lead to accelerated removal of channel

proteins, e.g. through the proteasome (Section 4.14.2 below).

3. Secondary effects, e.g. altering the activity of one ion channel can cause openings or closings of others in response to cellular ion imbalance and/or changes in membrane potential.

Oxidative stress can damage proteins involved in maintenance of essential ion gradients between cells and extracellular fluids. The **Na$^+$, K$^+$-ATPase system** (often called the **sodium pump**) in the plasma membrane uses energy released by ATP hydrolysis to export Na$^+$ and import K$^+$. It thus keeps intracellular K$^+$ high and intracellular Na$^+$ low, compared with levels in extracellular fluids. This enzyme contains catalytically-essential −SH groups that are susceptible to oxidative attack, and is readily inactivated by RS.[18] Potassium channels are also affected by RS and by aldehydes produced during lipid peroxidation, such as HNE (Section 4.12.5.3); K$^+$ channels are essential in generation of electrical activity in neuronal and cardiac cells, but are also important in a variety of other cell types such as T-lymphocytes, vascular smooth muscle cells and epithelial cells.[17,19] The effects of RS vary, depending on the channel and the RS used; sometimes a K$^+$ channel is opened, sometimes its function is inhibited.[20]

4.3.1.1 *Cell volume changes*
Alterations of cellular ion balance can produce changes in cell volume, which in turn affect cell function. For example, generation of H$_2$O$_2$ (e.g. by adding a substrate for monoamine oxidase) or infusion of *tert*-butyl hydroperoxide in isolated perfused rat liver leads to K$^+$ release (due to abnormal opening of K$^+$ channels) and hepatocyte shrinkage. Shrinkage stimulates several metabolic events, including proteolysis, glycogen breakdown, biliary GSSG release, and urea synthesis. It decreases others such as protein synthesis, lactate uptake, and actin polymerization.[19] Cells exposed to hypotonic conditions activate plasma membrane chloride channels in response to the swelling; in some cell types increased ROS production may be the signal for opening.[21] Hydrogen peroxide affects the Na$^+$/H$^+$ exchange system and can acidify the cytosol (Section 4.4.1.2 below).

4.3.2 Calcium[22]

4.3.2.1 *Keeping it low*
Normally, intracellular 'free' Ca^{2+} levels are low, around 0.1 μM or less. Total cell Ca^{2+} is far greater, but most is safely sequestered within mitochondria and the ER or bound to cytoplasmic proteins. Transient increases in free Ca^{2+} regulate many physiological processes, including cell proliferation and neurotransmitter release. Extracellular signalling molecules bind to cell surface receptors and lead to release of Ca^{2+} from the ER by stimulating synthesis of an intracellular messenger, **inositol triphosphate** (IP$_3$) (Section 4.5.6.2 below). This compound opens Ca^{2+} channels in the ER membrane and lets Ca^{2+} escape into the cytosol. However, uncontrolled rises in intracellular 'free' Ca^{2+} can lead to cell injury and death.

Low intracellular Ca^{2+} levels are maintained by the concerted operation of several systems:[11,22,23]

1. Plasma membrane ATP-dependent Ca^{2+}-extrusion systems (in most cells). In cells which make extensive use of Ca^{2+} signalling (e.g. muscle and nerve), Na$^+$–Ca^{2+} exchange transporters are additionally present. Extracellular Ca^{2+} levels are in the mM range in animals, so these Ca^{2+}-export systems need energy to export Ca^{2+} against a high concentration gradient. Energy comes from ATP hydrolysis, or by linking Ca^{2+} export to entry of extracellular Na$^+$ down its concentration gradient. The Na$^+$ is then ejected by the ATP-dependent sodium pump.

2. Uptake of Ca^{2+} into the ER lumen by an ATP-dependent pump.

3. Uptake of Ca^{2+} by mitochondria, driven by the energy of the proton gradient (Fig. 1.8). This system seems to be a 'back-up' to the others; it only operates at fairly high intracellular Ca^{2+} level.

4. Binding of Ca^{2+} to proteins, e.g. **calmodulins**, Ca^{2+}-binding proteins found in all eukaryotic cells. Calmodulins regulate many enzymes, including **calcineurin** (Section 4.5.5.3 below) and nitric oxide synthases (Section 2.5.6.6), and multiple cellular processes such as cytoskeletal assembly. Calmodulins are rich in methionine residues, and are a potential target of oxidative damage,[23] since methionine is easily oxidized by RS (Section 4.13.4.1

below). Binding of Ca^{2+} to high-affinity binding sites on calmodulin causes a conformational change which enables the calmodulin to bind to target proteins in the cell. These include the Ca^{2+}-ATPase in the plasma membrane (activated by calmodulin binding), and a family of Ca^{2+}/calmodulin-dependent **protein kinases** which phosphorylate serines and threonines in their substrate proteins, activating such processes as smooth muscle contraction, catecholamine synthesis in certain neurons and the breakdown of glycogen in muscle.

4.3.2.2 *Oxidative stress: pushing* Ca^{2+} *up*[22–24]

Oxidative stress dysregulates Ca^{2+} metabolism, generally causing a rise in intracellular 'free' Ca^{2+}. This can contribute to the pro-proliferative effects of low-level oxidative stress as well as to the cytotoxic effects of higher levels. Reactive species can damage the ER Ca^{2+}-uptake system and interfere with Ca^{2+} efflux through the plasma membrane, by leading to oxidation of essential −SH groups on the transmembrane channels. In addition, oxidative stress can open channels in the plasma membrane that allow Ca^{2+} to enter, for example by decreasing the membrane potential and opening the **voltage-gated Ca^{2+} channels**. In some cells (e.g. gut, lung, eye, lymphocytes, monocytes, neutrophils, pancreatic β-cells [Section 8.5.1] and certain neurons [Section 9.16.5]), RS such as H_2O_2 open the **TRPM2 cation channels** in the plasma membrane and let Ca^{2+} in. These channels are non-selective, also transporting Na^+ and K^+, so depolarizing the membrane and letting in even more Ca^{2+} by opening voltage-gated channels. Opening of TRPM2 channels requires NAD^+, which is hydrolysed to ADP–ribose by the channel protein itself. The ADP–ribose produced from PARP-1 can open the channel, and may account for some or all of the opening by RS.[24] The normal physiological function of these channels is uncertain, but their presence renders cells exceptionally sensitive to rises in 'free' Ca^{2+} in response to RS.

A common consequence of excessive (>5 µM) rises in extracellular Ca^{2+} is **membrane blebbing** (Fig. 4.4), caused by disruption of the cytoskeleton. Polymerization and reorganization of actin are involved in multiple cell functions and are controlled by a range of actin-binding proteins. Actin also associates with membrane-anchoring proteins located in **focal adhesion sites** where the cell attaches to the extracellular matrix. Signalling molecules such as **focal adhesion kinase** play a key role in their formation. Membrane blebbing is usually associated with loss of focal adhesions. Calcium ions can activate proteinases (**calpains; calcium-activated non-lysosomal proteinases**) that cleave actin-binding proteins such as **spectrin**, eliminating the plasma membrane 'anchorage' to the cytoskeleton and allowing it to 'bleb out'. Calpains are present in all mammalian cells and perform several essential functions, but their activity is normally tightly regulated. Over-activation of calpains has been implicated in many diseases, including muscular dystrophy and Alzheimer's disease. Oxidation of −SH groups on cytoskeletal proteins by RS, and falls in ATP (needed for maintenance of cytoskeletal integrity), also facilitate blebbing. Calpains are cysteine proteinases and so might themselves be subject to oxidative damage.

An abnormal rise in 'free' Ca^{2+} will stimulate eNOS and nNOS (Section 2.5.6.6) producing more $NO^{\bullet}$, which could lead to $ONOO^-$ formation if $O_2^{\bullet-}$ were also being produced. The rise in Ca^{2+} can indeed lead to a rise in $O_2^{\bullet-}$ production; in certain cells containing XDH, active calpains convert it to XO, generating more ROS (Table 1.16). Nitric oxide at high levels can also be directly toxic, for example by inhibiting cytochrome oxidase (Section 2.5.6).

Calcium additionally stimulates **phospholipase A_2**, an enzyme which cleaves membrane phospholipids to release arachidonic acid for synthesis of prostaglandins and leukotrienes (Section 7.12.3). Excess production of free fatty acids and eicosanoids thus occurs, as well as accumulation of the hydrolysis products of membrane lipids, causing disruption of membrane organization. Rises in Ca^{2+} also activate **Ca^{2+}-dependent endonucleases** in the nucleus to cause DNA fragmentation, an event important in apoptosis (Section 4.4.1 below). **Transglutaminases** can be activated by Ca^{2+}; they catalyse the crosslinking of proteins between side-chain amino groups of lysine residues and

(a)   (b)

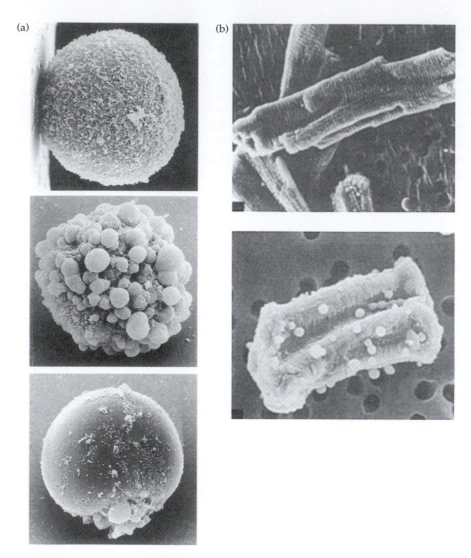

Figure 4.4 Bleb formation. (a) Hepatocytes were exposed to the quinone menadione, which leads to oxidative stress (Section 8.6). Top: untreated cell, showing microvillus surface structure. Centre: after exposure to 200 μM menadione for 30 min, showing multiple blebs. Bottom: a hepatocyte at a later stage, dominated by a single bleb which may soon rupture; the remainder of the original cell, with smaller blebs, can be seen at the bottom of the photograph. From *Trends Pharmacol. Sci.* **10**, 282, 1989 by courtesy of Professor Sten Orrenius and Elsevier Science Publishers. (b) Blebbing in rat cardiac myocytes treated with cumene hydroperoxide for 30 min. Top: normal myocytes. Bottom: myocytes after peroxide exposure. Photograph by courtesy of Dr A.A. Noronha-Dutra.

side-chain glutamine $-CONH_2$ groups to produce insoluble aggregates.

If blebbing proceeds to such an extent that bleb rupture occurs (Fig. 4.4) without immediate resealing, the cell loses its ion gradients and is effectively dead. Its contents are released into the surrounding area, that is necrotic cell death occurs. Death involving excessive rises in Ca^{2+} may be a common feature of multiple noxious stimuli, including intense oxidative stress and O_2 deprivation (Table 4.2).

4.3.2.3 Ca^{2+} and mitochondria

Excess Ca^{2+} can trigger the mitochondrial permeability transition (MPT), which opens pores in the inner membrane and collapses the membrane potential

Table 4.2 Some agents causing necrotic cell death in which excessive rises in intracellular Ca^{2+} have been implicated

Agent	Comments
O_2 deprivation. Inhibition of ATP-producing pathways (e.g. cyanide, rotenone, iodoacetate, mitochondrial uncouplers such as dinitrophenol)	Lead to severe fall in ATP; plasma membrane and ER Ca^{2+} pumps inoperative, no mitochondrial Ca^{2+} uptake (probably Ca^{2+} release). Metabolic inhibition potentiates cell damage by low levels of H_2O_2
A23187 (calcimycin)	Ca^{2+} ionophore, carries Ca^{2+} into the cell, raises Ca^{2+} to approaching extracellular levels
Quinones/ semiquinones	Can act by producing ROS and/or by binding to —SH groups, depleting GSH and inhibiting Ca^{2+}-sequestration systems (Section 8.6)
Some metal ions, e.g. lead, mercury, tin	Section 8.15
Excitotoxicity	Section 9.16.4

(Fig 1.9, legend). The MPT requires elevated Ca^{2+} levels plus another 'inducing agent'; effective agents include organic peroxides, agents oxidizing —SH groups, and $ONOO^-$. As solutes (including mitochondrial GSH and Ca^{2+}) escape from the matrix through the pore, osmotic imbalance occurs and the mitochondria swell. Pore opening can be blocked by **cyclosporin**, a drug used to prevent transplant rejection. It acts by binding to cyclophilin D (Fig. 1.9 legend). The MPT halts mitochondrial ATP synthesis and can lead to cell death by apoptosis (involving cytochrome c release from mitochondria; Section 4.4.1 below) or necrosis.

4.3.3 Iron

Oxidative stress interferes not only with Ca^{2+} but also with iron and copper metabolism; its overall effect is to increase the levels of potentially pro-oxidant metal ions (Fig 4.1). Mechanisms include:

1. *Raising extracellular iron.* Cell lysis, e.g. by traumatic injury or necrosis, releases metal ions into the surrounding environment. A simple illustration is that homogenates of tissues, especially brain, undergo lipid peroxidation faster than intact tissues, and this peroxidation is inhibited by iron chelators (Section 9.16.5).

2. *Increasing the size of the intracellular labile iron pool, LIP* (Section 3.15.1.3). Mechanisms include:

(a) superoxide releases iron from ferritin and iron–sulphur proteins (Section 3.6.2.2);

(b) peroxides release iron by degrading haem proteins (Sections 3.15.3);

(c) peroxynitrite can attack iron–sulphur proteins, releasing iron; the reported ability of excess $NO^\bullet$ to damage mitochondrial Fe–S centres is probably mediated, at least in part, via $ONOO^-$;

(d) increased uptake of iron, e.g. the cytotoxicity of adriamycin to some cells requires the activity of the transferrin receptor in increasing intracellular iron (Section 9.15.2); many cells readily take up 'low-molecular-mass' iron, e.g. released by cell lysis;

(e) a special case, UV irradiation of skin increases its iron content (Section 6.12.1.2).

Preincubating cells with permeant iron ion-chelating agents can therefore decrease oxidative damage, and cells deficient in SOD are hypersensitive to injury by H_2O_2 (Section 3.4.1 and 3.6.2.2). It is ironic (forgive the pun) that chelators designed for other metals can sometimes bind iron and alter rates of oxidative damage. For example, **Quin-2** was one of the first fluorescent 'probes' used to monitor intracellular Ca^{2+}. Unfortunately, it also binds iron and the ferric-Quin 2 complex can react[25] with H_2O_2 to form $OH^\bullet$. Another 'probe' for Ca^{2+} within cells is **ruthenium red**, which contains ruthenium (Ru) ions. Ruthenium (III) ions can react with H_2O_2[26] to form $OH^\bullet$.

4.3.3.1 *Measuring 'catalytic' iron*

The LIP size can be estimated by the calcein and phen-green assays (Section 3.15.1.3). Such assays only measure iron that these probes can access, not necessarily all the iron 'catalytic' for free radical reactions in the cell.

What about the extracellular environment? Several methods have been developed to measure 'catalytic' iron in body fluids. In terms of physiological relevance, perhaps the best is the **aconitase assay**.[27] Reassembly of iron clusters in aconitase requires a source of iron. The molecular form of this iron, at least in bacteria (Section 3.6.2.2), seems to be equivalent to iron able to catalyse free radical reactions. Thus the restoration of activity to aconitase is a measure of the levels of such iron in a body fluid.

Another approach is the **bleomycin assay**.[28] The antibiotic bleomycin requires iron salts to degrade DNA (Section 9.15.3). If other reagents are present in excess, the amount of DNA degradation is proportional to the amount of iron that can be bound by bleomycin (Fig. 4.5). Hence the assay measures **bleomycin-chelatable iron (BCI)**. Bleomycin has a fairly low affinity for iron, and at pH 7.4 cannot remove it from iron-containing proteins (e.g. lactoferrin, transferrin, ferritin, myoglobin, haemoglobin or catalase). Hence no BCI is present in freshly prepared serum or plasma from healthy animals (Table 4.3), because almost all iron is bound to transferrin, and the rest to ferritin. Some BCI is, however, present in lung lining fluid, some sweat samples and the plasma from patients with iron-overload (Table 4.3).

Bleomycin-chelatable iron appears to represent iron ions bound to low-molecular-mass agents such as citrate, or loosely bound to certain proteins, such as albumin (Table 4.3). Studies upon human body fluids show that the BCI level often (but not always) correlates with the ability of these fluids to stimulate free-radical reactions.[28,29] For example, plasma samples from iron-overloaded patients stimulate peroxidation of lipids *in vitro* (Section 3.15.5.4), and BCI levels were associated with increased oxidative protein damage in patients undergoing cancer chemotherapy. Application of the bleomycin assay to tissue homogenates also measures iron; if the tissue is first subjected to an insult (e.g. ischaemia–reperfusion), the levels of BCI measured in homogenates may increase (Table 4.3).

Other assays to measure 'catalytic' iron have been developed, also based on the chelation principle. Iron chelatable by bathophenanthroline disulphonate (BPDS),[30] desferrioxamine or nitrilotriacetate (NTA)[31] has been measured in some studies, by chromogen formation (BPDS) or HPLC analysis of the iron complexes (NTA, desferrioxamine). For example, ischaemia–reperfusion of rabbit kidneys prior to homogenization increased the amount of desferrioxamine-chelatable iron in the homogenates.[32] Nitrilotriacetate and desferrioxamine

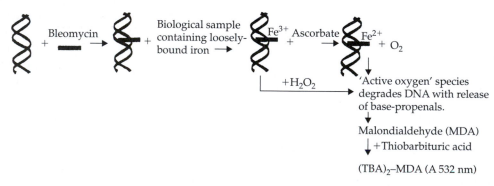

Figure 4.5 The bleomycin assay. Products of DNA degradation by bleomycin include base propenals that react, on heating with thiobarbituric acid (TBA) at low pH, to form a pink TBA–malondialdehyde adduct. The assay is highly sensitive and readily detects the iron contamination present in laboratory reagents and fluids for biomedical use (Table 4.4). Iron contamination of reagents can be partially removed by treating them with **Chelex resin**, which binds both iron and copper salts. However, there is little point in treating water with Chelex and then dissolving other reagents in it; commercial reagents (especially phosphates and phosphate esters) usually contribute much more iron than does the water (Table 4.4). In addition, Chelex usually makes the solution alkaline, which limits the treatment of most biological buffers. A more effective procedure (*FEBS Lett.* **214**, 362, 1987) to remove iron ions from buffers is to use columns or dialysis sacs containing iron-binding proteins, e.g. transferrin or (the cheaper) **conalbumin**. Careful control of pH in the bleomycin assay is essential (*Meth. Enzymol.* **233**, 82, 1994). A microwell version of the assay has been developed (*Clin. Chem.* **48**, 307, 2002). DNA damage can be measured by the loss of ability to enhance ethidium fluorescence instead of the TBA test (*Clin. Chem.* **100**, 239, 2001).

Table 4.3 Concentrations of bleomycin-chelatable iron (BCI) in body fluids

Sample	BCI concentration	Comments
Healthy humans or other animals (plasma)	0	Never present; plasma has considerable iron-*binding* activity due to unsaturated transferrin
Rheumatoid arthritis		
Plasma	0	Not present unless arthritis related to an iron-overload disease
Synovial fluid	$3.1\pm1.9\,\mu$M	About 40% of fluids show BCI if assayed at pH 5.3 (*Biochem. J.* **245**, 415, 1987)
Fulminant liver failure (plasma)	$2\pm2\,\mu$M	Possibly a consequence of iron release from failing liver and/ or its inability to make transferrin (*Free Radic. Res.* **20**, 139, 1994)
Acute lymphoblastic leukaemia, after chemotherapy (plasma)	Up to 1 μM	Transferrin saturation in patients prechemotherapy higher than normal, BCI sometimes but not usually present. Chemotherapy causes rise in total plasma iron; when transferrin saturation reaches 100% BCI appears (*Cancer Lett.* **94**, 219, 1995; *Clin. Chem.* **48**, 307, 2002)
Patients treated with cyclophosphamide and total body irradiation to kill bone marrow cells before transplantation	$0.1-1.1\ \mu$M	Found for $6-18$ days in all patients studied, with a peak on day 4 (*Br. J. Haematol.* **113**, 836, 2001). Injecting transferrin decreased the levels (*Br. J. Haematol* **119**, 547, 2002)
Patients with various cancers undergoing chemotherapy with bleomycin/etoposide/*cis*–platin or other regimes	$10.6\pm6.6\ \mu$M $1-4$ days after in treatment 64% of patients	None present before treatment or 2 months after treatment (*Clin. Sci.* **106**, 475, 2004). Levels of BCI correlated with severity of side-effects.
ARDS patients with multiorgan failure (plasma)	$0.5\pm0.2\ \mu$M	Represented 33% of ARDS patients in this study (*Thorax* **49**, 702, 1994)
Patients with autoimmune diseases administered iron–sucrose to treat anaemia, serum	$\sim0.5\ \mu$M	None in untreated subjects (*Kidney Int.* **66**, 295, 2004)
Lung lining fluid (bronchoalveolar lavage)		
Normal controls	$0.3\pm0.02\ \mu$M	A little BCI appears present normally in BAL fluid, which has low transferrin. In severe ARDS, excess entry of plasma proteins such as transferrin due to disruption of alveolar permeability barrier may bind the BCI (*Biochem. Biophys. Res. Commun.* **220**, 1024, 1996)
ARDS patients		
Survivors	$0.3\pm0.09\ \mu$M	
Non-survivors	0	
Cardiopulmonary bypass:		Perhaps released due to damage to blood cells or from anoxic/ reperfused tissues (*FEBS Lett.* **328**, 103, 1993; *Free Radic. Res.* **21**, 53, 1994; *Ann. Thoracic Surg.* **60**, 1735, 1995). Paediatric patients less than 5 years old at higher risk than adults (*Biochim. Biophys. Acta* **1500**, 342, 2000)
Extracorporeal blood circulation	$0.3\pm0.9\ \mu$M	
Blood cardioplegia (plasma)	$0.2\pm0.3\ \mu$M	
Mice deficient in transferrin synthesis (plasma)	$16.0\pm5.0\ \mu$M	Mice die unless transferrin periodically injected (*Biochim. Biophys. Acta* **1156**, 19, 1992)
Patients with iron overload due to idiopathic haemochromatosis (plasma)	$4.3\pm6.7\ \mu$M	At least some of the iron is bound to citrate (*Clin. Sci.* **68**, 463, 1985; *J. Biol. Chem.* **264**, 4417, 1989). Some BCI can exist even when transferrin *not* completely saturated (*Blood* **72**, 1416, 1988; *J. Hepatol.* **32**, 727, 2000). Plasma from thalassaemia patients can contain BCI (*Eur. J. Clin. Invest.* **32**, Suppl 1, 50, 2002)

Table 4.3 (*Cont.*)

Sample	BCI concentration	Comments
Umbilical cord blood plasma		
Newborn full-term babies	$0.3\pm0.6~\mu M^a$	Transferrin saturation is high at birth and may go over 100% in a few, apparently normal babies (*FEBS Lett.* **303**, 210, 1992)
Premature babies	$\sim$2–5 μM^b	*Free Radic. Res.* **16**, 285, 1995
Foetuses and babies with rhesus haemolytic disease, plasma	$\sim$0–44 μM	Very high levels in most cases. Higher in foetuses with complications (*Br. J. Obst. Gyn.* **111**, 303, 2004)
Kwashiorkor (plasma)	1.0–19.5 μM	BCI present in 58% of kwashiorkor patients (*Eur. J. Clin. Nutr.* **49**, 208, 1995)
Human sweat	$0.7\pm2.5~\mu M$ $4.6\pm3.0~\mu M$	BCI more often present in trunk sweat than arm sweat (*Clin. Chim. Acta* **145**, 267, 1985)
Urine, kidney reperfusion injury		
Before ischaemia–reperfusion	138 ± 54 pmol	
After ischaemia–reperfusion	1249 ± 506 pmol	*Kidney Int.* **34**, 474, 1988
Homogenized human tissues		
Cerebellum	26 ± 5 nmol/mg tissue	*FEBS Lett.* **353**, 246, 1994
Substantia nigra	51 ± 27 nmol/mg tissue	*Free Radic. Res.* **23**, 465, 1995
Arterial wall	$3\pm2.4~\mu M$	
Bacteria (five different strains)	0.003–1.046 μmol/mg protein	*Biochem. Int.* **8**, 89, 1984

[a] Only 6/25 positive.
[b] Most samples positive.

are stronger iron-chelating agents than bleomycin, and NTA in particular may be capable of removing iron from certain iron proteins. When six different methods were applied to serum from iron-over-loaded patients, six different answers were obtained, reflecting the unique chemistry of each assay.[31] The bleomycin method gave the lowest values.

Please remember that cell culture media, biochemical and clinical reagents are all iron-contaminated (Table 4.4), which must be allowed for in performing the above assays.

4.3.4 Copper

Oxidative stress can also increase the availability of copper. For example, caeruloplasmin is readily degraded by proteinases or on exposure to $ONOO^-$ (Section 3.15.2) to release copper, although it is fairly resistant to damage by peroxides. Copper ions are released when tissues are homogenized (Table 4.5).

In human blood plasma, most or all copper is bound to caeruloplasmin (Section 3.15.2.1). An assay for non-caeruloplasmin copper, the **phenanthroline assay**, has been developed, again based on the

ability of a chelating agent, **1,10-phenanthroline** (***o*-phenanthroline**; structure shown in Table 10.14) to degrade DNA in the presence of copper ions.[33] Degradation of DNA by copper-phenanthroline requires O_2 and conversion of Cu^{2+} to Cu^+ by an added reducing agent. This is followed by formation of $OH^{\bullet}$ that immediately attacks the DNA to release a product that can be detected in the TBA test. If other reagents are in excess, the technique measures copper that is available to the chelator, in other words **phenanthroline-chelatable copper (PCC)**. Reagents are treated with Chelex (Fig. 4.5 legend) to remove contaminating copper, and azide is added to inactivate catalase (H_2O_2 is involved in the $OH^{\bullet}$ formation). This assay detects copper bound to albumin and to amino acids such as histidine, but not copper on caeruloplasmin. Phenanthroline-chelatable copper has been found in numerous biological samples (Table 4.5). It is not present in plasma from healthy animals (which confirms that levels of copper–albumin and copper–amino acid chelates are low, or zero; Section 3.15.2.2).

The relationship of PCC to oxidative damage is unclear. Copper bound to albumin or histidine is

Table 4.4 Iron contamination of laboratory reagents and biomedical fluids

Solution analysed	Iron concentration
Laboratory reagents[a]	
Hydrochloric acid, 5.8 M	1–2 μM[b]
Saline buffer (67.5 mM Na_2HPO_4 + 4 mM KCl adjusted to pH 7.4 with HCl)	
Fresh	10 μM[b]
Old (stored in laboratory for several weeks in flask covered with Parafilm[c])	18 μM[b]
EDTA, 50 mM	8 μM[b]
Sodium formate, 0.5 M	9 μM[b]
Urea, 0.5 M	6 μM[b]
Thiourea, 0.5 M	3 μM[b]
Ascorbic acid, 20 mM	4 μM[b]
Biomedical fluids	
Albumin solutions for clinical use	15–32 μmol/mmol of albumin[d]
University of Wisconsin organ preservation fluid (used for preservation of heart and liver before transplantation)	1.9±0.4 μM[e]
Intralipid infusion for premature babies	0–0.6 μM[e]

[a] Solution were made up in double-distilled water that itself contained no detectable iron.
[b] Measured by atomic absorption.
[c] Parafilm can also contain the antioxidant butylated hydroxytoluene and release it into reaction mixtures (*Plant Cell Rep.* **16**, 192, 1996).
[d] Samples from six different manufacturers; also present were 1–7.9 μmol copper and 2.8–12.1 μmol vanadium per mmol albumin (*J. Pharm. Sci.* **81**, 611, 1992).
[e] Measured by the bleomycin assay (*Transplantation* **62**, 1046, 1996).

still redox-active, but the damage is largely directed to the ligand. Thus if, for example, the copper measured as PCC were bound to LDL (Section 9.3.5), DNA, or Na^+, K^+-ATPase (Section 2.4.6) it could be biologically significant, but if it was attached to albumin or histidine it might not matter.

4.4 Consequences of oxidative stress: cell death

A cell exposed to oxidative stress may die. Death can result from multiple mechanisms (e.g. PARP-1 activation; Section 4.2.4) and be measured by a variety of assays, each of which needs careful thought about what is really being measured (Table 4.6).

Cell death can occur by essentially two mechanisms, **necrosis** and **apoptosis**, although death by mechanisms with features of both pathways is often seen (Fig. 4.6). Necrosis and apoptosis result from many causes, including oxidative stress. For example, in mammalian cells, adding mM levels of H_2O_2 can cause necrosis, whereas lower levels can trigger apoptosis (Fig 4.1). During necrotic cell death, there is cell and organelle swelling, loss of integrity of mitochondrial, peroxisomal and lysosomal

membranes and eventual rupture of the plasma membrane, releasing cell contents into the surrounding area to affect adjacent cells. Contents can include antioxidants such as SOD, catalase or GSH, pro-oxidants such as haem, iron and copper ions, and other damaging agents, such as activated calpains (Section 8.10). Several constituents released from cells can provoke inflammation, especially the nuclear **high mobility group 1 protein (HMGB1)**.[34]

In apoptosis, the cell's own intrinsic 'suicide mechanism' is activated; apoptosing cells do not release their contents and so apoptosis does not, in general, affect surrounding cells. In particular, apoptotic cells do not release HMGB1; it remains bound to chromatin. Sometimes, however, peroxides generated during apoptosis (Section 4.4.1.2 below) can be released to a level that might affect surrounding cells,[35,36] and oxidized lipids might even act as antigens to provoke autoimmunity.[36]

4.4.1 Apoptosis

In apoptosis the earliest visible changes are cell shrinkage, and condensation and fragmentation of chromatin (Fig. 4.6). This is usually associated with

Table 4.5 Phenanthroline-chelatable copper in some biological materials

Material	Concentration	Comments
Healthy animals (plasma/serum)	0	Never detected in fresh samples. Amount of non-caeruloplasmin copper < 0.1 μM. Detected in *stored* samples, probably due to breakdown of caeruloplasmin.
Wilson's disease,[a] untreated (plasma)	2.7 μM	*Pediat. Res.* **37**, 219, 1995. Variably present in patients treated with copper-chelating agents.
Liver failure (plasma)	1–2 μM	May be due to metal release from failing liver and/or cessation of liver caeruloplasmin synthesis (*Free Radic. Res.* **20**, 139, 1994).
Sweat, human		
Arm	18.1±3.9 μM	Sweat also contains iron (Table 4.3) and may be an excretory route for both metals. Their presence facilitates bacterial growth in sweat (*Clin. Chim. Acta* **145**, 267, 1985).
Trunk	27.0±3 μM	
Homogenized human brain tissue		
Cerebellum	21±10 nmol/mg tissue	Levels of copper released on tissue homogenization broadly comparable to those of BCI (*FEBS Lett.* **353**, 246, 1994; *Free Radic. Res.* **23**, 465, 1995)
Substantia nigra	53±18 nmol/me tissue	
Arterial wall	4.9±2.8 μM	
Atherosclerotic material		
'Gruel' from advanced lesions	~4.0 μM	Copper ions are powerful catalysts of low-density lipoprotein (LDL) oxidation, which may contribute to atherosclerosis (*Biochem. J.* **286**, 901, 1992; *FEBS Lett.* **368**, 513, 1995). Atherosclerotic lesion extracts stimulate *in vitro* LDL oxidation.
Endarterectomy samples	0.3±0.1 nmol/mg protein	
Aneurysms	0.3±0.2 nmol/mg protein	

[a] A 'copper-overload' disease (Section 3.15.5.5).

DNA double-strand breaks in internucleosomal regions, so that the isolated DNA gives a 'ladder pattern' on gel electrophoresis; Fig. 4.7). Other features are the collapse of cytoskeletal structure, nuclear fragmentation, and eventual break-up of the entire cell into **apoptotic bodies**, without rupture of organelle membranes. Apoptotic bodies are phagocytosed by neighbouring cells or by phagocytes. Phagocytes use cell-surface receptors to recognize 'eat me' signals on the surface of apoptosing cells, one of which is the appearance of phosphatidylserine on the outer leaflet of the plasma membrane (Table 4.6). Binding of phosphatidylserine to the receptors (usually via 'bridging proteins') decreases macrophage production of proinflammatory cytokines, and increases that of anti-inflammatory ones.[37]

Cell death is essential during embryonic development, for example to eliminate thymocytes that recognize 'self-antigens', and unwanted cells during tissue remodelling. It is often then called **programmed cell death** (PCD), is usually induced by binding of ligands to specific receptors, and frequently occurs by apoptosis. Thus PCD and apoptosis are terms often used interchangeably, although cells can die during development by mechanisms other than apoptosis.

The apoptotic machinery exists in all cells except erythrocytes and can be triggered by a range of signals or by the removal of growth factors from the medium. Among insults that trigger apoptosis are interference with energy metabolism (e.g. partial inhibition of mitochondrial electron transport), oxidative stress, and the DNA-damaging effects of some drugs used in cancer chemotherapy (Section 9.15). However, these agents can also cause necrosis, depending upon the cell type studied and the level of stress

Table 4.6 Some popular methods used to detect cell death[a]

Method	Comments
Vital dyes, e.g. trypan blue, propidium iodide (PI), crystal violet, Hoechst 33258	Cannot penetrate intact plasma membrane but stain the cytoplasm or nucleus of cells with damaged plasma membranes. Measure loss of plasma membrane integrity. For PI, cells can be fixed and stained, allowing cell cycle analysis by flow cytometry or detection of chromatin condensation during apoptosis, by fluorescence microscopy.
Neutral red	Weak cationic dye that enters cells and targets lysosomes, cell injury decreases uptake if lysosomes are affected.
Tetrazolium salts (e.g. MTT, XTT)[b]	Reduced to coloured products (**formazans**) only by metabolically active cells. Measure loss of metabolic activity.
Alamar blue	Cell permeable, reduced by metabolically active cells to a fluorescent product.
Release of enzymes, e.g. lactate dehydrogenase (LDH), creatine kinase (CK), glutamate-oxaloacetate transaminase (GOT), glutamate-pyruvate transaminase (GPT), glucose-6-phosphate dehydrogenase (G6PDH)	Release of enzymes from cytosol or other subcellular compartments reveals plasma membrane damage. Used in diagnostic medicine to assess damage to liver (GOT, GPT), heart (LDH, CK), etc. Release also possible from reversible injury by the 'pinching off' of blebs, with the rest of the cell remaining viable. Be careful; released enzymes can sometimes be inactivated by certain RS, such as HOCl or $ONOO^-$, giving an underestimation of damage.
Calcein–AM	Cell-permeable, non-fluorescent compound, de-esterified by intracellular esterases to give the fluorescent dye calcein. Fluorescence is proportional to cellular esterase activity and can be used to determine cell viability. Calcein–AM is suitable for staining viable cells because of its low cytotoxicity. Using calcein–AM with cell impermeable DNA-binding fluorescent dyes such as PI or ethidium homodimer-1 allows discrimination between viable and dead/dying cells; viable cells stain with green fluorescence (calcein positive, PI negative) whereas dead cells stain with red fluorescence (calcein negative, PI positive). Dying cells show a mixture of green and red fluorescence.
^{51}Cr release	Cells must be preloaded with ^{51}Cr by incubation with labelled sodium chromate, which binds to intracellular proteins. Radioactive proteins released due to plasma membrane damage.
[^3H]thymidine release	Cells preloaded with tritiated thymidine, incorporated into DNA. Radioactive DNA release due to severe plasma membrane damage.
DNA laddering (Section 4.4.1)	Usually taken as evidence of apoptosis, but is insufficient evidence alone: ladder patterns might also be produced by internucleosomal attack by RS. For example, treatment of HepG2 cells with copper–phenanthroline chelates, which bind to DNA and generate OH•, gave a DNA ladder (*Biochem. J.* **317**, 13, 1996).
ATP	Commonly measured using luciferin–luciferase. The levels of ATP in cells correlate with cell viability. After loss of membrane integrity, cells lose the ability to synthesise ATP, endogenous ATPases destroy ATP and the levels of ATP fall rapidly.
Cell replication studies	Measure rate of cell replication (e.g. [^3H]thymidine incorporation, antibodies recognizing proteins involved in the cell cycle). Of course, cells no longer able to divide are not necessarily irreversibly injured, i.e. this is an index of cytostasis, rather than cell death.
Caspase activation	Used as an index of apoptosis. However, caspases are inactivated by several RS and their levels must be interpreted with caution. Various substrates hydrolysed to fluorescent products are commercially available.
Phospatidylserine membrane flipping (Annexin–V)	Can be used in parallel with PI to distinguish apoptotic from necrotic cells. Takes advantage of the fact that phosphatidylserine (PS) translocates from the inner (cytoplasmic) face of the plasma membrane to the cell surface soon after induction of apoptosis. Annexin V has a strong affinity for PS on the cell surface providing the basis for a staining assay.

[a] One of the simplest methods, often not used, is simply to look under the microscope and see what the cells are doing!

[b] 3-(4,5 dimethylthiazol-2-yl)-2,5-diphenyl-2*H*-tetrazolium bromide. Its reduction largely depends on mitochondrial function, but can also be achieved by other reducing systems and perhaps by certain ROS, e.g. $O_2^{•-}$. Always check that any agent you are adding to the culture medium does not directly reduce MTT. Several enzymes can also reduce MTT, including iNOS (*Diabetologia* **47**, 2042, 2004).

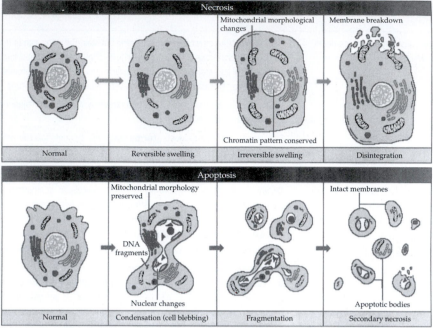

Figure 4.6 Apoptosis and necrosis: the basic differences. Adapted from *Guide to Cell Proliferation and Apoptosis Methods*, by kind permission of Boehringer Mannheim.

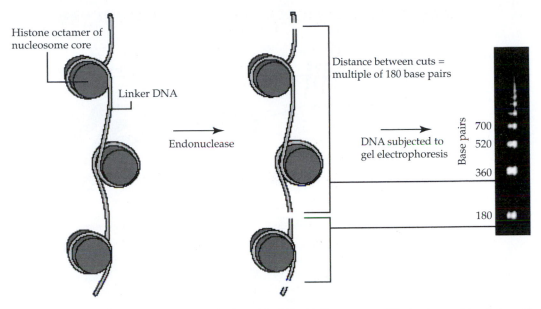

Figure 4.7 Internucleosomal cleavage of DNA. High molecular weight DNA, with histones arranged like beads on a string, is cleaved by a **caspase-activated DNAse (CAD)** which cuts between nucleosomes to give fragments of DNA that are multiples of 180–200 base pairs. When these fragments are separated by gel electrophoresis, a 'ladder' is seen. From *Guide to Cell Proliferation and Apoptosis Methods*, by courtesy of Boehringer Mannheim. The action of the DNAse is normally blocked by an inhibitor, **ICAD (inhibitor of caspase-activated DNAse)** which inhibits the DNAse activity and keeps the enzyme in the cytoplasm. This ICAD is destroyed by caspases-3 and -7, allowing the DNAse to translocate to the nucleus and cleave DNA.

applied (in general, higher stress levels are more likely to favour necrosis). Apoptosis plays a role in abnormal cell loss in certain diseases, such as the neurodegenerative diseases and some viral infections. By contrast, failure of cells with damaged DNA to undergo apoptosis can contribute to development of malignancy. **Anoikis**, apoptosis induced when cells detach from the extracellular matrix, is important in deterring tumour invasion and metastasis (Section 9.13.2).

4.4.1.1 *Molecular mechanisms of apoptosis*

Our knowledge of the mechanisms by which apoptosis occurs has increased exponentially in the past two decades. We confine ourselves here to the minimum information required to understand how apoptosis relates to RS and antioxidants.

Apoptosis depends on the activation of a family of proteinases with essential active-site cysteine residues, the **caspases**.[38,39] They cleave their protein substrates at aspartate residues, hence the name **cysteine-aspartyl-specific proteases**, abbreviated to caspases. Caspase activation can be triggered by at least four mechanisms. One is the binding of external ligands to **death receptors** (Fig. 4.8), which resemble receptors for tumour necrosis factors, TNF (Section 4.7 below). Ligands to them include members of the TNF family, such as TNFα, **Fas (fibroblast associated cell surface ligand L** (also known as **CD95L**) and **TRAIL (TNF-related apoptosis-inducing ligand)**. They bind to the death receptors (TNFα receptor, Fas, trail receptor 1 (DR4), trail receptor 2 (DR5), respectively) and cause them to aggregate into trimers. The cytoplasmic 'tails' of these receptors recruit other proteins such as **FADD** and **TRADD (TNF receptor-associated death domain)** (Fig. 4.9). These carry a **death-effector domain (DED)** that binds procaspase-8 and incorporates it into the **death-induced-signalling complex (DISC)**. Procaspase-8 is activated and in turn activates caspases-3, -6 and -7. Cellular mechanisms also exist to halt the pathway. For example, **FLIP** is a caspase-8

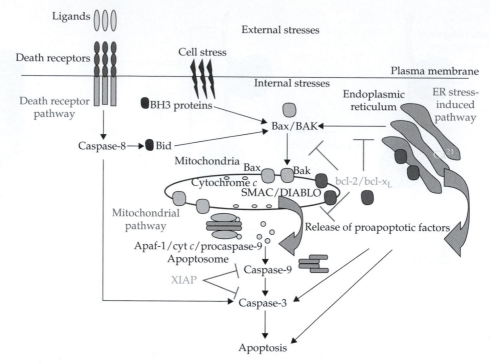

Figure 4.8 Molecular pathways leading to apoptosis. The diagram shows three of the pathways that can be activated when the cell encounters specific stresses. The cell-surface-mediated or death-receptor pathway involves the binding of a ligand to the TNF family of receptors (e.g. Fig. 4.9). Mitochondrial apoptosis is induced by many stresses that often increase Bax and Bak levels. These proteins then translocate to the mitochondrial membrane leading to release of apoptotic proteins. The endoplasmic reticulum (ER) pathway is induced by misfolded and aggregated proteins and other stresses in the ER that lead to the release of Ca^{2+} and activation of the mitochondrial apoptosis pathway and ER-associated caspases. Bid is a member of the proapoptotic BH3 subfamily. Bax and Bak are proapoptotic proteins containing multiple bcl-2 homology domains. SMAC/DIABLO, Apaf-1 and cyt c are among the apoptotic proteins housed in the mitochondria that are released upon loss of mitochondrial membrane integrity. XIAP is a member of the inhibitor of apoptosis protein family, which inhibits activation of downstream caspases. Abbreviations: Apaf-1, apoptotic proteinase activating factor-1; cyt c, cytochrome c; DIABLO, direct inhibition of apoptosis protein (IAP) binding protein with low pI; SMAC, second mitochondria-derived activator of caspases; XIAP, X-linked inhibitor of apoptosis. The IAPs are inhibitors of apoptosis proteins, which are inactivated by SMAC/DIABLO. Adapted from *Trends Biotechnol.* **22**, 174, 2004, by courtesy of Dr M.J. Betenbaugh and Elsevier. The proteasome may also play a role by degrading proapoptotic proteins such as SMAC/DIABLO; in turn, active caspases may attack the proteasome and impair its activity (*N. Engl. J. Med.* **351**, 393, 2004).

homologue that binds to FADD but does not cause caspase-8 activation, and some heat-shock proteins (Section 4.6) can inhibit apoptosis. Even the proteasome may play a role (Fig. 4.8).

Caspases are classified as **initiator caspases** (caspases-2, -8, -9 and -10) and **effector caspases**, such as -3, -6 and -7. Activation of the first type (often caspase-8 or -9) leads to activation of the effector caspases, which put in motion the cellular events characteristic of apoptosis. These include activation of the **caspase-activated DNAse** that fragments DNA (Fig. 4.7) and enzymes that remodel the cytoskeleton and cause blebbing. The

few hundred or so proteins that are cleaved by caspases during apoptosis include PARP-1 (cleavage inactivates it), DNA repair and cell-cycle regulatory proteins (including p53), and some proteins involved in signal transduction. Whereas PARP inhibition often protects cells against necrotic cell death (by blocking NAD^+ and ATP depletion), it rarely affects apoptosis.[15] Cell death resembling apoptosis can sometimes involve activation of calpains in addition to caspases, or occasionally instead of them.[40] A range of caspase and calpain inhibitors is commercially available but not all are specific; tin metalloporphyrin used

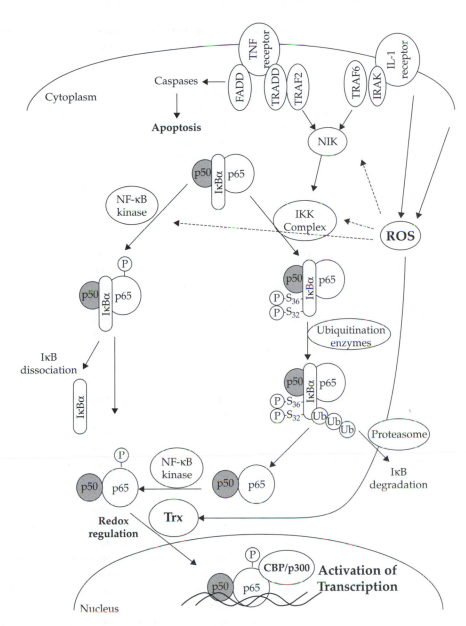

Figure 4.9 Pathways of NF-κB activation by TNFα and IL-1. These cytokines act via receptor-associated transducer proteins TRAF2 and TRAF6, which interact at the protein kinase NIK, NF-κB-inducing kinase. The IκB protein is directly phosphorylated by the IKKs 1 and 2 (sometimes called IKKα and *β*) in the IKK complex. Alternatively, NF-κB kinase phosphorylates on p65. Reactive species can facilitate kinase action by direct or indirect (e.g. phosphatase inhibition; affecting ubiquitination [Section 4.14.2 below]) mechanisms. Phosphorylation of IκB leads to its dissociation and sometimes, ubiquitination and destruction. Thioredoxin (Trx) keeps NF-κB in the nucleus in the reduced form required to promote transcription and, in at least some cell types, both NF-κB and thioredoxin comigrate to the nucleus. Modified from *Critical Reviews of Oxidative Stress and Aging: Advances in Basic Science, Diagnostics and Intervention* by courtesy of Drs Toshifumi Tetsuka and Takashi Okamoto and World Scientific Publishing. Endotoxin activates NF-κB by binding to **toll-like receptors**, which work through TRAF6 (*Science* **309**, 1854, 2005).

to inhibit haem oxygenases (Section 3.17) can also inhibit caspases-3 and -8.[41]

A second way of triggering apoptosis is to damage mitochondria (e.g. by MPT; Fig. 1.9).[42] This can lead to permeabilization of the outer mitochondrial membrane and release of factors from the inter-membrane space to the cytosol, including **apoptosis-inducing factor** (AIF), cytochrome c, and **SMAC** (alternative name **DIABLO**) (Fig. 4.8). The last is a protein that binds and inhibits endogenous caspase blockers (**inhibitors of apoptosis, IAP**). The overall result is activation of the caspase adaptor **Apaf-1 (apoptotic proteinase activating factor 1)** which binds ATP (hence apoptosis needs ATP) and cytochrome c to form a caspase-9-activating complex, the **apoptosome**. Caspase-9 then activates caspases-3 and -8. Apoptosis-inducing factor is a flavoprotein resembling bacterial NADH oxidases and can produce $O_2^{\bullet-}$ under appropriate assay conditions. This is probably irrelevant to its proapoptotic activity, but in some tumour cells it may be important in *suppressing* apoptosis (Section 4.4.1.2 below).[43]

The **Bcl-2 family of proteins** regulates the mitochondrial membrane potential, outer membrane permeability and hence the release of proapoptotic factors. It contains over 30 members. Some suppress apoptosis, such as Bcl-2, Bcl-X_L, Bcl-w and Bcl-B whereas others promote it, including Bax, Bak and Bcl-Xs. The balance of these various proteins controls the likelihood of mitochondria triggering apoptosis. There is an intimate link between caspase activation (triggered by any mechanism) and mitochondrial function. For example, caspase-8 cleaves the proapoptotic protein Bid, which moves to the mitochondria, binds to Bad and facilitates cytochrome c release. Caspase cleavage of a subunit of complex I plays a role in loss of mitochondrial membrane potential and ROS formation during apoptosis.[42]

A third way of triggering apoptosis is to introduce an agent that directly activates caspases and/or mitochondrial proapoptotic proteins. For example, **tributyltin** targets mitochondria, causing swelling and cytochrome c release.[44] **Natural killer** (NK) cells deliver a pore-forming protein (**perforin**) and a set of proteolytic enzymes (**granzymes**) into their target cells. Granzymes can cleave caspase-3, Bid and ICAD (Fig. 4.8).

The ER stress response (Section 4.6 below) can also lead to apoptosis (Fig. 4.8).

4.4.1.2 *Reactive species and apoptosis*[38,44]

Oxidative stress can lead to apoptosis, often by inducing the MPT and causing release of proapoptotic factors (Figs 1.9 and 4.8). Oxidation of the anionic phospholipid **cardiolipin** (Fig. 4.16 below) facilitates cytochrome c release from mitochondria and in turn cytochrome c can promote cardiolpin oxidation.[45] In contrast, the caspases have exposed $-SH$ groups and can be readily inactivated by H_2O_2, HOCl, $OH^{\bullet}$, $ONOO^-$ and other RS. Thus high levels of RS can delay or halt apoptosis, but often cell death continues by a necrotic or intermediate pathway. On the other hand, apoptosis triggered by other mechanisms (e.g. ligand binding to death receptors) is accompanied by oxidative stress. Release of cytochrome c, and caspase-dependent cleavage of complex I disrupt the mitochondrial electron transport chain, causing more $O_2^{\bullet-}$ formation.[42,45] The **p66**^{shc} protein may be involved in ROS production and could be a key player in inducing MPT (Section 10.3.1). Apoptosing cells show falls in GSH levels, because it is released into the medium.

Does this oxidative stress contribute to the cell death? To some extent yes; adding antioxidants often slows down apoptosis induced by a range of insults, although it is rarely completely prevented. Withdrawal of growth factors from the culture medium of many cells increases ROS production, and overexpression of antioxidant enzymes can delay the subsequent apoptosis. The externalization of phosphatidylserine during apoptosis is facilitated by its oxidation, a feature also promoting recognition of apoptosing cells by macrophages.[46] The fall in GSH can sometimes contribute to apoptosis by activating **sphingomyelinase** enzymes, that hydrolyse membrane spingolipids (Fig. 4.16 below) to liberate **ceramide**.[47] Ceramide can trigger apoptosis, in part by acting upon mitochondria, and it appears to contribute to apoptosis induced by cytokines and some other mediators in several cell types. Ceramide may be especially important in radiation-induced apoptosis and in COPD (Section 8.12.2). However ROS are not *essential* for apoptosis; apoptosis triggered by a range of insults can proceed in the absence of O_2.[48]

So are RS always proapoptotic? No; in some cell types, they can *prevent* apoptosis triggered by ligands to Fas/CD95 or by toxins affecting mitochondria.[49] For example, in the melanoma cell line M14, decreasing $O_2^{\bullet-}$ levels by overexpressing CuZnSOD *promoted* apoptosis, and decreasing CuZnSOD levels inhibited apoptosis. Generation of ROS by an NADPH oxidase was found to be an antiapoptotic, proliferative stimulus in pancreatic cancer cell lines[50] and the ability of AIF to oxidize NADH and make $O_2^{\bullet-}$ contributed to the viability of certain carcinoma cell lines.[43] **Leporipoxviruses** contain **decoy proteins** that bind the copper chaperone for SOD (Section 3.2.1) and cause a fall in cellular SOD levels, possibly to help suppress apoptosis in virally-infected cells.[51]

Elevated $O_2^{\bullet-}$ leads to a higher cytosolic pH that deters caspase activation. By contrast, H_2O_2 can promote apoptosis not only by damaging mitochondria but also by lowering the cytosolic pH (although it can also inactivate caspases, as discussed above). The actions of $O_2^{\bullet-}$ and H_2O_2 on cell pH seem to involve increasing or decreasing respectively the activities of a plasma membrane Na^+/H^+ exchange system.[49] Nitric oxide in excess can trigger apoptosis, for example by forming $ONOO^-$ that attacks mitochondria. Another mechanism is to nitrosylate G3PDH. This modified cytosolic enzyme then migrates to the nucleus, accompanied by an E3 ligase enzyme (Section 4.14.2.1 below). Once there, this ligase promotes the ubiquitin-dependent degradation of nuclear proteins and starts apoptosis.[52]

4.5 Redox regulation

4.5.1 What is it and how does it work?

Redox reactions are now thought to play key roles in intracellular signalling (e.g. in the response of a cell to hormones and growth factors, and in communication between nucleus and mitochondria), intercellular signalling (e.g. nitric oxide, cytokines) and in regulation of the organ and whole-body responses to stress. Some proteins are directly redox-regulated (e.g. some ion channels,[17] p53 [Section 9.13.5], aconitase) whereas for others their levels are controlled by altering gene transcription using redox-sensitive transcription factors.

In principle, there are at least two forms of redox regulation. One is the oxidation and reduction of −SH groups (either singly, or in pairs to form a disulphide). The second is the oxidation and reduction of iron ions, usually in [Fe–S] clusters. The latter is less common in animal cells, although the response of the IRPs to RS represents one example (Section 3.15.1.5) and human mitochondrial glutaredoxin has been reported to be a redox-regulated [Fe–S] protein,[53] forming a link between the two mechanisms. Our most detailed knowledge of physiologically important redox regulation comes from bacteria, so let us start there. Plants are considered in Section 7.11.

4.5.2 Bacterial redox regulation:[54] oxyR

Many bacteria respond to mild oxidative stress by becoming resistant to more severe oxidative stress. For example, when *E. coli* or *S. typhimurium* are exposed to moderate levels of H_2O_2, the synthesis of about 30 proteins increases and the cells become resistant to damage by higher levels of H_2O_2 (resistance to HOCl also increases). Some of these proteins are identical to those induced by heat shock (Section 4.6 below).

The levels of nine of these proteins are controlled by the product of one gene, *oxy*R. If two critical −SH groups within the oxyR protein are oxidized to a disulphide by H_2O_2, the oxidized protein acts as a transcription factor, promoting expression of the relevant genes. These nine proteins include several antioxidant defences: hydroperoxidase I (product of the *kat*G gene); fur (which controls iron uptake; Section 3.6.2.2); alkyl hydroperoxide reductase (*ahp*CF gene); glutaredoxin, and glutathione reductase (*gor* gene). Dps production is also increased by oxyR; Dps binds to DNA and protects it against oxidative damage. Deletion of the *dps* gene causes bacteria to become hypersensitive to H_2O_2 (Section 3.15.1.4).

How is the signal switched off? By reduction of the OxyR disulphide, probably involving glutaredoxin (Section 3.10). The *oxy*R system of *E. coli* maintains a steady-state intracellular H_2O_2 level of about $0.2 \mu M$ over a wide range of growth conditions. Strains lacking *oxyR* show increased spontaneous mutation rates, indicating its importance.

4.5.3 Bacterial redox regulation:[54] soxRS

Excess $O_2^{\bullet-}$ generation within *E. coli* leads to increased H_2O_2 formation that activates oxyR. The $O_2^{\bullet-}$ also activates transcription of ten or more additional genes, including those encoding MnSOD (but not FeSOD), a DNA-repair enzyme (**endonuclease IV**), fumarase C, aconitase A and G6PDH. Fumarase C and aconitase A seem to be 'back-up' enzymes insensitive to inactivation by $O_2^{\bullet-}$ (Section 1.6). The 'superoxide signal' is sensed by the protein encoded by the *soxR* gene. SoxR contains [2Fe–2S] clusters and is active only when they are in a fully oxidized, diferric state. SoxR protein oxidized by $O_2^{\bullet-}$ activates transcription of the *soxS* gene, whose product in turn accelerates transcription of the genes encoding the above proteins. Activation of the *soxRS* system also increases resistance of *E. coli* to several antibiotics, due to decreased synthesis of a membrane pore protein, **OmpF**. Oxidized SoxR is rapidly re-reduced at the expense of NADPH via a series of electron transfer proteins. The gene encoding MnSOD (*sodA* gene) has an iron box and expression is normally repressed by fur protein (Section 3.6.2.2), but this is over-ruled by soxS.

The *oxyR* and *soxRS* systems can also be activated by exposure of *E. coli* to excess $NO^{\bullet}$. It reacts with the SoxR [2Fe–2S] centres to displace sulphur and generate nitroso-iron-thiol complexes, which have some transcriptional activity.

B. subtilis uses a different mechanism to sense H_2O_2; the H_2O_2 reacts with an Fe^{2+} in the **PerR** protein to convert histidine to 2-oxohistidine and derepress the expression of antioxidant genes.[54A]

4.5.4 Redox regulation in yeast[55,56]

Anaerobically grown *S. cerevisiae* responds to the introduction of O_2 by activating the biosynthesis of haem, using a metabolic pathway that has two O_2-dependent enzymes (coproporphyrinogen III oxidase and protoporphyrinogen IX oxidase). The haem produced binds to and activates the transcription factor **Hap1**. This in turn accelerates transcription of genes encoding several antioxidants, including MnSOD, catalases and peroxiredoxins. Added haem activates Hap1 even in the absence of O_2; the synthesis of haem is the signal that O_2 is present.

As in bacteria, pretreatment of *S. cerevisiae* with modest levels of H_2O_2, organic peroxides or $O_2^{\bullet-}$-generating systems causes it to become resistant to higher levels. One gene involved is **YaP1** (which resembles the mammalian transcription factor AP-1; Section 4.5.10 below). The YaP1 protein (sometimes written as YaP1p) controls the expression of genes involved in the production and metabolism of GSH and thioredoxin, as well as other antioxidant and stress proteins, including SOD1, catalase and cytochrome *c* peroxidase. When cysteine residues in YaP1 are oxidized to a disulphide bridge, the protein migrates to the nucleus and increases gene expression. This occurs because oxidation leads to conformational changes that conceal YaP1's **nuclear export signal domain**, which normally keeps it out of the nucleus.

The Yap1 protein is not directly oxidized by peroxides; other proteins are involved. One is a yeast glutathione peroxidase homologue (**GPx3**) in which cysteine is present at the active site rather than selenocysteine. This is oxidized by peroxides and forms a disulphide bond with Yap1, which then converts to a Yap1 intramolecular disulphide bond. Reduced thioredoxin can reverse these processes: indeed Gpx3 can catalyse removal of peroxides using reduced thioredoxin as a substrate.

S. cerevisiae contains five peroxiredoxins; three in the cytosol, one in the nucleus and one in mitochondria. Two of the cytosolic forms (Prx1 and 2) also have chaperone-like activity (Section 4.6 below).[57]

4.5.5 Redox regulation in animals: kinases and phosphatases

4.5.5.1 *What is it about?*

Signal transduction describes the mechanisms by which cells sense and respond to their environment, from the detection of something (e.g. a growth factor or cytokine) by a receptor to the transmission of information through other molecules eventually to the nucleus, where gene transcription responds and eventually alters the behaviour of the cell. For example, binding of ligands to growth factor receptors activates protein tyrosine kinase domains on these receptors, that then phosphorylate and activate subsequent proteins in the signal cascade. In addition to intracellular signalling, all multicellular organisms require complex intercellular signalling networks to orchestrate and co-ordinate the functions of different cells to maintain homeostasis, defend against pathogens, repair injury, undergo development and tissue remodelling and deter malignancy.

4.5.5.2 Protein kinases[58]

The **mitogen-activated protein kinases (MAP kinases)** are a large family of enzymes that use ATP to phosphorylate their protein targets on serine or threonine residues. They are involved in cell proliferation (hence their name; they mediate cell responses to mitogens), differentiation and response to stress and usually lead to alterations in transcription factor activity to modulate gene expression. Three major subdivisions exist: the **p38 kinases**, the **extracellular-signal-related kinases (ERK kinases such as ERK-1 and ERK-2)** and the **c-Jun N-terminal kinases (JNK kinases)**. All are activated via overlapping signalling cascades involving other kinases that phosphorylate them (e.g. **MAP kinase kinase**, and **MAP kinase kinase kinase**). The ERK pathway is important in cell proliferation in response to growth factors, the p38 and JNK pathways more so in the response of cells to stresses such as cytokines, radiation, heat shock, osmotic stress and, of course, oxidative stress.

All three subfamilies can be activated when cells are exposed to RS. For example, addition of H_2O_2 to Jurkat T cells (a lymphocyte cell line) increased the phosphorylation of p38, ERK and JNK.[59] Addition of $ONOO^-$ to several cell types can also activate all three MAP kinase family members.[60] On the other hand, $ONOO^-$ can sometimes slow signalling by causing tyrosine nitration (Section 2.6.1). Activations of kinases by RS can lead (depending on the cell type and how much RS is added) to proliferation (e.g. low levels of H_2O_2 stimulated proliferation of alveolar type II cells by promoting ERK activation[61]), cytoprotection, (e.g. in endothelial cells treated with H_2O_2 activation of ERK was protective against membrane blebbing[62]), increased expression of cytoprotective stress

genes, growth arrest, or apoptosis. One general guideline (sadly over-simplistic[63] but still useful) is that, in response to stress, ERK activation tends to promote cell survival whereas prolonged JNK activation favours cell death, for example by apoptosis. Since both are usually activated, the balance between them is critical in determining cell fate.

We already mentioned the role of IP_3 in raising intracellular 'free' Ca^{2+} (Section 4.3.2). IP_3 is derived from phosphorylated forms of the membrane phospholipid **phosphatidylinositol** (Fig. 4.16). These phosphorylated forms, generated by **phosphoinositide-3-kinases (PI3-kinases)**, in turn activate **phosphoinositide-dependent kinases (PDK)** that phosphorylate and activate **Akt** (sometimes called **protein kinase B**). Active Akt is a serine/ threonine kinase that, like ERK, is important in response to growth factors and oxidative stress. For example, exposure of various cells to H_2O_2 increases phosphorylation of the epidermal growth factor receptor (EGFR), which in turn activates PI3K and hence Akt. Akt promotes cell survival, for example by phosphorylating and decreasing the activity of proapoptotic factors such as Bad and caspase-9 (Section 4.4.1).

Activation of Akt also leads to increased phosphorylation of the **forkhead transcription factors of class O (FOXOs)**. 'Forkhead' refers to a 'winged-helix' structural motif that all these proteins have, and the O to 'other', that is FOXO proteins are slightly structurally different from other forkhead proteins. Phosphorylation of FOXOs excludes them from the nucleus, so that they cannot promote gene transcription. Active intranuclear FOXOs promote cell cycle arrest and several other events (including increasing antioxidant defences), yet can paradoxically sometimes lead to apoptosis (Section 10.3.4), for example by increasing production of Fas ligand. Suppressing FOXO action requires the p66[shc] protein. Both p66[shc] and FOXOs play roles in regulating lifespan (Section 10.3.1). As usual, life's a bit more complicated—phosphorylation of FOXO4 at different sites by JNK tends to make it *enter* the nucleus, and H_2O_2 leads to JNK activation. Thus the cellular response to ROS involves a balance between signalling pathways that can switch off (Akt) and switch on (JNK) the nuclear transcriptional action of FOXOs.[64]

Phospho-phosphatidylinositols are cleaved to IP_3 and **diacylglycerol (DAG)** by **phospholipases C**, whose activity is stimulated by a **G-protein**.[a] Phospholipase C-γ1 (PLC-γ1) and PLC-γ2 are components of another growth-factor-receptor-mediated signalling system that responds to oxidative stress, whereupon they become phosphorylated. Phospholipase D, which hydrolyses phosphatidylcholine to phosphatidic acid, can also be activated by H_2O_2 in some cells.[66]

Protein kinases C[67] are another family of serine/threonine kinases involved in regulation of cell proliferation and response to stress. Most of them need Ca^{2+} and DAG, the second product of PLC action, for activity. The PKCs contain cysteine-rich regions susceptible to oxidation, causing loss of activity when high levels of RS are present. On the other hand, selective oxidation of the N-terminal regulatory domain can stimulate PKC activity by removing the requirement for DAG, which normally binds to this domain in the presence of Ca^{2+} to activate PKC. Peroxides can also activate PKCs by stimulating their phosphorylation. Hence PKCs are another target of redox regulation. They play a key role in phagocyte activation (Section 7.7.2.3) and are involved in cell adhesion, mitogenesis and regulation of apoptosis.

The **C-Abl** and **arg tyrosine kinases** (members of the **Abelson family** of kinases) are found in the cytoplasm of many cell types (i.e. they are not activated via receptors, so are sometimes called **non-receptor tyrosine kinases**). They can be activated by oxidative stress (e.g. added H_2O_2) which promotes their phosphorylation by a PKC. Their activation can promote apoptosis under certain conditions. These activated kinases can also bind to, phosphorylate and stimulate the activity of some antioxidant defence enzymes, including catalase and

[a] G-proteins are frequently found as cell surface receptors that respond to hormones, neurotransmitters and other signalling molecules. G-proteins are mostly trimers, but some are monomeric, the **small G proteins**. Binding of a ligand to the receptor activates the G-protein; it binds GTP and GDP is displaced. The 'switch' is turned off when the G-protein hydrolyses its bound GTP to GDP. G-proteins commonly use either Ca^{2+} or cyclic AMP as intracellular signalling molecules. They are important in ROS production by phagocytes and several other cell types (Section 7.7 and 7.10). GDP bound to G-proteins can be a target of attack by RS, which can sometimes promote GDP release and activate the protein.[65]

Gpx1.[68] Hence they play a dual role, promoting apoptosis in response to high levels of H_2O_2, but also allowing cells to adapt to lower levels. Phosphorylated catalase is targeted for ubiquitination and destruction by the proteasome (Section 4.14.2.1 below), however. Phosphorylation (by a different mechanism) also modulates activity of the peroxiredoxins, but this time decreasing it (Section 3.11.1).

4.5.5.3 *How do RS modulate signalling?*

Although some kinases can be directly affected by RS (e.g. PKC), in general RS tend not to stimulate phosphorylation directly. Instead, they increase net phosphorylation by inhibiting dephosphorylation. **Protein phosphatase** enzymes are constantly active in cells, and function to rapidly reverse protein phosphorylation and limit the extent and duration of signalling.[69] Phosphatase inactivation by RS usually occurs by oxidation of essential cysteine residues to cysteine sulphenic acid (cys-SOH), a reaction readily reversed by cellular thiols. These proteins are targets because the pKa value of their −SH groups is abnormally low. This allows ionization at physiological pH, to facilitate formation of a thiol-phosphate intermediate during catalysis. However, thiolate ions are more readily oxidized than are −SH groups; for example by $ONOO^-$, H_2O_2, other peroxides and HOCl. For example, when protein tyrosine phosphatase IB is oxidized, the sulphenic acid rapidly reacts with the amide nitrogen of an adjacent serine residue to give a **sulphenylamide** (S−N) species; it was proposed that this occurs to prevent further oxidation of the sulphenic acid to sulphonic ($-SO_3H$) or sulphinic ($-SO_2H$) species, which are more difficult to convert back to an active cysteine residue.[70] Inactivation of phosphatases can also occur by glutathionylation (Section 3.9.6).

In some other phosphatases such as **PTEN (phosphatase and tensin homologue)** ROS inactivate not by cys−SOH formation but by causing disulphide bridge formation.[71] The PTEN enzyme hydrolyses PIP_3, thus limiting activation of Akt (Section 4.5.5.2). Inactivation of PTEN can thus favour inappropriate cell survival via increased Akt phosphorylation. Indeed, PTEN knockout mice are prone to develop cancer, and PTEN is inactivated in some human prostate and endometrial cancers.[71] Another phosphatase sensitive to RS is **calcineurin**, a Ca^{2+}/calmodulin-dependent serine/threonine phosphatase particularly important in brain, cartilage and lymphocytes. Its inactivation occurs by a different mechanism, oxidation of iron irons at the active site,[72] and can be mediated by $O_2^{\bullet-}$.

Careful modulation of cellular H_2O_2-removing systems, especially the peroxiredoxins (Section 3.11.1),[70] allows 'bursts' of H_2O_2 (e.g. generated in response to extracellular signals; Section 4.5.6 below) to persist for a short time and trigger H_2O_2-dependent phosphatase inactivation and increased protein phosphorylation. Quickly however, the H_2O_2 is removed and the phosphatase activity restored.

Other mechanisms by which RS stimulate phosphorylation exist. For example thioredoxin binds to and inactivates **ASK1, apoptosis signal-regulating kinase-1**. Oxidative stress causes dissociation of the complex and the activated ASK1 can then phosphorylate and activate JNK and p38 kinases.[73]

4.5.6 Reactive species as mediators of the actions of signalling molecules?

Exposure of cells to RS activates a range of signalling pathways. But what about 'normal' signalling via binding of growth factors, cytokines and hormones to receptors? Their binding initiates protein phosphorylation and triggers signalling cascades. However, there is growing evidence that RS are also involved in the response of cells to these agents (Table 4.7). This suggests that ligand-binding and activation of receptor-linked protein kinases cannot produce enough phosphorylation to allow a full response; transient inactivation of phosphatases by RS may also be required. Strictly then, the RS are not 'second messengers' of the primary signal (the ligand), but 'secondary messengers', modifying the size or duration of another signal (i.e. receptor-binding-dependent phosphorylation).[69]

How are the ROS produced? Some authors[74] have suggested that EGF binding to its receptor (EGFR) generates ROS directly, but exactly how is not clear. One established mechanism for ROS production is for ligand binding to stimulate the PI3K pathway, which activates the small G protein **Rac1**, that in turn activates an NADPH oxidase, producing $O_2^{\bullet-}$. Such NADPH oxidases are widespread in plant and animal cells (Sections 7.10 and 7.11) and can produce $O_2^{\bullet-}$ in response to stresses (e.g. growth factor deprivation in neurons), hormones (e.g. angiotensin II in vascular smooth muscle cells), growth factors (e.g. **transforming growth factor-β1**, TGFβ1) and cytokines. Rises in Ca^{2+} can also increase RS, by increasing XO (in some cells), activating DUOX enzymes (Table 4.7, point 19), or stimulating $NO^{\bullet}$ production via eNOS or nNOS.

4.5.7 Intraorganelle communication?

Mitochondrial ROS production is often thought of as a nuisance, an unavoidable consequence of electron leakage under O_2. Indeed, the severe phenotype of MnSOD-knockout mice reveals the threat posed by too much $O_2^{\bullet-}$ in these organelles (Section 3.4.2). However, another view is that variations in mitochondrial H_2O_2 production are a signal that advises the cytoplasm and nucleus what the mitochondria are doing, leading to changes in nuclear gene transcription via activation of MAP kinases and other mechanisms.[75] Can this happen? Addition of antimycin A to cultured cells to partially block mitochondrial electron transport increased intracellular peroxide levels and the transcription of nuclear genes encoding mitochondrial proteins; both were antagonized by antioxidants.[76] Mice partially defective in mitochondrial MnSOD showed increased oxidative damage in *nuclear* DNA (Section 9.13.5.8). The increase in levels of antioxidants such as MnSOD in response to TNFα (Section 4.7.1 below) may be an example of mitochondria-to-nucleus signalling in which ROS are involved. However, how many ROS produced normally could escape the mitochondrial (Section 3.11.1) and cytosolic antioxidant defences to reach the nucleus? Not enough to cause oxidative damage to nuclear DNA, apparently.[77] In addition, overexpression of catalase in the mitochondria of heart and skeletal muscle decreased oxidative damage there and *increased* lifespan in mice (Section 10.4.2.1), implying that diminution of mitochondrial ROS production could be beneficial. On the other hand, more MnSOD and catalase in *Drosophila* shortened

Table 4.7 Examples of stimulatory effects of hormones, cytokines and growth factors involving reactive oxygen species in animal cells (*note that effects are usually described in cells or explanted tissues*)

---

1. Activation of NF-κB/AP-1 in response to several stimuli (Sections 4.5.8 and 4.5.9)
2. Response of cells to cytokines, especially TNFα (Section 4.7)
3. Epidermal growth factor-induced tyrosine phosphorylation in epidermoid cancer cells requires H_2O_2 (*J. Biol. Chem.* **272**, 217, 1997)
4. Angiotensin II raises $O_2^{\bullet-}$ production in blood vessels via a NOX (Section 7.10.3) leading to increased blood pressure
5. Activation of Akt by angiotensin II in vascular smooth muscle cells involves ROS (*J. Biol. Chem.* **274**, 22699, 1999)
6. PDGF receptor-induced phosphorylation of ERK, DNA synthesis and migration in smooth muscle cells involves H_2O_2 and is blocked by overexpression of catalase (*Science* **270**, 296, 1995)
7. Insulin-treated adipocytes and hepatoma cells show phosphatase inactivation involving H_2O_2 production; this may involve $O_2^{\bullet-}$ produced by a NOX4 enzyme (Section 7.10) (*Mol. Cell. Biol.* **24**, 1844, 2004)
8. Adhesion of NIH-3T fibroblasts generates ROS which promote phosphorylation of focal adhesion kinase (FAK) by inhibiting FAK tyrosine phosphatase (*J. Cell. Biol.* **161**, 933, 2003)
9. Basic fibroblast growth factor (FGF-2) induction of c-Fos in chondrocytes and lung fibroblasts requires ROS (*Am. J. Physiol.* **279**, L1005, 2000)
10. Synthesis of TIMP−3 by chondrocytes or of a contractile protein in smooth muscle cells in response to TGF-β1 involves ROS (*Free Rad. Biol. Med.* **37**, 196, 2004; *Arterio. Thromb. Vasc. Biol.* **25**, 341, 2005)
11. Cell division in explanted rat aortae in response to catecholamines is mediated via ROS, probably by activation of a NOX (*Circ. Res.* **94**, 37, 2004)
12. Shear stress induces generation of H_2O_2 in human arterioles in culture, which mediates flow-induced dilation (*Circ. Res.* **93**, 573, 2003) possibly via cyclooxygenase I (*Am. J. Physiol.* **285**, H2255, 2003)
13. Shear stress increased fluid-phase endocytosis in bovine aortic endothelial cells via increased ROS production by a NOX (*Free Radic. Res.* **40**, 167, 2006)
14. Cyclic stretch of lamb lung arterial smooth muscle cells increased TGF-β1, which increased ROS production via a NOX, leading to increased VEGF synthesis (*Am. J. Physiol.* **289**, L288, 2005)
15. Nerve growth factor-induced differentiation of PC12 cells is mediated by ROS (*J. Biol. Chem.* **275**, 13175, 2000)
16. Endothelin-1 activates ERK 1/2, PKB and protein tyrosine kinase 2 in vascular smooth muscle cells via ROS (*Free Rad. Biol. Med.* **37**, 208, 2004)
17. Insulin increases $O_2^{\bullet-}$ production in human skin fibroblasts via the PI$_3$ kinase pathway and NADPH, leading to ERK-1 activation (*Diabetes* **53**, 1344, 2004)
18. Thrombin-induced mitogenesis in vascular smooth muscle cells involves $O_2^{\bullet-}$ produced by a NOX (*J. Biol. Chem.* **274**, 19814, 1999)
19. Binding of antigen to receptors on a B lymphoma cell line raised intracellular Ca^{2+} which increased ROS production (by activating a DUOX enzyme; Section 7.10) and thus inactivated phosphatases (*Cell* **121**, 281, 2005)
20. TGFβ-induced cytoskeletal alterations in human umbilical vein endothelial cells involve ROS produced by a NOX (*Am. J. Physiol.* **289**, F816, 2005)
21. Exposure of cultured renal medulla cells to high osmotic pressure increased ROS production and raised COX-2 levels (*J. Biol. Chem.* **280**, 34966, 2005)

NOX, NADPH oxidase.

lifespan and made the insects somewhat unco-ordinated (Section 10.4.2). Mitochondrially targeted antioxidants (Section 10.6.11) may be useful tools to study physiological roles of mitochondrial ROS.

Some constituents of the electron transport chain are encoded in mitochondrial DNA, but the genes for most are in nuclear DNA. Hence nuclear and mitochondrial gene expression must be co-ordinated, both normally and in response to stresses, for example hypoxia. Two transcription factors, **nuclear respiratory factors-1 and -2**, **NRF1** and **NRF2**, help control expression of the nuclear genes encoding mitochondrial proteins. Binding of NRF2 (sometimes called **GA-binding protein, GA-BP**) to DNA is inhibited by ROS, apparently due to oxidation of essential −SH groups,[78] suggesting that redox changes can affect the supply of mitochondrial proteins. Luckily, oxidation is reversible by reduced thioredoxin. The NRFs can also be regulated by phosphorylation, itself modulated by ROS.

4.5.8 NF-κB[79–81]

NF-κB is an assembly of proteins that activates the transcription of multiple genes in response to a variety of stimuli. It belongs to the **Rel** family of transcription factors.

Active NF-κB is a heterodimer, usually containing proteins of relative molecular masses 50 000 and 65 000, referred to as **p50** and **p65**. NF-κB is present in almost all mammalian cells and in most of them spends much of its time in an inactive, cytoplasmic form. Cytoplasmic retention and lack of activity result from binding to the dimer of an inhibitory subunit, **IκB**. A wide range of stimuli such as endotoxin, mechanical stress, infection with viruses (Section 9.23) exposure to UV light, toxins (e.g. nickel, cobalt), γ-rays or certain cytokines (e.g. TNFα) lead to activation of NF-κB. Indeed, NF-κB is activated in a wide range of inflammatory diseases, from gastritis to rheumatoid arthritis (Chapter 9).

Activation results when IκB dissociates from the complex, usually caused by its phosphorylation on two serine residues by the kinases **IKK1** and **2**, which are themselves regulated by phosphorylation (Fig. 4.9). The IκB is then ubiquitinated and degraded by the proteasome (Section 4.14.2 below). The active NF-κB heterodimer moves into the nucleus, binds to DNA and increases expression of multiple genes, including those encoding several cytokines (IL-2, IL-6, IL-8, TNFα), acute phase proteins, iNOS, growth factors, adhesion molecules, cyclooxygenase 2 and cytokine receptors. Prompt resynthesis of IκB, also promoted by the activated NF-κB, shuts down the signal; it binds to nuclear NF-κB and helps push it back into the cytoplasm (Fig. 4.10). Activation of NF-κB can lead to inflammation, cell injury and apoptosis, but paradoxically it can also contribute to the resolution of inflammation (Section 9.13.6). NF-κB activation can also promote survival in several cell

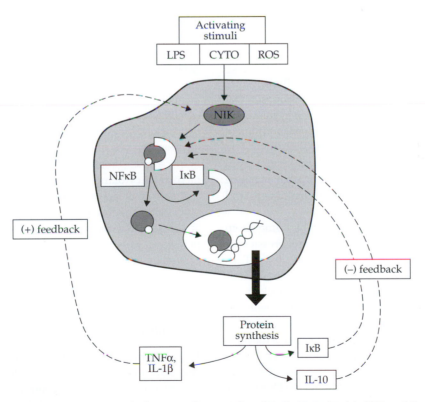

Figure 4.10 NF-κB regulation and its interaction with some cytokines. LPS, lipopolysaccharide (endotoxin); CYTO, proinflammatory cytokines; NIK, NF-κB inducible kinase; IκB, inhibitory protein. From *Br. J. Anaesthesia* **90**, 221, 2003 by courtesy of Drs J. Macdonald, N.R. Webster and H.F. Galley and the publishers.

types, by disfavouring apoptosis. This may be important (to the virus!) in virally-infected cells (Section 9.23). Whether NF-κB activation is bad or good depends on its extent, and on what else is activated or deactivated at the same time. Remember also that, overall, inflammation is usually beneficial to the body. Indeed, most NF-κB-activated genes are involved in what appears to be an early defence network against infection or injury. Glucocorticoid hormones decrease NF-κB activation; in some cell types this is achieved by increasing transcription of genes encoding IκB. Other agents that can inhibit NF-κB activation in certain cells are caffeic acid phenethyl ester[82] (a component of propolis; Section 3.22.4) and **acetylsalicylate** (aspirin).[83]

NF-κB is particularly important in the immune system. Imaging of NF-κB activity in whole mice showed it to be low in most tissues, except for lymph nodes, thymus and Peyer's patches in the intestine (also part of the immune system). Injection of cytokines or endotoxin increased activity in many organs.[80]

4.5.8.1 *ROS or no ROS?*

Since many stimuli that activate NF-κB also cause oxidative stress, Pahl and Baeuerle[81] proposed that ROS are a common second-messenger system used by all stimuli to activate NF-κB. Indeed, addition of micromolar amounts of H_2O_2, HOCl or ONOO$^-$ to the culture medium activates NF-κB in some (but not all) cell lines. Many data have been obtained using HeLa and Jurkat cells, both malignant (and thus somewhat abnormal) cell lines.

Further support for the concept came from experiments with antioxidants; overexpression of thioredoxin or GPx in the cells prevented NF-κB activation and several added antioxidants (including thiols, catechols and spin traps) blocked the activation of NF-κB by any stimulus. However, one should be careful in interpreting the effects of several widely used 'antioxidants' because they can have other actions. For example, *N*-acetylcysteine (Section 6.9.2) is a redox agent that raises cell GSH levels and can also block the binding of TNFα to its receptor.[84] **Pyrrolidine dithiocarbamate** is widely used as an antioxidant, but it also chelates metals and can interfere with ubiquitination of IκB.[84]

Another relevant factor may be the cellular iron status. For example, treatment of a liver macrophage cell line with endotoxin caused both a transient rise in the size of the LIP (Section 3.15.1.3) and activation of NF-κB; activation was blocked by iron chelators, iNOS inhibition or CuZnSOD, suggesting a role for ONOO$^-$. Indeed, direct addition of iron (or of ONOO$^-$) to these cells produced NF-κB activation.[85]

How could RS cause IκB dissociation and NF-κB activation? The trigger for IκB detachment is phosphorylation (Fig. 4.9). A likely mechanism therefore involves decreasing phosphatase activity. However, it's probably more complex than that. Also, as always in redox biology, there is a balance. Activation of NF-κB is but one step; to achieve biological effects the activated transcription factor must bind to DNA. Binding is modulated by phosphorylation and acetylation. It is also affected by redox state, being inhibited by oxidizing agents and potentiated by thiols, especially reduced thioredoxin, which may play a key role in keeping NF-κB reduced in the nucleus (Fig. 4.9). Hence the overall effects of redox state upon NF-κB-mediated gene expression can be variable. Too many RS may activate NF-κB, but inhibit binding of the active factor to DNA and in this case antioxidants (at a certain level) might *promote* NF-κB-dependent gene expression. For example, overexpression of catalase *increased* the NF-κB-dependent induction of iNOS in rat aortic smooth muscle cells treated with a mixture of cytokines and endotoxin.[86]

Agents that activate NF-κB frequently activate other cell signalling pathways, such as JNK. There is considerable cross-talk between these various pathways, in which they can co-operate (e.g. Akt activation promotes IκB phosphorylation) or antagonize each other's actions, depending on the cells studied and the signal applied.[87]

4.5.9 AP-1[88]

The transcription factor **AP-1 (activator protein 1)** also senses intracellular redox state and regulates the expression of multiple genes involved in stress response, growth and differentiation. It is a dimer of proteins of the **Fos** and **Jun** families, usually a c-Fos/c-Jun heterodimer. The activity of AP-1 is controlled both by regulating how much c-Fos and c-Jun the cell makes, and by phosphorylation of already-synthesized proteins (e.g. by MAP kinases). Various RS, such as H_2O_2, can alter both processes. The c-Fos and c-Jun proteins were originally described as products of proto-oncogenes (Section 9.13.4). c-Jun is phosphorylated by JNK (Section 4.5.5.2), and c-Fos by the ERK pathway. Both phosphorylations can be influenced by RS.

Binding of AP-1 to DNA is redox-regulated by a mechanism involving cysteine residues in the DNA-binding domain of Fos and Jun: oxidation decreases DNA binding. Oxidation can be reversed by thiols or by a cellular redox/DNA-repair protein called Ref-1 (**redox effector factor 1**), which interacts with reduced thioredoxin. This Ref-1 activity is located on an AP endonuclease protein involved in DNA repair (Section 4.10.3 below). Hence repair is closely linked to activation of transcription by AP-1.

4.5.10 The antioxidant response element[89]

Antioxidant response elements (ARE) are DNA sequences to which **Nrf1** and **Nrf2** proteins bind when xenobiotics are present. Binding allows increased transcription of genes encoding xenobiotic metabolizing enzymes such as NAD(P)H:quinone reductases (Section 8.6.4), GST (Section 3.9.5), HO-1 (Section 3.17), GI-GPx (Section 3.8) and γ-GCS (Section 3.9.3). These changes help to remove the xenobiotic, but can also render the cell resistant to oxidative stress.

How does this work? Many xenobiotics both induce oxidative stress and are, or can form, **electrophiles**, agents that react with sites of high electron density on proteins, DNA or lipids. An increase in oxidative/electrophilic stress can, for example, activate PKC (Section 4.5.5.2). This phosphorylates cytoplasmic Nrf2, causing it to fall away from the **Keap1** protein that normally keeps it inactive. The Nrf2 then migrates into the nucleus and binds to the ARE. The Keap1 functions not only to keep Nrf2 in the cytoplasm, but also to promote its destruction by the proteasome (Section 4.14.2). Other kinases may also phosphorylate Nrf2 and free it from Keap1. In addition, Keap1 is rich in cysteine residues and its direct modification by RS

and electrophiles, including cyclopentenone compounds and 4-HNE (Sections 4.12.3 and 4.12.5.3 below), could also release Nrf2.

Mice lacking Nrf2 are highly susceptible to the toxicity of such drugs as paracetamol (Section 8.10) and to cancer induced by benzpyrene (Section 9.14). Several dietary constituents modulate the ARE system (Fig. 10.6; Table 10.7).

4.5.11 Getting it together: co-operation and combination

The cellular response to oxidative, 'electrophile' or other stresses involves multiple signalling pathways, which can synergize or antagonize each other in dozens of ways. For example, the promoter of γ-GCS contains an ARE, an AP-1 binding site and an NF-κB-responsive site. Thus any, or any combination of, these transcription factors can raise cellular GSH levels. Reactive species can activate Nrf2 by direct attack on Keap1, indirect attack by aldehyde end products of lipid peroxidation, by stimulating PKC and/or by inactivating phosphatases and stimulating net Keap1 phosphorylation by this and other kinases.

In general (to use a gross oversimplification), activations of the heat-shock response (Section 4.6 below), AP-1, Nrf2, ERK, Akt and NF-κB promote cell survival after oxidative stress, whereas prolonged activations of JNK, p38 and p53 (Section 9.13.4) more often lead to apoptosis.[58] For example, the apoptosis induced by incubating HL-60 cells with desferrioxamine could be delayed by attenuating p38 kinase activation.[90]

4.5.12 Is it real? Physiological significance of redox regulation in animals

Evidence that redox regulation is physiologically important is very strong in bacteria and yeast (Sections 4.5.2 and 4.5.4) and reasonably strong in plants (Section 7.11). What about animals? Several redox regulation mechanisms were described earlier in this Chapter, but some are sceptical of their significance *in vivo*. Thus H_2O_2 leads to NF-κB activation in some cell types but not in many others; thus H_2O_2 cannot be a *universal* intracellular second messenger of NF-κB activation.[84] Similarly, most studies of redox regulation are upon cells in culture (Table 4.7). Here one must be careful, because cell culture imposes oxidative stress (Section 1.11). It is therefore possible that cultured cells adapt to use ROS to oxidize molecules and send signals that in the whole animal are sent in other ways.[91] For example, a signal normally sent by oxidation of −SH groups in a molecule via a network of thiol-containing proteins can also be sent (artefactually) by direct thiol oxidation by an RS. In the last edition of this book, we highlighted the need to move away from studies of isolated cells towards whole animals.

How far have we got? First, it is now clear that many cells *in vivo* contain NADPH oxidases that produce ROS (Section 7.10), consistent with a role for ROS *in vivo*. The properties of peroxiredoxins are consistent with a role for ROS in signalling (Section 3.11.1). Studies on NOX1-knockout mice and spontaneously hypertensive rats have revealed a role for $O_2^{\bullet-}$ in regulation of blood pressure (Section 7.10.3) and ROS mediate ischaemic pre-conditioning in some animal studies (Section 4.2.2). Transgenic mice overexpressing GPx1 and extra-cellular GPx showed less activation of NF-κB after ischaemia–reperfusion, consistent with some role for H_2O_2 in that activation.[92] They also showed less sensitivity to the deleterious effects of endotoxin, suggestive of an important role for H_2O_2 in inflammation,[93] and GPx1-overexpressing mice responded poorly to heat (Section 4.6 below). Mice with elevated SOD showed accelerated angiogen-esis after subcutaneous injection of basic fibroblast growth factor (bFGF) and abnormally high pro-duction of cytokines from macrophages during inflammation, suggesting that $O_2^{\bullet-}$ helps to modu-late angiogenesis and inflammation *in vivo*.[94]

However, these are mostly pathological situa-tions, indicating that ROS help co-ordinate response to injury (undoubtedly an important thing to do!). What about healthy animals? Mice with increased GPx1 showed mild hyperglycaemia and insulin resistance, apparently associated with impaired phosphorylation of insulin receptor in liver and Akt in liver and muscle. This supports a role for H_2O_2 in 'normal' insulin action *in vivo*.[95] Studies on dogs showed that both NO$^{\bullet}$ and H_2O_2 are involved in controlling vasodilator responses in coronary arteries, and H_2O_2 produced by vascular endothelium has been suggested to be a physiolo-gical vasodilator in several animals, including humans.[96] Both knockout and overexpression of EC-SOD (Section 3.16.3.1) affected hippocampal function in mice as measured by behavioural studies, leading to the suggestion that $O_2^{\bullet-}$ may play a role in hippocampus-dependent memory.[97] Mice lacking EC-SOD also show impaired ery-thropoietin synthesis under hypoxia, consistent with a role for ROS in regulating this process (Section 7.10.5). Exercise training in mice increased eNOS activity, an effect also seen in vascular endothelial cells treated with H_2O_2. Exercising mice overexpressing catalase did not show ele-vated eNOS, consistent with H_2O_2 being a physiological messenger.[98] Hydrogen peroxide may also mediate muscle adaptations to exercise in rats.[99] Nevertheless, more work must be done before we can be convinced that ROS are *major* players in signalling in the healthy animal.

4.5.13 Lessons from an amoeba

An interesting perspective is provided by the slime mould *Dictyostelium discoideum*, often called a 'social amoeba'.[100] It usually lives happily alone and feeds on bacteria, but when food runs out the amoebae aggregate to form a ball that produces a 'fruiting body' containing spores. The ball trundles to a 'better' location and releases the spores, each of which germinates to generate a fresh amoeba. At the onset of aggregation the cells release $O_2^{\bullet-}$ using a NADPH oxidase enzyme (Section 7.10); if $O_2^{\bullet-}$ levels are decreased by $O_2^{\bullet-}$ scavengers or over-expression of SOD, aggregation is inhibited. This use of $O_2^{\bullet-}$ in an amoeba as it converts from unicellular to multicellular raises the possibility of whether the same thing happened during the evolution of multicellular organisms, and whether they still retain aspects of ROS-dependent signal-ling. ROS seem also to be involved in differenti-ation in the slime mould *Physarum polycephalum*[101] and the fungus *Neurospora crassa*.[102] In both cases differentiation appears to be accompanied by increased oxidative stress, and changes in redox state may be the trigger for differentiation.

4.6 Heat-shock and related 'stress-induced' proteins, cross talk with ROS[58]

When cells are subjected to oxidative stress, it is not only antioxidant defences that can rise; levels of many other proteins increase as well, including some of the **heat-shock proteins (Hsp)**.[103] Production of other proteins (e.g. CYPs) may simultaneously decrease.[12] The Hsp are classified into six major families, denoted by their relative molecular mass (e.g. about 70 000 for **Hsp70**).

Heat-shock proteins were first identified by studies of the response to heat, hence the name. After a sudden increase in temperature all cells, from human to microbe, increase expression of genes encoding Hsp. Investigators soon found that cells produce Hsp when exposed to other stresses, including ischaemia–reperfusion, toxic metals, oxidative stress, cytotoxic aldehydes such as HNE, alcohol and other xenobiotics, and thus began to refer to them by a more general name, **stress proteins**. One can include metallothioneins (Section 3.16.1) and MnSOD in the general category of stress proteins, since their levels increase in response to many stresses.

Most Hsp act as **chaperones**, proteins that use energy from ATP to aid the folding and translocation of other proteins. Chaperones of the Hsp70 family act early in the life of a protein, before it leaves the ribosome, and then hand it over to **Hsp60** to help with later stages of protein folding. A special form of Hsp70, **BiP**, helps to fold proteins within the ER. Disturbances in ER Ca^{2+} homeostasis, inhibitors of protein glycosylation, oxidative damage to ER proteins or accumulation of misfolded proteins trigger the **ER stress response**.[104] This activates signalling pathways that decrease protein synthesis (to stop the problem getting worse), increase levels of BiP, other chaperones and PDI to help remedy the situation, and also speed up hydrolysis of proteins in the ER. Increased production of ROS by the Ero proteins (Section 3.10) may be involved in the ER stress response. Severe ER stress can lead to apoptosis (Fig. 4.8). Other chaperones are found in different subcellular compartments, including mitochondria, where some help to stabilize iron-containing proteins to deter release of redox-active iron.[105]

Cytoplasmic chaperones eventually 'hand over' proteins destined for organelles to the organellar chaperones; proteins enter organelles in a partially unfolded state and are then helped to fold correctly by the organellar chaperones.

Many stress-inducing agents cause protein damage, and the accumulation of partially denatured or abnormally folded proteins triggers the Hsp response. In animals, this involves activation of a **heat-shock transcription factor** (HSF), which binds to DNA sequences (**heat-shock *cis*-elements**) in the promoters of genes encoding Hsp, to activate transcription. In unstressed cells HSF is present in the cytoplasm and the nucleus (perhaps bound to Hsp70) as a monomeric form that has no DNA-binding activity. In response to stress, HSF is released from Hsp70 and forms a trimer that binds with high affinity to heat-shock gene promoters. The extra Hsp70 made as a result (hopefully!) facilitate the refolding (or removal of) damaged proteins. Chaperones collaborate with PDI (Section 3.10) and **peptidyl-prolyl isomerases** (which accelerate the *cis/ trans* isomerization of peptide bonds next to proline residues) to restore correct protein conformation. Elevations in Hsp70 and other Hsp enhance cell survival and decrease oxidative damage to lipids, proteins and DNA under a wide variety of stress conditions. For example, Hsp70 can antagonize JNK-mediated apoptosis in some cells. The Hsp 70 and 27 can inhibit key parts of the apoptotic pathway, including caspase activation, and Hsp 70 may deter the release of AIF from mitochondria.[106] Some yeast peroxiredoxins show chaperone activity,[57] as does human Prx2 after it has been exposed to H_2O_2.[107]

Certain Hsp have other roles. Thus the **ubiquitins**, a group of smaller (8500 molecular mass) Hsp, help to remove unwanted proteins via the proteasome (Section 4.14.2.1 below). Ubiquitin levels rise 5- to 7-fold after stress. The protein **Hsp32**, whose level increases in many tissues in response to haem administration, certain metal ions (e.g. cadmium) or oxidative stress, is identical to HO-1, which protects cells by degrading haem and generating bilirubin and CO (Section 3.17).

The action of oxidative stress in damaging proteins probably accounts for its ability to induce some Hsp. Similarly, Hsp induction by heat can involve ROS. Thermal induction of hsp70 in transgenic mice overexpressing GPx1 was subnormal, and the mice were less thermotolerant.[108] Adding catalase to U937 cells potentiated apoptosis induced by heat-shock, apparently by decreasing the levels of Hsp.[109]

Some plasma proteins may have limited chaperone-like activity, such as **clusterin**.[110] Haptoglobin (Section 3.16.3.4) can also exert some chaperone-like activity *in vitro*, in addition to its haemoglobin-binding action (Table 3.11).[110] However, it does not bind ATP nor can it refold proteins after denaturation.

4.7 Cytokines, hormones and redox-regulation of the organism[111]

Communication between distant cells in complex organisms is unlikely to be mediated by RS, since their lifetime is short. It is partly achieved by hormones such as insulin, thyroid hormones, adrenalin, oestrogen and testosterone, which are secreted into the plasma and affect many cell types in different ways, often including alterations of antioxidant defences (e.g. Section 3.19). Sometimes they work by making RS in their target cells (Section 4.5). Indeed, most of the redox regulation we have discussed so far has been at the cellular level. Can multicellular organisms use RS to transmit signals *between* cells? Nitric oxide is a clear precedent, but can other RS be similarly used? For example, if a cell is stressed, can it release RS that lead to increased defences in other cells and tissues? Yes it can; systemic acquired resistance is a good example in plants (Section 7.11). Reactive species may operate over short distances at sites of inflammation to trigger changes in adjacent cells, for example increased levels of adhesion molecules (Section 7.9) and sometimes cell migration. Intercellular communication can also occur through cell–cell contact (e.g. via gap junctions), which may allow information transfer about oxidative stress for example by changes in GSH/ GSSG ratio or the thioredoxin redox state.

Another (overlapping) localized signalling mechanism is provided by the cytokines. **Cytokine** is a loosely defined term that encompasses a wide range of polypeptides and glycoproteins. Their presence is usually transient and strictly controlled. Most cytokines are secreted, but some can be expressed in cell membranes. They act locally by binding to receptors on their target cells, exerting effects at low concentrations. Cytokines cross-talk; one cytokine affects the secretion and actions of others. When first discovered, cytokines were usually identified as products of single cell types, for example **monokines** from monocytes, **lymphokines** from lymphocytes and **interleukins** from leukocytes. The list expanded to include interferons, TNFs and cytokines affecting chemotaxis (**chemokines**) (Table 4.8). It was soon realized

Table 4.8 Some cytokines

Class	Examples
Interleukins	IL-1α, IL-1β, IL-2 to -7 and IL-9 to -17
Chemokines[a]	α-Chemokines, e.g. IL-8 (mainly act on neutrophils); β-chemokines (mainly act on monocytes/macrophages) e.g. monocyte chemoattractant protein 1 (MCP-1); monocyte inflammatory proteins (MIP-1α and 1β); RANTES (regulation-upon-activation, normal T-cell expressed and secreted)
Interferons	Interferons α, β and γ
Tumour necrosis factors	Cachectin (TNFα), lymphotoxins (TNFβ_1, β_2)
Colony-stimulating factors (CSFs)	Granulocyte CSF, macrophage CSF, granulocyte-macrophage CSF (GM–CSF)
Transforming growth factors	TGFα, TGFβ (several types), activins
Growth factors	Epidermal growth factor (EGF), fibroblast growth factor (FGF), hepatocyte growth factor (HGF), insulin-like growth factor (ILGF), keratinocyte growth factor (KGF), platelet-derived growth factor (PDGF), vascular endothelial growth factor (VEGF); VEGF expression can be upregulated by HIF-1α (Section 1.3.2)
Neurotrophic factors	Nerve growth factor (NGF); brain-derived neurotrophic factor (BDNF); ciliary neurotrophic factor (CNTF)

[a] Chemotactic cytokines.

that cytokines have multiple cellular sources, a broad (and often overlapping) range of biological activities and some redundancy in their effects; different cytokines often affect cells in the same way. In addition, most cytokines are **pleiotropic**, that is they exert different effects on various cells. One analogy is that cytokines are 'words' in the language of cellular communication; words mean different things depending on what other words surround them.

Cytokines play key roles in normal growth and development, inflammatory and other responses to injury, and tissue remodelling and repair (e.g. wound healing, angiogenesis). A complex balance between different cytokines regulates the final outcome. Thus some cytokines are regarded as proinflammatory (e.g. IL-1, IL-6, TNFα) whereas others are, overall, 'anti-inflammatory' (e.g. IL-1 receptor antagonist, IL-10). It is impossible to review all the cytokines here, but we briefly mention some that are particularly implicated in oxidative stress. Proinflammatory cytokines are often produced in response to oxidative stress, and act, in part, by causing oxidative stress in their target cells. For example, several cytokines are produced when NF-κB is activated (e.g. TNFα, IL-Iβ, IL-2, IL-6, IL-12, RANTES), and in turn this can increase NF-κB activation and cytokine production (Figs 4.9 and 4.10). By contrast, anti-inflammatory cytokines such as IL-10 suppress inflammation, in part by decreasing ROS formation (Fig. 4.10).

Thioredoxin plays a key role in regulating cellular redox state and how the cell responds to it (e.g. via NF-κB; Section 4.5.8) and has an intimate link with cytokine action. Thus secreted thioredoxin can act as a cocytokine with several interleukins, and a truncated thioredoxin (**TRX-80**) found in plasma is itself a mitogenic cytokine for monocytes.[111]

4.7.1 TNFα

Tumour necrosis factor alpha (TNFα), a protein of relative molecular mass 17 000, can be secreted by many cell types; monocytes, macrophages, B- and T-lymphocytes, mast cells, neutrophils and fibroblasts. It acts by binding to two different types of cell-surface receptors. The name TNF comes from its initial identification as a factor found in the serum of mice infected with *Bacillus Calmette Guerin* (a weakened form of the agent causing tuberculosis) that could cause haemorrhage and necrosis in tumours transplanted into the same mice. Over 100 years ago, Coley in New York observed that cancer patients repeatedly administered 'bacterial broths' could show haemorrhagic necrosis of their tumours. Later work showed that the active agent was endotoxin, which stimulates production of TNFα. Too much endotoxin causes severe injury, for example **endotoxic shock**, and over-production of TNFα is involved. TNFα was later found to be identical with **cachectin**, a 'body wasting factor' identified in seriously-ill cancer patients. It promotes mobilization of fat stores, and muscle cells treated with TNFα show ROS-dependent NF-κB activation and stimulated proteolysis.[112]

Tumour necrosis factor α is strongly proinflammatory, for example promoting increases in adhesion molecules that favour phagocyte adherence to vascular endothelium, stimulating cartilage degradation and bone resorption and priming phagocyte (especially neutrophil) ROS production as well as increasing iNOS levels. It is often portrayed as a 'bad guy', and indeed it probably is overall in endotoxic shock and some chronic inflammatory diseases (Chapter 9). However, it often plays a key part in host defence responses against injury and infection. For example, transgenic 'knock-out' mice lacking TNF receptors are *more* sensitive to brain damage by certain neurotoxins or by ischaemia–reperfusion.[113]

Tumour necrosis factor α increases oxidative stress both in its target cells and (via promotion of phagocyte ROS production) in surrounding cells. It is a powerful activator of NF-κB in many cell types, often (but by no means always) acting via H_2O_2 (Section 4.5.8). Increased ROS production, in at least some target cells, appears to involve effects of TNFα on mitochondria.[114] Activation of FOXO1 and ROS production by TNFα can trigger cell death,[115] but can alternatively result in cytoprotection related to increased levels of antioxidant, antiapoptotic and other defence proteins, including ferritin H-chains, thioredoxins, metallothioneins, Hsp, MnSOD in mitochondria, and sometimes uncoupling proteins (Section 1.10.6). Increased mitochondrial ROS production due to TNFα can lead to activation of nuclear genes, in part via NF-κB[114] and sometimes by JNK-mediated activation of FOXOs (Section 4.5.5.2). Thus pretreatment of animals with low levels of TNFα (or endotoxin) protects them against several subsequent insults, including radiation, some cytotoxic drugs and ischaemia–reperfusion. Too much and you get a very sick animal—the usual balance!

4.7.2 Interleukins

Interleukin-1 exists in two forms, IL-1α and IL-1β, and is a key mediator of the response to injury and infection (Section 4.7.3 below). It is generally proinflammatory and is secreted by monocytes, lymphocytes, macrophages, fibroblasts, keratinocytes and endothelial cells, among others. Often IL-1β is secreted in an inactive form which has to be cleaved by a cysteine proteinase **interleukin-1β converting enzyme** (ICE) to generate active IL-1β. Interleukin-1 is a major contributor to fever (TNFα also contributes), and excess IL-1 has been implicated in tissue damage in several diseases.

Interleukin-8 is a chemokine (Table 4.8) important in promoting migration, adhesion and activation of neutrophils. It is produced by monocytes, smooth muscle cells, endothelial cells, lymphocytes, fibroblasts and keratinocytes. Again, overproduction has been implicated in several chronic inflammatory diseases. Reactive species can stimulate production of IL-8 and other interleukins by some cell types (Section 7.9.2).

Interleukin-10, by contrast, can inhibit production of proinflammatory cytokines by a range of cell types, and acts to downregulate inflammation (Fig. 4.10). It also induces HO-1 in a range of cells, for example IL-10-mediated protection against endotoxin-induced sepsis in mice was diminished by administering an HO-1 inhibitor.[116]

4.7.3 The acute-phase response

The **acute-phase response** is a 'whole body' response of animals to infections and inflammation generally, and includes fever (triggered by IL-1 and other cytokines). Biochemical alterations include increased synthesis of certain proteins by the liver (**acute-phase proteins**), decreased synthesis of albumin by the liver (often thus called a **negative-acute-phase protein**), decreases in plasma iron and zinc level, and negative nitrogen balance (i.e. more nitrogen is excreted than taken in the diet). Some acute-phase proteins are involved in antioxidant defence (Table 4.9). 'Acute' signifies that many of the changes occur within hours of the precipitating event. Many features of the acute-phase response are also present in chronic conditions, such as 'low-grade' infections, rheumatoid arthritis (Section 9.10; Table 9.8) and many forms of cancer.

The acute-phase response differs from the heat-shock response in that it has evolved only in complex multicellular organisms, and presumably serves to help co-ordinate the responses of different cell types.

4.8 Mechanisms of damage to cellular targets by oxidative stress: DNA[117]

4.8.1 DNA structure

Reactive species are involved in the development of cancer, both by direct effects on DNA and by modulating signal transduction, cell proliferation, senescence, and cell death (Section 9.13.5). Here we focus on their ability to damage DNA directly, although indirect damage also occurs. For example RS can lead to activation of Ca^{2+}-dependent endonucleases (Section 4.3.2). Direct damage to DNA by RS can affect the purine (adenine, guanine) or pyrimidine (cytosine, thymine) bases, and/or the deoxyribose sugar.

The backbone of DNA consists of deoxyriboses linked by esterifying the −OH group on position 5 of one to that on position 3 of the next by a phosphate group (a **phosphodiester bond**). The presence of multiple phosphate groups gives DNA a substantial negative charge since phosphates are ionized at physiological pH. Hence DNA binds cations such as Na^+ and K^+. Iron and copper ions also bind readily to DNA: the DNA binding affinity of Fe(III) has been calculated to be about 2.1×10^{14} at pH 7.4 and that for Cu^{2+} as 2×10^4. Copper ions bind especially well to guanine, and to a lesser extent, adenine residues. Iron and copper may be associated with DNA inside the nucleus, but can

Table 4.9 Some acute-phase plasma proteins

Protein	Typical increase in concentration	Biological function
Caeruloplasmin	50%	Iron metabolism, antioxidant defence (Section 3.15.2)
C3	50%	Third component of complement; some other components also rise (Fig. 7.11)
Antiproteinases (e.g. α-antiproteinase)	2- to 4-fold	Inhibit proteolytic enzymes, such as elastase. (Section 2.6.3)
Haptoglobin	2- to 4-fold	Binds haemoglobin; antioxidant defence, some chaperone-like effects (Section 3.16.3.4)
C-reactive protein (CRP)	1000-fold or more (little present normally), synthesis induced in hepatocytes by IL-6 and IL-1β; contains five identical subunits arranged around a central 'pore'	Transgenic mice overexpressing CRP are resistant to endotoxin (*Proc. Natl. Acad. Sci.* USA **94**, 2575, 1997)
Serum amyloid A protein (SAA)	Several-hundred-fold	—
Coagulation proteins (fibrinogen, prothrombin, plasminogen, factor VIII)	<10-fold	—

The acute-phase response was first recognized in the 1930s. Patients with pneumonia caused by *Streptococcus pneumoniae* were found to have a protein in their plasma which bound to a polysaccharide (**C-polysaccharide**) from the bacterial cell wall. The protein was thereafter called **C-reactive protein** or **CRP**. Binding is Ca^{2+}-dependent. C-reactive protein is a widely used marker of inflammation (*Circulation* **109**, 1914, 2004) but its exact function is unknown. Studies of its function can be hampered by the fact that commercial products can contain azide as a preservative and endotoxin as a contaminant (*J. Cardiovasc. Pharm.* **45**, 193, 2005; *Circ. Res.* **97**, 135, 2005).

also become spuriously bound to it during DNA isolation, since cell homogenization readily releases iron and copper ions (Section 4.3).

In the centre of the DNA double helix, adenine hydrogen bonds to thymine, and guanine to cytosine. *E. coli* DNA contains 4.2 million base pairs and forms a continuous circle whereas human nuclear DNA is linear and has about 3.3 billion base pairs. In the nuclei of eukaryotic cells, DNA is packaged into **chromosomes** (46 in humans), each of which contains a single length of double-helical DNA. The chromosomes are paired: one in each pair is inherited from the male parent and the other from the mother. There are 22 pairs of **autosomes** (genes on them are **autosomally inherited**) and two **sex chromosomes** (carrying **sex-linked genes**). For example, in males a Y chromosome is inherited from the father and an X chromosome from the mother. Proteins (**histones**) rich in basic amino acid residues (which are positively charged at physiological pH) help in the packaging of DNA in chromosomes; DNA is wound around histones to form **nucleosomes**, arranged like beads on a string,

each containing about 147 base pairs of DNA, separated by flexible linker DNA (Fig. 4.7). The complex of DNA with histones and other proteins is called **chromatin**. In principle, the default state of DNA in chromosomes is to be assembled into nucleosomes. The non-nucleosomal regions are often sites at which gene transcription is initiated and are maintained as non-nucleosomal sites by transcription factors.

DNA is replicated by **DNA polymerases**, enzymes which use deoxyribonucleoside triphosphates (dATP, dGTP, dCTP and dTTP; Table 4.10) to add deoxyribonucleotides, e.g.

$$DNA + dATP \rightarrow (DNA-A) + pyrophosphate$$

$$(DNA-A) + dGTP \rightarrow (DNA-A-G) + pyrophosphate$$

to the 3'-OH terminus of a pre-existing DNA chain, the **primer**. They will not copy single stranded DNA unless a primer is present to give a 'starter point' for the second strand. Indeed, in DNA

Table 4.10 DNA bases, nucleosides and nucleotides; nomenclature as exemplified by guanine

Name	Compound
Guanine	A purine base
Guanosine	Guanine attached to ribose, the combination of base plus sugar is called a **nucleoside**
GMP	Guanosine monophosphate, a nucleoside phosphate (or **nucleotide**)
2′-Deoxyguanosine	A nucleoside, guanine attached to 2′-deoxyribose
8-Hydroxy-2′-deoxyguanosine, 8OHdG	A nucleoside, 8-hydroxyguanine attached to 2′-deoxyribose
8-Hydroxyguanosine, 8OHG	A nucleoside, 8-hydroxyguanine attached to ribose
GTP	Guanosine triphosphate (nucleoside plus 3 phosphate groups; nucleoside triphosphate)
dGTP	Deoxyguanosine triphosphate
8OHdGTP	8-Hydroxy-2′-deoxyguanosine triphosphate

Similarly for adenine (base), 2′-deoxyadenosine or adenosine (nucleosides with deoxyribose or ribose respectively), AMP or dAMP (nucleotides), ATP or dATP (nucleoside triphosphates), and so on for the other two DNA bases.

replication a short RNA primer is used and later removed. Polymerases can only copy from a double helix if the sugar–phosphate backbone of one strand is broken and the helix partly unravelled at the site where copying starts. DNA polymerases only catalyse formation of a phosphodiester bond when the base on the incoming nucleotide forms the correct hydrogen bonds with (is **complementary to**) the base on the strand being copied; guanine with cytosine, and adenine with thymine. Once a base has been inserted, most DNA polymerases 'double-check' it and excise it if it is wrong (the **proof-reading** or **error-checking function**).

The need for an RNA primer causes a problem; the new DNA molecule would have an incomplete 5′ end and should get shorter with every round of replication. This problem is avoided by having **telomeres** at the ends of chromosomes (Section 10.3.5).

4.8.2 Damage to DNA by reactive species

DNA is fairly stable, but does undergo 'spontaneous' chemical decomposition.[118] Loss of purines (leaving **apurinic sites**) has been estimated to occur 10^4 times per day in the human genome. Cytosine can slowly lose its amino group (**deaminate**) to generate uracil, whereas 5-methyl-cytosine in DNA can deaminate to thymine. Oxidative stress accelerates DNA damage, which may be measured as strand breakage and/or chemical modifications to the DNA bases or to deoxyribose (Section 5.13).

DNA isolated from archaeological materials (sometimes called **ancient DNA**) is usually fragmented, depurinated, deaminated, and oxidatively damaged, making it difficult to amplify by PCR.[118,119]

What RS can damage DNA? Some, but not all.[117,120] Physiologically relevant levels of $O_2^{\bullet-}$, $NO^{\bullet}$, H_2O_2 or organic peroxides do not react at significant rates with any of the DNA (or RNA) bases or with the deoxyribose (or ribose) sugars. However, $O_2^{\bullet-}$ and $NO^{\bullet}$ could react with radicals formed after DNA is attacked by more aggressive RS.

4.8.2.1 *Hydroxyl radical*[117,120]

As might be expected from the high reactivity of $OH^{\bullet}$, exposure of DNA (or RNA) to it generates a multitude of products. For example, $OH^{\bullet}$ can add to guanine at positions 4, 5 or 8 in the purine ring. Addition to C-8 produces a C-8 OH-adduct radical that can be reduced to 8-hydroxy-7,8-dihydroguanine, oxidized to 8-hydroxyguanine (Table 4.10 explains the nomenclature) or undergo ring opening followed by one-electron reduction and protonation, to give **2,6-diamino-4-hydroxy-5-formamidopyrimidine**, usually abbreviated as **FAPyG** (Fig. 4.11). Similarly, $OH^{\bullet}$ can add on to C-4, C-5, or C-8 of adenine. Pyrimidines are attacked by $OH^{\bullet}$ to give multiple products. Thus, thymine can suffer addition of $OH^{\bullet}$ to the ring, or $H^{\bullet}$ abstraction from the methyl group. The resulting radicals give rise to a variety of products including **thymine glycols** (5,6-dihydroxy-6-hydrothymines), **5-hydroxy-5-methylhydantoin, 5-formyluracil**, and **5-(hydroxymethyl)**

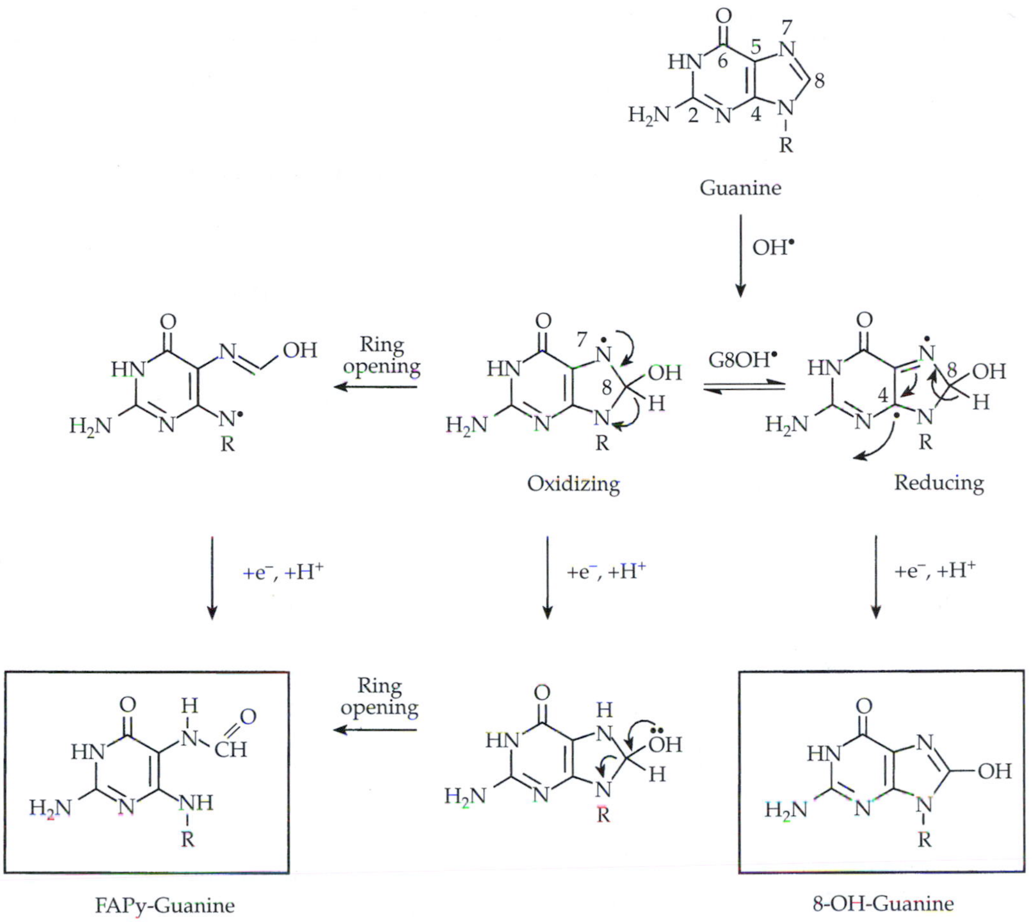

Figure 4.11 Guanine modification by hydroxyl radicals. Addition of OH• to C-8 of guanine in DNA generates an 8-hydroxyguanine radical (Remember the rule; *when a radical reacts with a non-radical, a new radical is formed*). 8-Hydroxyguanine radical can be oxidized (losing one electron) to 8-hydroxyguanine or reduced to give a ring-opened product. Thus to assess radical attack on C-8 of guanine, both 2,6-diamino-4-hydroxy-5-formamidopyrimidine (FAPyG) and 8-hydroxyguanine should be measured, since reaction conditions can affect the ratio between them, i.e. the same amount of OH• attack on guanine can lead to different levels of 8-hydroxyguanine. Attack of OH• at other positions upon guanine also occurs. Adapted from *Free Rad. Biol. Med.* **18**, 1033, 1995 by courtesy of Professor John Murphy, Dr Tony Breen and Elsevier Publishers.

uracil (Fig. 4.12). Cytosine similarly forms several products, including **cytosine glycol** and **5,6-dihydroxycytosine** (Figs 4.12 and 4.13). The presence of O_2 and/or transition metal ions affects the rate and mechanism of the radical reactions and hence the relative amounts of the various end-products obtained (Fig. 4.11; for a human example see Table 9.16). Thus the product distribution will vary depending on whether OH• is generated by radiation or by metal ion–H_2O_2 systems, and if the latter, which metal was used. For example, copper ions bind to GC-rich sequences in DNA;

subsequent reaction with H_2O_2 favours formation of guanine damage products.[121]

Deoxyribose and ribose are fragmented by OH•, yielding dozens of products. All positions are susceptible to hydrogen abstraction by OH•, forming carbon-centred radicals. In the presence of O_2 these convert rapidly to sugar peroxyl radicals, which undergo a series of reactions, including disproportionation, rearrangement, elimination of water and C–C bond fragmentation, to yield a variety of carbonyl products. Some sugar products remain within DNA or constitute end groups of broken

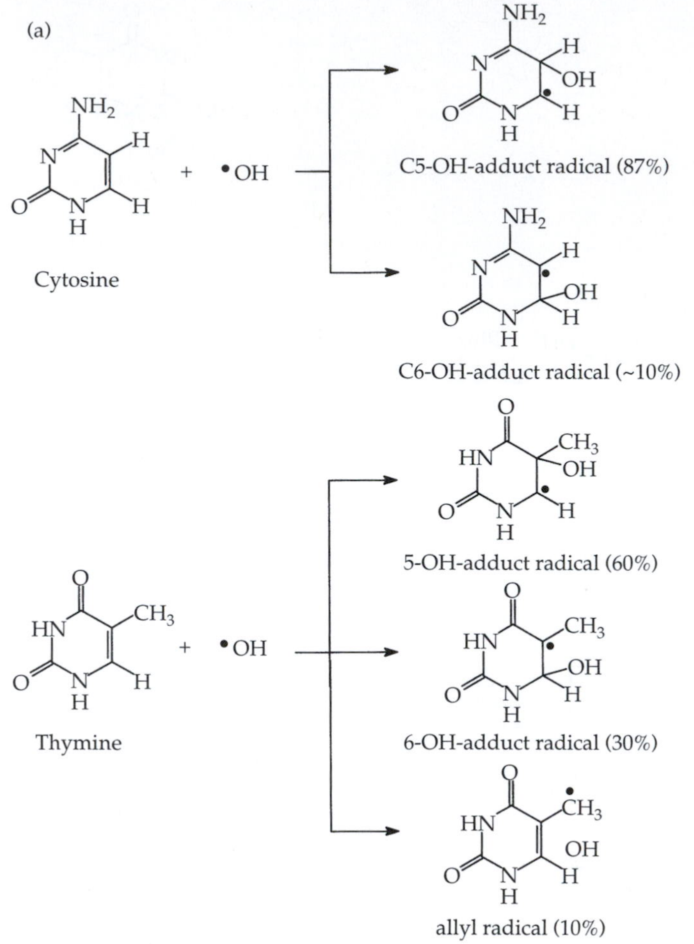

(a)

Cytosine + •OH →

C5-OH-adduct radical (87%)

C6-OH-adduct radical (~10%)

Thymine + •OH →

5-OH-adduct radical (60%)

6-OH-adduct radical (30%)

allyl radical (10%)

Figure 4.12 (a) Reactions of OH• with pyrimidines. (b) What happens next; some fates of the thymine radicals. From Ref.[120] by courtesy of Drs Evans, Dizdaroglu and Cooke, and Elsevier.

DNA strands, whereas others are released. Irradiated solutions of 2-deoxy-D-ribose produce carbonyls and dicarbonyls which are mutagenic to *Salmonella typhimurium* (in the Ames test). Malondialdehyde (MDA) is also produced. Like many carbohydrates, 2-deoxy-D-ribose binds iron, which makes it vulnerable to attack by OH• produced during Fenton reactions. Indeed, release of MDA from 2-deoxy-D-ribose is the basis of an assay for OH• (Section 5.3.3).

At low O_2 levels, the C5' radicals of deoxyribose can survive long enough to add on to C8 on purine rings in the same nucleoside, resulting in cyclised products, **8,5'-cyclo-2'-deoxyguanosine (cyclodG)** and **8,5'-cyclo-2'-deoxyadenosine (cyclodA)** (Fig. 4.13). Two stereoisomers (R and S) of each can form.

Nuclear proteins can be attacked by OH•. Protein radicals can cross-link to DNA base-derived radicals if the two meet in chromatin, giving **DNA-protein cross-links** that can interfere with chromatin unfolding, DNA repair, replication and transcription.[122] Alternatively, DNA base radicals can attack amino acid residues. For example, the allyl radical of thymine (Fig. 4.12a) can attack tyrosine residues to form a thymine–tyrosine cross-link. Treatment of rats with ferric-NTA, a renal carcinogen and promoter of Fenton chemistry (Section 3.15.4.2) increased levels of thymine–tyrosine cross-links in kidney chromatin.[123]

4.8.2.2 *Hydrogen peroxide*[124]
Addition of H_2O_2 to cells often produces increased DNA strand breakage within minutes accompanied

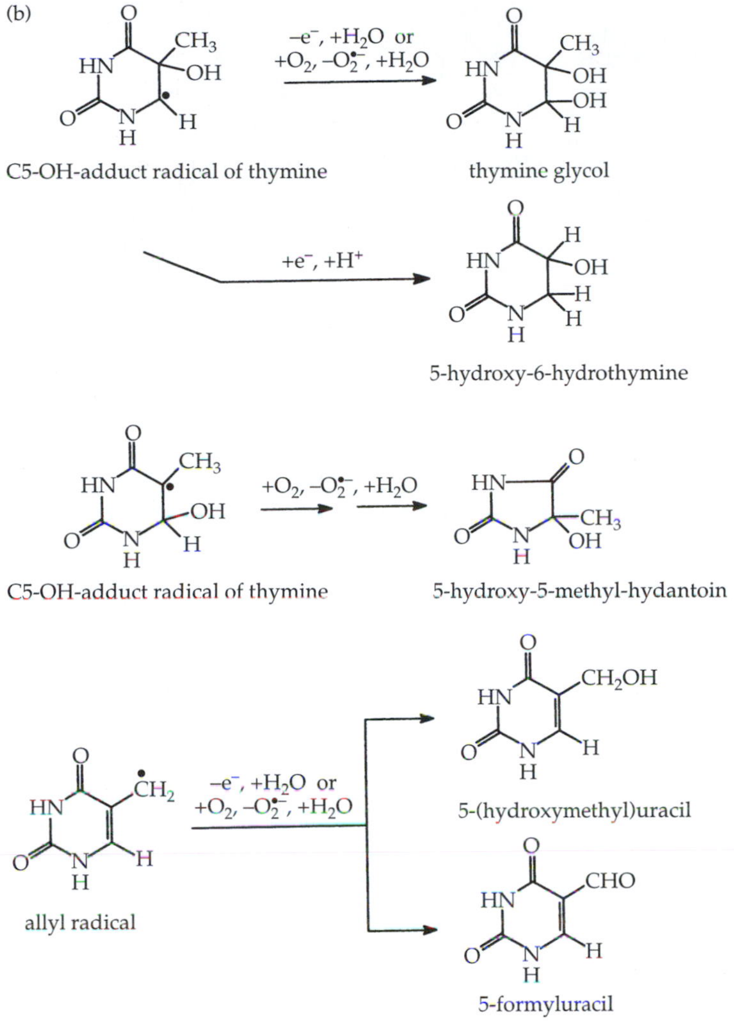
(b)
CH3
HN
OH
O
N
H
H
C5-OH-adduct radical of thymine
−e⁻, +H2O or
+O2, −O2•⁻, +H2O
thymine glycol
+e⁻, +H⁺
5-hydroxy-6-hydrothymine
+O2, −O2•⁻, +H2O
C5-OH-adduct radical of thymine
5-hydroxy-5-methyl-hydantoin
CH2OH
5-(hydroxymethyl)uracil
CH2
allyl radical
CHO
5-formyluracil

Figure 4.12 *(Cont.)*

by an increase in base modification products (Fig. 4.14). RNA can also be oxidized, sometimes more so than DNA.[125] Yet H_2O_2 does not damage DNA or RNA directly. The pattern of DNA damage (rises in the levels of multiple products from all four bases) indicates attack by $OH^{\bullet}$. If $OH^{\bullet}$ is attacking DNA, it must be produced very close to it since $OH^{\bullet}$ is too reactive to diffuse from its site of formation. The likely culprit is Fenton chemistry. Pretreatment of cells with certain metal ion chelating agents (such as *o*-phenanthroline) prevents damage to DNA by peroxides (Section 3.6.2.2). If Fenton chemistry generates $OH^{\bullet}$ in the nucleus, then the iron ions must be in close proximity to DNA. Copper/ H_2O_2 reactions may also generate DNA-damaging oxo-copper complexes in addition to $OH^{\bullet}$ (Section 2.4.6).

Are metals always bound to DNA *in vivo*? They might be; iron and copper are present in the nucleus, but this does not mean that they are in a molecular form that will cause $OH^{\bullet}$ formation. Another possibility is that oxidative stress causes release of intracellular iron and/or copper ions that then bind readily to DNA (Section 4.3), making it a target of H_2O_2 attack. In human lymphocytes, it

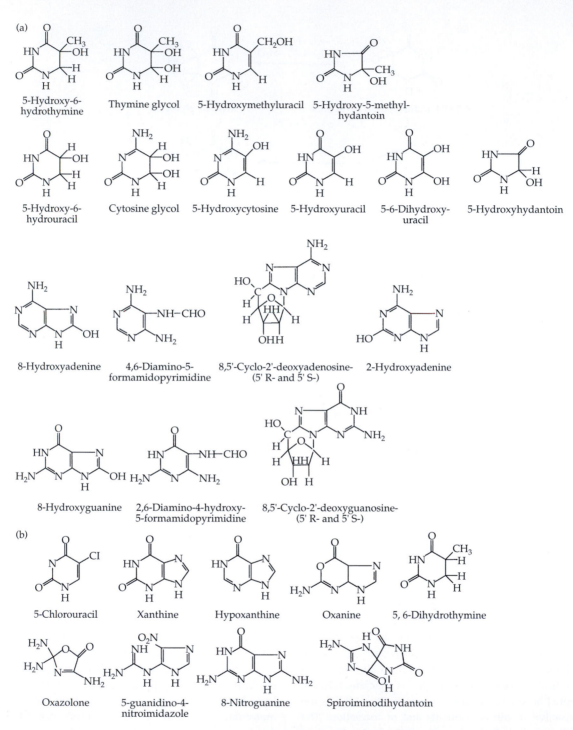

Figure 4.13 Some of the products resulting from attack of reactive species upon DNA bases. (a) Modified bases that can be formed by OH•. (b) 5–6-Dihydrothymine is a product of attack of H• or hydrated electrons upon thymine. 8-Nitroguanine is formed by reaction of DNA with ONOO⁻. Xanthine and hypoxanthine result from deamination of guanine and adenine respectively. 5-Chlorouracil is a chlorinated base produced when DNA is treated with HOCl and subsequently hydrolysed with acid; it probably results from breakdown of the initially formed chlorocytosine under acidic conditions (*Chem. Res. Toxicol,* **10**, 1240, 1997).

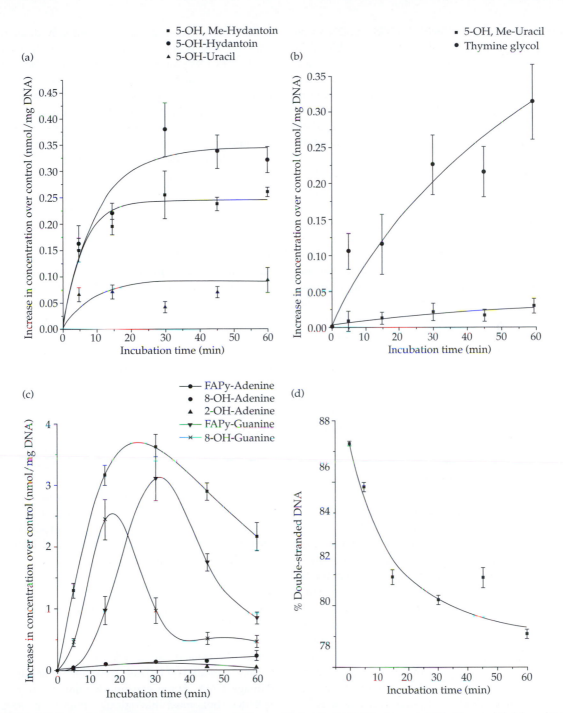

Figure 4.14 Rates of repair of oxidative DNA base damage. Human respiratory tract epithelial cells were treated with a non-lethal dose of H_2O_2 (100 μM). Note the formation of a wide range of base oxidation products, characteristic of attack by $OH^\bullet$, as well as the rapid onset of repair of some (c) but not all (a, b) base damage products. During repair, DNA strand breakage (d) continues to increase, since repair itself involves DNA strand breakage. Data by courtesy of Dr Jeremy Spencer.

was observed that the level of 8OHdG in DNA was positively correlated with that of the labile iron pool; the size of this pool is known to be increased by H_2O_2 addition (Section 3.15.1.3).[126] In cultured cells, raising the level of Fe^{2+} in the culture medium increases steady-state levels of oxidative DNA damage.[127] The damaging effects of H_2O_2 on *E. coli* also involve metal ion release and Fenton-type chemistry.[128]

Either way, the presence of metal ions on DNA favours 'site-specific' $OH^•$ generation, leading to DNA damage that '$OH^•$ scavengers' find it difficult to protect against. Another reason for lack of protection by scavengers is that some of the scavenger-derived radicals themselves cause DNA damage.[129] Radicals derived from formate, propan-2-ol, glycerol and (under anoxic conditions) dimethysulphoxide are able to cause single-strand breaks in DNA. The latter is due to methyl ($CH_3^•$) radicals; when O_2 is present $CH_3^•$ radicals react rapidly to give $CH_3O_2^•$, apparently less damaging.

DNA-associated copper ions might also react with certain phenols (e.g. 2-hydroxyoestradiol, 2-methoxyoestradiol, diethylstilboestrol and L-DOPA) to produce ROS and oxidized phenols. This could form a range of oxidative DNA lesions and phenol adducts to the DNA bases, which might contribute to the carcinogenicity of certain phenolic compounds (Section 9.14.1).[130]

4.8.2.3 *Use of iron and hydrogen peroxide for oxidative 'footprinting'*

Binding of transcription factors to DNA regulates gene expression and so it is important to identify the DNA sequence to which a given protein binds. This can be achieved by 'footprinting'. Essentially, the DNA–protein complex is treated with a DNA-degrading reagent such as a deoxyribonuclease. The bound protein protects the part of the DNA to which it is attached, which can then be isolated and sequenced. The high reactivity of $OH^•$ towards DNA has led to the development of alternative footprinting methods.[131] In one, reaction of Fe^{2+}-EDTA with H_2O_2 is used to produce $OH^•$. Iron(II)-EDTA has a negative charge at physiological pH, and so will not bind to DNA (also negatively charged). Any $OH^•$ produced by reaction of Fe^{2+}-EDTA with H_2O_2 that escape scavenging by the

EDTA enter 'free solution' and randomly damage sites in DNA. A bound protein blocks the cleavage of DNA by $OH^•$, allowing identification of the base sequence to which it was bound. Since $OH^•$ has no marked sequence preference, it does not have the specificity problems encountered with nuclease enzymes. It is also possible to attach Fe^{2+}-EDTA to compounds that intercalate into DNA at specific sites, allowing site-specific cleavage by $OH^•$. Some authors have used similar 'oxidative footprinting' techniques to analyse protein structure: the most 'accessible' parts of a protein will be targeted by $OH^•$ first.[131]

4.8.2.4 *Histidine, H_2O_2 and DNA damage*

Some amino acids present in cell culture media, especially histidine, enhance DNA damage by H_2O_2. Since this effect is usually decreased by metal ion chelators, it may involve metal binding.[132] Whether these effects are important *in vivo* remains to be ascertained, but histidine also promotes iron-dependent lipid peroxidation (Section 3.18.7).

4.8.2.5 *Singlet oxygen*

The singlet states of oxygen are far more limited in their attack on DNA than is $OH^•$. Singlet O_2 is inefficient at producing strand breakage and attacks only guanine, the base in DNA that is the easiest to oxidize. Singlet O_2 adds across the 4,8 bond of the imidazole ring to give unstable endoperoxides that generate various products[133] including 8OHdG; this is readily oxidized further by $^1O_2$ (Section 4.8.2.12 below).

4.8.2.6 *Carbonate radical*

This also generates 8OHdG from guanine in DNA.[134]

4.8.2.7 *Peroxyl and alkoxyl radicals*

Peroxyl and alkoxyl radicals have limited ability to damage DNA. Some can attack guanine to give 8OHdG, but most biologically important ones probably do not (Section 2.5.4).

4.8.2.8 *Hypochlorous acid*

This mainly targets pyrimidines in DNA, although there is some chlorination of adenine (to

8-chloroadenine). Major end-products formed include thymine glycol and 5-chlorocytosine.[135] The latter has been detected at sites of inflammation in rats, indicative of HOCl-mediated (or at least RCS-mediated) DNA damage *in vivo*.[136] Hypobromous acid (HOBr) can brominate cytosine and adenine residues.[137] Chloramines and bromamines formed by reaction of HOCl/HOBr with $-NH_2$ groups on the DNA bases are probably intermediates in formation of these other halogenated bases.

4.8.2.9 *Ozone*[138]

This can fragment DNA and oxidize bases (especially guanine and thymine) both directly and via formation of $OH^{\bullet}$ in aqueous solution (Section 2.6.5).

4.8.2.10 *Reactive nitrogen species*

Exposure of DNA to N_2O_3 or HNO_2 (probably via N_2O_3) can deaminate DNA bases, converting cytosine to uracil, 5-methylcytosine to thymine and adenine to hypoxanthine. Guanine, the preferred target of attack, is converted to xanthine and oxanine (Fig. 4.13).[139,140] Oxanine can cross-link to amino groups on nuclear proteins.[140] Peroxynitrite (probably via its reaction products with CO_2/HCO_3^-; Section 2.6.1.1) converts guanine into 8-nitroguanine (Fig. 4.13), which is rapidly lost from DNA by spontaneous depurination. A more stable end-product is **5-guanidino-4-nitroimidazole** (Fig. 4.13).[141] Some 8OHdG is formed when $ONOO^-$ attacks DNA, but it is rapidly oxidized by $ONOO^-$.

4.8.2.11 *Ultraviolet light*

UV light readily damages DNA. First, UV-C can convert H_2O_2 to $OH^{\bullet}$. Second (and more important), UV leads to covalent cross-linking of adjacent pyrimidines to give **cyclobutane pyrimidine dimers** and **6−4 photoproducts** (Fig. 6.24).

4.8.2.12 *Oxidation of oxidation products*

DNA base oxidation products are themselves subject to oxidation. This is especially true for 8OHdG, which is much more easily oxidizable than guanine, itself the most oxidizable of the four DNA bases. 8-Hydroguanine can be oxidized by singlet O_2, chromium salts (Section 8.15.4), HNO_2, $CO_3^{\bullet-}$, $ONOO^-$ and HOCl.[133,139,141] Singlet O_2 can oxidize it to cyanuric and oxaluric acid, $CO_3^{\bullet-}$ or singlet O_2

to **spiroiminodihydantoin** (Fig. 4.13) and $ONOO^-$ to a range of products including spiroiminodihydantoin, **oxazolone**, oxaluric and cyanuric acids. The product distribution varies enormously depending on how much $ONOO^-$ is added.[141]

4.8.3 Damage to mitochondrial and chloroplast DNA

In both plants and animals the genetic information encoding the vast majority of proteins is encoded in nuclear DNA. However, chloroplasts and mitochondria contain some DNA that encodes a few proteins.

Reactive species can damage mitochondrial and chloroplast DNA; mitochondrial DNA damage has been suggested to be important in several human diseases and in ageing (Section 10.4). Indeed, great excitement was generated by a report in 1988 that oxidative DNA base damage (measured as levels of 8OHdG) is several-fold higher in mitochondrial DNA than in nuclear DNA. This seemed logical because of the proximity of mitochondrial DNA to ROS generated during electron transport, and the fact that mitochondrial DNA is not protected by histones. It was also suggested that DNA repair in mitochondria is less rapid than in the nucleus and that oxidative damage could contribute to the deletions and other mutations in mitochondrial DNA that are known to accumulate with age. The mtDNA genome has no introns, so that a random 'hit' by a RS is more likely to damage a gene than it is for nuclear DNA.

However, ROS do not normally cause specific deletions in DNA, but rather point mutations (Section 4.9 below). It may be that some base oxidation products cause mitochondrial DNA polymerase (**pol γ**) to 'slip' on the DNA to generate deletions, and/or that oxidative damage to the polymerase diminishes its capacity for accurate replication.[124,142] Only recently have the difficulties in accurately quantitating oxidative damage in mitochondrial DNA been appreciated (Section 5.13). A review of the literature by Beckman and Ames concluded that the huge disparity between published measurements of oxidative damage makes it impossible to confidently conclude that mtDNA suffers greater oxidation than nuclear DNA.[143]

The high O_2 concentrations generated during photosynthesis (Section 6.8) would be expected to favour damage to chloroplast DNA, but little information is available on this topic. Plant nuclei contain DNA repair enzymes, but the rate of repair of UV-induced lesions (and probably of other lesions) appears slower in the chloroplast than in the nucleus.[144]

4.9 Consequences of damage to DNA by reactive species

4.9.1 Mutation[120,145]

Damage to DNA (oxidative or otherwise) usually halts DNA replication and cell division, by mechanisms involving p53 (Section 9.13.4.2), until repair is complete. Too much DNA damage can lead to cell death via p53-mediated apoptosis and/or NAD^+ depletion via PARP (Section 4.2.4). However, if not all base or sugar lesions are removed before DNA replication resumes or begins, error-prone **translesional DNA synthesis (TDS)** can occur. Polymerases normally involved in DNA replication have efficient error-correcting mechanisms, but in TDS they are transiently replaced by others with less fidelity until the lesion is bypassed (Fig. 4.15, Plate 7), increasing the mutation rate.[145]

Several modified DNA bases can mispair. For example, whereas adenine pairs with thymine, its deamination product hypoxanthine can pair with cytosine. Uracil pairs with adenine rather than guanine. Thus RNS cause **AT $\leftrightarrow$ GC transition mutations**, for example

$$G-C \xrightarrow[\substack{\text{deamination} \\ \text{of C}}]{\text{RNS}} G\text{---}U \xrightarrow[\text{replication}]{\text{DNA}} \begin{array}{c} G-C \\ + \\ A\text{---}U \xrightarrow[\text{replication}]{\text{DNA}} A-T \end{array}$$

$$A-T \xrightarrow[\substack{\text{deamination} \\ \text{of A}}]{\text{RNS}} HX\text{---}T \longrightarrow \begin{array}{c} HX\text{---}C \longrightarrow G-C \\ + \\ A-T \end{array}$$

8-Nitroguanine residues in DNA can cause G $\rightarrow$ T transversions as well as spontaneously

deaminate, leaving an AP site that might produce mutation. 5-Guanidino-4-nitroimidazole (Section 4.8.2.10) is also mutagenic, producing G $\rightarrow$ C transversions and G $\rightarrow$ A and G $\rightarrow$ T transitions.

The presence of thymine glycol is a strong block to DNA replication, but it can lead to T $\rightarrow$ C transition mutations (although most thymine glycol hydrogen bonds correctly with adenine). 5-Hydroxycytosine and 5-hydroxyuracil can mispair with adenine giving C $\rightarrow$ T transitions. 5-Hydroxymethyluracil mispairs (again with a low probability) to guanine. 8-Hydroxyguanine leads to **GC $\rightarrow$ TA transversion** mutations since it can hydrogen bond to adenine, although most 8-hydroxyguanine pairs correctly with cytosine.

$$G-C \xrightarrow{\text{RNS}} 8OHG-C \xrightarrow[\text{replication}]{\text{DNA}} \begin{array}{c} 8OHG\text{---}A \\ + \\ G-C \end{array} \xrightarrow[\text{replication}]{\text{DNA}} T-A$$

Some of the oxidation products of 8OHdG, such as oxaluric acid, oxazalone, cyanuric acid and spiroiminodihydantoin (Section 4.8.2.12) may be more mutagenic than 8OHdG.[146] 8-Hydroxyadenine has a low probability of mispairing with guanine, but mostly it pairs correctly with thymine and is less mutagenic than 8OHG. The ring-opened purines (FAPyG, FAPyA) are thought to block DNA replication. Some end-products of lipid peroxidation can also bind to DNA and cause mutations (Section 4.12.5 below).

One approach to examining the overall mutagenic effect of base changes in DNA is to expose cells to RS and look for mutations in the nuclear or mitochondrial genomes or in transfected DNA. For example, in one study[147] a plasmid was transfected into monkey cells. The cells were treated with H_2O_2 and then incubated to allow repair and replication of the plasmid, which was then isolated and sequenced. The mutations detected included deletions and base substitutions. Such studies reveal that the distribution of mutations induced by RS is not random; they cluster at so-called **hotspots**. This can be accounted for by several mechanisms, including accessibility of DNA to the RS and to repair enzymes (for example, internucleosomal DNA is more exposed than DNA

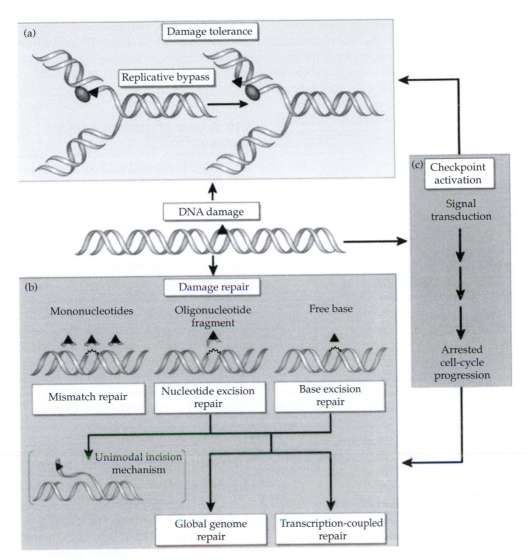

Figure 4.15 (see plate 7) Responses to DNA damage. DNA damage (▲) results in either repair or tolerance. (a) During damage tolerance, damaged sites are recognized by the replication machinery before they can be repaired, resulting in an arrest that can be relieved by replicative bypass (translesional DNA synthesis). (b) DNA repair involves the excision of bases and DNA resynthesis(〰〰〰), which requires double-stranded DNA. Mispaired bases, usually generated by mistakes during DNA replication, are excised as single nucleotides during mismatch repair. A damaged base is excised as a single free base (base excision repair) or as an oligonucleotide fragment (nucleotide excision repair). Such fragments are generated by incisions flanking either side of the damaged base. (c) The cell has a network of complex signalling pathways that arrest the cell cycle and may ultimately lead to apoptosis. From *Nature* **421**, 436, 2003 by courtesy of Dr EC Friedberg and the publishers.

within nucleosomes), the sequence around a particular base influencing its oxidizability, and patterns of transition metal ion binding. Similar studies have been done with $ONOO^-$; a range of mutations results, depending on how the $ONOO^-$ is added (bolus or slow steady generation).[141]

Among the mutations identified in such studies are CC → TT transitions, so-called **tandem mutations**,[148] which can also arise from damage by UV light (Section 6.12.1.2). However, the most common changes observed are C → T transitions, and G → C and G → T transversions. The G → T changes often involve 8OHdG, for example in cells exposed to singlet O_2 G → T was the most common mutation since singlet O_2 is selective for damage at guanine. However, none of the above mutations is unique to oxidative damage: they can also occur as a result of polymerase errors, spontaneous deamination of cytosine to uracil (or 5-methylcytosine to thymine), and the misreplication of certain DNA–carcinogen adducts.

4.9.2 Misincorporation

Nucleosides and nucleotides can be modified by RS *prior to* their incorporation into RNA or DNA, thus introducing mutagenic lesions directly. This can happen with bromodeoxycytidine, a product of attack of HOBr on cytosine nucleoside,[149] although most attention has been paid to 8OHdG (Section 4.10.2 below).

4.9.3 Changes in gene expression[120]

A mutation in an exon might lead to an altered protein. However, mutations in introns are not necessarily innocuous, for example they can affect mRNA splicing. Mutations in promoter regions could affect transcription factor binding and alter gene expression, as has been demonstrated in the ageing brain (Sections 5.13.8 and 10.4.5). For example, some studies report that replacement of G by 8OHdG in promoters alters binding of AP-1 or NF-κB. Another possibility is that oxidative base damage can interfere with methylation of CpG, an event which usually suppresses gene transcription. If so, aberrant gene expression might result.[150]

4.9.4 Having sex

The multicellular green alga *Volvox carteri* normally reproduces asexually, but abnormally high temperatures cause production of **sexual inducer**. This glycoprotein acts on the reproductive cells so that in the next generation both females (carrying eggs) and males (with sperm) are produced and sexual reproduction occurs. The 'heat stress' appears to act by raising levels of ROS, which trigger the sexual response.[151] The related unicellular alga *Chlamydomonas reinhardtii* responds similarly but to

a different stress, nitrogen deprivation. Was the need to cope with oxidative DNA damage one of the driving forces for sexual reproduction to evolve?[152] It's an interesting hypothesis.

4.10 Repair of oxidative DNA damage[118,120,153]

DNA repair is essential to allow aerobes to survive without excessive mutation. DNA damage by RS is not the only problem. The polymerases that replicate DNA show high fidelity because of their error-correcting function, but do make some mistakes, and **mismatch repair** is needed to remove mispaired bases. Spontaneous depurinations/ deaminations must be repaired, as must adducts of xenobiotics that find their way onto DNA. One advantage of the DNA double helix is that, if one strand is damaged, the information in the other strand can be used to help repair it accurately. Thus double-strand breaks are intrinsically more damaging because this information is not available.[154] In addition, in a double helix the DNA bases are less exposed to attack, and they undergo spontaneous deamination/depurination at lower rates.

4.10.1 Reversing the chemical change[155,156]

Direct reversal of changes in DNA can sometimes occur. For example, *E. coli* contains a **DNA photolyase**. This enzyme binds to pyrimidine dimers in DNA, absorbs light in the near-UV and blue spectral regions, and uses the energy to split the dimers back to the original DNA bases. Photolyases contain two chromogens. One is FAD and the other differs according to the source of the enzyme (in *E. coli* it is a folate derivative). The excited flavin is thought to transfer an electron to the dimer to generate a radical pair (FADH$^{\bullet}$ plus [pyr-pyr]$^{\bullet-}$). The dimer splits and the electron is returned to the flavin to regenerate the catalytically-active FADH^{-} form.

Why such an enzyme is present in an organism whose normal habitat is the dark recesses of the animal colon (or in the light-shielded brain of the opossum!) is an enigma. However, similar enzymes are found in many eukaryotes, including

Drosophila, plants (Section 6.8.10), the goldfish *Carassius auratus* and some mammals (the opossum, as already mentioned, and the kangaroo rat; both marsupials) but not humans. In the absence of light, the photolyase can still bind to pyrimidine dimers and it has been suggested that it can facilitate repair by other mechanisms as well. For example, *E. coli* DNA photolyase binds to DNA cross-linked by *cis*-platin (an anticancer drug; Section 9.15) and stimulates removal of the cross-link by excision repair (Section 4.10.3 below). In humans, proteins similar to photolyases have been identified (**cryptochromes**), but act instead to regulate circadian rhythms.

Methylation of guanine in DNA by certain carcinogens forms a mutagenic lesion, O^6-methylguanine. O^6-**Methylguanine-DNA-methyltransferase**, found in all species, is a 'suicide' enzyme that repairs DNA directly; it transfers the O^6-methyl group to a cysteine residue at its active site, simultaneously inactivating itself. Inactive enzyme is then degraded by the proteasome. Overexpression of this enzyme helps to protect mice from cancers induced by DNA-alkylating agents.

Thymine hydroperoxide is a substrate for GPx4 and GST enzymes (Section 3.8) although the biological significance of this (and of the alcohol product) are uncertain. Glutathione can 'repair' the initial radicals generated by attack of some RS on DNA, preventing formation of oxidation products (Section 8.19).

4.10.2 Don't let it in: sanitization of the nucleotide pool[157,158]

Just as DNA and RNA can be oxidized, so can their precursors (Section 4.9.2). Some years ago, mutation of the *mutT* gene in *E. coli* was found to increase the occurrence of AT ↔ CG transversions. The MutT protein was later identified as an enzyme that destroys oxidized dGTP. It recognizes dGTP containing 8-hydroxyguanine (**8OHdGTP**) and prevents its incorporation into DNA, by hydrolysing it to the monophosphate 8OHdGMP. MutT also acts on 8OHGTP, an oxidized ribonucleoside precursor of RNA. A similar enzyme, **MTH1 (mutT homologue 1)** occurs in mammalian (including human) cells. It

hydrolyses 8OHGTP, 8- and 2-OHdATPs and 8-chlorodGTP as well as 8OHdGTP, and thus has a broader substrate specificity than *E. coli* mutT (which does not act on oxidized adenine derivatives). In mice, exceptionally high MTH1 levels are found in embryonic stem cells: levels in mouse liver, thymus and large intestine are also high. The 8OHdGMP produced cannot be rephosphorylated and is further hydrolysed to 8OHdG, which is excreted in urine in animals, including humans (Section 5.13.3). The dGTP pool is the smallest of the DNA precursor pools and turns over rapidly—is this perhaps another strategy to minimize damage to it?[118]

E. coli has a second enzyme that can remove 8OHdGTP, **GTP cyclohydrolase II**, and human cells may also have an enzyme (**NUDT5 protein**) that hydrolyses 8OHdGDP (but not 8OHdGTP) to 8OHdGMP.[158]

4.10.3 Chop it out: excision repair[153,155]

In one type of excision repair (the only type used for bulky lesions such as pyrimidine dimers, propanodeoxyguanosine adducts [Section 4.12.5.3 below] and certain carcinogen adducts) the DNA is cut some distance on either side of the lesion, which is thus removed as part of an oligonucleotide (Fig. 4.15). A DNA polymerase fills the gap (using information from the undamaged strand) and a ligase seals the DNA. This process is called **nucleotide excision repair (NER)**, and occurs in two forms. **Global genomic repair** acts on the non-transcribed parts of the genome whereas **transcription-coupled repair** acts on the transcribed strand of active genes to remove mutagenic and 'blocking' (i.e. those that can halt transcription) lesions. Nucleotide excision repair is especially important in removing UV-induced damage in animals, but it may also help remove oxidative DNA lesions such as 8OdHG and cyclo-2′-deoxyadenosine (Fig. 4.13).[159] Nucleotide excision repair in mammals begins with damage recognition by a set of proteins including **XPC**, followed by unwinding of DNA by another protein complex (that includes **XPB** and **XPD**), and incision by enzymes, including **XPF**. Abnormalities in XP proteins cause the disease **xeroderma pigmentosum** (Section 4.10.8 below).

In the second type of excision repair, the one used most often to remove oxidative damage, the damaged base is removed directly (**base excision repair, BER**). **DNA glycosylase** enzymes hydrolyse the bond linking the abnormal base to the sugar–phosphate backbone (Fig. 4.15), removing the base and leaving an **apurinic** or **apyrimidinic** site (AP site) in DNA. These sites are mutagenic and block transcription and DNA replication; they also arise by spontaneous base loss in DNA, and depurination of 8-nitroguanine. Some glycosylases are **bifunctional**; as well as removing the base they cut the DNA at the AP site. Other glycosylases (the **monofunctional** ones) cannot, and cleavage is then by a separate AP endonuclease enzyme. After cleavage, a polymerase (usually **polβ**) removes the AP site and inserts the correct nucleotide, and the DNA is then sealed (**short patch BER**). Sometimes the gap is extended by two to eight nucleotides before final repair and ligase action (**long patch BER**). Short-patch BER is more common when dealing with oxidized bases, long-patch for spontaneous base loss.

Human **AP endonuclease-1 (APE1)** plays a key role in BER, and also activates AP1 transcription factors (Section 4.5.9), a process involving a cysteine residue in its N-terminal half. Thus it is sometimes called **redox effector factor 1 (Ref 1)**. This activity also promotes NF-κB binding to DNA and can reduce oxidized p53 (Section 9.13.5); the reduced state of APE1 is maintained by thioredoxin. Activation of PARP (Section 4.2.4) facilitates BER by causing accumulation of **XRCC1**, a **scaffold protein** that associates with automodified PARP-1 and then helps the various proteins involved in BER (such as APE-1, DNA ligase and polβ) to assemble correctly.

Examples of BER include removal of hypoxanthine from DNA by **hypoxanthine–DNA glycosylase** and removal of uracil by **uracil–DNA glycosylase** (a monofunctional glycosylase). Both are found in bacterial and human cells. The **OGG1** enzymes remove 8OHdG and FaPyG residues from DNA and are present in animals, humans and yeast. The human enzyme (**hOGG1**) is a bifunctional glycosylase with nuclear and mitochondrial isoforms. A genetic polymorphism at codon 326 (ser 326 to cys) has been described; the serine-containing form of the

enzyme has been suggested to be more active in removing 8OHdG from DNA.

DNA repair enzymes have usually been purified by assaying their ability to act upon a single base lesion. However, they are often found to have a broader specificity when tested against a range of lesions.[160] For example, human uracil glycosylase also recognizes three uracil derivatives generated by oxidative damage to cytosine (5-hydroxyuracil, alloxan and isodialuric acid), while *E. coli* endonuclease III (a glycosylase despite its name) releases a range of thymine and cytosine oxidation products. This enzyme has a [4Fe–4S] cluster at its active site. A **FAPy glycosylase** that removes formamidopyrimidines and 8OHdG from DNA has been found in both bacteria (e.g. in *E. coli* it is called **Fpg** or **MutM**) and in mammalian cells.

E. coli also contains **MutY**, a glycosylase that removes adenine from adenine: 8OHdG mispairs. A similar adenine–DNA glycosylase is found in humans and called **hMYH (human MutY homologue)**, sometimes written as **hMUTYH**. It can remove 2-hydroxyadenine residues from DNA and also adenine itself wrongly incorporated adjacent to 8OHdG, i.e. it is involved it is involved both in excision repair and in mismatch repair (Section 4.10.4 below).

4.10.4 Mismatch repair[155]

Nucleotide and base excision repair correct errors in DNA before replication, whereas mismatch repair acts after replication to remove wrongly-paired bases caused by polymerase errors or miscoding induced by any DNA base modifications that were not removed. A protein complex, **MutS**α, 'spots' base mismatches such as G/T, G/G, C/C or A/C, and recruits a nuclease to excise the mispaired base.

4.10.5 Repair of 8OHdG

To see how various mechanisms integrate, let us ask how cells are protected against the mutagenicity of 8OHdG. First, removing 8OHdGTP from the precursor pool deters its incorporation into DNA. Second, BER, usually short-patch BER, is normally the major removal path of 8OHdG from DNA.

However, NER can also remove it. Fourth, if 8OHG escapes repair and mispairs with adenine, mismatch repair removes the A from the 8OHG:A pair. Overall, 8OHdG is repaired faster than several other base lesions, at least in certain human cell types (Fig. 4.14), consistent with the view that it is an important mutagenic lesion that cells must remove quickly.

4.10.6 Repair of double-strand breaks[154]

Cells cope with DNA double-strand breaks in two ways. In **homologous recombination** the DNA ends are trimmed in the $5' \rightarrow 3'$ direction by nucleases and the 3'-single-stranded tails invade the double helix of an undamaged homologous DNA strand. DNA polymerase extends the strand using information from the intact partner. When extension is complete the two strands separate. The **Rad proteins** play key roles in organizing homologous recombination, and the protein kinase **ATM** (Section 4.10.8 below) is also important; when DNA damage occurs, ATM phosphorylates many proteins, including p53. In **non-homologous recombination**, a common pathway for repair of damage by ionizing radiation, damaged bases/ sugars are trimmed from the broken end, replaced (without the benefit of an intact strand as template) and resealing occurs. This is error-prone, and small deletions often occur. Severe errors can generate large abnormalities in DNA, visible on the chromosome (**chromosomal aberrations**), or can lead to loss of chromosome portions. A key component of the non-homologous system is a DNA-dependent protein kinase that recognizes free DNA ends and phosphorylates proteins involved in the repair process. Another is the **Ku protein** which binds to double-strand breaks and acts as an alignment factor.

4.10.7 Mitochondrial DNA repair[161]

Until recently it was thought that repair of damage to mtDNA is slow and inefficient. That view is changing, although our knowledge is less extensive than for nuclear DNA repair. The only DNA polymerase in mitochondria, **Pol**γ, serves both for replication and repair. Short-patch BER occurs in

mitochondria, and in humans MutY and OGG1 are present in both nucleus and mitochondria. 8-Hydroxydeoxyguanosine is removed from mtDNA as efficiently as from nuclear DNA. In addition, MTH1 is present in mitochondria, to deter incorporation of 8OHdGTP and other oxidized DNA precursors (Section 4.10.2) into mtDNA.

4.10.8 Is DNA repair important?[153,155]

4.10.8.1 *Bacteria to mice*

DNA isolated from aerobic microorganisms, plants and animals (including humans) contains low levels of DNA base damage products (Section 5.13), suggesting that repair enzymes do not achieve complete removal of modified bases. Damage recognition may be the rate-limiting step in repair, since in humans over 10^9 base pairs must be 'probed' for errors by limited numbers of repair enzymes (e.g. only about 50 000 hOGG1 molecules per human cell)[162] to locate what are rare (<1 in 10^5 bases) lesions. Defects in DNA that is being replicated or transcribed appear to be repaired more rapidly than in DNA in condensed chromatin. In part, this occurs because the DNA is more available to repair enzymes, but transcription coupled repair is also important (Section 4.10.3). Consistent with this limitation on DNA repair rates, the steady-state levels of one or more base damage products increase in many diseases associated with increased RS production (Chapter 9). In *E. coli* and many other bacteria, a rise in DNA damage rapidly increases the activity of repair enzymes (the **SOS response**).[163]

Hence interfering with DNA repair would be expected to cause problems. This is indeed the case. Mice lacking MTH1 (Section 4.10.2) show increased mutation rates and an enhanced rate of spontaneous tumorigenesis, especially in the lung and liver; so do mice deficient in mismatch repair. Mice lacking OGG1 are viable and show some elevations in 8OHdG, but have more limited increases in cancer development, for example they develop more skin cancer after UVB irradiation (Section 6.12.1.2). Mice without MUTYH show increased intestinal cancers. Knockout studies indicate an absolute requirement for APE1 and polβ for survival; homozygous knockouts die during embryonic development. Heterozygous APE^+/APE^- mice survive, but show elevated levels of oxidative stress.[164] *E. coli* lacking Fpg or MutY show increased spontaneous mutation rates, and rates are 600- to 1600-fold greater than normal if both genes are defective. *E. coli* lacking uracil DNA glycosylase or MutT also suffer more mutations. *Salmonella* strains with defects in DNA repair are susceptible to damage by low concentrations of H_2O_2 and less virulent to mice, confirming that DNA is an important damage target of H_2O_2.[165]

4.10.8.2 *Mice to men*

Several human diseases involve defects in DNA repair. **Xeroderma pigmentosum**, a rare condition in which the skin is severely damaged by sunlight and the risk of skin cancer is high, is usually caused by defects in NER, leading to inability to remove pyrimidine dimers. Error-prone polymerases bypass these lesions and mutations accumulate. At least seven different defects, affecting different XP proteins (Section 4.10.3), have been identified. **Cockayne syndrome** is characterized by photosensitivity, growth retardation and deficient neurological development and is caused by defects (in the **CSA** or **CSB** proteins) that impair transcription-coupled repair of pyrimidine dimers, 8OHdG, and 8OHdA.[166] Defective mismatch repair is responsible for **hereditary non-polyposis colon cancer**, one of the most common hereditary cancers. Inherited mutations in hMYH can also lead to colon cancer.

In **severe combined immunodeficient (scid)** mice and in patients suffering **ataxia telangiectasia**, there are defects in the repair of double-strand breaks. The latter disease is characterized by a high incidence of cancers, hypersensitivity to ionizing radiation, immune deficiencies, ataxia due to neuronal loss in the cerebellum and telangiectasias (dilated and tortuous small blood vessels in the eyes, ears and hands). The mutation affects the **ATM (ataxia telangiectasia mutated)** gene that encodes a kinase important in repair of double-strand breaks (Section 4.10.6) and in cell-cycle checkpoints (Section 9.13.1). Without active ATM protein, the cell cycle often proceeds despite the presence of damaged DNA. Both AT patients and ATM-knockout mice have higher levels of 8OHdG and lipid peroxidation.[167] In mice, the neurobehavioural defects can be diminished by treatment with EUK-189, an antioxidant that crosses the blood–brain barrier (Section 10.6.4).[168] Increased oxidative stress in these knockout mice also damages the bone marrow.[169] In **Bloom's syndrome**, marked by photosensitivity, dwarfism and mental retardation, there is a defect in the **BLM protein**, which appears to be a helicase involved in repair of double-strand breaks.

The above diseases illustrate the essentiality of DNA repair mechanisms, consistent with the inability of antioxidant defences to prevent oxidative DNA damage *in vivo* completely (Table 4.1). Polymorphisms in OGG1 (Section 4.10.3) and other DNA repair systems have been suggested to be linked with various types of cancer, such as lung, prostate and nasopharyngeal. However, larger population studies are required to confirm this.[170]

4.10.9 Oxidative RNA damage

RNA bases and ribose can also be targets of RS (Section 4.8.2.2). Indeed, RNA base oxidation products accumulate in some neurodegenerative diseases (Section 9.20). Since most RNA turns over rapidly, the significance of its oxidation in normal cells is unclear, nor is much known about repair processes. We commented in Section 4.10.2 that MTH1 can degrade 8OHGTP as well as 8OHdGTP, although the importance of this reaction *in vivo* is uncertain.

4.11 Mechanisms of damage to cellular targets by oxidative stress: lipid peroxidation

4.11.1 A history of peroxidation: from oils and textiles to breast implants

Lipid peroxidation was defined by A.L. Tappel as *the oxidative deterioration of polyunsaturated lipids*. Polyunsaturated fatty acids (PUFAs) are those that contain two or more carbon–carbon double bonds

$$>C=C<$$

Monounsaturated and even saturated lipids can also be oxidized; it's just more difficult to do it.

Oxygen-dependent deterioration, leading to **rancidity**, has been recognized since antiquity as a problem in the storage of fats and oils and was often dealt with by using antioxidant spices (Section 3.22.4). Rancidity is even more relevant today with the popularity of 'polyunsaturated' margarines and cooking oils, and the importance of paints, plastics, lacquers, waxes and rubber, all of which can undergo oxidative damage. Even oils within breast implants can oxidize.[171] Attempts to study oil oxidation began in 1820 when de Saussure used a simple mercury manometer to show that a layer of walnut oil on water absorbed three times its own volume of air over 8 months. This was followed by a second phase of rapid air-absorption, the oil taking up 60-times its own volume of air in 10 days. During the following 3 months, the rate of air uptake gradually diminished, and the oil eventually took up 145-times its own volume, becoming viscous and evil-smelling. Commenting on these experiments, the famous chemist Berzelius (who also discovered selenium) suggested that oil autoxidation might be involved in the spontaneous ignition of wool after its lubrication with linseed oil, a common cause of fires in textile mills at that time.

The sequence of reactions which is now recognized as the 'core' of lipid peroxidation was worked out in detail by scientists at the British Rubber Producers' Association research laboratories in the 1940s. The relevance of these reactions to biological systems was not appreciated until later,

however. Food scientists have also made substantial contributions to understanding lipid peroxidation.

4.11.2 Targets of attack: membrane lipids and proteins

4.11.2.1 *What's in a membrane?*

The membranes that surround cells and organelles contain large amounts of PUFA side-chains (Table 4.11). We are therefore at constant risk of going rancid.

The major constituents of biological membranes are lipid and protein, the amount of protein increasing with the number of functions that the membrane performs. In the myelin sheath, which serves largely to insulate nerve axons, only about 20% of the dry weight of the membrane is protein, but most membranes have 50% or more protein, and the inner mitochondrial and chloroplast thylakoid membranes (Section 6.8) are about 80% protein. Some proteins are loosely attached to membrane surfaces (**extrinsic proteins**), but most are tightly attached (**intrinsic proteins**), being either partially embedded in the membrane, located in the membrane interior or even traversing the membrane. Lipid peroxidation in most biological membranes is thus very likely to damage membrane proteins as well as lipids.

Membrane lipids are generally **amphipathic**, that is they contain hydrophobic regions that tend to cluster together away from water, together with polar parts that like to associate with water. In

Table 4.11 Some common, naturally occurring fatty acids

Shorthand name[a]	Common name	Examples of occurrence
16:0	Palmitic acid	Natural fats and oils, especially palm oil
18:0	Stearic acid	Natural fats and oils, especially beef fat
18:1 (*n*-9)[b]	Oleic acid	Natural fats and oils, especially olive oil
18:2 (*n*-6)	Linoleic acid	Widespread, many seed oils
18:3 (*n*-3)	α-Linolenic acid	Plant leaves, some seed oils, e.g. soybean, rapeseed, linseed oils
20:4 (*n*-6)	Arachidonic acid	Animal membranes
20:5 (*n*-3)	Eicosapentaenoic acid (EPA)	Fish oils
22:6 (*n*-3)	Docosahexaenoic acid (DHA)	Fish oils, mammalian brain, retina

[a] Number of carbons in chain: number of double bonds.

[b] The numbering system in parentheses (often used in the nutritional literature) identifies double bonds from the methyl, $-CH_3$, end of the chain. For nomenclature in the chemical literature see Fig. 4.17.

animal cell membranes the dominant lipids are **phospholipids**, esters based on the alcohol glycerol (Figs 4.16 and 4.17), the commonest in animal cell membranes being **lecithin (phosphatidylcholine)**. Some membranes, particularly plasma membranes, contain significant proportions of **sphingolipids** and **cholesterol** (Fig. 4.16). By contrast, the membranes of subcellular organelles such as mitochondria or nuclei rarely contain much sphingolipid or cholesterol. Mitochondrial inner membranes contain **cardiolipin** (Fig. 4.16); peroxidation of PUFAs in this lipid may contribute to age-related decline in mitochondrial function[172] and can facilitate cytochrome c release during apoptosis (Section 4.4.1.2).

The fatty-acid side-chains of membrane lipids in animal cells have unbranched carbon chains and contain even numbers of carbon atoms, usually 14 to 24 (Table 4.11), and the double bonds are *cis* configuration, causing 'kinks' in the structure (Fig. 4.17). Other organisms have different lipid compositions. The composition of bacterial membranes depends on the species, culture conditions and stage in the growth cycle. Membrane fractions usually contain 10 to 30% lipid. In Gram-positive bacteria (i.e. those that take up **Gram's stain**, used by microscopists) phophatidylglycerol is present, but phosphatidylethanolamine is more common in Gram-negative species (such as *E. coli*).

4.11.2.2 *Membrane structure*

As the number of double bonds in a fatty acid increases, its melting point drops. For example, stearic acid (18:0) is solid at room temperature whereas linoleic acid (18:2) is liquid. Since membrane lipids are amphipathic, on exposure to water they aggregate with their hydrophobic regions clustered together and their hydrophilic regions in contact with H_2O. How this is achieved depends on the relative amounts of lipid and water. When phospholids are shaken or sonicated in aqueous solution they form **micelles** (Fig. 4.18), but as more phospholipids are added **liposomes** result, bags of aqueous solution bounded by a **lipid bilayer**. Liposomes can be surrounded by a single bilayer (**unilamellar**) or several bilayers (**multilamellar**), as shown in Fig. 4.18. The interior of liposomes contains some of the aqueous solution in which they were made, so they are often used as 'parcels'

for transporting drugs (including antioxidant enzymes) to target tissues. Liposomes are frequently used in studies of lipid peroxidation.

The lipid bilayer (Fig. 4.18) is the basic structure of all cell and organelle membranes. In each half of the bilayer, protein and lipid molecules can diffuse quickly—indeed a lipid molecule in one half of a bilayer can move from one end of the 'average' cell to the other in a few seconds. This **membrane fluidity** is largely due to the presence of PUFA side-chains, which lower the melting point of the membrane interior so that it has the chemical nature and viscosity of a light oil. Damage to PUFAs tends to decrease membrane fluidity, which is essential for the proper functioning of biological membranes. By contrast, exchange of lipids between the two halves of the bilayer is rare.

4.11.3 Targets of attack: dietary lipids, and lipoproteins

Dietary fats have to be digested, absorbed and transported around the body. They can be oxidized during cooking and storage, and possibly in the gastrointestinal tract itself (Section 6.2). Lipoproteins involved in fat transport may contain small amounts of oxidized lipids from the diet (Section 9.3.8) and can undergo further oxidation *in vivo*, contributing to atherosclerosis. Fatty acids circulating in the blood are also potential targets for oxidation; albumin and albumin-bound bilirubin may help protect them (Section 3.18.1).

4.11.4 How does lipid peroxidation begin?

Initiation of lipid peroxidation can be caused by addition of an RS or, more usually, by hydrogen atom abstraction from a methylene ($-CH_2-$) group by an RS. In both cases, a carbon radical results. For example, OH$^{\bullet}$ can react by addition

$$>C=C< \ + \ OH^{\bullet} \longrightarrow \ >\!\!\overset{|}{\underset{OH}{C}}\!\!-\overset{\bullet}{C}\!<$$

or by H$^{\bullet}$ abstraction

$$-CH_2- + OH^{\bullet} \rightarrow -{}^{\bullet}CH- + H_2O$$

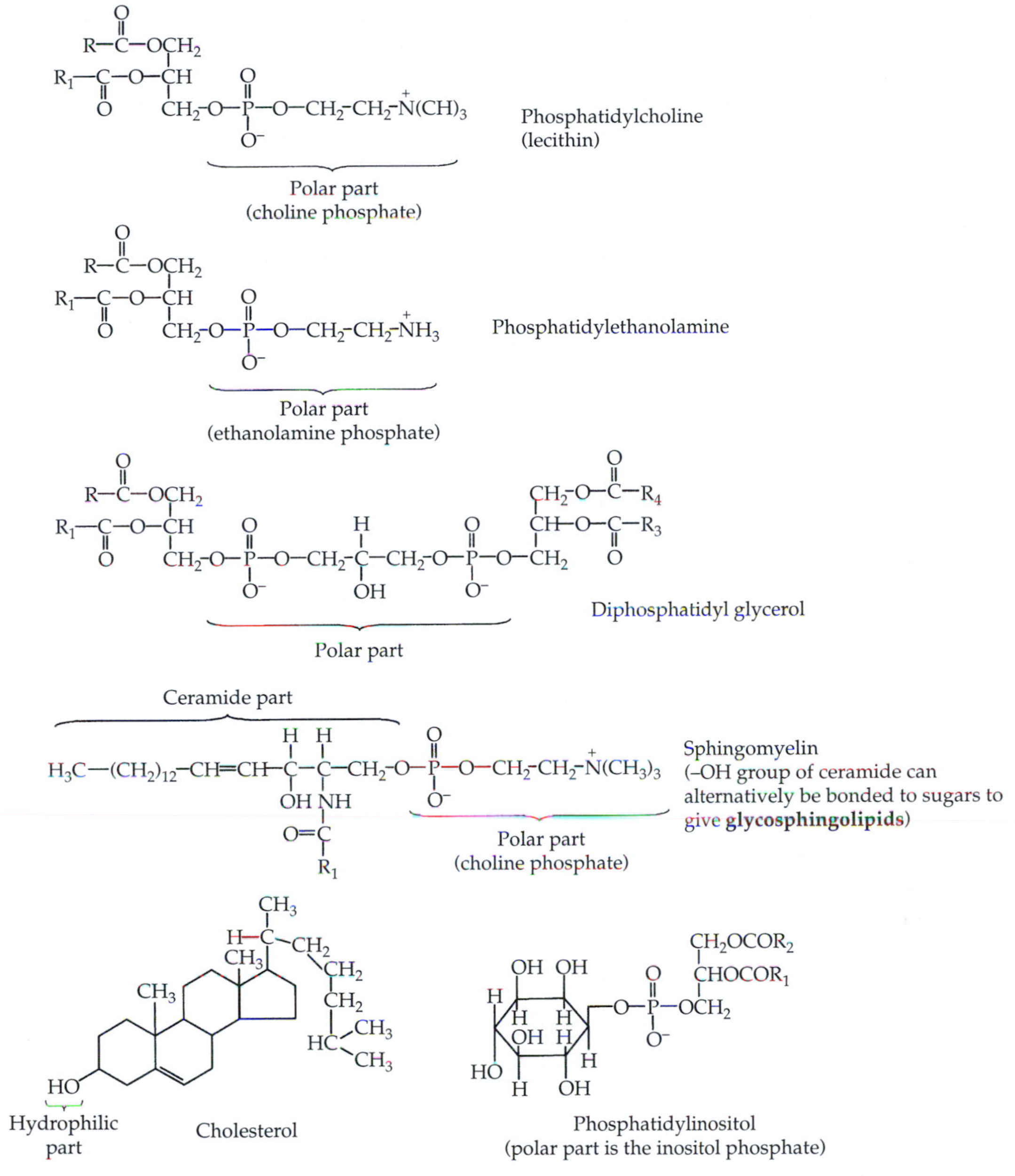

Phosphatidylcholine
(lecithin)

Polar part
(choline phosphate)

Phosphatidylethanolamine

Polar part
(ethanolamine phosphate)

Diphosphatidyl glycerol

Polar part

Ceramide part

Sphingomyelin
(–OH group of ceramide can
alternatively be bonded to sugars to
give **glycosphingolipids**)

Polar part
(choline phosphate)

Hydrophilic
part

Cholesterol

Phosphatidylinositol
(polar part is the inositol phosphate)

Figure 4.16 Lipid molecules found in animals. R_1, R_2, etc. represent long, hydrophobic, fatty-acid side-chains (for structures, see Table 4.11 and Fig. 4.17). In most lipids these are joined by ester bonds to the alcohol glycerol. In **sphingomyelins**, however, the fatty acids are attached to the $-NH_2$ group of **sphingosine**. All the lipid molecules shown contain a polar (hydrophilic) part that can interact with water, but in cholesterol this is very small (only an $-OH$ group) so that, overall, cholesterol is very hydrophobic. Diphosphatidyglycerol (**cardiolipin**) comprises about 20% of the phospholipids in the inner mitochondrial membrane.

Nitrogen dioxide can perform similar reactions (Section 8.11.2). whereas HOCl is more likely to chlorinate lipids by addition across double bonds (Section 2.6.3.1), although chloramines can form on $-NH_2$ groups on some lipids. Ozone directly oxidizes lipids, forming ozonides (Section 2.6.5).

A double bond weakens the bond energy of the C–H bonds present on the next carbon atom (the

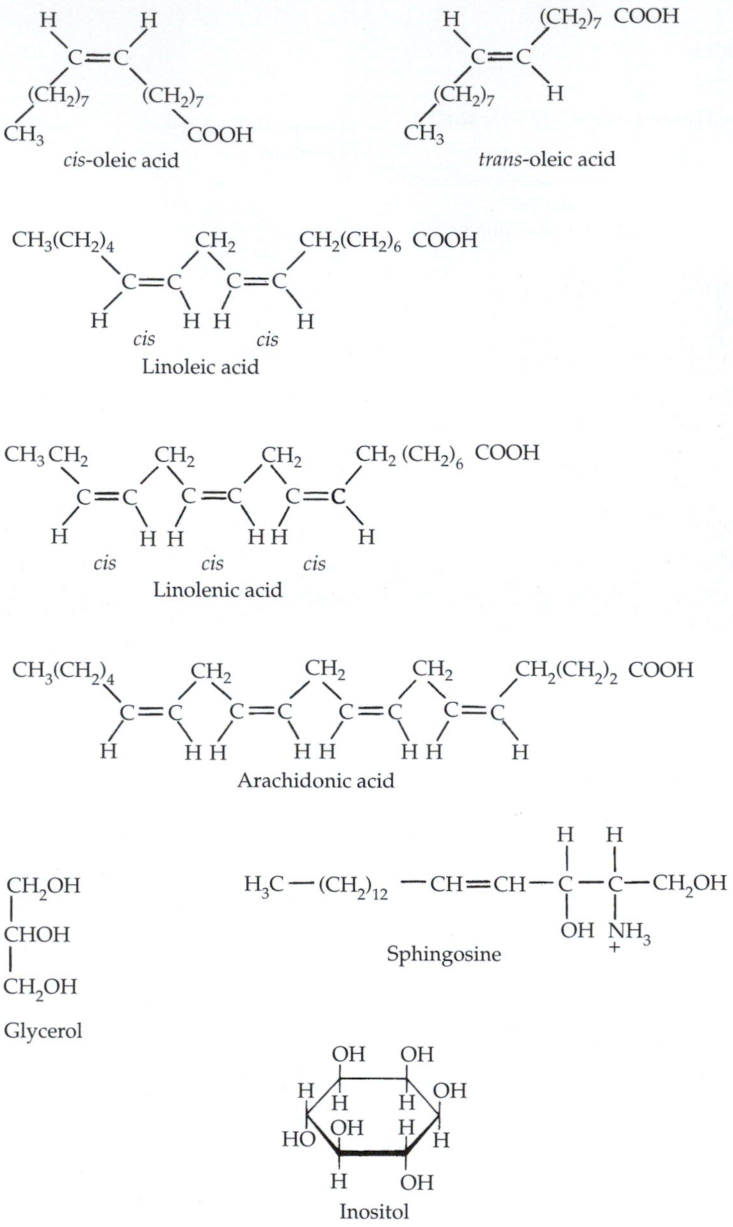

Figure 4.17 Fatty acids and other 'building blocks' of biological lipids. Phosphorylated inositols play key roles in signal transduction (Section 4.5.5). Top: *cis*- and *trans*-oleic acid ($C_{18:1}$). A double bond in a carbon chain prevents rotation of the groups attached to the carbon atoms forming it, so that they are forced to stay on one side of the double bond or the other, generating *trans* and *cis* configurations. Note the kink in the chain of the *cis* form. **Linoleic acid** (C_{18}) has two double bonds, at carbons 9 and 11 (where the carbon in the COOH group is counted as carbon number 1). **Linolenic acid** (C_{18}) has double bonds at carbons 9, 12 and 15. **Arachidonic acid** (C_{20}) has double bonds at carbons 5, 8, 11 and 14.

allylic hydrogens), especially if there is a double bond on either side of the C–H bond (Fig. 4.19), giving **bis-allylic** hydrogens. The reduction potential of a bis-allylic PUFA•/PUFA couple at pH 7 ($E°'$) has been estimated[173] as about 0.6 V. Hence OH•, HO$_2^{\bullet}$, RO• and RO$_2^{\bullet}$ radicals are

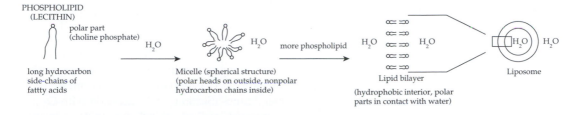

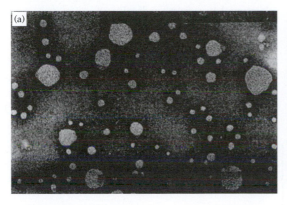
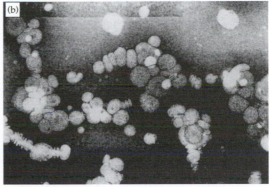

Figure 4.18 Formation of a lipid bilayer on mixing phospholipids with aqueous solutions. Top: general principles. Bottom: electron micrographs of preparations of (a) unilamellar and (b) multilamellar liposomes.

(thermodynamically at least) capable of oxidizing PUFAs (see Table 2.3) at allylic hydrogens. For example, the oxidizability of DHA or EPA (Table 4.11) *in vitro* is several times greater than that of linoleic acid. One consequence of this is that fish-oil supplements, widely advocated by health-food stores, undergo oxidation easily because they contain substantial amounts of these PUFAs. Clinical trials investigating the alleged benefits of fish-oil supplementation in various diseases have often given conflicting results: one reason may be the extent of oxidation of the preparation that was tested. However, there is no evidence for increased peroxidation of DHA *in vivo* in healthy subjects,[174] although it does occur in Alzheimer's disease (Section 9.20).

Hydroxyl radical readily initiates peroxidation of fatty acids, lipoproteins and membranes, although OH$^\bullet$ generated outside a membrane will also attack extrinsic carbohydrates and proteins (e.g. cell surface glycoproteins) and 'head groups' of phospholipids. Hence irradiation of biological material stimulates lipid peroxidation; this has been shown not only for membranes and lipoproteins but also for food lipids (a problem in attempts to sterilize or

preserve food by irradiating it). Radiation-induced peroxidation is inhibited to some extent by scavengers of OH$^\bullet$, such as mannitol and formate, which will compete with the lipids for any OH$^\bullet$ generated in 'free solution'. However, H$_2$O crosses membranes (Section 2.6.2) and any water undergoing homolysis within the membrane will generate OH$^\bullet$ not accessible to scavengers. The rate constant for reaction of OH$^\bullet$ with artificial lecithin bilayers has been measured[175] as about $5 \times 10^8\,M^{-1}s^{-1}$.

By contrast, neither NO$^\bullet$ nor O$_2^{\bullet-}$ is sufficiently reactive to abstract H from lipids; in any case, the charge of O$_2^{\bullet-}$ tends to preclude it from entering the lipid phase of membranes. Indeed, O$_2^{\bullet-}$ does not readily cross biological membranes, except where specific channels exist, nor does it appear to react with any membrane constituents on its passage through such channels (Section 2.5.3). However, HO$_2^\bullet$ is more reactive and can abstract H$^\bullet$ from some PUFAs, such as linoleic, linolenic and arachidonic acids (rate constants 1.2, 1.7 and $3.0 \times 10^3\,M^{-1}s^{-1}$ respectively).[176]

$$-CH_2- + HO_2^\bullet \rightarrow -\overset{\bullet}{C}H- + H_2O_2$$

Protonated $O_2^{\bullet-}$, being uncharged, should enter membranes more easily than $O_2^{\bullet-}$, and several papers have described $HO_2^{\bullet}$-dependent peroxidation of liposomes and lipoproteins. In addition, $HO_2^{\bullet}$ can stimulate peroxidation by reaction with preformed lipid hydroperoxides to generate peroxyl radicals.[176]

$$HO_2^{\bullet} + ROOH \rightarrow RO_2^{\bullet} + H_2O_2$$

4.11.5 Propagation of lipid peroxidation

Carbon radicals often stabilize by molecular rearrangement to form **conjugated dienes** (Fig. 4.19). If two carbon radicals collide within a membrane they might cross-link the fatty acid side-chains:[177]

$$R-\overset{\bullet}{C}H + R-\overset{\bullet}{C}H \longrightarrow R-CH-CH-R$$

However, the most likely fate of carbon radicals under aerobic conditions is to combine with O_2 (Section 2.5.4), especially as O_2 concentrates inside membranes (Section 1.1.3). Reaction with O_2 gives a **peroxyl radical**, $ROO^{\bullet}$ (or $RO_2^{\bullet}$), sometimes shortened to **peroxy radical**:

$$R^{\bullet} + O_2 \rightarrow ROO^{\bullet}$$

Of course, very low O_2 concentrations might favour self-reaction of carbon-centred radicals, or their reactions with other membrane components, such as $-SH$ groups on proteins. Hence the O_2

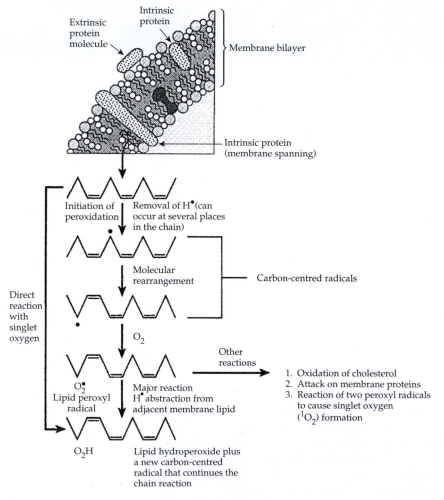

Figure 4.19 Idealized representation of the initiation and propagation reactions of lipid peroxidation. The peroxidation of a fatty acid with three double bonds is shown.

concentration affects the pathway of peroxidation, for this and other reasons (Section 4.12.3 below).

Peroxyl radicals can abstract $H^\bullet$ from an adjacent fatty-acid side-chain

$$ROO^\bullet + CH \rightarrow ROOH + C^\bullet$$

This is the **propagation stage** of lipid peroxidation. It forms new carbon radicals that can react with O_2 to form new peroxyl radicals, and so the **chain reaction** of lipid peroxidation continues (Fig. 4.19). The $RO_2^\bullet$ combines with the $H^\bullet$ that it abstracts to give a **lipid hydroperoxide** (ROOH). This name is sometimes shortened to **lipid peroxide**, although the latter term also includes **cyclic peroxides** (Fig. 4.20), which result when a peroxyl radical attacks another double bond in the same fatty acid residue (Fig. 4.20).

A single initiation event thus has the potential to generate multiple peroxide molecules by a chain reaction. The initial $H^\bullet$ abstraction from a PUFA can occur at different points on the carbon chain (Fig. 4.20).[178] Thus peroxidation of linoleic acid gives two hydroperoxides, that of linolenic acid four. Peroxidation of arachidonic acid gives six lipid hydroperoxides. Similarly, EPA can give eight hydroperoxides, and DHA ten. All these products are formed as racemic mixures of optical isomers, i.e. lipid peroxidation is not stereospecific. Cyclic and bicyclic peroxides can also form (Figs 4.20 and 4.21).

4.11.6 Transition metals and lipid peroxidation[180,181]

4.11.6.1 *Iron*

Interpretations of studies on the role of iron in lipid oxidation tend to be confused by the experimental conditions used by many scientists. Levels of 'free' metals *in vivo* are low, effectively zero in plasma and low μM in the LIP and in the plasma of patients with iron overload disease (Section 4.3.3). Yet many scientists add 50 to 100 μM Fe^{2+}, Fe^{3+}/ ascorbate or Fe^{2+}-ADP to their lipids to 'initiate' peroxidation *in vitro*, with considerable success. How does this work?

High concentrations of Fe^{2+} take part in electron-transfer reactions with O_2 to form $OH^\bullet$

$$Fe^{2+} + O_2 \rightleftharpoons (Fe^{2+}-O_2 \leftrightarrow Fe(\text{III})-O_2^{\bullet-}) \rightleftharpoons Fe(\text{III})-O_2^{\bullet-}$$

$$2O_2^{\bullet-} + 2H^+ \rightarrow H_2O_2 + O_2$$

$$Fe^{2+} + H_2O_2 \rightarrow Fe(\text{III}) + OH^- + OH^\bullet$$

Thus the addition of Fe^{2+} (or a ferric salt plus a reducing agent) to a peroxide-free unsaturated lipid in the presence of O_2 should initiate lipid peroxidation via $OH^\bullet$ formation. The resulting peroxidation should be inhibitable by H_2O_2-removing enzymes, scavengers of $OH^\bullet$, and chelating agents that bind iron and prevent its participation in free-radical reactions. Indeed, all these effects have been observed in several studies involving iron addition to dispersed lipid systems (e.g. fatty acids solubilized by detergents) or ultrapure lipids.

However, most scientists, including the authors, find that when catalase or scavengers of $OH^\bullet$ are added to lipids (e.g. microsomes, lipoproteins, liposomes) undergoing peroxidation stimulated by addition of iron ions, there is no inhibition, despite the fact that $OH^\bullet$ radicals can be detected in the reaction mixtures. Formation of $OH^\bullet$ *is* inhibited by H_2O_2-scavenging enzymes.[180] It follows that the $OH^\bullet$ being made from H_2O_2 is not *required* for the peroxidation. One might argue that the $OH^\bullet$ formation is 'site-specific', involving iron ions bound to the membrane, so that $OH^\bullet$ reacts immediately with the lipids and is not available for scavenging. However, H_2O_2-removing enzymes should still inhibit. The fact that they usually do not has led to proposals that initiation of lipid peroxidation by iron salts in the presence of O_2 is not due to $OH^\bullet$, but to other RS. Ferryl is one possibility, although ferryl formation by reaction of Fe^{2+} with H_2O_2 should still require H_2O_2. Perferryl ($Fe^{2+}-O_2 \leftrightarrow Fe(\text{III})-O_2^{\bullet-}$) could also be involved. However, perferryl may be insufficiently reactive to abstract $H^\bullet$ or to insert oxygen directly into fatty-acid side-chains. Studies of the kinetics of microsomal or liposomal lipid peroxidation in the presence of Fe^{2+} and/or $Fe(\text{III})$ salts have led to proposals that initiation requires a triple complex of $Fe(\text{III})/Fe(\text{II})/O_2$, or at least some specific critical ratio of Fe^{2+} to $Fe(\text{III})$. Attempts to characterize this complex have been fruitless, and the observation that some other metal ions can replace $Fe(\text{III})$ in

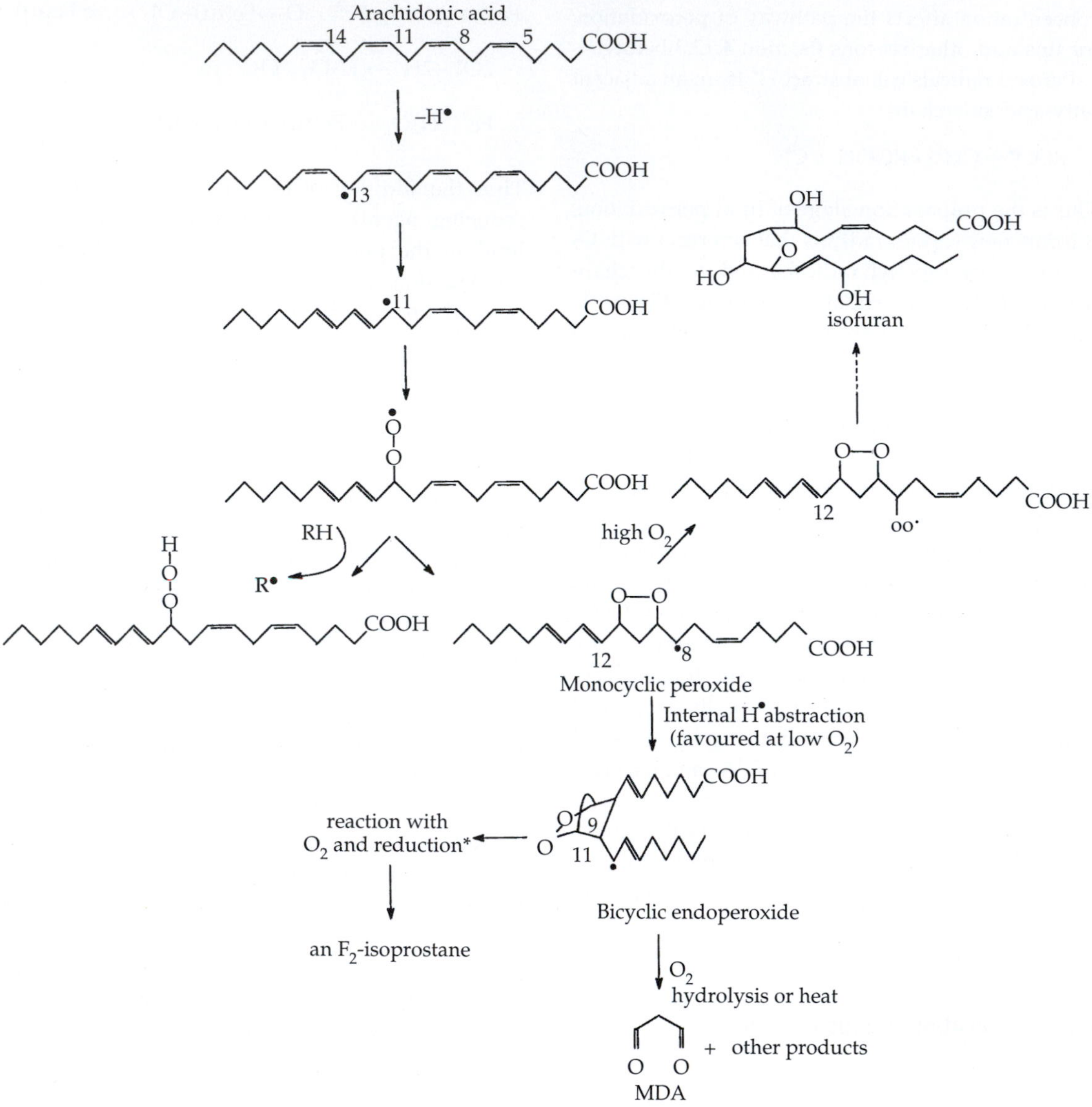

Figure 4.20 Formation of lipid hydroperoxides and cyclic peroxides from arachidonic acid. The chemistry is complex because abstraction of H$^\bullet$ can occur at different sites; for simplicity we show it only at C13. The RO$_2^\bullet$ radicals formed can generate hydroperoxides or cyclize to monocyclic peroxides. These result when peroxyl radicals attack a double bond in the same chain. Monocyclic peroxides can form bicyclic structures that can give rise to isoprostanes, or react with O$_2$, eventually producing **isofurans**. Unstable peroxides can decompose to aldehydes such as MDA (malondialdehyde). Even products containing bicyclic endoperoxide and cyclic peroxide groups in the same molecule (**dioxolane-isoprostanes**) can be generated (*J. Biol. Chem.* **279**, 3766, 2004). O$_2$ concentration affects the relative levels of isoprostanes and other products.∗ By GSH and other thiols.

stimulating Fe^{2+}-dependent peroxidation argues against a requirement for a specific Fe^{2+} − Fe(III) complex.

So how do we explain all this? It is not only the levels of iron used in many of these studies that are unphysiological, but also the state of the lipids, in that their peroxide content is abnormally high. Commercially available lipids are contaminated with peroxides, and so will be liposomes or micelles made from them. Sonication, often used to

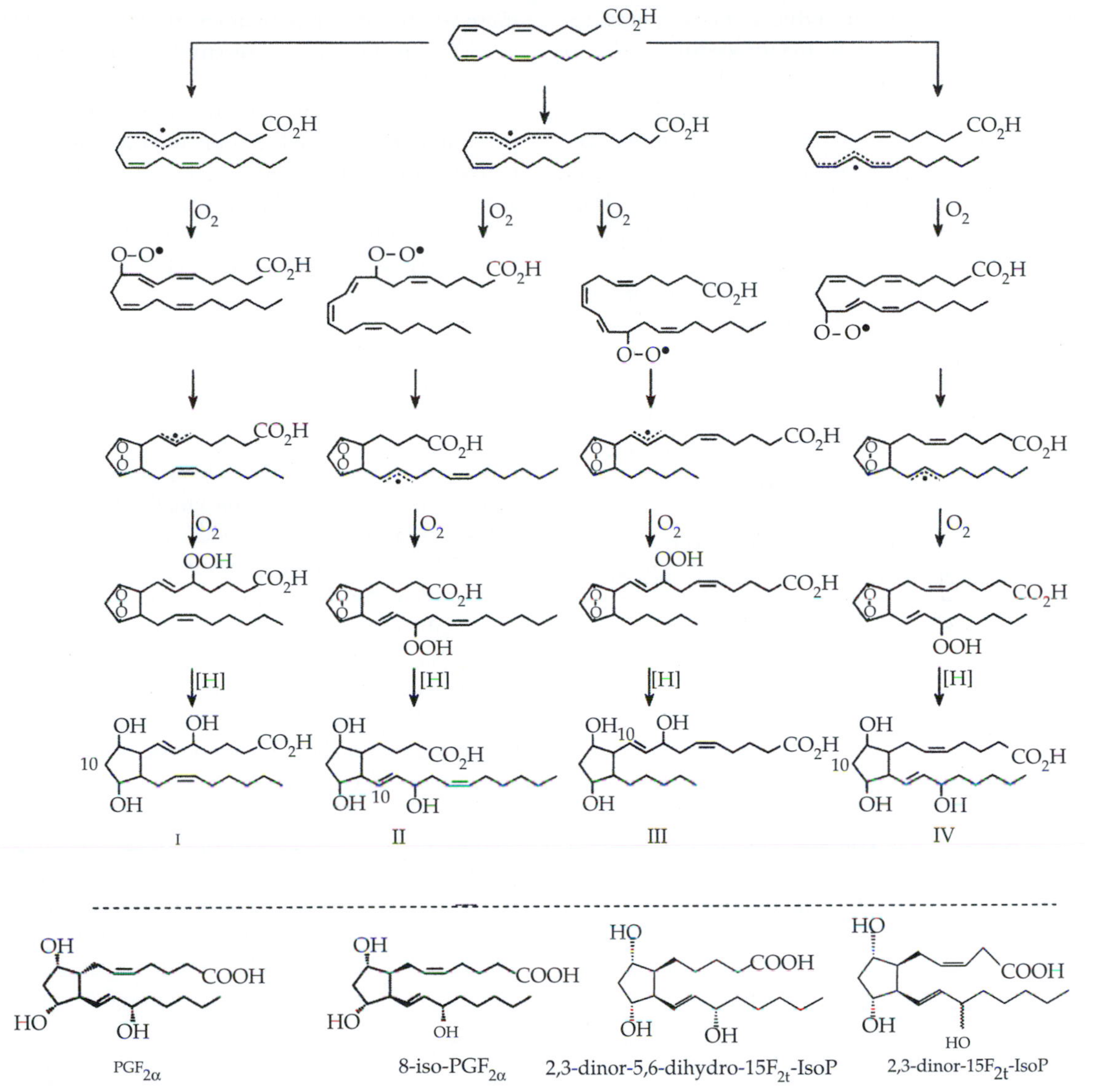

Figure 4.21 Formation of F_2-isoprostanes (IPs) from arachidonic acid. Above: free radicals can abstract H$^\bullet$ at three different positions. Four RO$_2^\bullet$ radicals are formed when O$_2$ reacts with the carbon-centred radicals. The RO$_2^\bullet$ attack double bonds in the same chain to cyclize the structure, a bicyclic structure forms by internal H$^\bullet$ abstraction (Fig. 4.20) and O$_2$ adds again to the new carbon radicals. Reduction gives four isomers (I–IV). If O$_2$ adds before bicyclization, isofurans can result (Fig. 4.20). For simplicity, stereochemistry is not indicated but each series potentially has 16 stereoisomers, giving 64 isomers in all. Below: these compounds are structurally isomeric with prostaglandin $F_{2\alpha}$, hence the name 'isoprostane'. Diagram by courtesy of Drs L. Jackson Roberts II and Jason Morrow. A systematic nomenclature for IPs has been proposed.[179] For example the 'official' name of the widely studied IP 8-*iso* PGF$_{2\alpha}$ is 15-F$_{2t}$-IsoP. Isoprostane is abbreviated to IP and different classes termed F$_2$-, D$_2$- etc as before. The former nomenclature (classes I–IV) is replaced by the location of the side-chain —OH group (5-, 12- etc). Thus regioisomer I is now a 5-F$_2$-IsoP, II is 8-F$_2$-IsoP, etc. The default absolute configuration of the side-chain —OH is *S*, if it is *R* the compound is called *epi*. If the ring —OH are oriented down (α), this is the default configuration, if up (β), the compound is designated *ent*. The favoured side-chain configuration of IsoPs is *cis* relative to the prostane ring, *epi* is used if they are *trans*. Subscripts c and t denote whether the side chains are oriented *cis* or *trans* with reference to the cyclopentane ring —OH groups. However the old names are still widely used, and yet another nomenclature has been proposed to enable differentiation of the regioisomers; thus 15-F$_{2t}$-IsoP is sometimes called iPF$_{2\alpha}$-III, 5-F$_{2t}$-IsoP as iPF$_{2\alpha}$-VI (*Prostaglandins* **54**, 853, 1997; *Trends Pharmacol. Sci.* **23**, 360, 2002).

prepare liposomes, introduces more peroxides (Section 2.5.1.1), as may the procedures used to isolate lipoproteins (Section 9.3.8). When tissues are damaged, lipid peroxidation is favoured (Section 9.2) and lipid peroxides are also formed enzymically in injured tissues by cyclooxygenase and lipoxygenase enzymes (Section 7.12).[181,182] Thus membrane fractions isolated from disrupted cells are enriched in lipid peroxides.

Pure lipid peroxides are usually stable at body temperature, but they decompose in the presence of transition-metal ions. Iron(II) and certain Fe^{2+} – chelates react with lipid peroxides in a similar way to their reaction with H_2O_2, splitting the O–O bond. This produces $RO^\bullet$, an **alkoxyl radical** (sometimes shortened to **alkoxy radical**).

$$ROOH + Fe^{2+} \rightarrow Fe(III) + OH^- + RO^\bullet$$
Lipid hydroperoxide   alkoxyl radical

Alkoxyl radicals can abstract $H^\bullet$ from PUFAs and from peroxides

$$RO^\bullet + L - H \rightarrow ROH + L^\bullet$$

$$ROOH + RO^\bullet \rightarrow ROO^\bullet + ROH$$

These reactions can continue propagation of lipid peroxidation. Alkoxyl radicals can sometimes attack their own PUFA chain, producing epoxy radicals.

Iron(III) and certain Fe(III) chelates can decompose peroxides to peroxyl radicals

$$ROOH + Fe(III) \rightarrow RO_2^\bullet + H^+ + Fe^{2+}$$
Peroxyl radical

Reactions of Fe^{2+} with lipid hydroperoxides are faster than reaction of Fe^{2+} with H_2O_2 (k_2 for $Fe^{2+} + H_2O_2$ is about $76\,M^{-1}s^{-1}$; that for $ROOH + Fe^{2+}$ is about $1.5 \times 10^3\,M^{-1}s^{-1}$), although the ligand to the metal affects these rates (see Table 2.4). Reactions of Fe(III) with hydroperoxides are usually slower than those of Fe^{2+}. Hence the rate of lipid peroxidation in the presence of Fe(III) can be increased by adding reducing agents, such as ascorbate or thiols, because peroxide decomposition is faster. Another factor is that Fe^{2+} salts are more soluble at pH 7.4 than Fe(III). Binding of $NO^\bullet$ to Fe^{2+} can decrease its reactivity with peroxides (Table 2.10).

Peroxyl radicals are efficient stimulators of lipid peroxidation. Thus when iron ions are added to peroxide-rich lipids, $RO_2^\bullet$ (and possibly $RO^\bullet$) account for the stimulation of peroxidation and $OH^\bullet$, although formed, is not required. Yet another complexity is that too much Fe^{2+} can *scavenge* radicals

$$RO^\bullet + Fe^{2+} + H^+ \rightarrow Fe(III) + ROH$$

$$RO_2^\bullet + Fe^{2+} + H^+ \rightarrow Fe(III) + ROOH$$

and so the ratio of $Fe^{2+}/LOOH$ is important in determining the peroxidation kinetics.[180,183]

Many iron chelates can stimulate lipid peroxidation (Table 4.12). For some proteins, such as ferritin, stimulation occurs because RS produced during lipid peroxidation release iron from the protein. Acceleration of peroxidation by myoglobin, haemoglobin and cytochromes can involve both peroxide-dependent release of haem and iron ions from the proteins, and reactions brought about by ferryl species and amino-acid radicals (Section 3.15.3).

What about $O_2^{\bullet-}$? It can contribute to the peroxidation in two ways. Hydroperoxyl radical can abstract some $H^\bullet$ and also convert ROOH to $RO_2^\bullet$. Superoxide can reduce Fe(III) to Fe^{2+}, although its effects are complex because it is also capable of oxidizing Fe^{2+} back to Fe(III) (Section 2.5.3.3).

4.11.6.2 *Copper*

Copper ions are powerful promoters of peroxide decomposition; for example Cu^{2+} is an excellent catalyst of LDL peroxidation (Section 9.3.8). Like iron, Cu acts mainly by decomposing peroxides

$$ROOH + Cu^{2+} \rightarrow Cu^+ + RO_2^\bullet + H^+$$

$$ROOH + Cu^+ \rightarrow RO^\bullet + Cu^{2+} + OH^-$$

$$ROOH + Cu^{2+} \rightarrow Cu(III) + RO^\bullet + OH^-$$

Again, the reaction rates depend on the ligands to the copper.

Table 4.12 Physiological forms of iron and their possible participation in RS formation

Type of iron	Will it decompose lipid peroxides to form alkoxyl and/or peroxyl radicals?	Can it form OH• by Fenton chemistry?
Iron ions bound to		
Phosphate esters (e.g. ADP, ATP)	Yes	Yes
Carbohydrates and organic acids (e.g. citrate, picolinic acid, deoxyribose)	Yes	Yes
DNA	Yes	Yes
Membrane lipids	Yes	Yes
Loosely bound to proteins, e.g. albumin	Yes	Yes
Iron bound to proteins		
(i) Non-haem iron		
Ferritin	Probably no[a]	No[a]
Haemosiderin	No[a]	No[a]
Lactoferrin	No[a]	No[a]
Transferrin	No[a]	No[a]
Tartrate-resistant acid phosphatase[d]	Yes (if iron is released)	Yes (if iron is released)
(ii) Haem iron		
Haem itself	Yes	Probably no[a]
Haemoglobin	Yes	Yes (when iron is released)
Leghaemoglobin	Yes	Yes (when iron is released)
Myoglobin	Yes	Yes (when iron is released)
Cytochrome *c*	Yes	Yes (when iron is released)
Cytochromes P450	Yes, especially CYP2E1	Yes (when iron is released)
Catalase[e]	Weakly[b]	No[c]

[a] Unless iron is released from it in the reaction mixture.
[b] Activity may be due to partial degradation of catalase: catalase subunits show greater peroxidase activity.
[c] Unless enzyme activity is lost and iron is released.
[d] See Section 3.15.4.2.
[e] Catalase can also photosensitize to cause lipid oxidation (Section 3.7.5).

4.11.6.3 *Other metals*

Certain cobalt(II) chelates can decompose lipid peroxides, whereas Zn^{2+} and Mn^{2+} do not. Some other metal ions cannot themselves stimulate lipid peroxidation, but appear to bind to lipids in a way that facilitates iron-dependent lipid peroxidation under certain reaction conditions; examples (Section 8.15.11) are aluminum(III) and lead(II). Their binding to the membrane surface may somehow produce a local 'freezing' of the motion of phospholipid molecules that facilitates propagation reactions. However, the physiological significance of these effects is unknown.

4.11.7 Microsomal lipid peroxidation

Microsomal fractions prepared from plant or animal tissues undergo rapid lipid peroxidation when incubated with Fe^{2+} salts, or Fe(III) salts plus ascorbate or NADPH.[184] This is a popular experimental system, although extremely complex, in part because 'microsomes' are a heterogeneous collection of lipid vesicles (Section 1.10.8) and contain variable amounts of endogenous antioxidants such as α-tocopherol and coenzyme Q. Often, iron is added as chelates with ADP, pyrophosphate or EDTA. During microsomal peroxidation, cytochromes b_5 and P450 are attacked, their haem being degraded.[185] Carbon monoxide is one product. Antibodies raised against NADPH-cytochrome P450 reductase inhibit NADPH/Fe(III)-dependent peroxidation by more than 90%. This enzyme can reduce some Fe(III) chelates, generating Fe^{2+} and stimulating peroxidation. Hence both CYPs and their reductases contribute to microsomal lipid peroxidation.

4.11.8 Acceleration of lipid peroxidation by species other than oxygen radicals

4.11.8.1 Singlet oxygen[186]

Unlike ground-state O_2, singlet $O_2^1\Delta g$ can react with carbon–carbon double bonds by an *ene* reaction to give peroxides (Section 2.6.4.6). Reaction of singlet O_2 with the double bond between C-12 and C-13 of linoleic acid gives two hydroperoxides:

12-hydroperoxide

13-hydroperoxide

9- and 10-Hydroperoxides result when $^1O_2$ reacts with the double bond between C9 and 10. Thus four products result when linoleic acid is exposed to singlet O_2. By contrast, free-radical peroxidation of linoleate gives mainly, but not exclusively, the 9- and 13-hydroperoxides.[182] Strictly speaking, singlet O_2 is not *initiating* peroxidation; unless the peroxides are decomposed (e.g. by metal ions) to give peroxyl and alkoxyl radicals, a chain reaction will not begin.

The lifetime of singlet O_2 in the hydrophobic interior of membranes is greater than in aqueous solution (Section 2.6.4). Hence illumination of lipids in the presence of sensitizers of $^1O_2$ formation induces rapid peroxide formation. Such reactions are important in the eye (Section 6.10) and in plants (Section 6.8). Cholesterol within membranes can also be oxidized by $^1O_2$, for example to its 5α-hydroperoxide. Singlet O_2 reacts with membrane proteins, on average faster than it does with lipids (Fig. 2.15, legend). However, a photosensitizer in a membrane can target the damage to lipids if it resides in a lipid-rich domain.

Singlet oxygen can *form* during lipid peroxidation and might then cause more lipid peroxide formation. A likely mechanism is the self-reaction of peroxyl radicals (Section 2.5.4), which can be regarded as a **chain termination** reaction, since it removes two peroxyl radicals. Singlet O_2 formation might account for some of the chemiluminescence

that accompanies lipid peroxidation (Section 5.14.10), but its overall contribution to lipid peroxidation is uncertain. Under most physiological/pathological (unless photochemically induced) conditions it seems likely to be small; the self-reaction of $RO_2^\bullet$ is unlikely to be favoured until they have accumulated to significant levels within the membrane, that is until peroxidation is already extensive.

4.11.8.2 Adding organic peroxides or azo initiators

Another way of stimulating lipid peroxidation *in vitro* is to add azo initiators (Section 2.5.4) or artificial organic hydroperoxides such as **tert-butyl hydroperoxide** or **cumene hydroperoxide**. Decomposition of these peroxides to alkoxyl or peroxyl radicals accelerates the chain reaction of lipid peroxidation.[187] Decomposition is facilitated by 'free' metal ions and haem proteins, including methaemoglobin and CYPs, CYP2E1 being especially effective. For example, for Fe^{2+}

tert–butyl hydroperoxide   alkoxyl radical

cumene hydroperoxide   alkoxyl radical

Both of the above alkoxyl radicals can form methyl radicals, for example for cumene hydroperoxide

$$PhC(CH_3)_2O^\bullet \rightarrow PhC(O)CH_3 + CH_3^\bullet$$

Rate constants for the reactions of cumene and *tert*-butylhydroperoxides with Fe^{2+}-ATP are about 3.1×10^3 and $1.3 \times 10^3\,M^{-1}s^{-1}$ respectively.

Cytochromes P450 can carry out both one-electron and two-electron oxidations of organic peroxides.[188] For cumene hydroperoxide, one-electron reduction of the O–O bond generates the alkoxyl radical, which can go on to form the ketone acetophenone and methane gas (via methyl radical, $CH_3^\bullet$). Two-electron reduction generates cumyl alcohol (–OOH reduced to –OH) plus a CYP oxo-iron species of capable of substrate hydro-xylation (Section 1.4.1).

Cumene and *tert*-butyl hydroperoxides are widely used as model peroxides to impose oxid-ative stress upon cells, because they are easy to obtain pure (e.g. Fig. 4.4). How far they mimic the actions of the lipid peroxides produced *in vivo* is, however, uncertain.

4.12 Lipid peroxidation products: bad, good or indifferent?

4.12.1 General effects

The overall effects[189] of lipid peroxidation are to decrease membrane fluidity, make it easier for phospholipids to exchange between the two halves of the bilayer, increase the 'leakiness' of the membrane to substances that do not normally cross it other than through specific channels (e.g. Ca^{2+}) and damage membrane proteins, inactivat-ing enzymes and ion channels. Cross-linking of membrane proteins decreases their lateral and rotational mobility.

Rises in Ca^{2+} induced by oxidative stress can activate phospholipase A_2, which releases arachi-donic acid from membrane phospholipids (Section 4.3.2.2); the free arachidonic acid can then undergo lipid peroxidation and stimulate eicosanoid syn-thesis, a pathway intimately linked to lipid perox-idation (Section 7.12). The **lysophospholipids** it leaves behind have mild detergent-like effects and can contribute to membrane disorganization if they accumulate in large amounts. Phospholipase A_2 can also cleave oxidized arachidonic acid residues from membranes and may show some degree of selectivity for them, although its degree of 'prefer-ence' is uncertain.[190]

Continued oxidation of fatty-acid side-chains and their fragmentation to produce aldehydes and hydrocarbons (Section 4.12.5.1 below) will eventu-ally lead to loss of membrane integrity. For ex-ample, rupture of lysosomal membranes will spill hydrolytic enzymes into the rest of the cell. Per-oxidation of erythrocyte membranes causes them to lose their ability to change shape and squeeze through the smallest capillaries (Section 6.4.1). Loss of viability of spermatozoa on prolonged incubation at 37 °C can involve lipid peroxidation (Section 6.11.1), as can the loss of the germinating ability of seeds stored under warm, damp condi-tions. In some bacteria, the DNA is close to or attached to the cell membrane and it can be damaged during peroxidation. Damage to ER or Golgi apparatus by peroxidation will decrease the ability of cells to synthesize and export proteins, as happens during CCl_4 toxicity (Section 8.2).

Peroxyl and alkoxyl radicals, aldehydes and singlet O_2 can damage receptors, enzymes such as glucose 6-phosphatase, the Ca^{2+}-ATPase of the ER, the Na^+, K^+-ATPase, and K^+ channels (Section 4.3.2). Since 'voltage regulated' K^+ channels play an essential role in generation of electrical activity in nervous tissue and heart, damage to them can result in irregularities in heartbeat, and death of neurons.[191] Within mitochondria, both matrix enzymes and constituents of the electron-transport chain can be damaged, ubiquinone destroyed, and mitochondrial DNA attacked.[192] Lipid oxidation in foods can change the taste, alter the texture of food proteins and destroy essential amino acids, a par-ticular problem in the storage of fish.[193]

4.12.2 Lipid hydroperoxides (ROOH)

Oral administration of large doses of peroxidized lipids to animals causes some injury, for example heart damage in rats, 'fatty liver' in rats and rabbits, and damage to the immune system in mice.[194] Spin-trapping has been used to detect lipid-derived radicals in such animals (Section 5.2). Overall, however, the toxicity is low, and animals can tolerate moderate amounts of oxidized lipids in the diet. Indeed, the toxicity may sometimes not be due to lipid peroxides at all, but to carbonyls formed by their decomposition in the stomach (Section 4.12.5 below).[195] Oxidized lipids can have effects on cells similar to those of H_2O_2 (Section 4.2); low levels can stimulate proliferation, higher levels block proliferation and yet higher ones induce apoptosis and necrosis.[196] Such events occur in atherosclerosis (Section 9.3) and maybe in the gastrointestinal tract (Section 6.2). Lipid chlorohydrins may also exert some toxicity.[197]

Products of lipid peroxidation can also have more specific effects. For example, some mimic the actions of **platelet activating factor** (PAF, 1-*O*-alkyl-2-acetyl-*sn*-glycero-3-phosphocholine), a phospholipid synthesized by several cells, including leukocytes, platelets, and endothelial cells. It exerts effects at concentrations in the 10^{-10} M range: these include activation of phagocytes, platelet aggregation and marked vascular (e.g. hypotension) and bronchial effects. While useful at physiological levels, overproduction of PAF contributes to tissue injury in several diseases, including asthma and ischaemia–reperfusion. Once secreted, PAF is rapidly destroyed by **PAF acetylhydrolase**, an enzyme present within plasma lipoproteins (mostly LDL). Peroxidation of phosphatidylcholine can generate fragments that bind to PAF receptors on target cells and exert PAF-like activity. Some of these phospholipid fragments are also substrates for PAF acetylhydrolase.[199] Oxidized 1-palmitoyl-2-arachidonoyl-*sn*-glycero-3-phosphorylcholine (**ox-PAPC**) can stimulate cytokine production in endothelial cells, but can *inhibit* activation of NF-κB by endotoxin and subsequent cytokine production, i.e. it can be anti-inflammatory under some circumstances. It can also increase levels of HO-1, a cytoprotective enzyme (Section 3.17), in endothelial cells. Indeed intraperitoneal injection of ox-PAPC allowed mice that had been treated with a normally-lethal dose of endotoxin to survive.[200,201]

Hence several specific lipid oxidation products act as signalling molecules and their actions are not always bad (also see Sections 4.12.3 and 4.12.4). We predict that more such roles will be found.

4.12.3 Isoprostanes, isoketals and cyclopentenone compounds[179,201]

Isoprostanes (IPs) are important products of lipid peroxidation, and their measurement is probably the best currently available assay of lipid peroxidation (Section 5.14.6). They are prostaglandin-like compounds (Fig. 4.20) formed from PUFAs with at least three double bonds, including linolenic acid, arachidonic acid (**F_2-isoprostanes**), EPA (**F_3-isoprostanes**) and DHA (**F_4-isoprostanes**, sometimes called **neuroprostanes**). Sixty-four F_2-IP isomers exist (Fig. 4.21). D- and E-ring IPs can also form by rearrangement of the cyclic peroxide precursors (Fig. 4.22) and similar products isomeric to the leukotrienes

(**isoleukotrienes**) also exist, although they appear to be formed in smaller amounts during peroxidation (Fig. 4.22). Dehydration of D_2- and E_2-IsoPs can generate **cyclopentenone IPs**, which are highly reactive with –SH groups (Fig. 4.22) and cytotoxic. They may not be all bad, however, since they can damp down the inflammatory response in macrophages exposed to endotoxin.[202] **Isoketals** can also form; they combine fast with –NH_2 groups and form adducts with lysine residues on membrane proteins or –NH_2 groups on phosphatidylethanolamine. Initially a Schiff base is formed, which then dehydrates to a pyrrole and reacts with O_2 to form **lactam** and **hydroxylactam** structures (Fig. 4.22). Protein cross-linking can also result. Hence both these and the cyclopentenone IPs can damage membrane proteins *in vivo*, cross-linking the lipids containing them to membrane proteins. Isoketal-protein adducts have been detected at μM levels in human plasma.[203]

Isoprostanes are generated *in vivo* by peroxidation of phospholipids, and most of them in tissues and plasma are esterified to phospholipids (a difference from prostaglandins, which are only generated by COX enzymes from free PUFAs). Increased formation of IPs is observed in many systems undergoing oxidative stress, such as in multiple human diseases (Chapter 9) and after exposure to a range of toxins (Chapter 8). They can be released in the free form by lipases, including PAF acetylhydrolase (Section 4.12.2). Free IPs turn over rapidly; their half-life in human blood is less than 20 minutes. They are both excreted and metabolized, for example 15-F_{2t}-IsoP (8-*iso* PGF$_{2\alpha}$) undergoes β-oxidation and reduction in humans to **2,3-dinor-5,6-dihydro-15-F_{2t}-IsoP** which is also excreted in urine; another metabolite is **2,3-dinor-15-F_{2t}-IsoP** (Fig. 4.21). Figure 4.23 summarizes the array of products formed from arachidonic acid peroxidation. The levels of O_2 and thiols influence the relative amounts of the various products generated (Figs 4.20 and 4.23), which include compounds with a tetrahydrofuran ring structure, called **isofurans**. At physiological O_2 levels IPs are the major products, although this may not be true in hyperoxia (Section 5.14.6).

Isoprostanes are also biologically active; 15-E_{2t}-IsoP, 15-F_{2t}-IsoP (Fig. 4.21) and its major metabolite 2,3-dinor-5,6-dihydro-15-F_{2t}-IsoP, are powerful

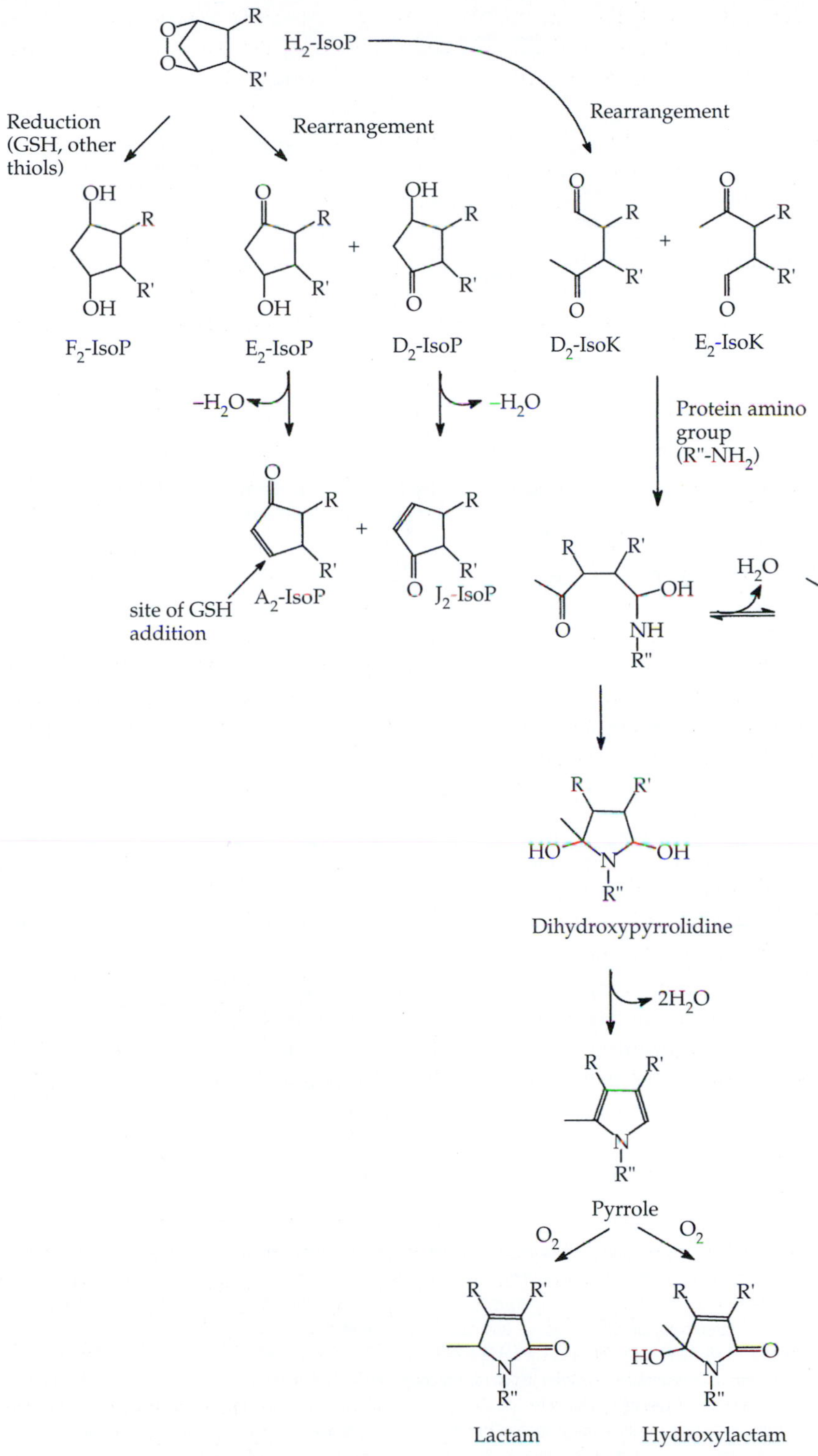
H2-IsoP
Reduction (GSH, other thiols)
Rearrangement
Rearrangement
F2-IsoP
E2-IsoP
D2-IsoP
D2-IsoK
E2-IsoK
–H2O
–H2O
Protein amino group (R''-NH2)
site of GSH addition
A2-IsoP
J2-IsoP
H2O
Schiff Base
Dihydroxypyrrolidine
2H2O
Pyrrole
O2
O2
Lactam
Hydroxylactam

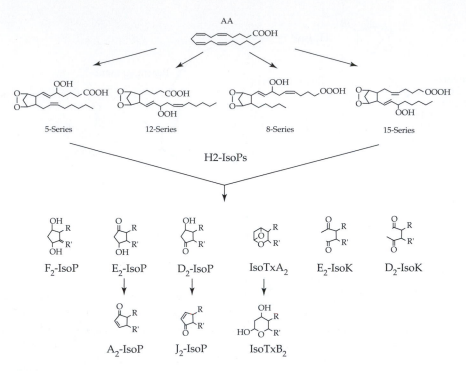

Figure 4.23 An array of products from the IsoP pathway of lipid peroxidation. From [201] by courtesy of Dr L. Jackson Roberts II and Elsevier. Each of the four regioisomers derived from arachidonic acid (AA) can give eight E_2-type and eight D_2-type isoketal diastereomers, 64 possible isoketals in total (*Chem. Phys. Lipids* **128**, 173, 2004). IsoTxA$_2$ and -B$_2$ are isoleukotrienes.

vasoconstrictors. 15-F_{2t}-IsoP provokes bone resorption, affects platelet aggregation induced by ADP or collagen, may provoke proliferation of smooth muscle cells (e.g. during atherosclerosis), and is involved in the toxicity of high glucose levels to embryos.[204] Many IPs exert vasoactive effects in the lung and act as endothelial 'contracting factors'. Several of these effects are due to binding of IPs to eicosanoid receptors. Renal vasoconstriction due to elevated F_2-IPs may contribute to the pathology of **hepatorenal syndrome**, a usually fatal disorder in which kidney failure develops in patients with severe liver disease.[205] Also, some IPs can rearrange at

body temperature to give 'real' prostaglandins (Section 7.12.5).

Neuroprostanes are formed in increased amounts in some neurodegenerative diseases (Section 9.20). Because DHA has more double bonds, eight regioisomers can be formed (Fig. 4.24). In addition E_4- and D_4-NPs can form, although at lower levels, as well as cyclopentenone structures (**A_4/J_4 neuroprostanes**), isoketal-like compounds (**neuroketals**) and isofurans (**neurofurans**).

Less attention has been given to the two classes of IPs that could arise from linolenic acid or the six

◀ **Figure 4.22** Formation of E- and D-ring isoprostanes (IPs) by rearrangement of F_2-IP precursors and their dehydration to cyclopentenone IPs. The availability of reducing agents such as GSH can affect the ratios of F_2-, E_2- and D_2-products. α-Tocopherol, if present at high levels, may also act as a reductant (*Biochem. Pharmacol.* **65**, 611, 2003). The same regioisomers of E_2- and D_2-IsoPs are formed as for the F_2-IsoPs (Fig. 4.21). The F_2-IPs appear to be the preferred products *in vivo*, presumably because thiols are abundant. For example in rats exposed to CCl_4 (Section 8.2) the liver levels of F_2-, E_2/D_2-IPs and isoleukotrienes were 672 ± 179, 161 ± 37 and 102 ± 30 ng/g respectively.[201] Dehydration of the E_2- and D_2-IsoPs can generate cyclopentenone isoprostanes (A_2-, J_2-IsoP) which rapidly conjugate with thiol groups to form adducts and are cytotoxic. Probably most react with GSH *in vivo* (a reaction that can be catalysed by GST A4-4; Section 3.9.5.2), but they might also form damaging adducts with $-$SH groups in membrane proteins. Yet another possibility is the formation of acyclic γ-ketoaldehydes (D_2IsoK, E_2-IsoK), the **isoketals** (sometimes called **isolevuglandins**). Figure adapted from[201] by courtesy of Dr L. Jackson Roberts II and Elsevier, and from *Cell Mol. Life Sci.* **59**, 808, 2002 by courtesy of Drs L. Jackson Roberts II and J.D. Morrow and Birkhauser, Basle.

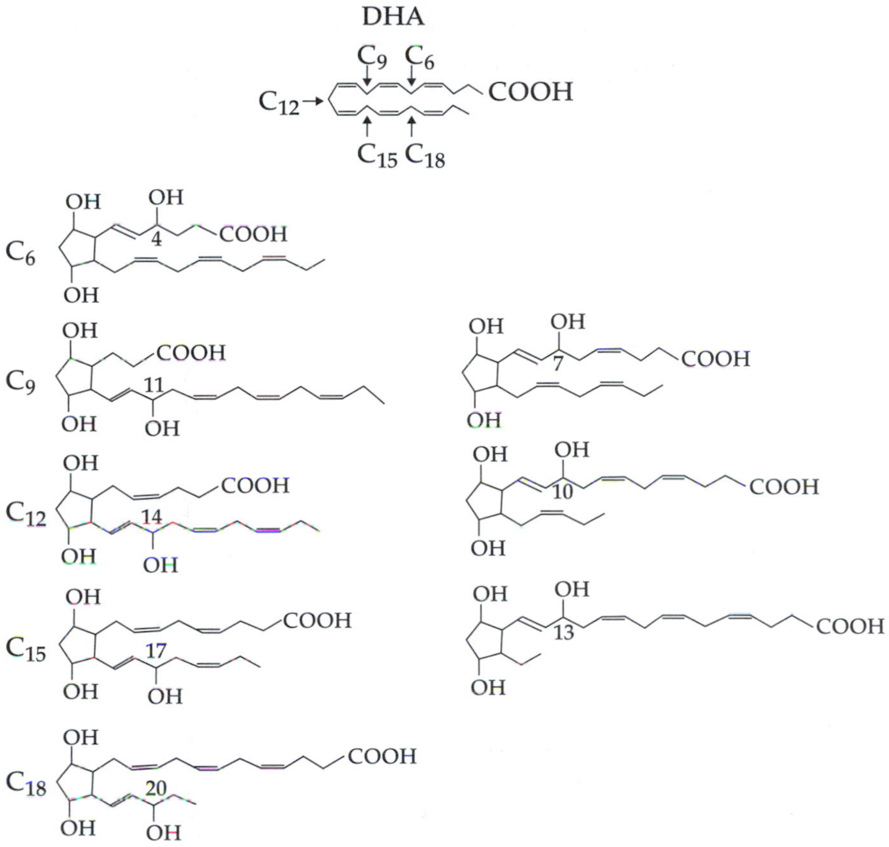

Figure 4.24 The neuroprostanes. The carbons from which H• abstraction occurs to result in regioisomer formation are shown. Abstraction of H• from C6, C9, C12, C15 or C18 gives 4-, 7-, 10-, 11-, 13-, 14-, 17- and 20- series neuroprostanes, giving a total of 128 isomers. The 4- and 20-series are more commonly formed than the others. From [201] by courtesy of Dr L. Jackson Roberts II and Elsevier.

classes from EPA, although linolenate-derived IPs (**phytoprostanes**) have been described in plants (Section 6.7).

4.12.4 Cholesterol oxidation products (COPs)[186]

Cholesterol in membranes and lipoproteins can be oxidized photochemically and during lipid peroxidation, generating a mixture of products (Fig. 4.25). Cholesteryl esters can be oxidized on the ring and/or on the esterified fatty acid (giving hydroperoxides, isoprostanes, etc) and some of these products have been detected in human plasma (Table 5.12). Reports on the cytotoxicity of COPs are conflicting, possibly because many studies have used complex mixtures rather than single products. For example, oxidation products of cholesterol have variously been claimed to stimulate or to suppress

atherogenesis. Several studies on isolated cells show that COPs can decrease cytokine production induced by endotoxin treatment, apparently by decreasing NF-κB activation,[206] but others report proinflammatory effects.

Cholesterol can be oxidized in foodstuffs, and some of the COPs absorbed through the gastro-intestinal tract.[207] Plant sterols (**phytosterols**) also undergo oxidation; since they are now being added to many foodstuffs the biological consequences of their oxidation products probably deserve more attention.[208]

4.12.5 Decomposition products from lipid peroxides: what do they do?

Decomposition of lipid peroxides by metal ions or by heating (e.g. of oxidized cooking oils) generates a

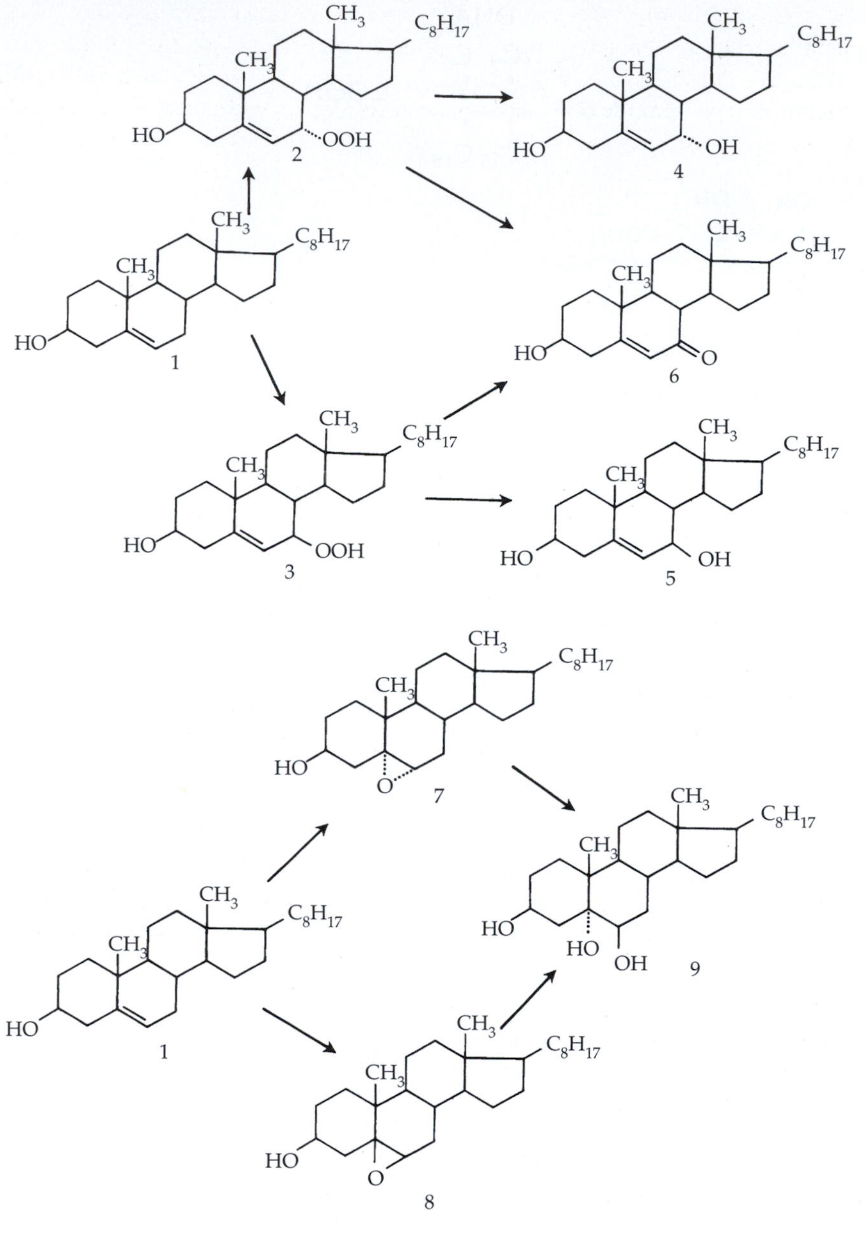

Figure 4.25 Cholesterol and some of its oxidation products. 1, Cholesterol; 2 and 3, cholesterol 7-hydroperoxides; 4 and 5, cholest-5-ene-3-β7-diols; 6,3β-hydroxycholest-5-en-7-one; 7 and 8, 5,6β-epoxy-5β- and 5,6α-epoxy-5α-cholestan-3-β-ols; 9,5α-cholestane-3β,5,6β-triol. Diagram modified from *Chem. Phys. Lipids* **44**, 87, 1987 by courtesy of Professor L.L. Smith and the publishers. Reaction of singlet O_2 with cholesterol yields primarily the 5α-hydroperoxide (Fig. 2.15) whereas free-radical oxidation gives 7β and 7α-hydroperoxides and the other products shown.[186]

hugely complex mixture of products, including epoxides, saturated aldehydes (e.g. **hexanal**), unsaturated aldehydes such as ***trans, trans*-2,4-decadienal**, ketones (e.g. butanones, pentanones, octanones), and hydrocarbons.[209] Thermal homolysis of the

O–O bond yield radicals, that can attack other PUFAs

$$ROOH \rightarrow RO^\bullet + OH^\bullet$$

Cleavage of aldehyde, hydrocarbon or other

fragments from peroxidized lipids still leaves an oxidized fragment attached to the parent lipid by an ester bond. It has been speculated that exposure to peroxide decomposition products in heated cooking oils during stir-frying could contribute to the high incidence of lung cancer in non-smoking women in Singapore and China.[210]

4.12.5.1 *Ethane and pentane*

Metal ions (especially iron and copper) and haem proteins can cause hydrocarbon formation from peroxides. For example, if Fe^{2+} reacts with a hydroperoxide on the fifth carbon from the methyl end of a PUFA, **pentane** can be produced. This can happen with linoleic and arachidonic acids

$$CH_3(CH_2)_4 - \overset{\overset{H}{|}}{\underset{\underset{OOH}{|}}{C}} - R \; + \; Fe^{2+} \longrightarrow Fe(III) \; + \; OH^- \; + \; CH_3(CH_2)_4 \overset{\overset{H}{|}}{\underset{\underset{O^{\cdot}}{|}}{C}} - R$$

(R, rest of molecule)   alkoxyl radical

$$CH_3(CH_2)_3CH_3 \xleftarrow[\substack{\text{from another}\\ \text{fatty-acid side-}\\ \text{chain}}]{\text{abstracts H.}} CH_3(CH_2)_3\overset{\cdot}{C}H_2 \; + \; \overset{\overset{H}{|}}{\underset{\underset{O}{\|}}{C}} - R$$

pentane   pentane radical

    (β-scission reaction, to the right of alkoxyl radical)

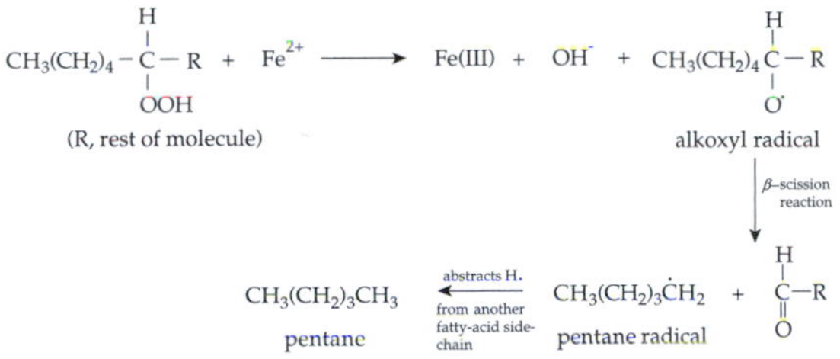

Ethane (C_2H_6) and **ethylene** (ethene, $H_2C=CH_2$) gases are produced in similar reactions form linolenic acid. *β*-**Scission**, shown above, is a well-known reaction of alkoxyl radicals. Formation of these gases has been used to estimate rates of lipid peroxidation *in vivo* (Section 5.14.8).

4.12.5.2 *Malondialdehyde*[209]

Malondialdehyde, sometimes called **malonaldehyde**, was a focus of attention in lipid peroxidation for years because it was commonly thought that the widely used thiobarbituric acid (TBA) assay measures free MDA. Sadly, it does not (Section 5.14.9). Also, MDA toxicity was over-estimated; it is less reactive than HNE (see below) and much less so than the levuglandins (Section 7.12.6) or isoketals (Section 4.12.3).

Malondialdehyde arises largely from peroxidation of PUFAs with more than two double bonds, such as linolenic, arachidonic and docosahexaenoic acids, but some is formed enzymatically during eicosanoid metabolism (Section 7.12). It exists in various forms, depending on pH (Fig. 4.26). At physiological pH most 'free' MDA will exist as an

enolate anion which has low reactivity toward most amino groups. As pH falls, reactivity increases and proteins can then be attacked by MDA, resulting in modification of several residues (especially lysine) and formation of intra- and intermolecular cross-links.

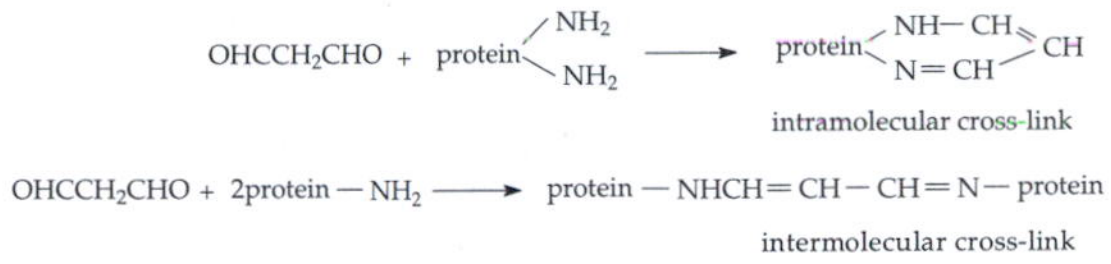

$$OHCCH_2CHO \; + \; \text{protein} \overset{NH_2}{\underset{NH_2}{<}} \longrightarrow \text{protein} \overset{NH-CH}{\underset{N=CH}{<}} CH$$

intramolecular cross-link

$$OHCCH_2CHO \; + \; 2\text{protein}-NH_2 \longrightarrow \text{protein}-NHCH=CH-CH=N-\text{protein}$$

intermolecular cross-link

Malondialdehyde also reacts with DNA bases (Fig. 4.27) and can introduce mutagenic lesions. Guanine is a preferred target. The contribution of MDA-DNA adducts to mutagenicity *in vivo* is uncertain: indeed, pure MDA is poorly mutagenic in several bacterial test systems. However, if DNA pretreated with MDA is expressed in *E. coli*, about a 10-fold increase in mutation frequency is observed: G → T transversions, A → G transitions and C → T transitions are predominant, but some frameshifts and deletions occur.[211] Such DNA is also mutagenic in human cells, causing large insertions and deletions as well as base-pair substitutions.[212]

Malondialdehyde is rapidly metabolized in mammalian tissues. Aldehyde dehydrogenases oxidize it to malonic semialdehyde, which decarboxylates to acetaldehyde, in turn oxidized by aldehyde dehydrogenases to acetate.

4.12.5.3 *4-Hydroxy-2-*trans*-nonenal (HNE) and other unsaturated aldehydes*[182,209]

The compound HNE is formed during the peroxidation of *n*-6 PUFAs, such as linoleic and arachidonic acids.[213] It is one of several unsaturated aldehydes (**alkenals**) formed during lipid peroxidation; others include decadienal and ***trans*-4-hydroxy-2-hexenal** (HHE), which is particularly damaging to mitochondria.[214] Indeed, HHE is the ultimate toxic product formed in the liver during the metabolism of pyrrolizidine alkaloids such as **senecionine**,[215] which are found in several plants that can poison livestock. Linoleic acid autoxidation during beer preparation generates **trans-2-nonenal**, excess of which leads to a stale, 'cardboard' flavour of the beer.[216]

Effects of HNE observed *in vitro* fall into three main categories, depending on its concentration:

1. 100 μM or above: toxic to most cell types, mitochondrial damage, cell death. These levels are generally above those that can occur *in vivo*.

2. 2 to 20 μM: inhibits DNA and protein synthesis, but stimulates phospholipase A$_2$. Generally inhibits cellular cell proliferation and toxic to many cells (especially neurons), may also inhibit nucleotide excision repair.[217,218] Can inhibit PARP-1, chaperone action (e.g. of Hsp72), and certain CYPs, for example CYP2E1 and CYP1AI. Such concentrations may be achievable *in vivo* during oxidative stress.

3. 1 μM or lower: may represent basal levels of HNE in healthy tissues (although probably protein-bound rather than free). *In vitro*, low μM

levels of HNE can stimulate phagocyte chemotaxis and the activities of several receptors and enzymes, including adenylate cyclase, guanylate cyclase, phospholipase C, PDI, and protein kinase C. These HNE levels can lead to increased synthesis of Hsp (including HO-1), and can act via Keap1 (Section 4.5.10) to elevate GST and γ-GCS activities. Hydroxynonenal has been implicated in liver fibrogenesis, by increasing collagen biosynthesis and levels of the profibrogenic and proinflammatory cytokine TGFβ$_1$ (Section 8.8).[218]

Hydroxyalkenals owe their chemical reactivity to three main features; the aldehyde group, the double bond and the −OH group (Fig. 4.28). Their ability to react rapidly with thiol groups at physiological pH accounts for much of their

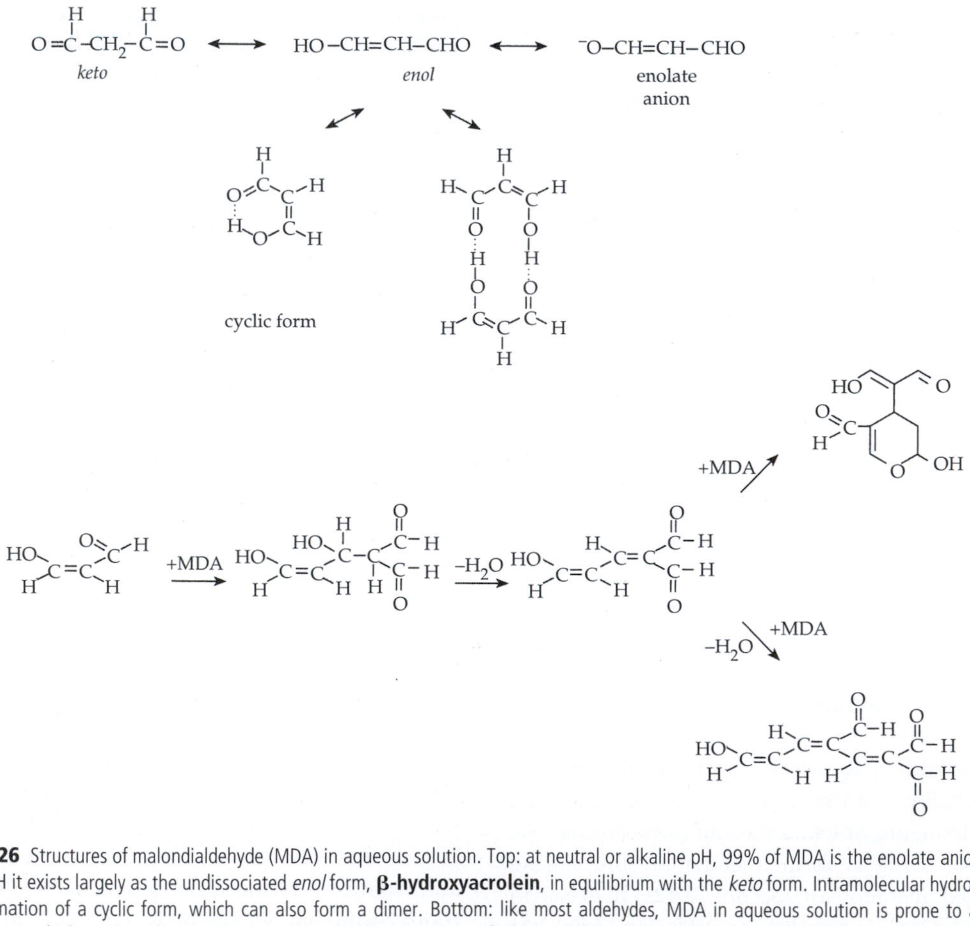

Figure 4.26 Structures of malondialdehyde (MDA) in aqueous solution. Top: at neutral or alkaline pH, 99% of MDA is the enolate anion whereas at acidic pH it exists largely as the undissociated *enol* form, **β-hydroxyacrolein**, in equilibrium with the *keto* form. Intramolecular hydrogen bonds favour formation of a cyclic form, which can also form a dimer. Bottom: like most aldehydes, MDA in aqueous solution is prone to aldol condensations which produce dimers, trimers and large polymers, many of which are fluorescent (excitation at 365–395 nm, emission at 490 nm). Data abstracted from *Free Rad. Biol. Med.* **11**, 81, 1991 by courtesy of the late Professor Hermann Esterbauer and Elsevier.

cytotoxicity. For example, GSH reacts with HNE to form a saturated aldehyde, followed by an intramolecular rearrangement to yield a five-membered ring (Fig. 4.28). Thiol groups on proteins as well as amino groups on DNA bases (Fig. 4.27), proteins (e.g. on lysine residues; histidine can also be attacked) and phospholipids (phosphatidylethanolamine and phosphatidylserine) can react with HNE. The products of reaction with aminolipids are fluorescent at 430 nm when excited at 360 nm, properties similar to those of peroxidized lipids.

When HNE is generated *in vivo*, it rapidly reacts with proteins and other biomolecules containing $-NH_2$ or $-SH$ groups and does not stay 'free'; this is one problem in assessing the biological significance of its effects at different 'levels' of addition, as indicated above. For example, HNE added to blood plasma (where GSH levels are low) rapidly binds to $-SH$ groups on albumin; some may attach to ascorbate (Section 3.20.1.3). **Fatty acid binding proteins**, found in epithelial cells,

have been suggested to absorb HNE and protect other cell constituents.[219] However, levuglandins (Section 7.12.6) and isoketals (Section 4.12.3) damage proteins faster than HNE. Etheno-adducts formed by HNE in DNA are mutagenic but can be removed by BER and NER (Fig. 4.27).

Cells can also catabolize HNE. It can be reduced to an alcohol by aldose reductase, oxidized to a carboxylic acid by aldehyde dehydrogenases (Fig. 4.28), or form GSH conjugates, both non-enzymically and catalysed by certain GSTs, especially GST A4-4.[220] Conjugates are degraded to mercapturic acids and excreted in urine. Aldehyde–thiol conjugates are in general about ten-fold less toxic than the parent aldehydes, although not completely harmless: they may be somewhat toxic in their own right and/ or act as a 'reservoir' that slowly releases HNE.

Acrolein, $H_2C=CHCHO$, is also formed during lipid peroxidation and reacts readily with $-SH$ groups, and with $-NH_2$ groups on proteins and

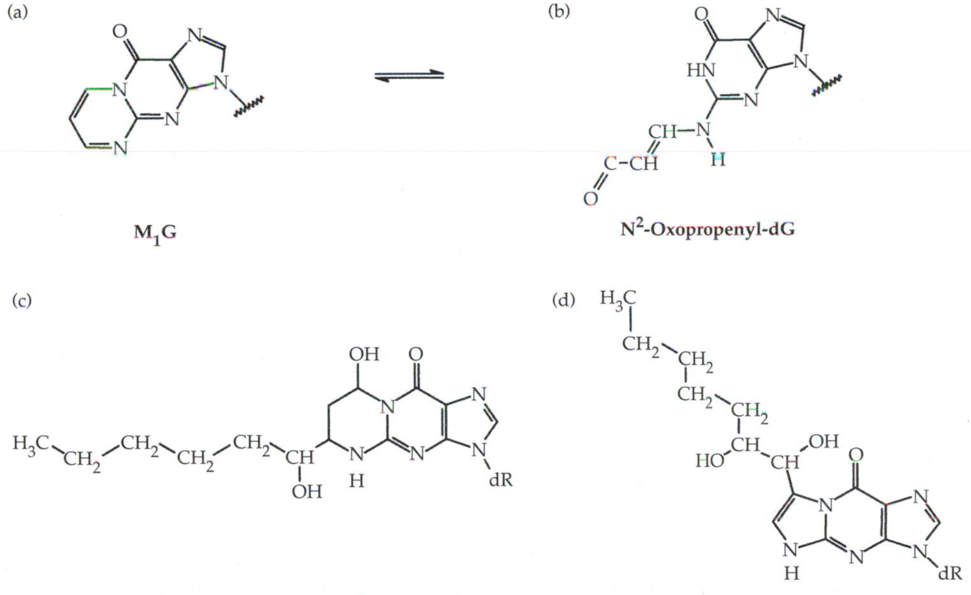

(a) M_1G

(b) N^2-Oxopropenyl-dG

(c)

(d)

Figure 4.27 Reaction of cytotoxic aldehydes with DNA bases. The major product of reaction of MDA with guanine in DNA at physiological pH is (a) pyrimido[1,2-α]purine-10(3H)-one (**M₁G**), shown as a nucleoside (dR = deoxyribose). This product has been identified in rat and human DNA at low levels. M₁G undergoes ring opening to **N²-oxopropenyl-G** (b) when positioned opposite C in double-stranded DNA (*J. Am. Chem. Soc.* **126**, 8237, 2004). It can also be formed in DNA from base propenals arising from oxidation of the C4¹ site on deoxyribose, for example by OH•, i.e it is *not* a specific marker of MDA damage to DNA (*J. Biol. Chem.* **280**, 25377, 2005). Hydroxynonenal reacts with all four DNA bases but G is a preferred target, an NH₂ group adding to the double bond of the aldehyde to give **1,N²-propano-2¹-deoxyguanosine** adducts (c). A substituted **1N²-ethenodeoxyguanosine** (d) is also formed in smaller amounts; its formation is favoured by the presence of high levels of H₂O₂. Nucleotide excision repair can remove these adducts from DNA (*Biochemistry* **43**, 7514, 2004).

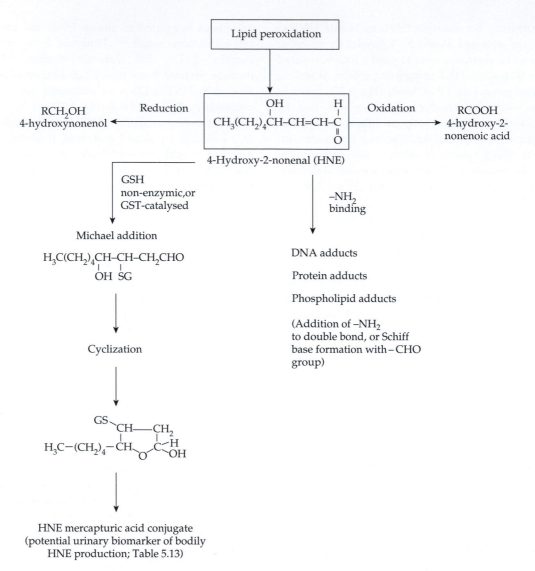

Figure 4.28 Toxicity and metabolism of 4-hydroxynonenal.

DNA bases, especially guanine.[221] Its reaction with DNA bases is faster than that of HNE.

4.12.6 Peroxidation of other molecules

PUFAs are not the only molecules that contain double bonds and can be peroxidized. Carotenoids can (Section 3.21.3). Retinal can be oxidized in the eye (Section 6.10). The retinal precursor **retinol (vitamin A)** can undergo peroxidation and

degradation,[222] as can some antibiotics that contain double bonds (Section 8.16).

4.12.7 Repair of lipid peroxidation

Peroxides within membranes can be reduced to alcohols by PHGPx (Section 3.8.1). Alternatively, they may be cleaved from membranes by phospholipase A_2 (Section 4.12.1), whereupon the released fatty acid peroxides can be acted upon

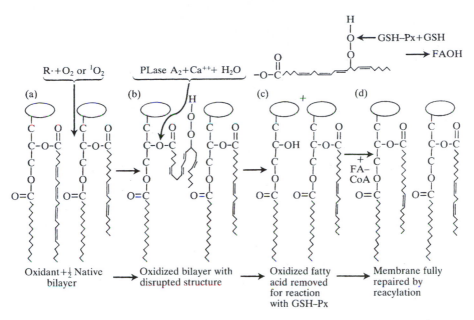

Figure 4.29 Model for the repair of lipid peroxides. Formation of peroxides in the membrane causes rearrangement as these more-polar species move to the surface. There they are cleaved by phospholipase A_2 (PLase A_2) in the presence of Ca^{2+}. Glutathione peroxidase (GSH-Px) in the surrounding fluid reduces the released fatty acid peroxides to alcohols (FAOH). Repair is completed by reacylation with a fatty-acyl-coenzyme A. Diagram adapted from *Trends Biochem. Sci.* **12**, 31, 1987 by courtesy of Dr van Kuijk and Elsevier. Phospholipase A_2 releases both oxidized and unmolested fatty acid side-chains from membranes.

by GPx1 (Fig. 4.29). PAF acetylhydrolases (Section 4.12.2) can remove aldehyde residues from partially-oxidized phospholipids.

When phosphatidylcholine hydroperoxide is added to human plasma, it is reduced to the alcohol, despite the fact that plasma GPx has almost no GSH available to it (Section 3.8.1). One enzyme contributing to loss of the hydroperoxide is **lecithin cholesterol acyltransferase** (LCAT), found in HDL. This enzyme reversibly transfers fatty-acid side-chains from phospholipids to cholesterol, generating cholesteryl esters for storage in the HDL core. It appears to reduce the phosphatidylcholine hydroperoxide to an alcohol, whilst generating a cholesterol ester hydroperoxide.[223]

4.12.8 Lipids as antioxidants? The plasmalogens

Plasmalogens are choline- or ethanolamine-containing phospholipids that have an ether rather than an ester bond at C1 of the glycerol backbone (Fig. 4.30). Several papers suggested that they might act as endogenous 'membrane antioxidants'. Plasmalogens are found at significant levels in red blood cells, heart, sperm and nervous tissue (Section 9.16.6.12). Cells lacking them are more rapidly killed by oxidative stresses, including generation of singlet O_2 by photosensitization. The double bond next to the ether group (Fig. 4.30) appears to be attacked especially rapidly by RS, so 'sparing' other membrane lipids. The products decompose rapidly into species that do not appear to propagate lipid peroxidation.[224] However, the cellular consequences of plasmalogen oxidation (e.g. do they form reactive aldehydes?) need to be better understood before this can be truly described as an antioxidant effect. Reactive chlorine and bromine species can oxidize and halogenate membrane plasmalogens, producing chloro- and bromoaldehydes that have been suggested to be chemotactic agents for phagocytes.[225]

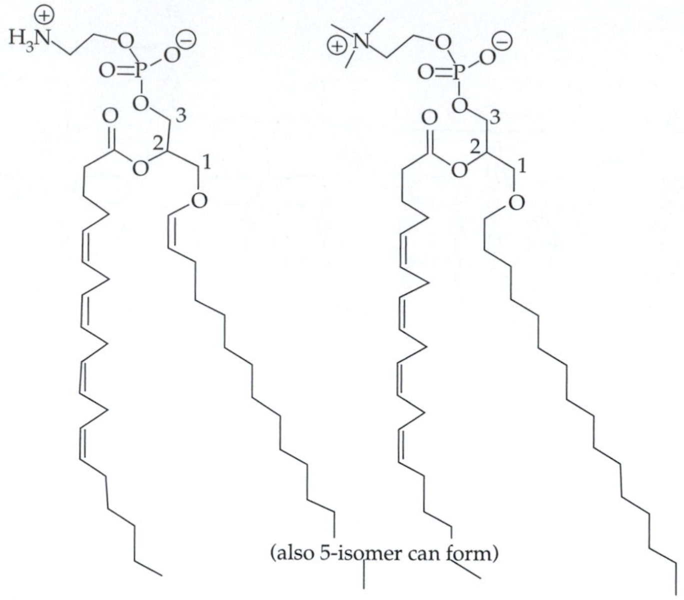

(also 5-isomer can form)

Plasmenyl-glycerophospholipid
Hexadec-1-enyl-2 arachidonoyl-sn-
glycero-3-phosphoethanolamine

Plasmanyl glycerophospholipid
1-O-hexadecyl-2-arachidonoyl-sn-
glycero-3-phosphocholine

Figure 4.30 Examples of plasmenyl and plasmanyl glycerol-based phospholipids found in membranes. Plasmenyl species are commonly referred to as **plasmalogens**, with a *cis* double bond adjacent to the O atom of the ether linkage to glycerol. Plasmalogens form about 15–20% of total phospholipids in many cell membranes and are about 5% of phospholipids in human lipoproteins. From *Chem. Res. Toxicol.* **14**, 463, 2001 by courtesy of Dr R.C. Murphy and the American Chemical Society.

4.12.9 Polyamines: antioxidants or pro-oxidants?

The polyamines

putrescine $H_3\overset{+}{N}(CH_2)_4N\overset{+}{H}_3$

spermine $H_3\overset{+}{N}(CH_3)_3NH(CH_2)_4N\overset{+}{H}(CH_2)_3NH_3$

and

spermidine $H_3\overset{+}{N}(CH_2)_4NH(CH_2)_3N\overset{+}{H}_3$

are positively-charged at physiological pH and bind readily to phospholipids and to DNA. Under certain circumstances, they can protect these biomolecules against oxidation, for example by deterring the binding of transition metal ions. Indeed, *E. coli* unable to make polyamines are killed by 95% O_2, a level tolerated by wild-type *E. coli*.[226] However, polyamine oxidation products might be cytotoxic. For example, during brain ischaemia polyamines can be converted to reactive aminoaldehydes such as **3-aminopropanal**, a potent neurotoxin.[227] Overall, the significance of polyamines as antioxidants *in vivo* is uncertain.

4.13 Mechanisms of damage to cellular targets by oxidative stress: protein damage

4.13.1 Does protein damage matter?

Oxidative protein damage occurs during X-ray crystallography (Section 8.9.10), but is also important *in vivo* because it can impair the functioning of receptors, antibodies, signal transduction and transport proteins and enzymes. For example hyperbaric O_2 damage to *E. coli* involves inactivation of specific enzymes (Section 1.6). Protein damage can lead to secondary damage to other biomolecules, for example by raising Ca^{2+} levels (Section 4.3.1) and activating nucleases. Damage to DNA repair enzymes raises oxidative DNA damage levels and increases mutation frequency, whereas damage to DNA polymerases may decrease their fidelity in replicating DNA. Oxidized proteins may be recognized as 'foreign' by the immune system,[228] triggering antibody formation and perhaps autoimmunity, for example in rheumatoid arthritis and scleroderma (Sections 9.9 and 9.10). In the pharmaceutical industry, oxidation can be a problem in the handling of protein/polypeptide drugs, methionine and cysteine residues being particularly prone to damage. For example, oxidation of methionine residues in cholecystokinin was a particular nuisance during production of this peptide.[229]

4.13.2 How does damage occur? Is it random or specific?

Damage to proteins can occur by direct attack of RS, or by 'secondary damage' involving attack by end-products of lipid peroxidation, such as iso-ketals, MDA and HNE. Proteins can also be damaged by glycation (Section 9.4). Some protein damage is reversible, such as peroxiredoxin inactivation (Section 3.11.1), methionine sulphoxide formation (Section 4.14.1 below), S-nitrosylation (Table 2.9), destruction of Fe–S clusters by $O_2^{\bullet-}$ (Section 3.6.1), glutathionylation (Section 3.9.6) and, possibly, nitration (Section 2.6). Other damage, for example oxidation of side-chains to carbonyl residues, appears irreversible and the protein is destroyed and replaced (Section 4.14.2 below).

When cells are subjected to oxidative stress, proteomic techniques reveal that often only a small number of proteins are damaged, although the mechanisms of this selectivity remain undetermined. For example, in E. coli treated with H_2O_2 **alcohol dehydrogenase E** (Section 7.3), elongation factor G, enolase, a heat shock protein, an outer membrane protein and oligopeptide-binding protein A were major targets.[230] In yeast, H_2O_2 treatment damaged mitochondrial enzymes, Hsp60, cytosolic fatty acid synthase, G3PDH, and peroxiredoxin.[231] In skin fibroblasts treated with H_2O_2, several proteins in the ER (including PDI; Section 3.10) were rapidly oxidized, triggering an ER stress response.[232] Specific proteins undergo oxidative damage during ageing (Section 10.4.5) and in

the brains of patients with Alzheimer's disease (Section 9.20).

4.13.3 Chemistry of protein damage[233,234]

Some radical-containing enzymes are attacked by O_2, forming peroxyl radicals that fragment and inactivate the protein (Section 7.3). However, most proteins in vivo are 'non-radicals'.

Attack of various reactive nitrogen and halogen species (e.g. $ONOO^-$, $NO_2^{\bullet}$, HOCl, HOBr and NO_2Cl) upon tyrosine (both free and in proteins) leads to production of 3-nitro-, bromo-, chloro- and dihalogenated tyrosines. Nitration of phenylalanine and tryptophan can also occur (Fig. 4.31). Attack of $OH^{\bullet}$ or singlet O_2 upon proteins generates a multiplicity of end-products; Figs 2.15 and 4.31). The chemistry of oxidative protein damage is even more complex than for DNA; instead of four bases and one sugar there are 20 or more amino acid residues, each capable of forming several oxidation products. Peptide bonds can also be attacked, for example $H^{\bullet}$ abstraction by $OH^{\bullet}$. By contrast, H_2O_2, $NO^{\bullet}$ or $O_2^{\bullet-}$ at physiological levels generally have little or no direct effect on proteins, although H_2O_2 can attack certain easily-oxidizable, accessible – SH groups, as in G3PDH (Section 2.6.2) and the caspases (Section 4.4.1.2).

In the early 1900s, Dakin, Tappel and their colleagues showed that a wide variety of carbonyls and peroxides is produced in irradiated protein solutions. Initial $OH^{\bullet}$ attack generates free radicals that combine with O_2 to give alkoxyl and peroxyl radicals, the latter capable of abstracting $H^{\bullet}$ and forming peroxides. Alkoxyl radicals can fragment by β-scission, releasing carbonyls from the proteins. Peroxides can form on the peptide backbone, and on the side-chains of amino-acid residues. Amino-acid peroxides, like lipid peroxides, are fairly stable at physiological temperature but can decompose to $RO^{\bullet}$ and $RO_2^{\bullet}$ radicals on heating or if transition-metal ions are added. Since many proteins bind metal ions, especially iron and copper, subsequent exposure of them to H_2O_2 generates $OH^{\bullet}$ which selectively damages the amino-acid residues at the binding site. For example, copper ions can bind to histidine residues on albumin (Section 3.16.3.5) and on apoprotein B of LDL (Section 9.3.8). Subsequent

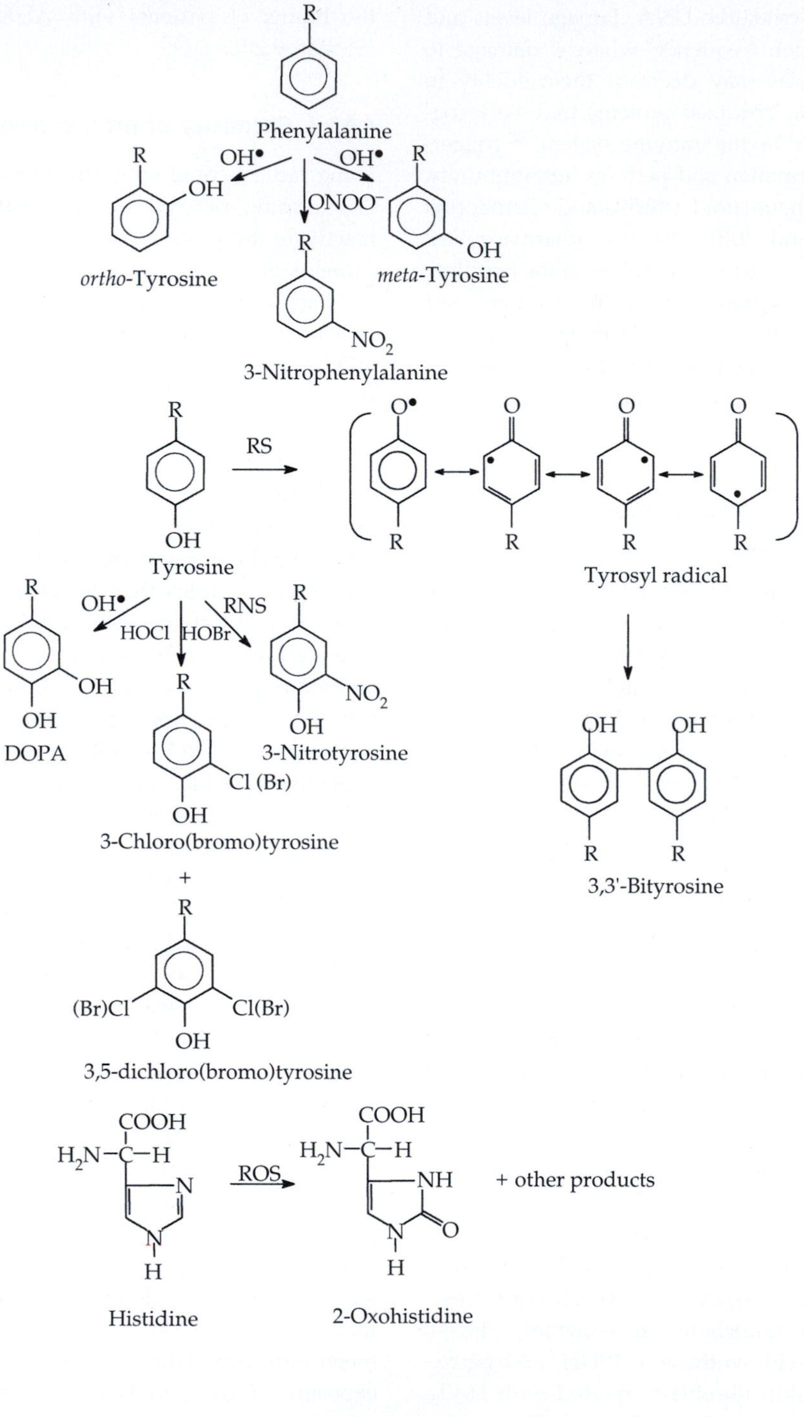

Figure 4.31 Some end-products of oxidative damage to amino-acid residues in proteins. Only selected products are shown; many others form, and some have not yet been identified.

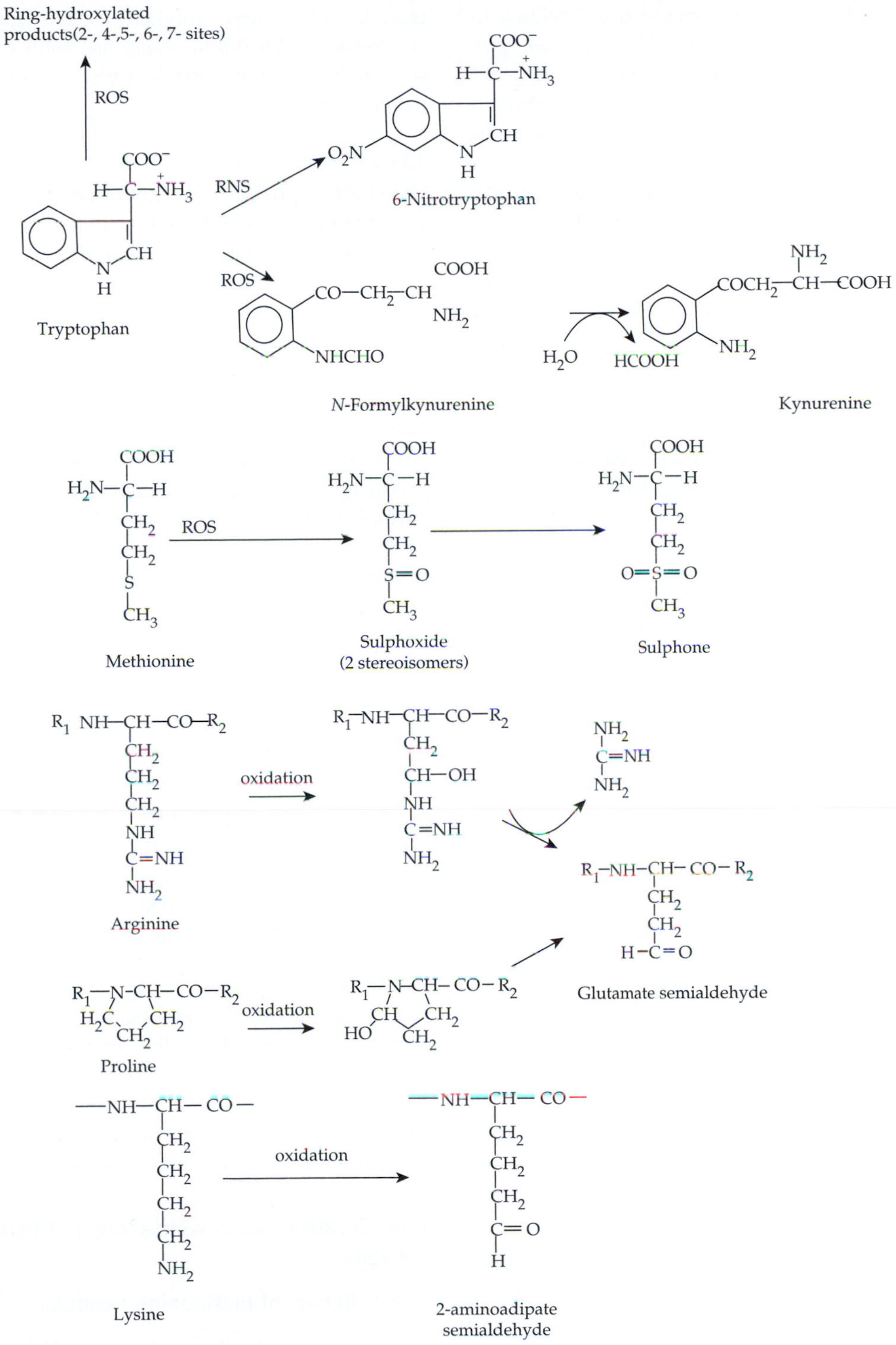

Figure 4.31 (*Cont.*)

addition of H_2O_2 causes conversion of histidine to 2-oxohistidine (Fig. 4.31). Like H_2O_2, protein peroxides can damage enzymes with delicate –SH groups, such as caspases.[235] Unlike H_2O_2, protein peroxides are hard to remove, not being substrates for catalase or GPx enzymes.

When amino-acid radicals are generated in a protein, electrons can 'migrate' to other residues, that is the final products observed need not necessarily represent the initial sites of RS attack upon the protein. For example, methionine radicals can oxidize tryptophan, and trytophan radicals can oxidize tyrosine: in terms of reduction potentials $E^{\circ\prime}$ for met$^{\bullet}$/met>trp$^{\bullet}$/trpH>tyrO$^{\bullet}$/tyrOH. Tyrosine radicals can react with several antioxidants and also with $O_2^{\bullet-}$. Thus, although $O_2^{\bullet-}$ rarely reacts directly with proteins, its presence can alter the distribution of products generated by exposure to more reactive species such as OH$^{\bullet}$. For example, if TyrO$^{\bullet}$ is generated, $O_2^{\bullet-}$ can decrease bityrosine formation; reaction with $O_2^{\bullet-}$ 'diverts' tyrosine radicals and diminishes their cross-linking. Protein radicals can combine to cross-link proteins, for example by bityrosine formation (Fig. 2.6 and 4.31), disulphide bridges or the joining of two carbon-centred radicals (favoured at low O_2).

4.13.4 Damage to specific amino-acid residues

4.13.4.1 *Cysteine and methionine*
Thiol groups are easily oxidized by RS and by transition-metal ions, forming thiyl radicals, disulphides and further oxidation products such as sulphones and sulphonic acids (Section 2.5.5). Methionine is readily oxidized by OH$^{\bullet}$, $^1O_2$, HOCl, chloramines and ONOO$^-$. Two electron oxidation produces **methionine sulphoxide**, which can undergo further oxidation to the sulphone (Fig. 4.31). One-electron oxidation (e.g. by OH$^{\bullet}$) generates a sulphur radical cation (**metS$^{\bullet+}$**) as an intermediate in sulphoxide formation. Methionine residues are often essential for protein function, for example for α_1-antiproteinase (Section 2.6.3), and oxidation of methionine decreases their activity.

4.13.4.2 *Histidine*
Damage to histidine residues in enzymes often leads to inactivation, one example being PerR

(section 4.5.3) and another *E. coli* glutamine synthetase.[233] Histidine reacts fast with OH$^{\bullet}$ and singlet O_2, forming several products, including 2-oxohistidine (Fig. 4.31).

4.13.4.3 *Proline, lysine and arginine*
Oxidation of proline and arginine residues can lead to **glutamate semialdehyde** whereas lysine can form **2-aminoadipate semialdehyde** (Fig. 4.31).

4.13.4.4 *Tryptophan*
Tryptophan residues are sensitive to damage by singlet O_2, RO$_2^{\bullet}$, RO$^{\bullet}$, OH$^{\bullet}$, and some other RS, generating ring hydroxylation products, peroxyl radicals, peroxides and eventually **N-formylkynurenine** and **kynurenine** as fluorescent oxidation products (Fig. 4.31). In mitochondria isolated from normal human heart, *N*-formylkynurenine was detected in multiple proteins, especially those of complexes I and V, suggesting ongoing oxidative protein damage in these organelles.[236]

4.13.4.5 *Tyrosine and phenylalanine*
Tyrosine residues in proteins can be attacked by RNS, reactive halogen species, OH$^{\bullet}$ and RO$_2^{\bullet}$/RO$^{\bullet}$ (Fig. 4.31). Attack of OH$^{\bullet}$ can hydroxylate tyrosine to **dihydroxyphenylalanine** (DOPA), although this product is easily further oxidized. Attack of OH$^{\bullet}$ upon phenylalanine generates intermediate radicals which can form *ortho-*, *para-* and *meta-*tyrosines. Phenylalanine can also be a target of attack by RNS, generating nitrophenylalanines (Fig. 4.31).

4.13.4.6 *Valine*
Valine hydroperoxides are readily formed when proteins are exposed to OH$^{\bullet}$, including β-hydroperoxyvaline, (2S, 3S)-γ-hydroperoxyvaline and (2S, 3R)-γ-hydroperoxyvaline. They can be decomposed by transition metals or acted upon by GPx. Products include **valine hydroxides**.

4.14 Dealing with oxidative protein damage

4.14.1 Repair of methionine residues[233,237]

Methionine sulphoxide reductases (MSR) play a key role in this. Methionine sulphoxide has R- and S-stereoisomers (Fig. 4.31). *E. coli*, *Neisseria* *gonorrhoeae* and many other bacteria, protozoa, yeasts, higher plants and mammalian (including human) tissues contain enzymes that reduce methionine sulphoxide in peptides/ proteins back to methionine and reactivate proteins inhibited by methionine oxidation. Both *S*- and *R*-specific reductases have been identified; **MsrA** (sometimes called **MsrS**) is specific for the *S*-isomer and **MsrB** (**MsrR**) for the *R*-isomer. The reducing power is supplied by thioredoxin (often replaced by the synthetic dithiol dithiothreitol in laboratory assays).

Methionine sulphoxide reductase A has an essential cysteine residue at its active site, which is oxidized by met sulphoxide and re-reduced by thioredoxin. In some animal MsrB enzymes, a selenocysteine plays the same role. Hence selenium deficiency can promote oxidative protein damage by interfering with MsrB activity (Section 3.11.2).

4.14.1.1 *A methionine cycle?*[233]

It has been suggested that methionine residues on a protein surface can act as 'sinks' for RS, since the resulting sulphoxide can readily be repaired, or even that reversible oxidation of methionine residues may play a role in redox signalling. Indeed, bacteria or yeast lacking MSR are hypersensitive to damage by H_2O_2 or RNS, whereas overexpression of MSR in *Drosophila* extended lifespan (Section 10.4.2). In animals MSR are present in both mitochondria and cytosol, and mice lacking MsrA have shortened lifespans, neurological symptoms (Section 9.16.6.9), decreased resistance to oxidative stress and increased accumulation of protein carbonyls with age, despite the presence of MsrB.

4.14.2 Removal: lysosomes and proteasomes[238,239]

When a protein is damaged *in vivo* by RS, it is often 'marked' for proteolytic removal. This is necessary because accumulation of proteins with incorrect conformation can lead to cell death, especially if it occurs in the ER (Fig. 4.8). By contrast, heavily oxidized proteins may resist proteolytic attack and form aggregates, a process which may decrease their toxicity by sequestering them in insoluble clumps.

There are several ways to destroy unwanted proteins. One is to dispatch them to the lysosomes, which contain hydrolytic enzymes, such as **cathepsins**. Erythrocytes have an oxidized protein hydrolase (Section 6.4.6). Lysosomes degrade proteins taken into the cell by endocytosis, and also take up some cytoplasmic proteins and organelles for destruction (**autophagy**). Another system is the **Lon proteinase**, an ATP-stimulated mitochondrial proteinase that degrades aconitase and several other mitochondrial proteins after they have become oxidized. It recognizes hydrophobic patches that appear on the surface of aconitase after oxidation.

However, most attention has been paid to the **proteasome**, a cytoplasmic and nuclear system in eukaryotic cells that removes unwanted proteins, including IκB (Section 4.5.8), HIF-1α (Section 1.3.2), phosphorylated catalase (Section 4.5.6), IRP-2 animal (Section 3.15.1.5), cyclins (Section 9.13.1), Keap1 (Section 4.5.10) and oxidatively damaged proteins. Bacteria such as *E. coli* do not contain proteasomes, although various non-ubiquitin-dependent 'chambered proteases' are present. However, the archaeon *Thermoplasma acidophilum* does contain a proteasome; studying it has told us a lot about how eukaryotic proteasomes operate.

The core of the animal system is the **20S proteasome**, named for its sedimentation coefficient when spun in an ultracentrifuge. It has a relative molecular mass of about 700 000, and is a cylindrical structure made of a stack of four rings, each containing seven protein subunits. The cylinder has three internal cavities: the central cavity contains proteolytic sites and access to it is controlled by gates from the two outer cavities, too narrow to admit folded proteins. The **chymotrypsin-like proteolytic sites** cleave proteins adjacent to hydrophobic amino acid residues (tyrosine or phenylalanine), the **trypsin-like sites** after basic residues (arginine, lysine) and the **peptidylglutamyl sites** after acidic residues (aspartate, glutamate). *In vivo*, however, the 20S proteasome is often assembled into a larger structure, the **26S proteasome**; the 20S cylinder plus additional groups of proteins (**19S cap complexes**) attached at each end.

4.14.2.1 *Any role for ubiquitin?*

The 26S proteasome recognizes many of its targets because they have been marked for degradation by attachment of **ubiquitin**, a 76 amino-acid Hsp (Section 4.6). **Ubiquitination** (attachment of multiple ubiquitin molecules) is ATP-dependent. It is catalysed by a group of enzymes that first attach ubiquitin to lysine residues on the target and then add more ubiquitins to lysines on the ubiquitin itself. A chain of at least four ubiquitins is usually needed for proteasomal degradation. **Ubiquitin-activating enzymes (E1)** use ATP to activate ubiquitin, which is transferred to several **ubiquitin conjugating proteins (E2)**. These co-operate with hundreds of **ubiquitin ligases (E3)**, each of which recognizes 'destruction signals' on its target protein and attaches ubiquitin. These E3 enzymes are largely responsible for the specificity of targeting proteins for degradation. Various **deubiquitinating enzymes** can remove ubiquitin residues and rescue proteins. If this does not happen, the cap structures recognize the polyubiquitinated protein, unfold it and feed it slowly into the proteolytic core using energy from ATP hydrolysis. Once inside, it is hydrolysed into short peptides. Simultaneously, polyubiquitin is removed, disassembled back into monomers by enzymes, including **ubiquitin C-terminal hydrolase (UCHL1)**, and the monomeric ubiquitin made available for the cycle to repeat. The 26S proteasome thus catalyses an ATP-dependent degradation of ubiquitinated proteins. The 20S protease will not attack ubiquitinated proteins; recognition requires the 19S cap complexes.

Several inhibitors of the proteasome have been described. For example the *Streptomyces* metabolite **lactacystin** inactivates the proteasome and is cytotoxic to dividing cells by interfering with cyclin-dependent regulation of the cell cycle. Other inhibitors include **epoxomycin, aclacinomycin A** and **MG132** (a synthetic inhibitor). Proteasome inhibitors such as **bortezomib** (**Velcade**®) are under test for cancer chemotherapy.[240] However, proteasome inhibitors that could enter the brain might be neurotoxic; indeed defects in the brain's ubiquitin–proteasome system are observed in Alzheimer's and Parkinson's diseases (Section 9.18). Proteasome inhibitors induce oxidative stress in cells (sometimes promoting RNS production[241]), and can cause apoptosis. Paradoxically, however, adding low levels of proteasome inhibitors can produce cytoprotection by increasing production of Hsp and of the proteasome itself.[242]

Lowering proteasomal activity (by chemical inhibitors or antisense oligonucleotides) increases levels of oxidized proteins in cells, suggesting that their degradation proceeds via this system.[241,243] However, the role of ubiquitination is uncertain; it appears that the 20S proteasome is sufficient to degrade oxidized proteins.[243] How? Possibly it recognizes partial unfolding of oxidized proteins to expose hydrophobic surface patches that somehow (sounds a bit vague!) 'open' the gates and allow the oxidized proteins to enter in the absence of ubiquitin. Such a mechanism is not without precedent, since the 26S proteasome can degrade a few proteins (e.g. p21 and ornithine decarboxylase) without ubiquitination being necessary. Another possibility is that Hsp such as hsp90 recognize oxidized proteins and deliver them to the 20S proteasome.[244]

The nuclear proteasome may help to remove oxidized nuclear proteins, and PARP-1 activation appears to enhance its function.[245] One exception to the tentative generalization that ubiquitin is not required to remove oxidized proteins is IRP-2, whose oxidized form is degraded by the proteasome (Section 3.16.1.5); the E3 ligase that attaches ubiquitin to it has been identified.[246] There may be other exceptions.[247]

4.14.2.2 *Clogging up the proteasome?*

Proteasome activity may decline with age, promoting accumulation of oxidized proteins (Section 10.4). In addition, some oxidatively-damaged proteins appear to inhibit proteasome function rather than being degraded by it. These include HNE-modified proteins[248] and proteins modified by isoketals; a single isoketal adduct slowed degradation by about 50%.[249] Thus these end-products of lipid oxidation could lead to further cell dysfunction via impaired proteasome activity.

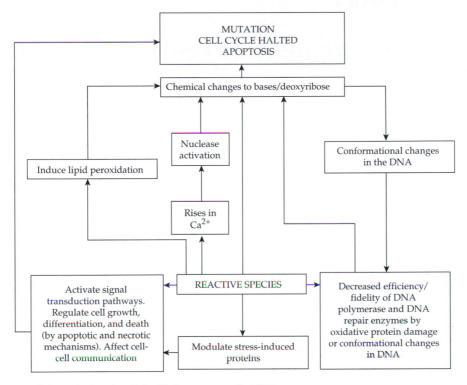

Figure 4.32 Some of the mechanisms by which oxidative stress can affect DNA.

4.15 Summary: oxidative stress and cell injury

Oxidative stress can produce injury by multiple pathways that overlap and interact in complex ways. For example, DNA can suffer direct oxidative damage, for example by OH•, indirect damage by binding of end-products of lipid peroxidation such as HNE and MDA, failure to repair it because of oxidative damage to polymerases and repair enzymes, inaccurate replication by damaged polymerases, and cleavage by nucleases activated by rises in intracellular free Ca^{2+} (Fig. 4.32).

Different antioxidants are needed to protect against these various events, and there is no universal single 'marker' of oxidative stress, as we explore in Chapter 5. For example, failure to find lipid peroxidation does not rule out the occurrence of oxidative stress: damage to DNA and proteins is often an important injurious event. Failure of a chain-breaking antioxidant such as α-tocopherol to protect is also inconclusive, for the same reason. Often, the only evidence that oxidative stress has occurred *in vivo* may be increases in antioxidant defence systems, indicating that the cell has responded and counteracted the damage.

CHAPTER 5

Measurement of reactive species

I often say that when you can measure what you are speaking about and express it in numbers you know something about it; but when you cannot measure it, when you cannot express it in numbers, your knowledge is of a meagre and unsatisfactory kind.

Lord Kelvin

It is difficult to find a black cat in a dark room, especially if there is no cat.

An old Chinese saying

5.1 Introduction

Reactive species (RS) play physiological roles (Chapters 4 and 7) and are involved in many diseases (Chapter 9) and in the actions of several toxins (Chapter 8). A major problem in ascertaining their importance is that these evanescent species are difficult to measure. How can we approach this? In essence, there are two direct ways, and several indirect ones.

5.1.1 Trapping

The only technique that can observe free radicals directly and specifically is **electron spin resonance (ESR)**, sometimes called **electron paramagnetic resonance (EPR)**. This technique is too insensitive to detect $O_2^{\bullet-}$ and $OH^{\bullet}$ directly in living systems: direct ESR of biological material only detects less-reactive radicals, such as ascorbyl radical. One approach to this difficulty has been **trapping**, in which a radical is allowed to react with a trap molecule to give one or more stable products, which are then measured. Mention of trapping usually brings to mind the technique of **spin trapping**, in which the radical reacts with a spin trap to form a more stable radical, which accumulates to a level that does permit detection by ESR. However, there are many other trapping methods,

as we shall see later. One fundamental point to appreciate is that *traps perturb the system under investigation*. For example, let us suppose that damage in a biological system is caused by $OH^{\bullet}$. Adding a molecule that traps $OH^{\bullet}$ should decrease the damage, provided that enough $OH^{\bullet}$ is trapped. Indeed, spin traps and other trapping molecules have often been shown to inhibit oxidative damage. In some cases, this has been a starting point to design therapeutic antioxidants (Section 10.6.5).

5.1.2 Fingerprinting: the biomarker concept[1]

An alternative to trapping is **fingerprinting** (one could also call it **footprinting**). The principle behind such methods is to measure not the RS themselves but the damage that they cause. If an RS attacks a biological molecule to leave a unique chemical 'fingerprint', then the presence of that fingerprint (which is of course an example of oxidative damage) can be used to infer that the RS was formed. Such **biomarkers of oxidative damage** can then be used to investigate effects of antioxidants or other agents on oxidative damage, hopefully leading to experimentally verifiable predictions of the likely effects of these compounds on oxidative stress-related diseases. Since the methods currently available for the direct measurement of RS are of limited applicability to humans (discussed below), most human studies focus on the measurement of oxidative damage biomarkers. This is to some extent logical, since it is the damage caused by RS that matters rather than the total amount of RS generated. For example, if $OH^\bullet$ are generated within a cell, many may react with unimportant targets. The fraction that reacts with DNA, with key proteins, or with lipids (initiating lipid peroxidation) may be the most important.

Table 5.1 summarizes the characteristics of an ideal biomarker. Validation of biomarkers requires two different steps. One is **analytical validation**, including development of procedures, analysis of reference materials, elimination of methodological artefacts and quality control. The second, more fundamental, is to demonstrate that changes in biomarkers do reflect the later development of disease. No currently used biomarker of oxidative damage has yet fulfilled this second criterion; the necessary experiments have not been done. It is sad that biomarkers were never built into the human intervention trials with antioxidants; they could have been of value in interpreting the confusing and conflicting results (Section 10.5). No currently available biomarker of oxidative damage meets all parts of criterion (B) in Table 5.1, but some are better than others.

Table 5.1 Criteria for an 'ideal' biomarker of oxidative damage

A. Fundamental criterion
  The biomarker predicts the later development of disease.
B. Technical criteria
  i. The biomarker should detect a major part, or at least a fixed percentage, of total oxidative damage to the target molecule *in vivo*.
  ii. It must employ validated measurement technology.
  iii. The coefficient of variation between different assays of the same sample should be very small in comparison with the differences between subjects or the effect of experimental manipulations (e.g. antioxidant supplementation) upon a subject.
  iv. It must not be confounded by diet.
  v. It should ideally be stable on storage, not being lost, or formed artefactually, in stored samples.
  vi. For human use, it is preferable if it can be measured in easily obtainable samples, e.g. blood, urine, saliva, skin biopsy.

5.1.3 Indirect approaches

5.1.3.1 *Vascular reactivity*
Nitric oxide plays a key role in vasodilation, but its action is antagonized by $O_2^{\bullet-}$ (Section 2.5.6). Some papers have claimed that high doses of infused or orally administered antioxidants (e.g. ascorbate) can scavenge ROS, restore $NO^\bullet$ bioavailability and ameliorate human endothelial dysfunction, although not all reports have confirmed this. The timing of antioxidant administration and the state of the vascular bed (healthy, mildly diseased or severely diseased) may be critical variables in explaining conflicting results.[2] Hence it is possible that examination of short-term vascular effects, which is easily achievable in human studies by measurements of forearm blood flow (a measure of the state of resistance of arterioles) or pulse wave analysis (which provides information on both structure and function of the arterial system and is particularly sensitive to $NO^\bullet$-mediated vascular effects), can gather evidence about *localized* scavenging of RS in blood vessel walls by antioxidants, unlike measurement of biomarkers in plasma or urine, which report on whole-body effects. However, it must not be assumed that any beneficial effects of antioxidants on vascular function are necessarily due to RS scavenging. Ascorbate may have a direct stimulating effect on eNOS activity by increasing endothelial tetrahydrobiopterin levels, for example (Section 3.20.1).

5.1.3.2 *Erythrocyte and plasma antioxidants*
Several other indirect approaches have been used to implicate RS in human disease. One is the measurement of changes in total antioxidant capacity (Section 5.17 below). Another is measurement of GSH and/or GSSG in human plasma, or levels of erythrocyte antioxidant defences. Careful procedures are needed for the former;[3] GSH is easily oxidized during plasma preparation and can be released from blood cells by haemolysis. In addition, plasma GSH is a 'transit pool' (Section 3.9.3) and changes in its level can be due to altered release by the liver as well as to altered consumption by γ-glutamyltranspeptidase (γGT) and/or by oxidative stress.[3] This enzyme is present not only on cell surfaces but also in plasma, and epidemiological studies suggest that plasma levels are correlated

with biomarkers of inflammation (e.g. C-reactive protein) and oxidative damage (e.g. F_2–isoprostanes) and with the later development of cardiovascular disease. Why this should be so is not clear, although pro-oxidant effects of cysteinyl–glycine have been suggested.[4] This dipeptide can oxidize to make ROS and sulphur radicals, and can thiolate proteins.[5]

What do changes in erythrocyte antioxidant enzyme levels signify? Erythrocytes cannot synthesize proteins and their antioxidant enzyme levels may drop as they 'age' in the circulation. Thus changes in enzyme levels are likely to reflect changes in the rates of red blood cell turnover. If this slows down, the circulating erythrocytes will be older on average and so levels of antioxidant enzymes in them will appear to fall. *Vice versa*, if an intervention accelerates red cell removal or increases erythropoiesis, levels of antioxidants in red cells will seem to rise. Hence, interpret such data with caution.

5.1.3.3 Changes in gene expression: ROS biosensors?
Exposing cells to oxidative stress alters the expression of multiple genes and the levels of many proteins, such as HO-1 (Section 3.17). In bacteria, the *soxR* and *soxS* systems are well-defined responders to ROS (Section 4.5). Several laboratories have linked the promoters of the relevant genes to easily detectable markers. For example, in many bioluminescent organisms light is produced by the action of a **luciferase** enzyme on a substrate (**luciferin**) (Section 7.6). Luciferase genes are widely used as 'reporter genes' for activation of transcription, because transcription of the gene and translation of the mRNA into luciferase protein is readily detected by measuring light when a luciferin is added. For example, the *E. coli* MnSOD, *katG* (Section 3.7.1) or *soxS* gene promoters, or the yeast Yap1 response element, can be attached to a luciferase gene. Any agent inducing *soxR* production should activate the *soxS* promoter, leading to luciferase production. Be careful though, luciferase itself can generate some ROS that can activate the *soxRS* system.[6] Another marker is **green fluorescent protein** (Section 7.6.1), which is autofluorescent and so does not require a substrate to be added.

One use of such technology is to develop bacterial or yeast 'biosensors', which generate light when exposed to environmental toxins that emit ROS and/or deplete antioxidant defences.[7] Another is the use of transgenic mice that express luciferase under the control of NFκB, allowing direct visualization of the activity of this transcription factor (Section 4.5.8).

5.2 ESR and spin trapping[8,9]

5.2.1 What is ESR?

ESR is a spectroscopic technique that detects unpaired electrons and so is specific for free radicals. An unpaired electron can have a spin of either +1/2 or -1/2 and behaves as a small magnet. If exposed to an external magnetic field, it can align itself either parallel or antiparallel (in opposition) to that field. It thus creates two possible energy levels, which vary with the magnetic field strength. If electromagnetic radiation of the correct energy is applied, it will be absorbed and used to move the electron from the lower energy level to the upper one. Thus an absorption spectrum is obtained, usually in the microwave region of the electromagnetic spectrum. The ESR spectrometers display **first-derivative spectra**, which show the rate of change of absorbance.

The fundamental equation is:

$$\Delta E = h\gamma = g\beta H$$

where δE corresponds to the energy of absorbed radiation, that is the energy gap between the two energy levels of the electron, h is Planck's constant, γ is the frequency of applied electromagnetic radiation, H the applied field strength and β is a constant, the **Böhr magneton**. The value of g (the **splitting factor**) for a free electron is 2.00232 and most biologically important radicals have values close to this. If the above equation is obeyed, an absorption spectrum results. For a single electron this can be represented in a stylized way as

but, if presented as its first derivative by an ESR machine it appears as:

Some atomic nuclei, such as those of hydrogen and nitrogen, also behave like small magnets and will align either parallel or antiparallel to the applied magnetic field. Thus in a hydrogen atom the single unpaired electron will be exposed to two different magnetic fields: the one applied plus that from the nucleus, or the one applied minus that from the nucleus. Thus there will be two energy absorptions and the ESR spectrum appears as

If the unpaired electron is close to two hydrogens, each can be aligned in the same way with the applied field, in opposite ways, or one in the same way and one opposite, that is

giving a three-line spectrum in which the intensities are in the ratio $1:2:1$, that is

For example, in **methyl radical** ($CH_3^•$) the unpaired electron on the carbon is close to three hydrogens. The field of each hydrogen nucleus can align with or against the applied magnetic field, and a 'tree' diagram can be used to predict the spectrum,

which therefore consists of four lines with intensity ratios $1:3:3:1$, or:

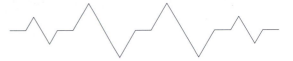

The number of lines in the ESR spectrum of a radical is called the **hyperfine structure** and can be large in radicals containing many nuclei. A radical can be identified from its ESR spectrum by looking at the g value, hyperfine structure and line shape. For example, Fig. 5.1 shows the ESR spectra of the ascorbyl and α-tocopheryl radicals. In spin-trapping experiments hyperfine splitting can be decreased if required, and sensitivity of detection increased, by using isotopically labelled traps. Thus replacing a H atom with deuterium abolishes doublet proton splittings, and using ^{15}N instead of ^{14}N, give doublet rather than triplet splitting.

The sensitivity of ESR is sufficient to detect species such as ascorbyl, α-tocopheryl and ubisemi-quinone radicals in biological material, as well as radicals produced by the mechanical disruption of fingernails, bone, cartilage and tooth enamel (Section 2.5.5.1). However, ESR is insufficiently sensitive to detect $O_2^{•-}$ and $OH^•$. One approach is to generate such radicals in a frozen, transparent solid matrix which prevents them from colliding and undergoing reaction. In 1969, a 'rapid freezing' ESR technique enabled the first identification of $O_2^{•-}$ production by an enzyme-catalysed reaction (XO and xanthine).[10] However, the spectra of immobilized radicals are often hard to identify in biological material, and so freeze-quenching techniques are not often used; spin trapping (Section 5.2.3 below) is more common.

X-band ESR is used in most studies, with an applied field frequency of about 9.5 GHz (gigahertz). At this frequency, sample penetration by the radiation is limited and only small samples can be examined. Lower frequencies can be used for bigger samples, such as whole organs or live rodents. For example **L-band ESR spectroscopy** uses 1 to 2 GHz or even lower, and it has been possible to image nitroxide radicals administered to whole animals.[11] However, use of lower frequencies decreases sensitivity.

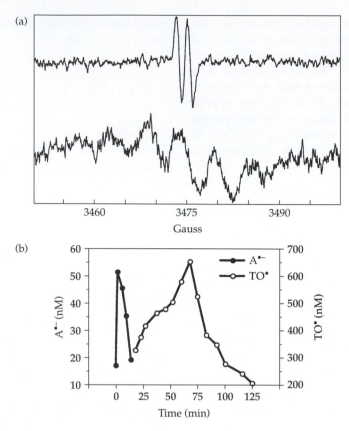

Figure 5.1 ESR spectra of ascorbyl and α-tocopheryl free radicals. Plasma was incubated with hypoxanthine and xanthine oxidase. (HX/XO), which generates $O_2^{\bullet -}$ and H_2O_2. Ascorbyl radical levels were initially low (<20 nM). Upon adding HX/XO, they rose rapidly but then fell as ascorbate was depleted (b). Not until ascorbate had almost disappeared did the vitamin E radical appear, consistent with a 'recycling' of this radical by ascorbate (Section 3.20.2.4). (a) Top: ascorbyl free radical spectrum measured at 1.5 min after adding HX/XO. Bottom: tocopheryl free radical measured at 70 min. Under these experimental conditions approximately 10 times more tocopheryl radical is needed to produce an ESR signal above the noise level, largely because it has a broad seven-line spectrum whereas ascorbyl radical is a narrow doublet. Data from *Free Rad. Biol. Med.* **14**, 649, 1993, by courtesy of Dr Gary Buettner and Elsevier.

5.2.2 Measurement of oxygen[12]

The ESR spectra of several free radicals are affected by O_2 concentration and so can be used to assess cellular and organ O_2 levels, by the method of **ESR oximetry**. Suitable probes include **triphenyl (trityl)-**based radicals and certain particulates that possess unpaired electrons (e.g. some coals). The latter often show a single ESR line whose shape is altered by pO_2. If small enough, they can be taken up by phagocytosis and report on intracellular O_2 concentrations. Several trityl probes are used *in vivo* as contrast agents in magnetic resonance imaging (MRI). Indeed, triphenylmethyl radical

$$Ph - \overset{\overset{\displaystyle Ph}{|}}{\underset{\underset{\displaystyle Ph}{|}}{C}}{}^{\bullet}$$

was the first stable free radical described, by Gomberg in 1900. Trityl probes can also be used to measure $O_2^{\bullet -}$ (Section 5.4.3 below).

5.2.3 Spin trapping[8,9]

In this technique, a short-lived radical reacts with a trap to produce a long-lived radical. Reaction of nitroso (R–NO) compounds with short-lived radicals can produce longer-lived **nitroxide** (sometimes called **aminoxyl**) radicals

$$R-N{=}O \ + \ R'^{\bullet} \longrightarrow \underset{\underset{R'}{|}}{\overset{\overset{R}{|}}{N}}-O^{\bullet}$$

reactive   nitroxide radical
radical   (fairly stable)

Their stability is associated with electron delocalization between the nitrogen and oxygen atoms

$$N-O^{\bullet} \longleftrightarrow \overset{\bullet+}{N}-O^{-}$$

Nitrone traps also produce nitroxide radicals

$$R-\underset{+}{\overset{\overset{H}{|}}{C}}{=}\overset{\overset{O^{-}}{|}}{N}-R' + R'^{\bullet\prime\prime} \longrightarrow R-\underset{\underset{R''}{|}}{\overset{\overset{H}{|}}{C}}-\overset{\overset{O^{\bullet}}{|}}{N}-R'$$

The ESR spectra of nitroxides have a main triplet $(1:1:1)$ splitting due to interaction of the unpaired electron with the nitrogen of the nitroxide group. Secondary splittings arise from magnetic nuclei in the trapped radical and sometimes from other magnetic nuclei in the spin trap. In nitroso traps the radical detected adds directly to the nitrogen, whereas with nitrones it adds to the adjacent carbon. With nitroso traps the trapped radical thus more easily influences the ESR spectrum and usually generates hyperfine splittings, whereas with nitrone traps the spectra tend to be broadly similar whatever the radical trapped. However, nitroso compounds often give less stable adducts than nitrones, especially when oxygen radicals are trapped, and they tend to be more toxic to animals and cells. Hence nitrones are more commonly used. Table 5.2 shows some of the trapping molecules that have been employed; **DMPO** and **PBN** are widely used and **DEPMPO** is increasingly popular.

The 'ideal' trap should react rapidly and specifically with the radical one wishes to detect, to produce a product that is chemically stable, not metabolized by living systems, and has a unique ESR spectrum. No currently available trap satisfies all these criteria and another area of concern is the presence of impurities in commercial spin trap preparations that can influence results.[13] For example, commercial PBN appeared to detect

radicals formed from Aβ peptides (Section 9.20.3), whereas pure PBN did not. Yet another factor to be considered is where the trap will localize in a biological system; for example, PBN is much more hydrophobic than DMPO (Table 5.2).

Nitric oxide has also been measured *in vivo* by ESR, using various traps (see Table 5.5 below).

5.2.4 DMPO, DEPMPO and PBN[13,14]

Spin trapping is often used to detect $O_2^{\bullet-}$ and $OH^{\bullet}$ in biological systems. For example, DMPO reacts with both $OH^{\bullet}$ and $O_2^{\bullet-}$ to form products with different ESR spectra (Fig. 5.2). The rate constants for the reactions are very different, however, at $<10^2\,M^{-1}s^{-1}$ for $O_2^{\bullet-}$ and $>10^9\,M^{-1}s^{-1}$ for $OH^{\bullet}$. Thus at equal concentrations of radicals $OH^{\bullet}$ is trapped much faster than $O_2^{\bullet-}$. Hence efficient trapping of $O_2^{\bullet-}$ requires high DMPO concentrations. Unfortunately, the product of reaction of DMPO with $O_2^{\bullet-}$ (DMPO–OOH) is unstable (half-time about 1 min) and decomposes to give several products, including DMPO–OH, the same product generated by direct reaction with $OH^{\bullet}$ (Fig. 5.2).

There are several solutions to this problem. One is to use DEPMPO, which reacts with $O_2^{\bullet-}$ and $OH^{\bullet}$ with rate constants comparable to DMPO but whose $O_2^{\bullet-}$ adduct is more stable. However, the spectra obtained are complex and need to be interpreted with caution.[14] The trap **EMPO** is another option (Table 5.2). A different strategy is to use DMPO but to employ $OH^{\bullet}$ scavengers to verify the source of the DMPO–OH adduct. If the DMPO–OH signal is due to trapping of $OH^{\bullet}$ by DMPO, then addition of excess ethanol should abolish it. Ethanol scavenges $OH^{\bullet}$ and competes with DMPO for $OH^{\bullet}$. In addition, reaction of ethanol with $OH^{\bullet}$ produces a **hydroxyethyl radical** (Fig. 5.2) which reacts with DMPO to give a new radical with a different ESR spectrum. This spectrum should appear as the DMPO–OH signal is lost. Dimethylsulphoxide (DMSO) can also be used: its reaction with $OH^{\bullet}$ produces a methyl radical that reacts with DMPO:

$$\underset{\text{DMSO}}{(CH_3)_2S{=}O} + OH^{\bullet} \longrightarrow \underset{\underset{OH}{|}}{CH_3S}{=}O \ + \ CH_3^{\bullet}$$

Thus if $OH^{\bullet}$ is really being trapped, addition of DMSO should scavenge $OH^{\bullet}$ and diminish the

Table 5.2 A selection of the 'spin-traps' that have been used in biological systems

Name	Abbreviation	Structure
tert-Nitrosobutane (nitroso-tert-butane)	tNB (NtB)	
α-Phenyl-tert-butylnitrone	PBN	
5,5-Dimethylpyrroline-N-oxide	DMPO	
5-Diethoxyphosphoryl-5-methyl-1-pyrroline-N-oxide	DEPMPO	
5-Ethoxycarbonyl-5-methyl-1-pyrroline-N-oxide[a]	EMPO	
tert-Butylnitrosobenzene	BNB	
α-(4-Pyridyl-1-oxide)-N-tert-butylnitrone	4-POBN	
3,5-Dibromo-4-nitroso-benzenesulphonic acid	DBNBS	

Table 5.2 (*Cont.*)

Name	Abbreviation	Structure
1,1,3-Trimethyl-isoindole *N*-oxide	TMINO	
Azulenylnitrone	AZN	

Spin traps vary in their hydrophobicity; for example, DMPO (octanol: water partition coefficient 0.08) or POBN (0.09) are less useful in trapping radicals within membranes or lipoproteins than PBN (partition coefficient 10.4). Lipophilicity can be increased by adding hydrophobic side chains to traps. For example the methyl group on DEPMPO can be replaced by a $PhCH_2CH_2-$ group (to give **DEPPEPO**) or a $-CH_3$ on DMPO by a *tert*- butoxy carbonyl group (to give **BMPO**).

[a] EMPO has been reported to give simpler EPR adducts than DEPMPO, although its $O_2^{\bullet-}$ adduct is less stable than that of DEPMPO, but still five-times more stable than that with DMPO. Various structural modifications can increase the stability of the $O_2^{\bullet-}$ adducts (*Biochem. Pharmacol.* **69**, 1351, 2005).

DMPO–OH signal in parallel with a rise in the DMPO–CH_3 signal. However, the $CH_3^{\bullet}$ radical reacts with O_2 faster than it reacts with DMPO (rate constants $\approx 3.7 \times 10^9$ and $10^6\,M^{-1}s^{-1}$, respectively) and so elevated O_2 will compete with DMPO for the $CH_3^{\bullet}$ produced.

Such approaches can work *in vivo*. For example, in animals coadministered DMSO and PBN, exposure to ionizing radiation to generate OH$^{\bullet}$ resulted in formation of a PBN–methyl radical adduct in the bile,[15] and PBN can detect radicals involved in liver damage by $CC1_4$ (Fig. 8.3). This trap reacts with OH$^{\bullet}$ but the adduct decomposes quickly and so DMPO or DEPMPO are better traps for OH$^{\bullet}$. However, PBN is rapidly metabolized *in vivo*.[16] Both PBN and DMPO bind to cytochromes P450, and PBN can inhibit various P450-dependent oxidations.[9]

5.2.5 *Ex vivo* trapping in humans

Spin traps such as PBN, DMPO, DEPMPO, EMPO and POBN are sufficiently non-toxic for short-term use in experimental animals, but cannot be administered to humans because of unknown toxicity at the high levels that are required for radical trapping *in vivo* (in order to allow the trap to compete with endogenous molecules for a reactive free radical). However, traps can be used on human body fluids and tissue samples. For example, PBN is able to detect free radicals when it is added to coronary sinus blood drawn during bypass surgery (Section 9.5.4). Of course, highly reactive radicals such as OH$^{\bullet}$ will not survive to be detected in *ex vivo* material, since OH$^{\bullet}$ reacts with whatever is in its immediate vicinity within microseconds. Trapping within *ex vivo* samples probably detects secondary radicals resulting from attack of highly reactive species (OH$^{\bullet}$, ONOOH etc) on biomolecules. Such secondary radicals can include protein- and lipid-derived radicals. For example, POBN is a good trap for lipid-derived carbon-centred radicals (Section 5.14.4.1 below).

The ability of spin traps to react with organic-solvent-derived radicals should be borne in mind when tissues or body fluids are treated with such solvents to extract lipophilic radicals for ESR studies. For example, chloroform/methanol mixtures are widely used to extract lipids, but methanol is easily oxidized by several RS, generating

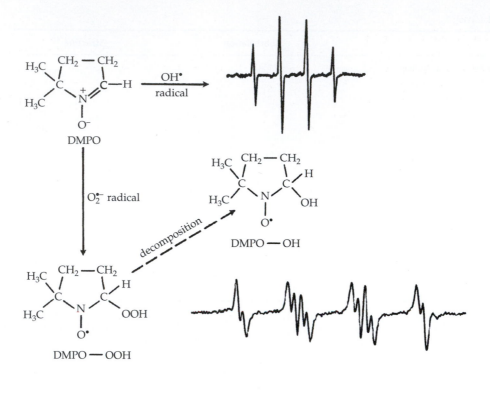

Figure 5.2 Reactions of DMPO with $O_2^{\bullet-}$, $OH^{\bullet}$ and ethanol radicals. The ESR spectra of the DMPO–OH and DMPO–OOH adducts are shown diagrammatically to illustrate the key differences between them. The spectrum of the DMPO–OOH adduct has 12 lines and results from complex interactions (*J. Org. Chem.* **70**, 1198, 2005). Spectrum by courtesy of Dr Paul Tordo and the American Chemical Society. It has also been suggested that the $O_2^{\bullet-}$ adducts of DMPO, EMPO and DEPMPO can decompose to release $NO^{\bullet}$ (*Org. Biomol. Chem.* **3**, 3220, 2005).

$^{\bullet}CH_2OH$ radicals. Hence trapped radicals can be artefacts of solvent extraction.[17] The anaesthetic **ketamine** can be metabolized to free radicals *in vivo* and should be avoided for anaesthesia of animals for spin trapping experiments.[18]

5.2.6 Further cautions in the use of spin traps

Nitroxide radicals are redox-active; they can be reversibly reduced to hydroxylamines

$$H^+ + e^- + R-N-O^{\bullet} \rightleftharpoons R-N-OH$$

or oxidized to oxoammonium cations,

$$R-N-O^{\bullet} \rightleftharpoons -R-\overset{+}{N}=O + e^-$$

both of which are **ESR-silent** (i.e. give no ESR spectrum) because there is no longer an unpaired electron. Indeed, cyclic hydroxylamines have also been used as probes for RS, which can oxidize them back to nitroxide radicals and an ESR signal appears. An example is **1-acetoxy-3-carbamoyl-2,2,5,5-tetramethylpyrrolidine**

This is hydrolysed by esterases to free the NOH group, which can then react with free radicals to generate a nitroxide. It has been used to detect ROS production in rat brain by following the appearance of an ESR signal.[19] A similar probe **bis(1-hydroxy-2,2,6,6-tetramethyl-4-piperidinyl)-decandioate**,

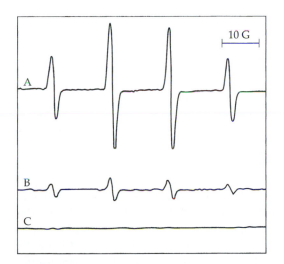

has been used to measure radicals in human blood and tissue samples.[20]

Nitroxide radical adducts of several spin traps are easily reduced by cellular reducing agents, such as ascorbate (Fig. 5.3), constituents of microsomal and mitochondrial electron transport chains and even by $O_2^{\bullet-}$ They can also be quenched by direct

addition of carbon-centred radicals in lipids. Indeed, $O_2^{\bullet-}$ reacts faster with the DMPO–OOH adduct (rate constant $>10^6\,M^{-1}s^{-1}$) than DMPO reacts with $O_2^{\bullet-}$. Reduction of nitroxides administered to animals can be observed by L-band ESR.[11] Haem ferryl species can *oxidize* nitroxides, again with loss of the ESR signal.[21] Caution should also be employed in using DMPO to trap $OH^{\bullet}/O_2^{\bullet-}$ in photochemical systems, since DMPO reacts with singlet O_2 to give products that include DMPO–OH and DMPO/ $HO_2^{\bullet}$ adducts.[22] Spin traps can often be oxidized by HOCl and ONOOH, the latter producing a variety of radical adducts.

5.2.7 Trapping thiyl radicals[23]

Spin trapping can be used to detect many radicals, including RS$^{\bullet}$ (Fig. 5.4 and Section 6.5.1). The DMPO adducts of different RS$^{\bullet}$ radicals are distinctive and the rate constant for reaction is high, $\sim 10^8\,M^{-1}s^{-1}$. The DMPO adduct of the glutathione thiyl radical, GS$^{\bullet}$, superficially resembles DMPO–OH, giving a four-line spectrum. However, the intensity pattern is usually $1:1:1:1$ rather than $1:2:2:1$. The trap PBN can also intercept thiyl radicals but forms less-characteristic spectra than does DMPO.

5.2.8 Spin trapping without ESR?

Spin traps can be used to detect radicals on proteins or DNA, the trap attaching to the protein- or DNA-bound radical. If the adduct is then

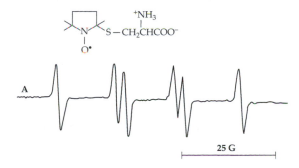

Figure 5.3 Reduction of the DMPO–OH spin adduct to an ESR-silent species by ascorbate. Hydroxyl radical was generated by reaction of Fe (III)–EDTA with H_2O_2. (A) Without ascorbate, (B) with 0.66 mM ascorbate, (C) a crystal of solid ascorbate added after the spectra had formed. Unpublished data of one of the authors (J.M.C.G.) with Lindsay Maidt, Gemma Brueggemann and Paul McCay. Caution should therefore be employed when attempting to use spin trapping to study the reactions of reducing agents with radicals; it is essential to show that the reductant does not simply destroy the trap–radical adduct. For example, the thiol-containing drug **captopril** reduces DMPO–OH to an ESR-silent species, which may have led to overestimates of captopril's ability to scavenge ROS (*Free Radic. Res.* **24**, 391, 1996).

Figure 5.4 ESR spectrum of the DMPO–cysteine thiyl radical adduct. The thiyl radical was formed by oxidation of cysteine using horseradish peroxidase. From *J. Biol. Chem.* **259**, 5606, 1984 by courtesy of Dr Ron Mason and the publishers.

oxidized to stabilize the linkage, the traps remain attached covalently at the point where the radical originally formed. Such adducts can be detected simply and sensitively (far more sensitively than by ESR) using antibodies directed against DMPO–protein or DMPO–DNA adducts.[21,24] Alternatively, protein mass spectrometry or DNA sequencing can be used to identify the site of DMPO attachment.

Another approach is to use traps that change colour. **Azulenyl nitrone** (Table 5.2) is green, but its nitroxide is purple, and breaks down to generate a red aldehyde. These products can be separated by HPLC and observed spectrophotometrically.[25] Azulenyl nitrones have been used as neuroprotective agents (Section 10.6.5). Finally, HPLC can be combined with ESR and/or mass spectrometry to identify all the products formed when a trap is added to a biological system, whether they give ESR signals or not.[26]

5.3 Other trapping methods, as exemplified by hydroxyl radical trapping

5.3.1 Aromatic hydroxylation[27–29]

Oxidation of aromatic compounds by metal ion–H_2O_2 mixtures has been known for over 100 years and, since the pioneering work of Merz and Waters in 1949, has generated an enormous chemical literature. In the case of the simplest aromatic compound, benzene, OH[•] addition produces a **hydroxycyclohexadienyl** radical (when a radical adds to a non-radical, the adduct must be a radical):

Two such radicals can join together to give a dimer, that may lose water to form **biphenyl**:

Hydroxycyclohexadienyl radical can alternatively be oxidized to phenol,

and can also disproportionate, one hydroxycyclohexadienyl radical being oxidized to phenol and the other reduced to benzene. The presence of O_2, Fe(III) or Cu^{2+} tends to increase the yield of hydroxylation products. Hence the amounts of these various end-products obtained from attack of a given amount of OH[•] upon benzene vary depending on reaction conditions. If substituted benzenes are attacked by OH[•], reactions become even more complex. For aromatic carboxylic acids, decarboxylation is favoured at low pH in the absence of metal ions, whereas hydroxylated product formation is favoured if metal ions are present.

Decarboxylation of benzoic acid, labelled with ^{14}C in the carboxyl group, has been used to detect OH[•] in biological systems. The assay is sensitive, since small amounts of [14]CO_2 can be trapped in alkaline solutions and measured accurately by scintillation counting. An alternative approach is to use benzoic acid labelled with ^{13}C in the carboxyl group and measure production of [13]CO_2 by mass spectrometry.[30] However, decarboxylation may be a minor reaction pathway under physiological conditions, and so only a small fraction of the OH[•] will be measured. Also, some $RO_2^{•}$ radicals appear able to decarboxylate benzoate.[30] Hence hydroxylated aromatic products are more often measured to detect OH[•]. Usually, hydroxylated products are separated by gas chromatography (GC) or HPLC and measured by electrochemical detection, fluorescence spectra or mass spectrometry. Suitable non-toxic aromatic 'detectors' must be chosen for use in biological systems. Salicylate (2-hydroxybenzoate) is popular; attack of OH[•] upon it produces two dihydroxylated products (2,3- and 2,5-dihydroxybenzoates), together with small amounts of the decarboxylation product catechol (Fig. 5.5). 4-Hydroxybenzoic acid can also be used, forming 3,4-dihydroxybenzoate. Attack of OH[•] upon phenylalanine produces three dihydroxylated products: 2-hydroxyphenylalanine (*o*-tyrosine), 3-hydroxyphenylalanine (*m*-tyrosine)

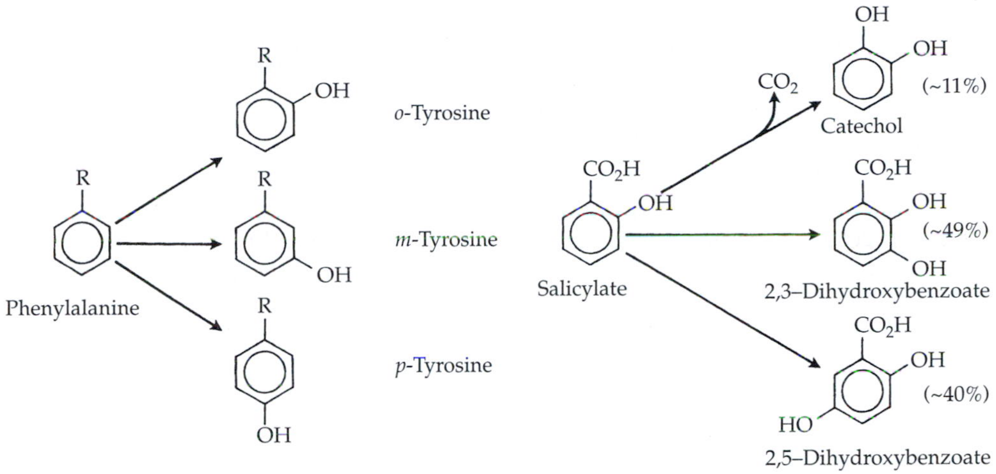

Figure 5.5 Products of the reaction of OH$^{\bullet}$ with aromatic compounds. A typical percentage distribution of salicylate hydroxylation products is shown but ratios of end-products vary depending on reaction conditions. Remember that the initial products of OH$^{\bullet}$ attack on aromatic rings are free radicals, that can have variable fates depending on what else is present in the reaction mixture.

and 4-hydroxyphenylalanine (**p-tyrosine**). *p*-Tyrosine is also formed from phenylalanine by the enzyme **phenylalanine hydroxylase**. Both D- and L-isomers of phenylalanine react with OH$^{\bullet}$ equally fast, but the D-isomer is not a substrate for phenylalanine hydroxylase.

5.3.1.1 *Points to ponder*

If an aromatic compound reacts with OH$^{\bullet}$ to form hydroxylated products that can be accurately measured in biological material, and one or more of these products is not identical to enzyme-produced hydroxylated products, then formation of the 'unnatural' product(s) can conceivably be used to assess OH$^{\bullet}$ formation *in vivo*. Success in such studies requires that the aromatic 'trap' be present at sites of OH$^{\bullet}$ generation at concentrations sufficient to compete with other molecules that can scavenge OH$^{\bullet}$. Given that all biological molecules react fast with OH$^{\bullet}$, it seems unlikely that a trap (whether aromatic or a spin trap) can intercept more than a small percentage of any OH$^{\bullet}$ generated *in vivo*. The method also assumes that any hydroxylated product is not metabolized. For example, dihydroxybenzoates are rapidly metabolized in perfused liver, so that salicylate is not a good detector of OH$^{\bullet}$ in this organ. On the other hand, it works well in the rat heart.[31] 2, 3-Dihydroxybenzoate can also be readily further oxidized, eg by HOCl or ONOOH.

Both salicylate and phenylalanine (Fig. 5.6) have been used as 'probes' for the generation of OH$^{\bullet}$ *in vivo*. Thus, 2,3-dihydroxybenzoate (2,3-DHB; Fig. 5.5) does not appear to be an enzyme-produced metabolite of salicylate in animals, whereas 2,5-DHB can be generated from salicylate by CYPs, i.e. 2,3-DHB is the preferred product to measure. For example, hydroxylation of salicylate to 2,3-DHB was used to show OH$^{\bullet}$ generation in the lungs of animals breathing silicate dusts.[32] Similarly, *o*- and *m*-tyrosines do not appear to be formed enzymically in humans. Low levels of *o*-, but not *m*-tyrosine were reported in human urine;[33] this *o*-tyrosine could originate from diet (Section 5.15.1 below) or from oxidative damage. Both salicylate and phenylalanine have been used to measure *ex vivo* OH$^{\bullet}$ formation in body fluids from patients with rheumatoid arthritis (Section 9.10) or in humans exposed to ozone (Section 2.6.5). Phenylalanine was used to detect OH$^{\bullet}$ formation in saliva (Section 8.12.6). Several human studies have used salicylate to detect OH$^{\bullet}$ *in vivo*, with some success. Examples include studies on diabetes, alcoholism and myocardial infarction.[28] Phenylalanine hydroxylation was used to detect OH$^{\bullet}$ formation in the colon of rats[34] and endogenous levels of protein-bound *ortho*- or *meta*-tyrosines have also been used to implicate OH$^{\bullet}$ formation *in vivo* (Section 5.15.1 below).

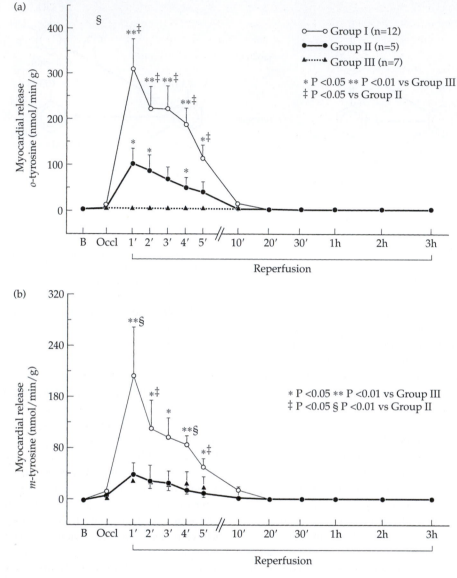

Figure 5.6 Use of phenylalanine hydroxylation to measure OH$^\bullet$ production after myocardial ischaemia–reperfusion *in vivo*. If part of the myocardium of an open-chest anaesthetized dog is made ischaemic for a brief period (too short to kill the tissue), subsequent reperfusion does not cause immediate return of contractile function. This **myocardial stunning** phenomenon can be attenuated by several antioxidants. The involvement of OH$^\bullet$ was confirmed using phenylalanine (Fig. 5.5). Animals were preloaded with L-phenylalanine. No *o*- or *m*-tyrosines were detected in the circulation since these are not normal metabolites of L-phenylalanine (unlike *p*-tyrosine, produced by the enzyme phenylalanine hydroxylase). However, *o*- and *m*-tyrosine, (a) and (b) respectively, *were* produced by the heart after ischaemia–reperfusion (group I animals, o). The amounts formed were decreased by antioxidants, including mercaptopropionylglycine (group II, •) and a mixture of SOD, catalase and desferrioxamine (group III, ▲) but not by inhibitors of NOS, i.e. NO$^\bullet$ (and, by implication, ONOO$^-$) were not involved in the OH$^\bullet$ generation. Data adapted from *Circ. Res.* **73**, 534, 1993, by courtesy of Dr Roberto Bolli and the publishers.

Some RS other than OH$^\bullet$ can hydroxylate aromatic compounds. Singlet O_2 hydroxylates phenol and aniline (to 4-hydroxyaniline). It also attacks salicylate,[35] but produces 2,5-DHB rather than 2,3-DHB (another reason why measurement of 2,3-DHB is preferable as an index of OH$^\bullet$ generation). Addition of ONOO$^-$ to salicylate or phenylalanine at pH 7.4 can generate hydroxylation products identical to those in Fig. 5.5. This may be due to generation of OH$^\bullet$ from decomposition of ONOOH, but could also involve direct attack of ONOOH on aromatic rings (Section 2.6.1.1).[27] Thus aromatic hydroxylation experiments must be interpreted with caution if ONOO$^-$ is being generated. However, addition of ONOO$^-$ (unlike OH$^\bullet$) generates nitration products from salicylate and phenylalanine, so measuring these can distinguish[27] hydroxylation due to ONOO$^-$ from that due to 'real' OH$^\bullet$.

5.3.2 Use of hydroxyl-radical scavengers

Inhibition upon addition of OH$^\bullet$ scavengers is often used as evidence that OH$^\bullet$ is responsible for a particular reaction (e.g. Table 5.3). In simple chemical systems this often works well, but in biological systems it is fraught with danger. Scavengers can be ineffective when OH$^\bullet$ is not generated in 'free solution' but is formed upon a biological target, for example when iron or copper ions bind to a protein or to DNA that is then exposed to H_2O_2. Reaction with the target is favoured over reaction with a scavenger in free

solution. This principle is illustrated by the deoxyribose assay (Fig. 5.7; Section 5.3.3 below) and the coumarin hydroxylation assay (Table 5.4). In addition, many OH$^\bullet$ scavengers are non-specific (e.g. the widely used **thiourea** and **dimethylthiourea** also react with $O_2^{\bullet-}$, H_2O_2, HOCl and ONOO$^-$ and chelate metal ions)[36] whereas several oxysulphur radicals can react with formate and ethanol (Section 8.11.3).

5.3.3 The deoxyribose assay[37]

Attack of OH$^\bullet$ on 2-deoxyribose produces a range of products (Section 4.8.2.1). On heating at low pH, some of them decompose to form malondialdehyde (MDA), which can be detected by adding thiobarbituric acid (TBA) to give a pink (TBA)$_2$–MDA chromogen. This can be used to detect OH$^\bullet$ production, although it is unclear whether or not some other ROS can degrade deoxyribose.

5.3.4 Measurement of rate constants for OH$^\bullet$ reactions

The definitive technique for studying the rate and mechanism of compounds reacting with OH$^\bullet$ is pulse radiolysis (Section 2.3.3.1), but many laboratories use other methods. For example, an OH$^\bullet$-generating system can be incubated with DMPO and the ESR signal of DMPO–OH observed. An added OH$^\bullet$ scavenger competes with DMPO for OH$^\bullet$ and decreases the ESR signal; a competition plot allows a rate constant to be calculated. The

Table 5.3 Formation of hydroxyl radicals during the oxidation of xanthine by xanthine oxidase in the presence of an iron chelate

Reagent added	Rate constant for reaction with OH$^\bullet$ ($M^{-1}s^{-1}$)	Percentage inhibition of hydroxylation
None	–	0
Mannitol (5 mM)	2.7×10^9	37
Sodium formate (5 mM)	3.5×10^9	52
Thiourea (5 mM)	4.7×10^9	76
Urea (5 mM)	$<7.0 \times 10^5$	0

Experiments were carried out at pH 7.4 using OH$^\bullet$ generated by reaction of $O_2^{\bullet-}$ and H_2O_2 (from oxidation of xanthine by XO) with ferric EDTA (*FEBS Lett.* **92**, 321, 1978). The OH$^\bullet$ formed was detected by measuring salicylate hydroxylation (colorimetrically). Hydroxyl radicals generated by iron–EDTA that escape reaction with iron–EDTA and the other reagents present (e.g. xanthine) are equally 'available' to the salicylate and to other added scavengers of OH$^\bullet$. Hence the amount of hydroxylation can be decreased by adding 'OH$^\bullet$ scavengers'. The faster these 'scavengers' react with OH$^\bullet$, the more they inhibit formation of hydroxylated products.

(a)

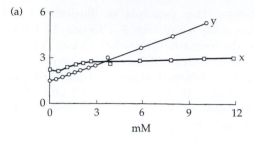

(b)

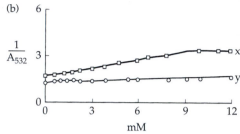

(c)

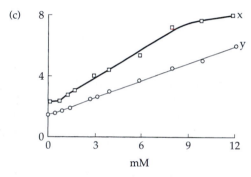

Figure 5.7 Examples of OH$^\bullet$ scavenging in the deoxyribose assay. (a) Double-reciprocal plot showing the ability of Hepes, a powerful OH$^\bullet$ scavenger, to inhibit deoxyribose degradation by OH$^\bullet$ generated by a mixture of Fe(III)-EDTA, H$_2$O$_2$ and ascorbate at pH 7.4 (line y). Rate constant for OH$^\bullet$ scavenging calculated from the slope of the line as $>10^9$ M^{-1}s^{-1}. Line x shows that Hepes is a much poorer inhibitor when EDTA is omitted. This is probably because Fe(III) then binds to the deoxyribose, OH$^\bullet$ generation becomes site specific and added OH$^\bullet$ scavengers cannot protect. (b) The same experiment using citrate. Line y shows that citrate is a poor OH$^\bullet$ scavenger (rate constant $<10^8$ M^{-1}s^{-1}). Line x shows it to be a good inhibitor of site-specific OH$^\bullet$ generation; citrate can chelate iron ions from deoxyribose and iron–citrate chelates are less redox active. (c) The same experiment, using ATP. ATP is a good OH$^\bullet$ scavenger (line y; rate constant $>10^9$ M^{-1}s^{-1}). Line x also shows its ability to chelate iron ions from deoxyribose, as would be expected from the presence of sugar and phosphate groups. The iron–ATP complex is redox active, but the ATP absorbs a large number of the OH$^\bullet$ produced, so that they do not escape into free solution. Calculation of rate constants from the slope of lines y is by the equation

$$\frac{1}{A} = \frac{1}{A^0}\left[1 + \frac{k_s[S]}{k_{DR}[DR]}\right]$$

deoxyribose assay can also be used; OH$^\bullet$ is generated by a mixture of ascorbate, H$_2$O$_2$ and ferric EDTA (Fig. 5.7).[37] Any OH$^\bullet$ not scavenged by the iron–EDTA or other reactants attacks the deoxyribose. An added OH$^\bullet$ scavenger competes with deoxyribose for the OH$^\bullet$, and inhibits generation of MDA. A competition plot can be used to calculate the rate constant for OH$^\bullet$ scavenging (Fig. 5.7).

These and similar methods require several controls:[37]

1. Check that the substance under test does not interfere with OH$^\bullet$ *formation*. For example, if OH$^\bullet$ is made by Fenton chemistry does the substance scavenge H$_2$O$_2$ or bind iron ions? The deoxyribose assay avoids the latter by binding the iron to EDTA.
2. Check that the substance does not interfere with measurement of products. For example, does it reduce the DMPO–OH adduct to an ESR-silent species (Fig. 5.3)? In the deoxyribose assay, does it interfere with the TBA test, or generate a false chromogen when it reacts with OH$^\bullet$?

If EDTA is omitted from the deoxyribose assay, some of the iron binds to deoxyribose.[37] The bound iron ions appear to participate in Fenton chemistry, but the OH$^\bullet$ immediately attacks deoxyribose. Hydroxyl-radical scavengers (such as Hepes, methanol or ethanol), at moderate concentrations, do not inhibit this site-specific deoxyribose degradation. The only substances that do inhibit are those that chelate iron ions well enough to remove them from deoxyribose (Fig. 5.7).

5.3.5 Other trapping methods for hydroxyl radical

Multiple other detector molecules for OH$^\bullet$ have been described, each with its own advantages and drawbacks (Table 5.4).

5.4 Detection of superoxide

Methods used to detect O$_2^{\bullet-}$ overlap with those used to assay SOD (Section 3.2.5). Spin trapping

---

where A is the absorbance in the presence of a scavenger S at concentration [S] and A^0 is the absorbance in the absence of scavenger. A plot of $1/A$ against [S] should give a straight line of slope $k_s/k_{DR}[DR]A^0$ with an intercept on the y axis of $1/A^0$. Hence the rate constant k_s for reaction of S with OH$^\bullet$ can be calculated. k_{DR} is 3.1×10^9 M^{-1}s^{-1} (*Anal. Biochem.* **165**, 219, 1987).

Table 5.4 Some methods for the detection of hydroxyl radicals

Method	Principle of method	Comments
Hydroxylation of antipyrine H_3C / HC=CH / HC–N–C=O / H_3C–N–phenyl	Metabolized *in vivo* in humans to 3-hydroxymethyl and 4-hydroxylated products. Attack by OH$^\bullet$ gives *ortho*- and *meta*-hydroxylation on the benzene ring: these are apparently not normal metabolites.	Used to study OH$^\bullet$ production during exercise and intermittent claudication (*Free Radic. Res* **35**, 435, 2001; *Metabolism* **50**, 1484, 2001).
Hydroxylation of terephthalic acid (benzene 1,4-dicarboxylic acid) COOH—(benzene ring, * marked)—COOH	Non-fluorescent; hydroxylated by OH$^\bullet$ at position marked* to fluorescent 2-hydroxyterephthalate (excitation 326 nm, emission 432 nm).	Only 1 isomer formed. Sensitive method, but to date not widely used in biological systems (*Free Radic. Res* **31**, 429, 1999; *Biomed. Chromatog.* **18**, 470, 2004), although was employed to detect OH$^\bullet$ in the brains of foetal sheep *in utero* (*J. Appl. Physiol.* **98**, 2304, 2005).
Hydroxylation of phthalic hydrazide	Non-fluorescent, forms fluorescent 3-hydroxylated product.	Used to study OH$^\bullet$ in fungal degradation of wood (*Holzforschung* **51**, 557, 1997).
Hydroxylation of phenethyl polyacrylate	A high molecular-weight polymer, cannot be taken up by cells.	Used to detect OH$^\bullet$ produced by brown rot fungi (*FEBS Lett.* **531**, 483, 2002).
Conversion of methional ($CH_3SCH_2CH_2CHO$) and related compounds (methionine or 2-keto-4-methylthiobutanoic acid, $CH_3SCH_2CH_2COCOOH$) into ethylene gas (H_2C=CH_2)	Measurement of ethylene by GC	Not specific for OH$^\bullet$; oxidized by $RO_2^\bullet$; decomposing ONOO$^-$ and some peroxidase enzymes (Section 7.5.4.3); confirmatory evidence for role of OH$^\bullet$ required.
Tryptophan method	Reaction of OH$^\bullet$ with tryptophan produces a characteristic set of products (*Bull. Eur. Physiopath. Resp.* **17**, 31, 1981).	Tryptophan also reacts with singlet O_2 but the products are different (Section 2.6.4).

Table 5.4 (*Cont.*)

Method	Principle of method	Comments
Coumarin fluorescence	Coumarin-3-carboxylic acid (CCA) is hydroxylated at position 7(*) to a fluorescent product.	This probe has been covalently linked to various biomolecules and fluorescence changes used to measure $OH^\bullet$ generation in their vicinity (*Int. J. Rad. Biol.* **63**, 445, 1993). For example, $OH^\bullet$ generation by copper ions bound to DNA could not be decreased by adding DMSO, methanol or ethanol but could be by histidine (which chelates copper). This is typical of a 'site-specific' reaction (Fig. 5.7) (*Free Rad. Biol. Med.* **18**, 669, 1995).
Measuring products of attack on cell wall polysaccharides	Hydroxyl radical attacks polysaccharides to give a wide range of products.	Used to implicate $OH^\bullet$ in cell wall softening during pear ripening (*Biochem. J.* **357**, 729, 2001)
Conversion of caffeine to 8-oxocaffeine	 Caffeine is hydroxylated at position 8; product analysed by HPLC with electrochemical detection.	Analogous to analysis of 8OHdG in DNA. Formation of 8-oxocaffeine from endogenous caffeine has been used to measure free-radical generation during roasting and brewing of coffee (*J. Agr. Food Chem.* **43**, 1332, 1995).
Dimethylsulphoxide (DMSO) method	Hydroxyl radicals react with DMSO, generating, in a complex set of reactions, methane gas, measured by gas chromatography (*Biochemistry* **20**, 6006, 1981), or formaldehyde, measured colorimetrically. $(CH_3)_2SO + OH^\bullet \rightarrow CH_3SO_2H + {}^\bullet CH_3$ ${}^\bullet CH_3 + O_2 \rightarrow CH_3OO^\bullet$ $2CH_3OO^\bullet \rightarrow HCHO + CH_3OH + O_2$ ${}^\bullet CH_3 + CH_3SO_2H \rightarrow CH_4 + CH_3SO_2^\bullet$ ${}^\bullet CH_3 + (CH_3)_2SO \rightarrow CH_4 + H_3SOCH_2^\bullet$	Not specific for $OH^\bullet$, e.g. oxidized by decomposing $ONOO^-$. Confirmatory evidence for role of $OH^\bullet$ required. Babbs *et al.* (*Free Rad. Biol. Med.* **6**, 493, 1989) have suggested that oxidation of DMSO to CH_3SO_2H, **methanesulphinic acid** (measured colorimetrically or by HPLC) is a means of detecting $OH^\bullet$ *in vivo*. Another approach is to trap the $CH_3^\bullet$ radicals (*Anal. Chem.* **69**, 4295, 1997). Levels of O_2 will affect the amounts of the various end-products since O_2 reacts with $CH_3^\bullet$ radicals.
Benzoate fluorescence	Reaction of benzoic acid with $OH^\bullet$ gives 3- and 4-hydroxybenzoates, which are fluorescent at 407 nm when excited at 305 nm.	Sensitive method (*Biochem. J.* **243**, 709, 1987); confirmatory evidence for role of $OH^\bullet$ required.

can be used (Section 5.2.3). Fluorescent probes such as dihydroethidium (DHE) and lucigenin are widely employed to detect $O_2^{\bullet-}$, but their chemistry is complex, although conversion of DHE to 2-hydroxyethidium may be a promising assay (Section 5.11 below). Often, $O_2^{\bullet-}$ is measured by its ability to reduce cytochrome c or nitroblue tetrazolium (NBT). The former reaction is simple

$$\text{cytochrome } c \text{ –Fe(III)} + O_2^{\bullet-} \rightarrow$$
$$O_2 + \text{cytochrome } c \text{ –Fe}^{2+}$$

However, many other substances reduce cytochrome c (especially ascorbate and thiols) and interfere with $O_2^{\bullet-}$ determination. Nitroblue tetrazolium is less often reduced by other cellular reductants, but the chemistry of chromogen formation is complex, and $O_2^{\bullet-}$ can be generated during it (Fig. 2.4). Thus addition of NBT to a biological system not making $O_2^{\bullet-}$ but able to reduce NBT can create an artefactual $O_2^{\bullet-}$ generation. Using XTT (Section 3.2.5) is somewhat better. Superoxide can also oxidize molecules such as adrenalin (to an adrenochrome chromophore), a reaction sometimes used to detect $O_2^{\bullet-}$ (Table 3.5). Again there are problems: once adrenalin has begun oxidizing (whether or not oxidation was started by $O_2^{\bullet-}$), $O_2^{\bullet-}$ is generated and oxidizes more adrenalin. Thus it is difficult to relate adrenochrome formation to the rate of $O_2^{\bullet-}$ generation by the system under test. Another detector molecule sometimes used is **Tiron** (1,2-dihydroxybenzene-3,5-disulphonate).[38] Like many diphenols (Section 2.5.3.5), it reacts with $O_2^{\bullet-}$ to give a semiquinone, which can be measured by ESR. For example, tiron semiquinone formation has been used to measure $O_2^{\bullet-}$ production by chloroplasts. One problem is that diphenols are oxidized by many systems, including peroxidases and $RO_2^{\bullet}$ radicals, so confirmatory evidence is needed that $O_2^{\bullet-}$ is being detected.[38] Tiron also chelates Ca^{2+}, and probably other metals.[39] Even inhibitions by SOD must be interpreted with caution in systems containing semiquinones (Section 2.5.3.5).

Superoxide electrodes have been described.[40] Some measure reduction of bound cytochrome c; usually SOD addition is used to show that reduction is $O_2^{\bullet-}$-mediated. Others electrochemically detect H_2O_2 from dismutation of $O_2^{\bullet-}$ by SOD attached to the electrode. Obviously, H_2O_2 from other sources can affect them. Cytochrome c-based sensors are also subject to interference by H_2O_2, which reacts with this protein (Section 3.15.3). Another approach is to detect redox changes in SOD's copper ions, a method less affected by H_2O_2.[40]

5.4.1 The aconitase assay[41]

Superoxide displaces iron from the $[4Fe–4S]^{2+}$ cluster of aconitase, causing loss of enzyme activity. The rate constant for reaction is about $2 \times 10^7 \, M^{-1}s^{-1}$ at 25°C, from which it was calculated that in SOD-deficient *E. coli* the $O_2^{\bullet-}$ concentration was $\sim$300 pM, as compared to 20 to 40 pM in normal *E. coli* (Section 3.4.1). The assay has also been used to calculate intramitochondrial $O_2^{\bullet-}$ levels in animal cells. For example antimycin addition to block mitochondrial electron transport increased $O_2^{\bullet-}$ from $\sim$6 pM to $\sim$15 pM in rat fibroblasts.

This is a sensitive assay, relevant to an important biological effect of $O_2^{\bullet-}$. One problem is that other RS (e.g. $ONOO^-$, N_2O_3) and the iron status of the cell can affect aconitase activity.

5.4.2 Rate constants for reactions with $O_2^{\bullet-}$

These are ideally obtained by pulse radiolysis (Section 2.3.3.1). However, pulse radiolysis is unsuitable for measuring many reactions of $O_2^{\bullet-}$ in aqueous solution, since the reaction rates are often lower than non-enzymic $O_2^{\bullet-}$ dismutation. Sometimes, simpler methods are adequate. For example, a mixture of hypoxanthine (or xanthine) and XO at pH 7.4 generates $O_2^{\bullet-}$, which reacts with cytochrome c and NBT with known rate constants, 2.6×10^5 and $6 \times 10^4 \, M^{-1}s^{-1}$, respectively. Any added molecule reacting with $O_2^{\bullet-}$ decreases the rates of cytochrome c or NBT reduction, and a competition plot allows calculation of an approximate rate constant. Essential controls[37] are as follows:

1. Check that the substance under test does not inhibit $O_2^{\bullet-}$ generation (e.g. by inhibiting XO).

Many compounds absorb strongly at 290 nm, making spectrophotometric assessment of urate production by XO inaccurate. HPLC determination of urate, or measurement of O_2 uptake by XO, are alternatives.

2. Check that the substance under test does not directly reduce cytochrome c or NBT.

3. Consider the possibility that a radical formed by attack of $O_2^{\bullet-}$ on a substance could itself reduce cytochrome c or NBT. This is often revealed as deviations from linear competition kinetics at high scavenger concentrations.

5.4.3 Triphenyl radical-based probes[42]

These probes show well-defined ESR spectra, sensitive to pO_2 (Section 5.2.2). Some can also react with $O_2^{\bullet-}$, to cause loss of the ESR signal. One of them, **TAMOXO63**, $R_3C^{\bullet}$ where R is

HOH$_2$CH$_2$C, HOH$_2$CH$_2$C — C — S ... S — C — CH$_2$CH$_2$OH, CH$_2$CH$_2$OH

reacts with $O_2^{\bullet-}$ (and/or with $HO_2^{\bullet}$ in equilibrium with $O_2^{\bullet-}$) with a rate constant of $3.1 \times 10^3 \, M^{-1} s^{-1}$ but is not reduced by GSH, NADPH or ascorbate. Simultaneous observation of the shape (Section 5.2.2) and loss of the ESR signal can be used to measure levels of both $O_2^{\bullet-}$ and O_2. The probe also reacts with $RO_2^{\bullet}$ radicals, apparently more slowly than with $O_2^{\bullet-}$, but not with $NO^{\bullet}$. Reaction with $O_2^{\bullet-}/HO_2^{\bullet}$ can also be followed by a fall in absorbance at 464 nm accompanied by a rise at 546 nm due to product formation.

5.4.4 Histochemical detection[43]

Histochemical methods to detect $O_2^{\bullet-}$ in tissues have been described. For example, perfusion with tetrazolium salts can lead to microscopically observable formazan precipitation at sites of $O_2^{\bullet-}$ generation. Figure 5.8 shows an animal example and Figure 7.17 a plant one. Another method employs conversion of **diaminobenzidine** (DAB) to an insoluble product. Tissues or organs are perfused with DAB and Mn^{2+} ions. Superoxide oxidizes Mn^{2+} to $Mn(III)$, which in turn oxidizes the DAB. This compound can be used to detect

H_2O_2 under different reaction conditions (Fig. 5.8, bottom, Plate 8).

5.5 Detection of nitric oxide[44]

Many methods have been developed to measure $NO^{\bullet}$. Some are trapping methods, involving reactions of $NO^{\bullet}$ or its derivatives with spin traps, dyes, haem compounds, other metal complexes or ozone (Table 5.5). An alternative approach is to implicate $NO^{\bullet}$ in a biological process if that process is blocked by NOS inhibitors. However, NOS inhibitors are not necessarily specific; often they can scavenge $OH^{\bullet}$, HOCl or ONOOH and so controls are needed (Table 5.5). Yet another technique is to examine end-products of $NO^{\bullet}$, the most common being NO_2^- (Table 5.5). For example it has been suggested that plasma levels of NO_2^- in humans are a measure of vascular endothelial $NO^{\bullet}$ synthesis.[45] However, NO_2^- is quickly oxidized to NO_3^- *in vivo* (Section 2.5.6.4).

Nitric oxide can oxidize to form such species as N_2O_3 and can also react with $O_2^{\bullet-}$ to give $ONOO^-$. All these species can interfere with $NO^{\bullet}$ detection by various methods (Table 5.5). For example, whereas $NO^{\bullet}$ under aerobic conditions eventually forms NO_2^-, breakdown of $ONOO^-$ generates mostly nitrate, NO_3^- (Section 2.6.1). Thus measurement of only NO_2^- in biological systems can underestimate the total amount of $NO^{\bullet}$ generated; both NO_2^- and NO_3^- should be measured.

5.5.1 Calibration

Regardless of the method used to measure $NO^{\bullet}$, it will need calibration. The direct methods (Table 5.5) can be calibrated using $NO^{\bullet}$ itself. This may be purchased as a gas, generated by acidification of nitrites or produced by the decomposition of 'NO$^{\bullet}$ donors', although their chemistry is complex and care must be taken in interpreting results obtained with them (Table 2.12).

5.6 Detection of peroxynitrite and other reactive nitrogen species

5.6.1 Probes for peroxynitrite

Generation of $ONOO^-$ by cells and tissues has been assessed by several mechanisms. For example,

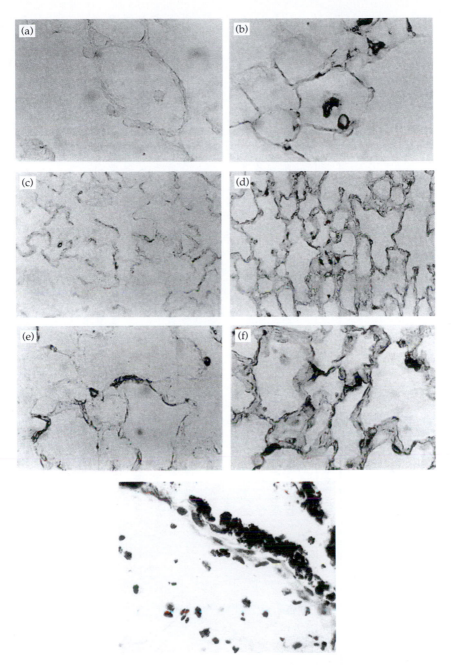

Figure 5.8 (see plate 8) Top panels: Detection of superoxide and nitrated proteins *in vivo*. Rats were injected with endotoxin to cause septic shock. There was an increase in iNOS in the lung. Staining of lung sections with an anti-nitrotyrosine antibody showed the presence of this modified amino acid. Perfusion with nitroblue tetrazolium was also carried out; $O_2^{\bullet-}$ reduces it to blue formazan. Lungs from untreated rats (A, C, E) or 48 h after endotoxaemia (B, D, F) were perfused with a phorbol ester to activate the respiratory bust and with nitroblue tetrazolium, and fixed. Sections were then stained with an anti-nitrotyrosine antibody (C, D, E, F) or control antiserum (A, B). (A) No staining; (B) formazan production suggestive of $O_2^{\bullet-}$; (C, E) control for anti-nitrotyrosine staining; (D, F) Increased nitrotyrosine and formazan in endotoxaemic animals. Magnification: ×1000 (A, B, E, F) or ×400 (C, D). Data from *J. Leuk. Biol.* **56**, 759, 1994, by courtesy of Dr Debra Laskin and the publishers. Bottom panel: histochemical detection of H_2O_2 production in a healing (3 day) rabbit, inflammatory skin lesion. The leukocytes in the crust are actively producing H_2O_2 (shown by the orange-brown colour). New epithelium is growing beneath the crust. The tissue section was fixed for 4 h at 4°C and stained with DAB for 5 h at 37°C. Photograph from *J. Leuk. Biol.* **56**, 436, 1994, by courtesy of Dr Arthur M. Dannenberg Jr and the publishers.

Table 5.5 Some methods for the detection of nitric oxide

Methods	Principle of method	Comments
A. *Direct methods*		
Light emission	Reaction of $NO^\bullet$ with O_3 produces light, via excited-state nitrogen dioxide $NO + O_3 \rightarrow O_2 + NO_2^\bullet$ (excited) $NO_2^\bullet \rightarrow NO_2^\bullet + $ light (excited)	Sensitive (nM range). Measures only gas-phase $NO^\bullet$. Potential interference by other light-emitting systems. $NO^\bullet$ must be displaced from the biological material into the gas-phase for analysis, e.g. by flushing with N_2, sometimes transfer is not quantitative.
$NO^\bullet$ electrodes	Several types. In **porphyrinic sensors** $NO^\bullet$ binds to a Ni^{2+}–porphyrin adsorbed onto an anode and is oxidized electro-chemically: $Ni(P) + NO^\bullet \rightarrow Ni(P)NO \rightarrow Ni(P)NO^+ + e^-$ Another method is an adaptation of the Clark O_2 electrode, in which O_2 diffuses through a membrane and is reduced. $NO^\bullet$ can be detected by changing the relative potentials of the silver and platinum electrodes.	Used to study $NO^\bullet$ exhalation in humans, and demonstrate elevated levels in asthma (*Thorax* **51**, 233, 1996), ~10 nM sensitivity. Easy to use, but several reports of interference by catecholamines. Clark probe is slower to respond to changes in $NO^\bullet$ than the porphyrinic probes and less sensitive. Insertion of a porphyrinic probe into a hand vein was used to detect $NO^\bullet$ *in vivo* (*Lancet* **346**, 153, 1995).
Haemoglobin trapping	Nitric oxide reacts with oxyhaemoglobin, eventually convert-ing it to methaemoglobin, ΔA is measured.	Sensitivity: ~µM. Simple to perform. Interference can occur with other oxidizing agents, e.g. $ONOO^-$ causes the same oxidation, as does NO_2^- (more slowly). Myoglobin can also be used. Haemoglobin addition often used to bind $NO^\bullet$ and block its effects in experimental systems.

Spin trapping

Various traps available, including

• Haemoglobin (ESR changes are an alternative to ΔA measurement)
• Other haem proteins (Fe^{2+} state)
• Fe^{2+}–dithiocarbamates (diethyldithiocarbamate often used)
• Fe^{2+}–thiosulphate

Nitric oxide is a good ligand to Fe^{2+} ions and the nitrosyl complexes produced have characteristic ESR spectra (e.g. HbNO, NOFe[DTC]$_2$, Fe[S$_2$O$_3$]$_2$[NO]$_2$). One must be aware that some or all of these Fe^{2+}–traps can react with H_2O_2 to form OH• and the ferric form can be reduced back by ascorbate or GSH (*Free Rad. Biol. Med.* **39**, 1581, 2005).

• Ribonucleotide reductase (removal of the tyrosyl radical at the active site by NO• abolishes the ESR signal). Depends on availability of enzyme, thus not widely used.

Attempts to use DMPO to trap NO• have given equivocal results. More success has been obtained with **nitronylnitroxides**, a group of organic compounds containing both nitrone and nitroxide groups. Nitronylnitroxides react with NO• to give iminonitroxides, detectable by ESR since they have different ESR spectra. The NNO **carboxy–PTIO** has also been used to antagonize the action of NO• in biological systems. Chelotropic agents such as 7,7,8,8-tetra-methyl-*o*-quinodimethane, have also been used to detect NO•. They bind NO• to generate a nitroxide radical, detectable by ESR (*J. Am. Chem. Soc.* **116**, 2767, 1994).

Formation of ESR-detectable nitrosylhaemoglobin in blood and tissues can be used as an index of NO• production, e.g. in ischaemia–reperfusion of organs and in animals with septic shock. Injected Fe^{2+}–dithiocarbamates have been used to detect NO• in animals with septic shock (*FEBS Lett.* **345**, 120, 1994). Nitrosothiolate ligand signals, probably involving non-haem iron–sulphur proteins, have been detected by ESR in NO•-exposed cells and tissues.

Reduction of nitroxides to ESR-silent species by ascorbate, GSH and sometimes $O_2^{•-}$ (Fig. 5.3) can be a problem in biological systems (e.g. *Free. Radic. Res.* **26**, 7, 1997).

Table 5.5 (Cont.)

Methods	Principle of method	Comments
4,5-Diaminofluorescein diacetate (**DAF-2-diacetate**) and related compounds (e.g. **DAF-2-FM**, a fluorinated derivative).	Enter cells and the acetyl group removed by esterases. Can accumulate to mM intracellular levels. React with NO^+ or N_2O_3 produced by $NO^{\bullet}$ oxidation to form a fluorescent product. Can be used to identify individual $NO^{\bullet}$-producing cells in tissue slices.	See *Nitric Oxide* **9**, 217, 2003 and *Free Rad. Biol. Med.* **39**, 327, 2005. Requires the $NO^{\bullet}$ to oxidize. Detection limit $\sim$5 nM. Can also react with $ONOO^-$ and peroxidase–H_2O_2 systems. Interference by ascorbate and dehydroascorbate reported.
Diaminoanthroquinone	Purple dye oxidized by NO-derived species (e.g. N_2O_3) to insoluble red fluorescent product.	Can be used to detect sites of $NO^{\bullet}$ production in tissues. Probably oxidized by several RNS (*Nitric oxide* **9**, 217, 2003).
B. Indirect methods NO_2^- measurement	Oxidation of $NO^{\bullet}$ generates mostly NO_2^- $4NO^{\bullet} + O_2 + 2H_2O \rightarrow 4NO_2^- + 4H^+$ In the **Griess reaction** NO_2^- reacts with sulphanilamide in an acidic solution of N-(1-naphthyl)ethylenediamine to give a coloured azo product (ΔA at 548 nm). Fluorimetry: reaction of NO_2^- with 2,3-diaminonaphthalene forms a fluorescent product, 3,3-naphthotriazole.	Sensitivity: μM. NO_2^- *in vivo* is rapidly oxidized to NO_3^-, which appears to be stable in body fluids. NO_3^- can be detected in the assay by using nitrate reductase enzymes or chemical reducing agents. Nitrate and NO_2^- can also come from diet (Section 2.5.6.5). Thus in one human study basal plasma NO_3^- was 29 ± 1 μM and rose to 205 μM 2 h after intake of NO_3^--rich food. Ranges of NO_2^- and NO_3^- in plasma samples are quoted as 1.3–13 μM and 4.0–45.3 μM in healthy people (*Clin. Chem.* **41**, 892, 1995). They can also be measured in urine. Inhaled $NO^{\bullet}$ is largely converted to NO_3^- in humans.
Measurement of other oxidation products	Based on formation of more-reactive species on the pathway from $NO^{\bullet}$ to NO_2^- in presence of O_2. Thus oxidizing $NO^{\bullet}$ oxidizes ferrocyanide to ferricyanide (ΔA at 420 nm) and the dye ABTS to the coloured $ABTS^{\bullet+}$ (ΔA at 660 nm). Nitrosation of sulphanilamide generates a coloured azo dye.	All simple spectrophotometric methods. Potential interference from other RNS, e.g. $ONOO^-$ or $NO_2^{\bullet}$.

| Use of NOS inhibitors | Can be 'general' inhibitors of all NOS isoforms or selective for a particular type. The former are generally analogues of the NOS substrate L-arginine, such as N-monomethyl-L-arginine (L-NMMA) or N-**nitro-L-arginine methyl ester** (L-NAME). Essential controls include showing that the D-isomers do not inhibit (e.g. both L- and D-forms are powerful OH$^\bullet$ scavengers; *Br. J. Pharmacol.* **122**, 1702, 1997) and that inhibition is reversed by adding excess L-arginine. More-selective inhibitors include aminoguanidine (iNOS) and **7-nitroindazole** (nNOS). | Subject to suitable controls, can provide evidence that NO$^\bullet$ (or species derived from it) are involved. However, NO$^\bullet$ can arise by reactions not involving NOS, e.g. decomposition of NO$_2^-$ by acid in the stomach or reaction of deoxyhaemoglobin with NO$_2^-$ (Sections 2.5.6.5 and 2.5.6.6). |

Adapted from Table 1, p. 278, *Analysis of Free Radical Reactions in Biological Systems* (Favier *et al.*, eds), Birkhauser–Verlag, Basle, 1995 by courtesy of Dr M. Fontecave and the publishers. Also see *Meth. Enzymol.* **268**, 1996 and *Antiox. Redox. Signal* **6**, 649, 2004.

$ONOO^-$ oxidizes the dye **dihydrorhodamine 123** (DHR 123) into **rhodamine 123**, which fluoresces at 536 nm when illuminated at 500 nm.[44] Oxidation does not require metal ions and is not inhibited by $OH^\bullet$ scavengers, but can be inhibited 60% by 100 mM HCO_3^- (which reacts with $ONOO^-$; Section 2.6.1). Oxidation of injected DHR 123 was observed in rats suffering from endotoxic or haemorrhagic shock and was decreased by administration of NOS inhibitors. However, DHR is not specific as a 'probe' for $ONOO^-$ (Section 5.11.2 below). Peroxynitrite also reacts with lumino1[44] (Section 5.11.4 below) to produce light, probably via $ONOOCO_2^-$ formation leading to $CO_3^{\bullet-}$ radical, since HCO_3^- addition enhances light production. Again, luminol is not a specific probe for $ONOO^-$.

5.6.2 Nitration assays[46]

Addition of $ONOO^-$ nitrates many aromatic compounds, including tyrosine, tryptophan and phenylalanine. Most attention has been paid to tyrosine: both the free amino acid and tyrosine residues within proteins (e.g. bovine SOD; Section 3.2.6) can be nitrated to give 3-nitrotyrosine (3-NT). Nitrations by $ONOO^-$ are accelerated by metal ions and certain metalloproteins, including CuZn-SOD, MnSOD and horseradish peroxidase. Tyrosine does *not* react directly with $ONOO^-$; it is first oxidized to tyrosyl radicals by RS generated from $ONOO^-$ (Section 2.6.1). The tyrosyl radicals can react with $NO_2^\bullet$ to generate 3-NT, or they can form bityrosine or react in other ways (Section 5.6.2.1 below). The presence of CO_2/HCO_3^- stimulates tyrosine nitration, possibly because $CO_3^{\bullet-}$ radical (Section 2.6.1) efficiently forms tyrosyl radical from tyrosine.

Nitration of tyrosine can be measured spectrophotometrically (3-NT is yellow at alkaline pH), or by amino-acid analysis after hydrolysis of modified proteins. Gas chromatography/mass spectrometry or HPLC with absorbance or electrochemical detection have also been used. HPLC analysis should be interpreted with caution because some tissues, especially brain, contain compounds[47] that coelute with 3-NT. Electrochemical detection (which has high sensitivity) is easier if the nitrotyrosine in biological samples is first reduced to **aminotyrosine**, which is oxidized at much lower voltages, by addition of the strong reducing agent dithionite. Aminotyrosine, unlike nitrotyrosine, has a characteristic fluorescence spectrum.

An alternative approach is the use of polyclonal or monoclonal antibodies directed against nitrated proteins. Although less-quantitative than the above approaches, these methods have the advantage that they permit the localization of nitrated proteins in tissues (Fig. 5.8). Essential controls include showing that the antibody binding is blocked by authentic 3-NT (or nitrated peptides/proteins) and/or by treatment of the sample with dithionite. Proteomic techniques have been used to identify which proteins are nitrated. Thus nitrated MnSOD was detected in rejected kidney transplants (Section 9.6), nitrated succinylcoenzyme A: 3-oxoacid coenzyme A transferase in a rat model of diabetes, β-enolase and creatine kinase in the skeletal muscles of old rats[48] and several proteins (including β-actin, α-enolase and triose phosphate isomerase) in the brains of patients with Alzheimer's disease (Section 9.20). Selectivity of nitration can be explained by several factors, including the relative abundance of the protein, its proximity to the RNS-generating systems, the amount of tyrosine it contains, the environment and location of those tyrosine residues, and the presence of metal centres that facilitate nitration.[46] Mass spectrometry can be employed to identify specific sites of nitration within a protein.

5.6.2.1 *Specificity for peroxynitrite?*[46,49]

Is 3-NT specific as a marker for $ONOO^-$? Nitric oxide does not nitrate aromatic compounds, but it can react rapidly with tyrosyl radicals, presumably to form nitroso adducts that could conceivably rearrange to nitro products, although this is probably uncommon. Nitrogen dioxide can nitrate tyrosine *in vitro* and in animals exposed to high levels of this toxic gas, but appears less efficient as a nitrating agent than $ONOO^-$, probably because it is not so good at converting tyrosine to tyrosyl radical. Mixtures of NO_2^- and HOCl can nitrate tyrosine, apparently by the intermediate formation of **nitryl chloride** (nitronium chloride), NO_2Cl. However, when NO_2^- and HOCl were added together to cells or cell lysates, no nitration was observed,[50] perhaps because HOCl reacts faster with other cell constituents than it does with NO_2^-. Myeloperoxidase (MPO), eosinophil peroxidase (EPO), and several other peroxidases can oxidize NO_2^- in the presence of H_2O_2 to a nitrating species, presumably $NO_2^\bullet$. They can also oxidize tyrosine to tyrosyl radical. If NO_2^- is simultaneously present, the enzymes can convert it to $NO_2^\bullet$, which reacts with tyrosyl and 3-NT is formed. For example, EPO-dependent nitration appears to occur in the airways of asthmatic patients.[51] Consumption of $NO^\bullet$ by MPO, and associated nitration of such extracellular proteins as fibronectin, may contribute to vascular dysfunction during inflammation.[52]

Alternative fates of tyrosyl radical are to dimerize to bityrosine, or react with $O_2^{\bullet-}$, GSH or ascorbate (Section 2.5.4). Nitrogen dioxide is also scavenged by ascorbate and GSH (Section 6.9.3). Hence the amount of nitration achieved *in vivo* when peroxidases oxidize tyrosine and NO_2^-, or when $O_2^{\bullet-}$ and $NO^\bullet$ react together, will depend on their relative ratios, the surrounding antioxidant levels, the presence of metals/metalloproteins and the CO_2/HCO_3^- levels. To summarize, observation of nitration *in vivo* should not be equated to formation of $ONOO^-$; it is more a general assay of RNS, and nitration levels are not a quantitative measure of RNS.[46,49]

5.6.2.2 *Reliability?*

The formation of nitrotyrosine in injured tissues is widespread (Table 5.6), although different antibodies, and sometimes the same antibodies in different laboratories, give different results for the intensity of 3-NT staining. Chemical measurement of nitrotyrosine in body fluids and tissues has been a controversial area, with claimed levels varying over two orders of magnitude. The best methods are based on mass spectrometry. It is essential to avoid exposure of biological material to low pH during sample work up, storage (even freezing phosphate-containing samples can cause low pH to develop) and the assay: at low pH traces of NO_2^- present can form nitrating species via HNO_2 and cause artefactual nitration. Addition of deuterated tyrosine can be used to check for this: there should be no deuterated 3-NT (easily distinguished from normal nitrotyrosine in the mass spectrometer) in biological materials.[53,54] Levels of free- and protein-bound

3-NT in human blood plasma from healthy subjects are in the low nanomolar range, and it is scarcely detectable (≤ 10 nM) in human urine.[54] Nitrotyrosine is metabolized to **3-nitro-4-hydroxyphenyla-cetate (NHPA)** in animals, which has sometimes been measured in urine as an estimate of 3-NT production *in vivo*. However, some (and perhaps most) urinary NHPA arises by other mechanisms,[55] making the assay questionable.

Nevertheless, provided that artefacts are avoided, measurement of 3-NT is a useful biomarker of protein damage by RNS and how it is affected by antioxidant or other interventions. For example, statin treatment decreased nitro-, chloro- and *ortho*-tyrosine levels in plasma of hypercholesterolaemic patients,[56] consistent with the view that hypercholesterolaemia is accompanied by oxidative stress (Section 9.3).

5.7 Detection of reactive halogen species

Hypochlorous acid is a powerful oxidizing and chlorinating agent (Section 2.6.3). It can even destroy 3-NT, and so its formation at sites of inflammation could lead to underestimation of tyrosine nitration.[57]

Several assays for HOCl have been described. Quenching of GFP was used to measure HOCl attack upon *E. coli* in phagocytic vacuoles (Section 7.7.3.3). The **taurine assay** is based on conversion of taurine to a chloramine

$$\text{Taurine}-NH_2 + HOCl \rightarrow \text{taurine}-NHCl + H_2O$$

which (like HOCl itself) oxidizes yellow thionitrobenzoic acid to a colourless oxidized product, 5,5′-dithiobis(2-nitrobenzoic acid) (DTNB, **Ellman's reagent**; Fig. 5.9). Chlorination of **monochlorodimedon** to dichlorodimedon, with loss of absorbance at 290 nm, has been used to assay HOCl production by MPO (Section 2.6.3). Since HOCl reacts fast with many biomolecules, these assays are not generally useful to measure it *in vivo*.

Exposure of free or protein-associated tyrosine to HOCl leads to production of some 3-chlorotyrosine and 3,5-dichlorotyrosine (Fig. 4.31), which have been suggested as biomarkers of HOCl generation.[58]

Table 5.6 Some of the conditions in humans and/or animal models in which increased formation of 3-nitrotyrosine has been reported

Cancer:
pancreas, oesophagus, lung, liver, colon, stomach (aggravated by *Helicobacter pylori* infection), cholangiocarcinoma, melanoma, murine mutatect tumours, glioblastoma

Lung disease:
transplant rejection, cystic fibrosis, chronic obstructive pulmonary disease, irradiation, bronchopulmonary dysplasia, pulmonary tuberculosis, respiratory failure, obliterative bronchiolitis, hyperoxic injury, radiation-induced acute lung injury, emphysema, asbestos inhalation, pneumonia, pulmonary fibrosis, pulmonary granulomatous inflammation, acute respiratory distress syndrome, nasal allergy, cigarette smoking, $NO^\bullet$ inhalation (some studies), influenza, asthma

Diseases of the nervous system:
amyotrophic lateral sclerosis, stroke, Parkinson's disease, hydrocephalus, AIDS dementia, multiple sclerosis, Pick's disease, diffuse Lewy body disease, progressive supranuclear palsy, Alzheimer's disease, thiamine deficiency, Lyme disease, sciatic nerve injury, Huntington's disease, encephalomyelitis, meningitis, chronic cerebral vasospasm, traumatic brain injury, spinal cord injury, diabetic neuropathy

Ischaemia–reperfusion:
organ transplantation, stroke, subarachnoid haemorrhage, graft rejection, septic shock, haemorrhagic shock

Cardiovascular:
giant cell arteritis, atherosclerosis, doxorubicin cardiomyopathy, myocardial infarction, myocardial stunning, transplant rejection, cardiopulmonary bypass, diabetes, atrial fibrillation, myocarditis, hypertension, nitrate tolerance

Muscle:
inclusion body myopathies, ischaemia–reperfusion, immobilization-induced stress

Eye:
glaucoma, uveitis, optic neuritis, retinitis, diabetic cataract

Inflammation:
hepatitis, carrageenan exposure, rheumatoid arthritis, coeliac disease, acute pancreatitis, hip replacement (loosening of the prosthesis), inflammatory bowel diseases, peritonitis, ileitis, influenza, systemic lupus erythematosus, scleroderma

Kidney and related:
glomerulonephritis, graft rejection, renal failure, diabetic nephropathy, obstructive bladder disease

Miscellaneous:
apo-E deficiency, foetal growth retardation, pre-eclampsia, chorioamnionitis, ageing, heat stress, skin lesions with anaphylactoid purpura, sickle cell anaemia, carbon monoxide exposure, osteoarthritis, ageing of normal cartilage, paracetamol hepatotoxicity, burns, UVB exposure, bone cysts, noise-induced hearing loss

For references see *Free Radic. Res.* **31**, 651, 1999; *Free Radic. Res.* **34**, 541, 2001 and [46]. Nitration can occur by several mechanisms, whose relative importance depends on the cell types present in the tissues and many other factors. For example, EPO plays a major role in respiratory tract protein nitration in a mouse model of asthma, but not in a model of peritoneal inflammation. Similarly, MPO-knockout mice show diminished nitration in some models of inflammation but not in others (*J. Biol. Chem.* **277**, 17415, 2002). The levels of nitrated proteins in 'normal' tissues are uncertain because of variations in the basal levels of antibody staining when using different procedures in different laboratories, but nitrated proteins have been detected in 'normal' tissues in several studies, including muscles of old rats.[48]

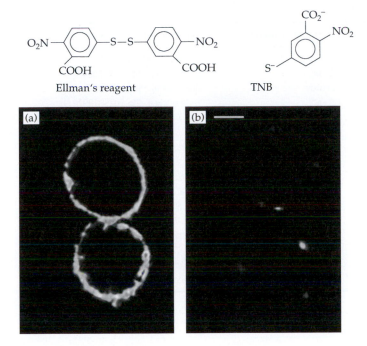

Figure 5.9 Loss of thiol groups after oxidative stress. Top: Ellman's reagent, 5,5′-dithiobis(2-nitrobenzoic acid) (DTNB) is widely used to measure −SH groups in proteins or 'total −SH' in cells (the sum of GSH, cysteine, protein−SH and any other −SH compounds). Thionitrobenzoate (TNB), absorbs strongly at 412 nm when ionized (pH ≥8) (See *Arch. Biochem. Biophys.* **82**, 70, 1959). Oxidation of TNB, with loss of absorption at 412 nm, has also been used in assays for HOCl and $ONOO^-$. Bottom: visualization of cell surface protein−SH groups by MPB-based immunofluorescence. Confocal laser scanning fluorescence imaging. (A) Control leukaemia cells, showing a ring of protein−SH group at the surface. (B) Loss of surface protein−SH following exposure to HNE. Bar: 10 μm. MPB; 3-(*N*-maleimidylpropionyl) biocytin. From *Histol. Histopathol.* **15**, 173, 2000, by courtesy of Professor A. Pompella and Jiménez-Godoy publishers, S.A. Murcia, Spain.

Similarly, HOBr brominates tyrosine. However, NO_2Cl also chlorinates tyrosine, so simultaneous measurement of nitrated and chlorinated products (e.g. by HPLC or MS after hydrolysis of proteins) can be useful in distinguishing effects of $ONOO^-$ (nitration), HOCl (chlorination) and NO_2Cl (both). Tyrosine chlorination is not a quantitative measure of the amounts of HOCl or NO_2Cl generated: these species react with multiple other targets, whose levels will determine how much tyrosine modification occurs *in vivo* (also see Section 5.15.2 below). Mass-spectrometric methods for simultaneous analysis of *ortho-*, *meta-*, bromo- chloro- and nitro-tyrosines have been developed[33,54] as have antibodies directed against bromo- or chlorotyrosine (Table 5.7). It is important to check the antibodies for specificity, for example do they recognize other halogenated tyrosines? One important tip: hydrolysis of proteins in HCl can lead to artefactual tyrosine chlorination—avoid it.

Halogenated tyrosines are natural constituents of some structural proteins in marine invertebrates and insects, for example chloro- and dichloro-tyrosine occur in the cuticle of the desert locust *Schistocerca gregaria*.[59] Chlorotyrosine can be oxidized to 3-chloro-4-hydroxyphenylacetate and to several dechlorinated metabolites (e.g. 4-hydroxyphenylacetate) *in vivo*.

5.8 Detection of hydrogen peroxide

Several methods exist (Table 5.8). To be useful in biological systems they must be sensitive, since rates of H_2O_2 production by cells and organelles are usually only in the nmol/min range (except for activated phagocytes). Steady-state concentrations of H_2O_2 in hepatocytes and mitochondria are estimated[41] as no more than 10^{-7} to 10^{-9} M. Commonly used assays employ the H_2O_2-dependent oxidation of substrates by horseradish peroxidase (HRP). Substrates include homovanillic acid, **Amplex red** or DCFDA (Table 5.8), oxidized to fluorescent products. By contrast, the fluorescent compound **scopoletin** is converted to a non-fluorescent product by HRP/H_2O_2.

It is essential to check that the reaction mixture does not contain compounds that are substrates for HRP, that could compete and cause an artefactual inhibition.[37] For example, ascorbate and thiols are oxidized by HRP, and can interfere with peroxidase-based assay systems. This can happen in the

Table 5.7 Some examples of the detection of chlorotyrosines *in vivo*

System	Method of measurement	Representative reference
Human pregnancy (placenta)	Antibody	*Lab. Invest.* **81**, 543, 2001
Alzheimer's disease	GC–MS	*J. Neurochem.* **90**, 724, 2004
Inflamed human kidney	Antibody	*Am. J. Path.* **150**, 603,1997
Human atherosclerotic lesions	GC–MS	*J. Clin. Invest.* **99**, 2075, 1997
Human lung lining fluid proteins after transplantation	HPLC/ECD	*Am. J. Resp. Crit. Care Med.* **161**, 2035, 2000
Sputum from cystic fibrosis patients	GC–MS	*Am. J. Physiol.* **279**, L537, 2000
Septic mice	GC–MS	*J. Clin. Invest.* **109**, 1311, 2002
Asthma patients	GC–MS	*Clin. Exp. Allergy* **34**, 931, 2004
Burn injury in rats	GC–MS	*Am. J. Path.* **162**, 1373, 2003
Preterm infants	GC–MS	*Pediat. Res.* **53**, 455, 2003
Dialysis patients	GC–MS	*Free Rad. Biol. Med.* **31**, 1163, 2001
Rheumatoid arthritis	GC–MS	*Arch. Biochem. Biophys.* **391**, 119, 2001
	HPLC	*Inflammation* **17**, 167, 1993
ARDS patients	GC–MS	*Crit. Care Med.* **27**, 1738, 1999
Churg–Strauss syndrome	GC–MS	*J. Allerg. Clin. Immunol.* **114**, 1358, 2004
Liver injury in mice (bile duct ligation)	Antibody	*Hepatology* **38**, 355, 2003

3-Bromotyrosine has also been measured in some systems (e.g. *J. Biol. Chem.* **277**, 17415, 2002 and *Clin. Exp. Allergy* **34**, 931, 2004).

assay of H_2O_2 production by mitochondrial preparations, for example.[41] Such a control is also essential when checking for the H_2O_2-scavenging activity of compounds by using HRP to measure the loss of H_2O_2: one must check that the test compound is not itself a substrate for HRP.[37] Superoxide decreases HRP activity (forming compound III; Section 3.13.4) and may compromise measurement of H_2O_2 in systems generating $O_2^{\bullet-}$. This can be avoided by adding SOD.[60]

Catalase is frequently used in assays of H_2O_2 production to check for specificity (Table 5.8). It can also detect H_2O_2 directly; observation of the spectral intermediates of catalase has been used to assess H_2O_2 production in organs (Fig. 5.11). Catalase can use H_2O_2 to oxidize methanol and formate (Section 3.7.4), and this has been made the basis of various assay systems, for example decarboxylation of ^{14}C-labelled formate to $^{14}CO_2$. Catalase is inhibited by **aminotriazole**, but only when H_2O_2 is present (Section 3.7.3). Hence the extent of inactivation of catalase by aminotriazole has been used to calculate H_2O_2 production in cells and organs. Various cytochemical stains for H_2O_2 have been developed (Table 5.8), often relying on

the ability of peroxidase to oxidize substrates such as DAB when H_2O_2 is present. Figure 5.8, bottom photograph, shows an example from animals and Fig. 7.17 one from plants.

Hydrogen peroxide has been detected at μM levels in human urine and arises in part by the autoxidation of excreted compounds (Section 2.6.2). It is simple to measure, but levels vary widely with time of day and between subjects, and it is uncertain to what extent urinary H_2O_2 might be a 'biomarker' of whole-body production[61] of ROS. Hydrogen peroxide can also be measured in exhaled air (Section 5.14.8 below).

5.9 Detection of singlet oxygen[62,63]

Singlet O_2 formed in biological systems (Section 2.6.4) is difficult to detect unambiguously. For example, photosensitization reactions can damage biomolecules by production of other ROS (e.g. OH$^{\bullet}$) and by direct interaction of excited states with the biomolecule (type I reactions). Hence it must never be assumed that $^1O_2$ is responsible for photochemical damage. One way to distinguish between type I and type II ($^1O_2$-mediated) damage

Table 5.8 Some methods for measuring H_2O_2 in biological systems

Method	Principle of the method	Examples of systems to which it has been applied
Observation of intracellular catalase compound I	See Fig. 5.10	Bacteria, organs (perfused and *in situ*), organ slices, homogenates.
Oxidation of [^{14}C]methanol or [^{14}C]formate by catalase compound I	See text	Difficult to use in whole animals as methanol can be oxidized by alcohol dehydrogenase and formate by formate dehydrogenase enzymes.
Cytochrome *c* peroxidase	Enzyme oxidizes reduced cytochrome *c* and is specific for H_2O_2. Forms a complex with H_2O_2 that absorbs at 419 nm (Section 3.13.1) whereas free enzyme absorbs at 407 nm.	Animal and plant mitochondria, protozoa, peroxisomes, microsomes (*Biochem. J.* **128**, 617, 1972). Assay often difficult to apply to biological systems because other cytochrome *c* reductases/oxidases and catalase present.
Horseradish peroxidase plus substrates	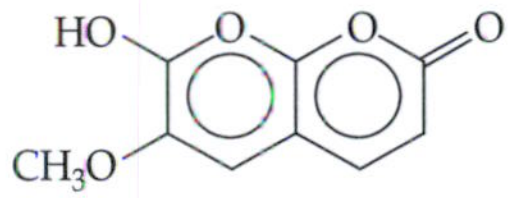 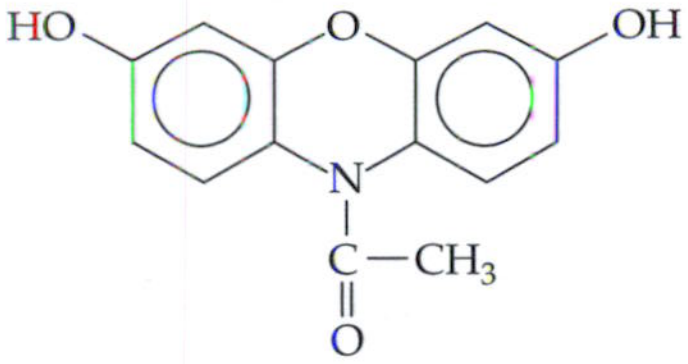	Animal and plant mitochondria, submitochondrial particles, phagocytes, protozoa, microsomes (*J. Biochem. Biophys. Methods* **18**, 297, 1989; *J. Bioeng. Biomemb.* **34**, 227, 2004; *Anal. Biochem.* **253**, 162, 1997), human urine, breath condensate (*Eur. J. Clin. Invest.* **33**, 274, 2003; *Anal. Chem.* **77**, 2862, 2005).

(7-hydroxy-6-methoxy-coumarin)

Scopoletin (structure above) is a popular substrate: others include homovanillic acid (3-methoxy-4-hydroxyphenylacetic acid) and **Amplex Red** (*N*-acetyl-3,7-dihydroxyphenoxazine),

which are oxidized to fluorescent products. Other possible 'H_2O_2 sensors' include fluorescent proteins that lose fluorescence when oxidized with HRP/H_2O_2.

Table 5.8 (*Cont.*)

Method	Principle of the method	Examples of systems to which it has been applied
O_2-electrode method	Add excess catalase and measure release of oxygen: $2H_2O_2 \rightarrow 2H_2O + O_2$	Chloroplasts, mitochondria. Also used to study rate constants for reaction of compounds with H_2O_2, by measuring residual H_2O_2. Not very sensitive but useful in turbid systems. Used to measure H_2O_2 in human urine (*Biochem. Biophys. Res. Commun.* **262**, 205, 1999).
H_2O_2 electrode	Uses membrane-coated Pt microelectrode, μM sensitivity. Some '$O_2^{\bullet-}$ electrodes' also detect H_2O_2 (Section 5.4)	Enzymes, neutrophils. Not very sensitive (*Free Rad. Biol. Med.* **31**, 894, 2001).
Inhibition by catalase	If a reaction requires H_2O_2, then it should be inhibited by catalase.	Catalase slow at destroying low concentrations of H_2O_2, so a large amount must be added. Often used to investigate the role of H_2O_2 in oxidative damage. Controls with inactive enzyme required. Commercial catalases often contaminated with SOD, thymol (a phenolic antioxidant) and endotoxin. Catalase poorly active at low or high pH.
Ferrithiocyanate method	H_2O_2 oxidizes Fe^{2+} to $Fe(III)$ which forms coloured products with ferrithiocyanate.	Simple, not very sensitive Microsomes, cells (*Eur. J. Biochem.* **25**, 420, 1997; *Free Rad. Biol. Med.* **15**, 57, 1993; *Circ. Res.* **84**, 1203, 1999). Would detect any oxidizing species; need control with catalase.
GSSG release	Section 3.9.4	Isolated organs. Measures GSH oxidation, not necessarily exclusively due to H_2O_2.
Aminotriazole inhibition of catalase	See text	Fungi, various bacteria, *Mycoplasma*, erythrocytes, other animal tissues.
Dichlorofluorescein diacetate (DCFH-DA)	Section 5.11.1	Widely used to measure H_2O_2 and other peroxides in cells but in fact reacts only slowly with them. Its oxidation by H_2O_2 plus horseradish peroxidase was introduced in 1965 as a sensitive fluorimetric assay for H_2O_2.

Table 5.8 (*Cont.*)

Method	Principle of the method	Examples of systems to which it has been applied
Decarboxylation of keto acids	Glyoxylate, pyruvate and α-ketoglutarate react non-enzymically with H_2O_2. Use of ^{14}C-labelled substrates permits sensitive measurement of $^{14}CO_2$ release.	Eye lens, human body fluids, peroxisomes (*Free Radic. Res. Commun.* **5**, 359, 1989).
Histochemical staining method	Several exist, e.g. in plants one method is based on oxidation of iodide to I_2 by H_2O_2, detected by formation of a blue complex with starch. More often in animals, the tissue is treated with Fe^{2+}-diethylenetriamine penta-acetic acid. This is oxidized by H_2O_2 to the ferric chelate which in turn oxidizes ciaminobenzidine to an insoluble chromogen.	Plant slices (*Plant Physiol. Biochem.* **36**, 817, 1998). Perfused organs, cells, animal tissue slices (*Methods Enzymol.* **233**, 619, 1994). Would presumably detect other oxidizing agents as well but if due to H_2O_2 catalase should inhibit.
Oxidation of dimethylthiourea (DMTU) to a dioxide product	DMTU is oxidized by $OH^\bullet$, $HOCl$, $ONOO^-$ and H_2O_2, but only H_2O_2 is reported to give the dioxide product.	Enzymes, neutrophils, lung. *Proc. Natl. Acad. Sci. USA*, **85**, 3422, 1988. Not widely used.
Titration with acidified potassium permanganate, $KMnO_4$	Measure loss of colour	Not very sensitive. Has been used in a few studies to measure reaction of molecules with H_2O_2.
Peroxyfluor-1 (PF1)	Oxidized by H_2O_2 to a fluorescent product	One of a series of boronate-based probes that respond to H_2O_2 by producing fluorescence. Reportedly less-sensitive to $O_2^{\bullet-}$, $NO^\bullet$, organic peroxides, $HOCl$, O_3, $OH^\bullet$ or singlet O_2 (*J. Am. Chem. Soc.* **127**, 16652, 2005).

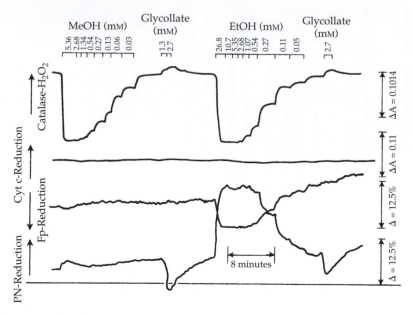

Figure 5.10 Production of H_2O_2 in rat liver perfused with a bicarbonate-saline solution containing 2 mM L-lactate and 0.3 mM pyruvate at 30°C. Light was shone through a liver lobe and the concentration of catalase compound I measured by dual-wavelength spectrophotometry. There is a steady concentration of compound I from which the endogenous rate of H_2O_2 production can be calculated as being about 82 nmol H_2O_2/min/g of liver, in livers from normally fed animals. Inclusion of methanol (MeOH) in the perfusion medium decreases compound I concentration because MeOH is a substrate for the peroxidatic action of catalase. Ethanol (EtOH) has a similar effect, but it also causes an increased reduction of pyridine nucleotides (PN) since it is a substrate for the alcohol dehydrogenases, which convert NAD^+ to NADH. There is also some reduction of flavoproteins (Fp). Infusion of glycollate raises the steady-state concentration of compound I because it is oxidized in the peroxisomes to form H_2O_2 by glycollate oxidase:
glycollate $+ O_2 \rightarrow$ glyoxylate $+ H_2O_2$
Cyt-c, cytochrome *c*. Data from *Arch. Biochem. Biophys.* **154**, 117, 1973, by courtesy of Professor Britton Chance and Academic Press. Also see [41].

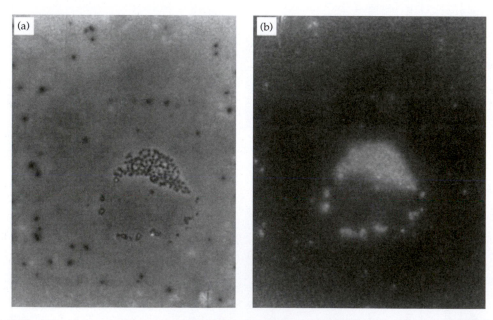

Figure 5.11 Fluorescence from neutrophils loaded with dichlorofluorescein diacetate, after stimulation to produce ROS by adding fMet-Leu-Phe, (a) light field and (b) fluorescence field. Excitation was at 500 nm; emission was measured at 530 nm. From *Biochem. J.* **248**, 173, 1987 by courtesy of Professor A.K. Campbell and the Biochemical Society.

to a target is by immobilizing the sensitizer on a solid support (e.g. a glass slide, suspended above a thin well of substrate solution), thus allowing the $^1O_2$ produced to diffuse a short distance to the target. Hence the target does not contact the excited-state photosensitizer. An alternative method is to pass a stream of O_2 over a bed of sensitizer and then into the test system.

5.9.1 Direct detection

Decay of $^1O_2$ yields two types of light emission: the weak **monomol** emission at 1270 nm and the **dimol** emission resulting from collision of two $^1O_2$ molecules, which produces light at 630 and 701 nm. The 1270 nm (infrared) emission has been much used to study $^1O_2$ chemistry, whereas the dimol emission wavelengths are prone to interference by other light-emitting reactions. The mere production of light does not implicate $^1O_2$ unless the correct emission spectrum can be demonstrated. This is because many other RS-related processes produce light, including Fenton reactions, reactions of haem proteins with H_2O_2 and the decomposition of dioxetanes, which produce excited-state carbonyls that emit light as they return to the ground state.

5.9.2 Use of scavengers and traps

Scientists have often relied on 'singlet-O_2 scavengers' and quenchers to implicate $^1O_2$ in biological systems. Popular compounds include DABCO, diphenylisobenzofuran, histidine and azide (Section 2.6.4). Addition of these should inhibit a reaction dependent on $^1O_2$. If, when added at high concentrations, they do not inhibit, one can usually conclude that $^1O_2$ is not required for that reaction. If they do inhibit, this does *not* prove a role for $^1O_2$, because these compounds are not specific for $^1O_2$. For example, they all react with $OH^\bullet$, often with a greater rate constant (usually $>10^9 \, M^{-1}s^{-1}$) than for reaction with $^1O_2$. For example, azide reacts with $OH^\bullet$ to give a reactive **azide radical**, $N_3^\bullet$

$$N_3^- + OH^\bullet \rightarrow N_3^\bullet + OH^-$$

β-Carotene and DABCO also react with $RO_2^\bullet$ radicals (Section 3.21.3.1).[64] Fortunately, the products of reaction of certain fatty acids, cholesterol and tryptophan with $^1O_2$ are different from those obtained on reaction with $OH^\bullet$, so isolation and characterization of them allows distinction. For example, observation of the 'ene' product, 5α-hydroperoxycholesterol, is considered good evidence for $^1O_2$ and has been used to detect it in skin (Section 6.12). β-Carotene may give unique products when oxidized by $^1O_2$. These approaches need skill in analytical chemistry, however, and the use of $^1O_2$ scavengers, like that of spin traps or $OH^\bullet$ scavengers, cannot be recommended to the chemically naive.

Another trap that has been employed is **9,10-diphenylanthracene** (or its water-soluble derivatives), to which singlet O_2 adds to form a fluorescent endoperoxide.

For example, oxidation of diphenylanthracene bound to glass beads was used to investigate $^1O_2$ production by phagocytes after engulfment of the beads into the phagocytic vacuole.[65] In reverse, decomposition of endoperoxides can be a source of $^1O_2$ (Section 2.6.4.5). An anthracene-based spin trap for $^1O_2$, **2-(9,10-dimethoxyanthracenyl)-*tert*-butylhydroxylamine** has been described, which is oxidized by $^1O_2$ to a nitroxide,[66] although it has not been widely used. ***Trans*-1-(2′-methoxyvinylpyrene)** has been used to detect $^1O_2$, by formation of an endoperoxide that emits light as it decomposes. It appears not to react with $OH^\bullet$, H_2O_2 or $O_2^{\bullet-}$.

$$\text{(pyrene-CH=CH-OCH}_3) \xrightarrow{^1O_2} \text{(dioxetane O—O with OCH}_3) \rightarrow \text{(pyrene-CHO}^a\text{)}$$

CL(Em = 465 nm)

[a] This equation is reproduced by courtesy of the Molecular Probes company, USA.

5.9.3 Deuterium oxide (D₂O)

Another approach, often employed in studying photodynamic effects, is to use D_2O. The lifetime of $^1O_2$ is longer in D_2O than in H_2O by a factor of 10 or 15 (Section 2.6.4). Thus if a reaction in aqueous solution is dependent on $^1O_2$, carrying it out in D_2O instead of H_2O should potentiate the reaction. Theoretically, a type I reaction would be unaffected.

5.10 Studies of 'generalized' light emission (luminescence/fluorescence)

Following early research in Eastern Europe, many scientists have used photomultipliers or luminometers to measure the light emitted by animal tissues, injured plants, whole organs and organisms such as protozoa or parasitic worms. Human breath shows low-level light emission (about 7000 counts per litre of breath per second), as do blood and plasma.[67,68]

This **low-level chemiluminescence** often increases in response to oxidative stress, for example elevated O_2 concentration or introduction of ROS-generating drugs. It is too weak to be seen by the naked eye (hence it is sometimes called **ultraweak chemiluminescence** or **dark chemiluminescence**) and its source is undefined. Light can arise from $^1O_2$, triplet excited states (e.g. carbonyls), reactions of $ONOO^-$, lipoxygenase action, haem protein/peroxide reactions and Fenton chemistry. Nevertheless, it has some potential as a non-invasive technique of 'general' ROS production.

5.11 Measurement of reactive species in cultured cells[28,44]

Many methods are available to identify RS in cells, and some have become widely used, although precise chemical information on what they really measure tends to be limited. An important first consideration is that *the cell culture process itself causes oxidative stress*, both by facilitating generation of ROS and by hindering adaptive upregulation of cellular antioxidants (Section 1.11). Trypsinization or serum deprivation of cells (even transiently, e.g. to allow loading of probes) increases ROS formation. In addition, results can be confounded by free radical reactions taking place in the culture media. For example, some reports of effects of ascorbate, flavonoids and dopamine[69] on cells in culture are artefacts caused by their oxidation in the culture media (Sections 3.20.1 and 3.22.3).

Some simple guidelines can help in understanding oxidative stress/oxidative damage in cell culture. Hydrogen peroxide can cross cell membranes (Section 2.6.2). Thus catalase added outside cells can lower intracellular H_2O_2, by removing extracellular H_2O_2 and establishing a concentration gradient that drains H_2O_2 out of the cell. By contrast, $O_2^{\bullet -}$ does not generally cross membranes, although it can do so through protein channels in some cells (Section 6.4). Thus if externally added SOD is protective against an event in cell culture, be wary; this could indicate extracellular $O_2^{\bullet -}$-generating reactions. Similarly, neither the iron-chelator desferrioxamine (Section 10.7) nor GSH enter cells easily, so again be wary if they have protective effects in short-term cell culture

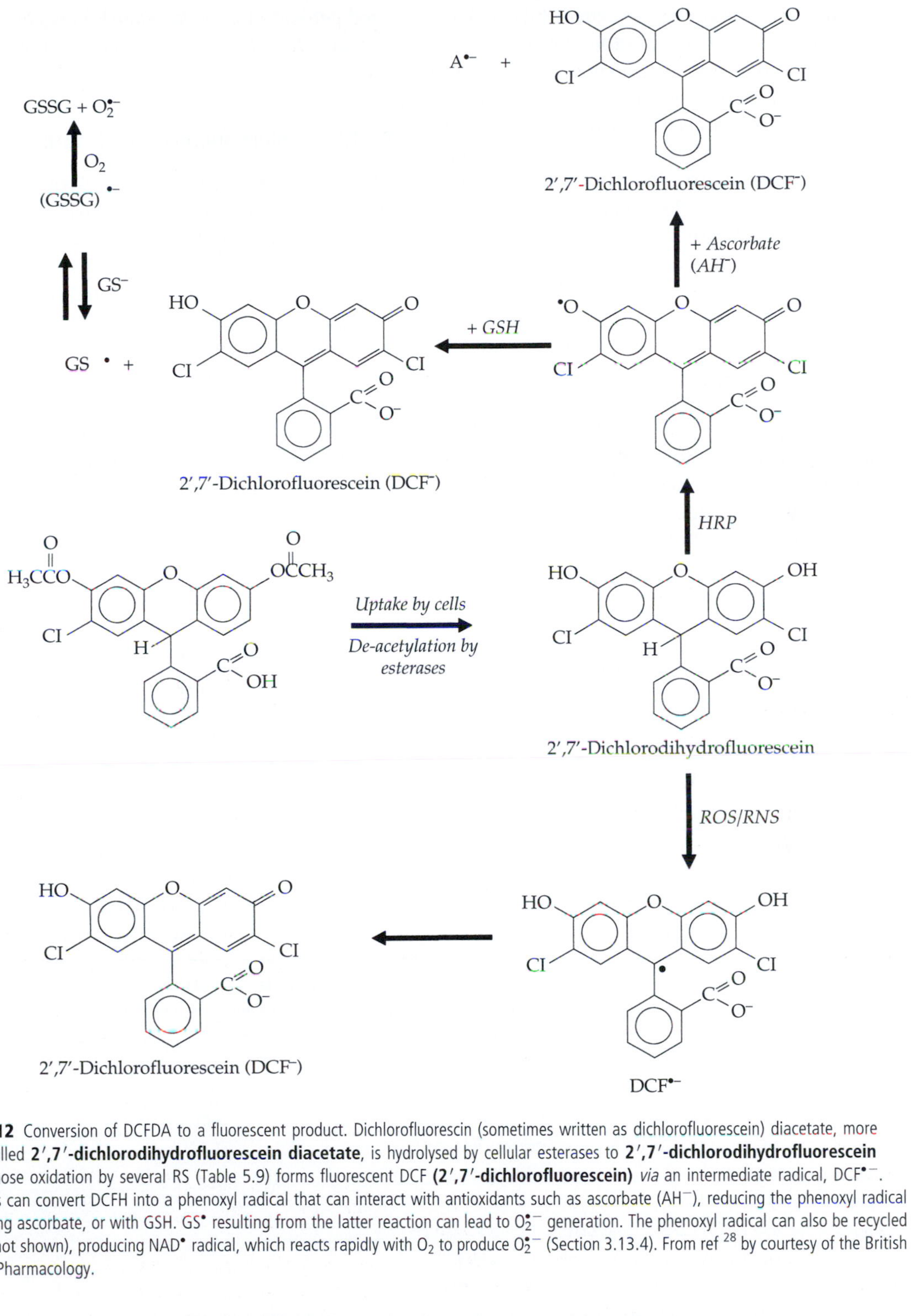

Figure 5.12 Conversion of DCFDA to a fluorescent product. Dichlorofluorescin (sometimes written as dichlorofluorescein) diacetate, more correctly called **2′,7′-dichlorodihydrofluorescein diacetate**, is hydrolysed by cellular esterases to **2′,7′-dichlorodihydrofluorescein** (DCFH), whose oxidation by several RS (Table 5.9) forms fluorescent DCF (**2′,7′-dichlorofluorescein**) *via* an intermediate radical, DCF$^{\bullet-}$. Peroxidases can convert DCFH into a phenoxyl radical that can interact with antioxidants such as ascorbate (AH$^-$), reducing the phenoxyl radical and oxidizing ascorbate, or with GSH. GS$^\bullet$ resulting from the latter reaction can lead to O$_2^{\bullet-}$ generation. The phenoxyl radical can also be recycled by NADH (not shown), producing NAD$^\bullet$ radical, which reacts rapidly with O$_2$ to produce O$_2^{\bullet-}$ (Section 3.13.4). From ref [28] by courtesy of the British Society of Pharmacology.

experiments: this may suggest extracellular actions. For example, in one study, added GSH protected cells against damage by dopamine by reacting with cytotoxic dopamine quinones/semiquinones generated *in the medium*.[69] Given long enough, however, everything can enter cells, including desferrioxamine (into the lysosomal system; Section 10.7) and SOD (by pinocytosis).

Production of RS in cells can be measured by aromatic compounds or spin traps, and oxidative damage by assaying products of damage to bimolecules (Sections 5.12–5.15 below). Spin traps have been used successfully in many cell studies, since a wider range of traps at higher concentrations can be used than is possible *in vivo*. Again, be aware of the possibility of reduction of free radical-spin trap adducts to ESR-silent species by non-enzymic antioxidants (such as ascorbate) and cellular enzymatic reducing systems (Section 5.2.6).

Often however, cellular production of RS is measured by various fluorescent 'probes'. Probes of lipid peroxidation/membrane RS are considered in Section 5.14 below, but let us now examine some of the others.

5.11.1 Dichlorofluorescin diacetate (DCFDA)[28]

This is the most popular probe, frequently used to measure putative 'cellular peroxides' (Fig. 5.12). Sadly however, it doesn't detect peroxides very well (the boronate-based probes may be more specific for H_2O_2 [Table 5.8] although more work is required to establish this). The DCFDA enters cells and accumulates mostly in the cytosol, where it is deacetylated by esterases to dichlorofluorescein (DCFH) and converted by various RS into DCF, which can be visualized by fluorescence at around 525 nm when excited at around 488 nm.

So what then does it measure? Neither peroxides nor $O_2^{\bullet-}$ oxidize DCFH rapidly, but $RO_2^{\bullet}$, $RO^{\bullet}$, $NO_2^{\bullet}$, $CO_3^{\bullet-}$, and $OH^{\bullet}$ radicals can, as can $ONOO^-$ (Table 5.9). It follows that DCFDA only detects

Table 5.9 Sensitivity of various probes to different reactive species

Reactive species	HPF	APF	DCFH
$OH^{\bullet a}$	730	1200	7400
$ONOO^{-b}$	120	560	6600
Hypochlorite[c]	6	3600	86
Singlet O_2[d]	5	9	26
Superoxide[e]	8	6	67
H_2O_2[f]	3	<1	190
$NO^{\bullet g}$	6	<1	150
$ROO^{\bullet h}$	17	2	710
Photochemical oxidation of the probe[i]	<1	<1	2000

Structures and full names of these probes are shown in Figures 5.13 and 5.14. Probes (final 10 μM; 0.1% DMF as a cosolvent) were added to sodium phosphate buffer (0.1M, pH 7.4). The fluorescence intensities of HPF, APF and DCFH were measured at excitation wavelength of 490, 490 and 500 nm and fluorescence emission wavelength of 515, 515 and 520 nm, respectively.

[a] 100μM of Ferrous perchlorate (II) and 1mM of H_2O_2 were added.

[b] 3μM (final) of $ONOO^-$ was added.

[c] 3μM (final) of NaOCl was added.

[d] 100μM of 3-(1,4-dihydro-1,4-epidioxy-1-naphthyl)propionic acid was added.

[e] 100μM of KO_2 was added.

[f] 100μM of H_2O_2 was added.

[g] 100μM of 1-hydroxy-2-oxo-3-(3-aminopropyl)-3-methyl-1-triazene was added.

[h] 100μM of 2,2′-azobis(2-amidinopropane)dihydrochloride was added.

[i] Solutions of probes were placed under a fluorescent lamp for 2.5 hours.

Adapted from *J. Biol. Chem.* **278**, 3170, 2003, by courtesy of Professor Tetsuo Nagano and the American Society of Biochemistry and Molecular Biology.

cellular peroxides efficiently if they are converted to radicals, for example by transition metal ions or haem proteins such as MPO, other peroxidases, or cytochrome c. Thus cellular levels of catalytic iron/copper ions and haem proteins are essential variables to consider when interpreting studies using DCFDA. Hence DCF fluorescence is an assay of generalized RS production rather than of any particular RS, and it is **not** a direct assay for H_2O_2, $NO^\bullet$, lipid peroxides, singlet O_2 or $O_2^{\bullet-}$. To avoid cytotoxicity, cells should be loaded with DCFDA at low concentrations (e.g. $1–10\,\mu M$ for $45\,min–1\,h$). Higher levels of DCFDA or high light intensities can cause artefactual photochemical oxidation to fluorescent products that can be mistaken for RS generation (Table 5.9).

One-electron oxidation of DCFH by various radicals or by haem proteins can produce intermediate radicals, including phenoxyl radicals, that can interact with GSH, ascorbate and NADH to create more free radicals (Fig. 5.13). The extent to which this contributes to the signal is uncertain but is another reason for using low DCFDA levels. Cytochrome c can catalyse DCFH oxidation, so using DCFDA to measure oxidative stress during apoptosis should be approached with caution; a rise in cytosolic cytochrome c levels could give a bigger signal without any change in ROS levels.[70] Several other oxidants, including chromium(v), can directly oxidize DCFH and cause an artefactual signal, and the possibility of direct oxidations must be checked before using DCFDA to measure oxidative stress in cells exposed to toxins. Variation in cellular esterase content could conceivably affect the use of DCFDA as a probe, but this issue has not been explored in the literature.

The probes HPF and APF (Table 5.9; Fig. 5.13) seem useful. Both fluoresce after reaction with $OH^\bullet$, $ONOO^-$ and peroxidase-derived species but only APF emits light after exposure to HOCl. Both are more stable to photochemical events than DCFDA and neither responds to $^1O_2$, $O_2^{\bullet-}$, H_2O_2, $NO^\bullet$ or $RO_2^\bullet$ radicals.

5.11.2 Dihydrorhodamine 123 (DHR)[44]

This compound is used to detect several RS ($OH^\bullet$, $ONOO^-$, $NO_2^\bullet$, peroxidase-derived species), but is poorly responsive to $O_2^{\bullet-}$, H_2O_2 or $NO^\bullet$. It is better

at detecting HOCl than is DCFDA. These various RS convert DHR to rhodamine 123 (Fig. 5.14), which is highly fluorescent around $536\,nm$ when excited at about $500\,nm$. Rhodamine 123 is lipophilic and tends to accumulate in mitochondria. At high levels, rhodamine 123 can *sensitize* mitochondrial singlet O_2 formation.

5.11.3 Dihydroethidium[71]

Dihydroethidium (DHE), sometimes called **dihydroethidine**, is frequently used as a probe for $O_2^{\bullet-}$, being oxidized to a fluorescent product, probably **2-hydroxyethidium** (Fig. 5.14), which can intercalate into nuclear DNA and fluoresces strongly. Although fairly specific for $O_2^{\bullet-}$ under most conditions (showing little oxidation by H_2O_2, $ONOO^-$ or HOCl), DHE readily spontaneously oxidizes and it can be oxidized by singlet O_2. In addition, it can undergo direct redox reactions with haem proteins such as haemoglobin and cytochrome c to generate fluorescent products, and possibly with MnTBAP and other SOD mimetics (Section 10.6.4).[44] Assays using HPLC with fluorescence detection have been developed to detect 2-hydroxyethidium as a putative measure of $O_2^{\bullet-}$ in cells and tissues.

This and other probes can be attached to triphenylphosphonium residues to target them to mitochondria (Section 10.6.11).

5.11.4 Luminol and lucigenin[44]

These two compounds (Fig. 5.13) are often used to assess production of RS by activated phagocytes, and sometimes other cell types, such as endothelial cells. A luminol analogue **L-012** (Fig. 5.13) was reported to be a more sensitive $O_2^{\bullet-}$ detector than luminol or DHE.

The use of luminol to detect $O_2^{\bullet-}$ is problematic. It does *not* react directly with $O_2^{\bullet-}$ but must first be oxidized (e.g. by $OH^\bullet$, $ONOO^-$, HOCl, or peroxidase plus H_2O_2). The resulting luminol radical reacts with $O_2^{\bullet-}$ to generate a light-emitting product. Unfortunately, the luminol radical can reduce O_2 to *generate* $O_2^{\bullet-}$, so that the presence of luminol plus an oxidizing agent can lead to artefactual $O_2^{\bullet-}$ generation. Hence luminol is a questionable probe; any oxidizing

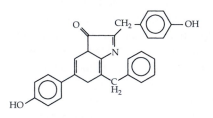

Almost non-fluorescent   Strongly fluorescent

X = O; HPF
X = NH; APF

Luminol

lucigenin (bis-*N*-methylacridinium)

2-methyl-6-(4-methoxyphenyl)-3,7-
Dihydroimidazo[1,2,-α]pyrazin-3-one]
(MCLA)

Cis-parinaric acid

4,4-difluoro-5-(4-phenyl-1,3,butadienyl)-
4-bora-3a,4a-diaza-s-indacene-3-
3-undecanoic acid (BODIPY®581/591 C11)

Coelenterazine

8-amino-5-chloro-7-phenylpyrido[3,4-d]pyridazine-
1,4-(2H,3H)dione (L-012)

Figure 5.13 Structures of some common probes used for detection of reactive species. HPF is 2-[6-(4′-hydroxyl)phenoxy-3H-xanthen-3-on-9-yl] benzoic acid and APF is 2-[6-(4′-amino)phenoxy-3H-xanthen-3-on-9-yl]benzoic acid.

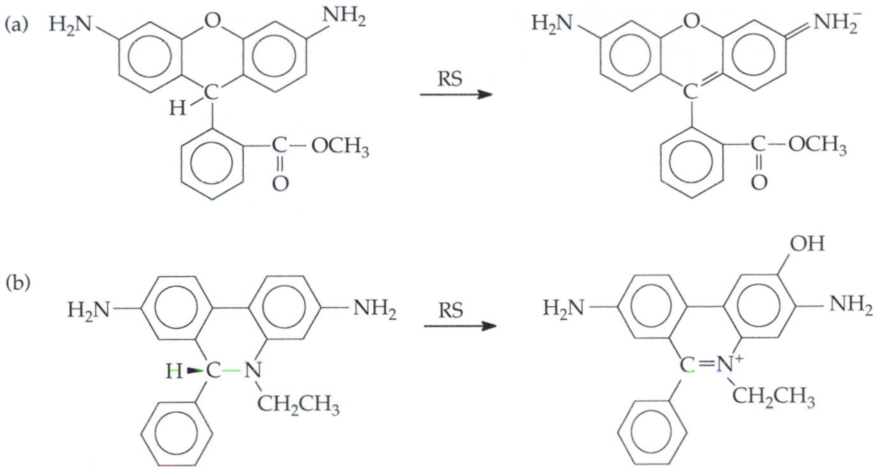

Figure 5.14 Conversion of (a) dihydrorhodamine 123 to rhodamine 123 and (b) of dihydroethidium to 2-hydroxyethidium.

agent that can remove one electron from it can cause light emission inhibitable by SOD, in which luminol is both the source and the detector of the $O_2^{\bullet-}$.

Lucigenin is often said to be more specific for the detection of $O_2^{\bullet-}$ than luminol, but again it does not react directly with $O_2^{\bullet-}$. Whereas luminol needs to be oxidized, lucigenin must first be reduced to lucigenin cation radical ($LC^{\bullet+}$). This reacts with $O_2^{\bullet-}$ to give an unstable dioxetane, which decomposes to a light-emitting species. Conversion of LC to $LC^{\bullet+}$ is not readily achieved by $O_2^{\bullet-}$, and usually involves other cellular reducing systems (e.g. XO, the mitochondrial electron transport chain or the phagocyte NADPH oxidase), introducing complexity in interpreting results. Even worse, $LC^{\bullet+}$ can reduce O_2 to $O_2^{\bullet-}$, so that addition of lucigenin can artefactually generate more $O_2^{\bullet-}$. The extent to which this artefact impairs accurate measurement of $O_2^{\bullet-}$ by lucigenin has been debated in the literature, but interference does appear to be significant in some cell systems.

5.11.5 Alternative fluorescent probes for superoxide

Alternative probes include **coelenterazine** (a lipophilic compound involved in light production in the aequorin system; Section 7.6), the luciferin analogue **MCLA** (Fig. 5.13) and several MCLA derivatives.[72] However, MCLA may also react with $RO_2^{\bullet}$ radicals and coelenterazine with $RO_2^{\bullet}$ and

$ONOO^-$. Both MCLA and coelenterazine compounds are highly photosensitive.

5.11.6 Measuring the light output of fluorescent probes

The simplest way is to use a fluorescence microplate reader, where data are presented as increases or decreases in relative fluorescence. Plate readers measure total fluorescence and do not distinguish between intracellular fluorescence and fluorescence from reactions in the culture medium. This is a potential problem with DCFDA, since DCFH and DCF can diffuse out of cells.

Flow cytometry allows one to measure the intracellular fluorescence, and the numbers of fluorescent cells. However, cells must be in suspension. **Confocal microscopy** is a powerful tool; cells can be loaded with fluorescent dyes and viewed in real time at 37°C. The intracellular location of RS can be visualized, and the role of mitochondrial, ER, or lysosomal events in oxidative stress can be visualized by coloading with **MitoTracker**, **ER Tracker** or **Lysotracker dyes** that associate with specific organelles. Caution must, of course, be used to ensure that the signal from the organelle tracker stain does not interfere with the measurement of that from the RS-sensitive dye. Overlapping of the tracker signal with the signal from the probes suggests involvement of a particular organelle in RS generation, but does not rigorously prove it.

Amyloid plaque formation in transgenic mice is associated with oxidative stress (Section 9.20). A recent paper used two probes to illustrate this (Fig. 5.15, Plate 9).

5.11.7 Effects of reactive species on other probes[28]

Many fluorescent probes are available to detect other cellular events, such as pH changes and ion movements. Some of these probes can be degraded by RS (HOCl, OH•, $^1O_2$ and ONOO$^-$ often being the culprits). Others can themselves generate ROS, including calcein and even MitoTracker Red. One must be alert for these effects when using a combination of probes in cells.

5.12 Biomarkers: the promise of urate oxidation?[28]

Several RS react in characteristic ways with biomolecules. The products can be regarded as fingerprints of oxidative attack, provided that they are unique, not generated by normal biological processes or originating from diet. For example, some groups have used ascorbyl radical, measured by ESR, as an indicator of oxidative stress (Fig. 5.1). Another approach (applicable only to primates) has been to detect allantoin and other products of RS attack upon urate (Section 3.18.6). Allantoin can be measured in human plasma and levels are elevated in conditions associated with oxidative stress, such as chronic inflammation, venous ulcers, diabetes, premature birth, iron overload, Down's syndrome, chronic heart failure and exercise. Allantoin can also be measured in urine, wound fluid and cerebral microdialysis fluid. Its levels rise in human muscle during exhaustive exercise, presumably due to oxidation of urate by RS. Allantoin measurement may be a promising method for human use, since human urate levels *in vivo* are high and it reacts with a range of RS. However, more validation is needed before it can be generally applied.

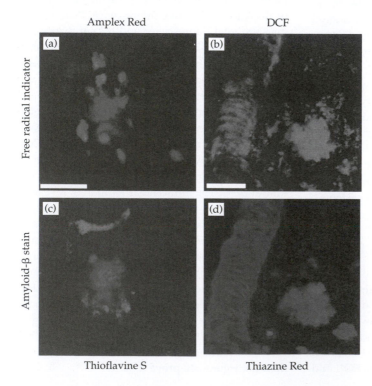

Figure 5.15 (see plate 9) Use of RS-detecting probes to show pro-oxidant effects of Aβ plaques in transgenic mice. The compounds DCFH and Amplex red were applied to the brains of living mice and imaged through cranial windows. Activation of Amplex red (A) and DCFH (B) by dense core plaques is shown. Histochemical markers of dense core plaques, thioflavine S (C) and thiazine red (D), respectively, were used to identify the plaques. Vessel-associated amyloid occasionally activated the probes (B), confirmed here with thiazine red (D). Autofluorescent lipofuscin was observed near plaques in multiple optical channels (A, orange). Fluorescein-containing blood vessels used to map sites for reimaging are shown in green in A and C. Scale bars: A, C, 10 µm; B, D, 25 µm. From *J. Neurosci.* **23**, 2213, 2003 by courtesy of Dr Brian Backsai and the publishers.

5.13 Biomarkers of oxidative DNA damage

5.13.1 Characterizing DNA damage: why bother to do it?

Oxidative DNA damage appears to occur continuously *in vivo*, in that low levels of 8OHdG (and, where measured, other oxidized bases) have been detected in DNA isolated from the cells of every aerobe examined. The presence of multiple oxidized purine and pyrimidine bases suggests that OH$^\bullet$ formation occurs within the nucleus *in vivo* (Section 4.8.2.2). However, if OH$^\bullet$ is attacking DNA, it must be made very close to the DNA. Background radiation may be one source, and Fenton chemistry another. Other potential sources of OH$^\bullet$ include ONOO$^-$ and the reaction of O$_2^{\bullet-}$ with HOCl, but when HOCl or ONOO$^-$ are added to cells, OH$^\bullet$ does not seem to contribute much to the DNA damage; direct reactions of these species with DNA predominate (Section 4.8.2). Low levels of the deamination products uracil, xanthine, and hypoxanthine are also detected in DNA from aerobes.

Many laboratories attempt to measure damage to DNA by RS. Why? It is widely thought that such damage contributes significantly to cancer (Sections 5.13.6 below). In other words, oxidative DNA damage may be a biomarker predictive (to some extent) of cancer later in life. If so, it can be used to evaluate what the effects of diet, lifestyle and supplements might be on later cancer incidence.

5.13.2 Characterizing DNA damage: what to measure?

Attack of RS on DNA can produce strand breakage, abasic sites, deoxyribose damage and modification of the purines and pyrimidines (Section 4.8). Multiple methods exist to measure strand breaks (Table 5.10 and Fig. 5.16, Plate 10) and some to detect abasic sites (Table 5.10). However, strand breakage and such sites also occur during DNA repair (Section 4.10) and so cannot be equated to oxidative DNA damage. Deoxyribose fragmentation generates multiple products. Probably more attention needs to be paid to them, since they may

well contribute to mutagenicity, both directly and via base propenal formation.[73,74]

Most attempts to 'fingerprint' oxidative damage to DNA have measured modified bases, most commonly the nucleoside **8-hydroxy-2′-deoxyguanosine**,[75] **8OHdG** (Table 4.10). This compound exhibits keto-enol tautomerism; the equilibrium favours the 6,8-diketo form, so some authors call it **8-oxo-7-hydro-2′-deoxyguanosine**, or **8oxodG** (Fig. 5.17). However, we stick with 8OHdG, for consistency. Its measurement has several advantages.

1. A sensitive assay (HPLC with electrochemical detection) is available.
2. It is formed in DNA by several RS, including $^1O_2$, OH$^\bullet$, CO$_3^{\bullet-}$ and some RO$_2^\bullet$ radicals.
3. It is a biologically important mutagenic lesion (Section 4.9); the multiple mechanisms employed to remove it (Section 4.10.5) suggest that cells 'perceive' it to be a threatening lesion which must be rapidly cleared.

Nevertheless, levels of 8OHdG are not a quantitative marker of DNA damage by RS. First, 8OHdG is only a minor product of attack on DNA by reactive nitrogen (e.g. ONOOH and nitrous acid) or chlorine (e.g. HOCl) species. Second, attack of singlet O$_2$ or OH$^\bullet$ upon guanine generates other products, such as FAPyG (Fig. 4.11). The ratio of 8OHdG to FAPyG is affected by the redox state of the cell (e.g. it is decreased at low O$_2$ concentrations) and by the presence of transition metal ions. Hence, changes in the amount of 8OHdG in DNA can result from changes in redox state and transition metal ion availability, not necessarily from changes in the rate of oxidative attack on DNA. In other words, the same amount of attack on DNA by RS could give different levels of 8OHdG (and of other bases; Fig. 4.12), depending on the environment. Third, 8OHdG is readily oxidized by RS, much faster than is guanine. Thus some authors have advocated that 8OHdG oxidation products be measured as well (Section 4.8.2.12).

Although assay of 8OHdG is useful and has provided important biological information,[75] it is intrinsically unreliable to measure a single product as an index of oxidative DNA damage. A better

Table 5.10 Some of the methods available to measure strand breakage in DNA

Method	Comment
[3H]thymidine incorporation	Cells are incubated with radioactive (tritiated) thymidine, which is incorporated into nuclear DNA. Production of radioactive fragments measured. Only useful for proliferating cells which can incorporate DNA precursors.
Incorporation of BrdU[a]	Non-radioactive alternative to [3H]thymidine. Incorporated into DNA. Fragments detected using antibodies against DNA containing BrdU.
Enzymatic labelling techniques	Free OH groups created by strand breakage are labelled with modified (e.g. fluorescent) nucleotides in the presence of enzymes, e.g. terminal deoxynucleotidyl transferase, TdT. The incorporated modified bases are detected fluorimetrically or using antibodies. A popular method is **TUNEL** (TdT-mediated X-dUTP nick end-labelling). Requires permeabilization of the cell to allow enzymes in.
Gel electrophoresis	For example used to measure internucleosomal DNA cleavage (Fig. 4.7).
'Comet' assay (single-cell gel electrophoresis)	Fig. 5.16
Alkaline elution	Cells are lysed above a filter and eluted by passing an alkaline buffer through. The high pH unwinds the helix and the smaller pieces pass through the filter quickly.
Alkaline unwinding	Cells are lysed and kept at high pH for a fixed time to denature the DNA. Unwinding begins from 'free ends' so is faster if strand breaks are present. The solution is neutralized and the fragments measured. Both elution and unwinding techniques can be combined with preincubation of the cell lysates with endonuclease/glycosylase enzymes to estimate the modified bases present (Section 5.13.5).
Use of supercoiled plasmid DNA	Strand breakage causes 'relaxation' to open circle and linear forms, measured as different migration on agarose gel electrophoresis or as increased fluorescence due to more intercalation of **ethidium bromide** in the relaxed DNA. Ethidium is a planar aromatic dye which readily intercalates between base pairs, although this is restricted in intact DNA by its resistance to distortion.
Cell DNA fragmentation ELISA	An antibody-based technique which detects histone-covered DNA fragments in cell cytoplasm; often used to study apoptosis, which generates DNA fragments inside cells.
Aldehyde reactive probe (ARP; N'-aminooxymethylcarbonylhydrazino-D-biotin)	ARP reacts with aldehyde groups which are the open ring form of the apurinic/apyrimidinic (AP) sites of damaged DNA. After the addition of ARP reagent, AP sites are tagged with biotin and quantified using avidin-biotin assay with colourimetric detection using peroxidase or alkaline phosphatase conjugates. Has also been used to measure M_1G (Fig. 4.27); see *Chem. Res. Toxicol.* **18**, 51, 2005. Abasic sites and deoxyribose degradation products can also be converted to oxime derivatives and measured by mass spectrometry.[74]

[a] 5-Bromo-2'-deoxyuridine

Most strand breaks detected by these techniques exist as such in the DNA. Others are *created* during the measurement, e.g. sugar damage can be converted into strand breakage on exposure of DNA to high pH during certain assays (**alkali-labile sites**).

approach is to measure multiple products (Fig. 4.13), which usually entails mass spectrometry. This can also give information about the damaging species. For example, the distinctive feature of OH• attack upon DNA is to produce *multiple* products from all four DNA bases. Several RNS can deaminate cytosine to uracil, guanine to xanthine, and adenine to hypoxanthine. Exposure to ONOO⁻ causes formation of 8-nitroguanine in DNA whereas HOCl generates chlorocytosine and pyrimidine oxidation products (Section 4.8.3). Mass spectrometry can distinguish these various product profiles as well as detect other lesions such as base–base and base–amino acid cross-links.

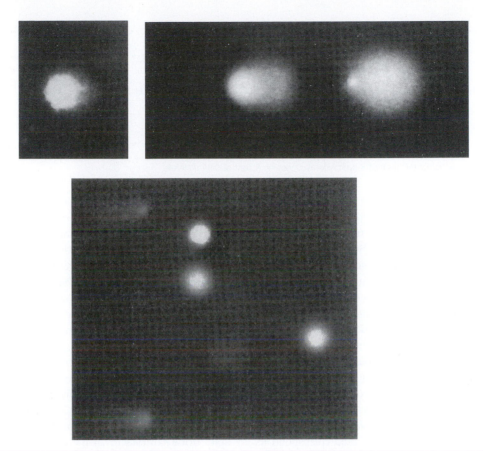

Figure 5.16 (see plate 10) The comet assay. Human lymphocytes or other cells (before or after H_2O_2 treatment) were suspended in low melting point agarose gel in buffer at 37°C and pipetted onto a microscope slide precoated with 1% high melting point agarose, similarly prepared in buffer. The agarose was allowed to set by incubating at 4°C for 10 min, and the slides immersed in lysis solution (1% Triton X-100, 2.5 M NaCl, 0.1 M Na_2EDTA, 10 mM Tris, pH 10.0) at 4°C for 1°h to remove cellular membranes, proteins, etc. and leave behind the DNA. Slides were then placed in a horizontal electrophoresis tank containing 0.3 M NaOH and 1 mM Na_2EDTA at 4°C for 40 min before electrophoresis in the same solution at 25 V for 30 min at 4°C (temperature of running solution not exceeding 15°C). DNA, being negatively charged, is attracted to the anode. The presence of breaks allows supercoiled DNA to relax and move faster to the anode to form a tail (hence the name comet assay), and the fraction of DNA in the tail reflects the frequency of breaks. The slides were washed three times for 5 min each with neutralizing buffer (0.4 M Tris-HCl, pH 7.5) at 4°C before staining. Above: the figure (left to right) shows increasing extents of DNA damage. Below: lymphocyte comets treated with H_2O_2 and stained with acridine orange, which stains double-stranded DNA yellow and single-stranded DNA red. Undamaged comets are yellow, whereas tailed comets are red. A modification of the comet assay permits detection of oxidized bases in addition to breaks. In this case, after lysis the slides were washed three times for 5 min each in buffer, drained, and the agarose covered with 50 µl of buffer containing endonuclease III, FAPy-glycosylase or other DNA repair enzymes, or buffer only, sealed with a coverslip, and incubated for 30 min at 37°C. Endonuclease III breaks the DNA at sites of oxidized pyrimidines and FAPy-glycosylase at 8OHdG and other oxidized purines. Alkaline treatment, electrophoresis and neutralization were carried out as before. Photographs by courtesy of Dr Andrew Collins.

5.13.3 Characterizing DNA damage: how to measure it

There are two types of measurement of oxidative DNA damage. **Steady-state damage**, the level measured in cellular DNA, reflects the balance between damage and repair. Hence a rise in its level could be due to increased damage, decreased repair, or both.

Attempts have also been made to estimate the **total oxidative DNA damage** *in vivo*, by measuring products of DNA repair that are excreted in urine. Several damaged bases are excreted in

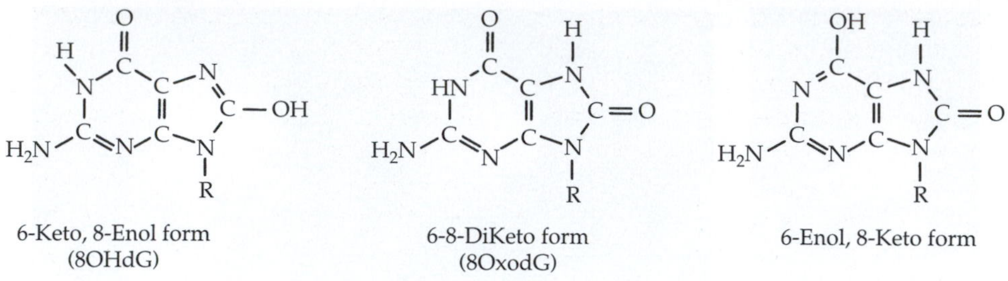

| 6-Keto, 8-Enol form | 6-8-DiKeto form | 6-Enol, 8-Keto form |
| (8OHdG) | (8OxodG) | (8OHdG) |

Figure 5.17 Keto-enol tautomerism of 8-hydroxydeoxyguanosine. R, rest of DNA molecule.

mammalian urine, including 8OHG, 8OHdG, thymine glycol, 5-hydroxymethyluracil, 8-hydroxyadenine and 7-methyl-8-hydroxyguanine.[76] The one most often measured is 8OHdG, usually by HPLC with electrochemical detection after concentration of the urine on columns,[75] although antibody- and MS-based techniques have also been described. Because urine contains thousands of compounds, sample preparation techniques are critical. Published urinary 8OHdG levels for humans seem fairly comparable between different laboratories, and are usually standardized against creatinine to allow for the concentration of the urine.[77–79] In a study of 169 adults in Denmark,[79] the average 8OHdG excretion was 200 to 300 pmol/kg body mass per 24 h, which would correspond to the not inconsiderable average of 140 to 200 oxidative modifications to the guanine in the DNA of each cell of the human body every day. Furthermore, 32 smokers in this study excreted, on average, 50% more 8OHdG than 53 non-smokers, suggestive of a 50% increased rate of oxidative DNA damage from smoking. Measurement of 8OHdG or other base products in urine gives no information about their tissue origin, although they can be measured in fluids from specific sites (e.g. saliva, synovial fluid, CSF) to give more 'local' information.

What do measurements of urinary DNA bases mean? The level of 8OHdG in urine seems to be (fortunately) unaffected by diet,[76,78] but some of the other products in urine could result from uptake of oxidized bases from the diet (e.g. after digestion of DNA damaged by cooking) and their excretion in the urine. Some (but not all)[78] studies have suggested that urinary 8OHG levels *are* influenced by diet (8OHG could in any case come from RNA, DNA or the RNA precursor pool). The question of

whether any 8OHdG is metabolized to other products in humans has not been fully addressed, although currently available data suggest that it is not.[76] A more worrying question is the source of the 8OHdG–does it arise from DNA, or from sanitization of the dGTP pool (Section 4.10.2)? Base excision repair pathways that remove 8OHdG from DNA liberate 8OHG and not 8OHdG (Section 4.10.3), although pathways that liberate 8OHdG probably also exist.[76,80]

Despite these problems, urinary 8OHdG measurement is widely used as an approximate index of how diet and lifestyle may influence 'whole body' oxidative damage to DNA and DNA precursors.[75–81] Comparable results seem to be obtained whether 'spot' urine samples or 24-h collections are used.[81]

5.13.4 Steady-state damage: the artefact problem[82–87]

Whereas there is approximate agreement between different laboratories on human urinary levels of 8OHdG, agreement on the levels of 8OHdG in isolated DNA is very poor—values vary over three orders of magnitude. It is even uncertain now whether mtDNA is more oxidized than nuclear DNA (Sections 10.4 and 1.10.5). Published values for nuclear DNA range from less than one 8OHdG per 10^6 guanines to over 100.[a] Which is correct? Possibly none of them. What is the problem?

---

[a] Comparisons between results from different laboratories may be aided by the following conversion factors (by courtesy of Dr Miral Dizdaroglu). x 8OHdG/10^5 deoxyguanosines is equal to $(x/4.65)$ 8OHdG per 10^5 DNA bases (since about 21.5% of bases are guanine in mammalian DNA) or $(x/33.6)$ nmol 8OHdG per mg of DNA. Similarly, 1 nmol of 8OHdG per mg of DNA is 156 8OHdG/10^5 deoxyguanosines or 33.6/10^5 DNA bases.

To measure oxidative DNA damage by most of the currently available methods, one must first isolate DNA. The isolated DNA is then hydrolysed and the hydrolysate prepared for analysis of oxidized bases. During isolation and preparation for analysis, DNA is exposed to ambient O_2 (hyperoxia compared with nuclear O_2 levels) and to transition metal ions that can catalyse oxidative damage. Metals can be present as contaminants in reagents (e.g. phenol) and equipment (e.g. dialysis membranes), and liberated during homogenization of tissues prior to DNA extraction (Section 4.3.3). In some analytical procedures, DNA is incubated for prolonged periods with digestion enzymes to liberate 8OHdG, or exposed to elevated temperatures (e.g. in hydrolysis using formic acid). Isolation, hydrolysis, and analysis all therefore have the potential to cause artefactual oxidation of DNA (especially of guanine residues), raising the apparent level of base oxidation products. If GC–MS is used, high-temperature derivatization in preparation for GC can cause extensive DNA base oxidation unless conditions are rigorously controlled. If the steady state level of 8OHdG in cellular DNA is less than one per 10^5 guanines, as some propose, it is easy to see how oxidation of <0.01% of unmolested DNA bases can invalidate the measurement.

Many laboratories are investigating better methods of isolating, hydrolysing and analysing cellular DNA. The unspoken criterion by which the results are judged seems to be that the lower the level of oxidized bases in cellular DNA that is obtained, the more likely it is to be correct. This is perhaps logical because one would expect organisms to 'perceive' oxidative DNA damage as a threat to the integrity of the genome, and so to minimize steady state concentrations of oxidized DNA bases using their plethora of DNA repair systems.[82] However, there are many surprises in biology; one must attempt to find the real answer rather than make *a priori* assumptions.

5.13.5 Overcoming the artefact[82–86]

Multiple approaches have been used. Many researchers avoid phenol in DNA extraction, since it is often metal ion-contaminated and oxidizes to generate ROS. Some add antioxidants or iron chelators such as desferrioxamine to the extraction solutions, or even attempt to extract DNA under nitrogen (tedious to do). Derivatization for GC–MS can be performed at room temperature in the presence of antioxidants, or the unmodified bases first removed by HPLC so that there is nothing to artefactually oxidize. One can avoid derivatization altogether and use liquid chromatography–MS instead. DNA can be digested with repair enzymes to remove oxidized bases, that can then be analysed by HPLC/MS, rather than digesting the whole DNA molecule. Of course, this assumes that the repair enzymes can remove all the lesions, which is uncertain. One interesting approach to evaluate work-up techniques is to use DNA containing some [^{18}O]-labelled 8OHdG, generated by exposing DNA to [^{18}O]-singlet O_2. The ratio of $8^{18}OHdG$ to $8^{16}OHdG$ in DNA during isolation should remain constant; if it falls, it suggests artefactual $8^{16}OHdG$ formation.[87]

Another approach is to bypass the problems of DNA isolation and preparation and measure damage in cells. Immunostaining methods using antibodies against 8OHdG or other oxidized DNA bases have been developed and proved useful in several studies (Fig. 5.18).[88] Perhaps the most widely used method is the **comet assay**, single cell gel electrophoresis. This measures DNA strand breaks (Fig. 5.16), but can be modified to allow an assessment of oxidative base damage—the cells are lysed and the slides exposed to DNA-repair enzymes. DNA is cleaved at sites of base modification, producing more strand breaks. Hence a comparison of the comets before and after enzymic treatment can estimate the oxidized bases present (Fig. 5.19).

The levels of oxidized bases measured by the comet assay in DNA are generally lower than those obtained by HPLC or MS techniques.[85] Is the comet assay more reliable, giving a lower value because artefactual DNA oxidation is minimized? Or does the comet assay simply underestimate damage? It seems unlikely that all the oxidized bases in tangled DNA can be recognized by exogenously applied enzymes, and two adjacent lesions may be recorded as a single strand break. Nevertheless, the comet assay is rapid, easy and uses only small amounts of material, although the numbers generated rely on semiquantitative assessments of the size of a 'tail'.

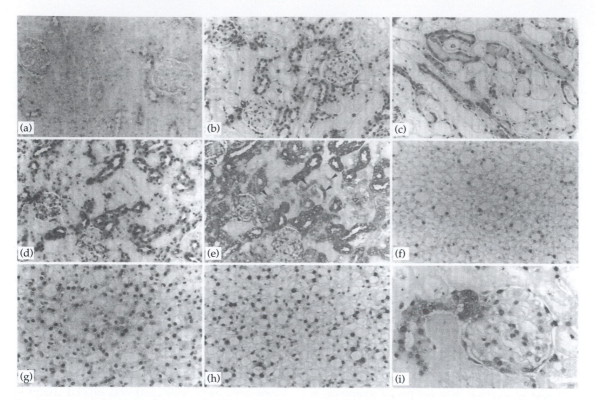

Figure 5.18 Immunohistochemical detection of 8OHdG and 4-hydroxy-2-nonenal (HNE)-modified proteins in the kidney of male Wistar rats treated with ferric nitrilotriacetate (Fe–NTA), a catalyst of Fenton chemistry (Section 3.15.4.2). (A) Renal cortex of control kidney. 8OHdG was visualized using N45.1, a monoclonal antibody. It can also detect 8OHG, albeit two orders of magnitude less effectively than 8OHdG, but not other oxidized bases. Faint nuclear staining of renal tubular cells is observed (original magnification, $\times$164). (B) Renal cortex 3 h after Fe–NTA treatment. Intense nuclear staining of proximal tubular cells without apparent degeneration is seen. *: Necrotic tubules (original magnification, $\times$164). (C) Renal cortex 24 h after treatment. Approximately half of the proximal tubular cells are necrotic. Moderate nuclear staining of both proximal and distal tubular cells is seen (original magnification, $\times$164). (D and E) Serial sections. Renal cortex 1 h after treatment immunostained with N45.1 and polyclonal antibody for HNE-modified proteins. Notably, almost the same tubules are stained. However, the distribution is nuclear for N45.1 and cytoplasmic for HNE-modified proteins. Whereas 8OHdG is found only in morphologically live cells, HNE-modified proteins also occur in the necrotizing degenerative cells (*arrows*: original magnification x164). (F) Renal medulla of control kidney. Nuclear staining is found in the collecting duct cells (original magnification $\times$249). (G) Renal medulla 1 h after Fe–NTA treatment. Intense nuclear staining of descending and ascending limbs of Henle's loop as well as collecting duct cells is observed (original magnification $\times$249). (H) Renal medulla 3 h after treatment. Nuclear staining is slightly decreased compared with that of 1 h (original magnification $\times$249). (I) Glomerulus 3 h after treatment (original magnification $\times$398). Nuclear staining of Bowman's capsule and some of the glomerular cells as well as proximal tubules is observed. All immunohistochemical specimens in Figure 2 are without nuclear counterstaining. From *Lab. Invest.* **76**, 365, 1997, by courtesy of Professor S. Toyokuni and Nature Publishing Group.

5.13.6 Interpreting the results: measure DNA levels or urinary excretion? What do the levels mean?

Some studies have combined both types of measurement. For example, administration of 2-nitropropane to rats led to elevated cellular 8OHdG. Levels subsequently decreased, accompanied by an increase in urinary 8OHdG excretion.[89] Cigarette smoking can raise both 8OHdG levels in human cells and 8OHdG excretion rates (Section 8.12). Hence, both nitropropane and cigarette smoke increase oxidative DNA damage *in vivo*. Repair (at least as indicated by 8OHdG excretion) also increases, but not to an extent that prevents a rise in the cellular 8OHdG. Measurements of only 8OHdG excretion rates should be interpreted with caution. For example, an agent that increases 8OHdG excretion might be interpreted as 'bad' (seemingly increasing DNA damage) but

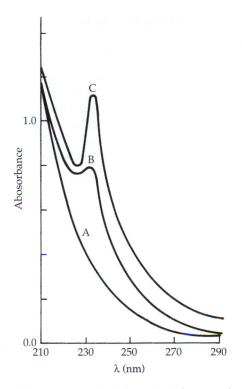

Figure 5.19 Lipid peroxidation followed by the formation of conjugated dienes. Ethyl linoleate (EL) was purified, and its absorbance spectrum is shown (plot A). Plot B shows EL after oxidation by air at 30°C for 8 h; and plot C, EL in which peroxidation was speeded up by adding nitrogen dioxide. In both cases the 'shoulder' of UV-absorbance due to conjugated diene formation is visible. Data by courtesy of Professor William Pryor.

might in fact be 'good' (if it stimulated repair and therefore decreased steady state 8OHdG concentrations in cellular DNA).

The ideal is thus to measure both cellular DNA damage levels and total damage (by urinary excretion rates). If only one measurement can be made, the steady state level is arguably preferable, because miscoding induced by oxidized bases is presumably what determines the risk of mutation and in turn the risk of cancer development. The repair process itself is not error free, however (especially if translesional DNA replication occurs; Fig 4.15), and can introduce mutations, so it could be argued that a greater 'throughput' of DNA base oxidation is deleterious even if it does not result in significant rises in the steady state concentrations of DNA damage products.

The problem with measuring cellular DNA damage is that the methods are not yet robust. Another problem (in humans) is the limited availability of tissues to obtain DNA from. Many studies are performed on DNA isolated from lymphocytes (or sometimes total white cells) from human blood. Most groups prefer to isolate lymphocytes, since total white cell DNA will include a major contribution from neutrophils. However, there is no obvious reason why levels of oxidative DNA damage in either cell type should reflect levels in other body tissues. Sperm, buccal cells, placenta, and biopsies of muscle, skin, colon, and other tissues are other potential sources of DNA, although biopsy samples often yield too little DNA for HPLC- or MS-based methods. Are we justified in assuming that changes in the amount of DNA damage in white blood cells caused, for example, by antioxidant supplementation, are reflected in the tissues in which cancer is most likely to develop later (e.g. breast, prostate rectum, and colon)? Are the basal amounts of oxidative damage in all body tissues the same? More data are needed. For example, a study in dogs showed that exercise decreased 8OHdG levels in lymphocytes and in colon, but not in other tissues.[90]

Nevertheless, it is encouraging to note that in smokers (Section 8.12), diabetics (Section 9.4) and rheumatoid arthritis patients (Section 9.10), increased 8OHdG can be detected by current methodology in both blood cells and urine. Elevated 8OHdG levels were also observed in leukocytes from subjects with liver inflammation caused by hepatitis C virus. In rats fed high-fat diets, oxidative DNA damage increased in both blood cells and mammary gland (reviewed in [91]).

Finally, are the levels of DNA base damage products found in cells biologically significant? They probably are in terms of cancer development, as discussed in Section 9.13.5.1.

5.13.7 Reactive nitrogen and chlorine species

Several RNS deaminate DNA bases and assays for the deamination products (including uracil, xanthine, and hypoxanthine) have been described. Peroxynitrite forms 8-nitroguanine (8NG) in DNA;

both this and 5-guanidino-4-nitroimidazole (Fig. 4.13) can be measured. For example, levels of both 8OHdG and 8NG (measured using an antibody-based method) were higher in the stomachs of patients infected with *H. pylori*[92] or in the livers of patients with hepatitis C infections (Section 9.12.3), and 8NG was increased in the lungs of mice infected with an influenza virus (Section 9.23). 8-Nitroguanine is detectable in urine, and smokers appear to excrete more.[93] 5-Chlorocytosine has been used as a biomarker of damage by RCS at sites of inflammation (Sections 4.8.2.8 and 9.9.1).

5.13.8 Gene-specific oxidative damage

Measurement of modified bases in nDNA does not tell us whether they are in active genes, inactive genes, telomeres or 'junk' DNA. Indeed, the GC-rich telomeres may be sensitive targets of oxidative damage because they are rich in guanine.[94] It is important to address the issue of localization; it is not only the level of damage but where it is that affects its biological importance. For example, one study[95] showed that oxidative damage is markedly increased in the promoters (and to a lesser extent the exons) of a limited number of genes whose expression is known to decrease with age in human brain cortex. How was this shown? The DNA was treated with FAPy-glycosylase and AP-lyase. The first removes an oxidized purine and the second creates a break at the apurinic site, which renders it resistant to amplification by the polymerase chain reaction (PCR). Hence DNA damage to specific sequences can be estimated by determining the ratio of intact PCR products in cleaved versus uncleaved DNA. The same promoters were selectively damaged when cultured human neurons were treated with iron and H_2O_2, causing decreased expression of the genes. A similar technique was used to show that oxidative DNA damage in *H. pylori*-infected human gastric mucosa is unevenly distributed between genes, being higher in those encoding p53 and TGFβ receptor type II, for example.[96] We need to combine molecular genetics with analytical chemistry to learn the true significance of oxidative DNA damage. Damage to promoters can affect transcription factor binding, for example (Section 4.9.3).

5.13.9 DNA–aldehyde adducts

Cytotoxic aldehydes are produced during lipid peroxidation (Section 4.12.5) and are additionally widespread in the environment. For example, cigarette smoke contains multiple aldehydes (Section 8.12) and bananas contain hexanal. If they reach DNA, aldehydes can bind to DNA bases (Fig. 4.27). Several assays to measure such adducts have been described, often employing GC–MS or HPLC–ECD after acid hydrolysis of DNA, or immunoassays, some of which can be applied to whole cells. For example, M_1dG (Fig. 4.27) has been detected in DNA from healthy animals. In one study, human liver DNA contained about five M_1dG per 10^8 bases. However, different analytical techniques can give different results.[97] This compound has also been detected in human colonic mucosa and the levels were influenced by diet.[98] M_1dG is metabolised rapidly to a 6-oxo product, which can be deleted in urine and is another potential biomarker.[98A] Reaction of HNE with DNA generates propano– and etheno–dG adducts (Fig. 4.27), which can also be measured.

However, there are caveats. M_1dG is not a specific marker of damage to DNA by MDA (Fig. 4.27). Tissue homogenates undergo peroxidation (Sections 4.3.3 and 9.16.5), leading to possible artefactual modification of DNA by aldehydes during the isolation process. Etheno–dG, etheno–dA, etheno–dC and dG–MDA adducts have been detected in human urine,[99] but a possible origin from diet (Section 5.14.9.4 below) is not ruled out.

5.14 Biomarkers of lipid peroxidation

Lipids can be oxidized, halogenated or nitrated by a range of RS (not including H_2O_2, $NO^\bullet$ or $O_2^{\bullet-}$, which are unreactive with lipids). Some RS initiate lipid peroxidation (e.g. $OH^\bullet$, $RO_2^\bullet$, $NO_2^\bullet$, ONOOH) whereas others oxidize lipids and do not directly start a chain reaction (e.g. singlet O_2, O_3, HOCl). Techniques for measurement of chlorinated and nitrated lipids are being developed, and nitrated PUFAs have been detected in blood plasma (Section 4.11). We await further studies on these compounds with interest.

5.14.1 Why measure lipid peroxidation?

Levels of certain end-products of peroxidation, especially the isoprostanes (IPs) and related compounds (Section 4.12.3), are elevated in many human diseases. Indeed, they are emerging as biomarkers of the extent of disease and possibly, in cases such as Alzheimer's disease (AD) and diabetes (Sections 9.4 and 9.20), as indicators predictive of later disease development.[100] Oxidation of lipids contributes to the actions of some toxins (Section 8.2). Lipid peroxidation is one of the commonest reasons for quality deterioration in processed foods, so food scientists are very interested in spotting it early and controlling it.

5.14.2 How to measure lipid peroxidation: general principles

Lipid peroxidation is a complex process that occurs in multiple stages. Hence many techniques are available for measuring it. Each measures something different, and no one method is an accurate, overall measure of lipid peroxidation. In addition, a number of studies have measured **peroxidizability** rather than peroxidation; they take a cell, tissue, membrane, body fluid or lipoprotein, expose it to oxidative stress *in vitro* and measure the amount of lipid peroxidation; they results. One example is the erythrocyte peroxide stress test (Section 6.4). Another is the incubation of lipoproteins with Cu^{2+} or AAPH *in vitro*, measuring the lag time before peroxidation

accelerates (Section 9.3.5). A third is the **D-Roms test**.[101] Plasma is exposed to acidic pH to liberate metals, which decompose peroxides and cause more peroxidation. The products are detected using N,N-diethyl-p-phenylenediamine. The values obtained are 250 to 300 Carratelli units (1 unit corresponds to 0.8 mg/l of H_2O_2) or about 5900 μM, much greater than 'real' levels of peroxides *in vivo* (Section 5.14.5 below). The peroxidizability of a system is a complex parameter determined by its fatty acid composition and antioxidant content, the type of oxidative stress used, and the assay employed to measure lipid peroxidation. Its biological significance is unclear; the fact that a tissue is more peroxidizable *in vitro* under heavy oxidative stress does not mean that it is oxidizing faster *in vivo*. To use an analogy, building A may be able to resist an explosion less well than building B, but this does not mean that building A is falling down.

5.14.3 Loss of substrates

Peroxidation causes loss of PUFAs, so a simple way to measure it (in principle) is to follow their disappearance (Table 5.11). The lipids are extracted from the system under study and hydrolysed to release fatty acids, which can then be measured by HPLC or converted into volatile products (e.g. by formation of esters with methanol) and separated by GC. Care must be taken to avoid peroxidation of fatty acids during the hydrolysis and extraction procedures: a common practice is to carry out the

Table 5.11 Loss of fatty acids during peroxidation of the red blood cell membrane

No. of carbon atoms in fatty acid	No. of $>C=C<$ bonds in fatty acid	% of total fatty acids in membrane	
		Normal	After lipid peroxidation
16	0	21	21
18	0	14	14
18	1	12	11
18	2	10	8
20	4	15	5
22	0	3	3
22	4	2	1

Data from one of the authors (JMCG). Erythrocytes were stressed by incubation with high levels of H_2O_2 in the presence of azide to inhibit catalase.

procedures under N_2. Information about which lipids are most affected can be gained by separating the different classes before hydrolysis.

The other substrate for peroxidation is O_2, so measurement of O_2 uptake is another index. De Saussure used this method in his studies on oxidation of walnut oil (Section 4.11.1). Today, rather than his simple manometer, we use O_2 electrodes. Most modern O_2 electrodes are Clark-type arrangements which measure dissolved O_2. Calibration is achieved by exposing them to known concentrations of dissolved O_2, although, strictly speaking, the electrode measures the 'activity' of O_2 and not concentration. It is usually assumed that air-saturated pure water has 0.258 µmol/ml of dissolved O_2 at 25°C and 1 atmosphere air pressure, although the presence of dissolved solutes decreases this solubility slightly (Section 1.1.3). Measuring O_2 uptake does not require sample preparation and is useful for complex matrices (e.g. food) that preclude the use of spectrophotometric methods. One disadvantage is poor sensitivity.

5.14.4 Measurement of intermediates

5.14.4.1 *Radicals*[102]
Spin traps such as PBN, DMPO and POBN can intercept radical intermediates in the chain reaction and are useful in mechanistic studies. The last is often used; POBN is good at trapping carbon-centred radicals. Traps that 'sit' at different places in the membrane have been developed, to help determine where radicals are located.[103] In some studies, lipid constituents were separated by HPLC, subjected to ESR and finally identified by mass spectrometry to gain detailed information about which lipids hosted the radicals.[104] Spin traps have been used in whole animals to detect carbon-centred, $RO^{\bullet}$ and $RO_2^{\bullet}$ radicals, and they can be added to body fluids to do the same (Section 5.2.5).

5.14.4.2 *Diene conjugates*
Oxidation of PUFAs forms conjugated dienes (Fig. 4.19) that absorb UV light at 230 to 235 nm (Fig. 5.19). Measurement of dienes is a useful index of peroxidation in pure lipids and isolated lipoproteins (Section 9.3.5) and has the advantage that it measures an early stage in peroxidation. Diene conjugation measurements can rarely be carried out

directly on tissues and body fluids because many other substances present absorb strongly in the UV. Extraction of lipids into organic solvents (e.g. chloroform: methanol mixtures) before measurement is a common approach to this problem.

Greater sensitivity for the diene conjugation method can be achieved by applying second-derivative spectroscopy. An absorbance spectrum plots absorbance (A) against wavelength (λ). A first-derivative spectrum plots rate of change of absorbance with wavelength ($dA/d\lambda$) against wavelength. The second derivative spectrum plots the rate of change of this rate of change ($d^2A/d^2\lambda$). Figure 5.20 applies this technique to linolenic acid oxidation; the changes in the second-derivative spectrum are much clearer than in the simple UV-absorption spectrum. Thus the 'hump' that appears in the absorption spectrum translates into a sharp minimum 'peak' at 233 nm in the second-derivative spectrum. The increased resolution of this technique can allow discrimination between different conjugated diene structures present.

Although conjugated diene measurements work well on isolated lipids and lipoproteins, their application to body fluids is problematic.[105,106] Separation of the UV-absorbing 'diene conjugate' material from human body fluids revealed that most or all of it is a non-oxygen-containing isomer of linoleic acid, **octadeca-9 (*cis*), 11 (*trans*)-dienoic acid**. It has nothing to do with lipid peroxidation and probably originates from both diet and microbial metabolism, involving bacteria in the gut, lung or cervical mucus. It can also be present in the calf serum used in cell culture media.[107] It follows that application of diene conjugation methods to body fluids, or to extracts of them, is a questionable index of lipid peroxidation. Of course, HPLC or GC–MS can be used to separate the 'real' conjugated diene products of lipid peroxidation from octadeca-9,11-dienoic acid.

The above compound and several isomers of it, known collectively as **conjugated linoleic acid**s (CLA), are often included in health supplements because of alleged anticarcinogenic and weight-reducing properties (based on animal studies and of unproven benefit in humans[108]). However, administration of CLA to humans was observed to *increase* levels of lipid peroxidation, as measured by F_2–IPs.[109]

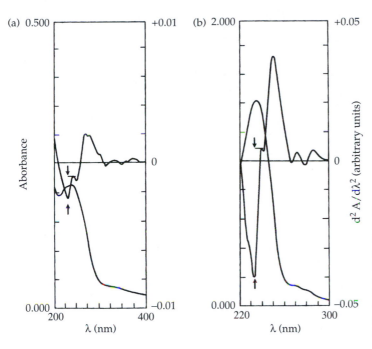

Figure 5.20 Second-derivative spectroscopy of conjugated dienes. (a) UV and second-derivative spectra of linolenic acid (allegedly pure but in fact slightly oxidized). In the second-derivative spectra the arrows show the height of the minimum peak at $\lambda = 233$ nm that is expressed as $d^2 2A/d\lambda^2$, in arbitrary units. (b) UV and second-derivative spectra of linolenic acid after 24 h of oxidation. The arrows show the height of the peak $d^2A/d\lambda^2$ at $\lambda = 233$ nm. Data by courtesy of Professor F. Corongiu.

5.14.5 Measurement of end-products: peroxides

Lipid peroxidation generates both hydroperoxides and various types of cyclic peroxides (Fig. 4.20) as well as cholesterol oxidation products (Section 4.12.4). Methods for peroxide measurement can be classified into those that measure 'total peroxides' and those that attempt separation of different peroxides (Table 5.12). The amount of peroxide present at a given time depends both on the rate of initiation of peroxidation and on how quickly peroxides are decomposing to give other products (e.g. if transition metals are added peroxides will decompose to carbonyls and other products) or are metabolized. Most assays reveal peroxide levels in human plasma to be in the low µM range, although some give lower values (Table 5.12), for reasons that have not been elucidated.

5.14.6 Measurement of end-products: isoprostanes, isofurans and isoketals[100,110]

Currently, the best available biomarker of lipid peroxidation appears to be the IPs (Section 4.12.3). Most work has been done on the F_2–IPs, which arise from arachidonic acid, but some data are available on isoprostanes from DHA and, to a lesser extent,

EPA. Isoprostanes are best measured by GC–MS or HPLC–MS techniques. Although immunoassay kits for F_2–IPs are commercially available, the reliability of some of them has been questioned by certain authors. Isoprostanes can be detected in foods, but luckily they do not appear to pass through the gut in sufficient quantities to affect plasma or urinary levels.[111] Reliable MS-based techniques have been established to detect IPs and their metabolites (e.g. 2,3-dinor-5,6-dihydro-15-F_{2t}-IsoP; Fig 4.21) in plasma and urine, although the 'work up' techniques prior to MS can be tedious. Correct sample storage is important: artefactual lipid oxidation and IP formation can occur in tissues and body fluids on standing in the laboratory in ice and (more slowly) at $-70°C$, unless antioxidants such as BHT are added. This is not a problem with urine, since there is no lipid to oxidize.

Even the IPs are not 'ideal' biomarkers. Several isomers tend to coelute during GC, so often groups claiming to measure a single product (e.g. 8-iso-$PGF_{2\alpha}$) are measuring a mixture.[100,110,112] Nevertheless, the levels reported in plasma and urine by different laboratories are broadly comparable; 0.1 to 0.4 ng/mg creatinine for urine and around 0.3 ng/ml for plasma.[112] Fasting tends to increase urinary IP levels[111,112] and so samples from fasted subjects

Table 5.12 Measurement of peroxides

Method	What is measured	Remarks
A. 'Total peroxide' measurements		
Iodine liberation	All peroxides	One of the oldest methods, widely used in the food industry; peroxides oxidize I^- to I_2. $ROOH + 2I^- + 2H^+ \rightarrow I_2 + ROH + H_2O$ In the presence of excess I^- the tri-iodide ion (I_3^-) can be measured at 358 nm. Useful for bulk lipids. Both H_2O_2 and protein peroxides also oxidize I^- to I_2. Method can be applied to extracts of biological samples if other oxidizing agents are absent. Peroxide levels in human plasma reported as 2.1–4.6 μM (*Anal. Biochem.* **176**, 360, 1989; *Anal. Biochem.* **176**, 353, 1989).
Methylene blue	All peroxides	Values in plasma reported as 8.6 ± 5.8 μM (*Atherosclerosis* **121**, 193, 1996; *Exp. Gerontol.* **22**, 103, 1987).
FOX (ferrous oxidation xylenol orange) assay	All peroxides	Simple, easy to use, works well *in vitro*, can be automated. Peroxides oxidize Fe^{2+} to $Fe(III)$, detected by xylenol orange (ΔA at 560 nm). Detects 3–5 μM 'lipid peroxide' in normal human plasma. 'Amplification' can occur in the assay since reaction of LOOH with Fe^{2+} will generate $LO^\bullet$ radicals that could propagate peroxidation. Antioxidants are often added to try and stop this. Sensitivity low μM range (*Anal. Biochem.* **220**, 403, 1994). Also detects H_2O_2 and protein peroxides. Addition of **triphenylphosphine** reduces lipid peroxides but not H_2O_2, and catalase can be added to remove H_2O_2. Use of perchloric acid allows distinction of protein and lipid peroxides (*Anal. Biochem.* **315**, 29, 2003).
Glutathione peroxidase-1 (GPx1)	Fatty acid hydroperoxides (GPx1 does not act on esterified peroxidized fatty acids within membranes or lipoproteins)	The GPx1 enzyme reacts with H_2O_2 and organic peroxides, oxidizing GSH to GSSG. Addition of glutathione reductase and NADPH to reduce GSSG back to GSH results in stoichiometric consumption of NADPH. Alternatively, GSSG can be determined directly; e.g. by HPLC (*Chem. Res. Toxicol.* **2**, 295, 1989; *Anal. Biochem.* **186**, 108, 1990). Cannot measure peroxides within membranes unless phospholipases are first used; in principle, PHGPx (Section 3.8) could be used to do this. Peroxide levels in plasma quoted as approx. 1 μM (*Chem. Res. Toxicol.* **2**, 295, 1989).
Cyclooxygenase (COX)	Lipid hydroperoxides, possibly cyclic peroxides	The rate at which COX oxidizes arachidonic acid is increased by adding lipid peroxides (Section 7.12.4). Thus stimulation of COX activity (usually assayed as O_2 uptake) can be used to measure peroxides in biological fluids (*Anal. Biochem.* **145**, 192, 1985; **193**, 55, 1991). Assay relates the presence of peroxides to one of their potential biological actions, stimulation of eicosanoid synthesis. Human plasma levels measured are ~0.5 μM. Values for 'total peroxide' depend to some extent upon which types are present, since different peroxides stimulate COX to different extents.
Diphenyl-1-pyrenylphosphine	All peroxides. Oxidation to the fluorescent oxide	Lipophilic, can be used to measure peroxides in oils, body fluids (*FEBS Lett.* **474**, 137, 2000), membranes and lipoproteins. A similar assay in which this compound is linked to a 7-hydroxycoumarin moiety has been described as more sensitive (*Biorg. Med. Chem.* **13**, 1131, 2005).

Similar probes include 3-perylene diphenylphosphine (*Biochem. Biophys. Res. Commun.* **338**, 1222, 2005).

B. Peroxide assays: separation of products[a]

Method	Peroxides detected
Haem degradation of peroxides (after HPLC separation)	All peroxides (HPLC allows separation of phospholipid, cholesterol and cholesterol ester peroxides)
Gas chromatography–mass spectrometry or HPLC–mass spectrometry	All peroxides (also aldehydes, isoprostanes, cholesterol/ cholesterol ester peroxides)
Thin-layer chromatography	All peroxides

Haem and haem proteins decompose lipid peroxides to form radicals that react with isoluminol to produce light. For example, **microperoxidase**, a haem-peptide produced by proteolytic degradation of cytochrome c, is often used. The HPLC methods measure ~40 nM levels of peroxides in human blood plasma (e.g. *Anal. Biochem.* **175**, 120, 1988; *Meth. Enzymol.* **233**, 319 and 324, 1994), even lower in some studies (*Lipids* **39**, 891, 2004). **Why this is lower than in other assays is unclear.** Other substrates for microperoxidase (e.g. ascorbate) might compete with isoluminol and interfere with the assay. Electrochemical or redox-dye detections of peroxides have also been described (e.g. *Free Rad. Biol. Med.* **20**, 365, 1996; *Anal. Biochem.* **343**, 136, 2005). Identity of peroxides after HPLC separation must be confirmed chemically and not based simply on retention time. **Diode array detection**, a technique which records the absorbance spectrum of each peak, is a useful validation method. Another means of detecting peroxides after HPLC is to react them with diphenyl-1-pyrenylphosphine to generate a fluorescent product (see above). Plasma cholesterol ester hydroperoxides reported as ~ 0.2μM in healthy subjects, rising to ~ 13 μM in patients with liver failure (*Lipids* **40**, 515, 2005).

Peroxides are extracted, usually reduced (e.g. by borohydride) to alcohols, separated by GC, and identified by mass spectrometry. Levels of 'total' hydroxy fatty acids usually in low μM range. Several methodological variations exist (e.g. *Meth. Enzymol.* **233**, 332, 1994; *Anal. Biochem.* **198**, 104, 1991; *J. Chromatog.* **B823**, 37, 2005). Controls are needed to show that the alcohols were not present in the system *before* reduction, e.g. alcohols are generated by GPx activity. Lipid hydroxides can be absorbed from the diet and so subjects need to fast before the assay (*Free Rad. Biol. Med.* **32**, 162, 2002). Some HPLC–MS methods not requiring reduction are available to measure peroxides and chlorohydrins (*Biochem. J.* **355**, 449, 2001). Methods to measure plasma or tissue COPs have been described (e.g. *Biochem. Pharmacol.* **58**, 1415, 1999; *Anal. Biochem.* **312**, 217, 2003; *Free Radic. Res.* **38**, 787, 2004; *Lipids* **40**, 515, 2005).

Separated peroxides detected by tetramethyl-*p*-phenylenediamine (*Anal. Biochem.* **327**, 97, 2004).

[a] All the assays listed under Section A could also be applied to separated peroxides.

should be regarded with caution. Whether this is due to release of IPs from fat stores or to an oxidative stress associated with fasting is uncertain.

Most IPs in tissues and plasma are esterified to phospholids. Eventually they are hydrolysed to free IPs, which are rapidly metabolized, turning over quickly. Thus a rise in plasma free IP levels could be due not only to increased formation, but also to slower metabolism. It is also important for published papers to identify whether they measured total IPs, free IPs, or both, in plasma. Measurement of IPs in plasma and urine is, of course, a 'whole-body' measurement; it is not always clear where they came from. Urinary IPs presumably arise from all body tissues, including kidney. Ideally both the F_2–IPs and their metabolites such as 2,3-dinor-5,6-dihydro-15-F_{2t}-isoP (which is not made in kidney) should be quantitated in urine. Isoprostanes can also be measured in fluids drawn from specific sites, such as CSF, synovial fluid, lung lavage fluid, seminal plasma, bile, pericardial fluid, wound exudates and exhaled air condensate (breath condensate).[113]

Another point to ponder, IP formation is influenced by O_2 concentration; the monocyclic peroxide precursors of IPs can alternatively react with O_2 to give isofurans (Fig. 4.20).[110] At normal tissue O_2 levels IPs are major products, but this may not be the case in hyperoxia. For example, in mice exposed to pure O_2, the isofuran levels in the lung increased whereas F_2–IPs did not. This problem could also affect measurements in cell culture, since cells are exposed to 95% air/5% CO_2. Studies on brain slices may also be affected; O_2 readily diffuses in from the air. Under such circumstances combined measurement of isofurans and IPs is recommended.[110] F_2–isoprostane precursors can rearrange to D_2– and E_2–IPs which dehydrate to cyclopentenone IPs, highly reactive with –SH groups (Section 4.12.3). The precursors can also form D_2– and E_2–isoketals, again highly reactive with proteins, at amino groups (Fig. 4.22). Isoketal–protein adducts have been measured by antibody methods in human plasma at approximately 4 μM levels, higher in subjects with atherosclerosis.[114] They can also be visualized by immunostaining (Fig. 5.21, Plate 11).

Increased levels of IPs in plasma and/or urine are observed in many animal and human conditions associated with oxidative stress, including renal, liver, cardiovascular, lung, and neurodegenerative diseases, diabetes, hypertension, *H. pylori* infection, brain trauma, cardiopulmonary bypass and angioplasty. Isoprostanes have been used to study effects of toxins (Chapter 8), antioxidant supplementation and dietary changes on lipid peroxidation (Section 10.2.2.2). They have also helped to reveal a gender difference in oxidative damage (Section 3.19).

Another advantage of IPs is that different PUFAs form different IPs, which provides a mechanism for following the peroxidation of individual PUFAs *in vivo*. Isoprostane 'biomarkers' arising from different PUFAs should be helpful in investigating the consequences of eating diets rich in various PUFAs, whether any increased peroxidation that results can be ameliorated by antioxidants, and, if so, how much antioxidant is needed. Isoprostane measurements have as yet given little evidence that EPA or DHA oxidize faster than arachidonic acid in healthy humans (Section 4.11.4), although data are limited.

5.14.7 Measurement of end products: aldehydes[115]

Many aldehydes and other carbonyls are generated during lipid peroxidation, including malondialdehyde (MDA) and 4-hydroxynonenal (HNE) (Section 4.12.5). For example, production of the saturated aldehyde **hexanal**[116] has been assayed (by GC) as a measure of LDL peroxidation. The food industry has developed 'electronic noses' to rapidly detect these and other volatile products in foods as indices of early spoilage by peroxidation.[117] Aldehydes can be reacted with dinitrophenylhydrazine to give dinitrophenylhydrazones, which can be separated by HPLC. Alternatively they can be converted into volatile products that can be separated by GC and identified by MS. A range of methods (Table 5.13) to measure MDA and HNE has been described.

Concentrations of 'free' aldehydes *in vivo* are probably low, because they readily conjugate to proteins. This can make their true levels difficult to assess, since the ability of the various HPLC- or GC-based methods that have been used (Table 5.13) to detect all the adducts formed is uncertain. Several

Table 5.13 Measurement of malondialdehyde (MDA) and 4-hydroxy-2-nonenal (HNE) in biological systems: some examples

Method	Sample	Measured/levels	Illustrative references
Nuclear magnetic resonance spectroscopy	Liposomes, oils, LDL	Several aldehydes, not very sensitive; useful to study effects of heating on cooking oils.	*Biochem. J.* **289**, 149, 1993; *Free Radic. Res.* **19**, 335, 1994
Thin-layer chromatography, HPLC, GC–MS	Omega-6 PUFAs; Omega-3 PUFAs	Several aldehydes	*Biochem. Biophys. Res. Commun.* **169**, 75, 1990
[U-^{14}C]arachidonic acid	NADPH-dependent microsomal lipid peroxidation	HNE comes mainly from arachidonic acid in polar phospholipids	*Biochim. Biophys. Acta* **876**, 154, 1986
HPLC, GC–MS	Synovial fluid of arthritic patients	0.54 µM HNE (rheumatoid arthritis); 0.24 µM (osteoarthritis)	*Ann. Rheum. Dis.* **51**, 481, 1992
HPLC	Isolated rat hepatocytes after anoxia/reoxygenation	1.4 µM HNE	*Free Rad. Biol. Med.* **15**, 125, 1993
	Human plasma	2.16 ± 0.29 µM total MDA (free and bound), mostly bound 25–38 nM	*Anal. Biochem.* **220**, 391, 1994 *J. Chromatog.* **742**, 315, 2000
HPLC	Rat liver	0.93 nmol/g HNE	*Free Rad. Biol. Med.* **15**, 281, 1993
	Plasma from Watanabe rabbits (hyperlipidaemic)	74 ± 10 nM HNE	*Biochem. Biophys. Res. Commun.* **199**, 671, 1994
	Plasma from control rabbits	47 ± 6 nM HNE	*J. Chromatog.B* **785**, 337, 2003
	Human plasma	The MDA was measured after derivatization with DNPH and heating with alkali to liberate bound MDA, 138 ± 132 µM (value seems high, other studies report much lower or zero, e.g. *Anal. Biochem.* **170**, 123, 1998)	
Monoclonal or polyclonal antibodies	A wide range, recognizing different MDA- or HNE-amino-acid residue adducts. For example several antibodies directed against MDA-modified LDL have been raised. The preferred antigen recognized by monoclonal anti-HNE antibody Ig4 is an HNE-histidine adduct		*FEBS Lett.* **359**, 189, 1995; *Free Radic. Res.* **25**, 149,1996; *Free Rad. Biol. Med.* **35**, 517, 2003

Table 5.13 (*Cont.*)

Method	Sample	Measured/levels	Illustrative references
GC–MS	Alveolar macrophages exposed to $NO_2^\bullet$;	1.3 ng/10^6 cells	*Free Rad. Biol. Med.* **18**, 553, 1995
	Plasma of ARDS[a] patients	HNE higher in ARDS (41 ± 2 μM) than in controls (21 ± 2 μM)	*Free Radic. Res.* **21**, 95, 1994; *J. Chromatog* **843**, 29, 1999
	Plasma of coronary bypass patients	Greater % increase in HNE when the plasma transferrin is fully iron-saturated	*Biochem. Mol. Biol. Int.* **34**, 1277, 1994
HPLC	Human plasma	Measurement of fragmented phospholipids, some of which have PAF-like activity (Section 4.12.5); 0.6 ± 0.2 μM short-chain oxidized phosphatidylcholine reported in human plasma	*J. Lipid Res.* **37**, 2608, 1996
Colorimetric (available as a commercial kit)	Body fluids	Both MDA and HNE react with *N*-methyl-2-phenylindole to give the same chromophore. Using different reaction conditions, MDA alone can be measured.	*Chem. Res. Toxicol.* **11**, 1176 and 1184, 1998
LC/MS, measuring HNE–GSH conjugates (Fig. 4.28)	Rat liver	Basal level of HNE–GSH was 20 pmol/g; treatment with ferric NTA raised levels 5-fold.	*Free Rad. Biol. Med.* **38**, 1526, 2005
Immunoassay (or LC-MS) of the major urinary metabolite 1,4-dihydroxynonane-mercapturic acid (Fig. 4.28)	Rat urine	Levels increased after treatment of animals with $BrCCl_3$ (Section 8.3.1).	*Free Rad. Biol. Med.* **40**, 54, 2006

[a] Acute respiratory distress syndrome (Section 9.7).

Aldehydes formed can rapidly bind to proteins: the ability of many of the HPLC– or GC–MS-based assays to detect all these adducts is uncertain. HNE-ascorbate adducts have also been proposed as a biomarker of oxidative damage (Section 3.20.1.3).

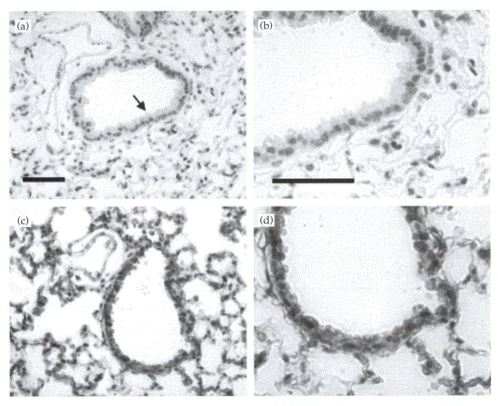

Figure 5.21 (see plate 11) Exposure of mice to >98% oxygen increases the levels of isoketals in airway and alveolar epithelium. Formalin-fixed, paraffin-embedded sections from airways of mice breathing either room air (21% O_2) or >98% O_2 for 7 h were stained with an antibody raised against a $15E_2$–isoketal peptide adduct. The presence of the antigen is indicated by the brown-colored DAB substrate. Sections were counterstained with hematoxylin. (A) Low-magnification photomicrograph of the airway epithelium of a mouse exposed to room air (bar = 50 μM). Arrow points to epithelial cells lining the airway. (B) High-magnification photomicrograph of the same airway (bar = 50 μM). (C) Low-magnification photomicrograph of the airway epithelium of a mouse exposed to >98% O_2 for 7 h showing immunoreactive airway epithelial cells and alveolar epithelial cells. (D) High-magnification photomicrograph of the same airway. Preadsorption with a peptide containing isoketal ablated the staining. From *Free Rad. Biol. Med.* **36**, 1163, 2004, by courtesy of Dr L. Jackson Roberts II and Elsevier.

methods use prolonged incubations to liberate bound aldehydes for analysis, running the risk of artefactually increasing peroxidation in the sample during processing. Aldehyde–protein conjugates are immunogenic and a range of antibody-based methods is available to detect them. The antibodies have variable specificity however, e.g. antibodies raised against HNE-conjugated proteins can recognize different HNE–amino acid residue adducts, so different preparations may give different results when applied to tissues or cells (Table 5.13).

Aldehydes arise by peroxide decomposition, which is often controlled by the availability of metal ions to decompose peroxides rather than by the rate of peroxide formation. Further, MDA, HNE and other aldehydes are metabolized by cells (Section 4.12.5). Hence their levels as a measure of lipid peroxidation should be interpreted with caution. It is also possible to measure aldehyde–GSH conjugates as a putative measure of HNE formation (Table 5.13).

5.14.8 Measurement of end products: breath analysis[113,118]

Air exhaled by humans and other animals consists of a gas phase containing O_2, $NO^•$, N_2, CO_2 and a little CO, plus a phase containing water vapour and non-volatile aerosol particles that can be condensed when the breath is cooled. F_2–isoprostanes, HNE-modified proteins, MDA, nitrated proteins (best measured by mass spectrometry, taking care to avoid artefacts; Section 5.6.2)[119] and H_2O_2 have all been measured in exhaled breath condensate. The gas phase contains a range of hydrocarbons, including ethane and pentane (Section 4.12.5.1). Constituents of the gas phase presumably originate from all over the body, whereas H_2O_2 and oxidative damage biomarkers in the condensate may come largely from the respiratory tract.[120,121]

Ethane is derived from (*n*-3) PUFAs and pentane from (*n*-6) PUFAs. The latter PUFAs predominate in the human body, suggesting that pentane would be produced in greater amounts if all PUFAs peroxidize equally. Both gases can be measured by GC; the expired breath is passed through an adsorbent at low temperature to bind and concentrate the hydrocarbons, which are then desorbed and assayed. However, hydrocarbons are minor end-products of peroxidation, and their formation depends on the presence of transition-metal ions to decompose peroxides. Hence an increased rate of gas production might reflect increased availability of such metal ions rather than increased initiation of peroxidation. Formation of hydrocarbons is also affected by O_2 concentrations, being favoured at low O_2. This is probably because the carbon-centred radicals that lead to hydrocarbon production (e.g. the pentane radical; Section 4.12.5.1) can also react with O_2 to form peroxyl radicals. In addition, some hydrocarbons are metabolized in the liver, for example pentane is hydroxylated by certain CYPs to pentanol. Hence agents that alter liver metabolism might affect pentane exhalation by altering its consumption by liver P450, and might mistakenly be thought to be altering the rate of lipid peroxidation *in vivo*.

Many GC columns used in the past did not separate pentane from **isoprene** (2-methyl-1,3-butadiene), a hydrocarbon present in large amounts in human breath, apparently a side-product of cholesterol biosynthesis. Thus several published 'breath pentane' levels are artefactually high and healthy humans exhale only low (picomolar) levels of pentane and other hydrocarbons. Given the problem of pentane metabolism, perhaps

ethane should receive more attention. Care must also be taken in experiments of this kind to control for hydrocarbon production from the bacteria always present on the skin (and fur) and in the oral cavity and colon. The air in large cities is contaminated with hydrocarbons from combustion processes, for example in motor vehicles and environmental tobacco smoke. Hydrocarbons partition into body fat stores and must first be flushed out by breathing hydrocarbon-free air before reliable measurements can be made. Nevertheless, techniques to avoid all these problems have been developed, and increased hydrocarbon exhalation with age, hyperoxia, smoking, scleroderma and some lung diseases has been demonstrated in several human studies.[118,122]

5.14.9 The TBA assay (thiobarbituric acid or 'that bloody assay')[123]

The TBA assay is one of the oldest and most frequently used methods for measuring peroxidation. It came originally from the food industry, being used to detect rancidity. It's amazingly easy: just heat some food, biological fluid or tissue with TBA in acid and a beautiful pink colour develops. Anyone can do it, and so they have, and filled the literature with masses of questionable data. Many people still believe that the TBA assay measures MDA in a sample. Unfortunately, the simplicity of performing the TBA assay belies its chemical complexity.

Small amounts of 'free' MDA are formed during the peroxidation of most membrane systems, especially microsomes. Malondialdehyde reacts in the TBA test to generate a coloured product, a $(TBA)_2$–MDA adduct.

In acid solution $(TBA)_2$–MDA absorbs light at 532 nm and fluoresces at 553 nm, and is readily extractable into organic solvents such as butan-1-ol. Construction of a calibration curve for the assay is complicated by the fact that MDA is unstable and must be prepared immediately before use by hydrolysing its derivatives, **1,1,3,3-tetramethoxy-propane** or **1,1,3,3-tetraethoxypropane**:

$$RO\!-\!\overset{\displaystyle RO}{\underset{\displaystyle RO}{}}CH\!-\!CH_2\!-\!CH\overset{\displaystyle OR}{\underset{\displaystyle OR}{}} \qquad R = C_2H_5 \text{ (ethyl)} \text{ or } CH_3 \text{ (methyl).}$$

In studying 'MDA' formed in this way, it is essential to ensure complete hydrolysis of these derivatives and to bear in mind that the solution will contain four molecules of ethanol (or methanol) per molecule of MDA. Some reports of enzyme inhibition, genotoxicity and carcinogenicity of 'MDA' may have originated from the biological activities of partially hydrolysed derivatives of the above compounds. For example, the ability of 'MDA' from tetraethoxypropane to inhibit XO was partly due[124] to the presence of **β-ethoxyacrolein**, ROCH=CHCHO. Malondialdehyde does bind to DNA, however, and probably is mutagenic *in vivo* (Section 4. 12.5).

So what's the problem with the TBA test? There are several.

5.14.9.1 *Problem 1: most TBARS (TBA-reactive substances) are generated during the assay*

Because the TBA assay is calibrated with MDA, the results are often expressed as 'MDA produced', giving the impression that the assay measures MDA in the sample. Indeed, the molar extinction coefficient of the $(TBA)_2$–MDA adduct ($1.54 \times 10^5 M^{-1} cm^{-1}$ at 532 nm) is often used to calculate the amount of 'MDA formed'. However, the amount of free MDA in most peroxidizing lipid systems is too low to give a substantial colour yield. It was shown as long ago as 1958, in studies with peroxidizing fish oil, that 98% of the MDA that reacts in the TBA assay was not originally present in the sample assayed but was formed by decomposition of lipid peroxides during the acid heating stage of the assay. Peroxide decomposition generates $RO_2^{\bullet}$ radicals that oxidize more lipid, i.e. the TBA test amplifies peroxidation and subsequent MDA formation. Peroxide breakdown is accelerated by iron ions in the sample or in the assay reagents, and removal of such iron decreases the TBARS detected. Conversely, antioxidants in the sample will decrease TBARS by interfering with this amplification. This can lead to errors in studies of the action of added antioxidants or metal-chelating agents on lipid peroxidation: they affect colour development in the TBA assay itself. Approaches to address these issues have included adding excess iron with the TBA reagents to maximize peroxidation, or (perhaps more logically) adding chain-breaking antioxidants (usually BHT) to suppress peroxidation. Table 5.14 illustrates how

Table 5.14 Variability of results in the HPLC-based TBA test depending on whether or not butylated hydroxytoluene (BHT) is added to the sample with the TBA reagents

Sample	TBA reactivity (μM MDA equivalents)	
	BHT not added	BHT added
Fresh human plasma		
Healthy subjects	0.45 ± 0.35 (12)[a]	0.10 ± 0.10 (12)
Hyperlipidaemic subjects[b]	0.88 ± 0.22 (17)	0.61 ± 0.25 (17)
Rat liver microsomes incubated with $FeCl_3$/ascorbate		
Peroxidizing for 5 min	12.0 ± 0.8 (4)	5.8 ± 0.9 (4)
Peroxidizing for 20 min[c]	14.7 ± 1.0 (4)	12.8 ± 1.0 (4)

[a] *n* values are given in parentheses.

[b] Elevation of TBARS persists even when expressed per unit cholesterol. Hyperlipidaemia is known to be associated with increased lipid peroxidation.

[c] By 20 min peroxidation was essentially complete: note how the absence of BHT appears to accelerate the rate of peroxidation as measured by TBARS. This is because of further peroxidation of the lipids during the assay, which is inhibited by BHT. When all the lipids have been oxidized the same TBARS values will result.

Data from *Free Radic. Res. Commun.* **19**, 51, 1991.

different assay conditions can affect the results obtained.

Thus the TBARS measured in a sample will differ according to the assay conditions used. The lack of specificity of the TBA assay when applied to plasma is exemplified by the work of Lands *et al.*; by the cyclooxygenase method (Table 5.12) they measured a peroxide level of around $0.5\,\mu M$ in human plasma, whereas expression of the results from a TBA assay on the same samples as 'peroxide equivalents' gave a mean value of $38\,\mu M$. MDA can be determined directly by HPLC or GC–MS and basal levels of free MDA in human plasma in most studies are far lower than values obtained by the TBA test (Table 5.13).

5.14.9.2 *Problem 2: false chromogens*

Several compounds other than MDA react in the TBA assay to give chromogens that absorb at, or close to, 532 nm. They include streptomycin, sialic acid and biliverdin. Measurement of TBARS at 532 nm could thus include contributions from them. For example, TBA tests on plasma from jaundiced patients can be confounded by bile pigments. However fluorescence measurements or examination of the full absorbance spectra can often distinguish the products they form from the 'real' $(TBA)_2$–MDA adduct.

5.14.9.3 *Problem 3: real chromogens but not from lipids*

An alternative approach to deal with Problem 2 is to separate the $(TBA)_2$–MDA adduct from other chromogens before measurement, usually by HPLC. However, exposure of several carbohydrates and amino acids to $OH^{\bullet}$, produced by ionizing radiation or metal-ion H_2O_2 systems, yields products that give a *genuine* $(TBA)_2$–MDA adduct on heating with TBA. They include deoxyribose, DNA base propenals and proline. Application of the TBA assay to human body fluids will also measure MDA produced enzymically during eicosanoid synthesis (Section 7.12.7).[125]

5.14.9.4 *Urinary TBARS*

Urinary TBARS has sometimes been used as an index of whole body lipid peroxidation, for example in nutritional studies. Unfortunately, there are major problems. First, diet has an effect; much of the TBARS in urine seem to arise from lipid peroxides or aldehydes (attached to lysine and other amino acids) in ingested food, presumably largely generated during cooking.[126,127] For example, a diet rich in cooked meat promotes urinary TBARS excretion, to an extent depending on the temperature at which the meat was cooked.[128] Asking subjects to eat lipid-poor diets or to fast for 24 h caused urinary MDA levels to drop, whereas levels of F_2–IPs increased during fasting.[111]

In any case, HPLC must be used to separate the real $(TBA)_2$–MDA adduct; much TBARS in urine is not even lipid-derived and some of the rest arises from aldehydes other than MDA,[129] although several MDA adducts are excreted (Fig. 5.22). When urinary 'MDA' was measured

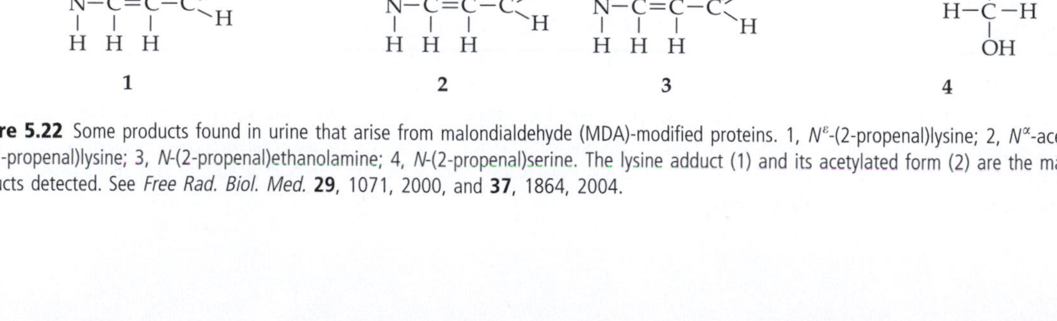

Figure 5.22 Some products found in urine that arise from malondialdehyde (MDA)-modified proteins. 1, N^{ε}-(2-propenal)lysine; 2, N^{α}-acetyl-N^{ε}-(2-propenal)lysine; 3, N-(2-propenal)ethanolamine; 4, N-(2-propenal)serine. The lysine adduct (1) and its acetylated form (2) are the major products detected. See *Free Rad. Biol. Med.* **29**, 1071, 2000, and **37**, 1864, 2004.

by HPLC after reaction with dinitrophenylhy-drazine, levels were 10-fold smaller than when an HPLC-based TBA assay was used. Excretion of HNE–mercapturic acid conjugates (Fig. 4.28) in urine might give some indication of HNE formation *in vivo*.

5.14.9.5 *Is the TBA assay useless?*

No; HPLC-based TBA assays eliminate much of the interference that plagues the simple TBA assay and are useful 'screening' methods for examining large numbers of biological samples for elevated perox-idation, to pick out these for more detailed study. The simple TBA test in the presence of BHT is useful in studying peroxidation of isolated lipids, lipo-somes, cells and subcellular fractions. However, the TBA assay cannot be used to compare levels of peroxidation between tissues with a different fatty acid composition, since MDA only originates from certain PUFAs (Section 4.12). We do not recommend urinary TBARS measurements until more work is done to investigate what the various assays are measuring, and the contribution of diet.[130]

5.14.10 Measuring lipid peroxidation: light emission

Several groups have used 'low-level chemilumin-escence' as an index of oxidative stress (Section 5.10) and some (but by no means all) of the light can come from lipid peroxidation. One source is singlet O_2 by the Russell mechanism

$$\text{>CHO}_2^{\bullet} + \text{>CHO}_2^{\bullet} \longrightarrow \text{>C=O} + \text{—C—OH} + {}^1O_2$$
$$\text{carbonyl}$$

The carbonyl compound produced might also be in an excited state and emit light as it decays to the ground state. Other possible sources of light are self reaction of alkoxyl radicals to give excited-state ketones:

$$\text{>CHO}^{\bullet} + \text{>CHO}^{\bullet} \longrightarrow \text{>C=O}^* + \text{—C—OH}$$

and the formation of dioxetanes by reaction of singlet O_2 with unsaturated fatty-acid side chains (Section 2.6.4): dioxetanes can decompose to give excited-state carbonyls

$$\text{>C=C<} + {}^1O_2 \longrightarrow \text{—C—C—} \longrightarrow \text{>C=O} + \text{>C=O}^*$$
$$\quad\quad\quad\quad\quad\quad\quad\quad\quad\;\; \text{O—O}$$

Measurements of light emission in cells or mem-brane fractions correlate reasonably well with results from other assays of lipid peroxidation, except that the peak light emission often occurs slightly later than the 'peak' recorded by other techniques. This is probably because maximum light production by the Russell-type mechanism only occurs during the later stages of lipid peroxidation, when enough $RO_2^{\bullet}$ are present in the membrane to increase their chance of colliding and reacting.

Some groups have measured generation of fluor-escent products as an index of lipid peroxidation in foodstuffs[117] and tissues;[131] the assay is sensitive but the chemistry is complex (of course, fluorescence is a sensitive way of detecting $(TBA)_2$–MDA). Fluores-cence is often thought to arise by reaction of carbo-nyl compounds with amino groups on proteins, phosphatidylserine, phosphatidylethanolamine or even DNA and RNA bases. However, there are other mechanisms. Aldehydes can polymerize into fluorescent products (Fig. 5.23). Reaction of MDA with –NH$_2$ groups at low pH can generate fluores-cent **aminoiminopropene Schiff bases**, but their contribution to the formation of fluorescent pro-ducts in peroxidizing membranes is unclear, since MDA has limited reactivity at pH 7.4 (Section 4.12.5.2). Other aldehydes, such as HNE, may be more important contributors. Even then, the role of Schiff bases has been questioned; **dihydropyridine dicarbaldehydes**[115,131] may be the major fluorescent products formed.

5.14.11 A summary: what is the best method to measure lipid peroxidation in tissues, cells and body fluids?

None is ideal, but some are better than others. On the basis of fairly rigorous chemical identification of products and broad general agreement between the values measured by different laboratories in plasma and urine, we recommend mass spectro-metric measurement of the F_2–IPs (combined with measurement of isofurans under certain circum-stances). Peroxide assays are also potentially useful (Table 5.12) although the effect of diet is uncertain

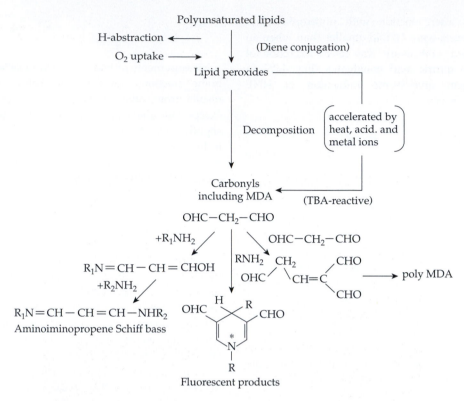

Figure 5.23 Formation of fluorescent products during lipid peroxidation. The starred product (*) is a 1,4-dihydropyridine-3,5-dicarbaldehyde. Malondialdehyde (MDA) can also condense with other aldehydes formed during peroxidation.

and the reasons for the discrepant values obtained by some of the methods need to be elucidated. Measuring aldehydes and hydrocarbons has some value, but if there is a shortage of metal ions to decompose lipid peroxides (and 'catalytic' metal ion levels are often low *in vivo*) there will be little formation of hydrocarbon gases, carbonyl compounds or their fluorescent complexes. Lack of formation of these products does not necessarily mean that there is no peroxidation. Also, measured levels of MDA and HNE vary widely between laboratories (Table 5.13).

Whatever method is chosen, one should think clearly about *what* is being measured and *how* it relates to the overall lipid peroxidation process.

5.14.12 Visualizing lipid peroxidation

There is nothing better than a nice picture to impress your audience, and the availability of staining reagents or antibodies that detect end-products of lipid peroxidation allows them to be visualized. Figure 5.18 shows one example, using anti-HNE. Figure 5.24 shows another, based upon the fluorescence of naphthoic acid hydrazide conjugates with carbonyl groups. Figure 5.21 shows a third: exposure of mice to >98% O_2 causes formation of protein-bound isoketals in the lung. It is essential when using antibody methods to check for cross-reactivity with other products and for non-specificity of staining, for example by adding the antigen (in free, protein bound or peptide form) and showing that the staining is blocked (Fig. 5.21, legend).

5.14.13 Probes of lipid peroxidation/ membrane reactive species

Several membrane-partitioning probes have been introduced to measure lipid peroxidation or RS within membranes. One is *cis*-**parinaric acid**

(Fig. 5.13). When incorporated into lipids undergoing peroxidation, it is rapidly oxidized, losing its fluorescence (emission at 413 nm, excitation 324 nm). Parinaric acid needs careful handling, because it is susceptible to non-specific oxidation, and it should be stored in the dark under a N_2 atmosphere. It can be added as the free acid or incorporated into specific phospholipids (**parinaroyl lipids**) and used to study their relative susceptibilities to oxidative damage within membranes.[132]

Another popular probe is **C-11-BODIPY**[581/591] (Fig. 5.13). Upon oxidation, its fluorescence shifts from red to green, so that the green/(red + green) ratio can be used as an estimate of membrane oxidation (Fig. 5.25, Plate 12). The BODIPY[581/591] molecule,

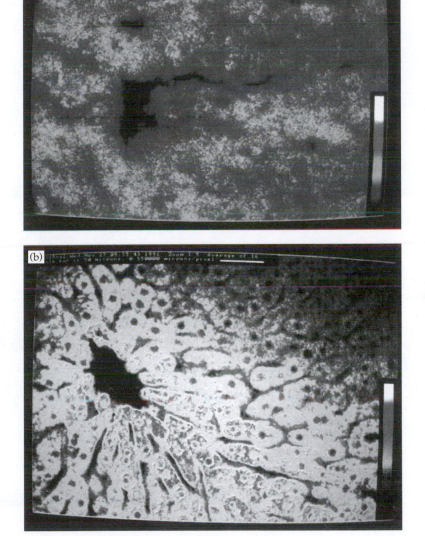

Figure 5.24 Imaging of oxidative stress by confocal laser scanning microscopy. Sections of liver from a control rat (a) or a rat treated with CCl_4 to induce lipid peroxidation (b) were stained with 3-hydroxy-2-naphthoic acid hydrazine reagent, which reacts with carbonyls to give a fluorescent product. Adapted from *Am. J. Pathol.* **142**, 1353, 1993 by courtesy of Professors Mario Comporti and A. Pompella and the publishers.

has a three-ring structure centred on a boron atom. Attack of RS on the diene 'linker' affects electron delocalization between the two ring structures to cause the colour change. Use of the ratio helps to decrease variations caused by heterogeneous probe distributions (cell thickness, uneven dye loading, compartmentalization etc). The BODIPY$^{581/591}$ probe responds to a range of RS (OH$^{\bullet}$, peroxyl, alkoxyl, ONOO^{-}, NO$_2^{\bullet}$), but not to O$_2^{\bullet-}$, NO$^{\bullet}$, H$_2$O$_2$, singlet O$_2$ or hydroperoxides. It may also detect tyrosyl radicals. Thus C-11-BODIPY$^{581/591}$ can be used to determine RS within membranes.[133] When added to cells, C-11-BODIPY$^{581/591}$ enters most membranes, with no apparent preference for any organelle.

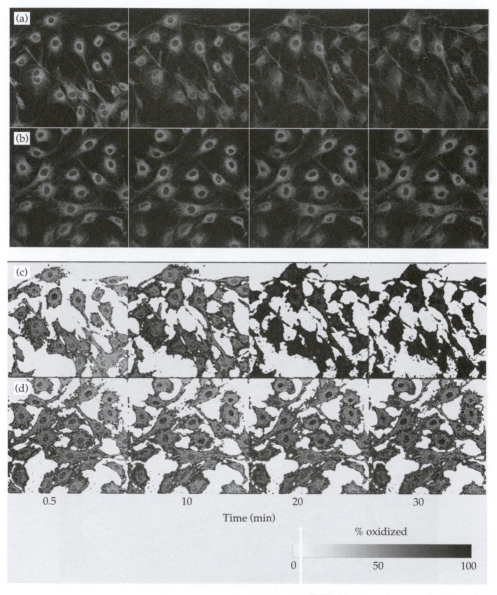

Figure 5.25 (see plate 12) Serial images of (A) rat fibroblasts loaded with C11-BODIPY$^{581/591}$ and exposed to 80 µM cumene hydroperoxide and 80 nM haemin. The green colour indicates RS attack on the probe. (B) The cells were preincubated with α- and γ-tocopherol for 16 h prior to exposure to the RS. In C and D, the fraction of oxidized C11-BODIPY$^{581/591}$ is presented. To obtain this fraction the green fluorescence is divided by the total fluorescence (green + red). From *FEBS Lett.* **453**, 278, 1999 by courtesy of Dr Karel Wirtz and Elsevier.

Of course, the presence of such probes can be expected to alter the rate, and perhaps the mechanistic pathway, of lipid peroxidation, as they trap various intermediates.

5.15 Biomarkers of protein damage by reactive species[134,135]

Proteins can be damaged by direct attack of RS, by binding end-products of lipid peroxidation such as HNE or isoketals, and/or by glycation/glycoxidation (Section 9.4.4). How can oxidative protein damage be measured?

5.15.1 Damage by reactive oxygen species

Analysing protein oxidative damage products is an order of magnitude more complex than dealing with DNA (Section 4.13.3). Some of the methods used are summarized in Table 5.15; loss of thiol groups or of tryptophan fluorescence and the carbonyl assay (Section 5.15.3 below) are popular methods that do not require the protein to be hydrolysed. Free radical attack on proteins can generate amino-acid radicals, which may cross-link or react with O_2 to give peroxyl radicals. Protein peroxyls may abstract H$^\bullet$, forming more free radicals and protein peroxides (Table 5.15) which can decompose in complex ways, accelerated by transition metal ions, to generate yet more radicals. Proteins can be oxidized during food cooking. Hence oxidized amino acids could conceivably be absorbed from the diet, which could confound measurements of them in body fluids as putative biomarkers of oxidative damage. Individual amino acid oxidation products (structures in Fig. 4.31) that have been measured in various human tissues include kynurenines (from tryptophan), valine and leucine hydroxides, L-DOPA, ortho-tyrosine, 2-oxohistidine, glutamate semialdehyde and adipic semialdehyde. For example, ortho-tyrosine has been measured in human lens proteins.[136] Altered tyrosines were measured in hair from 'Alpine man', Homo tirolensis,[137] although whether they were formed during life or after death as a result of exposure of the body to sunlight or transition metals (a corroded copper axe was next to the body) is unknown.

Bityrosine, easily detectable in human and other animal urines because of its intense fluorescence (Fig 2.6), formed by RS attack on a wide range of proteins, and apparently not metabolized, is a biomarker that may be worth further development for human use,[138] although a contribution from diet cannot yet be ruled out. For example, patients with sepsis showed increased urinary excretion of bityrosine, as did children with kwashiorkor, a disease believed to involve oxidative stress (Section 4.1). Bityrosine is present normally in the insect cuticle,[138] some fungal cell walls and the fertilization envelope of the sea urchin (Section 7.5.3). Tyrosine cross-linking is also important during bread making.[138] An immunohistochemical method to detect bityrosine in human brain has been described.[139]

An **acetyltyramine–fluorescein** probe to detect formation of tyrosine radicals in cells subjected to oxidative stress has been developed. If both the tyramine probe and tyrosine residues are oxidized by RS, the probe can cross-link to the protein tyrosyl residues, generating a stable cross-link similar to that in bityrosine. The fluorescein-labelled proteins can then be visualized, and identified if necessary by proteomic methods.[140]

5.15.2 Damage by reactive halogen and nitrogen species

Proteins are also attacked by reactive chlorine, bromine and nitrogen species, giving products such as 3-chlorotyrosine, para-hydroxyphenylacetaldehyde, 3,5-dichlorotyrosine, 3-bromotyrosine and 3-nitrotyrosine (Fig. 4.31), which can be detected by immunostaining or chemical analysis. Chlorotyrosines have been widely measured as an index of damage by RCS (Table 5.7), although they are minor end-products of damage (Section 2.6.3). When HOCl and HOBr are added to proteins, HOBr brominates tyrosine residues more readily than HOCl chlorinates them, since HOBr is less-well scavenged by cysteine and methionine residues. Hence if both halogenated tyrosines are measured, their ratio cannot be used to determine the relative amounts of HOCl and HOBr formed (HOBr will be over estimated).[141] 3-Nitrotyrosine is formed from tyrosine by a range of RNS

Table 5.15 Detection and measurement of oxidative damage to proteins: some methods

Method	Reaction/detection	Comments
A. General methods		
Amino acid analysis	Proteins hydrolysed and amino acids separated by ion-exchange chromatography	Gives an overall pattern of changes; measures loss of amino acids; can detect nitrotyrosine, chlorotyrosine, 2-oxohistidine etc.
Protein carbonyls	2-4-dinitrophenylhydrazine: absorbance at 360–390 nm (after removal of excess DNPH by organic solvent extraction or HPLC), fluorescence, radiochemically after reduction by tritiated borohydride or 'blotting'	Widely used 'general' assay; essential to remove nucleic acids when analysing tissues
Protein peroxides	Several methods, including iodometry and FOX assay	See Table 5.10
ESR of protein radicals	Often signals are broad and give limited structural information	Can be useful under some circumstances (*Free Rad. Biol. Med.* **36**, 1072, 2004)
Measurement of DMPO adducts	A sensitive alternative to spin trapping	Section 5.2.8
Increased susceptibility to proteolysis	Proteins more rapidly degraded by proteinases	May be a common feature of oxidized proteins (Section 4.14.2)
(1) Alanine formation	Alanine dehydrogenase/NAD$^+$	Red blood cells cannot synthesize alanine, and its release indicates protein degradation, which is accelerated as a result of oxidative damage
(2) Increased/decreased exposure of amino groups (e.g. as a result of hydrolysis, or after modification of lysines by aldehydes)	Fluorescamine: excitation 390 nm, emission 475 nm; *O*-phthalaldehyde: excitation 340 nm, emission 450 nm	As a protein is degraded, one mole of $-NH_2$ is exposed for each mole of amino acid released. Loss of $-NH_2$ can also occur, e.g. when HNE reacts with protein
Amide bands	Infrared spectroscopy of the amide bands in the region 1900–1400 nm; absorbances vary depending on secondary structure	Can measure changes in secondary structure due to oxidative damage (or other mechanisms)
B. Specific changes to individual amino acids		
Loss of –SH (thiol) groups	Ellman's reagent (Fig. 5.9) Staining for thiol groups	Measures available thiol (–SH) groups Allows visualization of their loss (Fig. 5.9)
Tryptophan		
(1) Loss of fluorescence	Fluorescence changes: excitation 280 nm, emission 342 nm	Loss of the native fluorescence of tryptophan
(2) Formation of tryptophan oxidation products	Fluorescence: (acid) excitation 360 nm, emission 450 nm; (alkaline) excitation 327 nm, emission 342 nm; HPLC	Products such as *N*-formylkynurenine are fluorescent (*Amino Acids* **3**, 184, 1992)

Tyrosine	Bityrosine: fluorescence excitation 315 nm in alkaline solutions, emission 420 nm; HPLC separation with fluorescence, or ECD detection, GC–MS. Hydroxylation product L-DOPA can be measured by HPLC (DOPA present naturally in some proteins). See Fig. 2.6.	Bityrosine is highly fluorescent, but interference problems can occur in biological matrices (*Methods Enzymol.* **233**, 363, 1994; *Amino Acids* **25**, 233, 2003; Punchard, NA and Kelly, FJ eds (1996) *Free Radicals: A Practical Approach*, p. 171. IRL Press, Oxford)
Methionine	Oxidation to methionine sulphoxide and sulphone (HPLC or GC–MS)	Specific enzymes repair methionine sulphoxide residues (Section 4.14.1)
Nitration of proteins	Antibodies, HPLC or GC–MS; usually measured on tyrosine, but nitration also occurs on phenylalanine and tryptophan	Provides evidence of damage by RNS
Chlorination/bromination of proteins	Chloro(bromo)tyrosine; antibodies, HPLC or GC–MS	Detects damage by RCS/RBS such as HOCl, HOBr or NO_2Cl
2-Oxohistidine	Attack of ROS (especially $OH^\bullet$) upon histidine, HPLC. Also detected in carbonyl assay	Levels rise in SOD inactivated by H_2O_2, suggesting ROS production at active site (Section 3.2.1.6). See also *FEBS Lett.* **332**, 208, 1993)
Phenylalanine	Hydroxylated by $OH^\bullet$ to *ortho-*, *meta-* and *para-*tyrosines; nitrated by $ONOO^-$ and probably other RNS	HPLC or GC–MS measurement
Valine/leucine	Peroxides or their reduction products (hydroxides) measured	*Biochem. J.* **324**, 41, 1997
Arginine/proline	Can be oxidized to γ-glutamate semialdehyde which on reduction and hydrolysis forms 5-hydroxy-2-aminovaleric acid	HPLC or GC–MS measurement (*Free Rad. Biol. Med.* **21**, 65, 1996), also see [135].

(Section 2.6.1). Nitro-, bromo- and chlorotyrosines can be measured as the free amino acid or in proteins after hydrolysis. Hereby lies a potential for artefact. Hydrolysis of proteins by HCl should be avoided if chlorotyrosine is to be measured. Traces of NO_2^- in most biological samples can generate RNS upon exposure to acid that can nitrate tyrosine (Section 5.6.2).

5.15.3 The carbonyl assay[135,142]

The **carbonyl assay** is a 'general' assay of oxidative protein damage. Several RS (including $OH^\bullet$, $RO_2^\bullet$, O_3, HOCl, $ONOO^-$ and singlet O_2) oxidize amino-acid residues in proteins to form products with carbonyl groups, which can be measured after reaction with 2,4-dinitrophenylhydrazine (DNPH). For example, $OH^\bullet$ converts histidine to 2-oxohistidine and singlet O_2 converts tryptophan to N-formylkynurenine (among other products). Glutamate and aminoadipic semialdehydes (Fig. 4.32) are significant ($\sim$50%) contributors to plasma and tissue protein carbonyl levels. Carbonyls are readily measured spectrophotometrically, by ELISA techniques, after reduction by tritiated sodium borohydride (the incorporation of tritium into the protein being measured; Table 5.15) and by cytochemical techniques using anti-DNPH antibodies. However, some carbonyls can be released from proteins by fragmentation and will be lost during the washing procedures of the assay.[143] Another approach is to use biotin hydrazide; carbonyls react with the hydrazine component and can then be isolated using biotin-binding columns or identified on gels using fluorescently labelled **avidin** (a protein that binds to biotin).[144]

The carbonyl assay is widely used and many laboratories have developed individual protocols for it (just as with the TBA assay). Indeed, tissue or plasma carbonyls are elevated in many diseases. Sometimes the assay procedures used are not specified precisely in published papers. This is important because there is a considerable variation in reported 'baseline' levels of protein carbonyls in cells and tissues, depending on how the assay is performed. For example, reported carbonyl levels for human brain cortex range from 1.5 to 6.4 nmol/mg protein.[145] By contrast, most groups seem to obtain broadly comparable values for protein carbonyls in mammalian plasma, of 0.4 to 1.0 nmol/mg protein.

The carbonyl assay as applied to tissues and body fluids measures the 'average' extent of protein modification, a steady state between generation of modified proteins and their removal, for example by the proteasome (Section 4.14.2). Separating and identifying the oxidized proteins often gives useful information; sometimes only a small number of proteins is oxidized. For example, in human plasma subjected to oxidative stress most carbonyls were found on fibrinogen.[146] In the brains of subjects who died with Alzheimer's disease, proteomic techniques showed only a few proteins to be highly oxidatively modified (Section 9.20). Experiments on chickens showed that dietary antioxidants affect the levels of carbonylation of different muscle proteins to variable extents.[147]

Direct measurements of glutamate and aminoadipate semialdehydes in human plasma proteins have also been used to assess the effects of alterations in antioxidant intake on protein oxidation.[148]

5.16 Is there a single biomarker of oxidative stress or oxidative damage?

The answer is probably no, although (as might be expected) biomarkers of damage to different molecules frequently rise in parallel in cells subjected to severe oxidative stress. Why is there little or no correlation between biomarkers in healthy tissues? For example, no correlation was observed between levels of plasma IPs and white cell oxidative DNA damage in healthy human subjects.[28] Levels of 8OHdG and other DNA base damage products are a balance between rate of oxidative DNA damage and rate of DNA repair, different lesions being removed at different rates (Fig. 4.14). Isoprostanes, once formed, are hydrolysed from lipids; once free, they are metabolized quickly. Oxidized proteins are degraded, mostly by the proteasome system, and appear to turn over more slowly. Thus even if all biomolecules are damaged, the extents and time courses of the biomarkers of such damage can be different.

5.17 Assays of total antioxidant capacity[149,150]

Increased generation of RS can deplete one or more antioxidants. Loss of individual antioxidants and/or generation of oxidation products from them (e.g. ascorbyl radical, GSSG, allantoin) can be measured as an index of oxidative stress. Antioxidant depletion does not necessarily mean that oxidative damage has taken place: it might simply signify that the defence mechanisms have removed the RS and protected the system.

Attempts have been made to assess the **total antioxidant capacity (TAC)** of body fluids rather than go to the trouble of identifying what has happened to each component of the complex antioxidant defence network. The first TAC assay used was the **TRAP (total (peroxyl) radical trapping antioxidant parameter) assay.**[151] A body fluid is incubated with AAPH (Section 2.5.4), which forms peroxyl radicals that react with antioxidants in the fluid. Only when antioxidants have been depleted will the $RO_2^{\bullet}$ radicals attack lipids (lipids in the fluid, or lipids added to it) to cause peroxidation. By measuring the lag period before onset of peroxidation (e.g. by O_2 uptake) and calibrating the assay with a known antioxidant (usually **Trolox C**), a value for TRAP can be obtained as the micromoles of peroxyl radicals trapped per litre of fluid. Each Trolox molecule can trap two $RO_2^{\bullet}$.

In human plasma, TRAP values are around $10^3\,\mu mol\ RO_2^{\bullet}$ trapped/litre; major contributors to TRAP are urate (35–65%), plasma proteins (10–50%), ascorbate (up to 24%) and vitamin E (5–10%) (Table 5.17). The known antioxidants do not account for all the measured TRAP, i.e. there is an 'unidentified' component. This could be due to antioxidants not yet identified, and/or to synergy between antioxidants such that they work better in combination than individually. It is essential to ensure that O_2 is not depleted during the TRAP assay because the carbon-centred radicals ($R^{\bullet}$) generated from AAPH can themselves react with certain antioxidants (Section 2.5.4).

Variations on the TRAP assay exist. One is to use lipid-soluble $RO_2^{\bullet}$ generators (e.g. AMVN; Fig. 2.7). Another is to use alternative detection methods, such as luminol-enhanced chemiluminescence (Table 5.16). Other TAC assays have been developed using various RS and different detector molecule (Tables 5.17 and 5.18). In several assays (e.g. ORAC, TRAP, ABTS), urate is a major contributor to the total antioxidant activity of plasma or saliva (Section 6.2.2.1). By contrast, human CSF has about four-fold higher ascorbate concentrations but lower urate concentrations than plasma, and so ascorbate is a more significant contributor to TRAP.[152] Total CSF TRAP values are lower ($\sim$237 μM) than those in plasma.

Total antioxidant capacity assays can be used to compare the antioxidant activities of different molecules, foods or beverages. Often ABTS is used, as in Table 5.18. Many other assays have been employed for antioxidant characterization; one of the first introduced uses **1,1-diphenyl-2-picrylhydrazyl** (DPPH; Fig. 5.26),[153] a stable free radical with a distinctive ESR signal. Its reactions with antioxidants can be followed by loss of either the ESR signal or of absorbance at 540 nm. Loss of the ESR signal from nitroxides was used to assess the TAC of beer, for example.[154]

5.17.1 What do changes in total antioxidant capacity mean?

Assays of TAC are useful in getting a global picture of relative antioxidant activities in different body fluids and how they change in clinical conditions. Results should be interpreted in the light of the chemistry of the assay (Table 5.16). For example, is the ability to reduce iron (as in FRAP) or copper (as in CUPRAC) really equal to the ability to scavenge $RO_2^{\bullet}$ or $ABTS^{\bullet+}$? Changes in various antioxidants can give misleading conclusions. For example, rises in urate could obscure depletions of ascorbate or other antioxidants. Urate levels go up in many human diseases because of alterations in purine metabolism, which explains why some studies have detected rises in plasma TAC in sick people. Several scientists have used TAC determinations to imply that consuming various foods (e.g. chocolate, fruits, vegetables) contributes specific phenolic antioxidants to plasma that increase its TAC. Often, however, eating these foods transiently raises plasma urate levels, which accounts for most or all of the changes.[155,156] Several assays show a greater plasma TAC in males than females (Section 3.19), perhaps due to higher urate levels.

Table 5.16 Some assays for total antioxidant capacity (TAC)

Method	Principle	Comments
TRAP assay	Peroxidation of endogenous or exogenous (e.g. added linoleic acid) lipids in body fluids on exposure to azo initiators.	Can measure O_2 uptake by O_2 electrode, or detect $RO_2^\bullet$ directly, e.g. by luminol-enhanced chemiluminescence (*Free Rad. Biol. Med.* **21**, 211, 1996), other chemiluminescence methods, or bleaching of pyrogallol red (*Free Radic. Res.* **39**, 729, 2005). Can be used to compare antioxidants as $RO_2^\bullet$ scavengers. Could also use proteins as targets, e.g. measure protein carbonyl formation or enzyme inactivation by $RO_2^\bullet$.
Phycoerythrin	Attacked by $RO_2^\bullet$ (or $OH^\bullet$) with loss of fluorescence (the **ORAC, oxygen radical absorbance capacity** assay). Usually uses emission 565 nm, excitation 540 nm and AAPH to generate $RO_2^\bullet$. Antioxidants cause decreased fluorescence loss. The reaction is usually taken to completion rather than allowed to run for a fixed time (e.g. as in the ABTS assay) or only a lag phase measured (e.g. as in the TRAP assay).	Phycoerythrin is a photosynthetic protein found in red algae. It carries 34 covalently-linked open-chain tetrapyrrole prosthetic groups, giving it high absorbance (λ_{max} 372, 497, 566 nm) and intense fluorescence (λ_{max} 578 nm) (*FASEB J.* **2**, 2487, 1988, *Free Rad. Biol. Med.* **27**, 1173, 1999). Other 'detectors' can be used in ORAC assays, e.g. DCFDA or fluorescein.
ABTS method	2,2'-Azinobis(3-ethylbenzothiazoline 6-sulphonate) is oxidized to a radical cation, $ABTS^{\bullet+}$, which absorbs at 660, 734 and 820 nm. Oxidation of ABTS to $ABTS^{\bullet+}$ can be achieved by metmyoglobin/H_2O_2, horseradish peroxidase/H_2O_2 or by simply adding MnO_2 or persulphate. Antioxidants decolorize the radical.	Rapid method, easily automated (*Redox Report* **2**, 161, 1996), measurement at high λ avoids interference from absorbance of most biomolecules. Can be applied to LDL. Better to preform the radical using persulphate (*Free Rad. Biol. Med.* **26**, 1231, 1999); otherwise some antioxidants (e.g. ascorbate) can interfere with its *generation* by peroxidase or metmyoglobin systems by competing with ABTS for oxidation.
FRAP (ferric reducing antioxidant power)	Measures ability of plasma antioxidants (vitamin E, urate, ascorbate, but not albumin) to reduce Fe(III) to Fe^{2+} at low pH. Pretreatment with ascorbate oxidase can be used to determine the contribution of ascorbate.	Easily automated; simple. Assumes reducing ability equates to free-radical scavenging (*Anal. Biochem.* **239**, 70, 1996).
Cyclic voltammetry	Uses variable voltage to oxidize and reduce components of the sample. Cyclic voltammogram can be used to identify antioxidants based on their oxidation potential as well as the total amount of reducing power present, a combination of the reducing power of each agent and its concentration.	Used to measure changes in TAC during various diseases and in ageing and to show that TAC is higher in the small intestine than in the colon (*Toxicol. Pathol.* **30**, 620, 2002). Equates reducing capacity to TAC.
Crocin method	Oxidation of crocin by $RO_2^\bullet$ radicals from AAPH causes bleaching of absorbance at 443 nm.	*Free Rad. Biol. Med.* **24**, 1228, 1998.
CUPRAC assay (Cupric reducing antioxidant capacity)	Ability to reduce Cu^{2+}–neocuproine	*Free Radic. Res.* **39**, 949, 2005. Equates reducing capacity to TAC.

In all these assays a radical is generated and scavenged by antioxidants. When the antioxidants are used up the radical reacts with a target molecule to produce a colour, fluorescence, chemiluminescence, loss or gain of an ESR signal or other observable change.

Table 5.17 Total antioxidant capacity of human blood plasma/serum by various assays

Method	Typical results (μM)	Reference
TRAP	~1000	See text
Crocin assay	~2000	*Free Rad. Biol. Med.* **24**, 1228, 1998
Enhanced chemiluminescence	829 ± 77	*Anal. Chim. Acta* **266**, 265, 1992
ORAC	$(3.1 \pm 0.49) \times 10^3$	*Free Radic. Res.* **33**, S59, 2000
Phycoerythrin assay (ORAC)	1162 ± 265	*Free Rad. Biol. Med.* **18**, 29, 1995
ABTS assay	~2000	Using persulphate-based assay: *Free Radic. Res.* **38**, 831, 2004
FRAP (ferric reducing antioxidant power of plasma)	612–1634[a] $(1.03 \pm 0.22)^b \times 10^3$	*Anal. Biochem.* **239**, 70, 1996 *Free Radic. Res.* **33**, 559, 2000

Note that different assays give different values, not surprisingly because the chemistry of each assay and the time-course over which it is conducted are different. Plasma and serum do not always give identical results. The anticoagulant used to prepare plasma can affect determination of TAC, since heparin stabilizes plasma against loss of TAC on standing better than EDTA (*Ann. Clin. Biochem.* **36**, 104, 1999). It is generally best to assay plasma samples immediately for TAC.

[a] Healthy Chinese adults.

[b] Caucasians. In general TAC values are higher in males than in females (*Ann. Clin. Biochem.* **36**, 104, 1999; *Arterio Thromb. Vasc. Biol.* **21**, 1190, 2001), although males tend to have higher oxidative damage levels by some assays (Section 3.19).

Table 5.18 Using the ABTS assay to determine the contribution of identified constituents to the total antioxidant activity of red wine *in vitro*

	Antioxidant activity[a] of pure compound	Concentration in wine (mM)	Contribution to total antioxidant activity
Catechin	2.4 ± 0.05	0.66	1.6
Epicatechin	2.5 ± 0.02	0.28	0.7
Gallic acid	3.01 ± 0.05	0.51	1.54
Cyanidin	4.42 ± 0.12	0.01	0.04
Malvidin-3-glucoside	1.78 ± 0.02	0.05	0.09
Rutin	2.42 ± 0.12	0.01	0.02
Quercetin	4.72 ± 0.10	0.02	0.09
Myricetin	3.72 ± 0.28	0.03	0.09
Resveratrol	2.00 ± 0.06	0.006	0.01
Caffeic acid	1.26 ± 0.01	0.014	0.02
Total contribution to antioxidant activity			4.2
Mean TEAC for red wines			16.7

[a] Expressed by comparison with Trolox as **Trolox equivalent antioxidant capacity (TEAC)**. Note the large TAC 'missing'.

Data by courtesy of Prof. C. Rice-Evans (also see *Free Rad. Biol. Med.* **20**, 933, 1996). Note the high *in vitro* antioxidant activity of red wines.

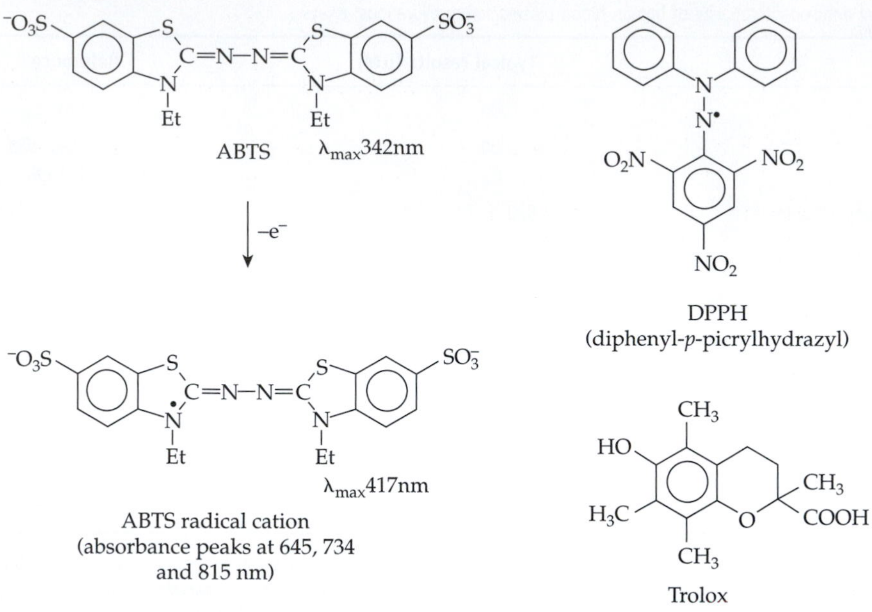

Figure 5.26 Some compounds used in 'total antioxidant capacity assays'. Both ABTS$^{\bullet+}$ and DPPH are nitrogen-centred radicals. Trolox, used to calibrate many assays, is a water-soluble form of α-tocopherol: the hydrophobic side chain is replaced by a $-$COOH group. One mole of Trolox can scavenge two $RO_2^{\bullet}$ radicals. Whereas ABTS is soluble in aqueous solutions, DPPH is dissolved in ethanol. Et, ethyl group.

Another problem is that body fluids, plant extracts and food contain a complex mixture of components that react with radicals at different rates. Hence the time over which the assay is conducted can influence the results. For example, reaction of ascorbate or trolox with ABTS$^{\bullet+}$ is complete within 1 to 2 min, but reaction of soy sauce with it continued for over 50 min.[157] Hence assays than are allowed to run to completion (e.g. ORAC) give different results from those run for a fixed time (as ABTS often is) or where a lag period is measured.

Reactive species can pose special problems needing special solutions: some examples

It's the free radicals, stupid!

Toren Finkel

6.1 Introduction

In earlier chapters we described the problems faced by aerobes in coping with O_2, and the usual ways in which they counter and repair oxidative damage. We have also seen a few 'special cases'. For example, the swim-bladders of some deep sea fish (Section 1.5.5) must tolerate high O_2 partial pressures (the effective O_2 concentration at 3000 m deep is 2500 times greater than ambient) yet the bladder remains undamaged. The fish as a whole cannot tolerate this pO_2, and so the bladder must be specially protected. How? We do not know. Maybe the bladder tissue has low metabolic activity and generates few ROS. The SOD activity of swim-bladders from several fish is higher than in other fish tissues examined, but there is nothing exceptional about their catalase or GPx activities.[1]

The purpose of this chapter is to discuss some other systems that have especially difficult problems of antioxidant defence. We also tackle the relationship of exercise to oxidative stress. The kidney has problems as well, but we defer them until Section 7.10.5.

6.2 The gastrointestinal tract[2]

6.2.1 Threatening your guts

The GI tract must absorb nutrients, keep bacteria and bacterial products (e.g. endotoxin) out of the body, and tolerate whatever we choose to eat, including carcinogens and pro-oxidants. Damage to it, for example by ischaemia, is life-threatening (Section 9.5.3). Animals are exposed to carbonyls in dietary lipids; for example, a range of aldehydes can arise from peroxidized cooking oils.[3] Cooked food of animal origin also contains isoprostanes, lipid hydroperoxides and cholesterol oxidation products (COPS). Oxidation products of plant lipids can also be ingested (Section 6.7 below). We may consume millimoles of these various oxidation products per day.[4] The systemic toxicity of lipid oxidation products is low (Section 4.12.2), probably because most are dealt with in the GI tract and do not enter the blood.[4] However, peroxidation can occur in the stomach, haem proteins being good catalysts.[5] Haem is fairly well absorbed, but an excess of it might reach the colon and exert pro-oxidant and proproliferative effects (Section 9.13.8). Transfer of aldehydes, lipid peroxides and COPS to the circulation appears limited, but some does occur.[4] However, the cells lining the GI tract will be exposed to the full force of these agents. For example, chronic dietary exposure to oxidized lipids decreased mucosal cell turnover in rat small intestine, whereas lower levels might be proproliferative.[4] DNA–aldehyde adducts are found in human colonic mucosa (Section 5.13.9).

Other sources of RS to which the mouth, oesophagus and stomach are exposed include:

1. Mixtures of iron and ascorbate, especially in the stomach and duodenum (Section 3.15.1), can catalyse lipid oxidation and promote OH$^\bullet$ generation. Diet-derived copper ions (e.g. in drinking water; Section 3.20.1.3) can generate OH$^\bullet$ and other RS from ascorbate. Multivitamin pills containing iron and/or copper plus ascorbate could conceivably be pro-oxidant.

2. Nitrite in saliva and foods being converted to HNO_2 by gastric acid, forming nitrosating and DNA-deaminating species (Section 2.5.6.5).

3. High (>100 µM) levels of H_2O_2 in certain beverages, especially coffee (Section 2.6.2). Hydrogen peroxide is also generated by oral bacteria (Section 3.13.3).

4. The presence in the diet of highly oxidizable pro-oxidant phenolic compounds, such as hydroxyhydroquinone (Section 2.6.2). Sometimes pro-oxidants are deliberately added to food, e.g. sulphite is widely used as a preservative but it can be oxidized by transition metal ions and the NADPH oxidase system of intestinal lymphocytes[6] to generate RS (Section 8.11.3).

5. The intestine contains part of the immune system and its resident phagocytes can respond to challenge with antigens in food or bacteria to produce RS.[6]

6. The cells of the GI tract may themselves release RS. Thus a $O_2^{\bullet-}$-producing NOX enzyme is found in colon (Section 7.10.1). A similar system, DUOX2, is found in salivary glands and perhaps throughout the GI tract, with some species difference in levels.[7] These systems may have antibacterial roles; adult *Drosophila* without active DUOX in the gut were much more prone to die from infections after eating microbe-contaminated food.[8] The ROS produced by NOX/DUOX systems could act directly against bacteria and/or by supplying H_2O_2 to peroxidases, such as lactoperoxidase (Section 3.13.3).

6.2.2 Defending your guts

Food with a high content of oxidized lipids tastes rancid, and we reject it. The GI tract is lined by mucus, a powerful scavenger of RS (Section 6.3 below). The colonic contents are usually anaerobic (although, of course, the cells of the colon are not). This may be fortunate, since exposure of faeces to air can cause substantial OH$^\bullet$ generation, probably due to bacterial H_2O_2 production interacting with unabsorbed transition metal ions.[9] However, transient aeration probably occurs frequently *in vivo*. Indeed, hydroxylated PBN and D-phenylalanine, as markers for OH$^\bullet$ (Section 5.2.4 and 5.3.1), were detected in the faeces of rats whose intestines were colonized with *Enterococcus faecalis*,[10] a facultative anaerobe that produces $O_2^{\bullet-}$ when exposed to O_2.

Like all animal tissues, the cells of the GI tract contain DNA repair enzymes, proteasomes that remove oxidized proteins, SOD, catalase, peroxiredoxins, GST and GPx, both GPx1 and the 'intestinal form', GPx2 (Section 3.8.1).[4] Some of the SOD and the GPx activities of the small intestine and colon appear to be located at the external cell surface, possibly to help detoxify RS from the food before they reach the cell surface. The GPx enzymes in GI cells may remove the bulk of peroxides present in absorbed lipids.[4] The gut is also rich in GSTs, which may metabolize peroxides and cytotoxic aldehydes. Several dietary constituents, including sulphoraphane (Section 10.5), can increase the levels of GSTs, GPx2 and other antioxidant defences in the GI tract via the ARE (Section 4.5.10).[11] Refeeding mice that had been starved for 48h activated HSF1 (Section 4.6) in both small intestine and liver (but not colon or stomach) leading to increased levels of Hsp in both tissues—does the gut somehow signal to the liver that xenobiotics in food may arrive shortly?[12]

6.2.2.1 *Saliva*

Saliva contains peroxidases (Section 3.13.3) and H_2O_2 added to it rapidly disappears, probably by the action of both peroxidases and catalase. The latter is liberated into saliva as the buccal cells lining the oral cavity turn over and are shed. The total antioxidant capacity (TAC) of saliva (Section 5.17) is lower than that of plasma; ascorbate levels are <10 µM and the major antioxidant present is urate.[13] The TAC of saliva varies depending on which of the salivary glands it came from.[13]

6.2.2.2 *Antioxidants from diet?*[2,5,14]

Foods and beverages deliver not only pro-oxidants, but also a complex mixture of antioxidants to the

GI tract. Some of these are absorbed well, others not so well, but even the unabsorbed ones might exert extracellular antioxidant protective effects in the GI tract. For example, flavonoids and some other phenolics are powerful scavengers of RS and inhibit lipid oxidation by haem proteins, but many *in vitro* studies showing this have employed concentrations much higher than are ever achieved in plasma or body tissues (Section 3.22.2). A similar caveat might be applied to the ability of carotenoids to scavenge RS *in vitro* (Section 3.21.3). However, when foods or beverages rich in phenolics and/or carotenoids are consumed, high (millimolar) levels of these antioxidants are delivered to the GI tract. The stomach probably encounters the highest levels, but there will be substantial exposure of the small intestine, and many flavonoids and carotenoids pass into the colon. Hence scavenging of RS within the GI tract is feasible. For example, nitrite from saliva and food forms nitrosating and

DNA-deaminating species, but damage by these *in vitro* is inhibited by flavonoids at levels similar to those that can occur in the gastric juice.[15] Of course, scavenging of various RS can generate oxidized, chlorinated, nitrosylated or nitrated products from the antioxidants, products that could themselves have biological effects, an area which remains to be explored. In addition, many phenolic compounds interact with iron, often in complex ways, although overall the effects are usually antioxidant (Section 3.22.2). Unabsorbed dietary iron and haem enter the faeces, where phenolics, by chelating iron and scavenging RS, may help to alleviate pro-oxidant actions (Fig. 6.1). Flavonoid levels in human faecal water can be up to $1 \mu M$, and much higher concentrations of monophenols (e.g. $>100 \mu M$ caffeic acid) are present.[14] As an interesting contrast, caterpillars may ingest so many phenols that they oxidize in the gut, catalysed by iron in the gut contents, and cause damage. Insects deal with

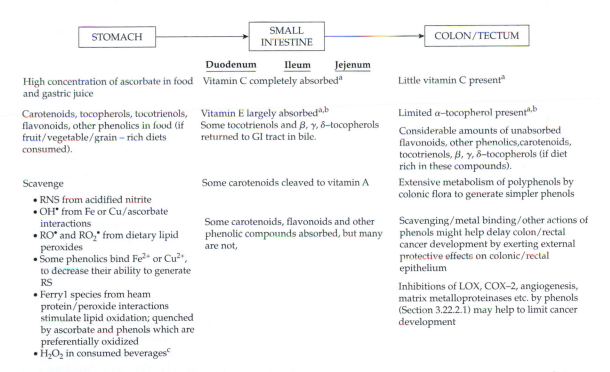

STOMACH	SMALL INTESTINE	COLON/TECTUM
	Duodenum Ileum Jejenum	
High concentration of ascorbate in food and gastric juice	Vitamin C completely absorbed[a]	Little vitamin C present[a]
Carotenoids, tocopherols, tocotrienols, flavonoids, other phenolics in food (if fruit/vegetable/grain – rich diets consumed).	Vitamin E largely absorbed[a,b] Some tocotrienols and β, γ, δ–tocopherols returned to GI tract in bile.	Limited α–tocopherol present[a,b] Considerable amounts of unabsorbed flavonoids, other phenolics, carotenoids, tocotrienols, β, γ, δ–tocopherols (if diet rich in these compounds).
Scavenge • RNS from acidified nitrite • OH$^{\bullet}$ from Fe or Cu/ascorbate interactions • RO$^{\bullet}$ and RO$_2^{\bullet}$ from dietary lipid peroxides • Some phenolics bind Fe^{2+} or Cu^{2+}, to decrease their ability to generate RS • Ferry1 species from heam protein/peroxide interactions stimulate lipid oxidation; quenched by ascorbate and phenols which are preferentially oxidized • H_2O_2 in consumed beverages[c]	Some carotenoids cleaved to vitamin A Some carotenoids, flavonoids and other phenolic compounds absorbed, but many are not,	Extensive metabolism of polyphenols by colonic flora to generate simpler phenols Scavenging/metal binding/other actions of phenols might help delay colon/rectal cancer development by exerting external protective effects on colonic/rectal epithelium Inhibitions of LOX, COX–2, angiogenesis, matrix metalloproteinases etc. by phenols (Section 3.22.2.1) may help to limit cancer development

Figure 6.1 Dietary antioxidants and the GI tract. [a] Except when supplements are taken. This diagram refers to normal dietary intake. [b] There is considerable intersubject variability in the efficiency of GI uptake of vitamin E (Section 3.20.2). [c] Much H_2O_2 may be removed in the oral cavity by saliva, and by its diffusion into the oral and oesophageal epithelium for rapid catabolism.

this by secreting high levels of ascorbate and GSH into the gut lumen and operating an ascorbate–glutathione cycle[16] similar to that in plants (Fig. 6.16 below).

The potential contribution of ascorbate and vitamin E in the GI tract must not be neglected (Fig. 6.1). Ascorbate can scavenge RS and decrease nitrosamine formation. When tocopherols and tocotrienols are absorbed from the GI tract, α-tocopherol is preferentially selected by the liver for incorporation into plasma lipoproteins (Section 3.20.2), whereas some of the other tocopherols are excreted in bile and returned to the GI tract. High concentrations of δ- and γ-tocopherols and tocotrienols are found in faecal matter compared with plasma levels;[14] they might be taken up by colonic cells as well as exert extracellular protective effects, for example γ-tocopherol scavenging RNS or inhibiting COX-2 (Section 3.20.2.7).

Protective effects of phenols, carotenoids etc. to the GI tract need not only be antioxidant; other mechanisms might be equally or more important (Fig. 6.1). Sadly, however, supplements of β-carotene, ascorbate and α-tocopherol do not protect against the development of human GI cancers; food is much more complex than these three compounds[17] (Section 10.5).

6.3 The respiratory tract

6.3.1 The challenges

The nasal passages, trachea, bronchi, bronchioles and alveoli are exposed to the full force of O_2 in inhaled air, unlike most body tissues (Fig. 1.4), yet alveolar type I cells are easily injured by too much O_2 (Section 1.5.2). Over an average human lifespan, about 3×10^8 litres of air are breathed. The respiratory tract must also tolerate oxidant gases in the inhaled air (Section 8.11). Those who smoke insult their own respiratory tracts and those of the people around them with a complex mixture of toxins (Section 8.12). The air is full of bacteria, viruses, fungal spores, plant pollen and other particulates, some of which can provoke alveolar macrophages to release RS, and/or promote the recruitment of neutrophils into the respiratory tract to do the same. Allergens in pollen can include nitrated

proteins (Section 8.11.2) and ROS-producing NADPH oxidases (Section 7.11). Allergens can recruit eosinophils to the lung, releasing such RS as HOBr (Section 7.8).[18] Over-activation of eosinophils contributes to airway damage in asthma, which is essentially an inflammatory disease of the airways. Indeed, lung tissue from asthmatic subjects shows increased levels of bromotyrosine.[18] Asthmatic patients also exhale more NO$^{\bullet}$ (probably due to increased levels of iNOS), have more H_2O_2 in their breath condensate,[19] and produce more isoprostanes.[20] Indeed, the airways of mice over-expressing CuZnSOD are less sensitive to allergens (Box 3.1), and SOD levels are reported to be lower in the asthmatic lung.[21] Paradoxically, however, CuZnSOD in pollen can act as an allergen.[22]

There is a constant production of NO$^{\bullet}$ in the respiratory tract, due to constitutive expression of iNOS in the epithelium, probably as an antibacterial mechanism (Section 2.5.6.6). In addition, pulmonary endothelial and smooth muscle cells contain NADPH oxidases (mostly the NOX4 type; Section 7.10). DUOX enzymes (Section 7.10) have been reported in some respiratory tract cells and levels may increase after cytokine treatment. Excessive $O_2^{\bullet-}$ production may contribute to asthma by scavenging this NO$^{\bullet}$ and forming ONOO$^-$, and possibly by causing abnormal proliferation of airway smooth muscle cells.[23] Indeed, protein nitration (including nitration of MnSOD) is elevated in asthma.[21] Of course, never assume that ONOO$^-$ is all bad; nitrosothiols formed by its reaction with GSH may be protective to the lung.[24]

The fluids lining the respiratory tract contain molecules essential to lung function. Excessive elastase activity can erode elastic fibres and interfere with lung expansion and contraction, leading to **emphysema**. Yet the α_1-antiproteinase (Section 2.6.3) in lung lining fluids that normally inhibits elastase is readily inactivated by ONOO$^-$, and by HOCl from activated neutrophils. The **surfactant** that maintains alveolar function (Section 1.5.2) can also be a target of oxidative damage, losing its ability to lower surface tension. The lipid component of surfactant (mainly the saturated lipid **dipalmitoylphosphatidylcholine**) is fairly resistant, but the proteins present can be damaged[25,26] by HOCl and ONOO$^-$. Indeed, nitration of surfactant proteins is observed in rats exposed to hyperoxia.[26] Despite the presence of some iron-binding proteins (Section 6.3.2 below), low levels of 'labile iron', measured by the aconitase assay (Table 4.3) have been detected in alveolar lining fluids.[27] The role (if any) of this iron is uncertain: it might result from a method of controlling lung cell iron levels by excreting it (probably via ferroportin; Section 3.15.1) for eventual clearance from the respiratory tract in the mucus. Indeed, isolated perfused rabbit lungs were observed to release iron into the perfusate. However, this 'free' iron could also be pro-oxidant.

6.3.2 Defending the respiratory tract

The cells of the respiratory system have the usual intracellular antioxidant defence and repair systems, including CuZnSOD, MnSOD, GPxs, catalase, peroxiredoxins, ascorbate, GSH and α-tocopherol. Plasma HDL seems to be the main source of α-tocopherol for type II pneumocytes.[28] Despite these defences, even a small rise in O_2 can cause oxidative stress; merely breathing 28% O_2 (7% above normal) for 1 h (a value too low to cause clinical symptoms) increased the levels of F_2-isoprostanes and IL-6 in exhaled air.[29]

There are also extracellular antioxidant defences. The upper respiratory tract is coated with a constantly renewed mucus layer, which helps trap bacteria, particulates and iron and remove them as the mucus is propelled upwards by the beating of cilia.[30] Mucus is a proteoglycan: a protein core with many carbohydrate side-chains attached. It has a high content of cysteine and disulphide bridges, which contribute to its viscosity. The mucus layer also contains materials (lipids, carbohydrates, proteins, DNA) originating from death and lysis of underlying epithelial cells during their normal turnover. Hence, as a whole, the mucus layer is a powerful scavenger of $OH^\bullet$, $ONOOH$ and $HOCl$ and may also absorb[30] some O_3 and $NO_2^\bullet$. Stimuli that promote mucus secretion can involve ROS in their mechanisms of action under certain circumstances (Sections 8.12.4 and 9.8).

Levels of antioxidants in respiratory tract lining fluids differ from those in blood plasma and vary between species (e.g. rat has higher ascorbate levels

than humans). Tables 6.1 and 6.2 show some values for humans. The most striking feature is that GSH levels are much higher than in plasma. Urate and albumin are lower, and ascorbate about the same.[30,31] Antioxidant defence enzymes are present, but at low levels. However, lung injury by O_2 or other toxic gases can allow leakage of plasma constituents into the lining fluid, replenishing ascorbate, urate and α-tocopherol and raising levels of albumin, perhaps thus augmenting antioxidant defences of the lung. Hence albumin transudation, often used as a marker of lung injury (e.g. as measurements of raised albumin levels in lung

Table 6.1 Approximate values for the concentrations of non-enzymic antioxidants in human plasma and lung lining fluid

Antioxidant	Concentration (μM)	
	Plasma	Lining fluid
Ascorbate	20–100	40–100
GSH	<5	40–200
Uric acid	160–450	90–250
α-Tocopherol	25	2.5
β-Carotene	0.4	trace
Albumin–SH	500	70

Values are approximate because lung lining fluid is sampled by washing out the lung (**bronchoalveolar lavage**). This causes considerable and variable dilutions, and the calculations used to obtain values for the 'undiluted' fluid *in vivo* make several assumptions and approximations. Other antioxidants in lung lining fluids include low levels of transferrin, caeruloplasmin, lactoferrin, EC–SOD, catalase and extracellular GPx. Antioxidant levels differ in different parts of the respiratory tract, e.g. alveolar lining fluid has more GSH than fluid lining the upper respiratory tract (Table 6.2). Data abstracted from *Environ. Health Perspect.* **106** (Suppl. 5), 1246, 1998 by courtesy of Professor Carroll Cross and the publishers.

Table 6.2 Approximate concentrations of some antioxidants in human nasal lining fluid compared with lung lining fluids

Antioxidant	Concentration (μM)	
	Nasal lining fluid	Lung lining fluid
Ascorbic acid	2–20	40–100
Uric acid	20–250	90–250
Glutathione	0–15	40–200
Albumin–SH	10	70

Data abstracted from *Environ. Health Perspect.* **106** (Suppl. 5), 1246, 1998 by courtesy of Professor Carroll Cross and the publishers. The values are approximate, for the reasons given in the legend to Table 6.1.

lavage fluid after pollutant exposure) may initially be beneficial (Section 3.16.3.5).

6.3.3 Asthma and antioxidants

Epidemiological studies show that the incidence and severity of asthma correlate with low plasma antioxidants, the data being especially clear for ascorbate.[32] Does the chronic inflammation of asthma use up antioxidants, or is a low intake a predisposing factor? If it is, is the benefit really due to the antioxidants and/or to other constituents of antioxidant-rich foods? Would supplements help? Despite the many papers published in this area, the answer to these questions is unclear as yet.[32] Often two issues get mixed together; the asthma itself and the aggravating effects of air pollutants such as O_3 on its symptoms. Thus it is possible that antioxidant supplements might modulate the latter but not the former.[33] In any case, we do not know to what extent antioxidant concentrations in the respiratory tract lining fluids increase with dietary intake; thus some studies suggest that nasal lining fluid levels of ascorbate correlate better with dietary intakes and plasma levels than do levels in alveolar lining fluids (ref[34] and F.J. Kelly, personal communication). The antioxidant OTC appeared to improve asthma in a mouse model (Section 10.6.9.1).

6.4 Erythrocytes

Red blood cells (also known as erythrocytes), are biconcave discs averaging about $7.7\,\mu m$ in diameter (Fig. 6.2). In humans, they lack a nucleus, mitochondria, and other organelles. Their average lifespan in the human bloodstream is around 120 days (Table 6.3) and about 200 billion new ones are produced per day. Each travels about 400 km during its lifespan.

Erythrocyte cytoplasm is rich in protein, of which about 33% is haemoglobin (up to 280 million molecules per erythrocyte). Adult males have 14 to 16.5 g of haemoglobin per 100 ml of blood, and females 12 to 15 g/100 ml. As the erythrocyte passes through the lung capillaries, the four haem groups of haemoglobin bind O_2 (Section 1.10.3). The haem iron in deoxyhaemoglobin is in the Fe^{2+} state, but when O_2 attaches, there is some electron delocalization (Section 1.10.3). Every so often a molecule of oxyhaemoglobin releases $O_2^{\bullet-}$, a water molecule or an OH^- replacing the O_2

$$haem-Fe^{2+} - O_2 \rightarrow O_2^{\bullet-} + haem-Fe(III)$$

The Fe(III) product, **methaemoglobin**, cannot bind oxygen.

6.4.1 What problems do erythrocytes face?

Erythrocytes must keep their membranes intact for long periods (Table 6.3) in the face of:

1. A constant flux of $O_2^{\bullet-}$ from oxyhaemoglobin. About 3 to 4% of oxyhaemoglobin is estimated to undergo oxidation every day.[35,36] Complete oxidation should thus occur in 33 to 34 days and the cell would be unable to carry O_2. Oxidation is accelerated by NO_2^-, which can be oxidized to NO_3^- or reduced to $NO^{\bullet}$ by haemoglobin (Section 2.5.6.5).

2. Carrying high concentrations of a pro-oxidant haem protein and O_2 inside a membrane rich in PUFA side-chains. Pro-oxidant reactions of haemoglobin, as well as its ability to bind $NO^{\bullet}$, have caused problems in the development of cross-linked haemoglobins as 'blood substitutes'. One attempt to overcome this has been to cross-link SOD and/or catalase with the haemoglobin.[37]

3. Erythrocyte cytoplasm may contain low molecular mass 'catalytic' iron in amounts increasing with age,[38] presumably arising from haemoglobin breakdown.

4. Repeated deformation and consequent physical stress upon red cell membranes as these cells squeeze through tiny capillaries at 37°C. Deformation can aggravate the effects of lipid peroxidation in causing leakage of ions across the membrane.[39]

5. No ability to synthesize new proteins (e.g. ferritin to sequester iron) or lipids to replace oxidized ones. Lacking mitochondria, red blood cells rely on glycolysis to make ATP, which is consumed mostly in ion transport (e.g. Na^+, K^+-ATPase) and GSH synthesis (red blood cells do make GSH; defects in GSH synthesis can lead to haemolysis [Section 3.9.4]). Of course, with no mitochondria, red blood

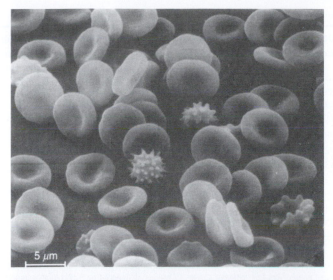

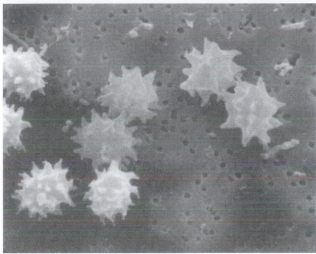

Figure 6.2 Top: erythrocytes. The membrane is about 44% lipid, 49% protein and the rest is carbohydrate. Bottom: echinocytes produced by peroxide treatment. Electron micrographs by courtesy of Dr David Hockley and Prof. C. Rice-Evans. Peroxide damage causes morphological change, increased membrane rigidity with consequent decreased deformability, lipid peroxidation and damage to membrane proteins, including spectrin and band 3. Peroxide-treated erythrocytes also show increased senescent antigen on their surfaces.

cells don't have to worry about mitochondrial ROS production, some consolation perhaps.

6.4.2 Solutions: antioxidant defences

Erythrocytes contain a lot of CuZnSOD; indeed, the bovine erythrocyte enzyme was the first CuZnSOD to be purified (Section 3.2.1). This SOD seems to keep intraerythrocyte $O_2^{\bullet-}$ levels[36] at around 10^{-13} M. No MnSOD is present, as there are no mitochondria. The CuZnSOD converts $O_2^{\bullet-}$ to H_2O_2, some of which can be removed by catalase and GPx1 (Fig. 6.3), the only GPx present. The relative importance of these two enzymes in catabolizing H_2O_2 may vary between species (Table 6.3); the conventional view for years, although periodically challenged, was that GPx1 is more important at low (physiological) fluxes of H_2O_2 whereas catalase, with its higher K_m for H_2O_2, becomes important at higher H_2O_2 levels (Section 3.11.1). Indeed, erythrocytes can act as sinks for extracellular H_2O_2 and $O_2^{\bullet-}$. Hydrogen peroxide crosses their membranes easily and the erythrocyte has an anion channel through which $O_2^{\bullet-}$ can move. This channel (**band 3 protein**) is involved both in

Table 6.3 Erythrocyte lifespan and antioxidant defence enzymes: a comparison between species

Species	Erythrocyte lifespan (days)	SOD (U/g Hb)	Glutathione peroxidase (U/g Hb)	GSH (μM/g Hb)	Catalase (IU × 10^{-4}/g Hb)	Glutathione reductase (IU/g Hb)
Homo sapiens	120–150	2352	32	6.7	14	7.8
Macaca mulatta (rhesus monkey)	100	2572	130	9.1	19	5.5
Canis familiaris (domestic dog)	115	2118	130	7.8	n.d.	3.2
Felis cattus (domestic cat)	77	2885	156	8.0	24	7.7
Oryctolagus cuniculus (rabbit)	67	3324	39	7.2	13	3.9
Ovis aris (sheep)	150	3132	124	8.9	2	1.2
Bos taurus (cattle)	175	3259	165	7.7	8	1.0
Rattus rattus (rat)	67	2967	141	8.0	11	1.8
Mus musculus (mouse)	51	3148	314	7.0	5	9.8
Misocricetus auratus (hamster)	79	2771	22	7.5	6	2.2

n.d., not determined; IU, international units.
Erythrocytes are long-lived cells in all animal species. SOD and GSH levels are broadly comparable between species, but activities of GPx and catalase vary widely, which in part helps to explain the variable susceptibility of erythrocytes from different species to haemolysis induced by H_2O_2 (another important factor is the peroxiredoxin system). Data abstracted from *Comp. Biochem. Physiol.* **106B**, 477, 1993 by courtesy of Dr M Suzuki and the publisher.

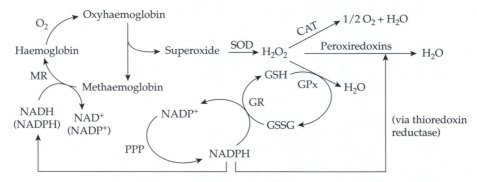

Figure 6.3 Protection of erythrocytes against oxidative damage. MR, methaemoglobin reductase systems; SOD, CuZn superoxide dismutase; CAT, catalase; GPx, glutathione peroxidase; GR, glutathione reductase; PPP, pentose phosphate pathway (first enzyme: glucose 6-phosphate dehydrogenase). MR uses both NADH and NADPH. Peroxiredoxins seem to be the major pathway of H_2O_2 removal, and their activity requires thioredoxin and thioredoxin reductase in the erythrocyte (*Biochem. Biophys. Res. Commun.* **26**, 217, 1995).

anchoring the cytoskeleton to the membrane and as an ion transporter. It normally exchanges HCO_3^- for Cl^-, but $O_2^{\bullet-}$ can pass through it as well, as can NO_2^- (Section 2.5.6.5). Indeed, similar **anion exchange proteins** are found in several tissues, including lung.[40] Even $ONOO^-$ can get through red blood cell membranes, probably through the same protein.[41] Once inside, $ONOO^-$ can react with erythrocyte GSH and with oxyhaemoglobin, yielding NO_3^-, methaemoglobin, some H_2O_2 (probably via $O_2^{\bullet-}$ dismutation), and some ferrylhaemoglobin.[41]

However, the GPx/catalase debate was, in retrospect, fruitless. Erythrocyte problems are rarely seen in knockout mice lacking GPx1 or catalase, or indeed in human acatalasaemic subjects. By contrast, mice lacking peroxiredoxins (Section 3.11) gradually develop severe haemolytic anaemia, preceded and accompanied by protein oxidation, haemoglobin instability, inclusion body formation, shortened erythrocyte lifespan, anaemia and spleen enlargement. Hence peroxiredoxins and their companions (thioredoxin and thioredoxin reductase), play an important role (Fig. 6.3). Indeed, peroxiredoxins are some of the most abundant proteins in red blood cells, with levels of 0.24 mM being quoted.[36,42] At least three types are present,

Prx1, 2 and 6. These various H_2O_2-removal systems keep internal levels down to about 10^{-11} M.

The NADPH needed for glutathione and thioredoxin reductases is provided by the pentose phosphate pathway, which also supplies NADPH for a **methaemoglobin reductase** enzyme that converts methaemoglobin to ferrous haemoglobin to permit continued O_2 transport. However, most methaemoglobin reductase activity in erythrocytes is NADH-dependent, using an enzyme system containing FAD and cytochrome b_5. Mutations affecting the reductase system can cause **hereditary methaemoglobinaemia**, accompanied by mild **cyanosis** (blue colour of the extremities due to poor O_2 delivery). There are two types of mutation, one affecting only the erythrocyte enzyme and the other affecting all tissues. In the second type, neurodegeneration occurs as well as erythrocyte abnormalities, since the enzyme is required for desaturation and elongation of fatty acids in tissues.[43]

6.4.3 Solutions: diet-derived antioxidants

Erythrocyte membranes contain α-tocopherol. Indeed, an early sign of inadequate α-tocopherol intake is the increased lysis of isolated red blood cells (**haemolysis**) when they are treated with millimolar (grossly unphysiological) levels of H_2O_2 in the presence of a catalase inhibitor (azide): the **peroxide stress haemolysis test**. Haemoglobin oxidation plays an important role in the haemolysis.[44] Pity the poor pheasant, its erythrocytes are more susceptible to lysis by H_2O_2 than are human ones, due to lower antioxidant defences.[45] Older erythrocytes in human blood contain a higher ratio of α-tocopherol to arachidonic acid residues than do younger ones, because the lipid content of the membrane decreases with age whereas α-tocopherol remains approximately constant.[46]

α-Tocopheryl radical is probably recycled to α-tocopherol in the membrane by cytoplasmic (or perhaps even extracellular) ascorbate. The NADH–cytochrome b_5 reductase can also recycle α-tocopheryl radical, *in vitro* at least. Ascorbate radical and dehydroascorbate (DHA) in the erythrocyte cytoplasm can be converted to ascorbate by GSH-dependent **dehydroascorbate reductase**,[47] although this activity is probably catalysed by glutaredoxin

and thioredoxin reductase (Section 3.11). Erythrocytes can take up DHA from plasma and convert it to ascorbate.[47] They can also reduce some extracellular electron acceptors, such as ferricyanide or ferricytochrome c, by the action of a transmembrane redox system. Electrons can come from NAD(P)H or from ascorbate in the erythrocyte cytosol. The function of this system is uncertain; one suggestion is that it participates in reducing ascorbyl radical generated in plasma.[47]

6.4.4 Erythrocyte peroxidation in health and disease

It is difficult to persuade red cells from healthy subjects to undergo lipid peroxidation; whether plasmalogens (Section 4.12.8) contribute to this is uncertain.[48] In the peroxide stress haemolysis test, some peroxidation can be measured (Table 5.11), as can the generation of oxidatively modified and cross-linked membrane proteins, but this test is a physiologically irrelevant insult to the cell (so no real need to pity the pheasant). Peroxidation of erythrocytes can also be induced by high levels of organic hydroperoxides, such as *tert*-butyl, or linoleic acid hydroperoxides. Figure 6.2 shows the **echinocytes** that can be produced under such conditions.

Susceptibility to lipid peroxidation is increased in erythrocytes from patients with several diseases, including thalassaemia (Section 3.15.5.3) and **sickle-cell anaemia**. Sickle-cell anaemia is an inherited defect in which a glutamate residue at position 6 in the haemoglobin β-chains is replaced by valine. The protein still binds O_2, but its deoxy form is unstable and tends to precipitate in the erythrocyte, interfering with its deformability and creating sickle-shaped cells (hence the name of the disease). The sickled cells can block capillaries, causing tissue ischaemia–reperfusion accompanied by increased production of ROS and RNS.[49] They haemolyse readily and are marked for destruction, leading to anaemia. Sickle-cell patients show elevated plasma XO activity, which generates $O_2^{\bullet-}$, forms $ONOO^-$, and worsens the problem.[49]

Unstable haemoglobins tend to precipitate on the erythrocyte membrane and may release haem and iron, setting the scene for site-specific, free-radical reactions that promote lipid peroxidation and damage to membrane proteins, decreasing 'deformability' even more.[50] Some other mutant haemoglobins impose oxidative stress on red cells by autoxidizing to produce $O_2^{\bullet-}$ faster than normal haemoglobin.[43] Infections can initiate haemolytic crises in carriers of unstable haemoglobins, possibly due to their faster oxidation and denaturation during the elevated body temperatures in fever.[51] Accelerated oxidation is also a problem with the isolated α- or β-chains that accumulate in thalassaemic patients (Section 3.15.5.3). Indeed, there has to be careful co-ordination of α- and β-subunit synthesis when haemoglobin is being made. An **α-haemoglobin stabilizing protein (AHSP)** transiently holds α-subunits and slows their oxidation and precipitation.[52] Knockout of AHSP in mice impairs erythropoiesis and produces red cells with increased oxidation and shortened lifespan.[52]

Erythrocytes undergo GSH oxidation and slow peroxidation when stored at 1 to 6°C in blood banks,[53] accounting for their finite 'shelf life'.

6.4.5 Glucose-6-phosphate dehydrogenase (G6PDH) deficiency

Almost 400 million people, principally in tropical and Mediterranean areas, have an inborn defect in the gene on the X chromosome that encodes G6PDH, the first enzyme of the pentose phosphate pathway. Indeed, G6PDH deficiency is the commonest human inborn error of metabolism. Different mutations cause variable decreases in enzyme activity in erythrocytes and elsewhere; rarely or never is all activity lost.[54] Indeed, complete loss may be embryonic lethal.[55] Often the mutations cause enzyme instability, which affects erythrocytes most because of their long lifespan and inability to replace proteins. Severe G6PDH deficiency can impair $O_2^{\bullet-}$ and $NO^{\bullet}$ production by phagocytes, perhaps explaining increased susceptibility to infections seen in some patients.[56] Humans are not alone in this problem; the African black rhinoceros can suffer from G6PDH deficiency, sometimes accounting for episodic, massive haemolysis in zoo animals.[57]

Deficiency of G6PDH sometimes accelerates oxidative damage to the erythrocyte membranes, but not usually enough to cause symptoms unless the rate of RS production in erythrocytes is increased, for example by certain drugs (Table 6.4). If H_2O_2 production exceeds the capacity of the residual enzyme to generate NADPH, then GSH/GSSG ratios fall and haemolysis may result, leading to anaemia and jaundice.[43,58] African-American patients with mild G6PDH deficiency have a tendency to worse outcome after severe injury, presumably due to lowered ability to tolerate injury-related ROS production (Fig. 9.1), and it has been suggested that low levels of G6PDH may predispose to the development of cardiovascular disease.[59]

6.4.6 Solutions: destruction

Erythrocytes can degrade oxidized haemoglobin and other abnormal proteins (e.g. H_2O_2-inactivated CuZnSOD), apparently by the 20S proteasome.[60] For haemoglobin, this 'solution' may be a problem if too much iron is produced (Section 6.4.1, point 3). An **oxidized protein hydrolase** enzyme that can remove damaged membrane proteins in red blood cells has also been described.[61]

Senescent erythrocytes are removed from the circulation and haemoglobin's iron recycled (Section 3.15.1). A **senescent cell antigen** (SCA) appears on the surface of old cells, binds immunoglobulin G and is then recognized by the Kupffer cells in the liver and sometimes by macrophages in the spleen, using 'scavenger' receptors, some of which also recognize oxidized LDL (Section 9.3.4).[62] In vitamin E-deficient animals, SCA appears earlier than usual (Section 3.20.2.8). This antigen arises by damage to the band 3 protein. Damage to this protein in other tissues (e.g. brain and lymphocytes) also generates the antigen.

6.5 Erythrocytes as targets for toxins
6.5.1 Hydrazines

Several agents cause haemolysis, including too much NO_2^- (Section 1.10.3). Two of the most

Table 6.4 Inborn deficiencies of erythrocyte enzymes in relation to drug and toxin-induced haemolysis

Abnormality	Prevalence	Usual clinical feature	Examples of drugs inducing haemolysis
Glucose-6-phosphate dehydrogenase deficiency (X-linked, recessive)	Common in patients in tropical or Mediterranean areas or their descendents, e.g. in African Americans	Some RBC damage is often detected in laboratory tests but severe haemolysis rare *in vivo*. Some patients show increased susceptibility to infections, but most do not.	Fava beans, furazolidone, nitrofurantoin, nitrofurazone, pamaquine, primaquine, sulphonamides. Sepsis may also provoke erythrocyte damage (*Am. J. Physiol.* **286**, H2118, 2004). Primaquine may cause damage by its conversion *in vivo* to 5-hydroxyprimaquine, which is readily oxidized in red cells (*J. Pharm. Exp. Ther.* **314**, 838, 2005).
Glutathione peroxidase (GPx1) deficiency	Rare	Usually none, occasionally severe haemolysis, infertility	Sulphonamides, nitrofurantoin
Glutathione reductase deficiency	Very rare, but lack of riboflavin in the diet can also decrease the activity (enzyme has FAD at the active site). The drug BCNU, used in cancer chemotherapy, is a powerful inhibitor of glutathione reductase and can cause erythrocyte damage	Often none, sometimes severe haemolysis, sometimes early cataract (Section 3.9.4)	Sulphonamides
Abnormal haemoglobins (e.g. Hb Torino, Hb Shepherd's Bush, Hb Peterborough, Hb Zurich)	Rare	Often some haemolysis seen related to protein instability; drug administration can cause a haemolytic crisis	Sulphonamides
Methaemoglobin reductase deficiency (autosomal recessive)	Rare	Can be severe, depends on type (Section 6.4.2)	Benzene derivatives, NO_2^-, antimalarials

Data are mostly taken from the article by Gaetani, GF and Luzzatto, L (1980) in *Pseudo-allergic Reactions. Involvement of Drugs and Chemicals*, Vol. 2 (Dukor, P *et al.*, eds), S Karger, Basle, Switzerland. Also see[43,58] and Section 3.9.4.

studied are **phenylhydrazine** and **acetylphenylhydrazine**.[35,48] Injection of them into animals causes haemolysis, and the bone marrow responds by putting immature erythrocytes into the circulation. Indeed **reticulocytes**, erythrocyte precursors, can be obtained for study by injecting animals with phenylhydrazine and removing reticulocyte-rich blood several days later. The animals suffer increased oxidative damage in the liver, however.[63]

Phenylhydrazine and its derivatives slowly oxidize in aqueous solution to form $O_2^{\bullet-}$ and H_2O_2, a reaction catalysed by transition metal ions. The first stages can probably be represented by the equations below, in which M^{n+} represents the metal ions and Ph the benzene ring (Fig. 6.4). A nitrogen-centred **phenylhydrazine radical** is formed.

$$Ph-NH-NH_2 + M^{n+} \rightarrow H^+ + Ph-NH-NH^\bullet$$
$$\text{phenylhydrazine radical}$$
$$+ M^{(n-1)+}$$

$$Ph-NH-NH^\bullet + O_2 \rightarrow H^+ + O_2^{\bullet-} + PhN=NH$$

Addition of SOD slows down oxidation.

However, the damage done by phenylhydrazine to erythrocytes is not prevented by SOD.[35] Methaemoglobin, acting as a peroxidase, oxidizes phenylhydrazine in the presence of H_2O_2. Oxyhaemoglobin also oxidizes phenylhydrazine, but H_2O_2 is not required. These oxidase and peroxidase reactions of haemoglobin form several radicals.

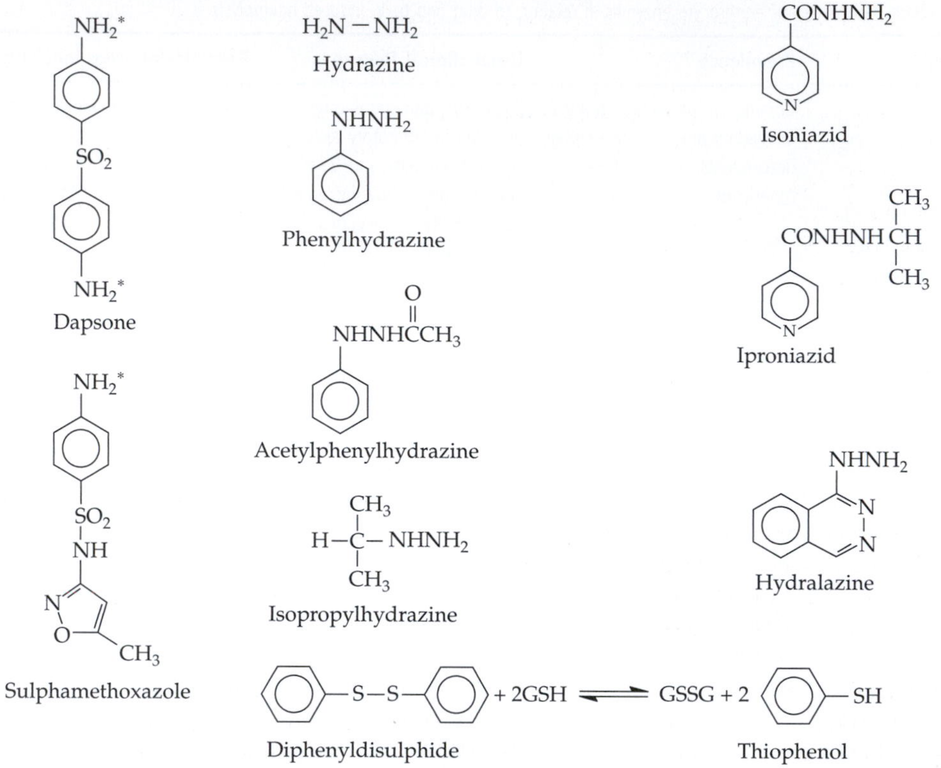

NH_2^*

SO_2

NH_2^*

Dapsone

NH_2^*

SO_2

NH

Sulphamethoxazole

H_2N-NH_2
Hydrazine

$NHNH_2$

Phenylhydrazine

O
‖
$NHNHCCH_3$

Acetylphenylhydrazine

CH_3
|
$H-C-NHNH_2$
|
CH_3

Isopropylhydrazine

$CONHNH_2$

Isoniazid

CH_3
|
$CONHNH\ CH$
|
CH_3

Iproniazid

$NHNH_2$

Hydralazine

Diphenyldisulphide $-S-S-$ + 2GSH ⇌ GSSG + 2 $-SH$ Thiophenol

Figure 6.4 Structures of some hydrazine and hydroxylamine-containing drugs. * $-NH_2$ groups that can be converted to hydroxylamines ($-NHOH$) *in vivo*.

$$Ph-NH-NH_2 \xrightarrow{\text{haemoglobin}} Ph-NH-NH^\bullet$$

$$\xrightarrow{\text{haemoglobin}} PhN=NH$$

$$PhN=NH + O_2 \longrightarrow Ph^\bullet_{\text{phenyl radical}} + O_2^{\bullet -}$$

$$+ N_2 + H^+$$

(via $PhN=N^\bullet$, **phenyldiazine radical**)

$$Ph^\bullet \xrightarrow{H^\bullet \text{ abstraction}} Ph-H \text{ (benzene)}$$

Hence end-products of the oxidation include benzene and nitrogen. The most damaging species seems to be phenyldiazine radical, which can denature haemoglobin to form intracellular precipitates (**Heinz bodies**) as well as deposits on the cytoskeleton and plasma membrane, causing eventual haemolysis. The haem group is converted into a green product; both cleavage of the ring and covalent binding of phenyl radicals to it occur. Some of the denaturation products of haemoglobin, as well as released iron, might catalyse OH$^\bullet$ formation. Indeed, when mouse erythrocytes are incubated with phenylhydrazine, there is a rapid release of 'catalytic' iron.[63] Lipid peroxidation plays little, if any, role in the haemolysis.[48]

Hydrazine derivatives are widely used in industry, as rocket fuels, and in medicine. Many can be oxidized, not only by haemoglobin but also by cytochromes P450. For example, **hydralazine** has been used to treat high blood pressure, but has several side-effects, and prolonged use can produce autoimmunity (lupus- and rheumatoid arthritis-like syndromes) (Section 9.10.6). Hydralazine is oxidized by haem proteins and transition metal ions to form $O_2^{\bullet -}$, H_2O_2, and nitrogen-centred radicals, which may participate in the side-effects.

The antituberculosis drug **isoniazid** (isonicotinic acid hydrazide) and the antidepressant **iproniazid** (Fig. 6.4) can similarly be oxidized, and the products again might contribute to their side-effects (also a risk of autoimmunity). Indeed, oxidation of isoniazid by a *M. tuberculosis* catalase–peroxidase enzyme (**KatG**) contributes to its antitubercular effect (since the oxidation product blocks an essential metabolic pathway), and mutations in this enzyme can result in isoniazid resistance.[64] Iproniazid can be metabolized in the liver to the hepatotoxic and haemolytic **isopropylhydrazine** (Fig. 6.4). Spin trapping with DMPO (Section 5.2.7) was used to identify haemoglobin thiyl radicals in the blood of iproniazid-treated rats.[65] An antioxidant used in the rubber industry, **N-isopropyl-N'-phenyl-p-phenylenediamine**, can cause oxidation and denaturation of haemoglobin (both free and in erythrocytes) about 40 times faster than phenylhydrazine.[35] Antioxidants designed by chemists are not always antioxidants in biological systems!

Hydroxylamine, NH_2OH, and its derivatives are used industrially, but can lead to haemolysis by oxidizing haemoglobin and causing free radical formation.[48,66] Similar reactions contribute to aniline toxicity (Section 8.6.9). Some drugs, such as **sulphamethoxazole** and **dapsone** (Section 6.12.1.3 below), are metabolized to hydroxylamines that may contribute to their side-effects (Fig. 6.4).[48]

6.5.2 Sulphur-containing haemolytic drugs[67]

Diphenyl disulphide administered orally to rats causes haemolysis. It can be reduced by GSH to thiophenol (Fig. 6.4), which is oxidized by oxyhaemoglobin to form methaemoglobin, $RS^\bullet$ radicals, $O_2^{\bullet-}$, and H_2O_2; all these species probably contribute to its haemolytic action. Garlic contains sulphur compounds that can be haemolytic under certain circumstances (Table 10.8).

6.5.3 Favism[58]

Many so-called 'haemolytic agents' have only minor effects when small doses are given to healthy animals. Greater effects can be seen in patients with inborn defects in erythrocyte defence mechanisms. For example, patients with G6PDH deficiency show little or no haemolysis normally, but it can be induced (often severely), by some drugs (Table 6.4) and by certain foods such as the broad bean, *Vicia faba*. *Vicia*-induced haemolysis, a condition known as **favism**, is common in certain Mediterranean countries such as Sardinia and Greece, in the Middle East and in parts of southeast Asia. Its distribution follows that of G6PDH deficiency, but not all patients deficient in the enzyme are sensitive to the bean, for unknown reasons.

Soon after ingesting the bean, the erythrocytes of susceptible patients show a rapid fall in $NADPH/NADP^+$ ratios and GSH levels. The chemicals in *V. faba* responsible for this are the pyrimidine derivatives, **vicine** and **convicine**, which are present at about 0.5% of the total weight of the bean. They are hydrolysed by β-glucosidase enzymes to give 'aglycone' products (Fig. 6.5) that react rapidly with O_2 to form both H_2O_2 and quinones. The quinones are re-reduced by GSH, leading to more H_2O_2 generation, haemoglobin oxidation and sometimes an increase in the 'catalytic' iron pool.[63]

Drugs that trigger haemolysis in G6PDH-deficient patients include the antimalarials **primaquine** and **pamaquine** (Table 6.4), again involving ROS production. Indeed, the **blackwater fever** observed in some troops given prophylactic antimalarials during World War II was probably related to G6PDH deficiency. The term 'blackwater' refers to the urinary discoloration produced by excretion of haemoglobin and its degradation products released from destroyed erythrocytes.

6.6 Bloodthirsty parasites: problems for them and for us

Several blood-dwelling parasites, including *Plasmodium* (Section 6.6.1 below), *Schistosoma* and *Angiostrongylus*, digest substantial quantities of haemoglobin, releasing haem and iron. Degradation occurs in a lysosome-type digestive vacuole. How do the parasites protect themselves against these potential pro-oxidants? One suggestion is

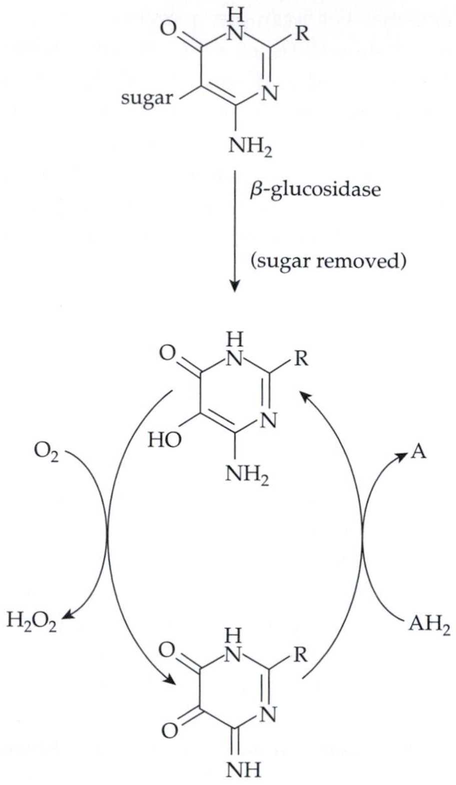

Figure 6.5 Compounds causing favism. Redox cycling of the aglycones derived from hydrolysis of convicine (R = OH) and vicine (R = NH$_2$) from *Vicia faba* seeds. The aglycone of convicine is called **isouramil**, that of vicine is called **divicine**. Diagram by courtesy of Prof. G Rotilio. AH$_2$ signifies a reducing system (such as GSH).

that, when dwelling in O$_2$-rich blood, they switch their metabolism to glycolysis, avoiding ROS production by aerobic respiration.[68] Some, including *Plasmodium*, lack haem oxygenase and convert the haem to a dark-brown insoluble aggregate (**haemozoin**, sometimes called **malaria pigment**) that is safely kept inside the digestive vacuole. These aggregates are not completely redox-inactive but less pro-oxidant than haem itself.[69] The antimalarials chloroquine and quinacrine (shown in Fig. 9.15) interfere with haem metabolism and have been suggested to cause a toxic build-up of haem that kills the malaria parasite.[70,71]

Bloodsucking insects have similar problems: they can consume several times their own weight in blood and digest it rapidly, loading the gut with

haem and iron. There is a rapid increase in ferritin in the gut to cope with this, and in the insect *Rhodnius prolixus* (an important vector of *Trypanosoma cruzi*) haemozoin is also produced there.[72] Haem also accelerates urate synthesis in this insect, perhaps as an antioxidant defence.[73]

6.6.1 Malaria, oxidative stress and an ancient Chinese herb

The prevalence of G6PDH deficiency, thalassaemia and sickle-cell anaemia in certain parts of the world has been suggested to be related to their ability to protect humans against malaria.[71] Deficiency of G6PDH in the black rhinoceros[57] may have similar advantages.

Malaria is caused by infection with protozoan parasites of the *Plasmodium* genus. Several species infect humans, but *P. falciparum* is the most virulent. Worldwide, malaria infects more than 500 million people, of whom over 1 million still die each year, and the problem of resistance to therapies is growing.[71] Malaria is transmitted by the bite of an infected female *Anopheles* mosquito, whereupon the parasites enter the subcutaneous tissue or a blood vessel, migrate to the liver, develop within hepatocytes and eventually leave to infect erythrocytes, wherein they proliferate and release progeny to infect new red blood cells. Infected red blood cells adhere to vascular endothelium and impair blood flow. Another mosquito sucks blood from the infected person, and the cycle repeats. *Plasmodium* must undergo a complex developmental cycle in the mosquito's salivary glands and midgut. Some *Anopheles* strains block the parasites' life cycle by enclosing it in a capsule in the midgut. Capsule formation involves tyrosine oxidation by ROS in the midgut, facilitated by the degradation of haemoglobin from the blood meal.[74] Sadly, other *Anopheles* strains don't use ROS in this useful fashion and transmit malaria to humans.

Evidence consistent with the 'malaria protection' hypothesis is provided by the observation that transgenic mice expressing the gene for the human β sickle-cell haemoglobin chain are protected against infection by murine *Plasmodium* species.[75] Studies in the south-western Pacific island of Espiritu Santo suggested increased incidence of a mild form of malaria, but decreased incidence of severe malaria in children with α-thalassaemia, a view supported by studies in Ghana and elsewhere.[76] But how does it work? Perhaps sickling of infected cells kills the parasite, and/or the abnormal haemoglobin cannot be digested properly. Or is it RS yet again? Malaria-infected erythrocytes seem to be under oxidative stress, showing significant lipid oxidation[77] and low GSH/GSSG ratios.[78] *Plasmodium* is readily damaged *in vitro* by systems generating RS, and by lipid peroxides, or cytotoxic aldehydes; although *P. falciparum* contains FeSOD, and GSH- and thioredoxin-dependent peroxide removal systems,[79] these may have limited activity.[80] Hence if oxidative stress were increased, for example by abnormal haemoglobins, without causing too much damage to the erythrocyte, the parasite might be killed. Increased formation of SCA (Section 6.4.6) by the combined pro-oxidant effects of parasitaemia and abnormal haemoglobin should also accelerate clearance of infected cells.

Consistent with this, inhibiting GSH synthesis with buthionine sulphoximine inhibited *P. falciparum* development in human red cells; malaria-infected red cells rapidly leak glutathione as GSSG, so it must be continually replaced.[78] Injection of alloxan (a ROS-producing agent; Section 8.5.1), phenylhydrazine, divicine or *tert*-butylhydroperoxide into malaria-infected mice killed the parasites.[81] The effects of alloxan or divicine were overcome by pretreatment of the mice with desferrioxamine, suggesting that ROS produced by these agents are interacting with iron (from haem degradation?) to kill the parasite.[81] A clinically important antimalarial agent that may act by imposing oxidative stress is found in a plant used in traditional Chinese medicine (Fig. 6.6). This compound, called **qinghaosu** or **artemisinin**, is a sesquiterpene endoperoxide. Desferrioxamine can interfere with artemisin action.[82]

Although chelating agents can, under some experimental conditions, protect malaria parasites against oxidative damage, they can also suppress parasite growth, by depriving them of iron. Growth of *P. falciparum* in isolated human erythrocytes is completely inhibited by only 30 μM desferrioxamine. However, this agent has not proved useful clinically.[83]

Some other protozoan parasites are sensitive to RS, a concept being exploited in drug design. *Trypanosoma brucei*, for example, cannot synthesize haem and lacks catalase. It can be killed by increasing intracellular ROS levels, for example by adding menadione (Section 8.6). The trypanothione/trypanothione reductase system (Section 3.12.1) is another target for drug intervention.

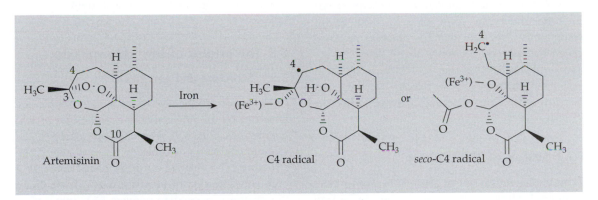

Figure 6.6 Structure of artemisinin. This drug was first isolated from *Artemisia annua* (sweet wormwood), an ancient Chinese herb (*quinghao*, the 'blue-green' herb) used for treatment of malaria. Written descriptions of the use of quinghao date back to 168 BC. The action of artemisinin involves interaction with haem and/or free iron to cleave the peroxide bridge, leading to haem modification and the generation of radicals that attack the parasite. One important target appears to be a parasite Ca^{2+}–ATPase that may be involved in regulating Ca^{2+} levels.[82] Artemisinin may also interfere with haemozoin formation (*Biochem. J.* **385**, 409, 2005). Several synthetic compounds with a similar endoperoxide bridge are being evaluated as antimalarials (e.g. see *Nature* **430**, 900, 2004). **Artemether** (a methyl ether) and **artesunate** (a sodium succinyl salt) are used in several countries. From *Nature* **424**, 887, 2003 by courtesy of Dr RG Ridley and the publishers.

Several ROS-producing nitro-compounds (Section 8.18) have antiparasite action.

6.7 Oxidation in plants: peroxides and phytoprostanes

Plants use peroxides and other RS (including $NO^{\bullet}$) for redox signalling and defence (Section 7.11) and expose themselves to high levels of these agents.[84–86] Nitric oxide may arise from nitrate reduction and/or from NOS-type proteins, which do not resemble animal NOS enzymes.[87] Indeed, rates of $NO^{\bullet}$ generation and basal levels of H_2O_2 and lipid hydroperoxides in plant tissues can be much higher than in animals.[84–89] Plants do not contain arachidonic acid, nor prostaglandins derived from it. However, some intermediates in the pathway of jasmonic acid biosynthesis (described in Fig. 7.20) are structurally similar to prostaglandin. The lack of arachidonic acid also means that plants do not make F_2-isoprostanes. However, non-enzymic oxidation of linolenic acid (the major PUFA in plants) can generate other isoprostanes (Fig. 6.7), for example the **phytoprostanes**, which arise from α-linolenic acid.[89] They have been detected in all plants analysed, often at high levels. Phytoprostane levels increase dramatically when plants are dried and stored, and they can be present in oxidized, plant-derived cooking oils.[89] Similar to other isoprostanes, phytoprostanes can form D_1-, E_1- and F_1-ring compounds. The D_1- and E_1- dinor isoprostanes can dehydrate and rearrange to J_1-, deoxy J_1-, A_1- and B_1-phytoprostanes (Fig. 6.8). Little is known as yet about their biological effects, but they may be involved in triggering defence responses (Section 7.11.1).

6.7.1 Sources of ROS in plants

Plant mitochondria can produce ROS, mainly from complex I. However, the rate appears to be kept low, both by uncoupling proteins (Section 1.10.6) and by an **alternative oxidase** system, a separate electron transport system that operates when the main one is over-reduced or inhibited.[90] Levels of plant uncoupling proteins may, like the animal ones, be increased[91] by $O_2^{\bullet-}$. Several oxidases in

plants generate H_2O_2, including peroxidases involved in lignification (Section 7.5.4) as well as amine, glycollate (Section 6.8.4 below) and oxalate oxidases; the last uses O_2 to oxidize oxalate to CO_2

$$\begin{array}{c} COOH \\ | \\ COOH \end{array} + O_2 \rightarrow H_2O_2 + 2CO_2$$

whereas plant amine oxidases contain copper and catalyse the reaction

$$RCH_2NH_2 + H_2O + O_2 \rightarrow H_2O_2 + NH_3 + RCHO$$

Several oxalate oxidases are manganese-containing proteins and some, for example the enzyme **germin**, found in the **apoplast** (the space between the leaf cuticle and the walls of the cells below it) show MnSOD activity *in vitro*.[92] Amine oxidases act on amines such as putrescine and spermidine (Section 4.12.9), which play important roles in plant growth and development and are involved in the response to pathogens (Section 7.11).

However, the biggest source of ROS in the light is the fundamental process that higher plants undertake in chloroplasts, photosynthesis. This process allows the authors and readers of this book to continue to live, providing both O_2 and food. Yet splitting water without destroying yourself is a fearsomely difficult process, since water is so stable. Indeed, that is one reason why there is so much of it on the planet. How is it done?

6.8 The origins of life: chloroplasts

6.8.1 Structure and genetics

Chloroplasts in the leaves of higher plants are bounded by an outer **envelope**, consisting of two membranes (Fig. 6.9). The envelope encloses the **stroma**, containing a complex internal membrane structure. The stromal aqueous phase contains a high concentration of proteins, most of which are the enzymes needed to convert CO_2 into carbohydrate by the **Calvin cycle**, a metabolic pathway requiring ATP and NADPH. The first enzyme in this cycle (**ribulose bisphosphate carboxylase**) catalyses reaction of the five-carbon sugar ribulose 1,5-biphosphate with CO_2 to form two molecules of phosphoglycerate.

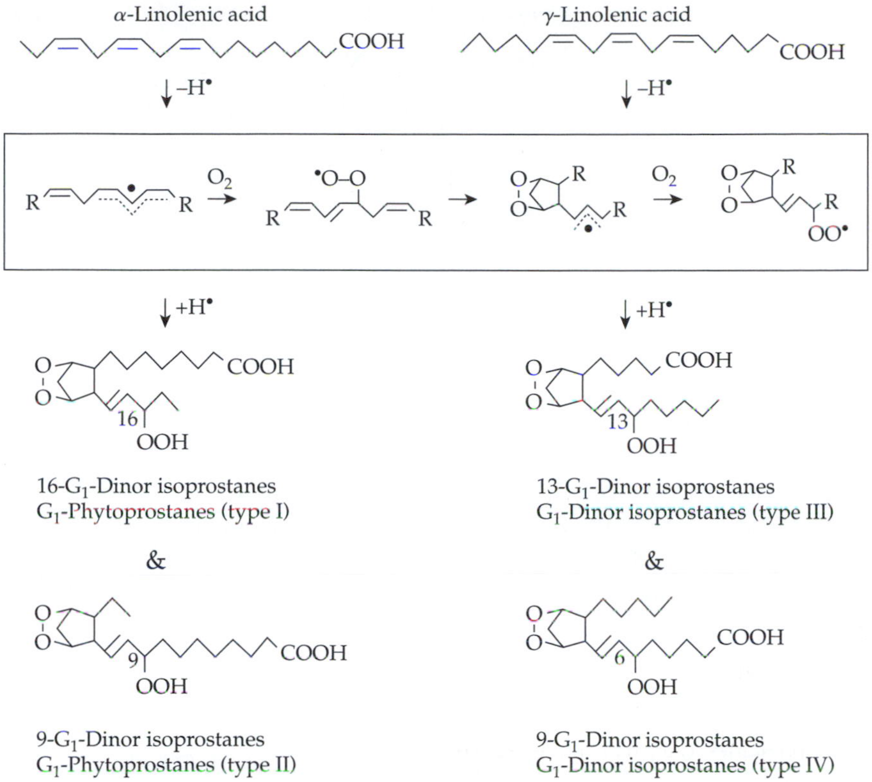

Figure 6.7 G_1-dinor isoprostanes in plants and mammals. Autoxidation and cyclization of α-linolenic acid (C18:3ω3) and γ-linolenic acid (C18:3ω6) yields structurally different G_1-dinor isoprostanes which can be classified with respect to the location of the side-chain hydroxyl group as 16-, 9-, 13- and 6-G_1-dinor isoprostanes or with reference to the ω-carbon as types I–IV G_1-dinor isoprostanes. Since α-linolenate is a major unsaturated fatty acids in plants and much less important in animals, the types I and II dinor isoprostanes have been termed **phytoprostanes**. From *Chem. Phys. Lipids* **128**, 135, 2004 by courtesy of Dr Martin Mueller and Elsevier.

The internal membrane structure of chloroplasts has two distinct features, regions of closely stacked membranes (**grana thylakoids**) interconnected by a three-dimensional network of membranes, the **stroma thylakoids**. Both contain photosynthetic pigments (chlorophylls *a* and *b*, green pigments that absorb light in the blue and red regions of the spectrum) together with **carotenes** and **xanthophylls** (yellow pigments absorbing blue light). The thylakoids produce the NADPH and, by the process of **photophosphorylation**, the ATP needed for the Calvin cycle and other chloroplast metabolic activities.

Chloroplasts contain DNA which encodes several proteins found in the thylakoid membranes, whereas most stromal proteins are encoded in the nucleus and imported when required. Among the proteins encoded in the chloroplast genome are the **D1** and **D2** proteins of photosystem II (Section 6.8.3 below), and the large subunit of ribulose bisphosphate carboxylase.

6.8.2 Trapping of light energy[93]

Absorption of light by chlorophyll causes electrons to move to higher energy states (**excited singlet states**). Blue light results in formation of a higher excited state than does red light, but this quickly loses its excess energy as heat, so that both red and blue light effectively produce the same first excited

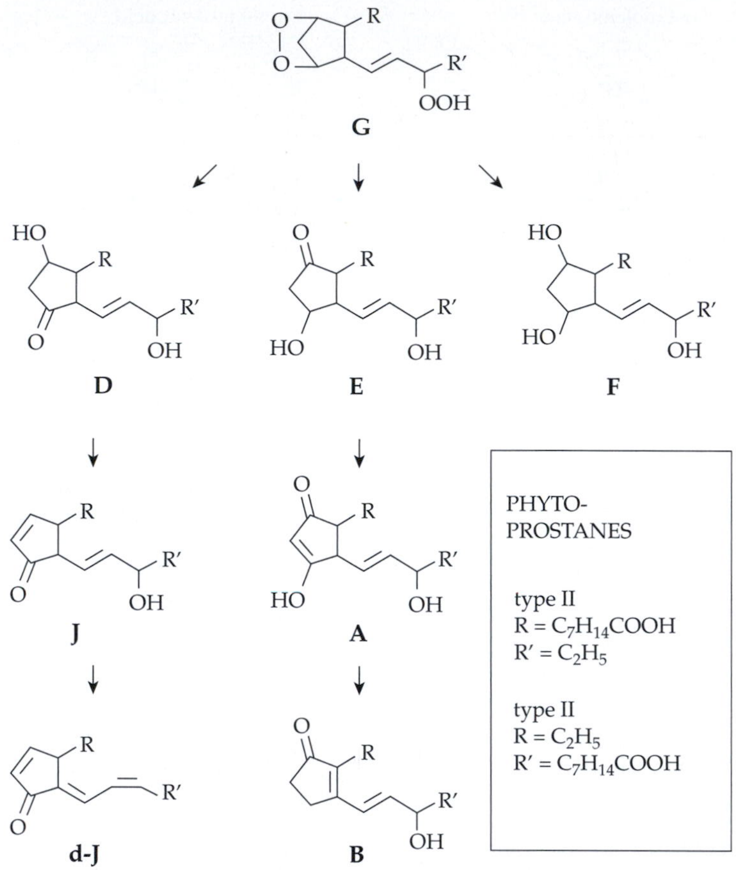

Figure 6.8 The phytoprostane pathway in plants. G_1-phytoprostanes rapidly decompose in aqueous solution. Non-enzymatic or enzymatic reduction of both peroxy groups yields stable F_1-phytoprostanes. In contrast, rearrangement of the endoperoxide group and reduction of the side chain hydroperoxy group of G_1-phytoprostanes yields D_1- and E_1-phytoprostanes which may dehydrate/isomerize to J_1- and deoxy-J_1-phytoprostanes or A_1- and B_1-phytoprostanes, respectively. From *Chem. Phys. Lipids* **128**, 135, 2004 by courtesy of Dr Martin Mueller and Elsevier.

state of chlorophyll. The excitation energy can be lost by re-emission of light to give **fluorescence**; it can be lost as heat (**thermal energy dissipation**) or it can be transferred to another molecule, for example an adjacent chlorophyll, the first molecule returning to the ground state, whilst the second becomes excited. The chloroplast carefully controls the distribution of energy between these three processes.

Special molecules of chlorophyll *a* in the thylakoid membrane (**reaction centre chlorophylls**) can, when excited, lose an electron to a neighbouring electron acceptor (A), producing a radical (chlorophyll$^{\bullet+}$ A$^{\bullet-}$) pair. This initial charge separation is the basic reaction of photosynthesis.

Light energy absorbed by other chlorophyll *a* or *b* molecules in the thylakoid membrane can be transferred to the reaction-centre chlorophylls, each of which is associated with a **light-harvesting array** of other pigment molecules that channel energy to it. Two different types of reaction centre contain two different forms of chlorophyll, known as **P700** and **P680**, each served by light-harvesting systems. The complexes containing P700 are called **photosystems I** (PSI) and those containing P680, **photosystems II** (PSII). Stroma thylakoids are rich in PSI whereas the stacked membranes are enriched in PSII.

Electrons ejected from the P680 chlorophyll of PSII pass to a **phaeophytin** *a* molecule and then to

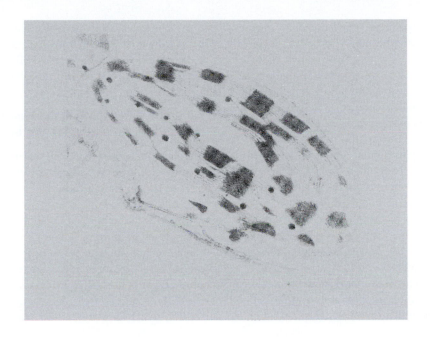

Figure 6.9 Top: electron micrograph of a chloroplast. Bottom: structure of chlorophylls.

acceptors Q_A (primary plastoquinone) and Q_B (secondary plastoquinone) (Fig. 6.10). Electrons then pass 'down' (i.e. to more positive reduction potentials) an electron transport chain that contains plastoquinone, plastocyanin and a cytochrome b–f complex, eventually entering PSI to replace the electrons lost on excitation of the P700 chlorophyll. Electrons ejected from PSI are transferred to chlorophyll, phylloquinone and then to an iron–sulphur cluster. They then pass to other iron–sulphur proteins bound to the membranes, and next to a soluble [2Fe–2S] iron–sulphur protein, **ferredoxin**. Reduced ferredoxin, in the presence of a reductase enzyme, converts $NADP^+$ to NADPH (Fig. 6.10, Plate 13). It also reduces thioredoxin (Section 6.8.10 below).

Alterations in the light-harvesting complexes can control the distribution of energy between PSI and PSII; a process which involves phosphorylation by a protein kinase activated by excess reduction of plastoquinone. When activated, it causes some redistribution of energy from PSII to PSI by realigning the light-harvesting complexes.[94]

6.8.3 The water splitting mechanism: a radical process and the reason for this book[93,95]

The electrons ejected from PSII reaction centres leave behind **chlorophyll radical cations** ($P_{680}^{\bullet+}$) that have a large positive reduction potential (greater than one volt). Electrons are replaced by the splitting of water, accompanied by O_2 evolution. The chemistry of water-splitting is complex and involves a cluster of four manganese ions and one Ca^{2+}. The radical $P_{680}^{\bullet+}$ oxidizes a tyrosine residue on the **D1 protein**, one of the two major protein constituents of the PSII reaction centre (the other is **D2**) to a tyrosyl radical, which in turn oxidizes the Mn_4Ca cluster.

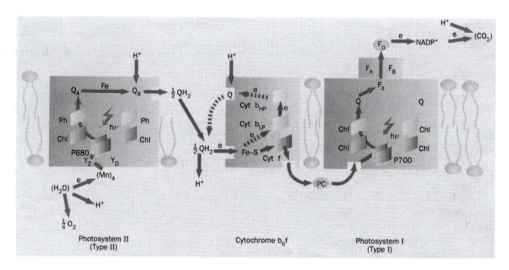

Figure 6.10 (see plate 13) The chloroplast electron transport chain. Reduction of plastoquinone (Q_A, Q_B, a quinone resembling ubiquinone) is driven by photosystems II, whereas photosystems I generate NADPH. Chl, chlorophyll a; Ph, phaeophytin a. The quinone (Q) in photosystem I is phylloquinone (a K vitamin; see Fig. 8.6 for more information). Fe, non-haem iron; F_X, F_A and F_B are iron–sulphur centres and F_D is ferredoxin. $(Mn)_4$, the cluster of four manganese ions involved in H_2O-splitting; Y_Z and Y_D are tyrosine residues, the former being on the main route of electron transfer. Y_D forms a tyrosyl radical during PSII operation, but is not directly involved in water splitting. Arrows show electron-transfer paths. Photosystems II and I are connected by the cytochrome b_6–f complex which oxidizes QH_2 (plastoquinol) and reduces a copper-containing protein, plastocyanin (PC). Because quinones can accept/donate two electrons/protons, the intermediate cytochrome complex accepts two electrons, one reducing an iron sulphur centre (Fe–S) and the other reducing a low potential b-type cytochrome (Cyt b_{LP}). The reduced Fe–S centre donates an electron to PC through a bound cytochrome f (Cyt f). The other electron participates in a quinone-dependent cycle involving high (Cyt b_{HP}) and low (Cyt b_{LP}) potential b-type cytochromes. As electrons flow from Q to PC, an electrochemical gradient (Fig. 1.8) is built up by proton movements and used to drive ATP synthesis from ADP and phosphate. Diagram adapted from *Nature* **370**, 33, 1994, by courtesy of Prof. Jim Barber and the publishers.

This cluster accumulates four oxidizing equivalents and enters increasingly higher oxidation states (sometimes called the S_1, S_2, S_3 and S_4 states) before water is split to O_2. Water binds to one Mn, which is oxidized to Mn(V), so that the ligated oxygen remaining after deprotonation of water can be attacked by the oxygen of the other water, which is bound to Ca^{2+} (Fig. 6.11).

6.8.4 What problems do green leaves face?

Green leaves, and especially their chloroplasts, are prone to oxidative damage for several reasons.[96]

1. Their internal O_2 concentration in the light will be greater than 21%, because O_2 is produced by PSII.
2. Lipids in the chloroplast envelope and thylakoids contain a high percentage of PUFA residues (mostly linoleate and linolenate), and are thus susceptible to peroxidation.
3. If the light energy absorbed by the chloroplast is not transferred efficiently to the reaction-centre chlorophylls, or lost as heat or fluorescence, **intersystem crossing** of the singlet state to the **triplet state** may occur. The triplet state can, in turn, transfer energy to O_2 to form singlet O_2, a powerful oxidant for chloroplast PUFAs.

Unlike humans, plants cannot go indoors if the sun gets too hot and they have to cope with any light they are exposed to. If too much energy is absorbed in relation to the demand for $NADP^+$, NADPH may pile up, the electron transport chain slows down and the reaction-centre chlorophylls may not be able to dispose of all their excitation energy. Hence singlet O_2 formation should increase. For example, in PSII $^1O_2$ could oxidize chlorophylls and damage proteins (especially D1). The D1 protein can be replaced (Section 6.8.10 below) but if it is damaged too quickly for replacement to keep up, inhibition of photosynthesis (**photoinhibition**) can occur. Damage to PSII proteins can liberate metal ions able to catalyse $OH^•$ formation, adding to the damage.[97]

4. The electron transport chain of chloroplasts can 'leak' electrons to O_2, a reaction favoured by the high O_2. Isolated illuminated thylakoids slowly take up O_2 in the absence of added electron acceptors, a process first observed by A.H. Mehler, and often called the **Mehler reaction**. One source of $O_2^{•-}$ is the reduction of O_2 to $O_2^{•-}$ by the electron acceptors of PSI. Addition of ferredoxin increases O_2 uptake, since it is rapidly reduced by PSI and reduced ferredoxin can, in turn, reduce O_2 (Fig. 6.12)

$$Fd_{red} + O_2 \rightarrow O_2^{•-} + Fd_{ox}$$

In vivo, however, reduced ferredoxin passes electrons on to $NADP^+$ via ferredoxin–$NADP^+$ reductase. If the supply of $NADP^+$ is limited, the rate of electron flow along pathway C (Fig. 6.12) should be decreased, and more $O_2^{•-}$ might be made by routes B and A. Superoxide can also result from direct reduction of O_2 by the electron acceptors of PSII (reduced pheophytin or Q_A), and can contribute to $OH^•$ production by Fenton chemistry in PSII at high light intensities.[97]

5. Oxygen has a direct effect on ribulose biphosphate carboxylase. The intermediate formed when the enzyme acts on ribulose bisphosphate can react

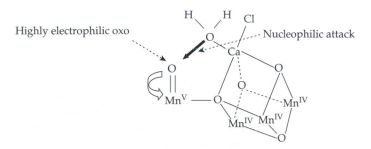

Figure 6.11 A possible water-splitting mechanism in PSII. From *Curr. Opin. Struct. Biol.* **14**, 447, 2004 by courtesy of Prof. Jim Barber and the publishers. Other mechanisms have been proposed (e.g. *Science* **310**, 1019, 2005).

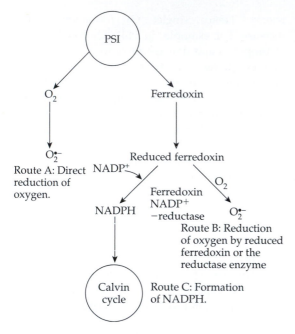

Figure 6.12 Routes of electron flow from reduced photosystem I (PSI). Reduced ferredoxin reduces oxygen to $O_2^{\bullet-}$ as well as passing electrons on to $NADP^+$. The electron acceptors of photosystem I can themselves slowly reduce O_2 to $O_2^{\bullet-}$. Electrons might also escape from the ferredoxin–$NADP^+$ reductase enzyme.

not only with CO_2, but also with O_2 (Fig. 6.13). Instead of forming two molecules of phosphoglycerate, this **oxygenase** activity of the enzyme forms one phosphoglycerate and one phosphoglycollate. The latter is hydrolysed to glycollate and further metabolized by a series of reactions known as **photorespiration**. The first step is **glycollate oxidase**, a peroxisomal enzyme that generates H_2O_2

$$\begin{array}{c} CH_2OH \\ | \\ CH_2OH \end{array} + O_2 \longrightarrow \begin{array}{c} CHO \\ | \\ CH_2OH \end{array} + H_2O_2$$

glyoxylate

If the catalase in peroxisomes fails in its job, glyoxylate can react non-enzymatically with H_2O_2, being oxidized to formate (Section 3.18.2). This may happen *in planta* under some circumstances. Usually, glyoxylate is further metabolized enzymatically, eventually forming CO_2. As a result of photorespiration, CO_2 previously fixed into the Calvin

cycle is released and has to be refixed, using more energy.

Luckily, the affinity of the carboxylase for CO_2 is so much greater than for O_2 that carboxylation is greatly favoured even at 21% O_2 and 0.03% CO_2, normal air levels. However, if O_2 is elevated and/ or CO_2 depleted, CO_2 fixation into the Calvin cycle is decreased and CO_2 loss by photorespiration increases. At some O_2/CO_2 ratio, a point is reached at which the leaf no longer achieves net CO_2 fixation, so plant growth stops. At higher O_2/CO_2 ratios there can be net loss of carbon from the plant as photorespiration exceeds CO_2 fixation, a lethal situation if continued for too long. Ribulose bisphosphate carboxylase is also a frequent target of oxidative damage in plants, as judged by protein carbonyl formation.[98]

6. Superoxide formed in chloroplasts can dismute to H_2O_2 non-enzymatically or by the action of SOD (Section 6.8.7.1 below). If peroxisomal catalase cannot cope with all the H_2O_2 generated by glycollate oxidase, some may escape and diffuse into chloroplasts. Hydrogen peroxide inactivates at least two Calvin cycle enzymes, **fructose bisphosphatase** and **sedoheptulose bisphosphatase**, apparently by oxidizing thiol groups essential for catalytic activity. Several iron-containing proteins in chloroplasts (e.g. cytochromes) could conceivably be damaged by excess H_2O_2, with release of 'catalytic' iron ions, although ferredoxin is resistant to H_2O_2.

7. Many higher plants produce photosensitizers, often to deter predators.[99] For example, marigolds produce **α-terthienyl** (Fig. 6.14), apparently as a 'photodynamic insecticide'. Plants can photosensitize themselves if not careful, or can be attacked in the same way. For example, *Cercospora* fungi attack a range of crops by producing **cercosporin** (Fig. 6.14). This generates singlet O_2 and other ROS in the presence of light to damage plant cell walls and allow fungal entry. The fungus is resistant to cercosporin and other photosensitizers; why is unknown[100] although a role for fungal pyridoxine (vitamin B_6) as a $^1O_2$ scavenger has been suggested.[101]

8. Hydrogen peroxide generated by PSII can form $OH^{\bullet}$ by Fenton chemistry,[97] but little else is known about the availability of metal ions 'catalytic' for

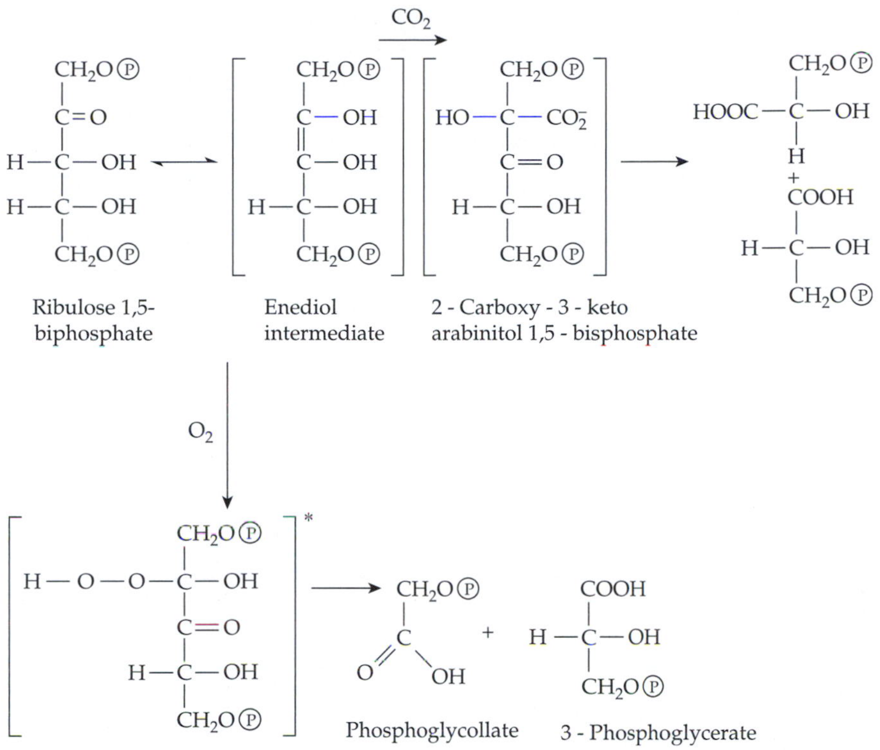

Figure 6.13 Oxygenase and carboxylase activities of ribulose biphosphate carboxylase, the first enzyme of the Calvin cycle. The peroxyketone (*) can decompose in a minor side reaction to generate H_2O_2 (*FEBS Lett.* **571**, 124, 2004).

free radical reactions in chloroplasts. Such iron could arise by H_2O_2-dependent breakdown of haem proteins (point 6 above). Chloroplasts often contain ferritin (**phytoferritin**)[102] from which $O_2^{\bullet-}$ could conceivably mobilize some iron. Ferritin levels in plants are increased by several stresses, including ozone and iron overload.[103]

6.8.5 Solutions: minimizing the problem[96]

We described photorespiration as a problem, but it could also be a solution; it may help to ensure that at high light intensity some CO_2 is always available, causing a demand for NADPH and preventing over-reduction of the electron transport chain. The phosphorylation process that alters the alignment of the light-harvesting complexes (Section 6.8.2) may also help alter electron transport from its normal mode, producing O_2, to one of cyclic electron flow around PSI.[94]

Carotenoids are not only light-harvesting pigments; they have an important antioxidant role. First, they quench singlet O_2 rapidly and scavenge many RS (Section 3.21.3). Second, they can absorb energy from the chlorophyll triplet states that would otherwise lead to singlet O_2 formation. Lutein and zeaxanthin (Section 6.8.6 below) are especially important, being intimately involved in the efficient transition of light harvesting complexes from an 'energy transfer to reaction centres' mode to an 'energy dissipation' mode.[94,104]

Considerable evidence supports this antioxidant role of carotenoids in plants.[96] For example, illumination of mutant plants unable to synthesize carotenoids causes rapid bleaching of chlorophylls and destruction of chloroplast membranes. Similar destructive effects are seen in normal plants if carotenoid biosynthesis is inhibited by certain herbicides, including **aminotriazole** (also a catalase inhibitor; Section 3.7.3), **pyriclor** and **norflurazon**.

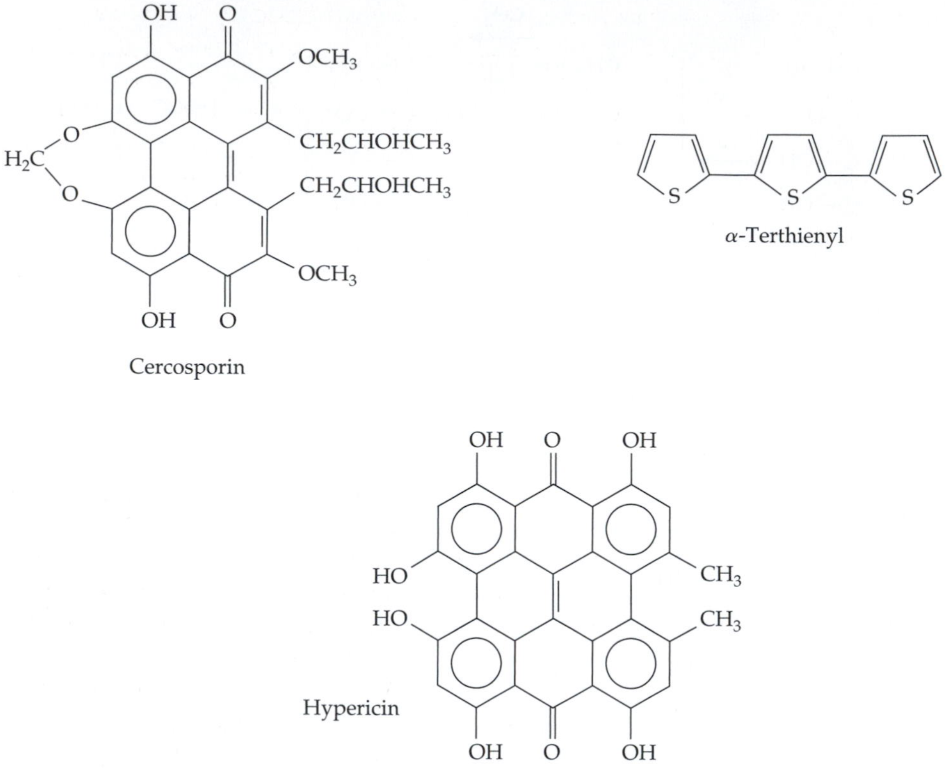

Cercosporin

α-Terthienyl

Hypericin

Figure 6.14 Structures of some plant-derived photosensitizers. Diagram from *Active Oxygen in Chemistry*, Vol. 2, 1995, by courtesy of Dr Chris Foote and Blackie Academic and Professional Publishers.

The *Dunaliella* group of green algae accumulate large amounts of β-carotene, both all-*trans* and 9-*cis*-β-carotene, apparently to protect against photodamage. Indeed, this alga has been used as a source of β-carotene for dietary 'nutritional supplements'.

6.8.6 The xanthophyll cycle[94]

This cycle (Fig. 6.15) functions to raise the level of zeaxanthin when needed. Under normal conditions, zeaxanthin is converted to **violaxanthin**, which does not dissipate energy well. Epoxidation of zeaxanthin to violaxanthin, via the intermediate **antheraxanthin**, is an O_2-dependent reaction that occurs in the thylakoids under both light and dark conditions. When there is excess light, the sequence is reversed; de-epoxidation is an ascorbate-dependent process that occurs only in the light, apparently because the de-epoxidase enzyme is located on the inner side of the thylakoid membrane and only functions at the low pH generated there when a proton gradient (Fig. 6.10) is established across the membrane. The accessibility of violaxanthin to the de-epoxidase also appears to be increased by light-dependent conformational changes in the membrane. Zeaxanthin can quench both $^1O_2$ and chlorophyll excited states and may be strategically located in the thylakoids to do this. It then rapidly loses the energy as heat. Zeaxanthin can also inhibit lipid peroxidation in chloroplast membranes. Thus a mutant of the green alga *Chlamydomonas* lacking both lutein and zeaxanthin underwent extensive lipid oxidation and loss of photosynthetic capacity at high light intensities. The lack of either carotenoid alone impaired growth, but was not lethal.[105]

6.8.7 Solutions: antioxidant defence enzymes control, but do not eliminate, reactive species

6.8.7.1 *Superoxide dismutases*[106]

Superoxide is capable of reducing plastocyanin (Section 2.5.3.2) and chloroplast cytochromes, but the significance of this *in vivo* is uncertain. Most, if not all, $O_2^{\bullet-}$ formed in plants is probably disposed of by SODs. Chloroplasts usually contain CuZn-SOD, some of which is bound to the thylakoids, and the rest free in the stroma, at concentrations up to 30 µM. Plants often also have one or more cytosolic (and sometimes peroxisomal) CuZnSODs. Copper is delivered to these proteins by a copper chaperone (Section 3.2.1).[107] There have been reports of MnSOD in chloroplasts, although the possibility of contamination of isolated chloroplast fractions by other organelles must be considered, since plant mitochondria and peroxisomes contain MnSOD. Leaf FeSOD, present in some plants (e.g. *Brassica campestris*, tomato, *Ginkgo biloba* and *Arabidopsis thaliana* leaves) is usually largely or entirely located in the chloroplast.

6.8.7.2 *Removal of hydrogen peroxide*

Most of the H_2O_2 produced by illuminated chloroplasts seems to arise from $O_2^{\bullet-}$. Like other CuZnSODs (Section 3.2.1.6), the chloroplast enzyme is slowly inactivated on prolonged exposure to H_2O_2, and FeSOD is even more sensitive (Section 3.2.5.1). Some Calvin cycle enzymes are rapidly inactivated by H_2O_2 (Section 6.8.4). Thus it is essential that the chloroplast removes H_2O_2.

How does it do this? Catalase is not present; leaf catalase is located in peroxisomes and helps dispose of the H_2O_2 generated by glycollate oxidase. This role is illustrated by the properties of a barley mutant deficient in peroxisomal catalase; it would not grow well at low CO_2 levels (favouring photorespiration), but grew normally at high CO_2.[108] The chloroplast also lacks selenoprotein GPx activity (indeed selenoprotein GPx enzymes are rare or absent in plants). In some plant species, GPx-like activity has been identified in chloroplasts and cytoplasm, and genes similar to those encoding GPxs in animals (most commonly resembling PHGPx genes) occur in several plant

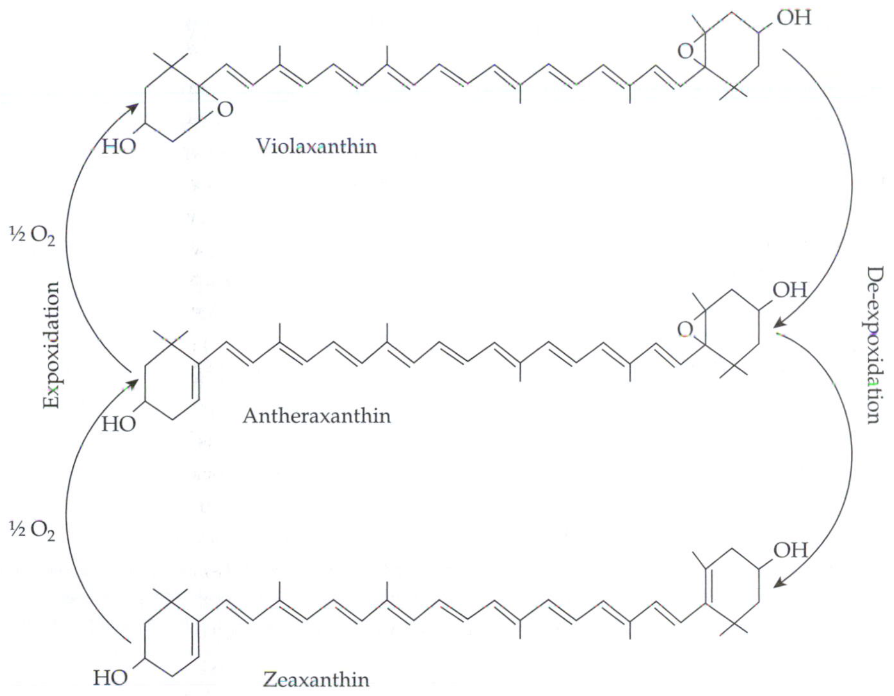

Figure 6.15 The xanthophyll cycle.

genomes.[109] Plant GPxs have cysteine rather than selenocysteine at the active sites, which decreases their catalytic activity as compared with seleno-protein GPx enzymes. Indeed, at least some of the plant enzymes may prefer thioredoxin to GSH as a substrate.[110] Glutathione-S-transferases, present in many plants,[111] can reduce organic hydroperoxides, but the physiological significance of this is uncertain.

A major chloroplast H_2O_2-metabolizing enzyme is **ascorbate peroxidase** (Section 3.13.7). In chloroplasts it is present in both stromal and thylakoid-bound forms; it is also found in the cytosol and in other plant organelles. Oxidized ascorbate can be regenerated by GSH (in the **ascorbate–glutathione cycle**) or by NAD(P)H or reduced ferredoxin (Fig. 6.16). Peroxiredoxins and thioredoxins (Section 6.8.10 below) may also play a key role in removal of H_2O_2 in chloroplasts and other parts of the plant.[112]

6.8.7.3 *Redox signalling*

Although it is important to minimize H_2O_2 levels in chloroplasts, plants in general accumulate higher levels of peroxides than animals (Section 6.7), both for defence and redox signalling. Examples of the latter include controlling light harvesting by regulating kinase activity and hence phosphorylation (Section 6.8.2), and signal-ling to the nucleus to control expression of genes

encoding chloroplast proteins. For example, ROS are involved in signalling to increase the syn-thesis of carotenoids in the fungus *Neurospora crassa* when it is exposed to light.[113] Our knowledge of the precise role of ROS in signal-ling is scanty, but the thioredoxin system is often involved.[114]

6.8.8 Ascorbate and glutathione

The stroma contains 1 to 5 mM GSH, and ascorbate at concentrations up to 25 mM. The ratios of reduced to oxidized forms (GSH/GSSG and ascorbate/dehydroascorbate) are normally high under both light and dark conditions. One reason for this may be because exposure of ascorbate peroxidase to H_2O_2 in the absence of ascorbate inactivates this enzyme.[115] Ascorbate and GSH might also act as RS scavengers in chloroplasts, for example millimolar ascorbate could contribute to removal of $O_2^{\bullet-}$. As in animals, GSH is involved in a range of processes in plants, including cell differentiation, detoxi-fication of xenobiotics and flowering.[116] It can also lead to protein glutathionylation, reversible by glutaredoxin (Section 3.9.6).

Apart from some dry seeds, ascorbate is pres-ent in all parts of plants, including the apo-plast.[114,117] The millimolar levels in the apoplast may help remove oxidizing toxins such as $NO_2^{\bullet}$

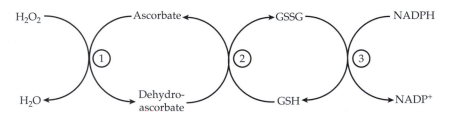

Figure 6.16 The ascorbate–glutathione cycle in chloroplasts. Enzymes involved: 1, ascorbate peroxidase; 2, dehydroascorbate reductase (reaction 2 can also occur non-enzymically at high pH—the pH of the stroma during photosynthesis may rise to as high as 8, due to formation of the proton gradient); 3, glutathione reductase. The first product of oxidation of ascorbate by ascorbate peroxidase is semidehydroascorbate (SDA); two SDA radicals can undergo disproportionation to form ascorbate and dehydroascorbate. NAD(P)H-dependent and ferredoxin-dependent mechanisms for reducing SDA also exist in chloroplasts. Indeed **monodehydroascorbate reductase** is the only type of enzyme known to use an organic free radical as a substrate. Thylakoid-bound ascorbate peroxidase can scavenge H_2O_2 as it is produced, and the resulting SDA can be reduced by electrons from photosystem I. The cycle shown above has been called the Foyer–Halliwell–Asada cycle after the names of the two scientists who first proposed it and the third who did much to establish evidence for its occurrence. However, this name ignores the contribution of Groden and Beck, who discovered ascorbate peroxidase in chloroplasts. The cycle also operates in plant mitochondria (*J. Biol. Chem.* **278**, 46869, 2003), the root nodules of leguminous plants (Section 6.8.11) and the intestines of some insects (Section 6.2.2.2).

and O_3 (Section 6.9.3 below) before they reach the underlying leaf cells. Ascorbate in the central vacuoles of leaf cells may co-operate with phenols to remove H_2O_2 (Section 3.22.2). As in animals, ascorbate in plants is involved in several metabolic processes, including hydroxylation of proline in cell wall proteins, and it is a precursor of oxalate and tartrate in some plants[117] as well as participating in the xanthophyll cycle (Fig. 6.15). **Ascorbate oxidases**, copper-containing enzymes that convert ascorbate to SDA whilst reducing O_2 to H_2O, are found in many plant tissues. They have usually been isolated from fruits and vegetables (squash, melon, cucumber, pumpkin etc.), where they are mainly associated with cell walls. Their function is uncertain, although a role in promoting cell wall growth has been postulated.[117] However, in some plants (such as tobacco) ascorbate oxidase can be present in the apoplast, and may help to regulate ascorbate levels there.[118]

Whereas the last step of ascorbate synthesis in animals generates H_2O_2 (Section 3.20.1), that in higher plants does not; most ascorbate arises from a pathway in which GDP-D-mannose is converted via GDP-L-galactose into L-galactono-1, 4-lactone. This is oxidized to L-ascorbate by **L-galactono-1,4-lactone dehydrogenase**, located on the outer side of the inner mitochondrial membrane and donating electrons to cytochrome c. This enzyme can be inhibited by the alkaloid **lycorine**.[117]

6.8.9 Plant tocopherols

Whereas non-green plant tissues contain a mixture of tocopherols, often γ-tocopherol predominating (Section 3.20.2.3), thylakoid membranes are enriched in α-tocopherol (indeed it is synthesized in the chloroplast).[119] It can inhibit lipid peroxidation (ascorbate could presumably regenerate tocopheryl radicals) and scavenge singlet O_2, although its role in the latter is thought to be less important than that of the carotenoids,[94] since α-tocopherol deficiency does not affect growth of *Arabidopsis* under normal light conditions.[120] However, this may be a premature conclusion, since levels of ascorbate and GSH in the mutant plant are increased, presumably to help compensate. Toco-

pherylquinone, a product of the reaction of tocopherol with singlet O_2 and other ROS (Fig. 3.29) has been detected in chloroplasts, and levels increase during illumination.[96] *Arabidopsis* mutants lacking violaxanthin de-epoxidase accumulated more α-tocopherol, further illustrating the likelihood of cross-compensation between antioxidant defence systems when one is missing.[120] However, in *Chlamydomonas* treated with the herbicide **pyrazolynate** to block α-tocopherol biosynthesis, illumination caused accelerated loss of α-tocopherol, D1 protein and PSII activity.[121]

As is the case for animals (Section 3.20.2.9), tocopherols in plants may not serve *only* as antioxidants. γ-Tocopherols may help plants to resist RNS such as $NO_2^{\bullet}$ from polluted air (Section 6.9.3 below). Tocotrienols are a major component of vitamin E in seeds of several plants, such as rice, oats, wheat and palm; genetic manipulation has been used to obtain plants that over-produce tocopherols and/or tocotrienols.[119]

The reduced form of plastoquinone (**plastoquinol**) can, like ubiquinol (Section 3.18.5), scavenge peroxyl radicals and inhibit lipid peroxidation *in vitro*.[122] Whether this occurs *in planta* is uncertain.

6.8.10 Solutions: repair and replacement

A large part of chloroplast protein synthesis in the light is devoted to replacing the D1 protein in photosystem II.[123] This protein is destroyed rapidly by singlet O_2 and other ROS and the inactive D1 is removed by proteinases associated with photosystem II.

Chloroplasts can repair some oxidative damage. DNA repair enzymes are present, the most important being **photolyases** that cleave UV-induced pyrimidine dimers (Section 4.10.1), since DNA damage by UV light is a major threat to plants.[124] Chaperones in chloroplasts assist protein folding, including their refolding after partial denaturation. Chloroplasts have several types of thioredoxin,[114] and reduced thioredoxin can reactivate several enzymes inactivated by ROS, such as the oxidized forms of fructose and sedoheptulose bisphosphatases. Thioredoxin is also involved in peroxiredoxin action and in regulating the activity of Calvin cycle and other chloroplast enzymes by thiol–disulphide interchange.

Methionine sulphoxide reductases, also thioredoxin-linked, are present in chloroplasts and cytoplasm to remove oxidized methionine residues.[125] The disulphide forms of thioredoxins in chloroplasts are reduced by **ferredoxin-dependent thioredoxin reductase**, a [4Fe–4S] enzyme.

Different thioredoxins are present in other plant organelles (mitochondria, endoplasmic reticulum and cytosol) and there the thioredoxin reductase is NADPH-dependent (as in animal tissues) rather than ferredoxin-dependent.

6.8.11 The special case of the root nodule

Some leguminous plants use symbiotic bacteria in root nodules to fix nitrogen (Section 1.2.1). The leghaemoglobin present keeps O_2 levels low, but is a potential threat because it can oxidize to generate $O_2^{\bullet-}$ as well as react with H_2O_2 to give ferryl species and/or to release iron (Section 3.15.3).[126] Nodules are rich in antioxidant defences, including GSH, CuZn-SOD, MnSOD, sometimes FeSOD, ascorbate, catalase, thioredoxins, and (sometimes) homoglutathione (Section 3.12) and they operate the ascorbate–glutathione cycle (Fig. 6.16). They also contain ferritin.

Eventually, nodules undergo senescence, as do we all. Antioxidant defences fall, leghaemoglobin degrades, 'catalytic' iron levels rise and oxidative damage increases (at least in soybean nodules, although maybe not in all other plants).[126,127] It would be interesting to find out which is the initiating event.

6.9 Plants as targets for stress and toxins

6.9.1 Inhibition of electron transport and carotenoid synthesis[96]

Many herbicides (e.g. **diuron** (DCMU) and **atrazine** [Fig. 6.17], which bind to the D1 protein of photosystem II) act by inhibiting the chloroplast electron transport chain. This stops light-dependent generation of ATP and NADPH and thus CO_2 fixation. Carotenoid destruction, chlorophyll bleaching, and membrane peroxidation occur subsequently, probably caused by excess singlet O_2 resulting from blocked energy dissipation.

Herbicide inhibitors of carotenoid biosynthesis have similar effects (Section 6.8.5).

The **diphenylether** herbicides (e.g. **oxyfluorfen**; Fig. 6.17) also damage plants by generating singlet O_2 and other ROS, resulting in lipid peroxidation and other oxidative damage. They act in a different way, by inhibiting the enzyme **protoporphyrinogen oxidase** in mitochondria and chloroplasts, leading to accumulation of the photosensitizer protoporphyrin IX;[128] a plant version of porphyria (Section 2.6.4.3), perhaps.

6.9.2 Bipyridyl herbicides

The bipyridyl herbicides **paraquat** and **diquat** are useful because they kill a range of weeds, but do not accumulate in soil, being destroyed by various microorganisms.[129] 'Bipyridyl' means that that the structure contains two pyridine rings, aromatic rings in which a carbon atom is replaced by nitrogen. The rings may be joined by their number-2 carbon atoms, or by their number-4 carbon atoms (the nitrogen counting as atom number 1), to give 2,2'-bipyridyl or 4,4'-bipyridyl respectively. The prime is used to indicate an atom in the second ring. In paraquat, a methyl group is attached to each nitrogen; its full chemical name is **1,1-dimethyl-4,4'-dipyridylium ion** (Fig. 6.17). In diquat, the two nitrogen atoms are joined by an ethylene group, to give **1,1'-ethylene-2,2'-dipyridylium ion**. Paraquat is usually manufactured as a chloride salt, diquat as a bromide.

4,4'-Bipyridyl compounds form coloured products upon reduction. Indeed, several such compounds, under the general name **viologens**, have been used for this reason to study redox reactions. Hence paraquat is sometimes called **methyl viologen**. The colour is produced by one-electron reduction to form a radical that has a characteristic ESR spectrum, and absorbs visible light (λ_{max} in the visible range is at 603 nm for paraquat). The added electron delocalizes over both rings with partial neutralization of the positive charge on each nitrogen atom.

6.9.2.1 Redox cycling[129]

Many years ago, it was observed that the killing of green plants by paraquat or diquat is accelerated

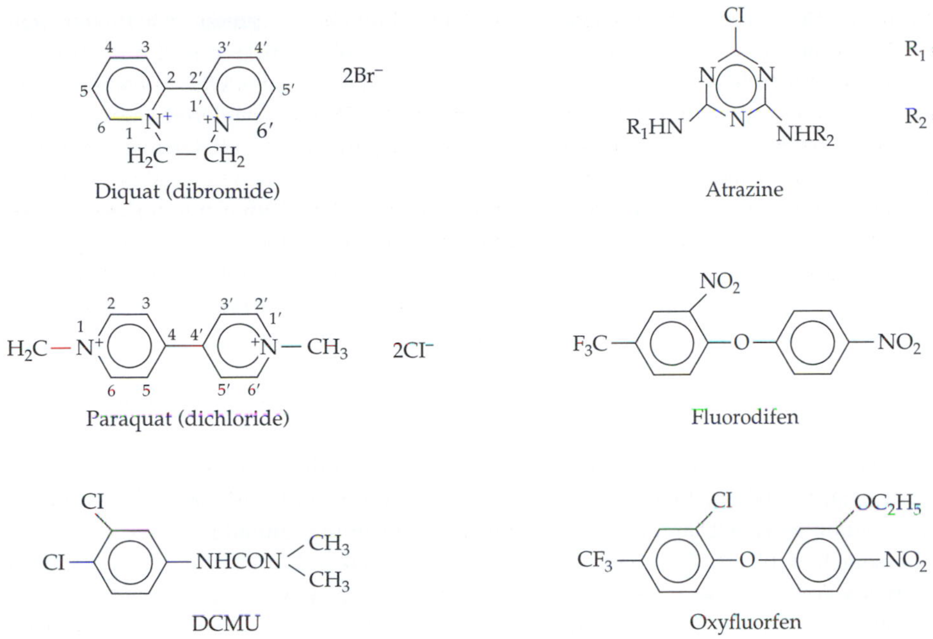

Figure 6.17 Structures of some herbicides.

by light, but slowed if O_2 levels are decreased by flushing with nitrogen. Later work showed that paraquat and diquat can cross the chloroplast envelope. Once inside, they accept electrons from the Fe–S proteins associated with PSI and also from the flavin at the active site of ferredoxin–NADP$^+$ reductase (Fig. 6.10), and are reduced to bipyridyl radicals. These radicals can be identified in paraquat-treated chloroplasts by their absorbance or ESR spectra if O_2 is absent. When O_2 is present however (as it usually is in chloroplasts!) the radicals disappear because they react fast with it. If BP^{2+} is used to represent a bipyridyl herbicide, the reactions are

$$BP^{2+} \xrightarrow[\text{chain}]{\text{electron transport}} BP^{\bullet+}$$

$$BP^{\bullet+} + O_2 \longrightarrow BP^{2+} + O_2^{\bullet-}$$

($k_2 = 7.7 \times 10^8$ M^{-1}s^{-1}, for paraquat)

Thus treatment of illuminated chloroplasts with paraquat or diquat leads to a rapid uptake of O_2 as they are continuously reduced and reoxidized to

generate $O_2^{\bullet-}$ in a **redox cycle**. Hence bipyridyl herbicides are examples of **redox-cycling** agents (Section 8.6).

Much of the $O_2^{\bullet-}$ will be converted into H_2O_2 by chloroplast SOD, and H_2O_2 can be dealt with by the ascorbate–glutathione cycle and peroxiredoxins. However the latter are susceptible to oxidation at high H_2O_2 levels (Section 3.11.1). In paraquat-treated chloroplasts, the load of H_2O_2 is such that GSH and ascorbate are quickly oxidized, inactivation of Calvin cycle enzymes occurs, and CO_2 fixation stops (Table 6.5). An additional reason for inhibition of CO_2 fixation is that diversion of electrons to the herbicides decreases the supply of NADPH for the Calvin cycle, and for glutathione reductase.

Inhibition of CO_2 fixation is followed by membrane damage and leakage of ions from the leaves, and lipid peroxidation. Electron microscopy reveals deterioration involving breakdown of thylakoids and eventually of other membranes, including the membrane surrounding the central vacuole of the plant cell. This vacuole contains hydrolytic enzymes, and often accumulates organic acids to a high concentration, so release of its contents into the rest of the cell will potentiate damage. Paraquat also causes oxidative protein damage.[130] For example, in paraquat-treated pea leaves there was rapid inactivation of several mitochondrial proteins, especially glycine decarboxylase, possibly by the action of end-products of peroxidation such as HNE.[131]

6.9.2.2 *Evidence that ROS are important in paraquat toxicity*

Much evidence supports a role for ROS in the damage to plants caused by bipyridyl herbicides. Some strains of ryegrass[132] are comparatively resistant to paraquat even though they still take it up, and their leaves contain more SOD and catalase than the leaves of sensitive plants. By contrast, tobacco plants with lowered catalase were more sensitive.[133] Although leaf catalase is located in peroxisomes, excess H_2O_2 might diffuse across the chloroplast envelope into the peroxisomes for removal. Potato plants overexpressing CuZnSOD were more resistant to paraquat,[106] as were *Arabidopsis* plants overexpressing ascorbate peroxidase[134] or methionine sulphoxide reductase[125] or tobacco plants overexpressing catalase, ascorbate peroxidase, MnSOD or FeSOD in the chloroplast.[135,136] The protective effects of SODs, ascorbate peroxidase or catalase suggest that $O_2^{\bullet-}$ and H_2O_2 are both involved in paraquat toxicity. Is this

via $OH^{\bullet}$? Probably; expressing a fungal gene in tobacco chloroplasts that raised the intrachloroplast mannitol (a putative $OH^{\bullet}$ scavenger) concentration to ~ 100 mM rendered the plants less sensitive to paraquat.[137] Desferrioxamine protects pea (*Pisum sativum*) leaves against damage by paraquat, consistent with a role for iron.[138] Such a role is supported by the increased paraquat resistance of tobacco plants overexpressing ferritin.[102] Indeed, the DMSO method (Table 5.4) detected $OH^{\bullet}$ in paraquat-treated plants.[139]

Paraquat and diquat are also toxic to non-green plant tissues. For example, they cause membrane damage in fungi such as *Aspergillus niger* and *Mucor hiemalis*. If this is due to redox cycling, how are the bipyridyl radicals formed? Several flavoproteins, including glutathione reductase,[140] can reduce paraquat and/or diquat; the herbicides take electrons from the flavin ring. Similar reactions can account for the (slowly developing) toxicity of paraquat to leaves in the dark. Indeed, tobacco plants expressing chloroplast MnSOD were more resistant to paraquat in the dark. However, increased resistance was also observed if MnSOD was overexpressed in the mitochondria, suggesting that 'dark' paraquat reduction can involve enzymes (e.g. glutathione reductases) present in both organelles.[135,136]

A major disadvantage of bipyridyl herbicides is that they poison animals, an action also mediated by ROS (Section 8.4).

Table 6.5 Effects of paraquat on illuminated spinach chloroplasts

Time after paraquat addition (min)	[GSH] (mM)	[GSSG] (mM)	GSH/GSSG ratio	[Ascorbate] in reduced form (mM)	Fructose bisphosphatase activity (U/mg chlorophyll)
0	6.5	0.25	26	13	62
2	3	3.2	0.9	8	20
5	3.1	1.5	2.1	6	8
10	3.0	0.8	3.8	4	0

Spinach-leaf chloroplasts were isolated and treated with paraquat in the light. The stromal contents of GSH, GSSG and ascorbate were measured, as was the activity of fructose bisphosphatase, an enzyme essential to the Calvin cycle. GSSG levels rise rapidly but some then disappears, possibly by glutathionylation of proteins. Such rapid changes are not seen if paraquat is added to darkened chloroplasts, since the electron transport chain is not active to reduce paraquat. Data selected from *Biochem. J.* **210**, 899, 1983 by courtesy of the Biochemical Society. Falls in ascorbate can allow the inactivation of ascorbate peroxidase.[115]

6.9.3 Environmental stress: air pollutants (ozone, sulphur dioxide, nitrogen dioxide)

Worldwide, ozone may cause more damage to crops and forests than any other air pollutant. Exposure of plants to O_3 causes direct oxidation of proteins and lipids (Section 2.6.5), aldehyde formation, lipid peroxidation, and DNA damage (e.g. levels of 8OHdG in chloroplast DNA rise if beans or peas are exposed to high levels of O_3).[141] Ozone can trigger the hypersensitivity response (Section 7.11.1), which, if not properly controlled, can cause serious damage. If the plant does control it however, it can paradoxically lead to the development of tolerance not only to O_3 but also to other toxins and to pathogens (Section 7.11.1). For example, limited exposure to O_3 can induce resistance to tobacco mosaic virus in tobacco plants and to *Pseudomonas syringae* in *Arabidopsis*.[142]

Antioxidants play a key role in the ability of plants to resist oxidizing air pollutants such as O_3 and nitrogen dioxide ($NO_2^\bullet$). Developing tolerance to O_3 can involve increased synthesis of ascorbate, GSH, catalase, phenolic compounds, methionine sulphoxide reductase,[125] ascorbate peroxidase, and glutathione reductase; indeed, tobacco plants low in catalase were more sensitive[133] to O_3 whereas they were more resistant if overexpressing MnSOD in the chloroplast.[106] The first 'line of defence' may be ascorbate in the apoplast, since ascorbate reacts fast with O_3. Indeed, lowering apoplastic ascorbate levels increased the sensitivity of *Arabidopsis* and tobacco plants to O_3.[143] Interestingly, different **vtc mutants** (for 'vitamin C') of *Arabidopsis* deficient in different enzymes of the ascorbate biosynthetic pathway showed variable increases in sensitivity to O_3 even though they lowered leaf ascorbate to about the same extent.[144] Levels of leaf antioxidants vary with leaf age and also seasonally,[106] and so pollution resistance can similarly vary. Another relevant compound may be **isoprene** (C_5H_8; **2-methyl-1,3-butadiene**), which is produced in the chloroplasts of several plants. Blocking its synthesis increases leaf damage by O_3. Whether it scavenges O_3 directly or exerts indirect effects is uncertain.[145] Isoprene, like many alkenes, reacts quickly with singlet O_2 and O_3.

Nitrogen dioxide is pro-oxidant (Section 8.11.2) and additionally contributes to the **acid rain** that is devastating trees in several countries. Acid rain damages plants both by its low pH, and by converting insoluble compounds of toxic metals in the soil (e.g. aluminium) into soluble metal ions that can be absorbed by the plant. Ascorbate and tocopherols help plants resist $NO_2^\bullet$. Thus, ascorbate readily reduces $NO_2^\bullet$ to NO_2^- (Section 3.20.1) and γ-tocopherol reacts with $NO_2^\bullet$ to form a nitro adduct (5-nitro-γ-tocopherol).[146] Stored grain in silos has been claimed to sometimes generate high levels of $NO_2^\bullet$ that can be scavenged by γ-tocopherol.

Sulphur dioxide can damage plants.[96] This toxic reducing gas dissolves in water to form sulphites and bisulphites, which can oxidize to generate $O_2^{\bullet-}$, sulphur-containing radicals, and H_2O_2 (Section 8.11.3). Hence antioxidants help protect against SO_2 toxicity. For example, growth of the alga *Chlorella* in the presence of sulphite raised SOD levels and rendered it more resistant to paraquat.[147] Similarly, a paraquat-resistant strain of *Conyza boriensis* (with elevated SOD) is more tolerant to SO_2 than the wild type, whereas the vtc1 mutants of *Arabidopsis* are more sensitive.[148]

6.9.4 Environmental stress: heat and cold

Exposure of leaves, or isolated chloroplasts, to high light intensities causes photoinhibition; photosynthesis slows down and the chloroplast is damaged. Photoinhibition is especially severe if illumination is performed in the absence of CO_2. Excessive loss of the D1 protein, due to damage by ROS faster than D1 can be resynthesized, is a key event. Catalase may also be inactivated at high light intensities.[149]

One major factor affecting the sensitivity of plants to photoinhibition is the extent to which they can alter the conformation of light harvesting complexes to switch them to an 'energy dissipation' mode, which is in turn partially related to their levels of carotenoids and xanthophyll cycle enzymes. Indeed, in hot dry summers (or icy winters with high light intensity; see below), many evergreen plants dissipate almost all of the energy they absorb.[94] High light intensity is often accompanied by heat and/or drought stress, and plants can respond by raising levels of chaperones and antioxidant defences such as α-tocopherol and the ascorbate–glutathione cycle.[150] Expression of a thermostable superoxide reductase enzyme (Section 3.3) in tobacco cells rendered them more resistant to heat,[151] suggesting involvement of $O_2^{\bullet-}$ in heat sensitivity. Isoprene production may also be somewhat protective. Plants can also be stressed by exposure to high salt levels, and apoplastic ascorbate may help to protect.[118]

At the other extreme, many temperate plants show depressed photosynthesis after exposure to low temperature for one or more days (**chilling injury**; Fig. 6.18, Plate 14). This probably initially involves changes in membrane structure as the lipids 'freeze' below their transition temperature, fluidity is decreased and electrons cannot pass properly through their normal paths. In addition, decreased activity of Calvin cycle enzymes at low temperature reduces the demand for NADPH. Chilling injury affects photosystem II via damage to D1, and ROS again play a role. For example, a strain of *Chlorella* resistant to chilling injury showed greater SOD activity than did a sensitive strain; increasing its SOD activity by pretreating *Chlorella* with paraquat conferred increased resistance to chilling.[152] Hydrogen peroxide accumulation and oxidative protein damage were observed in cold-exposed maize leaves.[130] Transgenic tobacco plants expressing pea CuZnSOD in the chloroplast (so raising total chloroplast CuZnSOD) are more resistant to chilling injury, as are transgenic cotton plants expressing MnSOD in the chloroplast (Fig. 6.18). By contrast, antisense 'knockdown' of catalase in tomato plants increased their susceptibility to chilling injury.[153]

Water deprivation induces oxidative stress in plants, frequently lowering SH/disulphide ratios and increasing oxidative protein damage.[154] Once antioxidants such as GSH are severely depleted on prolonged desiccation, the plant may be unable to recover.[154] In some species, there is an adaptive response involving increased levels of antioxidants such as SOD, thioredoxin, α-tocopherol, carotenoids and ascorbate peroxidase.[155] Transgenic alfalfa (*Medicago sativa*) plants overexpressing MnSOD tolerated water deficit better,[156] as did

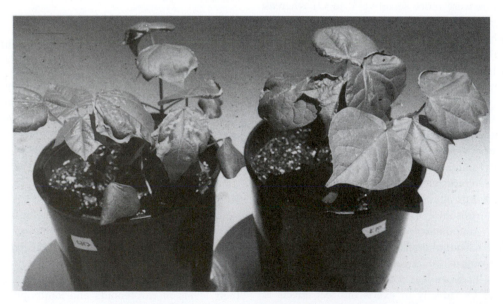

Figure 6.18 (see plate 14) Transgenic cotton plants that express chloroplast-localized MnSOD have increased tolerance to chilling-induced oxidative stress. Plants grown to the four-leaf stage in a growth chamber at 28 °C day and 15 °C night were exposed to chilling temperatures of 15 °C day and 4 °C night for 5 days. Immature leaves of wild-type cotton plants were visibly damaged (left), whereas those of transgenic cotton plants had no visible damage (right). Photograph from *Plant Physiol.* **107**, 1049, 1995 by courtesy of Dr R.D. Allen and *Plant Physiology*.

tobacco plants overexpressing catalase.[135] Chilling or water stress in pea plants causes lipid peroxidation and inactivation of mitochondrial glycine decarboxylase,[131] an effect resembling that of paraquat treatment (Section 6.9.2.1). The ability of many seeds to resist drying for long periods can involve accumulation of high levels of certain sugars, antioxidant defences (including thioredoxin)[157,158] and other protective proteins. Seed germination also involves ROS (Section 7.11.2).

Paradoxically, not only drought but also waterlogging can cause oxidative stress in plants. Submerged parts of plants may become hypoxic. Upon re-exposure to the air an 'ischaemia–reperfusion damage' involving excess ROS production can occur (Section 9.5.9).

6.9.5 Coral reef bleaching and toxic algal blooms: examples of plant-dependent oxidative stress?

Production of RS may be contributing to the degradation of the world's coral reefs. Many coral reef invertebrates accommodate endosymbiotic dinoflagellates (**zooxanthellae**) within their cytoplasm; the zooxanthellae photosynthesize and provide nutrients for their host and receive protection in return. However, the host has to suffer the O_2 production. If UV exposure and temperature rise, too many RS can be made, which can result in **coral bleaching**, death of the symbiont and degradation of its photosynthetic pigments. Damage to the host results, both by oxidative stress and by lack of nutrients.[159]

Overgrowth of certain unicellular marine organisms resulting from excess nutrients due to water pollution can result in the death of fish. The organisms produce toxins that attack the gills, causing the fish to die of anoxia. One of these toxins appears to be H_2O_2 and/or other ROS; this has been demonstrated in the toxic red tide planktons *Chattonella marina* and *Karenia mikimotoi*, which have killed many fish around Japan.[160]

6.10 The eye

The eye (Fig. 6.19) combines problems of lung (the cornea is exposed to 21% O_2), erythrocytes (long-lived proteins in the lens) and chloroplasts (the risk of damage by too much light). We already described **retinopathy of prematurity** (ROP) in premature babies (Section 1.5.3), but further problems arise at the other end of the age spectrum. One is **macular degeneration** (Section 6.10.1.1 below). Another is **cataract**, defined as a clinically significant opacity of the lens. These two account for most cases of blindness in the world. More than 17 million people worldwide are blind from cataract, and in the USA cataract removal is the most frequently performed surgical procedure on old people.

The outward-facing side of the lens is covered by a layer of metabolically highly active epithelial cells that undergo division, elongation and development to form the **lens fibres**, which synthesize the major proteins of the lens, the **crystallins**.[161] These account for about 90% of the soluble protein of the lens fibres and there are three main classes (**α-, β-** and **γ-crystallins**) in mammalian eyes. Newly formed fibres push the older ones towards the centre of the lens to form the **lens nucleus**. New fibre production is rapid in young animals, but soon decreases to a low constant level for the remainder of the lifespan. Thus the inner region of the lens is the oldest part. The nucleus, mitochondria and other organelles are lost during fibre maturation as the fibres become more transparent, so that fully differentiated lens fibres, which comprise a large proportion of the lens in adult animals, can no longer synthesize proteins to replace damaged ones. The lens epithelium actively transports Na^+ out of the lens, and K^+ into it, using an Na^+, K^+ATPase enzyme.[161]

6.10.1 What problems does the eye face?

1. The cornea is exposed to the 21% O_2 of ambient air, and to any pollutants and irritants in the air.
2. The lens contains photosensitizers of singlet O_2 formation, and too much light can thus damage and cross-link lens proteins. For example, UV light degrades tryptophan to *N*-formylkynurenine (Fig. 4.31), which sensitizes singlet O_2 formation (by contrast, some other tryptophan derivatives are protective; Section 6.10.2.1 below).[162] Lens proteins, especially the crystallins, have a long turnover time

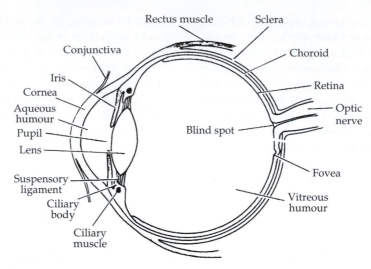

Figure 6.19 Structure of the mammalian eye. The **sclera** is a tough fibrous coat, inside which is the **choroid layer** containing a network of blood vessels that supply food and O_2 to the eye. The choroid is highly pigmented with melanin. The **aqueous humour** is a watery fluid whereas the **vitreous humour** is more jelly-like. Pressure of these fluids outwards on the sclera maintains the shape of the eye. Any marked variation in the pressure of the humours can alter blood flow in the eye. For example **ocular hypertension** (too much pressure) can restrict blood flow and cause ischaemic damage (Section 9.5.8); **glaucoma** is the name of a group of diseases in which this occurs and has been associated with increased oxidative DNA damage (*Arch. Ophthalmol.* **123**, 458, 2005) and protein nitration. Another contributor to glaucoma (and to retinal damage by ischaemia–reperfusion) is the release of excess glutamate and subsequent excitotoxicity (Section 9.16.4; *Am. J. Pathol.* **163**, 1997, 2003). The cornea, lens and conjunctiva obtain nutrients and O_2 by diffusion from the aqueous humour—they contain no blood vessels. The **lens** is suspended in position by ligaments and covered by a collagenous capsule. The **retina** contains neurones specialized to recognize light. These photoreceptors are of two types, **rods** and **cones**. The light-absorbing material in rods and cones is an aldehyde, **11-*cis*-retinal** attached to proteins called opsins, giving **rhodopsin**. Upon exposure to light, 11-*cis*-retinal isomerizes to all-*trans*-retinal, falls off the protein, and must then be reconverted to this *cis* form (Fig. 6.20). 11-*cis*-Retinal is synthesized from vitamin A. Only the cones are sensitive to coloured light, but the rods are more responsive to dim light (hence the diminished perception of colour as light intensity decreases). The **macular region** (*macula* in Latin means 'spot' or 'stain'), about 6 mm diameter in humans, is the area of greatest visual acuity. It surrounds the **fovea**, a depression in the middle of the retina highly enriched in cones. In humans and other primates, the macular region is yellow because of the presence of lutein and zeaxanthin.

and so damage is cumulative. Their normal organization maintains the transparency of the lens: denaturation, oxidation and aggregation decrease transparency. To some extent, α-crystallin may act as a 'chaperone', helping to protect the other crystallins from thermal insult and oxidative cross-linking.[161]

Thus prolonged exposure to sunlight or other UV sources (or to ionizing radiation) is a risk factor for cataract. Indeed, proteins isolated from cataractous lenses contain elevated amounts of such oxidative damage products as methionine sulphoxide, tryptophan degradation products, *meta*-tyrosine, *ortho*-tyrosine, L-DOPA, and leucine hydroxide.[163] Cataractous lenses show elevated H_2O_2 but decreased GSH levels.[164] The hyperglycaemia of diabetes (Section 9.4) can lead to

glycation and oxidation of lens proteins, which contributes to diabetic cataract. A major component of normal and diabetic cataractous lenses is glucosepane (Fig. 9.10).

3. The vitreous humour (Fig. 6.19) contains hyaluronic acid. This can be depolymerized by $OH^•$, causing loss of viscosity (Section 9.10). Normal H_2O_2 levels in lens have been estimated by some as 20 to 30 μM, but other scientists have challenged the validity of the assays used, and the possibility of *post mortem* H_2O_2 generation in eyes must not be ignored. A more realistic value may be around 1 μM normally, higher in cataract.[164] Nevertheless, even these levels of H_2O_2 can generate sufficient $OH^•$ to cause damage if metals are present to allow Fenton chemistry. Indeed, introduction of iron ions or haem proteins into the eye leads to retinal and lens damage (sometimes sufficient to cause blindness)[165]; this can happen as a result of penetration by iron objects or by haemorrhage. The potential of iron to cause damage is further illustrated in mice lacking caeruloplasmin or hephaestin (Section 3.15.1); they suffer retinal iron overload followed by retinal degeneration.[165] Metal ion availability may also increase as a result of tissue damage, as in maculas undergoing degeneration[166] and in cataractous lenses.[167]

4. Lens epithelial cells are readily damaged by peroxides, showing DNA strand breakage and abnormalities of ion transport, e.g. damage to the Na^+, K^+ATPase.[164,168]

5. The retina has a high rate of O_2 uptake because of the intense energy demand for both neurotransmission and the synthesis and recycling of molecules involved in vision (Fig. 6.20). Even brief ischaemia can lead to irreversible vision damage. However, a high rate of O_2 uptake may equate to a high rate of ROS production. The lipids present in the membranes of retinal rods and cones (Fig. 6.19) contain a high percentage of PUFA side-chains, especially of docosahexaenoic acid (DHA), and are thus highly susceptible to peroxidation. Indeed, F_2-isoprostanes are present in an esterified form in human retina[169] and aqueous humour,[170] although F_4-isoprostanes do not appear to have been measured. Sadly, the 'visual pigment' rhodopsin and its product A2E (Fig. 6.20) readily sensitize formation of singlet O_2, and photoreceptor outer segments contain rhodopsin alongside the highest DHA level of any cell in the human body.[171] Hence exposure of isolated retinas or animal eyes to high light intensities induces lipid oxidation. Retinal proteins can also be oxidatively damaged, both by peroxidation products such as HNE and by direct photooxidative damage. One important target is **ABCR**, a transporter involved in the recycling of all-*trans*-retinal.[172]

Lipid peroxides are also increased in the retina after exposure of animals to elevated O_2 or to ionizing radiation, and injection of preformed lipid peroxides into eyes causes severe retinal damage.[173] Deficiencies of selenium and α-tocopherol in the diet of rats cause loss of PUFAs and

accumulation of fluorescent products in the retinal pigment epithelium.[174]

6.10.1.1 *Macular degeneration, lipofuscin and singlet oxygen*

Age-related macular degeneration (deterioration of the retina around the macular region) is the leading cause of permanent blindness in the elderly in advanced countries (e.g. over 1.6 million persons in the USA suffer advanced macular degeneration). There is atrophy of the **retinal pigment epithelium** (RPE), a layer of cells between the photoreceptors of the retina and the choroid capillary network.

The RPE supplies the retina with O_2 and nutrients (which pass through it from the capillaries) and phagocytoses worn out photoreceptor membranes, that are constantly shed and replaced. Indeed, RPE cells may be the most active phagocytes in the healthy human body. The RPE often accumulates a yellow pigment (**lipofuscin**) with age. Its formation begins when all–*trans*-retinal reacts non-enzymically with phosphatidylethanolamine followed by further reactions, including oxidation, to generate products that cause light-dependent (absorption maximum at 425 nm) injury to the RPE by promoting oxidative damage and lysosomal destabilization. These events occur in the photoreceptor outer segments if all-*trans*-retinal is formed faster than it can be recycled to 11-*cis*-retinol (i.e. at high light levels). The final product (**N-retinylidene-N-retinylethanolamine**, or **A2E**) accumulates in lysosomes of the RPE after phagocytosis of rod/cone membranes, forming a major component of lipofuscin. Oxidative damage to the ABCR protein makes things worse,[172] a concept illustrated by patients with **Stargardt's disease**. They have a defective ABCR, accumulate pigment in the RPE at an early age and suffer accelerated onset of macular degeneration. The A2E chromogen not only sensitizes singlet O_2 formation, but can also react with it to form epoxides that are directly cytotoxic to RPE cells, inducing oxidative DNA damage.[175]

Degeneration of the RPE leads to the death of its associated rods and cones. The defective RPE can no longer absorb waste products, resulting in

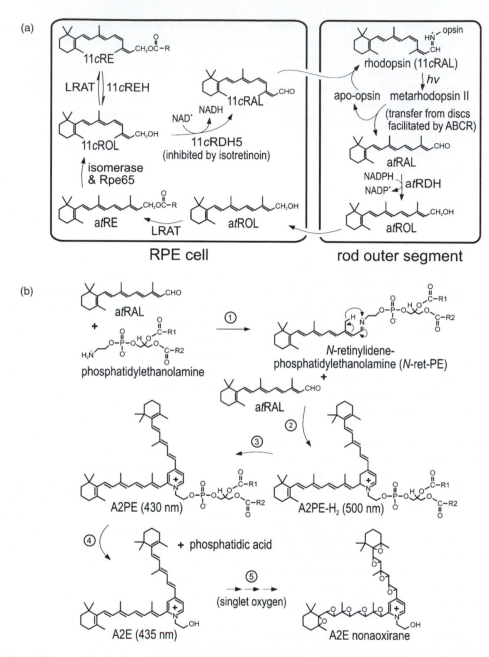

Figure 6.20 (a) *The normal visual cycle mediating rhodopsin regeneration.* Absorption of light (*hv*) by rhodopsin in a rod outer segment disk induces photoisomerization of the 11-*cis*-retinal (11cRAL) chromophore, yielding activated metarhodopsin II. After several seconds, metarhodopsin II decays to yield apo-rhodopsin and free all-*trans*-retinal (atRAL). The ABCR transporter accelerates removal of *at*RAL from the interior of outer segment discs to the cytoplasmic space. The *at*RAL is then reduced to all-*trans*-retinol (atROL; vitamin A) by all-*trans*-retinol dehydrogenase (atRDH). The *at*ROL is released from the outer segment and taken up by an adjacent RPE cell where it is esterified by lecithin retinol acyl transferase (LRAT) to form an ester, *at*RE. Isomerization is effected by an isomerase that uses *at*RE as a substrate, in conjunction with Rpe65. The resulting 11-*cis*-retinol (11cROL) is oxidized by 11*c* RDH (a dehydrogenase) to form 11*c*RAL again. 11*c*ROL may also serve as a substrate for LRAT to form 11-*cis*-retinyl esters. The final step is recombination of 11*c*RAL with aporhodopsin in the outer segment to form a new molecule of rhodopsin. (b) *When it goes wrong: synthesis of A2E.* Newly released *at*RAL condenses reversibly with phosphatidylethanolamine to *N*-ret-PE (step 1). Sometimes, a second molecule of *at*RAL will condense with *N*-ret-PE to form A2PE-H_2 (step 2), which absorbs light maximally at 500 nm.

abnormal deposits (**drusen**) in the retina. They contain oxidized proteins and lipoproteins and a range of other products, including complement and Aβ (Section 9.20.6). Drusen are often present (in much smaller numbers) in the eyes of elderly people.

6.10.2 Solutions

6.10.2.1 *Screening and prevention*

No blood vessels enter the lens; it derives food and O_2 by diffusion. Hence intra-lens O_2 levels are low, which perhaps helps to minimize oxidative damage. Rapid narrowing of the iris at high light intensity helps to protect the retina. As for the cornea, it has no blood vessels either, and its external surface is bathed in tear fluid, which contains ascorbate, urate and several proteins;[176] all of these can help to absorb such air pollutants as O_3, $NO_2^{\bullet}$ and SO_2. Lactoferrin in tear fluid (present in most animals, although in the rabbit transferrin replaces it)[177] can chelate iron safely and the protein **lipocalin** can bind not only iron complexed to bacterial siderophores (Section 3.15.4.1) but also lipid peroxides, including F_2-isoprostanes.[179] Any irritation increases tear flow, to wash away the offending agent and replenish the antioxidant supply. Hence human tears are powerful inhibitors of iron-dependent free-radical reactions (so don't cry over failed free-radical experiments: it will make things worse). Proteins in the cornea can absorb substantial amounts of UV light, especially **aldehyde dehydrogenase type 3**, which forms about 40% of the soluble protein there. It can also reduce end-products of lipid peroxidation[161] such as HNE.

Various tryptophan metabolites accumulate to millimolar levels in the human lens, including **4-(2-amino-3-hydroxyphenyl)-4-oxobutanoic acid *O*-glucoside** and **3-hydroxykynurenine glucoside**, and can help absorb UV light,[180] although at high UV levels the latter compound may turn into a photosensitizer. Melanin is present in the RPE[174] and choroid (Fig 6.19); it can absorb some UV light

and scavenge $^1O_2$. Melanin may also bind zinc ions, which have been suggested to contribute (in a way yet undefined) to maintaining RPE function. Consistent with a protective role for melanin, albinism (Section 3.18.9) is associated with poorer vision.

6.10.2.2 *Antioxidants in the eye*

Corneal epithelial cells contain the usual complement of antioxidants, including ascorbate, GSH, SOD and H_2O_2-removing enzymes. Ferritin is present; in addition to its usual iron sequestration role, it has been postulated to help protect DNA from UV damage. Exposure to UV light causes ferritin to move from the cytoplasm to the nucleus, carried by a protein called **ferritoid**.[181] The concentration of GSH in the lens of several mammals is as high as in the liver, being at especially high levels in the lens epithelium, although levels are lower in the lens nucleus.[168] GSH helps to protect the thiol groups of crystallins, preventing them from aggregating to form opaque clusters. Indeed, injection of buthionine sulphoximine, to inhibit GSH synthesis (Section 3.9.3), into newborn rats and mice causes them to develop cataract, an effect also seen in mice lacking γ-glutamyl transpeptidase (Section 3.9.4). The ability to synthesize GSH may decrease with age in the human lens, which would predispose to cataract. This may be, in part, due to loss of the ability to convert methionine to the GSH precursor cysteine.[182] Mice lacking GPx1 seem to develop more severe cataract as they age than controls.[183]

Oxidative stress can cause S-thiolation of lens proteins, which if not too severe can be reversed by glutaredoxin.[184] The GSH/GSSG ratio is normally kept high in the eye by glutathione reductase, which obtains NADPH from the pentose phosphate pathway. Glaucoma (defined in the legend to Fig. 6.19) decreases the supply of glucose to the lens, interferes with this pathway and so restricts NADPH supply. Glutathione peroxidase, peroxiredoxins,[184] and catalase are present in all parts of

---

Within the acidic and oxidizing environment of RPE phagolysosomes, A2PE-H$_2$ is oxidized to A2PE ($\lambda_{max} = 430$ nm) (step 3). Hydrolysis of the phosphate ester yields A2E ($\lambda_{max} = 435$ nm) and phosphatidic acid (step 4). Double bonds along the polyene chains of A2E may react with singlet O_2 to form a series of one to nine (nine is shown) oxiranes (step 5). Abbreviations: RPE, retinal pigment epithelium; *N*-ret-PE, *N*-retinylidene-phosphatidylethanolamine; A2E, *N*-retinylidene-*N*-retinylethanolamine; A2PE-H$_2$, dihydro-*N*-retinylidene-*N*-retinyl-phosphatidylethanolamine. From *Proc. Natl. Acad. Sci.* **101**, 5928, 2004 by courtesy of Dr GH Travis and the US National Academy of Sciences. Other fluorophores can also form.

the eye but, as in other cells (Section 3.11.1), high levels of H_2O_2 can inactivate ocular peroxiredoxins. Glutathione S-transferases are also present; their contribution to aldehyde and lipid peroxide metabolism is unclear, but might be significant.[185]

Superoxide dismutase is present in all eye tissues, mostly CuZnSOD, and the RPE additionally contains high levels of mitochondrial MnSOD.[174] In mice lacking MnSOD (Section 3.4.2), there were significant decreases in the photoreceptor layer depth and the optic nerve cross-sectional area, implying that absence of this enzyme accelerates cell death in these parts of the eye.[186] Copper–zinc SODs are susceptible to inactivation by glycation (e.g. in diabetes[187]) and by H_2O_2. Indeed, feeding aminotriazole to rabbits raises H_2O_2 concentration in the lens, induces cataract and causes a decrease in lens CuZnSOD activity. Hence, as usual, SOD activity has to be balanced with enzymes that remove H_2O_2.[168]

Rod outer segments and RPE are rich in α-tocopherol;[174] cell damage and lipofuscin accumulation in the RPE are accelerated in tocopherol-deficient animals or those lacking tocopherol transfer protein (Section 3.20.2.6). Feeding extra α-tocopherol decreases the severity of the cataracts caused by aminotriazole administration to rabbits. In premature babies, ocular α-tocopherol levels are subnormal (a factor predisposing to ROP) (Table 6.6). The fatty acid binding protein (Section 4.12.5.3) is also present in RPE and may help to protect[188] against damage by HNE.

Ascorbate is present not only in tear fluid but also at high concentrations in the lens, cornea, RPE, and aqueous and vitreous humours of human, monkey and many other animals (e.g. 1 to 2 mM in human lens and aqueous humour).[189] Corneal epithelial cells have the highest levels. Unlike the case for α-tocopherol, premature babies have *higher* retinal ascorbate levels (Table 6.6). Ascorbate in the cornea might help absorb UV light. Consistent with this, nocturnal animals (e.g. lynx, domestic cat, rat) have lower ascorbate concentrations in the eye.[190] Ascorbate's ability to recycle α-tocopheryl radical, interact with GSH, and scavenge $O_2^{\bullet-}$, singlet O_2, $OH^{\bullet}$ and other ROS may be important in the eye. For example, placing guinea pigs on a vitamin C-poor diet for several months decreased not only retinal ascorbate levels but also those of GSH and α-tocopherol.[191]

On the other hand, it has been suggested that light-induced degradation of ascorbate in the aqueous humour may be a *source* of H_2O_2. Once it has started to oxidize, ascorbate can cause 'glycation-type' reactions on proteins, including crystallins (Section 3.20.1.3).[192] Nevertheless, epidemiological data (Section 6.10.5 below) tend to support the view that the overall effect of ascorbate in the eye is beneficial, or at least not harmful.

6.10.2.3 *Sequestration of metal ions*

Lipocalin and lactoferrin in tears can bind iron (Section 6.10.2.1), but what about inside the eye? Ascorbate can be pro-oxidant if mixed with transition-metal ions. Indeed, incubation of crystallins with ascorbate plus iron ions *in vitro* produces oxidative changes resembling those seen in old human lens.[192] Exposure of rats to high light intensities increases levels of HO-I in the retina,[193] presumably an antioxidant response (removal of haem, formation of biliverdin, but also creation of 'free' iron). Bleeding can also raise HO-1. In the

Table 6.6 Levels of α-tocopherol and vitamin C in retina from adult humans or premature babies

Source of retina	α-Tocopherol		Vitamin C	
	nmol/mg DNA	nmol/cm^2 retina	nmol/mg DNA	nmol/cm^2 retina
Premature babies (vascular region)[a,b]	1.4±1.1	0.47±0.32	244±38	71.3±15.2
Mature retinas[c] (central region)	10.9±6.0	3.04±1.34	162±33	38.3±8.8

[a] Levels of α-tocopherol but not vitamin C were lower in avascular regions.
[b] 22–33 week's gestation.
[c] 13 samples, age range 1 month to 73 years.
Data abstracted from *Invest. Ophthalmol. Vis. Sci.* **29**, 22, 1988, by courtesy of Dr R E Anderson and the publishers.

healthy eye, iron-dependent damage may be minimized by the presence of transferrin in aqueous and vitreous humours.[194] Melanin can also bind iron and render it less redox-active. Retina contains ferritin, metallothionein, and the haem-binding protein haemopexin, whereas the photoreceptor cells express haptoglobin.[195]

6.10.2.4 *Repair of damage*

Methionine sulphoxide reductases are present in the lens[196] and function (in co-operation with thioredoxin) to repair oxidized methionine residues. Partially oxidized crystallins can be degraded in lens epithelial cells by the proteasome, but highly oxidized/cross-linked proteins can no longer be degraded and so accumulate. Proteasome activity may decrease with age, another factor predisposing to accumulation of oxidized proteins.[197]

6.10.3 Toxins, inflammation and the eye

Diquat (Section 6.9.2) causes cataract in rats, apparently by producing $O_2^{\bullet-}$ and H_2O_2 after its reduction to a bipyridyl radical by lens enzymes, including glutathione reductase.[140] Inflammation of the eye induced by infection or irritation can increase production of ROS and of $NO^\bullet$, resulting in $ONOO^-$ formation. Indeed, nitration and inactivation of MnSOD were observed in the eyes of rats with endotoxin-induced inflammation.[198]

6.10.4 The thorny question of ocular carotenoids: a Chinese herb good for the eyes?

β-Carotene and several other carotenoids are important to vision as precursors of vitamin A (Section 3.21), which in turn yields the chromophore of rhodopsin (Fig. 6.20). Indeed, lack of vitamin A is a major cause of blindness in the world. Carotenoids might also play direct protective roles (as light absorbers and/or $^1O_2$ quenchers) in the eyes of some species.[199] For example, in the compound eye of the housefly, a carotenoid is present in large amounts (four to ten molecules per rhodopsin). Carotenoid has also been reported in the lateral eye of the crab *Limulus*. The corneas of puffer fishers are clear in the dark but become

yellow in the light, owing to the migration of carotenoid pigment in chromatophore cells.

What about humans? The macula of primates is enriched in some carotenoids, especially lutein and zeaxanthin.[200] Their role in the eye is uncertain; they might act as blue-light filters and/or singlet O_2 and $RO_2^\bullet$ scavengers. Such roles are feasible, since their macular levels can be hundreds of micromolar.[200] However, there are large interindividual variations in levels in humans, probably dependent on dietary intake; ocular levels of lutein and zeaxanthin rise if more are present in the diet.[200] There is no evidence that persons with higher levels see better, but then again the question has not been investigated in detail. The Chinese frequently use in cooking a small red berry, *Lycium barbarum* (**wolfberry**), thought to be good for the eyes. It has been shown to be rich in zeaxanthin—a coincidence or something meaningful?[201] Foods rich in lutein include spinach, kale, broccoli, peas and brussels sprouts, whereas for zeaxanthin eat egg yolk, corn, orange peppers and honeydew melon. Genetically engineered plants with a disabled xanthophyll cycle, so that zeaxanthin accumulates, have been proposed for sale.[202] **Canthaxanthin** (Fig. 3.32) was once used as an oral skin-tanning agent; sadly, it can enter the eye and even crystallize there if too much is taken. Hence it is now banned in many countries.

6.10.5 Antioxidants, cataract and macular degeneration

Epidemiological studies have attempted to relate antioxidant intake, or blood antioxidant levels, to the incidence of cataract or macular degeneration. Several have suggested that high intakes of ascorbate, lutein, or zeaxanthin are associated with lower risk of both conditions[202,203] but the conclusions are tentative, in part because of the limitations associated with interpreting epidemiological data (Section 10.5). Patients with cystic fibrosis (Section 9.8) show low serum and macular levels of lutein and zeaxanthin, but see normally.[200] The results of intervention studies have been variable, some claiming decreased risk of cataract or macular degeneration after supplementation with mixtures of antioxidants, and others not. The **Age-Related Eye Disease Study (AREDS)**[202] reported that in elderly (55–80 years old) subjects a daily supplement of 500 mg vitamin C, 400 units α-tocopherol (sadly the dl-form was used), 80 mg zinc (plus 2 mg copper, since high-dose zinc can impair copper absorption) and 15 mg of β-carotene markedly decreased the progression of macular degeneration in subjects showing its early or intermediate stages. Both zinc alone and the antioxidant mixture showed positive effects, but the combination was more effective. It is not clear why β-carotene was used, since it does not enter the eye. Even worse, high doses may decrease intestinal uptake of lutein and zeaxanthin. Also, 80 mg of zinc daily is a lot (although the oxide used, ZnO, may not have had high bioavailability). Copper was supplied as CuO–it is also unclear if this can be absorbed. The zinc ± antioxidant supplements showed no effects on cataract development in the subjects.

Photodynamic therapy (Section 2.6.4.4) has been used to treat macular degeneration; the agent usually used is **verteporfin**, sometimes called **Visudyne**, a porphyin derivative.[204]

6.11 Reproduction and oxidative stress

All aspects of reproduction, from sex (Section 4.9.4), fertilization, embryonic development, normal pregnancy, complications of pregnancy, birth and the first weeks of life (indeed all of life!) involve RS, and can be affected if the balance of RS and antioxidant defence/repair systems goes awry. Let us examine some cases.

6.11.1 Preconception: spermatozoa have problems[205]

The first indication that oxidative stress could affect sperm came in 1943, when it was observed that human sperm rapidly lose motility when incubated under elevated O_2, and that adding catalase offers some protection. Indeed, sperm are quite susceptible to oxidative damage. Antioxidants in the seminal plasma normally help protect them (Section 6.11.3 below) but the washing of sperm (e.g. in preparation for *in vitro* fertilization) can remove this protection, especially if the

washing and resuspension fluids are contaminated with transition-metal ions (as they usually are). Attempts have been made to counter this by adding chelating agents and/or antioxidants to washing fluids.[206] Peroxidation can be further accelerated by prolonged storage of frozen sperm, or repeated freeze–thaw cycles.[207]

Why are sperm prone to oxidative damage? Their lipids are rich in PUFA side-chains: almost 50% are DHA residues. This high content of PUFAs gives the sperm plasma membrane considerable fluidity, needed for it to participate in the membrane fusion events associated with fertilization. In peroxidized sperm, fluidity decreases and the capacity to fertilize is diminished. Oxidative stress also causes rises in intracellular free Ca^{2+} (Section 4.3.2), depletions of ATP (interfering with sperm motility) and damage to sperm DNA, forming 8OHdG. Several studies suggest that high levels of 8OHdG correlate with poor fertility.[208]

Seminal fluid can generate ROS. The major source appears to be neutrophils, present in the ejaculate.[209] An additional source of RS might be sperm themselves, which appear to generate $O_2^{\bullet-}$, although there is disagreement about how much they make.[205,209] Superoxide production may involve an NADPH oxidase system of the NOX5 (Section 7.10) type.[205] Low-level $O_2^{\bullet-}$ generation has been proposed to play an important role in normal sperm function; it may contribute to **capacitation**, a collective term for the changes in sperm properties, needed to achieve successful fertilization, that occur as they pass through the female reproductive tract. These changes include development of the hyperactivated movement needed to achieve penetration of the membrane that surrounds the oocyte. These ROS might also contribute to the **acrosome reaction**, a membrane fusion event involving the outer acrosomal and plasma membranes of the sperm. The acrosome reaction causes release of the acrosomal contents, including proteinases that are thought to facilitate passage of the sperm into the egg. The ROS may facilitate these various events by increasing net protein phosphorylation (Section 4.5.5.3). Low levels of $ONOO^-$ can also promote capacitation in isolated sperm.[210] Hence, there is the usual fine balance: some RS are helpful to sperm, but too many are bad.

Sperm production requires the testes to be at a lower temperature than the rest of the body; warming them up impairs sperm production. It has been proposed that ROS are involved in this.[211]

6.11.2 The female story

As for the other gender, ROS have been suggested to be involved in oocyte maturation and regression of the corpus luteum during the normal mammalian ovarian reproductive cycle.[212] However, too many are bad; female mice lacking CuZnSOD show decreased fertility due to increased embryonic death, whereas male CuZnSOD⁻-mice are as fertile as usual.[213] Prostaglandins from both COX1 and COX2 play important roles in most aspects of reproduction[214] and so the role of ROS in regulating 'peroxide tone' and COX activity (Section 7.12.4) may be important.

6.11.3 Spermatozoa: the solutions[205,215,216]

Sperm contain SOD, the peroxiredoxin system, catalase, GPx, plasmalogens (Section 4.12.8), glutathione reductase and GSH, as well as ascorbate and α-tocopherol. However, they have limited biosynthetic capacity, making it difficult to replace any molecules that undergo damage. A PHPGPx produced in the testis plays a key role in sperm maturation (Section 3.8.1).

The enzymic antioxidants may be concentrated in the midpiece of the sperm, leaving the large expanse of membrane overlying the head and tail less protected. Hence the seminal plasma is important in protecting sperm against damage by ROS generated by the sperm themselves and by phagocytes in the ejaculate. This fluid contains SOD (mostly CuZnSOD, some EC–SOD), iron-binding proteins (lactoferrin and transferrin),[217] urate, GPx (mostly GPx3), GSTs, low (1–2 μM) levels of GSH, and higher levels of ascorbate (up to 400 μM) than in plasma. Hypotaurine (Section 7.7.3) is present and may help to scavenge several RS, including HOCl. The levels of 8OHdG in sperm DNA were found to be inversely correlated with seminal fluid ascorbate levels in some studies (Table 6.7). In rats, a selenium-independent GPx5 is present in epididymal fluid, but it may not be functional in humans (Section 3.8.1).

6.11.4 Spermatozoa as targets for toxins[205]

The testis is a site of intense cell division and relies heavily on ribonucleoside diphosphate reductase and thioredoxin (Section 7.2). Hence it is susceptible to agents that target dividing cells. Spermatozoa are readily damaged during inflammation of the reproductive tract, in part by RS generated by activated phagocytes (e.g. Section 8.1.3). Excessive damage can lead to infertility.[218] Cigarette smoke can also damage sperm DNA (Section 8.12.2).

Gossypol is a yellow polyphenol found in cotton plants; it has been tested (and abandoned) as a male oral contraceptive. Its toxic effects on sperm have been suggested to be due to ROS production (Section 3.22.3),[219] probably not via lipid peroxidation, since gossypol is a powerful chain-breaking antioxidant (Fig. 3.33). Gossypol inhibits the phosphatase calcineurin (Section 4.5.6) and could interfere with signal transduction.[220] The organic solvent **toluene** (methylbenzene) has many toxic effects, including causing reproductive dysfunction.

Table 6.7 Dietary ascorbate intake, semen ascorbate levels and 8-hydroxy-2′-deoxyguanosine (8OHdG) in DNA from sperm of human volunteers

	Ascorbate intake (mg/day)	Semen ascorbate (μM)	8OHdG (fmol/mg DNA)
Baseline	250	399±55	34.0±2.4
Depletion	5	203±72	66.9±8.5
Marginal	10 or 20	115±25	84.4±22.3
Repletion	60 or 250	422±100	53.8±16.8

Human volunteers were maintained on controlled diets supplemented with various amounts of ascorbate. Dietary ascorbate was decreased from 250 mg/day to 5 mg/day, and then repleted after 28 days. Data abstracted from *Proc. Natl. Acad. Sci. USA* **88**, 11003, 1991, by courtesy of Prof. Bruce Ames and the US National Academy of Sciences.

It has been hypothesized that this involves its oxidation products, such as methylcatechol, undergoing redox cycling to generate ROS in the reproductive tract.[221]

6.11.5 Problems of the embryo

The increasing popularity of assisted conception techniques in humans and other animals has focused attention on the problems of handling fertilized eggs and early embryos. Interestingly, newly fertilized eggs are capable of repairing oxidatively damaged sperm DNA.[222] This is fortunate, since sperm can suffer DNA damage when they are washed and handled.

During the preimplantation period prior to establishment of pregnancy (about 7 days in humans), the fertilized egg spends about 3 days in the oviduct and the rest in the uterus. Cell division gives a two-cell, four-cell and then up to 16-cell stage (Fig. 6.21). Compaction of the cells occurs at about the eight- to 16-cell stage; they flatten down upon one another, becoming wedge-shaped rather than spherical. Eventually a mature **blastocyst** is formed, consisting of an outer layer of polarized cells (**trophectoderm**) surrounding a fluid-filled cavity (the **blastocoel**) containing a cluster of cells, the **inner cell mass**. The embryo proper arises from some of the latter cells, whereas the remainder of the inner cell mass and the trophectoderm give rise to extraembryonic structures such as the **placenta**.

Preimplantation development is initially controlled by mRNA from the egg: expression of the embryonic genome begins at the four- to eight-cell stage in humans, but at the two-cell stage in mice. Eggs and embryos contain the usual complement of antioxidant defences, including ascorbate, α-tocopherol, SOD, GSH, GPx, catalase and metallothionein (levels of the last are increased after exposure to zinc or cadmium).[222] Severe depletion of oocyte GSH blocks embryonic development. Mouse eggs cultured *in vitro* often cease division at the two-cell stage, a phenomenon called the **two-cell block**. It can be overcome by placing the cells back into the oviduct, or by incubating in culture media containing EDTA and glutamine but lacking glucose. The two-cell block is representative of a series of 'blocks' that occur if one attempts to grow fertilized eggs in culture. Thus a four- to eight-cell block is often seen for human and cow eggs, and an eight- to 16-cell block for sheep and goat eggs. Pyruvate is the preferred metabolic substrate of the early stages of embryonic development, with glucose uptake increasing as the blastocyst is formed.

Several papers have suggested that oxidative stress is involved in the 'cell blocks', especially if eggs are kept under 21% O_2. This is hyperoxic for them since O_2 levels in the uterus and oviduct are only 11 to 60 mmHg.[223] The use of lower O_2 tensions or the addition of antioxidants (including catalase, transferrin, SOD, thioredoxin or even whole erythrocytes, which can absorb ROS) have been reported[224,225] to facilitate embryonic development *in vitro*. Pyruvate could conceivably act as a H_2O_2 scavenger (Section 3.18.2) as well as a nutrient. As with spermatozoa, however, there are suggestions that ROS play useful roles, for example by being involved in the apoptosis of unwanted cells during embryonic development.[226] Rabbit blastocysts have been reported[222] to contain a cell-surface NAD(P)H oxidase that generates $O_2^{\bullet-}$. Thus embryonic development may need just the right level of ROS, both too many and too few being deleterious. This could help to explain why over 50% of fertilized human eggs appear not to survive past the early embryonic stages, even in the protective environment of the reproductive tract.

Oviductal lining fluid has a low O_2 concentration and may contain several antioxidants, including SOD, ascorbate, hypotaurine and GPx, but its antioxidant defences have not been fully characterized, nor have those of uterine fluids or the amniotic fluid that surrounds the baby.[222] Indeed, amniotic fluid has been suggested to contain non-protein-bound iron.[227]

6.11.6 Problems of pregnancy: normal and abnormal O_2

The placenta delivers O_2, nutrients, and antioxidants from the mother to the baby, including iron, copper, ascorbate, cysteine and cystine for GSH synthesis, and *RRR*-α-tocopherol. Placental transfer of the last is fairly slow, which results in lower levels of α-tocopherol in babies than in

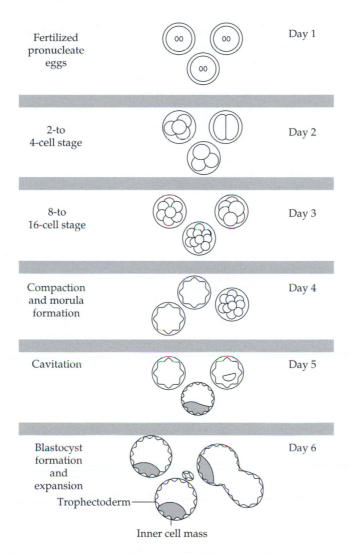

Figure 6.21 Embryonic development in humans. Diagram by courtesy of Drs MJ Conaghan, K Hardy and HJ Leese and the Biochemical Society (*The Biochemist*, April/May 1994, p. 9).

adults. Nevertheless it is important; placentas of mice lacking tocopherol transfer protein are abnormal, and the embryos die at midgestation (Section 3.20.2.6).[28] Indeed, vitamin E was first recognized as a 'factor' needed for normal reproduction in rats (Section 3.20.2.2). The human placenta has been reported to make 'extracellular' GPx (GPx3) and secrete it into the maternal circulation.[228]

Human placentas have low O_2 tension (<20 mmHg) and low antioxidant levels for about the first 10 weeks of gestation.[223] Oxygen levels rise to about 50 mmHg at 11 to 14 weeks as the maternal intraplacental circulation becomes fully established. Just at that time, there is a 'burst' of ROS production, which is accompanied by increased synthesis of CuZnSOD, GPx and MnSOD and may be physiologically useful in promoting correct cell differentiation, although it can cause damage if too large and/or prolonged.[223] Abnormally early onset of the full maternal circulation of the placenta is associated with many miscarriages, and oxidative stress may contribute. Indeed, levels of lipid per-oxides and 3-nitrotyrosine are elevated in placentas from miscarriages.[223] However, chlorinated and nitrated proteins, and lipid oxidation products (including HNE) are also present, to variable extents, in the healthy placenta, which is rich in macrophages[229,230] Nitric oxide plays a role in maintaining normal placental blood flood, but its presence means that there is a risk of excessive $ONOO^-$ formation if $O_2^{\bullet-}$ levels are raised. As in other tissues (Section 3.16.3.1), placental EC–SOD is involved in regulating the $O_2^{\bullet-}/NO^\bullet$ interaction.

Disruptions of placental blood flow later in pregnancy can cause **pre-eclampsia**, the leading cause of maternal death in advanced countries and a major cause of maternal morbidity and foetal growth restriction. It affects up to 2.8% of preg-nancies in developed countries, and more in developing ones. Impaired blood flow through the placenta causes severe hypoxia and release of **pre-eclamptic factors** into the systemic circulation. These promote vasoconstriction and hypertension as well as neutrophil and platelet activation in the maternal vascular system. The baby must be delivered as soon as possible to reverse the syn-drome, even if it is too premature to survive.[231,232]

Supplementation of 'at risk' women with 400 units/day of α-tocopherol plus 1 g/day of vit-amin C has been shown in some (but by no means all) studies to decrease the numbers who develop pre-eclampsia, suggesting that oxidative stress is involved and that low body levels of nutritional antioxidants may sometimes be a risk factor. However, the more studies that are done, the less impressive the effects seem.[231] Vitamin C supple-ments also protected some women against prema-ture rupture of the chorioamniotic membranes during pregnancy, perhaps because the subjects studied were sufficiently vitamin C-deficient to impair collagen synthesis.[233] However, attempts to demonstrate systemic oxidative stress in pre-eclampsia by measuring such biomarkers as plasma F_2-isoprostanes (F_2-IPs) have given variable results in different laboratories.[231,234,235] For example, one study showed plasma F_2-IPs to be higher in healthy pregnant women than in non-pregnant controls, but not further increased in pre-eclampsia.[236] However, increased oxidative damage to DNA (as 8OHdG), lipids (e.g. as HNE

and F_2-IP formation) and proteins, including 3-nitrotyrosine formation, has been shown in the pre-eclamptic placenta.[230,232,237] Presumably such localized damage is not always reflected in plasma biomarkers. Sources of ROS in the damaged placenta may include XO produced as a result of ischaemia–reperfusion, mitochondrial dysfunction and an NADPH oxidase system.[232,237] Foetal growth retardation may also be associated with elevated F_2-IP levels in amniotic fluid.[238]

Thus pregnancy is the usual balance; some ROS are needed for the placenta to work properly, but too many impair its function.

6.11.7 The embryo/foetus as a target for toxins[239]

The increased risk of foetal malformations observed in mothers with poorly controlled diabetes may involve oxidative stress, including toxic effects of F_2-IPs.[240] Indeed, induction of diabetes (by streptozo-tocin treatment; Section 8.5.2) in pregnant mice produced embryonic malformations, but fewer were seen if the embryos overexpressed CuZnSOD.[241] Hypercholesterolaemia in mothers can lead to atherosclerosis in foetal arteries (Section 9.3.2). Exposure of pregnant females to certain xenobiotics can cause embryonic death, lethal foetal malforma-tions or birth defects (**teratogenesis**). Teratogenicity can sometimes be latent, for example an increased risk of cancer development in the offspring after the mother was exposed to toxins, one example being **diethylstilboestrol**. Several teratogens have been suggested to act, in whole or in part, by imposing oxidative stress. They include the anticonvulsant **phenytoin** (diphenylhydantoin, Dilantin), hydro-xyurea (Section 7.2.2), and possibly cocaine (Section 8.9). **Thalidomide**, notorious for causing birth defects, has an antiangiogenic effect and causes severe foetal hypoxia; a role for ROS in its effects has been claimed but not fully substantiated.[242]

Fortunately, the maternal drug-detoxification systems (CYPs, glucuronidation, GSTs) and the barrier action of the placenta do an excellent job in protecting against most potential insults. Of course, CYPs can convert a few chemicals (including phe-nytoin and cocaine) to more reactive forms, but levels of CYPs in the placenta and foetus are low, probably with good reason (e.g. Section 8.2.2).

6.11.8 Birth

6.11.8.1 A cold hyperoxic shock

Birth involves hypoxia–reoxygenation complicated by an interruption of the nutrient supply until feeding is established. Newborns face a sudden transition from a warm, fluid-filled environment to a cooler, air-breathing environment, with exposure of the lung to O_2 concentrations much greater than those experienced *in utero*. Often, severe hypoxia occurs during birth itself, making the eventual exposure to 21% O_2 even more of a shock. Preparations for birth occur in the later stages of development *in utero* and include rises in the levels of such antioxidants as EC–SOD, other SODs, GSH, catalase, GPx and peroxiredoxins in the lung. The forkhead transcription factor **Foxa2** (Section 4.5.5) plays a key role in controlling these events, and the synthesis of surfactant.[243] There are marked interspecies differences in the time courses and extent of changes in antioxidants[244] and so one must wary of extrapolating studies on other animals to humans. Also, rat and mouse lungs do not have alveoli at birth, unlike human lungs. In human lung some antioxidants appear early in gestation (e.g. MnSOD and CuZnSOD) whereas others (e.g. catalase, thioredoxin) not until the last four weeks of pregnancy.[244]

Increased ROS production at birth may trigger important adaptations. *In utero*, the baby is not breathing and blood bypasses the pulmonary circulation through a foetal artery, the **ductus arteriosus.** This rapidly closes at birth, first by immediate vasoconstriction. Within a few days cell migration into the lumen makes the closure irreversible. How does this artery know when to close? One suggestion is that a 'redox sensor' (possibly mitochondria) responds to elevated O_2 by generating H_2O_2, which blocks K^+ channels, depolarizes the membrane, opens Ca^{2+} channels and causes vasoconstriction.[245] As the ductus arteriosus closes, pulmonary vascular resistance falls and blood flows through the lungs. Sometimes this fails to occur properly, lung resistance remains high and **persistent pulmonary hypertension of the newborn** results. Studies on animals suggest that this can involve excess $O_2^{\bullet-}$ production by lung NADPH oxidases.[246]

Newborns have low activities of methaemoglobin reductase in erythrocytes, and so are more prone to develop problems when exposed to agents that can oxidize haemoglobin, such as nitrite (Section 1.10.3).[43]

6.11.8.2 Prematurity

Premature babies face special problems: improvements in neonatal care have increased their survival rate, but often requiring respiratory support (with exposure to elevated O_2) for many weeks. Indeed, plasma F_2-IPs are higher than adult values in normal term babies, and even higher in premature babies. Placental esterified F_2-IPs were also higher for premature births.[247] Exposure of premature babies to excess O_2 contributes to the development of ROP and brain damage, including haemorrhage and **periventricular leukomalacia**, localized cell necrosis and damage to the precursor cells of oligodendrocytes.[248] A role for ROS in this damage has been proposed, since F_2-IPs are elevated and are toxic to the precursor cells.[248,249] Oligodendrocytes form the myelin sheath (Section 9.16), and severe undermyelination resulting from damage to their precursors can result in cerebral palsy. Another problem is **bronchopulmonary dysplasia** (BPD); BPD involves lung injury and fibrosis that resemble acute respiratory distress syndrome (Section 9.7) and is a significant cause of morbidity and mortality in premature babies. BPD is accompanied by increased oxidative damage, for example rises in allantoin/uric acid ratios (Section 5.12), protein carbonyls, lipid peroxidation, and urinary 8OHdG excretion.[244,250] The immature lung is deficient not only in certain antioxidants but also in surfactant (Section 1.5.2), and what surfactant there is can be damaged by RS. Synthetic surfactants (often more resistant to oxidative damage)[25] have found some role in the treatment of BPD.

Some authors have grouped ROP, BPD and brain damage together as different manifestations of **oxygen-radical diseases of prematurity**.[251]

6.11.8.3 Antioxidants

Babies, especially premature ones, have low levels of α-tocopherol in plasma and tissues (Table 6.6); the low levels in erythrocytes can predispose to haemolysis (Section 3.20.2.8). Tissue and plasma α-tocopherol levels rise fast after birth as it is taken in from milk; the earliest breast milk (**colostrum**) is especially enriched in α-tocopherol and coenzyme Q.[252] Plasma levels of vitamin C in babies are generally higher than in adults, but fall after a few days. Levels of plasma caeruloplasmin (and thus ferroxidase I activity), albumin, and α1-antiproteinase tend to be lower than in adults, whereas plasma XO is higher; any hypoxia will increase plasma hypoxanthine levels and potentiate ROS generation.[253]

Several papers have reported beneficial effects of antioxidants against hyperoxia-induced lung injury in premature animals of various species. For example, protections were seen using intraperitoneal GSH in rabbits, intraperitoneal N-acetylcysteine in guinea pigs, AEOL 10113 (Section 10.6.4) in baboons and intratracheal recombinant human CuZnSOD in piglets. However, attempts to use antioxidants therapeutically in human infants have been disappointing, neither N-acetylcysteine (aiming to raise lung GSH levels) nor recombinant human CuZnSOD being effective in preventing, or decreasing the severity of, BPD.[254,255] The SOD-treated infants also showed no fall in incidence of ROP or haemorrhage. However, at 1 year of age they did show fewer lung problems;[255] more work is needed to confirm this and explore the mechanisms behind it.

Healthy newborn animals of several species are more tolerant to hyperoxia than adults, because they can rapidly induce lung antioxidant defences. There is no evidence that this is the case in humans, sadly (Section 3.4.5).

6.11.8.4 *Iron metabolism*

Plasma ferritin levels, and the percentage saturation of transferrin with iron, are higher in newborn babies than in adults. In about 40% of low birthweight ($<1.5\,\text{kg}$) premature babies, and in a smaller percentage of apparently healthy full-term babies, transferrin is saturated and non-transferrin-bound iron (NTBI) is present in the plasma. *In vitro* studies show that this iron is capable of catalysing $OH^{\bullet}$ generation and peroxidation of lipids, including surfactant lipids.[256,257] Blood transfusions can increase NTBI levels, possibly helping to explain

why they are a risk factor for the development of ROP and BDP.[258] In addition, NTBI was found more often in babies who had experienced asphyxia at birth, especially so in those who developed neurological impairment, and NTBI levels in CSF were correlated with the degree of impairment.[259,260] There were also elevations in *ortho*- and *meta*-tyrosine levels (suggestive of $OH^{\bullet}$ production) and in F_2-IPs in CSF from these damaged babies.[260]

Why should there be more iron at birth? The foetus receives iron from the mother, especially during the last 3 months in utero. About 80% of foetal iron is in haemoglobin, most of the rest in ferritin. Birth is associated with a virtual cessation of red blood cell formation that persists for at least 6 weeks. Hence iron is not used up in erythropoiesis whilst red blood cell degradation continues. Foetal erythrocytes differ from those of adults:[261] they are larger, present in higher numbers per unit volume of blood, and contain predominantly haemoglobin F. Haemoglobin F, like adult haemoglobin, is a tetramer but the β chains are replaced by γ chains (i.e. $\alpha_2\gamma_2$ rather than $\alpha_2\beta_2$). Haemoglobin F has a higher affinity for O_2 under physiological conditions, optimizing transfer of O_2 from the maternal to the foetal circulation. Foetal erythrocytes are more susceptible to oxidative stress[261,262] than adult ones and they produce more $O_2^{\bullet-}/H_2O_2$, due both to a higher content of haemoglobin per cell and to higher autoxidation rates of haemoglobin F. Their membrane lipids have lower levels of linoleic and oleic acid esters than adult erythrocytes, but concentrations of arachidonic acid and DHA are higher. α-Tocopherol (both on a micromolar basis and per unit lipid), GPx1, catalase, methaemoglobin reductase and CuZnSOD are all lower in foetal erythrocytes than in adult ones.[261]

It is possible that the increased oxidative susceptibility of foetal erythrocytes contributes to their rapid destruction (Fig. 6.22). One result is increased plasma bilirubin levels. Although high bilirubin levels are toxic, more moderate 'physiological jaundice' may be beneficial if bilirubin acts as an antioxidant (Section 3.18.1).

6.11.8.5 *Parenteral nutrition*

Parenteral nutrition has been used in the management of low-birth-weight babies for years, but

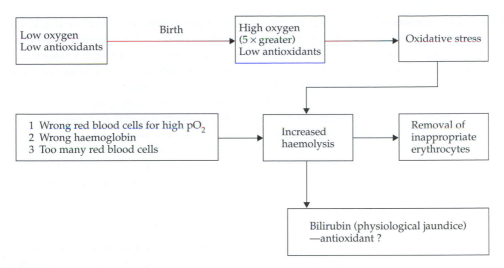

Figure 6.22 Oxidative stress: is it a mechanism for destruction of foetal erythrocytes?

sadly the lipids present in the infusions are often partially oxidized and contain aldehydes and lipid peroxides,[263] not good if there is 'catalytic' iron in the plasma. The fluids can also be iron contaminated themselves (Table 4.4). The amino acid/vitamin/mineral mixtures (especially those containing ascorbate; Section 3.20.1.3) that are often added to infusions can generate H_2O_2 on exposure to light. Indeed, urinary levels of H_2O_2 were elevated in babies infused with such mixtures.[264] Prolonged parental nutrition has been associated with oxidative stress in adults as well.[265]

6.11.8.6 *Antioxidants, PUFAs and iron*

Optimal development of the brain and nervous system in children requires an adequate dietary intake of all major nutrients, including antioxidant vitamins, copper, iron, and PUFAs. Nutritional antioxidant deficiency in the mother may lead to similar problems in the foetus, perhaps rendering the baby more sensitive to the 'oxidative stress' of birth.[266] Anaemia in children can lead to impaired mental development. Hence maternal iron deficiency should be avoided during pregnancy, although the widespread use of iron supplements for pregnant women in advanced countries may be unnecessary.

An adequate supply of PUFAs, especially DHA, is needed for development of the brain and nervous system. Infants have some capacity to synthesize DHA from linolenic acid but may need more from the diet. Supplementation of infant formulas with DHA must take into account the ease of peroxidation of this and other PUFAs, especially if simultaneous iron fortification is attempted. Breast milk is better; it is a good source of α-tocopherol and PUFAs and contains little, if any, 'catalytic' iron because of the lactoferrin present. Indeed, breast-fed babies (low-birthweight, or normal, 1 month old) showed lower urinary 8OHdG excretion than formula-fed ones.[267]

6.12 The skin

Mammalian skin has two major layers, **dermis** and **epidermis**. The dermis contains multiple cell types, including fibroblasts and **melanocytes** (melanin-producing cells), embedded in a fibrous network of connective tissue containing proteoglycans, elastin and collagen. Unlike the dermis, the epidermis has no blood vessels. Where it meets the dermis is a layer of actively dividing cells; cells from this layer (**keratinocytes**) migrate upwards in the epidermis and undergo differentiation, in the process of **keratinization**, sometimes called **cornification**. The uppermost layer of the epidermis (**stratum corneum**) represents the final stage of this process and consists of dead anucleate cells (**corneocytes**) embedded in a keratin- and lipid-rich matrix, forming a barrier. Transglutaminases (Section 4.3.2) are important in cross-linking proteins during corneocyte formation. These cells are constantly shed and are a major contributor to household dust. They provide food for house dust mites, to which many people are allergic.

Keratinocytes can produce low levels of $O_2^{\bullet-}$ by the action of a NOX system;[268] its physiological function is uncertain, but it could be involved in the regulation of cell proliferation after skin injury (Section 6.12.3 below).

6.12.1 Problems of the skin

The skin, like the lung and cornea, is directly exposed to atmospheric O_2, although the streateum corneum may hinder O_2 diffusion to the lower layers. The skin plays a role in heat exchange; vasodilation to lose heat and vasoconstriction to conserve it can deliver too much or too little O_2 to the skin respectively. Skin must also put up with air pollutants, deodorants (e.g. many antiperspirants are acidic and contain aluminium salts), other applied chemicals (e.g. in creams, lotions, cosmetics, greases, soaps, shower gels, shampoos, oils), industrial chemicals (which can include organic peroxides), water-borne toxins (e.g. chlorine, dissolved metal ions), UV light, other radiation, products from skin bacteria (Fig. 6.23), and fungi (e.g. fungal MnSOD can provoke an immune response in subjects with dermatitis, who may then develop an autoimmune reaction to their own MnSOD[269]), and agents excreted in sweat. Sweat is rich in transition metal ions capable of catalysing free-radical reactions and promoting bacterial growth.[270] Skin responds to many xenobiotics by increasing its content of cytochromes P450, for example CYP1A1 levels rise in response to carcinogenic hydrocarbons in coal tar (Section 9.14). **Retinoic acid**, widely used in the treatment of skin diseases, decreases CYP1A1 levels, an effect which contributes to its chemopreventative effect in skin cancer models.

Let us examine a few of these insults in more detail.

6.12.1.1 *Photosensitization*
The skin is at risk of photo-oxidative damage, both by type I reactions and by generation of singlet O_2, $OH^{\bullet}$, H_2O_2 and other ROS. Photosensitizers are found in some cosmetics or as ingested photosensitizing drugs that reach the skin, including some

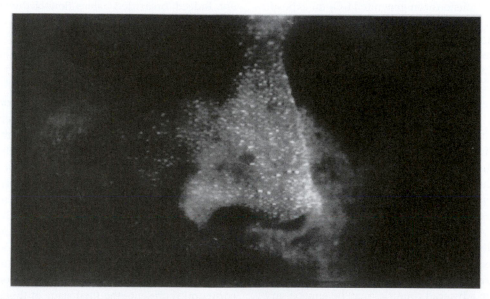

Figure 6.23 Fluorescence of *P. acnes*-derived coproporphyrin III on human skin as seen under UV light. This technique has been used to monitor the distribution of *P. acnes*, a bacterium more prevalent in acne patients. Photograph from *Biochem. Biophys. Res. Commun.* **223**, 578, 1996 by courtesy of Dr Kumi Arakane and Academic Press. Acne has sometimes been treated by careful exposure to blue light (405–420 nm), whereupon *P. acnes* can photosensitize and damage itself with its own coproporphyrin III (*J. Cosmet. Laser Ther.* **5**, 111, 2003). Since *P. acnes* contributes to inflammation, this can diminish the severity of acne.

phenothiazines (used as tranquillizers), as well as fluoroquinolone and tetracycline antibiotics (Sections 2.6.4.3 and 8.16). The skin also contains endogenous photosensitizers, including catalase (Section 3.7.5) and **pyridinoline**, a compound present in the cross-links of collagen.[271] Some people consume preparations of **St. John's wort** (*Hypericum hirsutum*) to treat depression. Do not consume too much and sunbathe however; this plant produces **hypericin** (Fig. 6.14), a photosensitizer, and the skin damage will make you even more depressed. This property of St. John's wort was recognized over a century ago by Arab herdsmen, who painted their white horses with henna or grazed only black sheep on pastures containing this plant.

Celery, parsnips and parsley contain **psoralens**; a patient undergoing photodynamic therapy (Section 2.6.4.4) suffered severe skin damage, apparently by the additive effects of the psoralens in the vegetables she ate and those given during the therapy.[272] **Porphyria** patients can suffer photo-oxidative damage, as do animals consuming **sporidesmin** (Section 2.6.4.3). *Propionibacterium acnes*, a normal inhabitant of the skin, produces coproporphyrin (Fig. 6.23). Several inks used in tattoos are photosensitizers that can damage the skin, and often also the tattoo will fade with time upon exposure to sunlight (a process accelerated when lasers are used to remove tattoos).[273]

6.12.1.2 Ultraviolet light

The biggest problem that the skin (and eye) face is light exposure, especially UV light. Exposure to sunlight is a risk factor for skin cancers (basal cell carcinoma and malignant melanoma) in humans, and a major contributor to the ageing of skin. Skin photo-ageing is accompanied by wrinkling, loss of elasticity, increased skin fragility, and slower wound healing.

In the UV region of the solar spectrum, it is only UV-A (320–400 nm) and some UV-B (290–320 nm) that reach the surface of the earth. Fortunately, the more damaging UV-C (190–290 nm) is filtered out. The major barrier to UV-C (and largely to UV-B) is the ozone layer in the stratosphere. Depletion of this layer (Section 2.6.5) may result in more UV-B reaching the Earth, with a corresponding increase in photochemical damage to both aquatic (e.g. fish,

amphibians) and terrestrial organisms, including plants and humans. It has been estimated that each 5% depletion of stratospheric O_3 will raise UV-B flux at ground level by 10%. Up to 10% of UV-B light falling on the skin can penetrate the epidermis to reach the dermis. The UV-A has greater penetration (e.g. about 20% at 365 nm). Whereas UV-B is much more damaging to skin than UV-A if equal exposures are carried out, the deeper penetration of UV-A and its greater abundance in sunlight (about 95% UV-A, 5% UV-B) suggest that it can also be a significant contributor to damage.

In contrast to X-rays and γ-rays, UV light does not deposit sufficient energy in water molecules to fragment them. However, if H_2O_2 is available, UV-B forms $OH^\bullet$

$$H_2O_2 \xrightarrow{\text{UV}} OH^\bullet + OH^\bullet$$

that can damage DNA directly.[274] More significant than this is the absorption of UV-B by thymine or cytosine, creating excited states that can react with water to form pyrimidine hydrates, or with an adjacent pyrimidine to produce cross-links (Fig. 6.24).[274] It has been suggested that sunlight passing through the skin can even cause DNA damage in white cells circulating through skin capillaries,[275] but the greatest damage is within the skin cells, including damage to dermal mitochondrial DNA; UV exposure leads to more deletion mutations.[276] Ultraviolet light also leads to oxidation of PUFA side chains and cholesterol in skin lipids;[277] generation of aldehydes such as acrolein and HNE from peroxides can damage proteins and DNA.[278]

DNA damage by these and other mechanisms contributes to skin ageing and cancer induced by UV; indeed patients (or mice)[279] with defects in DNA repair are often prone to skin cancer (Section 4.10.8.2). Pyrimidine dimers can cause $CC \rightarrow TT$ tandem double-base transition mutations in DNA (cytosine dimers are more mutagenic than thymine dimers). Mutations in the tumour suppressor gene **p53** (Section 9.13.4) appear to be early events in skin cancer development, and double transition mutations are much more common in mutated p53 genes from skin cancers than in cancers from internal organs, consistent with the role of sunlight.[280]

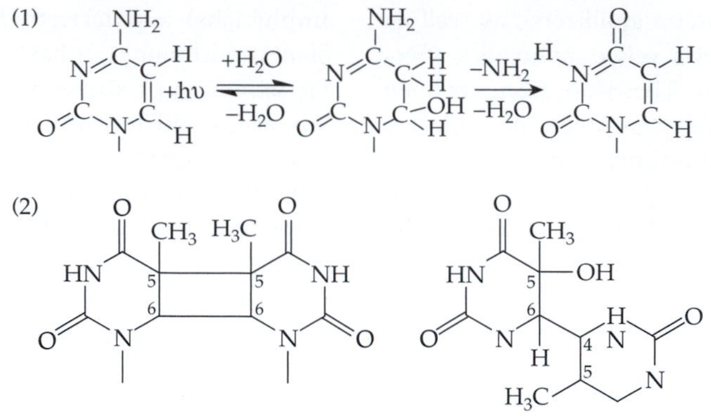

Figure 6.24 Examples of damage to DNA by UV light. (1) Reversible addition of H_2O to cytosine is shown, with the possibility of deamination to uracil. (2) Two types of pyrimidine dimer; (A) the **cyclobutane dimer** and (B) the **pyrimidine(6–4)pyrimidone dimers** (sometimes referred to as the **6–4 photoproducts**). Thymine dimers (shown above) are the main lesion in UV-exposed DNA, although they can be repaired efficiently and cytosine dimers (less well repaired) are considered more mutagenic. The cyclobutane dimers appear to contribute more to cancer risk and inflammation than the 6-4 photoproducts (*Curr. Biol.* **15**, 105, 2005). Cytosine within dimers undergoes accelerated deamination to uracil. Thymidine dimers, presumably arising from nucleotide excision repair (Section 4.10) have been detected in increased amounts (*J. Invest. Dermatol.* **117**, 263, 2001; *Cancer Epidemiol. Biomark. Prevent.* **14**, 2868, 2005) in urine after subjects were exposed to sunlight.

Ultraviolet-A or -B induce activation (sometimes via peroxides or singlet O_2 as signalling molecules)[281] of a wide range of transcription factors in skin cells, including AP-1 and NF-κB. This can increase production of matrix metalloproteinases (Table 7.2) that can degrade collagen and other connective tissue components. Levels of cytokines and iNOS also increase (Section 4.5.8), causing excess $NO^\bullet$ production and $ONOO^-$ generation. Iron liberation in photodamaged skin contributes to oxidative damage and activation of transcription factors.[282] Indeed, chronic exposure of hairless mice to low levels of UV-B increases the non-haem iron content of the skin; increases in iron with age and sun exposure are also observed in human skin. Topical application of certain iron ion chelators (e.g. 1,10-phenanthroline) to the skin of hairless mice appeared to delay the onset of UV-B-induced damage.[283]

6.12.1.3 *Inflammation*

Damage by UV causes an inflammatory response, including recruitment and activation of lymphocytes and neutrophils, to make ROS. Hydrolysis of phospholipids to liberate arachidonic acid, and the subsequent production of prostaglandins and leukotrienes are also important.[284] Several skin diseases involve inflammation, including acne (Fig. 6.23) and psoriasis. The latter affects up to 3% of the population

of advanced countries and is characterized by increased keratinocyte proliferation and abnormal keratinocyte differentiation; TNFα may be an important proinflammatory agent.[285] The skin is affected in many autoimmune diseases (Section 9.9).

Dapsone (Fig. 6.4) is a drug used to treat several skin diseases. It is metabolized to a hydroxylamine (and possibly to nitroxide radicals) *in vivo*, although the contribution of these to its therapeutic effects is uncertain.[286]

6.12.1.4 *Air pollutants*

Exposure to O_3 causes oxidation of proteins and lipids in the stratum corneum, whereas excess $NO_2^\bullet$ can nitrate them. Hopefully, the corneocytes are acting to absorb these toxic gases and protect deeper skin cells.[287]

6.12.2 The solutions

The best solution to UV is avoidance; stay out of the sun or use a sun block. Sadly, some constituents of sun creams (such as **titanium dioxide**, TiO_2) can themselves generate ROS upon illumination.[288] Tocopherols, vitamin C (often as hydrophobic esters such as ascorbyl palmitate), and flavonoids are now being added as protective agents to skin creams. However, their ability to penetrate deep into the skin is limited, and a better way of raising antioxidant levels in the dermis is to consume more of them in the diet. α-Tocopherol absorbs UV-B, but is photo-oxidized to a range of products, including an α-tocopherol dimer and a **spirodimer** in which the two ring –OH groups have been oxidized to quinones.[289] Indeed, tocopherol may photosensitize some singlet O_2 formation (Fig. 3.29). The epidermis contains *trans* urocanic acid,

which may absorb some UV light, dissipating energy as it isomerizes to the *cis* form.[290]

Sunlight induces the synthesis of melanin, which has a broad absorbance spectrum that ranges through the UV-B, UV-A and visible ranges. Melanin is made in melanocytes, which then transfer it to keratinocytes and to hair. Eumelanin is protective against photodamage[291] but this is not always true of pheomelanin (Section 3.18.9). In the disease **vitiligo** there is patchy depigmentation of the skin, decreased catalase activity, and accumulation of peroxides, although the relationship of these events to the origin of the disease is unclear.[292] Skin contains carotenoids at levels that correlate with blood levels. β-Carotene and lycopene are rapidly degraded in skin exposed to sunlight, and their overall photoprotective effect is probably small.[293]

Keratinocytes and skin fibroblasts contain millimolar levels of GSH, the usual complement of antioxidant defence enzymes (including peroxiredoxins), α-tocopherol, ascorbate (essential for skin collagen synthesis), and DNA repair enzymes, although repair of pyrimidine dimers in skin seems fairly slow.[294] In general, keratinocytes are more resistant than most animal cells to killing by H_2O_2, organic peroxides or peroxynitrite. The skin also contains 8OHdGTPase, which 'sanitizes' the DNA precursor pool (Section 4.10.2). In mice, levels of catalase, GPx, glutathione reductase, α-tocopherol, ubiquinol, ascorbate and GSH (but not SOD) are higher in epidermis than in dermis. Ascorbate, GSH, SOD, catalase and ubiquinol are depleted in both dermis and epidermis in UV-B-exposed skin,

and ascorbyl radicals can be detected.[295] The stratum corneum also contains some antioxidants, especially α-tocopherol, ascorbate, GSH and urate, the last being a good scavenger of O_3.[30] α-Tocopherol may be introduced to the skin surface as a constituent of the sebum secreted by the sebaceous glands.[296] Metallothionein (Section 3.16.1) may also be important; mice lacking MT-1 and MT-2 were more sensitive to UV-induced skin injury.[297]

In cultured human skin fibroblasts, UV-A induces synthesis of heat-shock proteins, including HO-1, coincreased with ferritin.[281] Ozone can also raise HO-1 in skin.[287] Keratinocytes are unusual in that they express Hsp72 constitutively, although levels rise under UV light. By contrast, keratinocytes have higher basal levels of haem oxygenase (HO-2), but little inducible (HO-1) activity. Given that skin fibroblasts are covered by the epidermis, it seems reasonable that they would have an inducible response to UV whereas the poor keratinocytes are directly 'in the firing line' and may need to keep HO around all the time.

Damaged proteins in the epidermis can be degraded by the proteasome system, provided that aggregation has not gone too far. Proteasome activity seems to decline with age, perhaps contributing to the photoageing phenomenon. In addition, accumulation of HNE-modified proteins during UV exposure[278] may inhibit the proteasome (Section 4.14.2.2).[298]

6.12.3 Wounds and burns

The skin can suffer cuts, abrasions and burns, and the resulting cell death and breakdown of red blood cells can release haem and iron, generating a pro-oxidant environment around the wound.[299] Is this bad? Not necessarily; ROS may play an important part in wound healing. First, they are produced by activated phagocytes to deter infection (Section 7.7), and haem accumulation may aid phagocyte recruitment.[299] Second, ROS may aid healing, for example by promoting fibroblast proliferation (Section 4.2.1) or by increasing the production of VEGF by keratinocytes[300] (remember that these cells contain an NADPH oxidase). Collagen synthesis is accompanied by H_2O_2 production; lysyl oxidase produces H_2O_2 as it catalyses collagen cross-linking.[301] Of course, too much fibroblast proliferation can produce excessive scarring. Some authors have reported that ascorbate and GSH are depleted in wounds, perhaps to allow the ROS leeway to act (Fig. 5.8).[302] By contrast, others report that levels of peroxiredoxin, HO-1, SOD, GPx1, PHPGx and catalase are increased in proliferating keratinocytes of injured mouse skin.[303] Whether applying antioxidants would promote or impair wound healing is a question that deserves more study, and the answer may depend on the wound. For example, wound healing is slower in diabetic mice; therapy with genes encoding eNOS or MnSOD accelerated healing, suggesting that a correct ratio of $O_2^{\bullet-}$ to $NO^{\bullet}$ is important.[304] α-Tocopherol was also reported as beneficial.[305] In ulcers, for example, the balance might be too far in favour of the ROS, so that they are causing harm.[306] Indeed wound dressings containing desferrioxamine have been developed, to decrease iron-dependent oxidative damage in wounds.[307] Remember, however, that iron is essential for cell proliferation, so chelation must not be overdone.

Burns also result in phagocyte activation, iNOS induction, protein nitration, oxidative damage to the skin and, in severe cases, systemic oxidative stress that may sometimes involve increased levels of XO in plasma (detected in both rats and humans).[308,309] Again, the question of using antioxidants in burn treatment is an open one, although some animal studies have suggested benefit of lipsomally encapsulated SOD[310] or of the antioxidant raxofelast (Table 10.13).[311] Severe burns can lead to extensive fluid loss, ARDS (Section 9.7) and shock syndrome, and administration of SOD or allopurinol to mice before severe thermal skin injury increased their survival times.[312]

6.13 Exercise: a cause of or a protection against oxidative stress?

It is often said that about 1 to 5% of the O_2 taken in by aerobes forms ROS. During exercise, bodily O_2 consumption can increase by as much as 10- to 15-fold, and O_2 uptake in the active skeletal muscle may go up 100-fold. If the same percentage for ROS formation holds true, exercise should lead to a large increase in total body ROS burden, and an even larger increase in the working muscles. This would be expected to cause muscle oxidative damage. Yet levels of SOD, catalase, GSH and GPx in muscle are only modest (Tables 3.4, 3.6 and 3.7). Skeletal muscle generates $NO^{\bullet}$ (from nNOS; Section 2.5.6.6), which could form $ONOO^-$ if $O_2^{\bullet-}$ production was elevated.

6.13.1 Exercise, lack of exercise and oxidative damage

Does exercise increase oxidative damage? Before answering that, let us step back a bit to remind ourselves that *lack of exercise* does. Obesity, related to too much food and lack of exercise, is associated with raised F_2-IP levels (Section 10.2.2.2). In caged mice, inactivity was associated with increased endothelial $O_2^{\bullet-}$ production and vascular dysfunction.[313] A striking example is provided by **disuse atrophy**. Immobilization of muscles causes wasting, accompanied by increases in protein carbonyls, 'catalytic' iron and $OH^{\bullet}$ production.[314] Similar problems occur in spaceflight and in patients mechanically ventilated (atrophy of the diaphragm).

So back to the question 'does exercise cause oxidative damage'? Exercise to an extent that causes severe muscle damage does. As long ago as 1982 it was found that severe, forced physical exercise in rats results in muscle damage, seen as a decrease in mitochondrial respiratory control, loss of structural integrity of sarcoplasmic reticulum and increased levels of lipid peroxidation.[315] α-Tocopherol-deficient rats had markedly lower endurance capacity for exercise. Later work showed increased protein carbonyls and 'catalytic' iron levels in the muscle. Protection against oxidative damage was offered by careful endurance training; such training increased the activities of GPx, glutathione reductase, catalase and SOD in rat heart and skeletal muscle.[316]

Are these observations relevant to humans? Vigorous prolonged exercise, especially in untrained individuals, produces muscle damage, demonstrable histologically or by measuring release of myoglobin or of muscle enzymes (such as **creatine kinase**) into the circulation. Prolonged strenuous exercise (e.g. running a marathon) increases the number of circulating neutrophils and may produce some features of an acute-phase response, such as falls in plasma zinc and iron, rises in IL-1, TNFα and C-reactive protein, and mild fever.[317] It can also (in severe cases) increase gut permeability, allowing endotoxin to enter the circulation and potentiate inflammatory changes (Section 9.5). But the muscle adapts to some extent; elevated temperature in exercising muscle is likely to trigger the heat shock response and endurance exercise has been reported to raise SOD and catalase levels in human muscle.[318,319] Regular moderate exercise improves vascular function, and induction of antioxidant enzymes may be involved (Section 9.3.3).

Hoards of papers have claimed increased oxidative damage after exercise in humans, but many have used unreliable biomarkers such as TBARS or diene conjugates. Nevertheless, there are data showing rises in better biomarkers, such as F_2-IPs.[319–321] Strenuous (but not moderate) exercise in humans or dogs[322,323] increased urinary excretion of 8OHdG; this could reflect more DNA damage (a bad thing) or activation of DNA repair processes (a good thing). This question was addressed in the dogs; levels of 8OHdG in lymphocytes and colon decreased after exercise, consistent with increased repair.[322] Indeed, moderate exercise increased the expression of mRNA encoding hMTH1 (Section 4.10) in leukocytes of sedentary humans.[324]

However, other papers have not found significant rises in oxidative damage or repair after exercise.[320,325] Why? First, the extent of any rise may depend on the intensity of the exercise.[323,326] Second, oxidative damage that occurs locally may not always be reflected systemically. For example urate can be oxidized by ROS to form allantoin within exercising muscle.[327] Urate may be beneficial in intercepting ROS, in that infusion of it into humans decreased rises in F_2-IPs caused by severe exercise.[328] One factor to consider is that prolonged vigorous exercise alters plasma volume; this must be corrected for in attempts to assess the significance of changes in antioxidant levels or oxidative damage biomarkers in plasma.

So where are we? Excessive exercise causes muscle damage, and injured tissues are likely to show elevated oxidative damage secondary to the injury (Section 9.2). Thus the extent of muscle damage may be one factor determining whether or not elevated lipid, DNA or protein oxidation can be detected in exercising humans. Another factor is that muscles produce ROS for useful purposes. Skeletal muscle sarcoplasmic reticulum contains a NOX system, and contractions of skeletal muscle were reported to increase extracellular levels of $O_2^{\bullet-}$, which might contribute to regulation of Ca^{2+} metabolism.[329,330] Indeed, $O_2^{\bullet-}$ generation can be detected even in resting muscle.[329] Reactive species might also be the 'trigger' for upregulation of antioxidant defence enzymes.[331] However, too much ROS produced in the muscle during exercise might be bad, generating $ONOO^-$ and causing injury. Indeed, mice with 50% of normal MnSOD levels showed reduced exercise endurance.[332]

6.13.1.1 Antioxidant supplements and exercise

Is antioxidant supplementation of athletes beneficial, either in minimizing oxidative damage secondary to vigorous exercise or in accelerating healing of damaged tissues? The question is open. N-acetylcysteine administration was claimed to decrease muscle fatigue in humans.[333] α-Tocopherol might increase recovery after injury, possibly (as some but certainly not all studies have suggested)[321,334,335] by modulating the inflammatory response. Overall, the effects of antioxidants vary in different studies from modest to non-existent, and in a few studies (e.g. ref 336) they worsened some parameters of damage. One factor may be the starting antioxidant levels of the subjects studied—if it were subnormal then a benefit might be more likely to be seen.

6.13.2 Exercise, health and free radicals

Regular physical activity in humans has positive effects, including improved cardiovascular function and glucose tolerance and lowered risks

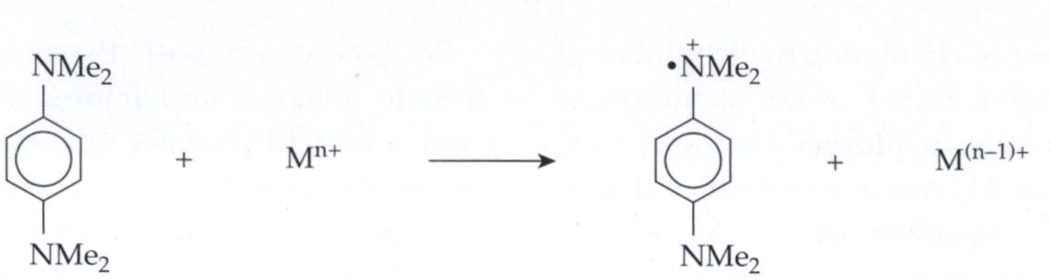

Figure 6.25 A suggested mechanism by which tetramethylphenylenediamine causes oxidative stress. Oxidation is catalysed by traces of metal ions. Damage to rat muscle by a series of *N*-methylated *para*-phenylenediamines was correlated with their rates of oxidation. From *Toxicology* **57**, 303, 1989 by courtesy of Dr Rex Munday and the publishers.

of obesity, hypertension, dementia, diabetes and certain infections (by contrast, hard-training athletes are more susceptible to certain infections, in part because lymphocyte numbers transiently decline). Exercise might even increase neurogenesis in the brain.[337] The extent to which the benefits of moderate exercise might be related to up-regulation of antioxidant defence systems in vascular endothelium, muscle, heart and elsewhere is unknown. They might also involve decreased ROS production in mitochondria (e.g. by upregulation of uncoupling proteins) or simply by accelerating electron transport by increasing the ADP supply: mitochondria tend to make fewer ROS when the electron transport chain is running fast. Regular moderate (but not low- or high-intensity) exercise appears to increase vascular endothelial $NO^{\bullet}$ production.[326]

6.13.3 Muscle as a target for toxins

Several toxins damage muscle. For example, the ***para*-phenylenediamines** are used in the rubber, dyestuff and photographic industries. Some of them cause necrosis of skeletal and cardiac muscle in animals and their oxidation to nitrogen-centred radicals may be involved (Fig. 6.25).

Inhibition of acetylcholinesterase in muscle, for example by organophosphates, delays the clearance of the neurotransmitter acetylcholine and causes excessive contractions, muscle damage and sometimes necrosis. Rises in F_2-IPs in the damaged muscle were blocked by the antioxidant U78517F (Section 10.6.8), which also decreased the number of necrotic fibres. Hyperactivity apparently led to muscle damage and lipid peroxidation, which contributed to further muscle injury.[338]

CHAPTER 7

Reactive species can be useful: some more examples

Everything that happens happens as it should, and if you observe carefully you will find this to be so.

Marcus Aurelius Antoninus

7.1 Introduction

We have already met (or will later meet) several examples of reactive species (RS) serving useful purposes, including ferryl at the active sites of cytochromes P450 (Fig. 1.10) and haem peroxidases (Section 3.13.4), water splitting during photosynthesis (Section 6.8.3), the flavin and pyrimidine radicals that can be present in DNA photolyase (Section 4.10.1), the tryptophan radical in cytochrome c peroxidase (Section 3.13.1), the multiple physiological roles of $NO^{\bullet}$ (Section 2.5.6), the roles of ROS as signalling molecules (Section 4.5.6) and the involvement of HOCl in antibiotic synthesis (Section 8.16). In Chapter 7, we examine some more such cases.

7.2 Radical enzymes: ribonucleotide reductase and its colleagues

First, let us consider a few more enzymes that use active-site free radicals to bring about their actions. In general, enzymes use such radicals to remove hydrogen atoms from unreactive positions in substrates.[1] This is chemically difficult, and the enzymes must control the radicals carefully to prevent damage to themselves.

Deoxyribonucleosides, the precursors of DNA, are made from ribonucleoside diphosphates by **ribonucleoside diphosphate reductase** enzymes, sometimes called **ribonucleotide reductases** and

often abbreviated to **RNR**. They replace the —OH group at position 2 on ribose by hydrogen, generating 2′-deoxyribose (Fig. 7.1).

7.2.1 The enzyme mechanism[2]

At least four types of RNR are known. **Class I RNRs** are found in both eukaryotes and microorganisms, whereas the other classes are found only in microorganisms.

In aerobically-grown *E. coli* and in animal cells the class I enzymes have four subunits, two α and two β. The α_2 dimer is called **protein R1** and contains the active sites, whereas **protein R2** is the β_2 dimer. The reducing power required usually originates from thioredoxin (Fig. 7.1). Each subunit of R2 contains two moles of Fe(III) connected by oxygen. The R2 dimer gives an ESR signal that arises from a tyrosine phenoxyl radical, derived by loss of hydrogen from a tyrosine residue in each amino acid chain. Tyrosine radicals are stable in 'resting' RNR, being buried inside the tertiary structure. The presence of TyrO$^{\bullet}$ is closely linked to the presence of iron; the radical is lost on removal of iron from the enzyme. It reforms on incubation of R2 with Fe^{2+} (or Fe(III) plus a reducing agent) in the presence of oxygen. Once present on R2, the two Fe^{2+} ions are oxidized by O_2 to create the diferric centre and form TyrO$^{\bullet}$. The overall

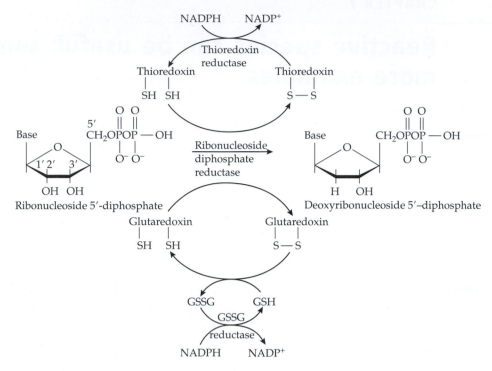

Figure 7.1 Reduction of ribonucleoside diphosphates by class I ribonucleotide reductases. Thioredoxin is the major electron donor. Glutaredoxin can supply reducing power in *E. coli* and possibly in animal cells, but is generally thought to be less important *in vivo*.

reaction is

$$\text{protein} - \boxed{\text{TyrOH}} + 2Fe^{2+} + O_2 + e^- + H^+$$
$$\rightarrow \text{protein} - \boxed{Fe(\text{III}) - O^{2-} - Fe(\text{III})TyrO^\bullet} + H_2O$$
$$\text{diferric oxygen bridge}$$

The electron required can be supplied from external sources (e.g. Fe^{2+}) or from within the protein itself.

Substrate binding and reduction occur on R1. The R2 tyrosyl radicals act as chain initiators, but do not come near the substrate. Instead, an electron-transfer process occurs through the protein, eventually reaching the active sites, which contain three cysteine residues. One is transiently converted into a thiyl radical, which abstracts $H^\bullet$ from the ribose, initially at position 3 on the sugar ring. The ribose radical rapidly shifts to position 2 and $-OH$ is displaced. The other two cysteines reduce this transient sugar radical, and are oxidized to a disulphide, which is then reduced by thioredoxin (Fig. 7.1). Thiyl radical is only generated when the substrate is in place, and substrate can only bind when the enzyme is in the reduced form, so that the sugar radical can be immediately reduced. In mutant enzymes lacking one of the reducing cysteines, the sugar radical forms but then the substrate degrades.

7.2.2 Inhibitors of RNRs

Hydroxyurea, $(H_2N\overset{\overset{\displaystyle O}{\|}}{C}NHOH)$, a widely used inhibitor of RNRs (and hence of DNA synthesis and cell proliferation), inactivates RNRs by reducing the tyrosine radical.[2] Hydroxyurea is sometimes used in cancer chemotherapy and in the treatment of sickle-cell anaemia. High levels of $O_2^{\bullet-}$ and $NO^\bullet$ can inactivate RNRs by the same mechanism (Sections 3.6.1 and 2.5.6.2). Reaction of tyrosyl radicals with $O_2^{\bullet-}$ probably reversibly forms a tyrosine peroxide and with $NO^\bullet$ a nitroso-tyrosine species. By contrast, $ONOO^-$ destroys the tyrosine radical, inactivates RNR and nitrates the tyrosine,[3] possibly by addition of $NO_2^\bullet$. In the R2 component of RNR from *Chlamydia trachomatis* (**class IV RNR**) the tyrosine is replaced by phenylalanine, which cannot generate a phenoxyl radical as the ring has no −OH group. Instead the iron cluster itself acts as the radical source.[4] It has been hypothesized that this variant mechanism protects the enzyme from inactivation by $NO^\bullet$ and thus helps it to survive antibacterial defences (Section 7.9.6 below).

Depletion of cellular iron (e.g. by incubation with iron chelators such as desferrioxamine; Section 10.7.1) can also inhibit RNR.

7.2.3 Class III ribonucleotide reductases and other 'sons of SAM' enzymes[5]

Under anaerobic conditions, *E. coli* uses a different RNR, although an iron centre is again used to form a radical. *S*-**Adenosylmethionine** (SAM) binds to the enzyme and undergoes one-electron reduction, causing it to fragment into a **5′-deoxyadenosyl radical** and methionine. The former abstracts hydrogen from a glycine residue to form a **glycyl radical**. The glycyl radical leads to modification of the substrate, again via an intermediate thiyl radical. This only works when O_2 is absent; O_2 reacts fast with glycyl radical to cause enzyme inactivation (Section 7.3 below). Class III enzymes use formate as a hydrogen donor rather than thioredoxin or glutaredoxin, the formate being oxidized to CO_2.

Another 'radical SAM' enzyme in *E. coli* is the O_2-independent coproporphyrinogen III oxidase (Section 1.3.1). An iron cluster cleaves SAM, leading to oxidation of the propionate side-chain on coproporphyrinogen III (Fig. 2.14). Others include biotin synthase and lipoate synthase, enzymes which insert sulphur into ring structures.

7.2.4 Class II ribonucleotide reductases and other cobalamin radical enzymes[2,6]

Ribonucleotide reductases from some other bacteria use a different source of 5′-deoxyadenosyl radical, **5′-deoxyadenosylcobalamin. Cobalamin**, otherwise known as **vitamin B_{12}**, consists of a **corrin** ring with a central cobalt ion. The radical is formed by homolytic cleavage of the fairly weak bond between the cobalt and the $-CH_2$ group in deoxyadenosylcobalamin (Fig. 7.2).

Cobalamin radicals are used by several other enzymes, including **methylmalonyl-CoA mutase**, which converts methylmalonyl coenzyme A to succinyl coenzyme A, a reaction important in bacterial fatty-acid metabolism. Others include **ethanolamine ammonia-lyase, lysine-2,3-aminomutase**, and **diol dehydratase**. The cobalamin radicals abstract $H^\bullet$ from substrates. The substrate radicals rearrange to product radicals, which then recreate radicals on the enzyme and form the product (Fig. 7.2).

7.3 Pyruvate–formate lyase: a similar mechanism[2,7]

The enzyme pyruvate–formate lyase (**PFL**) is found in many anaerobic bacteria, including anaerobically grown *E. coli*. It converts pyruvate to acetylSCoA:

$$CH_3COCOOH + HSCoA \rightleftharpoons CH_3COSCoA$$
$$+ \text{formate}$$

A glycyl radical is required for activity. This is generated by an activating enzyme, **PFL-activase**, a 'radical SAM' protein which uses reduced **flavodoxin** (an iron–sulphur protein) to supply electrons. The SAM is cleaved to 5′-deoxyadenosyl radical, which abstracts hydrogen from Gly734 on the PFL protein. The $Gly^\bullet$ radical in turn causes thiyl radicals to form and attack the pyruvate. Oxygen inactivates PFL within seconds; a peroxyl radical forms,

$$\text{serine} \overset{733}{\underset{}{-}}\text{NH}-\overset{734}{\underset{\bullet}{C}H}-\text{CO}-\text{NH}-\quad\overset{O_2}{\longrightarrow}$$

$$\text{serine} \overset{733}{-}\text{NH}-\underset{O_2^\bullet}{\overset{|}{C}H}-\text{CO}-\text{NH}-$$

followed by fragmentation of the backbone between serine-733 and the glycine, leaving an oxalyl (HOOC−CO−NH−) residue.

E. coli also contains a **PFL-deactivating system**, which reduces the glycyl radical and suppresses PFL activity. It may serve to prevent the above fragmentation during transition to aerobic conditions, preserving the enzyme for later use if O_2 disappears again. At least part of this PFL-deactivation activity is contributed by **alcohol dehydrogenase E (AdhE)**, an enzyme which also contributes to fermentation of

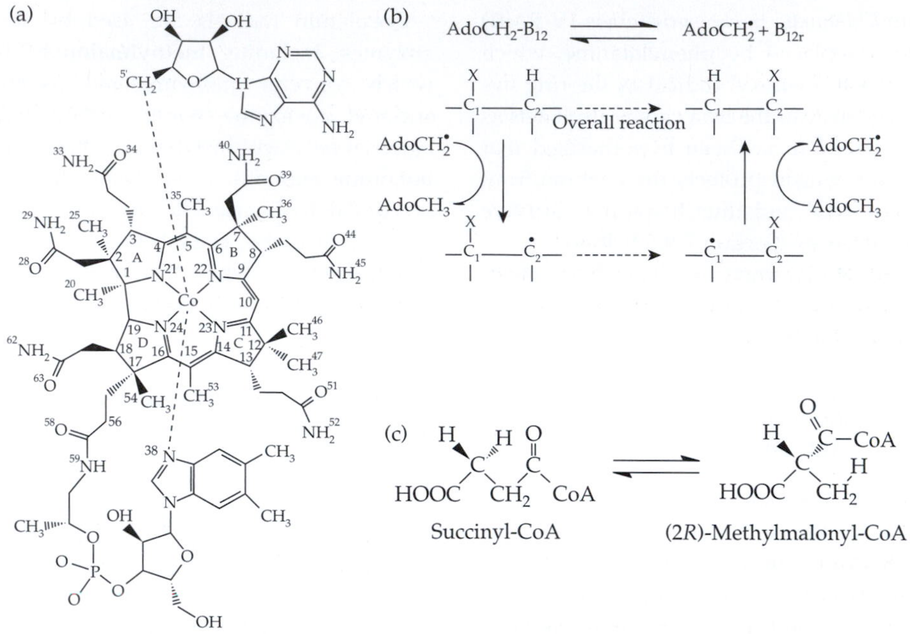

(a)

(b)

$$AdoCH_2\text{-}B_{12} \rightleftharpoons AdoCH_2^{\bullet} + B_{12r}$$

(c)

Figure 7.2 Vitamin B_{12} and its derivatives. Co is cobalt, a transition metal. The corrin ring has four nitrogen atoms co-ordinated to cobalt. The fifth co-ordination position is used to attach a derivative of dimethylbenzimidazole which is also attached to a side-chain of the corrin ring. The sixth co-ordination position of the cobalt can be occupied by several ligands, including cyanide, to give **cyanocobalamin** (cyanide is introduced during the isolation procedure and is not present *in vivo*). The cobalt atom in cobalamin can have a $+1$, $+2$ or $+3$ oxidation state. In **hydroxycobalamin**, OH^- occupies the sixth co-ordination position and the cobalt is in the Co(III) state. This form, called B_{12a} is reduced by a flavoprotein enzyme to $B_{12r}(Co^{2+})$ which is reduced by a second flavoprotein to give $B_{12s}(Co^+)$. NADPH is the donor in both cases. B_{12s} is the substrate for a reaction with ATP that yields **5′-deoxyadenosylcobalamin** (structure shown in a). This molecule is almost unique in living organisms in having a carbon–metal bond (CH_2–Co). Impaired absorption of cobalamin from the human diet results in **pernicious anaemia**. (b) Mechanism of coenzyme B_{12}-dependent rearrangements. Ado-CH_2-B_{12} is 5′-deoxyadenosylcobalamin, Ado-CH_2 and Ado-CH_3 are respectively the 5′-deoxyadenosyl radical and 5′-deoxyadenosine. X is the transferred group. (c) An example of (b): the rearrangement reaction catalysed by methylmalonyl-CoA mutase. The thioester group ($O = C$–CoA) is the group that migrates. From *Structure* **4**, 339, 1996 by courtesy of Dr Philip Evans and Current Biology Ltd.

sugars by *E. coli* under anaerobic conditions, helping to convert acetylSCoA to ethanol. Bacteria lacking the *adhE* gene show impaired growth[8] and increased ROS production in the presence of O_2. Interestingly, AdhE is one of the major targets of damage when H_2O_2 is added to *E. coli* (Section 4.13).

7.3.1 Pyruvate–ferredoxin oxidoreductase[9]

Another pyruvate-metabolizing enzyme used by anaerobic bacteria and some parasitic protozoa is **pyruvate–ferredoxin oxidoreductase** (PFOR). It catalyses a reversible reaction:

$$HSCoA + pyruvate + 2ferredoxin_{ox} \rightleftharpoons$$
$$acetylSCoA + CO_2 + 2ferredoxin_{red}$$

These enzymes contain Fe–S clusters and thiamine pyrophosphate (TPP). The reaction mechanism involves hydroxyethyl radicals attached to the TPP ($CH_3 - \overset{\bullet}{C}OH - TPP$) and *possibly* sulphur radicals from the coenzyme A ($^{\bullet}SCoA$). Hydroxyethyl radicals attached to TPP may also be involved in the pyruvate oxidase enzyme of *L. plantarum*, which converts pyruvate to acetyl phosphate, CO_2 and H_2O_2.[10]

7.4 Assorted oxidases

7.4.1 Galactose oxidase[11]

Galactose oxidase (GO) is a monomeric protein containing a single copper ion. It is released extracellularly by various *Fusarium* fungi and catalyses a two-electron oxidation of the $-CH_2OH$ group on galactose to $-CHO$, O_2 being reduced to H_2O_2. In the Cu^{2+} (oxidized) form of GO, the copper is liganded to two histidine residues, and to tyr 495 and tyr 272. The tyr 272 is covalently bonded to the sulphur of cys-228 to form a **cysteinyl–tyrosine**, in which the tyrosine is present as a tyrosyl radical. Of the two electrons abstracted from the substrate, one quenches the tyrosyl radical and the other reduces the copper to Cu^+. Oxygen then reoxidizes the enzyme to give Cu^{2+} and regenerate the $tyrO^\bullet$ radical.

Galactose oxidase is initially produced as a precursor protein without the cysteinyl–tyrosine but containing an extra 41 amino acids at the N-terminus. Part of this leader sequence is removed in the ER during preparation for secretion, and the rest during activation of the enzyme by Cu^+ and O_2, which can occur in the ER or Golgi apparatus or even outside the cell. During activation, the tyr–cys bond is created, the $tyrO^\bullet$ radical formed and the rest of the N-terminal peptide cleaved off. The precise chemistry of these events remains to be elucidated.

7.4.2 Indoleamine dioxygenase[12]

Indoleamine dioxygenase (IDO), a haem-containing enzyme, inserts oxygen into the ring structures of tryptophan and its derivatives, such as 5-hydroxy-tryptophan and tryptamine. This enzyme catalyses the first step in the kynurenine pathway, the major catabolic route for tryptophan in mammals (Fig. 7.3). Purified IDO is an inactive ferric enzyme, which must be reduced to the Fe^{2+} form to permit catalysis. This can be achieved *in vitro* by various chemical reducing agents as well as by $O_2^{\bullet-}$. Treating rabbit intestinal cells with the CuZnSOD inhibitor DDTC (Section 3.2.1.4), or the xanthine oxidase substrate hypoxanthine, increases tryptophan dioxygenation, suggestive of an interaction with $O_2^{\bullet-}$ in intact cells.

Levels of IDO in many tissues increase in response to infections and other pathological situations. Enzyme synthesis is usually promoted by the cytokine interferon γ, and is thought to be a defence and immunomodulatory response. This could theoretically involve a contribution to scavenging of $O_2^{\bullet-}$ if levels of IDO become sufficiently high (although the

Fe^{2+} enzyme can readily oxidize to the Fe(III) form and release $O_2^{\bullet-}$ again), and/or to the antioxidant abilities of such molecules as 3-hydroxyanthranilic acid and 3-hydroxykynurenine (Fig. 7.3). More work is needed to validate these suggestions.

7.5 Useful peroxidases

Glutathione-, ascorbate-, thioredoxin-dependent, and cytochrome *c* peroxidases are important H_2O_2-removing enzymes (Sections 3.8, 3.11 and 3.13). 'Non-specific' peroxidases may contribute to H_2O_2 removal in bacteria and plants, as well as being involved in such processes as auxin destruction (Section 3.13.4). In animals, non-specific peroxidases are less common, but important examples include myeloperoxidase (Section 7.7.3 below) and salivary peroxidase (Section 3.13.3). Let us look at some more.

7.5.1 Thyroid hormone synthesis

Formation of thyroid hormones requires iodination of tyrosine residues in the protein **thyroglobulin**, and coupling of the iodinated tyrosines to form **iodothyronines** (Fig. 7.4). Both processes are catalysed by **thyroid peroxidase**, an enzyme located in the ER of thyroid gland cells. It catalyses a *two-electron* oxidation (unusual for peroxidases)[13] of iodide ion (I^-), probably to form **iodonium ion** (I^+), which iodinates the tyrosines. It then catalyses one-electron oxidation of di-iodotyrosine to tyrosyl radicals which combine to form dimers. The H_2O_2 it requires is generated by a Ca^{2+}-dependent flavoprotein NADPH oxidase system, mutations in which cause congenital hypothyroidism, the most common congenital endocrine disorder.[14] A balance must be struck *in vivo* to allow thyroid peroxidase enough H_2O_2 to work yet prevent damage to the thyroid gland by excess H_2O_2. Peroxiredoxins help with this.[15]

Thyroxine and tri-iodothyronine are phenols (Fig. 7.4). As such, they show chain-breaking antioxidant activity *in vitro*, including increasing the 'lag period' of LDL oxidation (Section 9.3.5). However, the levels needed to achieve such effects are greater than physiological. Hence the biological significance of their 'antioxidant activity' is uncertain, especially as in plasma both compounds are almost entirely protein bound.

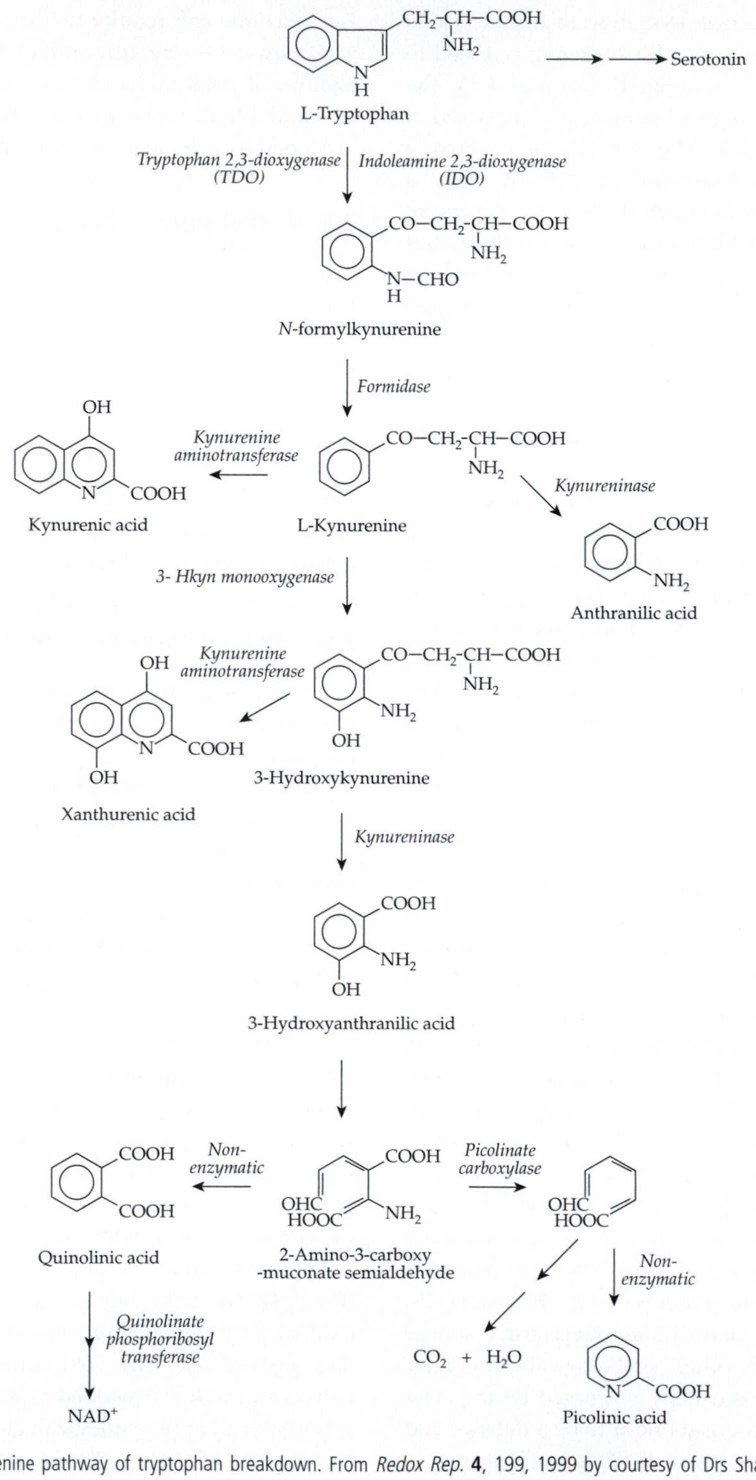

Figure 7.3 The kynurenine pathway of tryptophan breakdown. From *Redox Rep.* **4**, 199, 1999 by courtesy of Drs Shane Thomas and Roland Stocker and Maney publishers. The TDO enzyme catalyses the same reaction as IDO but is mainly found in liver. Quinolinic acid can act as an excitotoxin in the brain (Section 9.16.4), an effect which can contribute to the pathology of cerebral malaria (*Infect. Immun.* **73**, 5249, 2005).

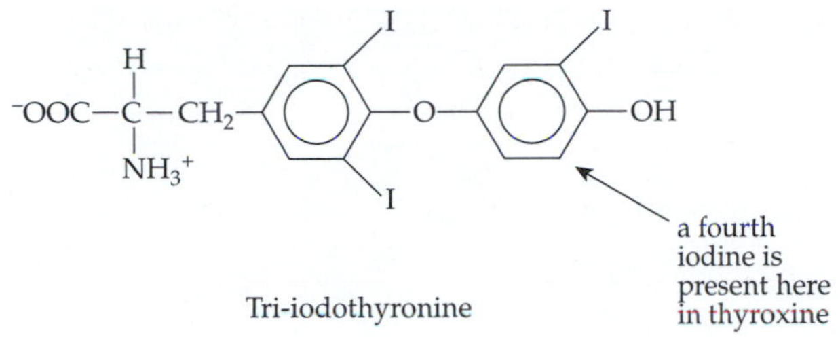

Figure 7.4 Structure of the thyroid hormones. They act on many cell types by binding to receptors and affecting gene transcription.

7.5.2 An 'antimolestation' spray

The ability of peroxidases to oxidize phenols into quinones in the presence of H_2O_2 is made use of by **bombardier beetles**, which attack their enemies by spraying them with hot, quinone-containing fluid (Fig. 7.5). A sac near the insect's 'ejection mechanism' contains a 25% aqueous solution of H_2O_2 plus 10% hydroquinone, and the spray is generated when the contents of the sac are pushed into a reaction chamber containing catalase and peroxidase. The hydroquinones are explosively oxidized to semiquinones and quinones, and part of the H_2O_2 is decomposed to O_2 by catalase. These events cause the temperature to rise up to 100°C and the pressure to build up, driving ejection of the hot spray to scare off whatever disturbed the beetle.

7.5.3 Thick coats[16]

Upon fertilization, eggs of the sea urchin *Strongylocentrotus purpuratus* rapidly form a 'fertilization envelope', to block further sperm from entering and to protect the developing embryo. This envelope contains cross-linked tyrosine residues. Their formation requires a peroxidase released from the egg, **ovoperoxidase**, which catalyses H_2O_2-dependent formation of tyrosyl radicals. Fertilization is accompanied by a 'burst' of O_2 uptake by a Ca^{2+} -dependent NADPH oxidase, which generates the necessary H_2O_2.

Any toxic effects of H_2O_2 produced at fertilization may be minimized both by the action of the usual H_2O_2-removing enzymes and by **ovothiol C** (Fig. 7.6), a thiol present at millimolar levels in sea-urchin eggs. The histidine ring facilitates ionization of the −SH group to increase its reactivity with H_2O_2. Oxidized ovothiol may be regenerated by reaction with GSH. Ovothiols are present in other marine organisms and some parasites (Fig. 7.6).

7.5.4 Making and degrading lignin[17]

Wood is one of Nature's toughest substances, and can last for centuries. Yet a few fungal strains have managed to harness the power of RS to break wood apart. One type is the **white rot fungi**, which degrade both **lignin** (a major constituent of wood) and cellulose. The wood becomes paler as lignin is destroyed, hence the name. **Brown rot fungi** mainly attack cellulose, leaving a residue of brownish, partially oxidized lignin.

7.5.4.1 *Making lignin*

Lignin arises from the oxidation and polymerization of phenolic alcohols synthesized from phenylalanine and tyrosine (Fig. 7.7).[18] Their oxidation to the phenoxyl radicals that polymerize (Fig. 7.7) is achieved by peroxidase enzymes bound to the plant cell wall. The source of the required H_2O_2 is not entirely clear, but it is likely that the cell wall peroxidases simultaneously oxidize NADH to generate $O_2^{•-}$, and H_2O_2 (Section 3.13.4). Another source may be NADPH oxidase enzymes, resembling these in animals (Section 7.10 below).[19] Diamine oxidase enzymes (Section 6.7.1) might sometimes contribute H_2O_2. The polymerization is not completely random; it is 'guided' by **dirigent proteins** in the cell wall (from Latin *dirigere*, to align or guide) that bind the radicals and only allow them to couple in certain ways.[18] **Laccases**, copper-containing enzymes that use O_2 to catalyse one-electron oxidation of phenols to semiquinones, also participate in lignin synthesis to a limited extent.[20]

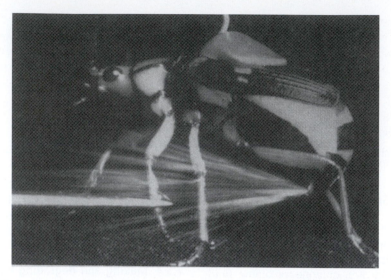

Figure 7.5 A bombardier beetle in action. Photograph by courtesy of Thomas Eisner and Daniel Aneshansley (also see *Experientia* **39**, 366, 1993 and *Science* **248**, 1219, 1990).

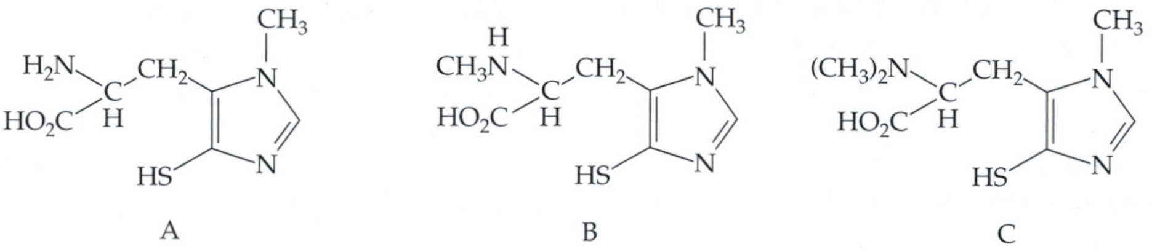

A   B   C

Figure 7.6 Structure of ovothiols, thio-histidine derivatives. **Ovothiol C** and related compounds have been detected in sea urchins and other marine invertebrates. Ovothiols A and B have been found in the eggs of trout and salmon. Ovothiol A has also been found in the parasites *Crithidia fasciculata* and *Leishmania donovani*, although the trypanothione pathway (Section 3.12.1) may be more important to them in removing peroxide (*Mol. Biochem. Parasitol.* **115**, 189, 2001). Diagram adapted from *Biochemistry* **29**, 1953, 1990 by courtesy of Dr Paul Hopkins and the publishers.

7.5.4.2 *Breaking lignin down*

Some wood-destroying fungi release both H_2O_2 and peroxidases extracellularly to aid lignin degradation. These peroxidases are much more oxidizing than horseradish peroxidase. For example, the white rot fungus *Phanerochaete chrysosporium*, can oxidize 60 to 70% of lignin to CO_2 and water, leaving the rest as small molecular fragments. This fungus produces at least two types of extracellular peroxidase. One is **lignin peroxidase**, a haem-containing glycoprotein that resembles HRP (Section 3.13.4), in that it has compound I, compound II and less active compound III states. Lignin peroxidase catalyses H_2O_2-dependent oxidation of **veratryl alcohol** (Fig. 7.7), a metabolite of the fungus. Oxidation forms a radical cation ($VA^{\bullet+}$) which diffuses into the wood and attacks the lignin. The peroxidase may additionally directly oxidize surface phenolic residues in the wood, generating other radicals to propagate depolymerization. Unlike HRP, the lignin peroxidase of *P. chrysosporium* uses a trp171 radical cation during its catalytic cycle, which is able to oxidize veratyl alcohol.[21]

The second type of peroxidases, also haem enzymes, oxidizes Mn^{2+} to Mn(III) in a 'classical' peroxidase reaction sequence:

$$\text{peroxidase} + H_2O_2 \rightarrow \text{compound I}$$
$$\text{compound I} + Mn^{2+} \rightarrow \text{compound II} + \text{Mn(III)}$$
$$\text{compound II} + Mn^{2+} \rightarrow \text{peroxidase} + \text{Mn(III)}$$

The Mn(III) binds to an organic acid, such as tartrate or oxalate, and the chelate is then believed to attack the lignin. In essence, both types of enzyme produce 'reactive species' ($VA^{\bullet+}$ or Mn (III)–chelates) that diffuse away from the peroxidase and attack lignin. Peroxidase–Mn(III) systems may also oxidize fungal lipids to generate $RO_2^{\bullet}$ radicals that could assist lignin breakdown.[22] Some fungi, for example *Bjerkandera adusta*, produce **versatile peroxidases** that can oxidize both veratryl alcohol and Mn^{2+}, getting the best of both mechanisms. A tryptophan radical is involved in the catalysis.[23]

From where do these various peroxidases obtain their H_2O_2? Several sources. One is an **aryl alcohol oxidase**. Another is a secreted **glyoxal oxidase**, which oxidizes several aldehydes to acids. Two substrates for this enzyme, glyoxal and methylglyoxal, are found in the extracellular environment of the fungi. Glyoxal oxidase converts glyoxal to oxalate and contains copper and a cysteinyl–tyrosine residue at its active site, rather like galactose oxidase (Section 7.4.1). Intracellular glucose oxidase enzymes can generate H_2O_2, which diffuses out of the fungus. An extracellular **cellobiose dehydrogenase** enzyme attacks cellulose in the wood, using quinones and metal chelates as electron acceptors. However, it can sometimes behave as a **cellobiose oxidase**, generating $O_2^{\bullet-}$ and H_2O_2.[17]

7.5.4.3 *A role for hydroxyl radical?*[24]

In the early days of research into lignin degradation by white rot fungi, it was suggested that free $OH^{\bullet}$ radicals were involved, because $OH^{\bullet}$ 'traps' such as methional and 4-methylthio-2-oxobutyrate (Table 5.4) were oxidized to ethene. However, these compounds can be oxidized directly by peroxidases, an illustration of the potential artefacts in their use as $OH^{\bullet}$ detectors. Nevertheless, some $OH^{\bullet}$ *can* be formed when H_2O_2 reacts with transition metals in the wood; metals can be reduced both by cellobiose dehydrogenase and by semiquinones generated during lignin oxidation.

It has been suggested that $OH^{\bullet}$ plays a greater role in wood degradation by brown rot fungi (e.g. *Gloeophyllum trabeum*) that do not produce lignin-degrading enzymes. These fungi release oxalic acid, which binds iron ions to give chelates that react with H_2O_2 to give $OH^{\bullet}$. Oxalate can be oxidized by $OH^{\bullet}$ to $CO_2^{\bullet-}$, which reduces O_2 to $O_2^{\bullet-}$ (Section 2.3.3.1). Some brown rot fungi also secrete hydroquinones to help keep iron in the reduced state. Hydroxylation techniques have been used to detect $OH^{\bullet}$ from brown rot fungi (Table 5.4).

7.6 Light production[25]

Still on the topic of wood, a peroxidase plays a role in light emission by the wood-boring mollusc *Pholas dactylus* (the common piddock). In many bioluminescent systems (e.g. in fireflies), light is produced when an enzyme (a **luciferase**) acts on a low-molecular-mass substrate (a **luciferin**) to generate an excited state, which produces light as it decays. However, *P. dactylus* luciferin is itself a protein, and can be induced to emit light when exposed to several systems generating ROS, such as Fe^{2+} in the presence of O_2, or a mixture of XO and hypoxanthine. Indeed, light emission from *P. dactylus* luciferin (often called **pholasin**) has been used as a sensitive method to detect ROS production by activated phagocytes. Bioluminescent marine scale worms also contain a protein (**polynoidin**) that emits light when exposed to ROS.

The *P. dactylus* luciferase is a glycoprotein with peroxidase activity, but it contains copper ions rather than haem. Similarly, luciferase from the earthworm *Diplocardia longa* (a luminescent earthworm several inches long found in Georgia, USA) contains copper and exerts peroxidase activity.

7.6.1 Green fluorescent protein: another example of autocatalytic oxidation

Oxidation reactions are involved in light production by the jellyfish *Aequorea victoria*. When this organism is disturbed, its intracellular Ca^{2+} levels change and cause emission of blue light by the protein **aequorin** (widely used in the laboratory as a Ca^{2+} detector). The chromagen is **coelenterazine**; light production from it involves formation of hydroperoxide and dioxetane intermediates (Fig. 7.8). Coelenterazine has been used to detect $O_2^{\bullet-}$ (Section 5.11.5) and both it and its oxidation product **coelenteramine** have been proposed to act

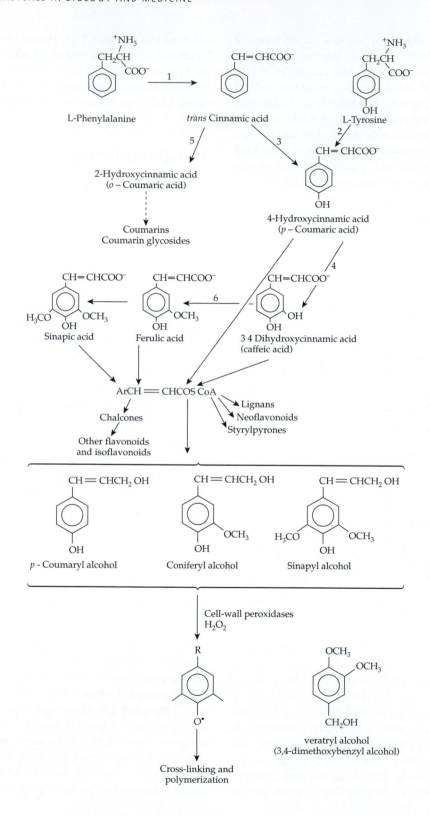

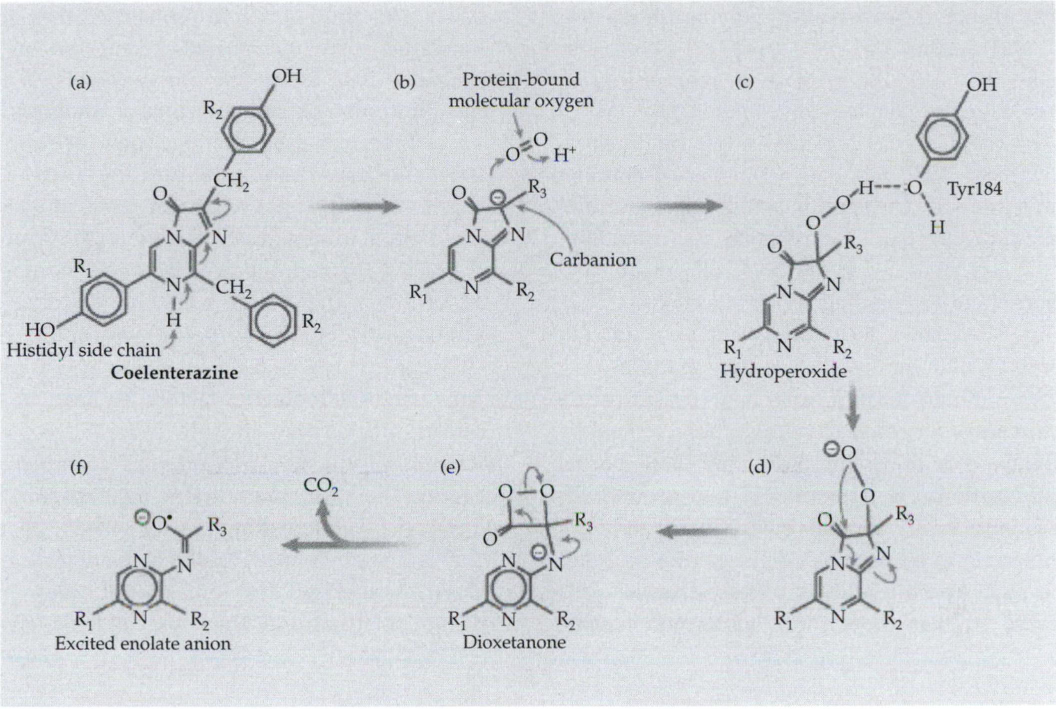

Figure 7.8 Possible chemical reactions underlying bioluminescence of aequorin. (a) Distortion of the ground state of coelenterazine by the aequorin protein leads to the formation of a reactive carbanion. (b) The carbanion attacks protein-bound O_2, leading to the hydroperoxide (c), which is stabilized primarily by hydrogen bonding to a tyrosine residue at position 184. (d) Binding of Ca^{2+} to aequorin induces a conformational change which allows attack by the hydroperoxide anion on the reactive carbonyl, leading to transient formation of an unstable dioxetanone (e). This undergoes scission to CO_2 and an enolate anion (f) in an excited state, which returns to the ground state by emission of a photon of blue light. From *Nature* **405**, 291, 2000 by courtesy of Dr Franklyn G Prendergast and the publishers. Also see *Nature* **405**, 372, 2000.

as antioxidants[26] in marine organisms by scavenging $O_2^{\bullet-}$ and other RS.

The blue light produced by aequorin is absorbed by another protein, **green fluorescent protein (GFP)**, which emits a bright-green flash. When first synthesized, GFP rapidly generates its own chromogen: a serine–tyrosine–glycine sequence (residues 65–67) in the protein undergoes autocatalytic oxidation to produce a chromophore. Adding extra –SH groups to the surface of GFP generates 'probes' that respond to cellular redox state by changes in fluorescence.[27]

7.7 Phagocytosis[28–30]

The phagocyte killing mechanism is probably the thing that comes immediately to mind when one is asked to name 'useful' roles for RS. The Russian scientist Metchnikoff was the first to report (in the late 1800s) the engulfment of bacteria by cells from the bloodstream of animals. This process is called **phagocytosis**–the cells 'flow around' the foreign particle and enclose it in a plasma membrane vesicle, which is then internalized (Fig. 7.9).

Most of the phagocytes in the human bloodstream are **neutrophils** (Table 7.1), which have a multilobed

Figure 7.7 An outline of the biosynthetic pathways of phenylpropanoid compounds in plants. Enzymes involved: 1, phenylalanine ammonia lyase (found in a wide range of plant tissues); 2, tyrosine ammonia lyase (found in some grasses); 3, cinnamate hydroxylase; 4, p-coumarate hydroxylase; 5, o-coumarate hydroxylase; 6, caffeic acid methyltransferase. Enzymes catalysing the later steps in the pathways are not shown in detail. Adapted from *Chloroplast Metabolism*, 2nd edition, Oxford University Press, 1984.

nucleus (hence they are called **polymorphonuclear cells**) and several different types of cytoplasmic granules (Fig. 7.9). The **primary** or **azurophil** granules contain the enzymes myeloperoxidase (MPO) and lysozyme, several proteinases (e.g. cathepsin G and elastase; Table 7.2), and a number of **granular cationic proteins**. The **specific** or **secondary granules** contain a protein that binds vitamin B_{12} (**cobalophilin**), the enzymes lysozyme and collagenase, and lactoferrin, an iron-binding protein (Section 3.15.1.2). A series of enzymes, including gelatinase (Table 7.2) is housed within the so-called **tertiary granules**.

When animal tissues are injured, an **acute inflammatory response** develops, characterized by swelling, warmth, pain, reddening and partial immobilization. The arterioles in and around the injured area relax, so that the capillary network becomes engorged with blood (hence the heat and redness). The permeability of the blood vessel walls increases so that more fluid leaks out, causing oedema. This fluid is rich in protein. As they enter the inflamed area, neutrophils often stop on the endothelial cells lining the blood vessels, a phenomenon known as **pavementing** or **margination**. Even in the normal circulation, some neutrophils loosely and transiently adhere to the vessel wall and roll along it. However, neutrophils at sites of inflammation adhere firmly, push out pseudopodia and squeeze through the gaps between endothelial cells, crossing the vessel wall and entering the inflamed area (Fig. 7.10). Some neutrophils may even pass *through* endothelial cells. Migration is induced by **chemotactic factors** formed in the inflamed area. These include *N*-formyl-peptides (bacterial products), products of complement activation (Fig. 7.11), leukotriene B_4 (Section 7.12.7 below), platelet-activating factor (PAF; Section 4.12.2) and chemokines. Platelet-activating factor is rapidly synthesized by endothelial cells after exposure to histamine, thrombin or leukotrienes.

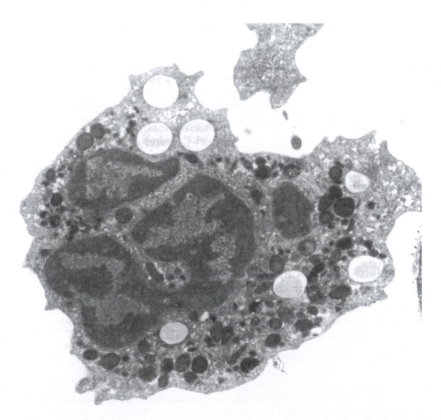

Figure 7.9 A neutrophil as seen under the electron microscope. The cell is phagocytosing opsonized latex beads (the white circles). Some are being taken up by the cell flowing around them and others are already present internally in vacuoles ($\times$ 18 000). Photograph by courtesy of Professor Anthony Segal.

Table 7.1 Cells in human blood

Type of cell	Cells/ μl blood	Function
Erythrocytes	5×10^6	Transport O_2 and CO_2; regulate pH; catabolize $NO^\bullet$, NO_2^-, and possibly H_2O_2 and $O_2^{\bullet-}$
White blood cells (leukocytes)		
Neutrophils	2500–7500	Phagocytosis
Eosinophils	40–400	Antiparasite; allergic and hypersensitivity responses
Basophils	0–100	Hypersensitivity reactions; release histamine
Mononuclear cells		
Monocytes	200–800	Precursors of macrophages
Lymphocytes		
B cells	~200–400	Make antibodies[a]
T cells	~1000	Kill virus-infected cells, regulate activities of other leukocytes
Natural killer (NK) cells	~100	Kill virus-infected and some cancer cells
Platelets	~3×10^5	Blood coagulation

Leukocytes, monocytes, and lymphocytes differ in morphology and function; for example, eosinophils differ from neutrophils in having larger cytoplasmic granules and often a nucleus with only two lobes. An abnormally high content of white cells in the blood (>11 000/μl) is called **leukocytosis**, whilst a decrease below 4000/μl is termed **leukopaenia** or, since neutrophils constitute such a high proportion of white cells, **neutropaenia**. Most eosinophils reside in the tissues rather than circulating in the blood. All these cell types, and red blood cells, derive from the same **haematopoietic stem cells** in the bone marrow.

[a] The principal function of B lymphocytes is to synthesize and secrete antibodies (**immunoglobulins**). When B cells are stimulated by encountering a foreign antigen, they undergo several cycles of cell division and then differentiate into specialized antibody-secreting **plasma cells**. The immune system can produce antibodies to almost any antigen encountered. When an animal comes into contact with an antigen, many B cells are stimulated. Each B cell carries on its surface immunoglobulin molecules with different antigen-binding sites. These act as the receptors for antigen and the secreted immunoglobulin of each cell has the same antigen binding site (specificity) as the membrane-bound immunoglobulin. Each B cell will divide to produce a **clone** of daughter cells, all producing immunoglobin with the same specificity. Since many B cells bind the antigen, the serum of the immunized animal will contain a mixture of the antibodies produced by many clones; **polyclonal antiserum**. (A **monoclonal antibody** is produced when a lymphocyte is fused with an immortalized cancer cell, producing a single clone which secretes monospecific antibody.)

T lymphocyte function involves direct contact with other cells, e.g. engaging death receptors, and/or production of cytotoxic proteins such as the pore-forming **perforin** protein and granzymes that can cause caspase activation (Section 4.4.1).

In general, the α-chemokines, including IL-8, act on neutrophils whereas the β-chemokines act on monocytes and macrophages (Table 4.8).

At a later stage of inflammation, monocytes (Table 7.1) leave the circulation and enter the inflamed area. These cells are less mobile and phagocytic then neutrophils, but once in the inflamed area they undergo differentiation into **macrophages**. This involves increases in their content of lysosomal enzymes, metabolic activity, motility and phagocytic and microbicidal capacity. Macrophages (a name derived from two Greek words—*macros* (big) and *phagos*, eater) are present normally in the lymph nodes and spleen, and as scattered cells in brain, bone, mammary gland, peritoneum and elsewhere (**resident macrophages**). For example, the **alveolar macrophages** lie on the alveolar walls, and help defend the lung against inhaled bacteria and other particles (Fig. 7.12). The **Kupffer cells**, which form part of the lining of the liver sinusoids, are macrophages, as are retinal pigment epithelial cells (Fig. 6.17). The term **mononuclear phagocyte system** is often used to encompass blood monocytes, their bone marrow precursors and tissue macrophages.

Macrophages phagocytose not only microorganisms but also host cells, for example erythrocytes and dead neutrophils. They can also ingest large amounts of insoluble material and retain it for months or years (Fig. 7.12). Uptake of too many erythrocytes by macrophages can depress their function, possibly by haem- and/or iron-dependent oxidative damage.[31]

7.7.1 Phagocyte recruitment, adhesion, activation and disappearance[28,32]

7.7.1.1 Getting to the right place
Recruitment of phagocytes to sites of tissue injury/ inflammation involves interactions between

Table 7.2 Animal proteinases[a] and antiproteinases and their response to reactive species: a summary

Type of proteinase	Comments	Effects of ROS on the proteinases/proteinase inhibitors
Serine at active site (serine proteinase)	Inhibited by organophosphates: endogenous inhibitors include α_1-antiproteinase (formerly called α_1-antitrypsin) and α_1-antichymotrypsin; often called **serpins** (serine proteinase inhibitors). Examples of serine proteinases are elastase, trypsin, chymotrypsin, cathepsin G and tryptase (Section 7.8).	Serine proteinases generally fairly resistant to RS, but α_1-AP can be inactivated by OH$^\bullet$, HOCl, ONOO$^-$, RO$_2^\bullet$ (Section 2.6.3; *J. Biol. Chem.* **275**, 27258, 2000) and cathepsin G by HOCl (*J. Biol. Chem.* **280**, 29311, 2005).
Cysteine at active site	Inhibited by –SH modifying reagents and leupeptin. Endogenous inhibitors include cystatins and α_2-macroglobulins (which inhibit a range of proteinases including elastase). Examples are cathepsins B, H, L and S. Caspases play key roles in apoptosis (Section 4.4.1).	Most are readily inactivated by a range of RS, sometimes including H_2O_2 and LOOH (especially caspases). α_2-Macroglobulin is inactivated by HOCl (*Biochemistry* **35**, 13983, 1999) and probably by ONOO$^-$.
Aspartic acid at active site	Inhibited by pepstatin. Examples are cathepsins D and E.	Probably fairly resistant to RS.
Metal ions at active site	Usually inhibited by EDTA. For example, the **matrix metalloproteinases** (MMPs) are a family of zinc-containing enzymes response for turnover and remodelling of the extracellular matrix. They include **collagenases** (MMP-1, -8, -13), **gelatinases** (MMP-2, -9), **matrilysin** (MMP-7), **stromelysins** (MMP-3, -10, -11) and **macrophage elastase** (MMP-12). Most are secreted as latent proenzymes, requiring proteolytic (or other) activation. Endogenous inhibitors include α_2-macroglobulin and **tissue inhibitors of metalloproteinases (TIMPs)**.	Complex effects; RS (especially HOCl) can activate the proenzymes but inhibit the activated proteinases (e.g. *J. Biol. Chem.* **278**, 28408, 2003). Some RS may promote increased expression of genes encoding MMP, e.g. in vascular smooth muscle cells (e.g. *Circ. Res.* **92**, e80, 2003) and skin (Section 6.12). Expression of genes encoding MMPs is frequently upregulated by cytokines, and ROS are sometimes involved in the mechanism (Section 4.7).
Ca^{2+}-dependent cysteine proteinases (calpains)	Section 4.3.2.	

[a] 'Proteinase' and 'protease' tend to be used interchangeably in the literature—we have standardized on the former.

proteins (**adhesion molecules**) on both phagocyte and vascular endothelial cell surfaces. As Metchnikoff said in 1893, 'next to leukocytes, the vessels and their endothelial lining play the most important role in inflammation'. Varying the levels of adhesion molecules (e.g. in response to different cytokines) determines which phagocytes are recruited and how tightly they stick. Agents that increase levels of adhesion molecules on endothelial cells include TNFα, IL-1, endotoxin, histamine, thrombin, leukotrienes and H_2O_2. Indeed, endothelial cells contain an H_2O_2-producing amine oxidase (**vascular adhesion protein 1, VAP1**) that may play some role in promoting adhesion.[33] Agents increasing the numbers of adhesion molecules on phagocyte surfaces include IL-8, TNFα, endotoxin, PAF and leukotrienes. Hypoxia also increases expression of adhesion molecules on both

phagocytes and endothelium, a process involved in ischaemia–reperfusion injury (Section 9.5.4). This process involves HIF-1 (Section 1.3.2); mice whose phagocytes lack HIF-1α show a decreased inflammatory response, perhaps because HIF-1 is needed for phagocytes to generate sufficient ATP by glycolysis in hypoxic regions of injured tissues (Section 7.7.2.1 below).[34]

A transient phagocyte contact with the endothelium (rolling along the vessel wall for a short time) is usually mediated by a member of the **selectin** family. Selectins are cell-surface proteins that have a carbohydrate-binding (**lectin**) domain on the end of a protein 'stalk' extending out from the cell surface. L-Selectin (CD62L)[a] is expressed by phagocytes and

[a] CD stands for 'cluster of differentiation': a cell surface marker that is recognized by a particular group of monoclonal antibodies is given a CD number.

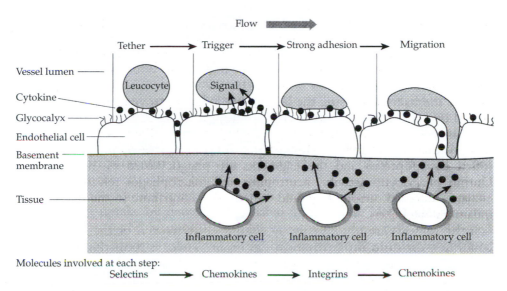

Figure 7.10 Steps in adhesion of leucocytes to endothelium. First, the leucocyte contacts the endothelial cells (**tethering**) by selectin-mediated interactions. Tethering allows any cytokines—often members of the chemokine family—present on the endothelial surface to bind receptors on the leucocyte and trigger integrins, which results in strong adhesion to the vessel wall. Subsequent migration into tissue is directed by cytokines (especially chemokines; Section 4.7) that are secreted by inflammatory cells beneath the endothelium and transported to the endothelial surface or released by the endothelium itself. For simplicity, the figure shows one cytokine triggering adhesion and directing migration, although many co-operate to regulate recruitment. From *Lancet* **343**, 832, 1994 by courtesy of Dr David Adams and the publishers. These processes are very important in the development of atherosclerosis (Fig. 9.5) and in many other diseases.

binds glycoproteins on the endothelial cell surface that are expressed at sites of inflammation. P-Selectin (CD62P) and E-selectin (CD62E) on the endothelial cell surface bind to carbohydrate on specific glycolipids or glycoproteins on neutrophils. E-Selectin levels are increased by elevated gene expression in response to cytokines (e.g. TNFα and IL-1), whereas P-selectin is stored in cytoplasmic granules, from which it is translocated to the plasma membrane when needed.

This initial selectin-mediated 'loose' binding allows a phagocyte to monitor the local environment; if it senses chemotactic factors it sticks more tightly to the endothelium and flattens out (Fig. 7.10). The chemotactic factors bind to receptors that activate **integrin** proteins on the phagocyte surface to change shape in preparation for binding to endothelial cell ligands. For example, **lymphocyte function antigen 1** (LFA-1) on neutrophils binds to **intercellular adhesion molecules 1 and 2** (ICAM-1 and -2) on endothelial cells, whereas integrin $\alpha_4\beta_1$ binds to **vascular cell adhesion molecule 1** (VCAM-1).

Migration of phagocytes between endothelial cells involves adhesion molecules as well,

including **platelet–endothelial cell adhesion molecule 1** (PECAM-1), present on endothelial cells at intercellular junctions and on phagocytes. It enables the phagocytes to interact with the endothelial cells as they pass through the junctions. Production of RS by phagocytes (Section 7.7.2 below) must be carefully regulated as they pass, to minimize endothelial damage. Adhesion usually deters RS production, but this can be over-ridden by high levels of TNFα, GM-CSF and PAF, which can thus promote endothelial damage.[35]

Matrix metalloproteinases, especially **matrilysin** (**MMP-7**; Table 7.2) play a role in phagocyte migration. They can digest matrix to facilitate movement, but can also limit inflammation by degrading some of the chemokines.[28] Sometimes they have more specific roles. For example, in mice injected with bleomycin (Section 9.15.3) there is inflammation of the lung lining cells. Neutrophils cross the capillary walls and the lung epithelium, and enter the alveoli. In mice lacking MMP-7, the neutrophils leave the blood vessels but do not cross the epithelium. The injured epithelial cells secrete a chemokine, which binds to the extracellular matrix.

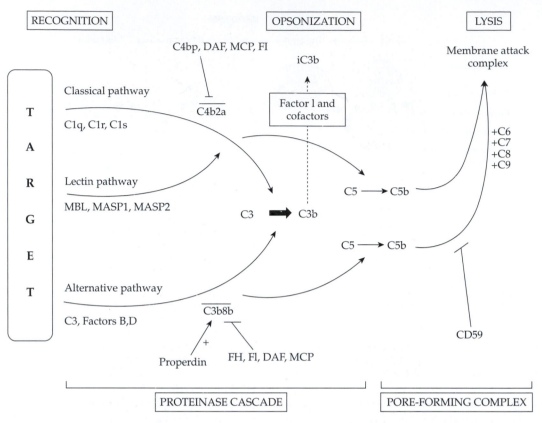

Figure 7.11 The complement cascade, a system evolved to destroy infectious microorganisms and damaged host cells. The cascade can be activated by at least three pathways, the **alternative pathway (AP)**, the **lectin pathway (LP)** and the **classical pathway (CP)**. The AP is activated by the continual slow cleavage of C3 and involves the deposition of thousands of copies of C3b onto a microbial target, a process called **opsonization**. Opsonization facilitates destruction of the target by allowing its recognition and engulfment by phagocytic cells via the C3b receptors on the phagocyte cell surface. The deposited C3b can also associate with either AP or CP C3 convertases (C3bBb and C4bC2a respectively) to form the **C5 convertases** (C3bBbC3b and C4bC2aC3b) that lead to formation of the **membrane attack complex (MAC)** and subsequent microbial cell lysis by forming pores ~100 Å in diameter. These pores are formed by polymers of between 12 and 18 molecules of C9 in the target membrane. The LP allows activation of complement through the recognition of carbohydrate structures on the surface of some yeasts, bacteria, and viruses by **mannose binding lectin (MBL)**. In the CP, the recognition molecule, C1q, binds to antigen–antibody complexes, in particular to the Fc regions of clustered immunoglobulins G or M (IgG or IgM) and to lipid A of Gram-negative bacteria. All pathways ultimately lead to the formation of multicomponent serine proteinases (C3 convertases) that allows these three routes to converge to the activation of C3. Thus unwanted organisms are destroyed by oposonization/phagocytosis and/or MAC formation. How are normal cells protected? Various membrane-bound glycoproteins on host cells protect against the destructive action of complement. From *Chem. Rev.* **102**, 308, 2002 by courtesy of Dr Pauline Rudd and the publishers.

The matrix is digested by MMP-7 to release the chemokine, provoking the neutrophils to cross.[28]

7.7.1.2 *What must phagocytes do?*
Three things: *recognize* foreign organisms, *engulf them*, and *kill* them. The fluid leaking into the inflamed area often contains antibodies that can bind to microorganisms. Both neutrophils and macrophages have surface receptors that recognize immunoglobulin G and the C3b component of reacted complement. The complement system plays a key role both in allowing recognition of foreign material by phagocytes and in killing microorganisms directly (Fig. 7.11). Coating of microorganisms with host-derived proteins, known collectively as **opsonins**, enables neutrophils and macrophages to

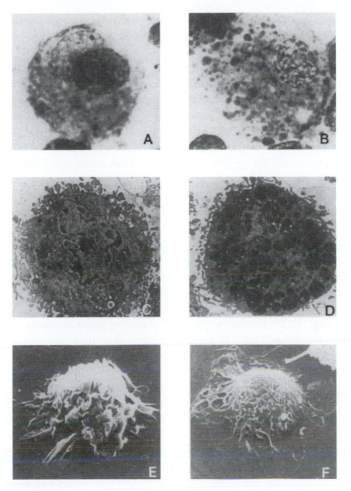

Figure 7.12 Human pulmonary macrophages, from the lungs of healthy volunteers. A, C and E are from non-smokers, and B, D and F from smokers. A and B are light micrographs. The cells vary from 15 to 50 μm in diameter. C and D are electron micrographs ($\times$ 6175); and E and F are scanning electron micrographs which show the surface of the cells. Large numbers of vesicles are present. Cigarette smoke causes marked changes in the cells, which contain characteristic 'smokers' inclusions', these include 'needle-like' or 'fibre-like' structures. These needle-like structures consist of kaolinite, an aluminium silicate present in cigarette smoke that the macrophages can engulf. Cigarette smoking increases the number of alveolar macrophages (Section 8.12.2). Photographs by courtesy of Professor W.G. Hocking.

recognize them, although a few species have coats that can be recognized directly. Once the foreign organisms have been engulfed, various cytoplasmic granules fuse with, and dump their contents into, the vacuole containing the engulfed particle (the **phagocytic vacuole** or **phagosome**). The engulfed particles are then killed and, if possible, digested within the phagocytic vacuole.

After the invading organisms have been destroyed (or, if injury was caused by another mechanism such as heat or chemicals, after the insult ceases) there is usually reversal of the inflammatory changes. The vessel walls regain their normal permeability. The emigrated neutrophils die (usually by apoptosis) and the fragments are phagocytosed by macrophages. If there was loss of tissue (e.g. in a wound), repair takes place, involving collagen synthesis and fibroblast proliferation. During phagocytic activity, neutrophils and macrophages release lysosomal enzymes into the surrounding fluid, where they contribute to the digestion of inflammatory debris.

If the bacteria are not completely eliminated, or the tissue injury continues, or something goes wrong with the normal mechanisms promoting resolution of inflammation (e.g. hyaluronic acid fragments persist; Section 9.10.4.1), **chronic inflammation** can result. Bacteria likely to cause chronic inflammation include those responsible for syphilis and tuberculosis; chronic lung inflammation can be induced by inhaled silica dust or silicate fibres (Section 8.14). Excess fibrous tissue produced during chronic inflammation causes loss of function. Chronic inflammatory lesions are rich in macrophages, several of which may fuse together to give **giant cells** with multiple nuclei. The function of giant cells is not clear, but they retain some phagocytic ability. One important factor influencing susceptibility to infection, the time course and severity of infection and the risk of developing chronic inflammation is the relative amounts of proinflammatory (e.g. TNFα) and anti-inflammatory (e.g. IL-10) cytokines produced in response to tissue damage. This is to some extent genetically determined.[36]

7.7.2 How do phagocytes kill?[29,37–39]

7.7.2.1 *Phagocytes show a respiratory burst*
Most studies on the biochemistry of phagocytosis have been carried out on neutrophils, fewer on monocytes, eosinophils and macrophages. Studies on the last are often done on alveolar macrophages since they can be readily obtained from humans (by washing them out of the lungs in the technique of **bronchoalveolar lavage**).

Resting neutrophils consume little O_2, since they rely mainly on glycolysis for ATP production and are rich in stored glycogen. By contrast, macrophages possess more mitochondria, rely more on oxidative phosphorylation and hence consume more O_2. At the onset of phagocytosis, however, all four types of phagocyte show a marked increase in O_2 uptake, called the **respiratory burst**. It is a bad name, since the extra O_2 uptake is not due to increased respiration and is not prevented by inhibition of mitochondrial electron transport. The increase in O_2 uptake during the respiratory burst can be 10 to 20 times the 'resting' O_2 consumption of neutrophils. As O_2 uptake increases, so does consumption of glucose by phagocytes, largely due to activation of

the pentose phosphate pathway (Section 3.8.3.1). The respiratory burst can be triggered by opsonized microorganisms, **opsonized zymosan** (a preparation of yeast cell walls used in the laboratory to activate phagocytes) and several chemicals. These include phorbol esters such as **phorbol myristate acetate** (**PMA**) (Section 9.13.3), aluminium fluoride, peptide 'mimics' of parts of certain bacterial proteins (such as *N*-formylmethionylleucylphenylalanine; **fMet–Leu–Phe**), unsaturated fatty acids and **concanavalin A**, a lectin. There is considerable person-to-person variation in the extent and time course of O_2 uptake by neutrophils isolated from human blood and activated *in vitro*, and activation can sometimes occur during the isolation procedures.[40] Neutrophil responsiveness also varies when these cells are obtained from the same person at different times.

Similarly, the size of the respiratory burst shown by macrophages depends on how, and from which tissue site, they are obtained. Resident macrophages tend not to be very active and need prior exposure to priming agents (Section 7.7.2.2 below) before they can mount a vigorous respiratory burst. This is often achieved experimentally by infecting animals with microorganisms such as the tuberculosis bacillus or by injecting irritating materials such as thioglycollate. The antibacterial behaviour of the macrophages obtained by these different procedures is variable and papers concerning, for example, the relative importance of ROS or RNS in killing by macrophages should be read with this in mind. Many cytokines affect macrophage RS production; macrophages are also a rich source of cytokines, such as IL-1, IL-6 and TNFα.[30] Macrophages are capable of secreting hundreds of other substances, including eicosanoids, proteinases (e.g. collagenase and macrophage elastase, an enzyme that has properties very different from neutrophil elastase and is not inhibited by α_1-antiproteinase), growth factors, enzyme inhibitors (e.g. α-macroglobulin; Table 7.2), some components of complement, angiogenesis factors and PAF.[30]

7.7.2.2 *Priming of the respiratory burst*[41]
Phagocytes can be 'primed' by prior exposure to certain agents; primed cells produce a more

Free Radicals in Biology and Medicine

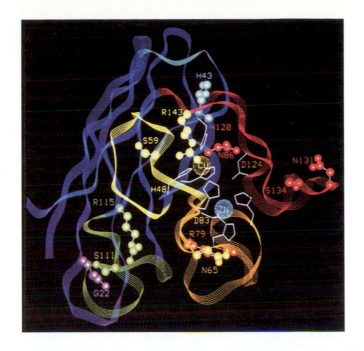

Plate 1 See Fig. 3.3.

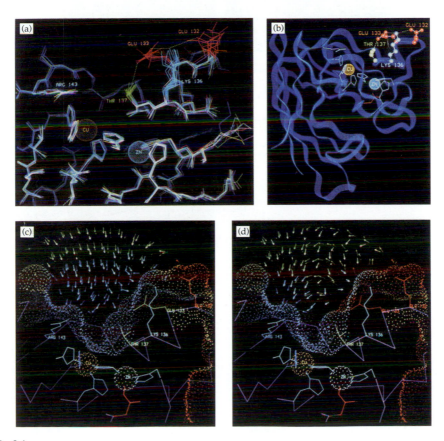

Plate 2 See Fig. 3.4.

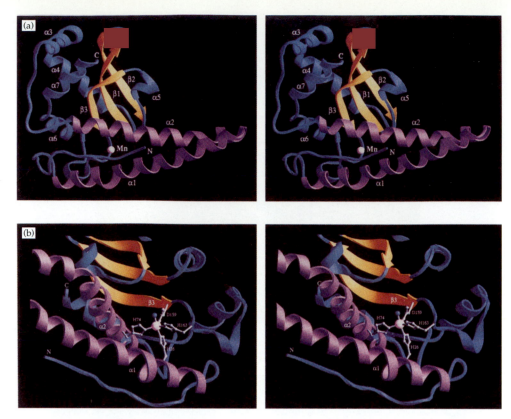

Plate 3 See Fig. 3.6.

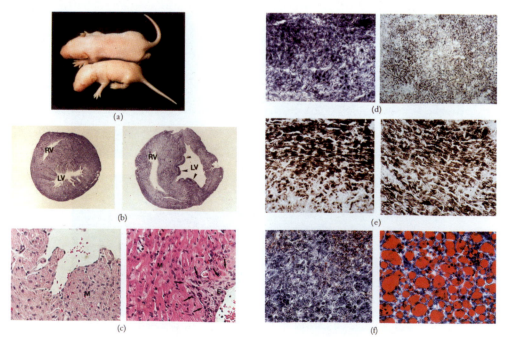

Plate 4 See Fig. 3.8.

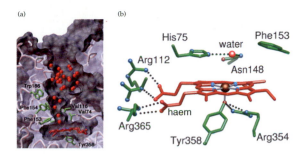

(a)　(b)

His75　water　Phe153

Arg112

Asn148

haem

Arg365　Tyr358　Arg354

Plate 5 See Fig. 3.10.

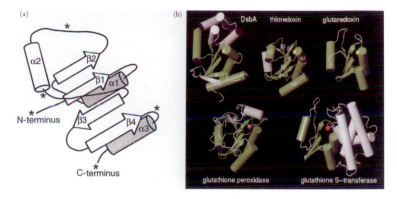

(a)

α2

β2

β1　α1

N-terminus

β3　β4　α3

C-terminus

(b)

DsbA　thioredoxin　glutaredoxin

glutathione peroxidase　glutathione S–transferase

Plate 6 See Fig. 3.16.

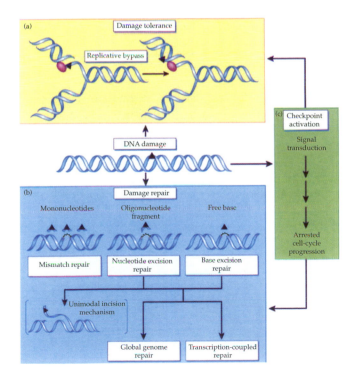

(a)　Damage tolerance

Replicative bypass

(c) Checkpoint activation

Signal transduction

DNA damage

Arrested cell-cycle progression

(b)　Damage repair

Mononucleotides　Oligonucleotide fragment　Free base

Mismatch repair　Nucleotide excision repair　Base excision repair

Unimodal incision mechanism

Global genome repair　Transcription-coupled repair

Plate 7 See Fig. 4.15.

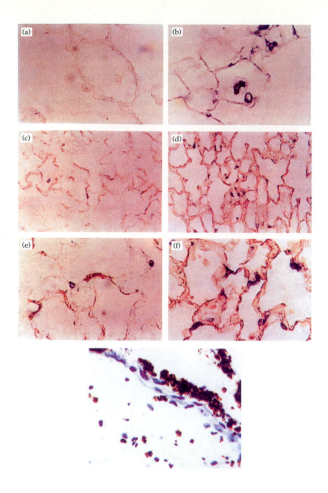

Plate 8 See Fig. 5.8.

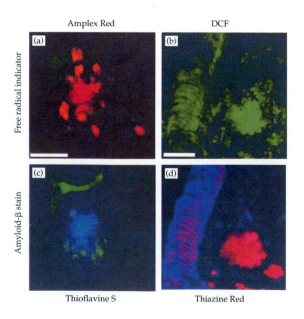

Amplex Red   DCF

Free radical indicator

Amyloid-β stain

Thioflavine S   Thiazine Red

Plate 9 See Fig. 5.15.

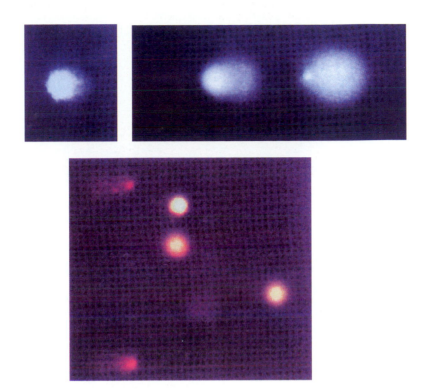

Plate 10 See Fig. 5.16.

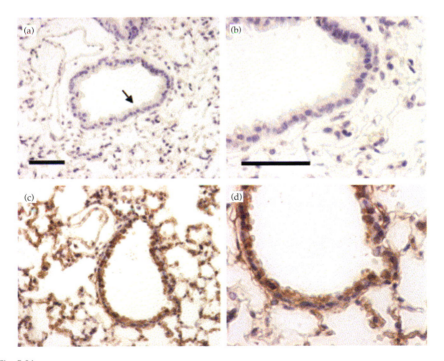

Plate 11 See Fig. 5.21.

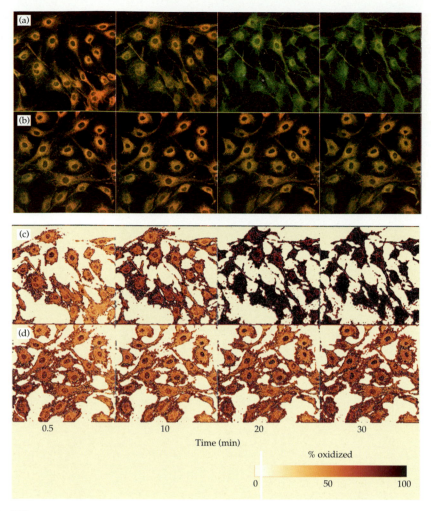

Plate 12 See Fig. 5.25.

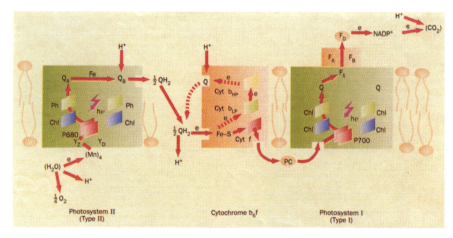

Plate 13 See Fig. 6.10.

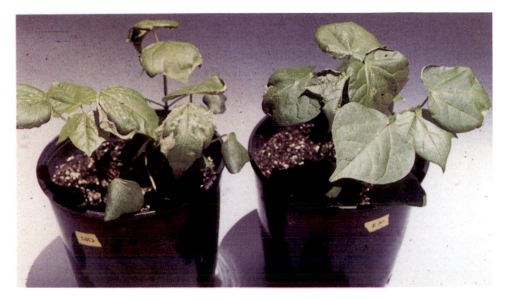

Plate 14 See Fig. 6.18.

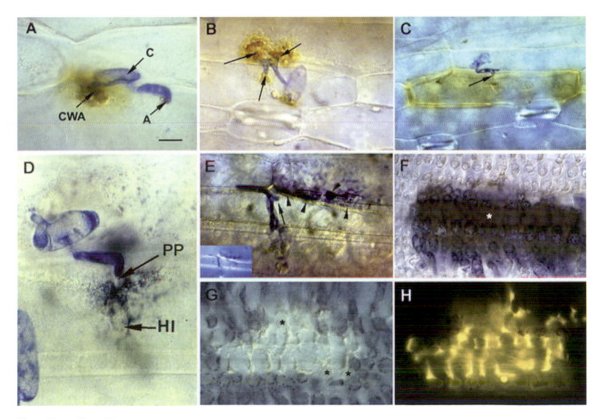

Plate 15 See Fig. 7.17.

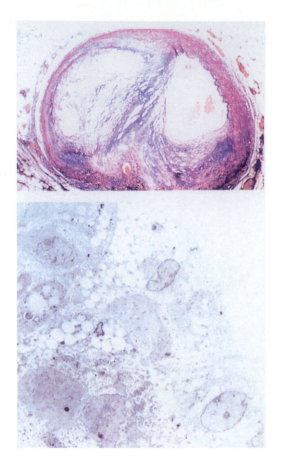

Plate 16 See Fig. 9.4.

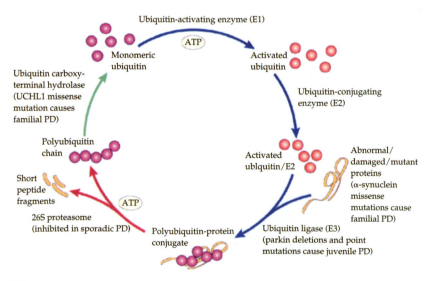

Ubiquitin-activating enzyme (E1)

ATP

Monomeric ubiquitin

Activated ubiquitin

Ubiquitin-conjugating enzyme (E2)

Ubiquitin carboxy-terminal hydrolase (UCHL1 missense mutation causes familial PD)

Polyubiquitin chain

Activated ubiquitin/E2

Abnormal/ damaged/mutant proteins (α-synuclein missense mutations cause familial PD)

Short peptide fragments

ATP

26S proteasome (inhibited in sporadic PD)

Polyubiquitin-protein conjugate

Ubiquitin ligase (E3) (parkin deletions and point mutations cause juvenile PD)

Plate 17 See Fig. 9.31.

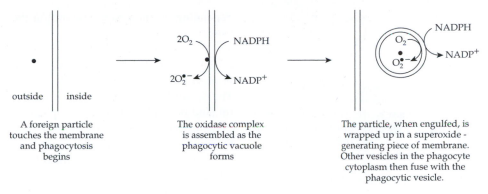

Figure 7.13 A schematic representation of the respiratory burst. The engulfed particles are exposed to a flux of $O_2^{\bullet -}$ inside the phagocytic vacuole. Activation of the oxidase involves translocation of proteins from the cytosol to the membrane.

vigorous respiratory burst on subsequent stimulation and have enhanced levels of adhesion molecules and receptors to fmet–leu–phe. Priming agents include interferon γ, PAF, IL-8, GM-CSF (Table 4.8), TNFα and bacterial endotoxin. The priming agents themselves (at *in vivo* levels) usually induce little or no respiratory burst.

7.7.2.3 *The respiratory burst makes superoxide*

Oxygen uptake during the respiratory burst is due to the activation of an enzyme complex in that part of the plasma membrane that forms the phagocyte vacuole. The activated complex oxidizes NADPH (largely provided by the pentose phosphate path-

b_{558} is present in the plasma membrane; the rest is in the cytoplasm, in secretory vesicles and specific granules, which can supply more of it to the plasma membrane upon activation of the respiratory burst. Activation of the neutrophil NADPH oxidase requires several proteins normally present in the cytosol of 'resting' neutrophils, especially **p47**^{phox}, **p67**^{phox}, **p40**^{phox} and **rac2**. They translocate to the membrane and help assemble the active complex. The suppression of neutrophil $O_2^{\bullet -}$ production that usually occurs as these cells pass through the endothelium (Section 7.7.1.1) occurs by modulation of rac2 activity.[35] Once the active complex is assembled an electron transport system operates.

NADPH → oxidized FAD		2 reduced cytochrome b	$2O_2^{\bullet -}$
H$^+$ + NADP$^+$ ← reduced FAD		2 oxidized cytochrome b	$2O_2$

approximate reduction potentials at pH 7   −320 mV   −280mV   −245mV   −160mV

way) into NADP$^+$, releasing two electrons that are used to reduce $2O_2$ to $2O_2^{\bullet -}$ (Fig. 7.13).

$$NADPH + 2O_2 \rightarrow NADP^+ + H^+ + 2O_2^{\bullet -}$$

The NADPH oxidase complex contains a **b-type cytochrome** (**cytb$_{558}$**) with a sufficiently low reduction potential to be able to reduce O_2 to $O_2^{\bullet -}$. It is a dimer, with a large β subunit (**gp91**^{phox}) that contains FAD and a smaller α (**p22**^{phox}) subunit.[b] Usually, less than 30% of neutrophil cytochrome

This system is arranged vectorially in the membrane so that electrons pass across it from the NADPH-oxidizing site to the O_2-reducing site (Fig. 7.13). NADPH-dependent $O_2^{\bullet -}$ formation can be inhibited by **diphenylene iodonium** and related compounds, although sadly they are not specific (Fig. 7.14). Movement of electrons across the plasma membrane is accompanied by outward movement of H$^+$ through proton-conducting channels to prevent excessive acidification of the cytosol by H$^+$ released by NADPH oxidation. The channels open when the oxidase is activated.

[b] *Phox* denotes phagocyte oxidase, *p* means protein, and *gp* glycoprotein.

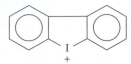

Figure 7.14 Structure of diphenylene iodonium (DPI). This and related compounds inhibit $O_2^{\bullet-}$ production by the phagocyte NADPH oxidase, although they are far from specific, inhibiting several other flavoproteins as well (e.g. NOS, cytochrome P450 reductase, XO, and mitochondrial NADH–CoQ oxidoreductase). Diphenylene iodonium intercepts an electron from the flavin and is converted to a radical, which then forms an adduct with the flavin, haem or amino acid residues to inactivate the protein (*Biochem. J.* **290**, 41, 1993; *J. Biol. Chem.* **277**, 19402, 2002).

The signal transduction pathways leading to activation of the oxidase by physiological stimuli contain membrane receptors, a small G protein[c] (Rac2 is human neutrophils, usually Rac1 in monocytes and macrophages), a phosphatidylinositol-specific phospholipase C and a protein kinase C (PKC). The Rac proteins are cytosolic and upon activation of the respiratory burst they bind GTP and migrate to the membrane to facilitate activation by interacting with p67^{phox}. Hydrolysis of phosphatidylinositol 4,5 bisphosphate produces inositol 1,2,5-triphosphate (IP$_3$) and diacylglycerol (DAG). The former enters the cytoplasm and raises intracellular free Ca^{2+} (Section 4.5.5.2) whereas DAG participates in the activation of PKC, leading to phosphorylation of many proteins, including p47^{phox} (on serine). This phosphorylation by PKC (other kinases may contribute) promotes translocation of p47^{phox} to the membrane and contributes to activation of the oxidase. Production of arachidonic acid also helps; it seems to increase the affinity of cytochrome *b* for O$_2$ and promote its interactions with the phox proteins.

Receptor-dependent oxidase activation is short lived; the oxidase rapidly 'switches off', in part by dephosphorylation of p47^{phox}, unless the signal is continual. Phorbol myristate acetate stimulates the respiratory burst by activating PKC directly; hence the resulting phagocyte response is unphysiological in that it is Ca^{2+}-independent and much more prolonged. There is still considerable debate over the precise sequence of events in activation and the roles of different receptors and kinases, which vary

[c] For an explanation of G proteins please see Section 4.5.5.

depending on the phagocyte and on the stimulus used.

7.7.2.4 *Superoxide is required to kill some bacteria*[29,37,39]

The K_m for O$_2$ of the activated oxidase complex in rat (and probably human) neutrophils is within the range of O$_2$ concentrations in body fluids, and so the amount of $O_2^{\bullet-}$ produced might be affected by O$_2$ concentration.[42] Carbon dioxide levels also affect $O_2^{\bullet-}$ and cytokine production, apparently by altering intracellular pH.[43]

If the respiratory burst of neutrophils is prevented by placing them under N$_2$, their killing of many bacterial strains is not impaired. Many of these bacteria are anaerobes, and the neutrophil would not be expected to rely upon an O$_2$-dependent killing mechanism for species that it is likely to encounter only at low O$_2$. Their killing is presumably achieved by the contents of the various granules as they empty into the phagocytic vacuole. For example, the enzyme **lysozyme** digests cell wall constituents of various bacteria, especially Gram-positive strains. Several of the granular cationic proteins have bactericidal activity, for example by acting as proteinases or by opening 'channels' across bacterial cell membranes and dissipating ion gradients. Lactoferrin binds iron essential for the growth of bacteria, and has been reported to kill a few bacterial strains directly. Elastase and cathepsin G are important in bacterial killing (Section 7.7.2.10 below); indeed, adding proteinase inhibitors can decrease bacterial killing by phagocytes. Neutrophil elastase degrades *Shigella* virulence factors, for example. Neutrophils release some of their granule contents extracellularly, forming sticky protein complexes that can trap and damage bacteria.[44]

However, the killing of other bacterial strains by neutrophils is decreased under anaerobic conditions. Indeed, patients suffering from **chronic granulomatous disease** (CGD), a collective term for inherited conditions in which phagocytosis is normal but the respiratory burst is absent, show persistent and multiple infections by some of these bacteria (Table 7.3). Hence superoxide production is essential for killing them. Why? Before attempting to answer that, it is worth mentioning that sometimes other sources of ROS contribute to killing. For example, a trypanocidal protein isolated from plasma of cape buffalo (*Syncerus caffer*) in Kenya turned out to be XO,[45] and the toxic agent was H_2O_2. Upon infection, blood hypoxanthine levels rise whereas catalase activity declines, preserving H_2O_2 to attack the parasite. In knockout mice lacking phagocyte oxidase, removal of *Burkholderia* (Table 4.3) was decreased; clearance of this organism was further decreased by injecting allopurinol,[46] suggesting an ancillary role for XO. A human salivary peptide, **histatin 5**, is taken up by *Candida albicans* and helps kill this fungus by causing excess ROS generation from its mitochondria.[47]

7.7.2.5 So how does superoxide kill? Via H_2O_2?

Several microorganisms are quickly killed by H_2O_2, formed from $O_2^{\bullet-}$ by non-enzymic or SOD-catalysed dismutation. Unlike $O_2^{\bullet-}$, H_2O_2 crosses bacterial envelopes. It can be toxic to bacteria by causing damage directly, or by forming $OH^{\bullet}$ within the bacterium. For example, increasing the intracellular iron content of bacteria sensitizes them to H_2O_2 (Section 3.6.2.2). Indeed, dimethylsulphoxide, a scavenger of $OH^{\bullet}$ that can penetrate into cells, partially protects *Staphylococcus aureus* against killing by human neutrophils. During these experiments, the formation of methane, a product of the reaction between dimethylsulphoxide and $OH^{\bullet}$, was observed.[48] The variable sensitivity of different bacteria to H_2O_2 is probably due to their different levels of H_2O_2-metabolizing systems, their varying ability to raise these levels quickly (e.g. via oxyR; Section 4.5.2) and to the different intracellular availabilities of transition-metal ions, which can be affected by the growth media used.

7.7.2.6 Via hydroxyl radical?

Although bacterial killing by H_2O_2 may involve intracellular $OH^{\bullet}$ formation, killing by converting H_2O_2 into $OH^{\bullet}$ in the phagosome is intrinsically unlikely; extracellular $OH^{\bullet}$ would probably attack the bacterial cell wall and do little damage.

Nevertheless, several scientists have detected $OH^{\bullet}$ in suspensions of activated neutrophils using a range of techniques, including deoxyribose degradation, benzoate decarboxylation, oxidation of methional to ethene gas, and spin trapping

(Chapter 5). How does it arise? Some may be artefactual. When neutrophils are isolated, they are separated from their normal environment and suspended in laboratory buffers, most or all of which are iron contaminated (Table 4.4). Neutrophil-derived $O_2^{\bullet-}$ and H_2O_2 can react with such iron to form $OH^{\bullet}$. Lactoferrin is secreted into the phagocytic vacuole of activated neutrophils, and also released from them. Its affinity for iron is high, the bound iron is not redox active, and lactoferrin needs to be at a pH below 3 for the iron to be rendered labile (Section 3.15.1.2). Lactoferrin secretion by neutrophils may thus help to *minimize* iron-dependent $OH^{\bullet}$ generation, by binding any available iron ions at sites of inflammation.

Activated neutrophils make both $O_2^{\bullet-}$ and hypochlorous acid (Section 7.7.3 below); interaction of these species (Section 2.6.3.1) could explain $OH^{\bullet}$ formation. Just to remind you, the reaction is:

$$HOCl + O_2^{\bullet-} \rightarrow O_2 + OH^{\bullet} + Cl^-$$

7.7.2.7 Via singlet O_2?

Singlet O_2 can arise from HOCl; we consider its importance (apparently not very great) in Section 7.7.3 below.

7.7.2.8 Via ozone?

Antibody-coated neutrophils activated by PMA were reported to produce ozone, known to be a highly bactericidal species.[49] The antibodies are thought to catalyse production of O_3 from H_2O by a $^1O_2$-mediated process (Section 2.6.5.1). Since neutrophil $^1O_2$ production appears limited, the significance of this pathway remains to be determined.

7.7.2.9 Via peroxynitrite?

Rat, mouse and some other animal neutrophils and macrophages (especially if primed) readily generate $NO^{\bullet}$. Nitric oxide at micromolar levels can kill certain bacteria and parasitic protozoa, both directly (e.g. by inhibiting respiratory chain function) and indirectly, by reacting with $O_2^{\bullet-}$ and generating $ONOO^-$ which attacks iron–sulphur proteins, essential –SH groups, and many other targets (Sections 2.5.6 and 2.6.1). Indeed, mice lacking iNOS are more susceptible to certain pathogens (Table 2.11). Thus iNOS induction and

Table 7.3 Chronic granulomatous disease

Incidence	1 in 250 000 to 1 in 500 000 (no ethnic differences)
Male:female ratio	6:1 (due to predominance of X-linked form; no gender difference in autosomal forms)
Inheritance	~60% X-linked (gp91^{phox} in b-type cytochrome defective); rest mostly autosomal recessive; defects in gp22^{phox} of b-type cytochrome, or in p47^{phox} or p67^{phox}, or in rac2 (the last types have normal cytochrome b levels)
Carrier state	Seen in X-linked CGD in mothers and sisters, usually asymptomatic
Age of onset	Congenital, first symptoms usually at <1 year of age (80%), rarely adult onset
Clinical manifestations	a. Recurrent bacterial and fungal infections; b. Sequelae of chronic inflammation (failure to thrive, anaemia, enlarged spleen, etc.); c. Obstruction due to granuloma formation
Diagnosis	Absence of $O_2^{\bullet-}$ and H_2O_2 production by activated phagocytes, e.g. failure to detect blue formazan production from NBT under the microscope
Organ involvement[a]	a. Lung (80%)—pneumonia (*Staphylococcus aureus, Aspergillus*) abscess, chronic changes; b. Lymph nodes (75%)—suppurative lymphadenitis (*S. aureus*), adenopathy; c. Skin (65%)—infectious dermatitis, abscesses; d. Liver (40%)—abscess (*Staphylococcus aureus*); e. Bone (30%)—osteomyelitis (*Serratia*); f. Gastrointestinal tract (30%); g. Sepsis and meningitis (20%); h. Genitourinary (10%)
Prognosis	Variable: death in infancy to middle age
Treatment	Prophylactic antibiotics

CGD is a defect in phagocyte $O_2^{\bullet-}$ production. Different defects exist, e.g. patients with X-linked CGD have a defective b-type cytochrome. Non-X-linked CGD can affect the b-type cytochrome or other proteins involved in assembling the respiratory burst complex. Adapted from *Current Clinical Topics in Infectious Disease* **6**, 138, 1985 by courtesy of the late Professor Bernie Babior and the publishers. Also see *Cell. Mol. Life Sci.* **59**, 1428, 2002. Other organisms that can cause problems in CGD patients include *Pseudomonas* and *Burkholderia cepacia*. The problems in CGD involve both failure to clear organisms properly and dysregulation of the immune response, e.g. RS sometimes are anti-inflammatory agents (Section 7.9.5).

[a] Transgenic mice lacking phagocyte oxidase constituents also show increased susceptibility to *S. aureus, Aspergillus, Burkholderia* and *Listeria monocytogenes* infections (*J. Immunol.* **158**, 5581, 1997; *Infect. Immun.* **68**, 2374, 2000).

the respiratory burst of phagocytes represent both parallel and overlapping (via ONOO⁻) defences. Indeed, knockout mice lacking both gp91^{phox} and iNOS died of spontaneous infections unless reared under pathogen-free conditions.[50] But be cautious when reading about knockouts that seem more susceptible to infection. Always ask 'what did the animals die of'? Was it overwhelming proliferation of the invader? Or a badly dysregulated immune response that killed the animal (Section 7.9.5 below)? Sometimes it's not clear.

Some are sceptical about the relevance of killing by RNS to humans, since it is difficult to persuade human neutrophils or macrophages to make NO$^{\bullet}$ *in vitro*.[51] Phagocyte NO$^{\bullet}$ generation mostly involves increased production of iNOS in response to cytokines, and human phagocytes can express iNOS if given the right cytokine mixture.[52] Indeed,

RNS production (as assessed by NO_2^-/NO_3^- levels, or nitrotyrosine production), is markedly elevated in many human diseases, showing that there is increased NO$^{\bullet}$ generation *in vivo*.

Although ONOO⁻ is bactericidal and virucidal *in vitro*, its importance in killing *in vivo* in humans is not yet clear. Engulfed bacteria in the phagosome of human neutrophils were reported to be chlorinated but not nitrated, suggesting limited exposure to RNS.[53] This is not surprising, since neutrophils isolated from healthy people rarely make NO$^{\bullet}$.

7.7.2.10 *By facilitating the action of other microbicidal agents?*[39]

Mice deficient in neutrophil elastase and/or cathepsin G (Table 7.2) show impaired killing of some bacterial species, even though $O_2^{\bullet-}$ production by their neutrophils is normal. Superoxide consumes

H^+ as it dismutates in the phagocytic vacuole, raising the pH, despite the entry of acidic constituents from the fusing granules. There is an influx of K^+ from the cytosol into the vacuole to partially compensate for the loss of H^+, and Cl^- movements also occur. Both this and the accumulation of bacterial degradation products make the vacuole hypertonic. This rise in ionic strength facilitates release of proteinases from the cationic granules, and the high pH is optimum for their action (Fig. 7.15). In this mechanism, $O_2^{\bullet-}$ and species derived from it have no direct killing role; they simply help to create the environment for the proteinases to operate. The K^+ crosses the phagosome membrane through Ca^{2+}-activated K^+ channels, and inhibitors of this channel do indeed decrease bacterial killing.

7.7.2.11 *Interference with quorum sensing*[54]
Some bacteria (e.g. *S. aureus*) communicate with each other by secreting small molecules. When the levels of these reach a certain threshold indicative of the necessary 'quorum' of bacteria, they trigger changes in bacterial gene expression that result in increased virulence. The quorum sensing molecules of *S. aureus* can be inactivated *in vitro* by HOCl and $ONOO^-$. Bacterial virulence was greater in mice treated with *N*-acetylmethionine to scavenge HOCl and $ONOO^-$, suggesting that this mechanism is relevant *in vivo*. Indeed, mice deficient in NADPH oxidase or (to a lesser extent) MPO, were unable to suppress quorum sensing properly.

7.7.2.12 *Fitting it all together*
Is the only function of the respiratory burst to create optimum conditions for proteinases to operate (Fig. 7.15)? Probably not; evidence indicates that phagocytes do use H_2O_2, HOCl, $ONOO^-$ (and possibly $OH^{\bullet}$ and O_3) to promote direct killing of some organisms. For example, a mutant of *E. coli* defective in the oxyR system (Section 4.5.2) was more susceptible to neutrophil killing. Indeed genes regulated by oxyR are strongly expressed upon phagocytosis by normal, but not CGD, neutrophils.[55] *H. pylori* unable to repair DNA properly were highly sensitive to killing either by ROS or by activated macrophages, and were less infectious in mice.[56] *S. typhimurium* lacking periplasmic CuZnSOD (Section 3.2.1) survived less well in macrophages and was less virulent in mice.[57] *Staphylococcus aureus* is so-named because of its golden-yellow colour, due to carotenoids which appear to have antioxidant action. Blocking carotenoid synthesis enhances killing by phagocytes, whereas expressing them in the normally non-pigmented *S. pyogenes* conferred resistance to killing and increased virulence.[58] These are a few of the many papers showing that microorganisms with disabled antioxidant defences are more sensitive to phagocytic killing, and they indicate a role for RS, which can also help to suppress quorum sensing. We need more experiments to dissect out the various contributions of all the killing pathways described above, using a range of microorganisms and phagocytes from different species. The relative importance of killing mechanisms may differ between species and for each microorganism that the phagocyte encounters.

7.7.3 The enigma of myeloperoxidase[38]

7.7.3.1 *Hypochlorous acid production*
Once the phagocytic vacuole is formed, other granules in the neutrophil cytoplasm fuse with it to deliver, among other things, the enzyme MPO, which comprises 2 to 5% of total neutrophil protein. This enzyme is also present in monocytes but not usually in macrophages, although it can appear under some circumstances in tissue macrophages, for example in AD (Section 9.20.3) and in human atherosclerotic lesions (Section 9.3). Myeloperoxidase is also found in leukaemic cell lines, which is worth bearing in mind when such cell lines (e.g. **HL60**) are examined for their sensitivity to RS. Peroxide-induced apoptosis in HL-60 cells may, for example, involve HOCl.[59]

Myeloperoxidase was first purified in 1941 from large volumes of pus and named **verdoperoxidase**, meaning a 'green peroxidase'. Indeed, it is MPO that gives pus and other infected body fluids their green tinge. It is a haem-containing enzyme that shows 'non-specific' peroxidase activity, being able to oxidize a wide range of substrates. It contains four subunits, two each of molecular weights $\sim$60 and 15 kilodaltons, formed by post-translational cleavage of an 88-kilodalton protein. The haem is covalently linked to the protein by two ester bonds

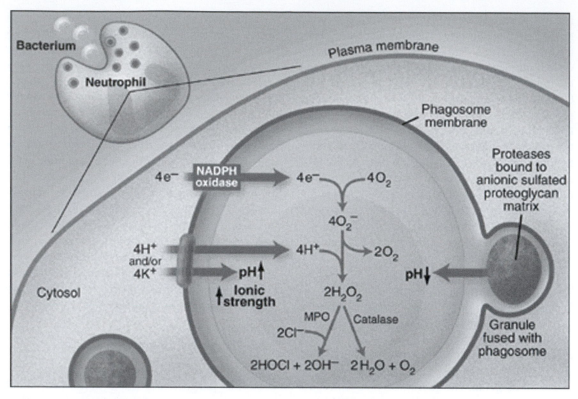

Figure 7.15 In the belly of the phagocyte. Within the small space between an ingested bacterium (shaded area) and the membrane of the phagosome, O_2 is reduced to $O_2^{\bullet -}$ by the NADPH oxidase. This charge transfer is compensated by an influx of protons (H^+) and K^+. The protons are used to convert $O_2^{\bullet -}$ to H_2O_2, which can be broken down to O_2 and water, or can combine with Cl^- to form HOCl, both reactions catalysed by myeloperoxidase; Section 7.7.3. The pH rises to about 8, despite the release of acid contents from granules in the cytoplasm that fuse with the phagosome. The influx of K^+ raises the osmotic pressure and facilitates solubilization of proteinases that are tethered to the proteoglycan matrix of the granules, and the high pH is optimum for their action. As a result, ingested bacteria within the phagosome are killed. From *Science* **296**, 670, 2002 by courtesy of Drs Dirk Roos and Christine Winterbourn and the USA National Academy of Sciences.

(with glutamate and aspartate residues) and a sulphur bond (to a methionine residue).

In the presence of H_2O_2, and chloride or iodide ions, MPO kills many bacteria and fungi *in vitro*. Since much more Cl^- than I^- is present in the phagocyte cytoplasm and in extracellular fluids, it is generally thought that MPO kills by oxidizing Cl^- into **hypochlorous acid**, HOCl. The enzyme can oxidize Br^- to **hypobromous acid**, although this probably does not matter much *in vivo*. Hypochlorous acid is highly reactive, able to oxidize (directly or via chlorine gas) many biological molecules (Section 2.6.3). Bacterial targets include membrane transport proteins, ATP-generating proteins, DNA, and iron–sulphur proteins. Indeed, killing of *S. aureus* by isolated human neutrophils could be decreased by MPO inhibitors

and was slower in MPO-deficient neutrophils. A popular MPO inhibitor is **4-aminobenzoic acid hydrazide**, which is oxidized by MPO into a radical that inactivates the enzyme.[60] Thirty percent or more of the H_2O_2 made (via $O_2^{\bullet -}$ dismutation) by activated neutrophils is used by MPO to make HOCl and, if the HOCl were allowed to accumulate, it could reach concentrations $>50\,\mu M$ in an hour. Both MPO and HOCl (Section 2.6.3) can oxidize SCN^- into hypothiocyanite, $OSCN^-$, which also has antibacterial effects (Section 3.13.3).

Hypochlorous acid reacts with various amines to produce chloramines, which are also good bactericidal agents[61] but less reactive with host biomolecules (Section 2.6.3). One such amine is **taurine (2-aminoethanesulphonic acid)**, present in plasma, neutrophils, other phagocytes, and several other tissues (e.g. heart and nerves). Taurine is an end-product of the metabolism of sulphur-containing amino acids (Fig. 7.16) and intracellular concentrations in human neutrophils have been estimated as 10 to 50 mM.[61] Proposals that the biological role of taurine is to act as an antioxidant are unlikely to be true, since it is a poor antioxidant even *in vitro*,[62] and taurine chloramines can still oxidize some biomolecules. Hypotaurine is a much better antioxidant, and may contribute to antioxidant defence in phagocytes, and in the reproductive system (Section 6.11).

7.7.3.2 *Singlet O_2 from MPO?*

Hypochlorous acid reacts with $O_2^{\bullet-}$ to give $OH^\bullet$ and with H_2O_2 (at alkaline pH) to form singlet O_2 (Section 2.6.3). However, the latter reaction is slower at pH 7.4 and the amount of singlet O_2 made by neutrophils is uncertain. In addition, HOCl reacts faster with many other biomolecules than it does with H_2O_2. Attempts to measure $^1O_2$ using 'probes' for this species have been frustrated by the fact that HOCl oxidizes a number of them directly, including DABCO, 2,5-diphenylfuran, histidine and β-carotene. However, some $^1O_2$ has been detected in activated neutrophils and macrophages (how it is formed in the latter is uncertain) using a 9,10-diphenylanthracene probe (Section 5.9.2). Singlet O_2 production may be more significant in eosinophils (Section 7.8 below).

7.7.3.3 *Does MPO matter?*

Measurement of HOCl levels within *E. coli* using GFP (the protein present within the bacteria after transfection of the GFP-encoding gene loses fluorescence on exposure to HOCl) showed that, after phagocytosis by human neutrophils, the bacteria were exposed to levels of HOCl that should be sufficient to kill them.[63] Given that HOCl *in vitro* is a powerful antibacterial, antifungal and antiviral agent, then MPO must be an important phagocyte killing mechanism? Sadly, no; humans with inborn deficiencies of MPO show only minor decreases in resistance to infection, implying that MPO is less important[64] in bacterial killing than is $O_2^{\bullet-}$. Only occasional increased susceptibility to *Candida* infection has been noted; MPO-knockout mice are also more susceptible to *Candida* (as well as *Klebsiella*) infections. Several different mutations in the MPO gene have been identified. Indeed, MPO deficiency is a common defect in humans (about 1 in 2000–4000 people).[64] Polymorphisms in the gene promoter region that alter MPO levels have also been described, and suggested (without strong evidence as yet) to affect susceptibility to lung and some other cancers (Section 9.14.1).

So where does MPO fit in? One must realize that, in CGD patients, phagocytes do not make $O_2^{\bullet-}$ and so no H_2O_2 is provided for MPO, i.e. there is a dual defect in generation of RS. One study[65] examined the fate of *E. coli* engulfed by human

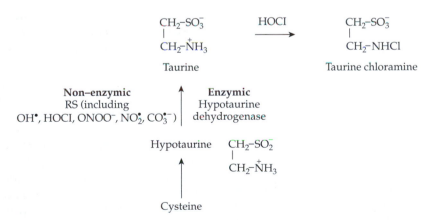

Figure 7.16 Structure of taurine and its reaction production with HOCl and other RS. Taurine is one product of attack of certain ROS on hypotaurine (also see *Biochem. J.* **389**, 233, 2005). Taurine chloramine breaks down to **sulphoacetaldehyde**, $^-SO_3CH_2CHO$ (*Biochem. J.* **330**, 939, 1998).

neutrophils. The bacterial envelope was quickly perforated and bacterial enzymes inactivated. Perforation was slower in neutrophils from patients with CGD. However, neutrophils from MPO-deficient patients showed a normal rate of perforation, but a lower rate of enzyme inactivation. Thus HOCl from MPO might help to destroy bacteria after they have been damaged, but does not, at least in this case, appear responsible for the initial damage. *E. coli* internalized by human neutrophils showed marked increases in their content of 3-chlorotyrosine, a biomarker for RCS, that paralleled killing,[53] but correlation does not, of course, imply causation.

7.7.3.4 *The MPO reaction mechanism*[66]
Oxidation of Cl^- or SCN^- by MPO occurs by compound I formation:

$$MPO-Fe(III) \text{ haem} \xrightarrow{H_2O_2} \text{compound I (Fe(IV)}$$
$$-\text{haem plus haem radical cation)}$$
$$\text{Compound I} + Cl^- \rightarrow OCl^- + Fe(III)-MPO$$

Hydrogen peroxide also converts compound I to compound II, a haem ferryl without the cation radical; this process releases $O_2^{\bullet-}$. Compound II is insufficiently oxidizing to convert Cl^- to HOCl, so it is essentially inactive until an 'easier' electron donor comes along, such as NO_2^- or ascorbate (Section 7.9.1 below). Similarly, $ONOO^-$ can convert MPO to compound II directly. Hydrogen peroxide can also convert compound I back to MPO with O_2 release. Thus under certain circumstances MPO has catalase-like activity (Fig. 7.15).

Myeloperoxidase, like HRP (Section 3.13.4), reacts quickly (rate constant $2 \times 10^6 M^{-1}s^{-1}$) with $O_2^{\bullet-}$ to form an 'oxyferrous' enzyme, compound III:

$$\text{enzyme}-Fe(III) + O_2^{\bullet-} \rightarrow \text{enzyme}-Fe^{2+}-O_2$$

Superoxide can also react with compound I, reducing it to compound II plus O_2.

The extent to which these various reactions occur in the phagocytic vacuole has yet to be established. They are all affected by pH, and their complexity means that the enzyme's behaviour is hard to predict under biological conditions. How MPO fits into the scheme in Fig. 6.15 is uncertain.

7.7.3.5 *Nitration by MPO*
MPO catalyses co-oxidation of tyrosine and NO_2^- to form nitrotyrosine, a major pathway for generation of this species *in vivo* (Section 5.6.2), although not much nitration seems to happen in the human neutrophil phagosome.[53] Nitric oxide can inhibit MPO activity by binding to the Fe(III)–haem. On the other hand, it can be oxidized by compound II (as can NO_2^-) and so recycle MPO into a form active in HOCl production.[67] This process consumes NO• in the vessel wall (Section 7.9.4 below).

7.7.3.6 *Similar defensive peroxidases*
Some *Anopheles* strains cannot transmit malaria because they 'seal up' the parasites in the gut (Section 6.6). *Anopheles stephensi* goes one better; it induces both iNOS and a peroxidase in the gut, the latter using RNS from the former to catalyse nitration and inactivation of the parasite.[68] The squid *Euprymna scolopes* contains an MPO-like enzyme that makes HOCl. It may use it to regulate symbiotic associations with bacteria, such as the luminous species *Vibrio fischeri*.[69]

7.8 Other phagocytes: similar but different

Formation of $O_2^{\bullet-}$ by a respiratory burst occurs not only in macrophages, monocytes, eosinophils, and neutrophils but also in the microglia in the brain, the osteoclasts of bone, the Kupffer cells of liver, basophils and mast cells. Isolated human monocytes show a more marked respiratory burst than do 'unprimed' macrophages, although it is not as large as in neutrophils. Eosinophils can also be highly active in $O_2^{\bullet-}$ production when stimulated.[70]

Most eosinophils are found in tissues, especially the bone marrow and intestinal mucosa. Their numbers in blood are usually low (Table 7.1), but increase in allergic conditions, such as bronchial asthma and hay fever, and during infestations by some parasites. Eosinophils are important in defence against parasites, which they can damage by producing ROS, by release of an eosinophil peroxidase (EPO), and by various cytotoxic proteins including **eosinophil cationic protein**. Whereas activated neutrophils engulf a target and direct toxins into the phagocytic vacuole, eosinophils release their toxins (since their parasite target is usually too large to phagocytose). Indeed, eosinophils account for much of the 'intestinal peroxidase activity' described in some papers. Eosinophil peroxidase has a catalytic mechanism similar to MPO, except that it prefers bromide (Br^-) as a substrate and generates HOBr, despite the fact that Cl^- levels in body fluids are much greater (140 mM Cl^- versus 20–100 μM Br^-). Indeed, bromotyrosine has been detected in the airways and sputum of asthmatic patients.[71] The peroxidase can also oxidize SCN^- to $OSCN^-$. Both HOBr and HOCl can react with H_2O_2 to form singlet O_2.

$$HOBr + H_2O_2 \rightarrow HBr + H_2O + {}^1O_2$$

The reaction with HOBr is faster, and HOBr is less quickly removed by other biomolecules (Section 5.15.2), so production of ${}^1O_2$ by eosinophils may be greater than by neutrophils, although its role in killing is uncertain.[72,73] Eosinophil peroxidase can also convert tyrosine and NO_2^- into nitrotyrosine.[74] However, human EPO deficiency, like that of MPO, appears asymptomatic.[75]

Basophils and mast cells present in connective tissue are rich in **histamine**, and both may be activated by allergens which combine with immunoglobulin E (IgE) bound to their surface. Such activation causes release of several mediators, including $O_2^{\bullet-}$, histamine and 5-hydroxytryptamine.[76] The last two products contribute to the symptoms observed when patients with allergies are exposed to the allergen that their bound IgE recognizes, such as pollen in the case of hay fever, or the house dust mite in many cases of bronchial asthma. Histamine has variable effects on phagocyte $O_2^{\bullet-}$ generation, depending on its concentration. At physiological levels, it may decrease the respiratory burst of macrophages and neutrophils.[77] Release of the serine proteinase **tryptase** by mast cells is thought to be involved in allergy; interestingly, MPO inhibits this enzyme.[78]

Dendritic cells, antigen presenting cells, can also release $O_2^{\bullet-}$ if exposed to endotoxin.[79]

7.9 What do phagocyte-derived reactive species do to the host?

Phagocyte-derived RS are important in killing foreign organisms, but they can damage host tissues as well. Nevertheless, inflammation usually resolves and the tissue heals—in other words, the benefit of removing the invading organism outweighs any tissue damage. Yet during chronic inflammation there is extensive tissue damage and often an increased risk of cancer. Is this due to RS?

7.9.1 Extracellular RS: what can they do?

During neutrophil activation, some $O_2^{\bullet-}$, H_2O_2, and MPO may be released extracellularly. The last can consume $NO^{\bullet}$, nitrate tyrosine residues, and react with H_2O_2 and Cl^- to form extracellular HOCl, leading to chloramines. Taurine chloramines, HOCl, and $ONOO^-$, inactivate α_1-antiproteinase and α_2-macroglobulin (Table 7.2) *in vitro*, favouring proteolytic action. Whereas elastase within neutrophils is microbicidal (Section 7.7.2.10), released elastase can hydrolyse connective-tissue components such as elastin and collagen; over-activity of extracellular elastase may contribute to the tissue damage caused in emphysema (Section 8.12), acute respiratory distress syndrome (Section 9.7) and in certain skin diseases, such as psoriasis. Elastase can also cleave receptors on the surface of macrophages to interfere with phagocytosis of apoptotic neutrophils.[80]

Do these inactivations of antiproteinases happen *in vivo*? It depends on what else is present. Hypochlorous acid or $ONOO^-$ added to plasma tend not to damage the antiproteinases because these RS react preferentially with albumin, present at 50 to 60 mg/ml (as compared with 1–3 mg/ml for α_1-antiproteinase).[81] In some other biological fluids (e.g. cerebrospinal, synovial or lung lining fluids) albumin concentrations are lower, and attack is conceivable. For example, inactivated chlorinated α_2-macroglobulin can be present in inflamed human rheumatoid joints.[82] Ascorbate can also scavenge ONOOH and HOCl, and the concentrations present in extracellular fluids (40–100 μM in plasma, alveolar lining fluid and synovial fluid, more in CSF) can protect α_1-antiproteinase against these species, at least until the ascorbate has been depleted.[83] Ascorbate reacts with MPO, but its effects on HOCl production are complex.[84] It can be oxidized by compound II, regenerating compound I and accelerating HOCl production. But it also acts as a competing substrate with Cl^- for compound I. GSH, present at high levels in alveolar lining fluid, can scavenge HOCl and ONOO⁻ and protect α_1-antiproteinase.

If left unscavenged, HOCl might additionally favour proteolysis by activating two enzymes present within neutrophils in a latent form— collagenase (which digests native type I collagen) and gelatinase (which attacks denatured collagen and native types IV and V collagen; Table 7.2). It's not that simple, however; HOCl can *inactivate* matrilysin and several other neutrophil enzymes, including lysozyme and MPO itself, as well as destroy chemotactic factors for neutrophils. Peroxynitrite can convert MPO to the less-active compound II. Thus the overall tissue-damaging effects of MPO, HOCl and ONOO⁻ at sites of inflammation are difficult to predict and may be minor.

7.9.2 Signalling

Reactive species released at sites of acute inflammation may play a role in signalling. They can increase levels of MMPs (Table 7.2) and stimulate fibroblast proliferation both directly (Section 4.2.1) and/or as intermediates in the action of cytokines (although if proliferation happens too much fibrosis results). For example, Fig. 5.8 shows the presence of H_2O_2 in a healing wound, not preventing (and possibly facilitating) the healing process (Section 6.12.3).

Many years ago, Del Maestro *et al.*[85] found that perfusion of a hamster cheek pouch with $O_2^{\bullet-}$-generating systems caused increased leakage of material from the vascular network and adherence of neutrophils to the vessel walls. Leakage was decreased by adding SOD or catalase to the perfusion medium. We now know that ROS facilitate phagocyte adherence to endothelium, by increasing expression[33,86] of such adhesion molecules as E-selectin, ICAM-1 and VCAM-1. Activation of their synthesis by ROS or by cytokines (which sometimes occurs via ROS) often involves NF-κB (Section 4.5.8). By contrast, NO$^{\bullet}$ can decrease expression of adhesion molecules and deter phagocyte adherence (under certain conditions), in part by decreasing NF-κB activation. Superoxide modulates this by removing NO$^{\bullet}$ and forming ONOO⁻. Initial adhesion of phagocytes

deters ROS production, but high levels of cytokines can over-ride this (Section 7.7.1.1).

Reactive oxygen species have been reported to stimulate synthesis of the chemokine MIP-1α by macrophages, and of IL-8 by fibroblasts and epithelial cells.[87,88] In other words, ROS can promote chemotaxis as well as adhesion. By contrast, ROS seem to impair IL-8 production by human neutrophils; neutrophils from CGD patients produced more.[89] Taurine chloramine was reported to decrease IL-8 production by rat neutrophils by interfering with activation of NF-κB,[90] whereas μM levels of ONOO⁻ increased production of IL-6 and TNFα by human monocytes by activating NF-κB.[91] Several aldehyde end-products of lipid peroxidation, including HNE, are chemotactic agents,[92] and chemotactic aldehydes are produced when HOCl and HOBr oxidize amino acids or lipids.[71,93] The effects of any RS on phagocytes are likely to be biphasic, depending on the RS level; too many will damage the phagocyte (Section 7.9.3 below). Reactive species also interact with the eicosanoid pathway (Section 7.12.1 below).

There are checks and balances however; increased blood flow rapidly replenishes α_1-antiproteinase and antioxidants such as ascorbate at sites of injury. Concentrations of several acute-phase antioxidant proteins (e.g. haptoglobin, caeruloplasmin) increase during inflammation (Table 4.9), and caeruloplasmin can inhibit MPO.[94] The nucleoside **adenosine** (adenine-ribose), released by a variety of normal, stimulated, and injured cells (including endothelium, platelets and leukocytes) decreases the respiratory burst in response to fmet–leu–phe, zymosan and TNFα, and diminishes phagocyte adherence to endothelium. Adenosine is a potent biological mediator that affects several cell types and exerts its effects by binding to at least four different types of receptor.[95]

7.9.3 Damage to the phagocyte

Reactive species can attack the phagocytes generating them. Indeed, oxidation of methionine residues to the sulphoxide,[96] DNA strand breakage, glutathionylation (Section 3.9.6) and DNA base oxidation and deamination occur within activated phagocytes.[97] The DNA damage probably reflects diffusion of RNS and H_2O_2 (to form $OH^•$ close to DNA) into the nucleus. During phagocytosis of *S. aureus* by human neutrophils, 94% of the chlorination occurred on neutrophil proteins rather than bacterial ones.[98]

Such damage to neutrophils probably matters little, since they are destined to die at sites of inflammation.[99] Once they leave the bone marrow, neutrophils are separated from the 'survival factors' there and undergo apoptosis within 24 hours. Cytokines (e.g. GM-CSF) and other factors (e.g. endotoxin, fmet–leu–phe) at sites of inflammation block apoptosis, but this is over-ridden by RS, which trigger apoptosis, for example by the ceramide pathway (Section 4.4).[100] Nevertheless, phagocytes do have antioxidant defences. They contain CuZnSOD, a MnSOD in the mitochondria, catalase, methionine sulphoxide reductase, peroxiredoxins and GPx, together with ascorbate and GSH at millimolar concentrations.[101] Activated phagocytes show higher rates of GSH turnover. Indeed, neutrophils deficient in glutathione reductase activity are more rapidly inactivated during phagocytosis than normal. Catalase seems less important in protection of phagocytes against H_2O_2, although activities vary between species. For example, human and guinea pig neutrophils contain more catalase than cells from rats and mice.[102]

Reactive species can have variable effects on the respiratory burst. For example, low levels of $ONOO^-$ or H_2O_2 can inhibit protein phosphatases and promote phosphorylation, associated with increased neutrophil adhesion, and activation of NADPH oxidase (Section 7.7.2.3).[41,103] However, production of $NO^•$ and other RNS (and possibly ROS) by phagocytes can impair the proliferative response of T-lymphocytes to mitogens or antigens. T-Lymphocytes play a key role in inflammation; they can produce ROS (Section 7.10.4 below) but can undergo apoptosis if RS levels are too high.[104] This could be good if it damps down inflammation, or bad if it happens too much and causes immunosuppression.[105,106] The effect of $NO^•$ can be modulated by $O_2^{•-}$, which removes $NO^•$. Oxidized phospholipids decrease the activity of dendritic cells in antigen presentation, again an effect that could be either good or bad, depending on degree.[107]

Thus the complex mixture of cell types producing RS and cytokines at sites of inflammation could conceivably result in every possible outcome. However, tissue 'damage' by RS is probably limited during the 'normal' acute inflammatory response. So what goes wrong when the inflammation does not go away? Persistent stimulus, e.g. by failure to clear hyaluronic acid fragments (Section 9.10.4.1), or the wrong mixture of cytokines (Section 7.7.1), perhaps. But sometimes too many ROS, or even *too few* RS. Let us see how.

7.9.4 Damage by phagocytes can be severe: the tragedy of chronic inflammation

Growing evidence links persistent inflammation to the development of cardiovascular and many other diseases,[108] and recent attention has focused on MPO.[109,110] This cationic protein readily binds to anionic sites, for example endothelial cell glycosaminoglycans in blood vessel walls. Here it can oxidize, chlorinate and (if NO_2^- is present) nitrate proteins such as the extracellular matrix glycoproteins,[111,112] and possibly initiate lipid peroxidation and deplete nitric oxide.[100,113,114] Many papers suggest a role for MPO in vascular (Section 9.3.5.2), and neurodegenerative (Sections 9.19 and 9.20) diseases. For example, when MPO-knockout mice were injected with thioglycollate followed by zymosan to induce peritonitis, they showed less formation of F_2-isoprostanes and nitrotyrosine.[113] However, it is best to be cautious before concluding MPO is a baddie; MPO-knockout mice showed *greater* lung injury after bone marrow transplantation,[104] *more* brain damage after ischaemia–reperfusion[115] and *less* atherosclerosis (Section 9.3.5.2) in some studies, although antibodies formed against MPO can aggravate inflammation.[116]

Persistent inflammation causes significant tissue damage. For example it increases the risk of cancer development; excessive DNA damage by RS may be the culprit (Section 9.13.6). Silica and asbestos provoke persistent phagocyte activation (Section 8.14) leading to serious lung damage. In 1968, it was discovered that within the first few minutes of blood dialysis, leukopaenia (Table 7.1) occurs. Contact of plasma with cellophane in the dialyser activated the complement system, leading to accumulation, aggregation, and activation of neutrophils and monocytes in the lung. This caused damage by interfering with blood flow, and by producing RS. Even modern kidney dialysis methods cause some phagocyte activation and plasma antioxidant depletion.[117] Some studies have tried to minimize this using membranes coated with α-tocopherol, but reports of clinical benefit range from substantial to zero.[118] Reactive species are involved in the rejection of transplanted organs, a process involving chronic inflammation (Section 9.6.1). The potential for damage by excess RS/proteinases is dramatically illustrated by the ability of activated phagocytes to corrode plastics, a process which can damage implanted biomedical devices such as heart valves and joint prostheses if inflammation develops around them.[119]

7.9.5 What does it all mean? Are RS both pro- and anti-inflammatory?

As Hazlitt said, 'When a thing ceases to be a subject of controversy, it ceases to be a subject of interest.' Life is complex. Evolution does not retain things that overall do harm (or at least did no harm under the conditions in which humans evolved, which are different from those under which we live now[120]). Thus inflammation, and its associated RS production, is beneficial overall in protecting us against pathogens. But are too many RS bad or good? Bad, because they can contribute to cancer. This may not matter to evolution—better to have a robust immune response that kills pathogens and stops you dying young from infections before you have children; if it gives you cancer late in life (after your reproductive years), who cares? But not always bad in the short term; joint inflammation induced by intra-articular injection of zymosan in mice was *more* severe if NADPH oxidase was knocked out (Section 9.10.5). This was accompanied by greater osteoclast activity and increased synovial expression of TNFα, IL-1 and matrix metalloproteinases. In this case, the RS seemed to damp down inflammation (e.g. by causing lymphocyte apoptosis) rather than aggravate it.[121] Similarly, mice lacking NADPH oxidase showed greater gastric damage by *H. pylori* (Section 9.12.2), whereas mice overexpressing CuZnSOD showed

increased intestinal inflammation in a model of inflammatory bowel disease (Section 9.11). Mice lacking both NADPH oxidase and iNOS died after exposure to *Candida albicans*, but apparently because of an excessive and abnormal inflammatory response rather than of inability to kill this fungus.[122] For balance, here are two cases where increased RS levels seemed to be proinflammatory. NADPH oxidase-knockout mice challenged with *E. coli* to induce sepsis showed increased recruitment of neutrophils into the lung and decreased bacterial clearance, associated with elevated levels of the chemoattractant MIP-2.[123] Mice lacking EC-SOD suffered worse tissue damage, apparently related to elevated cytokine production, during collagen-induced arthritis.[124]

The literature is complex and confusing. The authors use two guidelines in trying to make sense of it

1. Be careful in generalizing from studies with isolated activated phagocytes, separated from complex biological environments.
2. Be even more careful in extrapolating data from a single model (one animal species, one bacterium or other challenge, one type of damage measured for one period only) to make sweeping statements about what is or is not important to the organism as a whole.

7.9.6 Defeating the system: bacterial and fungal avoidance strategies[125–127]

Several bacterial strains swim away from environments containing H_2O_2, HOCl or chloramines, which may help them evade phagocytosis.[125] Other strategies to resist phagocytic killing include production of toxins that inactivate phagocyte RS production (e.g. the disulphide **gliotoxin**[128] by several pathogenic fungi) or halt phagosome maturation (e.g. in *N. gonorrhoeae* and *Mycobacterium tuberculosis*), rapid induction of bacterial heat shock proteins (e.g. in *Salmonella* and *M. tuberculosis*), high endogenous levels of antioxidant defence enzymes (e.g. SOD in *Mycobacterium leprae* and *M. tuberculosis*, or catalase and methionine sulphoxide reductase in *N. gonorrhoeae*; Section 3.5.1) and/or an ability to rapidly raise antioxidant levels as soon as

RS are sensed (e.g. by OxyR and soxRS systems). Peroxiredoxins and flavohaemoglobins that can scavenge RNS (Sections 3.11 and 1.10.3) are also important. Other strategies include generation of capsules that not only hinder recognition of the organism by the phagocyte but can also absorb RS (*P. aeroginosa* is an example), production of haem oxygenase to destroy the haem that phagocytes require to make the *b*-type cytochrome, and the replacement of RNS-sensitive enzymes by resistant ones (Section 7.2.2). The fungus *Cryptococcus neoformans* produces melanin as an antioxidant (Section 3.18.9) as well as high levels of intracellular mannitol; as an OH$^{\bullet}$ scavenger the latter could conceivably protect against phagocyte killing.[129] *Anaplasma phagocytophilum* suppresses the respiratory burst by blocking not only assembly of the oxidase but also the transcription of genes encoding gp91^{phox} and rac2, and even manages to multiply in neutrophils.[127] *H. pylori* seems to alter assembly of the NADPH oxidase so that most O$_2^{\bullet-}$ is released extracellularly instead of into the phagocytic vacuole (Section 9.12.2).[130]

Sometimes antioxidant proteins are present in the periplasmic space (Section 3.2.1.1) or even extracellularly. Thus several parasites (Section 3.16.3.2) and *M. tuberculosis* secrete antioxidant enzymes around themselves.[131]

7.10 NAD(P)H oxidases in other cell types[132]

For many years it was believed that only phagocytes produce RS 'deliberately', and that RS release by other cells was a deleterious 'accident of chemistry', a response to injury or toxin exposure, or even an artefact of the measurement methods. We now know that many other cell types do release ROS, and that NAD(P)H oxidase (**NOX**) systems are widespread. We have already seen four examples, spermatozoa (Section 6.11.1), lung (Section 6.3), adipose tissue (Table 4.7) and the thyroid NADPH oxidase (Section 7.5.1). Even the humble slime mould (Section 4.5.13) contains a NOX, to help it socialize.[133] Insects contain **haemocytes** to help defend against infection, and they produce O$_2^{\bullet-}$ by mechanisms similar to those of mammalian phagocytes.[134]

Many other mammalian cells possess oxidase components resembling those in phagocytes, such as p22^{phox}, gp91^{phox} (sometimes called **NOX2**), p47^{phox}, and p67^{phox}. Sometimes all are present, whereas in other tissues only some of these components occur (although probably other proteins take over their functions to allow O$_2^{\bullet-}$ to be made). At least seven members of the NOX family are known, **NOX1** to **NOX5**, **DUOX1** and **DUOX2** (some authors write these in capitals, as we do here, others in lower case). Sometimes NOX are present at a specific developmental stage, for example **NOX3** is found in foetal tissues and may play a role in signalling during development. It is also found in the inner ear; why is unknown, although mice lacking it have problems with balance (Section 8.17). In other cases NOX appear in response to cytokines, hormones or cell injury. For example, castration of rats led to increased levels of NOX1, NOX2 and NOX4 in the prostate. This was accompanied by decreased levels of SOD and H$_2$O$_2$-metabolizing enzymes and increased oxidative damage. All these events contributed to apoptosis and prostate shrinkage[135] and were partially ameliorated by testosterone administration. Thus castration increases ROS in the prostate; by contrast, testosterone aggravates pulmonary O$_2$ toxicity whereas castration decreases it (Section 1.5.3). Depriving neurons of growth factors leads to NOX activation and ROS-dependent apoptosis.[136] Treatment of airway smooth muscle cells[137] with TNFα increased NOX and produced more O$_2^{\bullet-}$. Hypoxia can increase levels of NOX in the retina, and the ROS produced may contribute to excessive VEGF production and thus to ROP (Section 1.6).[138]

Some NADPH oxidases (e.g. NOX1, NOX3, NOX4) closely resemble NOX2 (gp91^{phox}) in their structure. In general, NOX5 is similar, but has extra amino acid sequences, that make its activity Ca^{2+}-dependent. The DUOX1 and DUOX2 families are Ca^{2+}-dependent and contain N-terminal peroxidase domains that can use H$_2$O$_2$ generated by the oxidase domains, hence the name **DUOX** for **du**al **ox**idase. They provide H$_2$O$_2$ for thyroid peroxidase (Section 7.5.1), but their innate peroxidase activity might also contribute to iodination. Thus they are sometimes called **THOX1 (thyroid oxidase 1)** and **THOX2**, but DUOX are also found in placenta, brain, GI tract, testis, salivary ducts and lung. They can produce H_2O_2 in salivary ducts, and on tracheal, gut mucosal and bronchial epithelial cell surfaces, possibly for antibacterial actions (Section 3.13.3).[139]

The $O_2^{\bullet-}$ production by NOX/DUOX systems is often regulated differently from that of the phagocyte oxidase and does not respond to the same stimuli, for example NOX1 in colon (Section 7.10.1 below) does not respond to PMA. However, rac proteins are involved in regulation of most, if not all, NOX systems.[140] Let us look at some NOX systems in more detail.

7.10.1 The gastrointestinal tract[132]

A DUOX2 is often found in the GI tract (Section 6.2). In addition, NOX1 (previously called **MOX1, mi**togenic **ox**idase 1) is present in the epithelium of the colon and several other tissues (prostate, uterus, vascular smooth muscle). This NOX1 and its associated components form a functional NADPH oxidase that generates $O_2^{\bullet-}$ even in normal colon cells.[141] The physiological function of NOX1 may be as an antibacterial agent (at least in *Drosophila*, Section 6.2.1). However, interest in it has been raised in relation to carcinogenesis, since overexpression of NOX1 in NIH-3T3 cells followed by their introduction into mice caused the formation of highly vascularized tumours; coexpression of catalase prevented the effect. Although questions have been raised about these studies, they could relate to the ability of ROS to suppress apoptosis in tumour cell lines (Section 4.4.1.2). However, if NOX4 is expressed in NIH-3T3 cells, it produces $O_2^{\bullet-}$ but does *not* promote proliferation, rather senescence.[140,142] In other words, different NOX forms at different levels may have different cellular effects (as one expects from RS!). But is NOX1 increased in human colon cancer? It's not clear as yet (Section 9.13.5.8).

7.10.2 C. elegans[143]

This worm contains two genes that appear to encode DUOX proteins. One of these proteins, **Ce-DUOX1**, stabilizes the cuticle; H_2O_2 generated in the oxidase domain is used by the peroxidase domain to catalyse cross-linking of tyrosine resi-dues. The peroxidase segment resembles sea urchin ovoperoxidase (Section 7.5.3).

7.10.3 Blood vessel walls[144]

All major cell types in vessel walls (endothelial cells, smooth muscle cells and fibroblasts) express NOX and can release $O_2^{\bullet-}$ and H_2O_2. First, endothelial cells. Several sources contribute to their extracellular ROS production. Amine oxidases produce H_2O_2 (Section 7.7.1.1). Xanthine oxidase, which can bind to endothelial cell surfaces,[145] generates $O_2^{\bullet-}$ and H_2O_2. Endothelial NOS makes $O_2^{\bullet-}$ under certain circumstances (Table 1.4). In addition, NOX1, 2 and 4 can be present, as are $p47^{phox}$, $p22^{phox}$ and $p67^{phox}$. The physiological significance of extracellular endothelial $O_2^{\bullet-}$ production is uncertain; it might be that $O_2^{\bullet-}$ and $NO^{\bullet}$ antagonize each other's actions as part of a normal vasoregulatory mechanism, a view supported by the fact that NOX1-knockout mice have decreased blood pressure.[146] Of course, the resulting $ONOO^-$ would have to be disposed of safely. However, it is still unclear if endothelial cells make $O_2^{\bullet-}$ all the time *in vivo* or only after ischaemia–reperfusion, shear stress, other insults, or exposure to certain hormones or to cytokines. Be careful; the stresses of cell isolation and culture might artefactually increase NOX levels.

Vascular smooth muscle cells and fibroblasts have also been found to contain NOX1, 2 and 4, $p22^{phox}$, $p67^{phox}$, rac and $p47^{phox}$. For both these cell types and endothelial cells, there are tissue and species differences between the NOX forms present. Subcellular locations may also be different, for example NOX1 and 4 seem differently located within vascular smooth muscle cells, presumably indicative of different functions.[147] Fibroblasts and smooth muscle cells can respond to ROS by proliferation (Section 4.2.1), causing hypertrophy of the vessel wall. The cytokine TGFβ can accelerate fibroblast proliferation, and thrombin (Section 7.10.6 below) stimulates smooth muscle cell proliferation; ROS are involved in both processes.[148]

The concept that $O_2^{\bullet-}$ plays a role in normal vasoregulation is strengthened by the observation that **angiotensin II**[d] stimulates $O_2^{\bullet-}$ production by all three cell types, in part by increasing phosphorylation of $p47^{phox}$ and promoting oxidase assembly. Angiotensin II administration to animals increases plasma levels of F_2-isoprostanes, indicative of increased oxidative stress.[149] Decreasing NOX activity in animals by knockout or inhibitors decreases the hypertensive effect of angiotensin II.[146] Vascular $O_2^{\bullet-}$ production is increased in **spontaneously hypertensive rats (SHR)**, a strain whose blood pressure becomes abnormally high after 4 to 5 weeks of age. Transfer of the gene encoding EC-SOD to vessel walls using viral vectors (Section 10.6.3.1), administration of heparin-binding SOD (Section 10.6.3) or other $O_2^{\bullet-}$ scavengers, or of cocktails of nutritional antioxidants, decreases the animals' blood pressure and the vessel wall levels of nitrotyrosine.[150,151] These rats may in addition suffer excess production of $O_2^{\bullet-}$ in the part of the brain involved in controlling blood pressure, another reason for the hypertension,[152] and the kidney is involved as well (Section 7.10.5 below). However, antioxidants have given variable (often no) effects in lowering blood pressure when administered to human hypertensive patients, and F_2-IP levels are elevated in only some patients.[149]

Vascular $O_2^{\bullet-}$ production is increased in hypercholesterolaemia, and contributes to atherosclerosis (Section 9.3). Studies of knockout mice show it to be involved in angiogenesis stimulated by VEGF at sites of tissue injury (also see Section 1.6).[153] Hypertension can not only result from excess ROS but can itself *cause* more $O_2^{\bullet-}$ formation; excessive mechanical stress on vessels increases NOX levels and leads to falls in tetrahydrobiopterin, a process to which ROS from NOX may contribute.[154] Lowered tetrahydrobiopterin then facilitates $O_2^{\bullet-}$ production by eNOS (Table 1.4).

7.10.4 Lymphocytes

B-lymphocytes contain all the NADPH oxidase components found in phagocytes, but some 10- to 30-fold less abundant. The system can be activated by PMA and is defective in CGD patients (whereas other NOX systems generally are not). Its physiological role is unknown.[155] T-lymphocytes also

appear to produce ROS (probably by a NOX) during antigen-induced expansion, probably for signalling purposes.[156]

7.10.5 Reactive species, renal function and oxygen sensing

The kidneys consume about 10% of basal O_2 uptake in humans and are a ready target of damage by RS. For example, kidney injury by gentamicin may involve RS (Section 8.16.3), as does renal injury by myoglobin (Section 3.15.3). F_2-IPs can constrict renal blood vessels; particularly worrying since plasma F_2-IP levels and several other biomarkers of oxidative damage (e.g. protein carbonyls, HNE, AGE products) are elevated in patients with chronic kidney disease on dialysis.[157] Deposition of antigen–antibody complexes in the glomeruli can lead to complement activation and infiltration of neutrophils. In addition, resident phagocytic (**mesangial**) cells in the glomeruli can respond to complement activation by secreting eicosanoids, proteinases and ROS. Accumulation of MPO, and protein chlorination, are frequently observed in renal inflammation, for example MPO and chlorinated proteins colocalize in glomerular basement membranes in human membranous glomerulonephritis.[158] These membranes are easily damaged by HOCl.[159] Antibodies that develop against circulating MPO and other neutrophil granule components contribute to renal injury by binding to the membranes and provoking phagocyte attack.[158,159]

However, RS at more moderate levels may be involved in regulating renal function. Kidney contains NOX, $O_2^{\bullet-}$ from which may help control both renal blood flow (especially in the kidney medulla), and Na^+ uptake in the renal tubules.[160,161] For example, knockout of $gp91^{phox}$ in mice raised renal blood flow and lowered renal vascular resistance.[162] The levels of NOX can be increased both by angiotensin II and by high salt intake, leading to renal vasoconstriction and contributing to hypertension;[160] the effects of angiotensin II were less marked in the $gp91^{phox}$ knockout mouse.[162] Levels of renal NOX are abnormally high in the SHR rat (Section 7.10.3), although XO may also contribute to the excess $O_2^{\bullet-}$ generation. Hence more ROS are made in the kidney of hypertensive animals,

---

[d] Angiotensin II, a peptide which affects many body tissues and raises blood pressure, is produced from angiotensin I by the action of **angiotensin converting enzyme, ACE**. Inhibitors of ACE, such as **captopril** and **ramipril** are widely used clinically.

perpetuating the problem. Infusion of angiotensin II into rats led to nitration and inactivation of renal MnSOD.[163]

Oxygen sensing by the whole organism involves the carotid body and the neuroepithelial cells (Section 1.3.2). The action of the latter involves a NOX; newborn mice lacking gp91^{phox} breathe faster and more shallowly than control mice and do not respond properly to hypoxia.[164] When HIF is activated, one of its actions is to stimulate erythropoietin (EPO) production in liver and kidney. It has been suggested that NOX4, expressed in renal tubules (sometimes called **RENOX**, although NOX4 is by no means unique to the kidney), has a role in regulating HIF-directed EPO synthesis. One suggestion is that ROS normally repress EPO synthesis; in hypoxia less ROS are made and the EPO gene expression increases. Consistent with this, mice lacking EC-SOD show an impaired EPO response to hypoxia.[165]

7.10.6 Platelets[166,167]

Platelets are vital in decreasing blood loss from injured vessels; they rapidly adhere to collagen exposed when endothelial cells are damaged and form a 'platelet plug'. Simultaneously, blood coagulation occurs to form a fibrin-rich clot. The two pathways cross-talk, for example **thrombin**, a serine proteinase liberated during the blood coagulation cascade, promotes platelet aggregation. Adhesion and aggregation of platelets are triggered by changes in surface adhesion molecules, and by the release of proaggregatory mediators, including ADP (released from the 'dense granules' of the platelets), and thromboxane A_2 (Section 7.12.7 below). Aggregation involves thiol–disulphide exchanges in surface proteins and can be modulated by plasma GSH/GSSG ratios. Exposure of platelets to ROS potentiates aggregation induced by thrombin or collagen. Indeed, platelets themselves generate some $O_2^{\bullet-}$ via a NOX, and the rate is increased by collagen or thrombin. It has been suggested that $O_2^{\bullet-}$ and H_2O_2 produced by platelets, or cells around them, may synergize with other stimuli to promote aggregation. These ROS may also regulate thromboxane A_2 production by platelets. On the other hand, NO$^{\bullet}$ produced by platelets during aggregation

can deter further aggregation, possibly in part by helping to scavenge $O_2^{\bullet-}$. Indeed, nitration of platelet proteins has been detected during platelet activation by collagen.[166] However, too much H_2O_2 or ONOO$^-$ can damage platelets.

The physiological importance of platelet $O_2^{\bullet-}$ formation is uncertain, but it plays at least one pathological role. Patients with HIV infection can develop antiplatelet antibodies that bind to surface glycoproteins and cause platelet fragmentation. This requires activation of the platelet 12-lipoxygenase (Section 7.12.7 below), which in turn leads to increases in NOX activity, and ROS generation. Fragmentation can be blocked by antioxidants, for example catalase.[168]

7.10.7 Osteoclasts[169]

In these cells, both NOX2 and NOX4 are present and the $O_2^{\bullet-}$ produced may be involved in bone resorption (Section 9.10.2).

7.10.8 Other redox systems

There are many descriptions in the literature of NAD(P)H oxidases in the plasma membranes of multiple cell types, including erythrocytes (Section 6.4), adipocytes and renal brush border membranes. These oxidases have often been identified by using artificial electron acceptors such as ferricyanide (Fe(CN)$_6^{3-}$), or indophenol, and more work is required to elucidate their chemical nature, and physiological function.[170] Some may be involved in metal ion uptake (Section 3.15.1), others in regenerating NAD$^+$ for glycolysis by reoxidizing NADH in cells with limited mitochondrial function, and yet others in ascorbate metabolism (Section 6.4). In some cells, the plasma membrane NADH–ferricyanide reductase has been identified as **VDAC1, a voltage-dependent anion selective channel**. This protein also occurs in the outer mitochondrial membrane, where it is sometimes called **porin 1**.[171]

7.11 Even plants use reactive species[172]

Plants generate high levels of RS and oxidative damage products and must take special care with their antioxidant defences (Section 6.7). Nevertheless, they employ RS for useful purposes just as often as animals do, if not more so. Let us examine how.

Homologues of animal NOX enzymes have been identified in a wide range of plants, and are called **respiratory burst oxidase homologues (Rboh** proteins). They resemble NOX5 (Section 7.10), having extra N-terminal peptides, and Ca^{2+}-binding sites. In the plant *Arabidopsis thaliana* (At) there are at least 10 Rboh proteins with different functions. Thus **AtrbohC** is involved in the production of root hairs – the ROS it produces cause increased cytosolic Ca^{2+} levels, needed for the tip of the hairs to continue growth. The root hairs of plants lacking AtrbohC do not elongate; addition of ROS (at the right level!) restores growth, but in random directions, since the ROS are no longer focused to the root tip.[173] Similarly, **AtrbohD** and **AtrbohF** aid closure of leaf stomata in response to the plant hormone abscisic acid, by promoting fluxes of Ca^{2+} across the plasma membrane.[174] Other oxidases promote growth of cells in the shoot. Even plant pollens contain NOX enzymes, production of ROS by which when inhaled into the respiratory tract can contribute to their allergic effects in sensitive subjects.[175]

Rises in Ca^{2+} may increase catalase activity in plants by calmodulin-dependent reactions,[176] presumably to limit H_2O_2 levels (by contrast animal or bacterial catalases are unaffected by Ca^{2+}/calmodulin). Inactivations of peroxiredoxins (Section 3.11) may additionally regulate H_2O_2 signalling.

7.11.1 The hypersensitive response[172,176–178]

Sometimes infection of an animal leads to abscess formation: microorganisms and phagocytes battle it out in a walled-off area, stopping the pathogen from spreading. An analogy in plants is the **hypersensitive response**. It is triggered by signal molecules (**elicitors**) originating from the invading organism or synthesized by the plant itself. An early effect produced by elicitors is the rapid generation of ROS and RNS at the cell surface by the **plant oxidative burst** (Fig. 7.17, Plate 15). The H_2O_2 produced helps to kill pathogens and the plant cells harbouring them, but it also promotes other events. These include the synthesis of **phytoalexins** (small molecules with antimicrobial

activity), the strengthening of cell walls to 'wall in' or 'wall out' the pathogen (e.g. by cross-linking of proteins and more lignin synthesis), the death of cells ahead of the invader to stop it spreading, and the upregulation of defences (including GST and GPx enzymes) in other cells that render the plant resistant to attack by the same (and often other) pathogens, sometimes for weeks or months (**systemic acquired resistance**, SAR). At least three hormones, salicylate, ethylene and **jasmonic acid**, are involved in the regulation of ROS-induced cell death. Salicylate and ethylene sensitize plant cells to apoptosis induced by ROS; the ability of salicylate to bind to catalase and decrease its activity may contribute somewhat but is by no means the whole story. This localized cell death limits the spread of the invading pathogen, but, to avoid too much damage to the plant, jasmonic acid produced by dying cells exerts opposing effects and slows the death of plant cells, in part by raising the level of ascorbate and GSH. Ascorbate has a paradoxical effect; the *A. thaliana vtc* mutants (Section 6.9.3) are more sensitive to O_3 but less sensitive to certain pathogens. Jasmonic acid also plays a role in the wound response (Section 7.11.4 below). Another player is the phytoprostanes (Section 6.7), which can trigger increases in antioxidant and other 'antistress' defences in plant cells.[178] Lipoxygenase-catalysed reactions (Section 7.11.3 below) may also sometimes participate.

Production of ROS in the plant oxidative burst can involve diamine oxidases (Section 6.7) and peroxidases, but the major source is NADPH oxidases. For example, knockout of **AtrbohD** and **AtrbohF** in *Arabidopsis* prevents extracellular ROS production in response to pathogens, as does downregulation of **NtrbohD**[e] in tobacco. Activation of these rboh proteins involves Ca^{2+} ions, rac-type proteins and phosphorylation reactions, for example by a serine/threonine kinase produced by the *OXI1* gene in *Arabidopsis*,[174] and by MAP kinases. The OXI1 kinase is activated in response to H_2O_2 and helps activate the MAP kinases. Ozone exposure also activates NOX enzymes and can trigger the hypersensitivity response (Section 6.9.3).

Just as some fungi that infect animals accumulate mannitol, putatively to protect against

---

[e] Tobacco is *Nicotiana tabacum*, hence Nt.

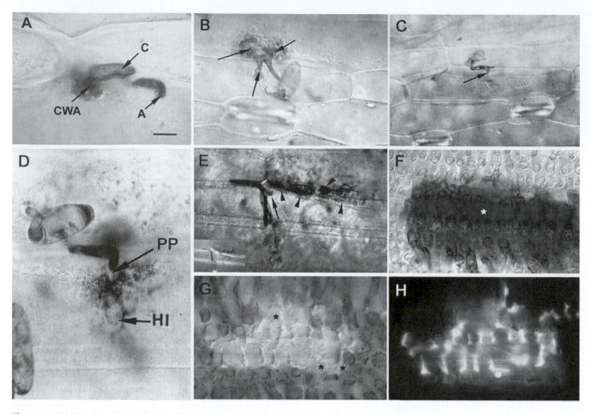

Figure 7.17 (see plate 15) Production of ROS during attack of the powdery mildew fungus *Blumeria graminis* f.sp. *hordei* (*Bgh*) on barley (*Hordeum vulgare*). (A) H_2O_2 accumulation in late phase I (12 h after spore landing). Starting from its conidium (*C*) the fungus has built a primary germ tube and an appressorium (*A*). Barley has built a cell wall apposition (CWA) beneath the primary germ tube where H_2O_2 accumulation is visible (reddish-brown DAB staining); bar 8 μm. (B) H_2O_2 accumulation phase II during formation of CWAs beneath three fungal penetration attempts (*arrows*). (C) H_2O_2 accumulation phase III during the HR of *Mla12* barley. The fungus penetrated successfully (*arrow*) and triggered whole-cell H_2O_2 accumulation (30 h after spore landing). (D) Superoxide accumulation phase I. Originating from the appressorium, *Bgh* formed a penetration peg (*PP*) and a haustorium initial (*HI*). Superoxide accumulation is indicated by dark-blue NBT staining around the penetration site. (E) Superoxide accumulation phase II. HR (UV-autofluorescence image in the left corner) of an attacked (*arrow*) cell is accompanied by $O_2^{\bullet-}$ accumulation in the neighbouring cell. Superoxide is visible at the nucleus and along the anticlinal cell wall (*arrowheads*). (F) NBT–DAB double staining showing H_2O_2 accumulation phase III and superoxide accumulation phase II associated with an HR (*asterisk*). (G, H) Superoxide phase II during multicell mesophyll HR in *Mla12* barley. Dark-blue NBT staining indicates superoxide in tissues around dead cells that are free of stain. Cells immediately before collapse (*asterisks*) also do not show NBT staining. Blue-light excitation reveals yellow autofluorescence of dead cells. From *Planta* **216**, 891, 2003 by courtesy of Dr Ralph Hückelhoven and the publishers.

ROS from phagocytes (Section 7.9.6), some fungi that attack plants make it to help them deal with plant-derived ROS.[179] Nitric oxide is also involved in the hypersensitive response but exactly how it is made and participates is not clear.[180]

7.11.2 Germination and senescence

Numerous papers have shown that adding H_2O_2 promotes germination of the seeds of several plants and that ROS (especially H_2O_2) are produced during germination and cause oxidation of selected proteins.[181] Sources of H_2O_2 can include peroxidases and oxalate oxidases. How ROS relate to promotion of germination is currently unclear, but they may be important since some antioxidants slow germination, and hormones affecting germination seem to act, at least in part, by regulating ROS production.[182] Mechanisms by which ROS could contribute to germination include loosening of the seed coat and activation of the pentose phosphate pathway, providing NADPH to reduce thioredoxin, an important protein in the regulation of germination and in antioxidant defence of seeds.[183]

Fruit growth, ripening, and plant senescence are also oxidative processes.[184] Fruit growth requires cell expansion, permitted by a loosening of cell walls in which peroxidases, H_2O_2 and possibly[185] even OH•, appear involved. Fruit ripening is usually promoted by ethylene and involves increases in peroxidase activity and oxidation products. For example, as pears ripen, the concentration of –SH groups in the fruit decreases, and there is an accumulation of H_2O_2 and lipid peroxides.

Senescence of plant tissues is characterized by a breakdown of chlorophyll, proteins, lipids, nucleic acids and cell walls. It can be speeded up by treatments that stimulate formation of H_2O_2 within the tissue (e.g. with abscisic acid), and OH• may be involved in cell wall degradation.[184,185] Membrane fluidity decreases in plasma and organelle membranes from many senescing plant tissues, and lipoxygenases (Section 7.11.3 below) are activated during senescence.[186]

7.11.3 Plant lipoxygenases[186,187]

Many plants contain **lipoxygenases** (LOXs), enzymes that catalyse reaction of PUFAs with O_2 to give 13- and/or 9-hydroperoxides (Fig. 7.18). The first LOX to be purified was from soybean. It is now known as **soybean lipoxygenase 1**, since other LOXs were later found in this plant. It has a pH optimum of 9 and its preferred substrate is linoleic acid, upon which it acts to produce mostly the 13-L-hydroperoxide (Fig. 7.18). Other LOXs have different pH optima, substrate specificity and produce different ratios of products. For example, soybean LOX 2 has a pH optimum of 6.8 and prefers arachidonic acid as a substrate, but will also convert linoleic acid into approximately equal amounts of the 13- and 9-hydroperoxides.

Although at least one manganese-containing LOX is known, from the fungus *Gaeumannomyces graminis*,[188] plant LOXs usually contain one (non-haem) iron ion per molecule. It must be in the Fe(III) state to allow the enzymes to function. Lipoxygenases abstract a hydrogen atom from a

PUFA in a stereospecific manner, the Fe(III) becoming Fe^{2+} and a carbon-centred PUFA radical forming. Bond rearrangement and O_2 insertion follow to give a peroxyl radical. Iron(II) reduces this to a peroxyl anion (LOO⁻) which protonates to a peroxide, and the active Fe(III) enzyme is regenerated.[189]

$$L{-}H \xrightarrow{\text{enzyme}} L^\bullet \xrightarrow{\ O_2\ } LOO^\bullet \xrightarrow{\text{enzyme}} \underset{\text{product}}{LOOH}$$

The action of LOXs on PUFAs can produce a 'co-oxidation' of other substrates such as thiols, carotenoids and chlorophylls. Indeed, LOXs are employed commercially to oxidize, and thus bleach, wheat-flour carotenoids during bread making. This happens when the intermediate peroxyl radicals that are normally reduced to hydroperoxides during the catalytic cycle instead attack the cosubstrate. Oxidation of linoleic acid by soybean LOX isoenzymes 2 and 3 is reported to be accompanied by singlet O_2 production, which could conceivably contribute to co-oxidations. It probably results from self reaction of peroxyl radicals (Section 2.6.4). Nitric oxide produced by plants might help to regulate LOX, by scavenging intermediate peroxyl radicals and decreasing product formation.[190]

7.11.4 The injury response and oxylipid signalling[187]

Many fruits, tubers, seeds (Fig. 7.19) and leaves respond to damage by initiating a cascade of reactions. First, hydrolytic enzymes attack membrane lipids and release PUFAs and other fatty acids. Linoleic and linolenic acids are the main PUFAs in plants, for example they represent about 75% of the total fatty-acid side-chains in potato tuber lipids. The released fatty acids are acted upon by LOXs, and the resulting hydroperoxides can be cleaved, both non-enzymically in the presence of metal ions and by the action of **hydroperoxide lyases**, specialized cytochromes P450. Several products result, including volatile aldehydes, alcohols and hydrocarbon gases, such as ethane and pentane. The 'wound hormones' jasmonic acid (Section 7.11.2), **traumatin, traumatic acid** and **phytodienoic acid** are also produced from hydroperoxides (Fig. 7.20). Traumatin and traumatic acid are growth promoters, whereas jasmonic acid and its methyl ester are involved in plant defence responses. All these products (Fig. 7.20) are often described as **oxylipins**, that is biologically active products of PUFA oxidation.

Some of the aldehydes produced have characteristic smells which contribute to the aroma of damaged plant tissues, such as new-mown grass and sliced cucumbers (legend, Fig. 7.19). The odour of crushed green leaves is caused by similar processes and involves generation of several products, including 2-hexenal (**leaf aldehyde**) and 3-hexenol (**leaf alcohol**).[191] The sequence shown in Fig. 7.19 can be fast: over 30% of the lipids in potato tuber slices are hydrolysed in less than 15 min even at 3°C. Hence slicing a potato greatly increases its uptake of O_2, both by LOX and in the subsequent metabolism of fatty acid products. Indeed, such oxidations of disrupted plant material give rise to problems of rancidity and 'off flavours' during food processing and storage, that have to be controlled by the use of antioxidants and/or LOX inhibitors. Lipoxygenases are inhibited by several antioxidants, such as propyl gallate, certain flavonoids and nordihydroguiaretic acid. These compounds may act by scavenging peroxyl radicals formed during the catalytic cycle and/or by reducing Fe(III)-lipoxygenases to the inactive Fe^{2+} state.[189]

The reaction sequence shown in Fig. 7.19 overlaps with the hypersensitivity response (Fig. 7.20). Thus salicylic acid can inhibit LOX and decrease formation of jasmonic acid during the early stages of the response. Non-enzymic lipid peroxidation also generates aldehydes and other products, including phytoprostanes (Section 6.7). Indeed, in some plants phytoprostane levels increase during the hypersensitivity response, and may contribute to MAP kinase activation and phytoalexin synthesis.[192] They may also increase synthesis of phenylalanine ammonia lyase, the first enzyme in lignin biosynthesis (Section 7.5.4).[192]

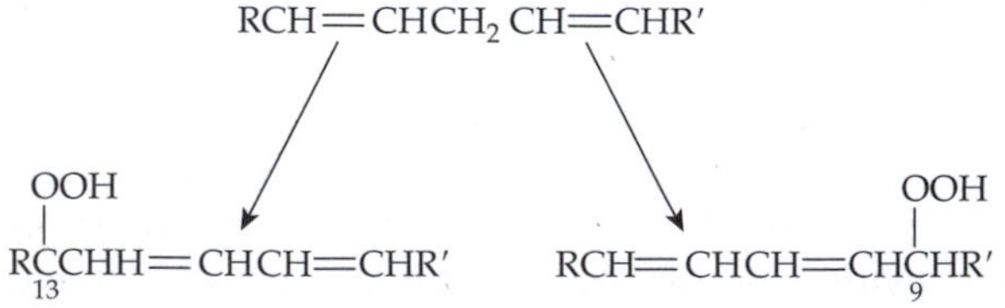

7.12 Animal lipoxygenases and cyclooxygenases: stereospecific lipid peroxidation[193]

Lipoxygenases are important in animals as well. For example, activation of a 15-LOX (Section 7.12.7 below) initiates the degradation of mitochondria that occurs as rabbit reticulocytes mature into erythrocytes.[194] Lipoxygenases also lead to leukotriene production.

7.12.1 Eicosanoids: prostaglandins and leukotrienes

Prostaglandins and **leukotrienes** are derived from PUFAs by insertion of O_2, brought about by stereospecific free-radical reactions at the active sites of enzymes. Prostaglandins and leukotrienes regulate numerous physiological processes and play key roles in inflammation. They, and other related substances such as the **thromboxanes** and various families of hydroxy-fatty acids, are often

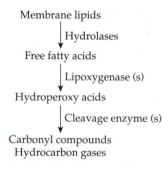

Figure 7.19 Breakdown of membrane lipids induced by wounding plant tissues. The volatile products from the 9-hydroperoxides of 18:2 and 18:3 fatty acids are ***cis*-3-nonenal** and ***cis*-3-, *cis*-6-nonadienal** respectively. These are the two main components of the odour of sliced cucumbers. The 13-hydroperoxides give **hexanal** and ***cis*-3-hexenal**. Several aldehydes have antibacterial and antifungal activity and can repel insects (*Proc. Natl. Acad. Sci. USA* **98**, 8139, 2001).

$$RCH = CHCH_2 CH = CHR'$$

OOH		OOH
RCCHH = CHCH = CHR' 13		RCH = CHCH = CHCHR' 9
13, L-hydroperoxide		9, D-hydroperoxide

Figure 7.18 Plant lipoxygenases catalyse stereospecific peroxidation of fatty acids with a *cis, cis*-1,4-pentadiene structure. For example, linoleic acid may be converted into 13-L- or 9-D-hydroperoxy derivatives or both, depending on the enzyme.

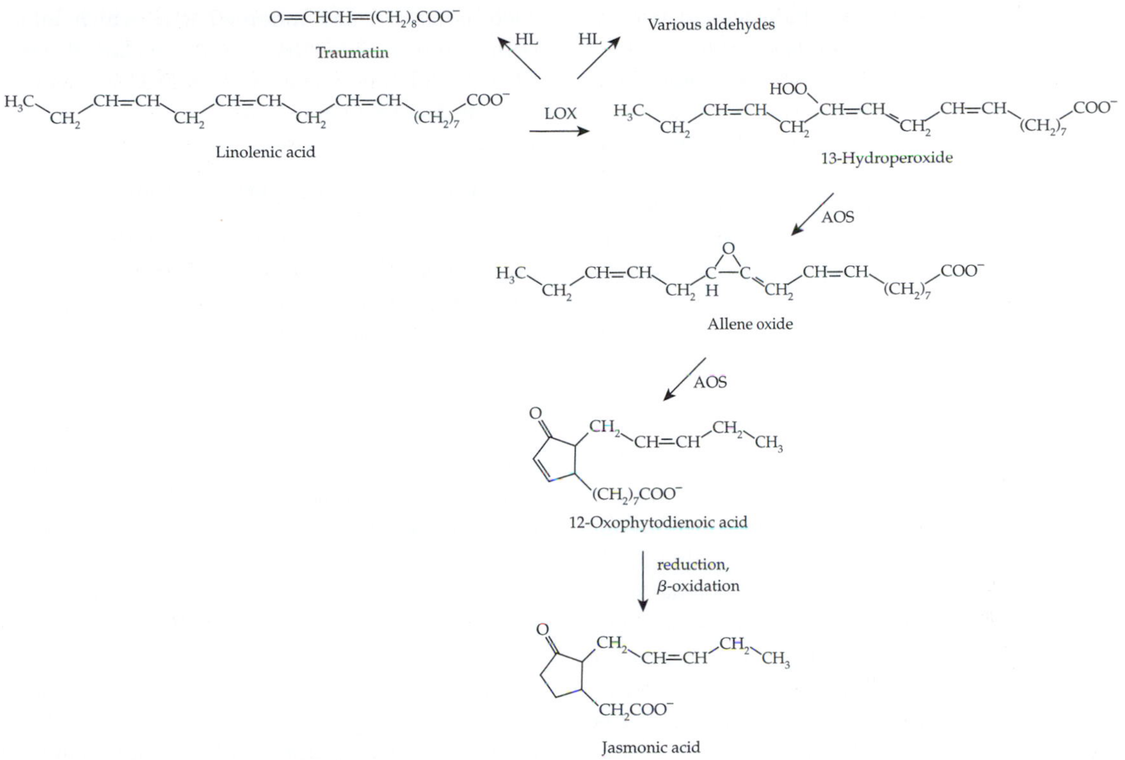

Figure 7.20 Some plant oxylipins derived from linolenic acid. Several steps in the conversions are omitted for simplicity. LOX, lipoxygenase; AOC, allene oxide cyclase; AOS, allene oxide synthase; HL, hydroperoxide lyase. Traumatin can arise by similar pathways from linoleic acid. Oxylipins can also form by the phytoprostane pathway. In **traumatic acid** the aldehyde of traumatin is oxidized to a carboxyl group. The methyl ester of jasmonic acid is often used in perfumes.

collectively called **eicosanoids**, because they are usually synthesized from PUFAs with 20 carbon atoms (*eikosi* is Greek for 20). The eicosanoids act as local hormones, effective at low concentrations. They are synthesized and released from cells in response to stimuli, interact with receptors on adjacent target cells and are quickly destroyed.

7.12.2 Prostaglandins and thromboxanes

Prostaglandins and thromboxanes (sometimes collectively called **prostanoids**) arise from PUFAs by insertion of O_2 to form a ring structure (Fig. 7.21). The term 'prostaglandin' was coined in the 1930s to describe compounds present in semen that could affect blood pressure in animals, and cause contraction of smooth muscle. In fact, 'prostaglandin' is a misnomer, because they arise from the seminal vesicle, not the prostate gland. The seminal vesicle

is the richest known source of prostaglandin-synthesizing enzymes, and seminal fluid is the only biological material in which prostaglandins accumulate to a substantial level. However, every body tissue (except erythrocytes) can make them. The first prostaglandins to be isolated were the stable species PGE_2 and PGF_2 (Fig. 7.21), but better analytical techniques soon identified unstable prostanoids such as PGG_2, PGH_2, thromboxane A_2 (TXA_2) and PGI_2 (**prostacyclin**).

Structurally, prostaglandins may be regarded as derivatives of **prostanoic acid**, a C_{20} acid containing a saturated five-membered (**cyclopentane**) ring. Different prostaglandins are distinguished by the chemical nature and geometry of the groups attached to the ring; these variations in chemical structure affect biological activity. Prostaglandins are synthesized *in vivo* from fatty acids that contain *cis* double bonds at positions 8, 11 and 14. The most important in humans is arachidonic acid (eicosatetraenoic acid, *cis* double bonds at positions 5, 8, 11 and 14), but others include 8,11,14-eicosatrienoic acid ($C_{20:3}$) and 5,8,11,14,17-eicosapentaenoic acid ($C_{20:5}$). This last fatty acid is unusually prevalent in the blood and membrane lipids of Eskimos, probably due to their fish-rich diet. It is thought that the relatively low incidence of coronary heart disease shown by Eskimos might, in part, be due to the formation of antithrombotic prostanoids from this $C_{20:5}$ fatty acid. However, we will confine further discussion to products derived from arachidonic acid.

7.12.3 Prostaglandin synthesis

The first step in eicosanoid formation is to provide a fatty acid precursor. Release of arachidonic acid from phospholipids can occur by activation of phospholipase A_2, or from hydrolysis of DAG (Sections 4.3.2 and 4.5.6). Hence agents increasing intracellular free Ca^{2+} concentrations can increase eicosanoid production, and lipase activity must be carefully controlled in the cell.

Once arachidonic acid is available, the haem-containing enzyme **cyclooxygenase 1** (sometimes called **prostaglandin G/H synthase 1**) adds O_2 to form the peroxide PGG_2, which it then reduces to the alcohol PGH_2. Cyclooxygenase 1 (**COX-1**) is constitutively present in almost all mammalian tissues. It can be inactivated by aspirin, which acts by acetylating a serine residue at the active site. A second type of cyclooxygenase, **prostaglandin synthase-2** (**COX-2**) can occur in many cells, but usually only after its synthesis is promoted by exposure to such agents as PAF, IL-1, TNFα or endotoxin. However, some cells in brain, kidney and a few other tissues produce COX-2 constitutively, and this enzyme is important in renal development and function. Levels of COX-2 increase at sites of inflammation and may be responsible for much of the prostaglandin production there, whereas COX-1 may synthesize the prostaglandins needed for normal tissue function. Hence selective COX-2 inhibitors have been proposed to be efficacious in controlling inflammation without the side-effects (e.g. renal damage and gastric ulceration) commonly seen with drugs

such as aspirin and indomethacin, which inhibit both enzymes. Side-effects limit the clinical use of COX-2 inhibitors, however. A third COX has been described in brain and heart.[193]

7.12.4 Regulation by 'peroxide tone'[195]

If PUFAs are treated with GSH and GPx to remove lipid peroxides, they are not immediately oxidized by COX-1: there is a lag period before rates of oxidation reach maximum. The lag is shortened or abolished by adding PGG_2. Other peroxides are also effective, including those formed by the action of LOX (Section 7.12.7 below) and during non-enzymic lipid peroxidation. Commercially available arachidonic acid usually contains peroxides at variable levels, and different batches can therefore produce different initial rates of reaction when used in COX-1 assays. Cumene hydroperoxide and $ONOO^-$ can activate COX, as can H_2O_2, although higher concentrations of the latter are required. For example, the spawning of abalones (marine snails) was induced by adding 5 mM H_2O_2 to their sea water, apparently by stimulation of prostaglandin synthesis.[196] Peroxynitrite only works over a limited concentration range; too much will inactivate the enzyme (Section 2.6.5).

Hence there is a bell-shaped relationship between lipid peroxidation, $ONOO^-$ production and prostaglandin metabolism. Efficient peroxide/$ONOO^-$ removal, or prevention of their formation, by antioxidants will slow down prostaglandin synthesis, at least until sufficient PGG_2 is formed to activate COX-1. By contrast, too many lipid peroxides or too much $ONOO^-$ can inactivate COX. Many years ago, it was suggested that the **peroxide tone** of the cell (i.e. its content of lipid peroxides, determined by the balance between peroxide generation by enzymic and non-enzymic mechanisms and the rate of peroxide removal) can control COX activity and hence prostaglandin synthesis. Indeed, one assay for lipid peroxides is based on their ability to activate COX-1 (Table 5.12). Although the supply of arachidonic acid may be the main regulatory mechanism in normal cells, peroxide tone could be important at sites of inflammation. It should be noted that peroxides formed enzymically by COX and LOX enzymes can be decomposed to

(a)

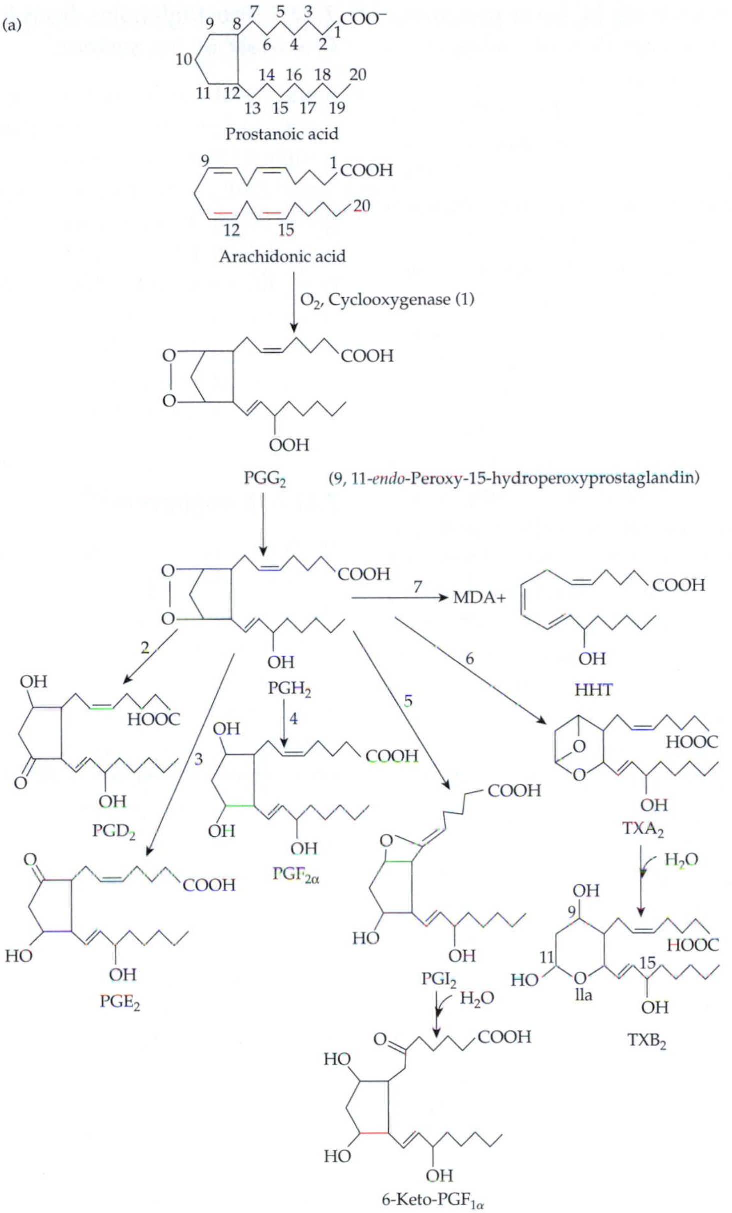

Prostanoic acid

Arachidonic acid

O_2, Cyclooxygenase (1)

PGG$_2$ (9, 11-*endo*-Peroxy-15-hydroperoxyprostaglandin)

MDA+

HHT

PGH$_2$

PGD$_2$

PGF$_{2\alpha}$

PGE$_2$

TXA$_2$

H_2O

PGI$_2$ H_2O

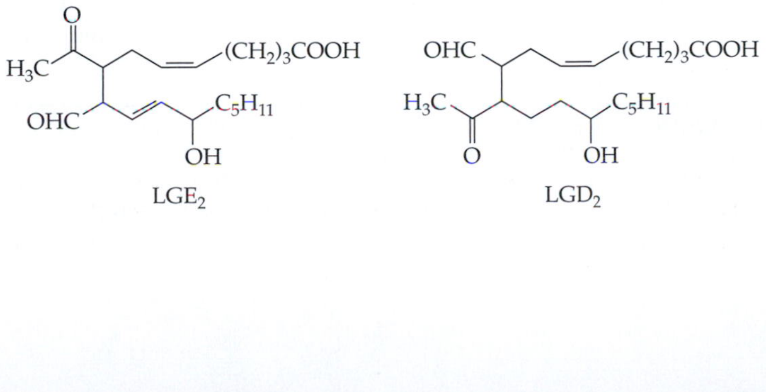

TXB$_2$

6-Keto-PGF$_{1\alpha}$

(b)

LGE$_2$

LGD$_2$

various radicals, for example by haem proteins or free metal ions, that can then stimulate non-enzymic lipid peroxidation.

What do the peroxides do to COX? They convert ferric COX into an intermediate containing ferryl haem and TyrO• radical (Fig. 7.22); the latter then stereospecifically abstracts hydrogen from arachidonic acid. The PGG_2 eventually produced can 'seed' the COX further, being converted to PGH_2. The COX enzymes also oxidize other substrates that can access the active site (Fig. 7.22). For example, during PGG_2 oxidation *in vitro*, COXs can co-oxidize adrenalin, methional (into ethene), and diphenylisobenzofuran (another example of the lack of specificity of this compound as a 'singlet O_2' scavenger), activate several aromatic amines to mutagenic products, convert the carcinogen benzpyrene into a quinone (Section 9.14.1.1), oxidize 13-*cis*-retinoic acid, cause the emission of light from luminol, and oxidize bisulphite ion (HSO_3^-) into sulphite ($SO_3^{•-}$) radical (Section 8.11.3). The metabolic significance of these co-oxidations is unclear, however.

If activated COX is not provided with a substrate to oxidize, the ferryl and tyrosine radicals can inactivate COX itself. Thus appropriate concentrations of phenols, adrenalin or other cosubstrates enhance prostaglandin synthesis in some experimental systems, by preventing this self-inactivation. Certain anti-inflammatory drugs, for example sulindac and 5-aminosalicylate, might exert some of their actions *in vivo* by acting as substrates for COX (Section 9.10.6).

Thus antioxidants can have variable actions on prostaglandin synthesis, not only by regulating 'peroxide tone' and $ONOO^-$ levels but also by preventing self-inactivation of COX. Peroxide tone affects COX-1 and COX-2 differently. COX-2 needs lower 'seeding peroxide' levels and so might be able to function under conditions where COX-1 activity is impaired.[195]

7.12.5 Prostaglandins from isoprostanes? Cross-talk of the systems[197]

Some IPs are unstable and can undergo rearrangement to produce prostaglandins, except that (unlike COX products) they are non-stereospecific. Thus $15-E_{2t}$-IsoP forms PGE_2, and $15-D_{2C}$-IsoP gives PGD_2. Indeed, racemic PGE_2 and $-D_2$ have been detected in animal tissues as well as in urine from humans and other animals. Urinary levels were up to 10% of the total prostaglandins detected and even higher in animals subjected to oxidative stress. Production of prostaglandins in this way should be unaffected by COX inhibitors.

7.12.6 Levuglandins[198]

If PGH_2 is not quickly metabolized, it can undergo ring cleavage to form ketoaldehydes (Fig. 7.21), **levuglandins E_2 and $-D_2$ (LGE_2, LGD_2)**. These highly reactive molecules rapidly form adducts with amino groups on nucleic acids, lipids or proteins, and can inactivate enzymes. Both levuglandins and cyclopentenone prostaglandins (Section 7.12.7 below) could mediate tissue injury if too much PGH_2 is formed during inflammation.

7.12.7 Prostacyclins and thromboxanes

The compounds PGG_2 and PGH_2 are usually rapidly transformed into other products such as PGE_2, PGD_2, $PGF_{2\alpha}$, TXA_2 and **prostacyclin** (Fig. 7.21), to an extent depending on the tissue. For example, platelets form predominantly TXA_2 and 12-hydroxy-5,8,10-heptadecatrienoic acid (HHT) whereas endothelial cells generate predominantly prostacyclin. Just as reactive cyclopentenone isoprostanes can form (Section 4.12.3), so can cyclopentenone prostaglandins. Thus PGE_2 can dehydrate to PGA_2, which binds to –SH groups and is rapidly conjugated with GSH, both

Figure 7.21 (a) Structure of prostanoic acid, and of thromboxanes and prostaglandins derived from arachidonic acid. Enzymes involved: 1, prostaglandin endoperoxide synthases (cyclooxygenases) convert AA to PGG_2 and then reduce the peroxide to an alcohol, giving PGH_2. The PGG_2 can also be reduced to PGH_2 by GPx and GSH. 2,3, Non-enzymic and/or catalysed by GSTs; 4, prostaglandin endoperoxide reductase; 5, prostacyclin synthetase; 6 and 7, prostaglandin endoperoxide: thromboxane A isomerase (thromboxane synthetase). (b) The levuglandins LGD_2 and LGE_2 formed non-enzymically from PGH_2.

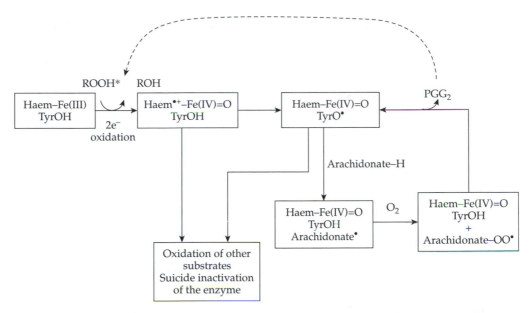

Figure 7.22 A model of the cyclooxygenase active site chemistry. Note its resemblance to peroxidase chemistry. The 'seeding peroxide' is reduced to an alcohol as it oxidizes the haem-Fe(III) enzyme to give a ferryl species plus haem cation radical (**compound I**). The cation radical converts an adjacent tyrosine to TyrO$^\bullet$ (**compound II**), which abstracts H$^\bullet$ from arachidonic acid, followed by O$_2$ binding to the resulting carbon-centred radical (arachidonate$^\bullet$). The tyrosine donates H$^\bullet$, PGG$_2$ is released and the cycle repeats. Cyclooxygenases can also catalyse peroxidase-type reactions. Compound I can accept one electron from a substrate to give ferryl haem enzyme, which can accept a further electron to restore ferric haem. Adapted from *J. Biol. Chem.* **271**, 33157, 1996 by courtesy of Dr William Smith and the publishers. Also see *Biochemistry* **41**, 15451, 2002.* ROOH denotes PGG$_2$ or other lipid peroxides. ROH denotes PGH$_2$ or other lipid alcohols.

non-enzymically and catalysed by GST enzymes. Similarly, PGD$_2$ can form PGJ$_2$ and several other products, which can again target biomolecules containing –SH groups. Cyclopentenone prostaglandins (unless swiftly removed using GSH) can damage proteins, including thioredoxin reductase[199] and the proteasome.[200] Damage to the latter will impair cellular protein turnover.

Although a detailed discussion of the tissue-specific complexities of prostaglandin biosynthesis is not appropriate here, it is worth saying a little about platelets and endothelial cells to understand the relationship of the pathways to redox biology. Thromboxane A$_2$ is formed upon platelet activation and promotes their aggregation; it is also a potent vasoconstrictor. Thromboxane A$_2$ is unstable (half-life about 20 s under physiological conditions) and quickly forms the stable, biologically inactive thromboxane B$_2$ (TXB$_2$; Fig. 7.21). Aspirin prolongs bleeding time after vessel injury by inhibiting COX and decreasing TXA$_2$ production. Thromboxane A$_2$ is also produced by activated neutrophils. The

enzyme **thromboxane synthase** (Fig. 7.21) cleaves PGH$_2$ to HHT, producing malondialdehyde (MDA). Prostaglandin endoperoxides decompose to MDA under the acid-heating conditions of the TBA test. Hence application of the TBA assay to tissues synthesizing prostaglandins can overestimate non-enzymic lipid peroxidation (Section 5.14.9).

The vascular endothelium synthesizes prostacyclin (PGI$_2$), which dilates blood vessels and inhibits platelet aggregation. Its actions complement those of NO$^\bullet$ but oppose those of TXA$_2$, and the relative amounts of these various molecules (which differ from species to species and blood vessel to blood vessel) help control platelet-vessel wall interactions and local blood flow. For example, NO$^\bullet$ counteracts COX self-inactivation,[201] and can also activate by forming ONOO$^-$ (up to a point). Both LOX (Section 7.12.7 below) and COX enzymes can, in the presence of peroxides, oxidize NO$^\bullet$, and platelet COX may be a significant 'sink' for NO$^\bullet$ *in vivo*.[202] Prostacyclin is unstable (half-life of minutes), decomposing to give 6-*keto*-PGF$_{1\alpha}$ (Fig. 7.21). Prostacyclin has many other

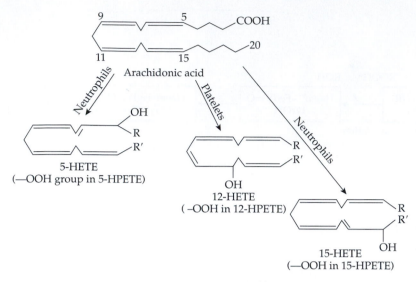

Figure 7.23 Some products of arachidonic acid metabolism by mammalian lipoxygenases. Until recently LOX enzymes were classified as 15-, 12- or 5-LOXs, but sequence studies and differences between species have complicated the picture (Section 9.3.5.3).

important effects, for example to regulate fluid transport in the kidney and gut, and gastric acid secretion. It also contributes to pain and swelling at sites of inflammation.

7.12.8 Leukotrienes and other lipoxygenase products

In Section 7.11.3, we described plant LOX enzymes as initiators of 'controlled lipid peroxidation', a process known for almost a century. It took until 1974 to discover a LOX enzyme in platelets, and later in many other mammalian cells. Animal LOXs contain non-haem iron, act by a mechanism similar to the plant enzymes and are involved in atherosclerosis (Section 9.2.5).

Platelet LOX acts upon arachidonic acid to form 12-hydroperoxy-5,8,11,14-eicosatetraenoic acid (**12-HPETE**), a reactive unstable peroxide that can be reduced to the 12-hydroxy derivative (**12-HETE**). Reduction involves GPx plus GSH; 12-HETE formation is thus decreased in the platelets of selenium-deficient animals. Platelet 12-LOX is involved in the antibody-induced lysis of platelets in patients with HIV infection (Section 7.10.6). Lipoxygenases present in other tissues introduce oxygen at different places in the carbon chain (Fig. 7.23 gives some examples), for example formation

of 12-HETE in skin, 5-HETE and 15-HETE in rabbit and human neutrophils, plus various 5,12-DHETEs (stereoisomers of 5,12-dihydroxy-6,8,10,14-eicosatetraenoic acids).

Lipoxygenases, like COXs, are affected by the $ONOO^-$ level and 'peroxide tone' of the cell; peroxides can oxidize any inactive Fe^{2+} enzyme that forms to active Fe(III) enzyme. They can also consume[190] $NO^\bullet$. Several phenolic antioxidants (e.g. some flavonoids) are LOX inhibitors, but the relationship between this ability and their antioxidant and iron-reducing properties has not been fully elucidated.[203]

The HPETEs are precursors of the **leukotrienes**, which differ from prostanoids in that they have no cyclopentane ring. Instead they have a conjugated triene structure (three double bonds separated form each other by single bonds). Figure 7.24 shows the leukotrienes that arise from 5-HPETE, but others arise from different HPETEs. Leukotriene A_4 is an unstable reactive epoxide which, in some tissues, is converted to leukotriene B_4 (LTB$_4$), a powerful chemotactic agent for neutrophils which also promotes the respiratory burst. Neutrophils themselves make LTB$_4$, helping to attract more of them to a site of inflammation. Leukotrienes C_4 and D_4 increase vascular permeability. Macrophages

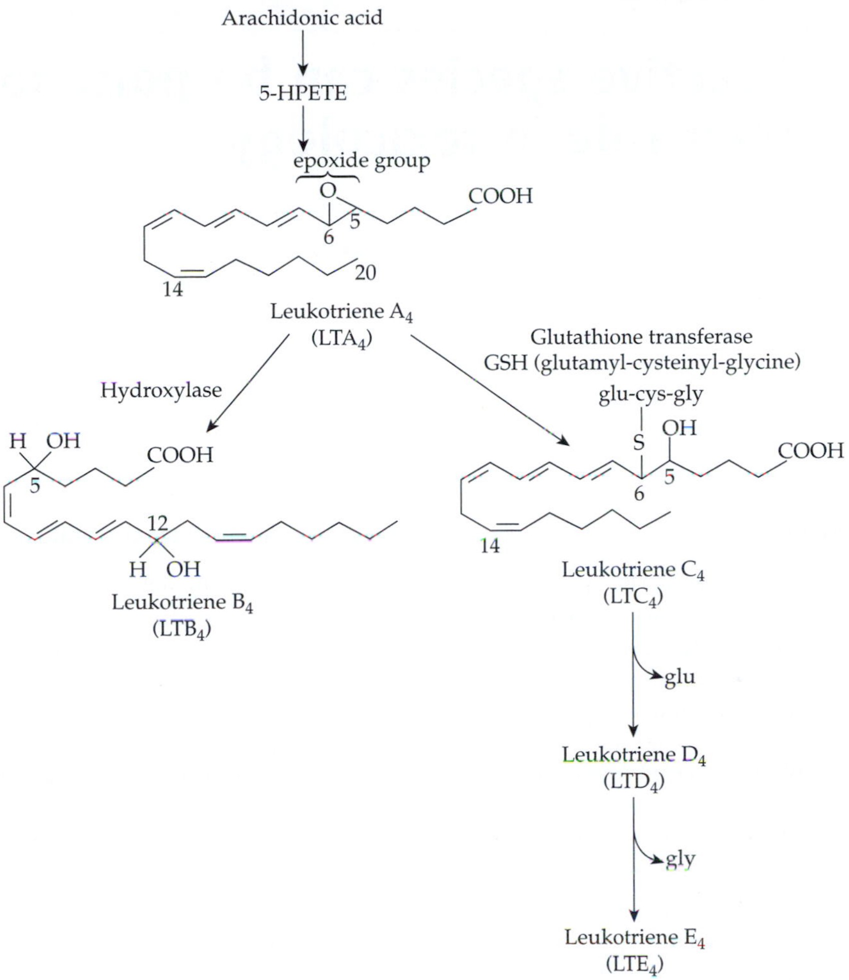

Figure 7.24 The leukotrienes. Leukotriene A_4 (LTA$_4$) is a reactive epoxide (full name: 5,6-epoxy-7,9,11,14-eicosatetraenoic acid) capable of forming adducts with DNA (*Arch. Biochem. Biophys.* **379**, 119, 126, 2000). It can be converted enzymatically into leukotriene B$_4$ (LTB$_4$; 5,12-dihydroxy-6,*cis*-8,*trans*-10,*trans*-14,*cis*-eicosatetraenoic acid) or non-enzymically to other 5,12- and 5,6-dihydroxy acids. Only LTB$_4$ is shown for simplicity. Alternatively, LTA$_4$ can be converted by GST-catalysed conjugation with GSH into LTC$_4$, which is exported from cells. γ-Glutamyltranspeptidase then acts to form LTD$_4$ and LTE$_4$ in the extracellular environment by successive removal of amino acids. Inborn deficiencies in γGT thus impair LTD$_4$ and LTE$_4$ synthesis (*J. Lipid Res.* **45**, 900, 2004). Another group of products is formed by initial oxygenation of arachidonic acid at C-15; for example, incubating neutrophils with 15-HPETE generates the **lipoxins**. Oxidation of 5-HETE can form **5-oxo-ETE** (5-oxo-6,8,11,14-eicosatetraenoic acid), a powerful chemoattractant for eosinophils (*Prog. Lipid Res.* **44**, 154, 2005).

produce LTB$_4$ and other leukotrienes, as do many other cell types, including mast cells. These mediators contribute to the inflammation and bronchial constriction seen in allergic asthma (along with other mediators such as PGD$_2$, PAF,

5-oxoETE [Fig. 7.24] and histamine). Leukotriene C$_4$ (LTC$_4$) is formed by conjugation of leukotriene A$_4$ (LTA$_4$) with GSH. Removal of a glutamate residue yields LTD$_4$, which is further degraded to the less biologically active leukotriene E$_4$.

CHAPTER 8

Reactive species can be poisonous: their role in toxicology

List of examples do not add up to understanding.

Carl Nathan

8.1 Introduction

Nathan's comment is particularly appropriate to this Chapter; hundreds of papers have demonstrated the formation of free radicals and other reactive species (RS) in cells, organs or whole animals exposed to a range of toxins. Yet for only a few toxins has a key role for RS in causing their toxicity been established. Let us first examine the basics.

8.1.1 What is toxicology?

Toxicology is concerned with the mechanisms of injury to living organisms by exogenous chemicals (**xenobiotics**). Although endogenous molecules often cause injury if present in excess (e.g. glucose, $O_2^{\bullet-}$ and $NO^{\bullet}$), we use the term **toxins** in the present chapter to mean exogenous injurious molecules. Modern medicine and agriculture use a range of toxins to control unwanted organisms (bacteria, fungi, insects, rodents, weeds, etc.). We are exposed to some toxins deliberately (e.g. therapeutic or recreational drugs) and others because they are present in the environment. The side-effects of some drugs may involve RS (Section 9.10.6). Some toxins can cross the placenta and damage the foetus (Section 6.11.7). Plants and bacteria synthesize many toxins that can injure humans, such as aflatoxins (Section 9.14) and photosensitizing agents (Section 6.12.1).

8.1.2 Principles of toxin metabolism

Most xenobiotics are metabolized by enzymes with broad substrate specificity; in general, they detoxify xenobiotics by converting them into molecules that are more soluble in water and thus easier to excrete. Metabolism often involves two types of process. **Phase I** reactions add (or sometimes unmask) a polar functional group onto the toxin. This is often done by cytochromes P450 (CYPs), but sometimes other enzymes are involved, such as esterases (e.g. for aspirin, Fig. 8.1), monoamine oxidases and alcohol dehydrogenases. Cytochrome P450 levels vary widely between tissues, the liver having the highest. Substantial levels are also found in adrenal gland, kidney, small intestine, and the **Clara cells** (non-ciliated bronchiolar epithelial cells) of the lung.

Phase II reactions involve conjugation; an endogenous molecule is added to the phase I reaction product, or sometimes directly to the xenobiotic. Examples of phase II reactions already discussed are conjugations with GSH catalysed by **glutathione transferases** (Section 3.9.5) and with glucuronic acid, catalysed by **glucuronyl transferases** (Section 3.18.1). Other examples of phase II reactions are sulphation (addition of a sulphate group, catalysed by **sulphotransferases), methylation** (addition of a methyl group, usually provided by S-adenosyl-methionine), **acetylation** (catalysed by N-acetyltransferases, an example being acetylation of the terminal amino group in

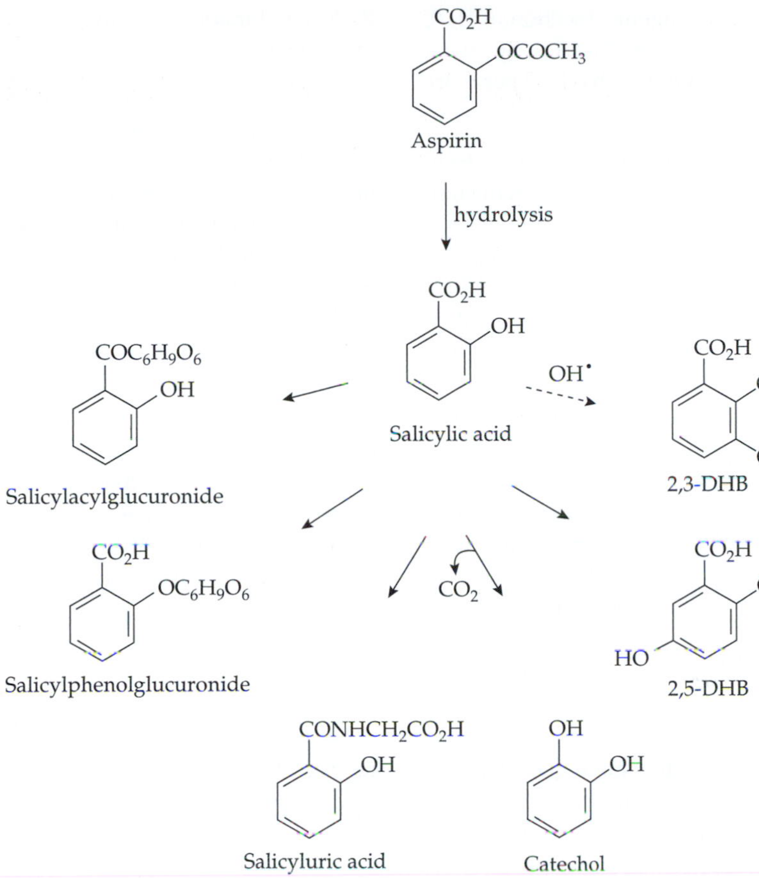

Figure 8.1 Metabolism of aspirin. Aspirin inhibits cyclooxygenases by acetylating them (Section 7.12.3). However, aspirin is rapidly deacetylated by esterase action *in vivo*. Metabolism of salicylate by CYPs produces 2,5-dihydroxybenzoate. 2,3-Dihydroxybenzoate does not appear to be metabolically produced and has been used as a 'biomarker' of OH$^•$ production (Section 5.3.1). Diagram by courtesy of Dr H. Kaur.

isoniazid; Fig. 6.4) and **glycine conjugation**. For example, benzoic acid is excreted in humans as a conjugate with glycine. The fate of **aspirin** (acetylsalicylic acid) in humans illustrates how a drug can be metabolized by several pathways (Fig. 8.1).

Genetic variations often affect activities of drug-metabolizing enzymes, especially CYPs and GSTs (Section 3.9.5). For example, the activity of CYP2D6 affects the metabolism of the antihypertensive drug **debrisoquine**. Most people are 'extensive metabolizers' but a few are 'poor metabolizers' because of low enzyme activity. Exposure to some toxins affects the metabolism of others, for example barbiturates and ethanol can raise levels of certain CYPs whereas xenobiotics in the diet can inhibit them (Table 10.7). Hyperoxia decreases CYP

synthesis in some organisms. There is growing evidence for redox regulation of the activity of some enzymes metabolizing toxins, as well as of the expression of the genes encoding them (Section 4.5.10). For example, rat liver **arylsulphotransferase IV** can be activated[1] by oxidation. A cysteine residue forms a disulphide bridge with another cysteine in the same enzyme, or with added GSSG, to stimulate activity.

8.1.3 How can reactive species contribute to toxicity?

Reactive species have been suggested to be involved in the actions of many toxins. Examples already discussed include haemolytic drugs

(Section 6.5), teratogenic agents (Section 6.11.7), and photosensitizers (Section 2.6.4.1). By what mechanisms could RS be involved? There are several:

1. The toxin itself is a RS, e.g. oxygen itself, nitrogen dioxide ($NO_2^\bullet$) or the peroxide artemisinin (Section 6.6.1).

2. The toxin is metabolized to a RS, e.g. carbon tetrachloride (Section 8.2 below).

3. The toxin undergoes **redox cycling**, i.e. it is reduced by a cellular system and the reduction product is then reoxidized by O_2, producing $O_2^{\bullet-}$ and regenerating the original compound. The cycle then repeats. An example is paraquat (Section 6.9.2.1).

4. The toxin interferes with antioxidant defences. Many toxins are metabolized by conjugation with GSH; a large dose may deplete GSH and lead to secondary oxidative damage by failure to adequately remove endogenous RS. The liver supplies GSH to other body tissues (Section 3.9.3); hence a toxin damaging the liver can lead to falls in GSH elsewhere.

5. The toxin stimulates endogenous generation of RS, e.g. by affecting mitochondrial electron transport, inducing iNOS or CYP2E1 (a 'leaky' form of P450; Section 8.8 below), or activating phagocytes. For example, inhibitors of mitochondrial electron transport (e.g. nitropropionic acid, MPP^+, cyanide) primarily injure cells by interfering with ATP production. However, the 'back up' of electrons they cause by slowing electron transport leads to increased $O_2^{\bullet-}$ formation, which contributes to the injury.[2] Several other toxins target mitochondria, sometimes inducing the mitochondrial permeability transition (Fig. 1.9), ROS production, cytochrome *c* release and apoptosis. **Clofibrate** (Section 9.14.2.1) is one example. Exposure of rats to **methyl chloride** (CH_3Cl), a widely used industrial gas, causes an acute inflammation of the epididymis and sperm defects, possibly because RS produced during the inflammation damage sperm DNA (Section 6.11.4).[3]

6. Some toxins and/or their metabolites can bind to biomolecules to create new antigens, provoking an immune response involving increased RS production.

7. A combination of any or all of the above mechanisms, e.g. for cigarette smoke (Section 8.12.2 below).

'Free-radical reactions' have been implicated in the actions of many toxins, but published reports often take insufficient care to distinguish between cases in which RS formation causes the toxicity, and others in which RS formation is a later stage in the process of cell injury or is peripheral to it. Oxidative damage proceeds faster once a tissue is injured, even if the damage was not started by RS (Section 9.2). A key point: *The fact that a toxin can be demonstrated to form RS in vivo does not mean that RS cause the injury.* Even when increased RS formation *is* an important toxic mechanism, one should ask what are the key molecular targets of oxidative damage. Answering this question is often difficult because mechanisms of cell injury are complex and inter-related (Fig. 8.2), and it is hard to disentangle primary from secondary events. Low levels of oxidative stress may also inhibit communication between adjacent cells.[4]

Let us examine the actions of some xenobiotics, to see how far the claims that 'free-radical mechanisms' are involved can be justified.

8.2 Carbon tetrachloride[4-6]

This was the first xenobiotic shown to cause injury largely or entirely by RS production. It is a colourless liquid, immiscible with water, used in industry as an organic solvent, for example as a degreaser. It was formerly employed as a dry-cleaning agent, but this use is now banned in many countries because of hepatotoxicity. When first introduced into medical practice (in 1847), CCl_4 was enthusiastically promoted as an anaesthetic (soon phased out in favour of chloroform after several deaths due to liver failure) and an antiliver-fluke agent.

8.2.1 Carbon tetrachloride synthesis: a free-radical chain reaction

CCl_4 can be generated by reaction of Cl_2 gas with methane, one of the first reactions encountered by a

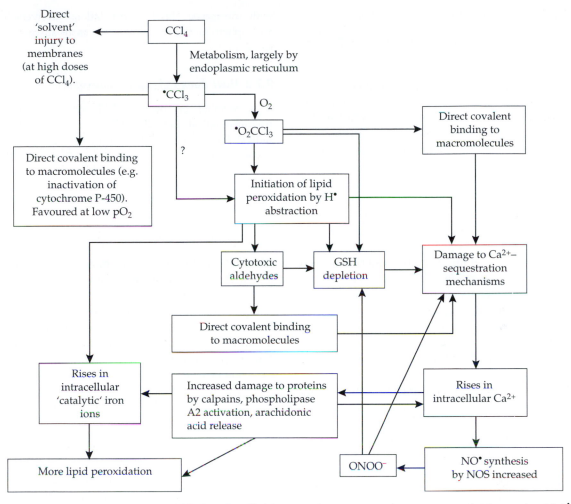

Figure 8.2 Mechanisms of hepatotoxicity of CCl$_4$. Several possible links are not shown. In organic solvents, O$_2^{\bullet-}$ can attack CCl$_4$ to produce CCl$_3$O$_2^{\bullet}$ and other products (Section 2.5.3.6): whether this contributes to CCl$_4$ hepatotoxicity is uncertain (see *J. Biol. Chem.* **263**, 12224, 1988). Carbon tetrachloride treatment activates the transcription factors AP-1 and NF-κB in rat liver (*Drug Metab. Disp.* **24**, 15, 1996). Nitric oxide may contribute to damage by CCl$_4$ (*Mol. Pharmacol.* **46**, 391, 1994). The CCl$_3^{\bullet}$ and CCl$_3$O$_2^{\bullet}$ radicals are capable of forming adducts to DNA bases (e.g. cytosine), yet CCl$_4$ seems only weakly mutagenic. Metal ions, XOR and activated calpains released from dying hepatocytes can cause systemic damage.

student of organic chemistry. Reaction of CH$_4$ and Cl$_2$ requires UV light, which provides sufficient energy to cause homolytic fission of the covalent bond in Cl$_2$. A radical chain reaction results.

Initiation:
$$Cl_2 \rightarrow Cl^{\bullet} + Cl^{\bullet}$$

Propagation reactions:
$$Cl^{\bullet} + CH_4 \rightarrow CH_3^{\bullet} + HCl$$
$$CH_3^{\bullet} + Cl_2 \rightarrow CH_3Cl + Cl^{\bullet}$$
$$Cl^{\bullet} + CH_3Cl \rightarrow HCl + {}^{\bullet}CH_2Cl$$
$${}^{\bullet}CH_2Cl + Cl_2 \rightarrow CH_2Cl_2 + Cl^{\bullet}, \text{etc.}$$

Termination reactions:
$$CH_3^{\bullet} + Cl^{\bullet} \rightarrow CH_3Cl$$
$$CH_3^{\bullet} + CH_3^{\bullet} \rightarrow C_2H_6 \text{(ethane)}$$

Hence CH$_4$ is successively converted into chloromethane (CH$_3$Cl, methyl chloride), dichloromethane (CH$_2$ Cl$_2$), trichloromethane (CHCl$_3$, **chloroform**), and CCl$_4$. Similar reactions occur with bromine, but more slowly.

8.2.2 Toxicity of CCl$_4$

The lipid solubility of CCl$_4$ allows it to cross cell membranes, and any CCl$_4$ ingested is distributed to all organs. However, its main toxic effects are shown on the liver. It causes fat accumulation due to a blockage in export of the lipoproteins that carry lipids away from the liver (Section 3.20.2.6). The hepatocyte endoplasmic reticulum (ER) becomes distorted, protein synthesis slows down and the activity of enzymes located in the ER, such as glucose-6-phosphatase and CYPs, declines, as does the ability of the ER to sequester Ca^{2+} ions (Section 4.3.2). Hence rises in intracellular 'free' Ca^{2+} occur (Fig. 8.2). The nuclear membrane is attacked more slowly. Eventually there is necrosis of hepatocytes in the central areas of the liver lobes, and liver fibrosis.

Although damage *in vivo* involves the ER, CCl$_4$ does not damage it directly. Instead, it is converted to the damaging product(s) by the P450 system. Indeed, neonatal animals have low CYP levels (Section 6.11.7) and are fairly resistant to the hepatoxicity of CCl$_4$. When NADPH is provided for the P450 reductase, CCl$_4$ induces rapid peroxidation of ER lipids accompanied by enzyme inactivation, including destruction of CYPs (thus CCl$_4$ hepatotoxicity can self limit sometimes). Fatty-acid side-chains attached to phosphatidylserine are especially prone to attack, perhaps because this lipid is adjacent to P450 *in vivo*. Pretreatment of animals with **phenobarbital**, or other agents, which raise CYP levels in liver, renders them more susceptible to CCl$_4$.

Elevated peroxidation is readily demonstrable *in vivo*,[7] shown histochemically in Fig. 5.23. Levels of F$_2$-isoprostanes (F$_2$-IPs) increase up to 50-fold in the liver, plasma and urine of animals given CCl$_4$; these increases are bigger in rats pretreated with phenobarbital. Large rises in liver IP levels precede those in plasma; smaller rises are seen in kidney, lung and heart, and F$_2$-IPs can be measured in bile from CCl$_4$-exposed rats. Such rats also exhale more pentane and ethane (Section 5.14.8), and levels of aldehydes such as HNE are greatly increased in their livers.

Does this lipid peroxidation contribute to the damage caused by CCl$_4$? Yes it does—administration of several antioxidants (including α-tocopherol and propyl gallate) decreases CCl$_4$ toxicity in parallel with decreased lipid peroxidation. Conversely, α-tocopherol-deficient animals are more susceptible to CCl$_4$.

8.2.3 How does CCl$_4$ cause damage?

It is metabolized by the P450 system to give **trichloromethyl radical** (CCl$_3^{\bullet}$), a carbon-centred radical detectable by spin trapping *in vivo* (Fig. 8.3). Several CYPs are involved, including CYP2E1 (Section 8.8 below).

$$\text{CCl}_4 \xrightarrow[\text{P450 system}]{\text{one-electron reduction}} {}^{\bullet}\text{CCl}_3 + \text{Cl}^-$$

The CCl$_3^{\bullet}$ radical might attack biological molecules directly, causing covalent modification (Fig. 8.2) and/or by abstracting H$^{\bullet}$ from membrane lipids to initiate lipid peroxidation. Indeed, CCl$_4$-treated rats exhale chloroform vapour, conceivably produced by combination of CCl$_3^{\bullet}$ with H$^{\bullet}$ abstracted from a lipid. Hexachloroethane, another product of CCl$_4$ metabolism, could arise by the reaction

$$\text{CCl}_3^{\bullet} + \text{CCl}_3^{\bullet} \rightarrow \text{Cl}_3\text{CCCl}_3$$

Promethazine, an inhibitor of lipid peroxidation, decreases peroxidation in liver cells and prevents loss of glucose 6-phosphatase activity, but not that of CYPs. Probably CYPs are directly attacked by CCl$_3^{\bullet}$ or other radicals derived from it, whereas the inactivation of glucose-6-phosphatase is brought about by products of lipid peroxidation.

However, CCl$_3^{\bullet}$ may only persist to cause damage in hypoxic regions of the liver; like most C$^{\bullet}$ radicals, it reacts fast with O$_2$

$$\text{CCl}_3^{\bullet} + \text{O}_2 \rightarrow \text{CCl}_3\text{O}_2^{\bullet} \quad k_2 = 3.3 \times 10^9\,\text{M}^{-1}\text{s}^{-1}$$

The product, **trichloromethylperoxyl radical**, is highly reactive (Section 2.5.4); the halogen in the side-chain increases the oxidizing capacity beyond that of most peroxyl radicals. Indeed, CCl$_3$O$_2^{\bullet}$ reacts fast with arachidonic acid ($k_2 = 7.3 \times 10^6\,\text{M}^{-1}\text{s}^{-1}$), linolenic acid ($k_2 = 7.0 \times 10^6\,\text{M}^{-1}\text{s}^{-1}$), thiol compounds and the tyrosine and tryptophan residues of proteins.

Essentially therefore, CCl$_4$ causes hepatic damage by initiating lipid peroxidation via its

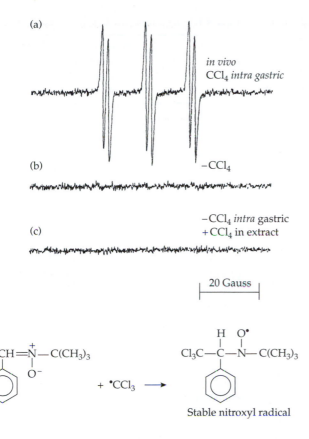

(a) *in vivo* CCl_4 *intra gastric*

$-CCl_4$

(b)

$-CCl_4$ *intra gastric* $+CCl_4$ in extract

(c)

20 Gauss

Stable nitroxyl radical

Figure 8.3 Trapping of trichloromethyl radical by the spin-trap PBN. From *Free Radicals: A Practical Approach* (Punchard, N.A. and Kelly, F.J., eds), p. 19, IRL Press, Oxford, by courtesy of Professor R. P. Mason and Oxford University Press. (a) ESR spectrum of a chloroform/ methanol extract of liver from a rat 1 h after administration of 0.8 ml/kg CCl_4 (intragastric) and 70 mg/kg PBN (intraperitoneal). (b) ESR spectrum of the extract of liver from a control rat given only the PBN. (c) As in (b), but liver was homogenized in a chloroform/ methanol mixture to which 25 μl of CCl_4/g of liver tissue had been added; this is an essential control to check for radical formation during solvent extraction.

metabolism to radicals. Subsequent damaging events include rises in intracellular Ca^{2+}, GSH depletion and iron release (Fig. 8.2). Liver injury by CCl_4 (or by almost any mechanism) can provoke activation of macrophages (**Kupffer cells**) resident in this organ. Recruitment of neutrophils from the circulation can also occur; production of RS by both types of phagocyte might contribute to injury by CCl_4. End-products of lipid peroxidation such as HNE and F_2-isoprostanes can promote fibrosis in the damaged liver (Section 8.8 below).

8.3 Other halogenated hydrocarbons[5]

Since the role of free radicals in CCl_4 toxicity is well established, it has often been proposed that they are involved in the toxicity of other halogenated hydrocarbons. For some, such as **1,2 dibromoethane** (ethylene dibromide), the anaesthetic **halothane**, **trichloroethylene**, **bromobenzene** (C_6H_5Br) and **vinyl chloride**, the evidence is not

compelling. For example, the toxicity of bromobenzene is largely associated with P450-dependent formation of an epoxide, which can react with GSH and protein thiols or be further metabolized to bromophenol. Nevertheless, the antioxidant Trolox C (Section 10.6.6) offered some protection against liver necrosis induced by toxic doses of bromobenzene in mice, and desferrioxamine was also protective. It may be that GSH depletion and rises in Ca^{2+} due to damage of Ca^{2+}-sequestering systems lead to 'secondary' RS production.[8]

Halothane, 2-bromo-2-chloro-1,1,1-trifluoroethane

is frequently used as an inhaled anaesthetic gas. It is generally safe, although about 20% of patients exposed to it show very mild liver dysfunction, as detected by laboratory tests (**halothane hepatitis** type I). About one in 35 000 patients given halothane shows severe liver damage, leading to necrosis and liver failure (**halothane hepatitis type II**). Re-anaesthesia of patients previously exposed to halothane can produce severe liver damage in a greater number of cases (about one in 3700). Increased levels of IPs have been observed in humans and animals exposed to halothane,[9] and various radicals can be spin trapped by PBN when halothane is incubated with liver microsomes plus NADPH *in vitro*. However, the major toxicity is by the binding of products of halothane metabolism to proteins to form **trifluoroacetylated proteins**, which appear to provoke a severe immune response in susceptible individuals.[10]

Perchloroethylene (tetrachloroethylene), $Cl_2C=CCl_2$, is widely used in dry cleaning, but can cause kidney damage if inhaled to excess. Free radical formation has been suggested, but not proven, to contribute to its toxicity.[11]

8.3.1 Chloroform and bromotrichloromethane[5,12]

Chloroform, a liquid at room temperature, was the first anaesthetic to be widely employed in surgery, introduced by Sir James Young Simpson in 1847. It is no longer used as an anaesthetic, but is still widely employed in industry as a solvent, and small amounts are sometimes added to cough mixtures and mouth washes. Traces may contaminate chlorinated drinking water.

Trichloromethane may be less harmful than CCl_4 because it induces lipid peroxidation much less effectively, possibly because the energy required to produce $CCl_3^\bullet$ from $CHCl_3$ is greater than for CCl_4. Consistent with this argument, compounds in which homolytic fission is easier, such as **bromotrichloromethane** ($BrCCl_3$) induce peroxidation faster than CCl_4 (Table 8.1). Nevertheless, liver damage is still a significant problem in humans exposed to excessive chloroform and several deaths from liver failure occurred in the early days of chloroform anaesthesia. The toxicity again involves metabolism by the P450 system, and agents raising CYP levels potentiate $CHCl_3$ toxicity.

Table 8.1 Lipid peroxidation induced by halogenated hydrocarbons

Homolytic fission reaction	Energy needed for homolytic bond fission (kcal/mol)	Relative rate of lipid peroxidation (%)
$CCl_4 \rightarrow Cl^\bullet + {}^\bullet CCl_3$	68	100
$CHCl_3 \rightarrow H^\bullet + {}^\bullet CCl_3$	90	7
$BrCCl_3 \rightarrow Br^\bullet + {}^\bullet CCl_3$	49	3650

Peroxidation induced in rat-liver microsomes in the presence of NADPH was measured by the TBA assay. Results are expressed relative to the effect of CCl_4. Data selected from *Biochem. J.* **123**, 805, 1971, by courtesy of the late Professor TF Slater.

Administration of $BrCCl_3$ (Table 8.1) to rats produced a different toxicity: damage to the Clara cells of the lung,[13] apparently by lipid peroxidation. As already mentioned, Clara cells are richer in CYPs than other lung cells.

8.3.2 Pentachlorophenol and related environmental pollutants

Pentachlorophenol (PCP) is used as a wood preservative, herbicide and insecticide, but can cause liver cancer in some strains of mice and rats. The major metabolite of PCP, **tetrachlorohydroquinone** (TCHQ),

can form mutagenic adducts with DNA and may be the toxic species. Several studies have shown increased levels of 8OHdG in the livers of animals fed PCP, and TCHQ exposure can increase 8OHdG in isolated cells and in the livers of mice.[14] It has thus been hypothesized that oxidative stress, perhaps involving $O_2^{\bullet-}$ formation during oxidation of TCHQ (a diphenol) to a semiquinone and on to tetrachlorobenzoquinone (TCBQ), causes additional oxidative DNA damage that leads to cancer. The TCBQ might also be able to form DNA adducts itself as well as generate OH$^\bullet$ (Section 2.5.1.1). Further work is needed to support this hypothesis since rises in 8OHdG may be a common feature of all carcinogenic agents (Section 9.13.5) rather than evidence that RS are major players in the carcinogenicity.

Other environmental contaminants that might cause oxidative stress include the chlorinated dioxin **TCDD (2,3,7,8-tetrachlorodibenzo-*p*-dioxin)**, a carcinogen that is more effective in female than in male, or ovariectomized female, rats. Its toxicity involves binding to an intracellular receptor protein (the **aryl hydrocarbon receptor, AHR**) and subsequently altering the transcription of multiple genes (including genes encoding several CYPs).[14] Giving high doses of TCCD to animals can increase mitochondrial ROS production (although exactly how is uncertain), lipid peroxidation, and oxidative DNA damage.[15] A relationship exists between TCCD toxicity and iron; iron-deficient animals show less injury. Increased levels of 8OHdG were detected in the livers of female rats chronically treated with TCCD: elevations were less marked in ovariectomized rats.[15,16] The significance of these observations is unclear; one possibility is that raising CYP levels increases the metabolism of oestrogen to catechol oestrogens, which can oxidatively damage DNA under certain circumstances (Section 8.6.5 below).

The fungicide **hexachlorobenzene** causes liver damage and interferes with haem biosynthesis, leading to a syndrome of liver damage and photosensitivity called **porphyria cutanea tarda**. Both the inherited version of this disease and the hexachlorobenzene-induced disease are aggravated by iron overload and are associated with inhibition of the hepatic uroporphyrinogen decarboxylase enzyme (Fig. 2.14). Unfortunately, TCCD can have similar effects.[17]

8.4 Redox-cycling toxins: bipyridyl herbicides

8.4.1 Toxicity to bacteria

The toxicity of bipyridyl herbicides to plants involves redox cycling (Section 6.9.2). So does their toxicity to bacteria and animals. Low concentrations (0.1–1.0 μM) of paraquat halt the growth of *E. coli* (a bacteriostatic effect), whereas higher (>100 μM) concentrations are required to kill.[18] Paraquat is taken up by *E. coli* and rapidly reduced to a bipyridyl radical, which can be detected by its absorbance or ESR spectrum under anaerobic conditions. Reduction is catalysed by several enzymes, including thioredoxin reductase and NADP$^+$: ferredoxin oxidoreductase.[19] In the presence of O_2, paraquat radical disappears, and $O_2^{\bullet-}$ is generated. Addition of paraquat to aerobically grown *E. coli* induces rapid synthesis of MnSOD, the same enzyme induced by elevated O_2 (Section 3.5.4). *E. coli* whose SOD activity is increased by paraquat pretreatment are more resistant to elevated O_2. *Vice versa*, cells with raised SOD due to previous exposure to hyperoxia or to transfection with SOD genes, are more resistant to paraquat. If increased production of MnSOD by *E. coli* is prevented, either by adding puromycin (an inhibitor of protein synthesis) or by a poor growth medium, then the toxicity of paraquat increases.

Damage to *E. coli* by paraquat probably involves $O_2^{\bullet-}$-dependent damage to [Fe–S] cluster enzymes (Section 3.6.1); released iron contributes by promoting Fenton chemistry.[20] Some paraquat radical can leak out of the bacteria and generate $O_2^{\bullet-}$ in the growth medium.[21]

8.4.2 Toxicity to animals

A major problem in the agricultural use of paraquat and diquat is that they are poisonous to animals, including fish, rat, mouse, cat, dog, sheep, cattle and humans. There have been many cases of children drinking paraquat carelessly stored in soft-drink bottles, and it is sometimes used in suicide attempts. Bipyridyl herbicides can also be absorbed slowly through the skin.

Oral intake of paraquat initially causes local effects—irritation of the mouth, throat and oesophagus, and sometimes vomiting and diarrhoea. Fortunately, gut absorption of bipyridyl herbicides is slow, and life may often be saved by washing out the stomach and intestines repeatedly with saline solutions or suspensions of clays that absorb the herbicides (e.g. bentonite or fullers' earth). Dialysis of blood can also be employed.

The major organ affected by paraquat in animals is the lung. The type I cells that line the alveoli (Section 1.5.2) begin to swell and are eventually destroyed, leading to oedema, capillary congestion and inflammation. Type II cells (Section 1.5.2) are also damaged and surfactant synthesis decreases. Oedema and loss of surfactant hinder gas exchange. In animals that survive, fibrosis often causes permanent interference with lung expansion.

8.4.3 Why is paraquat toxic to the lung?

The answer is simple; first, lung has a high pO_2. Second, several lung cell types actively accumulate paraquat, taking it up against a concentration gradient.[22] The diamino compound **putrescine** ($H_3N^+(CH_2)_4N^+H_3$) blocks this uptake in isolated rat lung slices, because paraquat 'rides on' a diamine transporter. Other tissues, including liver and kidney, are damaged by paraquat, but more slowly, because they do not concentrate it. By contrast, although large doses of diquat affect the lung, it is not the major target tissue (intestines and liver often suffer more). The 'targeting' of paraquat to lung by active transport means that poisoning can occur by inhaling paraquat droplets from crop spraying. Paraquat has allegedly caused lung damage in the USA to 'pot' smokers who obtained their marijuana from paraquat-treated Mexican plants.[23]

Microsomal fractions from lung (and most other animal tissues) reduce paraquat in the presence of NADPH, and the paraquat radical then reacts with O_2 to form $O_2^{\bullet-}$. Reduction is achieved by NADPH–cytochrome P450 reductase, since antibody directed against this enzyme inhibits paraquat reduction by microsomes *in vitro*. Indeed, intravenous injection of paraquat into rats causes a rapid activation of the pentose phosphate pathway in lung, presumably as SOD converts $O_2^{\bullet-}$ to H_2O_2 and NADPH is consumed by glutathione and thioredoxin reductases. NADPH is also required for the biosynthesis of fatty acids (needed to replace damaged membrane lipids and for surfactant), so that fatty acid synthesis is decreased in the paraquat-treated lung. There is an accumulation of 'mixed disulphides' formed between protein –SH groups and GSSG.[24] Oxidative protein

damage, lipid peroxidation, Fenton chemistry, and oxidative DNA damage may all make some contribution to paraquat toxicity. In the absence of O_2, $PQ^{\bullet+}$ can reduce Fe(III) chelates to Fe^{2+}, and reductively mobilize iron from ferritin,[25] although the relevance of these reactions in the lung, where O_2 is abundant, are uncertain. The powerful reducing ability of $PQ^{\bullet+}$ ($E^{o'} \sim -0.45\,V$) has caused problems in using desferrioxamine to study paraquat toxicity. Some authors have reported protective effects, but others have clamed an aggravation of paraquat toxicity.[26] Desferrioxamine prevents $O_2^{\bullet-}$-dependent $OH^{\bullet}$ formation because it binds Fe(III) tightly, and the Fe(III) chelate cannot be reduced by $O_2^{\bullet-}$ (Section 10.7.1). However, it is possible that the $PQ^{\bullet+}$ radical *can* reduce the Fe(III)–desferrioxamine complex, leading to Fe^{2+}–desferrioxamine. This compound, or Fe^{2+} released by it, could lead to $OH^{\bullet}$ generation by reaction with H_2O_2.

Cellular injury by paraquat raises intracellular free Ca^{2+} levels, which could increase $NO^{\bullet}$ production and the activity of calpains that can convert xanthine dehydrogenase to XO (Section 4.3.2). Indeed, there are reports that rises in XO contribute to lung damage by paraquat[27] and that NOS inhibitors offer some protection against lung damage in paraquat-treated animals.[28] However, NOS enzymes can reduce paraquat to $PQ^{\bullet+}$, an alternative explanation of why NOS inhibitors might offer some protection.

The damaging effects of paraquat to bacteria or animals are potentiated at high O_2 concentrations, consistent with a key role for reaction of paraquat radical with O_2. Indeed, overexpressing SOD in animal cells usually decreases the toxicity of paraquat to them. Pretreatment of adult rats with endotoxin increases catalase, SOD, G6PDH and GPx activities in the lung; such rats are resistant both to elevated O_2 (Section 3.4.5) and to paraquat.[29] Selenium-deficient rats are more sensitive to paraquat, which suggests that thioredoxin reductase and/or GPx enzymes protect, presumably by facilitating H_2O_2 removal (Section 3.8.2). Indeed, mice lacking peroxiredoxin 6 are hypersensitive to paraquat.[29A] Selenoprotein P could also contribute to protection.[30]

The toxicity of bipyridyl herbicides to tissues other than the lung is probably also mediated by redox cycling, involving NADPH–cytochrome

P450 reductase (which is widely distributed) and/or other flavoproteins, such as glutathione reductase (Section 6.10.3); reduction by this enzyme might account for the haemolysis sometimes seen in paraquat-poisoned humans. Paraquat is neurotoxic if it reaches the brain, with some degree of selectivity for cells in the substantia nigra (Section 9.19.3).

8.5 Diabetogenic drugs

8.5.1 Alloxan

Another redox-cycling toxin is **alloxan**; injection of it into animals causes degeneration of the β-cells in the islets of Langerhans of the pancreas. Since these cells synthesize insulin, alloxan is diabetogenic. Two-electron reduction of alloxan gives **dialuric acid** (Fig. 8.4), a cytotoxic pyrimidine[31] whose structure resembles that of the haemolytic agents divicine and isouramil (Section 6.5.3), although alloxan is not a haemolytic agent. An intermediate radical, formed by one-electron reduction of alloxan (or one-electron oxidation of dialuric acid), also exists.[32] Dialuric acid is unstable and readily

oxidizes back to alloxan, accompanied by reduction of O_2 to $O_2^{\bullet-}$. Its oxidation is accelerated by transition metal ions, which often also catalyse $OH^{\bullet}$ formation.

Any body tissue that can take up and reduce alloxan will be at risk of oxidative stress (and it can pass through the glucose transporters), so why are the islets a target? When alloxan is injected into rats, it accumulates both in islets and liver. Whereas liver contains high activities of antioxidant defence enzyme, activities in the β-cells are lower (Table 3.3, 3.4 and 3.6).[33,34] Further, isolated rodent β-cells reduce alloxan to dialuric acid at a high rate: reduction may involve GSH, thioredoxin and/or glutaredoxin.[31,35] Finally, islet cells contain the TRPM2 cation channel (Section 4.3.2.2) which means that they are highly susceptible to excessive rises in intracellular free Ca^{2+} when exposed to RS.[36] It is probably this combination of factors that makes β-cells a target. Note however that human islet cells are less sensitive to oxidative damage (e.g. by alloxan) than the commonly used rodent cells, perhaps because they have higher levels of SOD, catalase, heat-shock proteins and DNA-repair

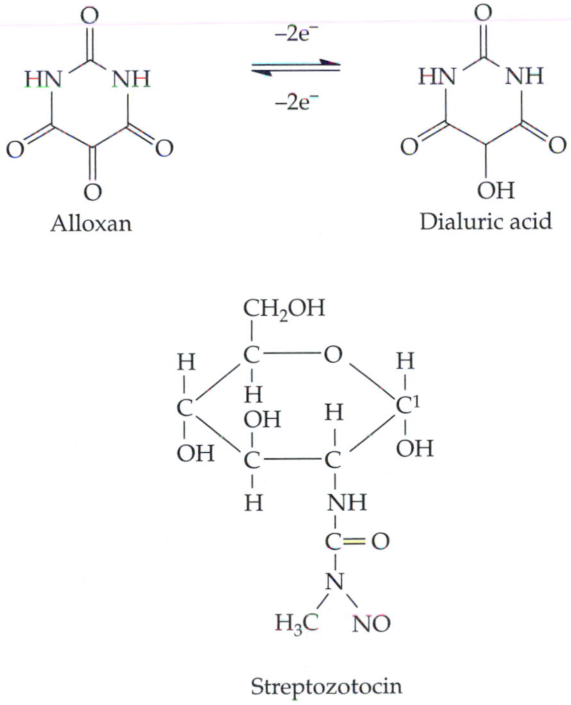

Figure 8.4 Diabetogenic agents. The α form of streptozotocin (N-methylnitrosocarbamylglucosamine) is shown; in the β form the arrangement of the −H and −OH groups on carbon 1 is reversed. The drug is normally a mixture of α and β forms.

enzymes.[37] The toxic effects of alloxan on rodent β-cells can be decreased[38] by adding SOD, catalase, OH• scavengers (including mannitol and dimethylsulphoxide) or iron chelators such as DETAPAC (in interpreting some of this older data, bear in mind the caveats described in Section 5.11; dialuric acid could oxidize in the cell culture media). DNA strand breakage is a key event in cell injury and is accompanied by activation of PARP-1 (Section 4.2.4). It may result from generation of OH• by transition metals bound to DNA (Fig. 8.5).

Are observations upon isolated β-cells relevant *in vivo*? Probably. Injection of CuZnSOD, attached to a high-molecular-mass polymer to reduce its clearance by the kidneys, into mice protected them against the diabetes normally induced by

a subsequent injection of alloxan, as did the iron-chelator DETAPAC.[38] EDTA, which (unlike DETAPAC) allows rapid $O_2^{•-}$-dependent reduction of iron bound to it, was not protective. ICRF-187 (Section 9.15.2) and 1,10-phenanthroline also protect against alloxan, presumably by chelating iron.[39,40] Transgenic mice overexpressing CuZn-SOD in islets were more resistant to alloxan than controls.[41]

As with paraquat (Section 8.4.3), there are conflicting reports on the ability of desferrioxamine to protect animals against alloxan. Some scientists reported protective effects in short-term experiments, but others find that desferrioxamine aggravates alloxan-induced diabetes *in vivo*.[38] The spin trap PBN can protect mice against alloxan-induced diabetes, possibly by trapping

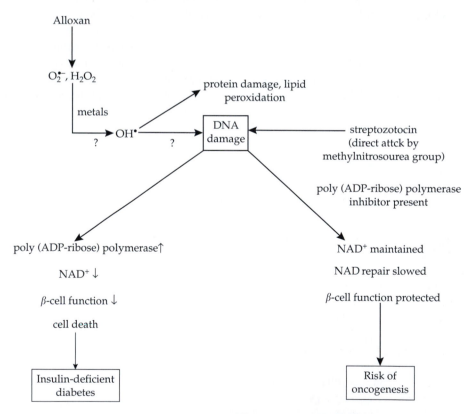

Figure 8.5 Mechanisms of the diabetogenic actions of streptozotocin and alloxan. Adapted from *BioEssays*, **2**, 19, 1985 by courtesy of Professor H. Okamoto and the publishers. Inhibitors of PARP-1 that protect against these agents include **benzamide, 3-aminobenzamide** and **theophylline**. The effects of excess NO• on islet cells may also involve DNA damage. Knockout mice lacking PARP-1 are resistant to streptozotocin (*Nature Med.* **5**, 314, 1999).

alloxan radicals,[32] but remember that PBN has multiple biological effects (Section 10.6.5).

8.5.2 Streptozotocin

Although it is not a redox-cycling agent, it is convenient to discuss here another drug often used to induce diabetes in animals. **Streptozotocin** (Fig. 8.4) is a nitrosourea compound produced by *Streptomyces achromogenes*. It induces DNA strand breakage in β-cells, probably by direct attack on DNA (Fig. 8.5). However, RS could play some role in streptozotocin action, since mice with increased levels of MnSOD and catalase in their islets showed much less damage by this agent.[42] How the RS might be produced is unclear as yet.

Inhibitors of PARP are protective, but treatment of rats with both streptozotocin and PARP-1 inhibitors led to the development of tumours of the β-cells (**insulinomas**) in a few animals. This is consistent with the concept of lethal NAD^+ depletion (Section 4.2.4); PARP-1 activation leading to severe NAD^+ depletion may help the organism by killing cells with excessive levels of DNA damage, so minimizing the occurrence of harmful mutations (Fig. 8.5).

8.6 Redox-cycling toxins: diphenols and quinones

Many quinones exist (Fig. 8.6); examples we have already met include TCHQ (Section 8.3.2), ubiquinone (Fig. 1.8) and plastoquinone (Section 6.8.2). Indeed, the medicinal properties of rhubarb and senna are probably due to quinones. Some quinones are used to repel predators, as in the bombardier beetle (Section 7.5.2), or to deter competitors, for example the walnut tree (Fig. 8.6 legend). Quinones are present in cigarette smoke (Section 8.11 below) and are used in cancer chemotherapy (Section 9.15.2) and as antibiotics (Section 8.16.2 below). How do these agents interact with RS?

8.6.1 Interaction with O_2 and superoxide

Superoxide can exist in equilibrium with diphenols and quinones, with the intermediacy of semiquinone radicals (Section 2.5.3.5 and Fig. 2.5). Hence diphenol/quinone systems can act as scavengers of $O_2^{\bullet-}$ or generators of $O_2^{\bullet-}$, depending on the position of equilibrium and the pH, since the degree of protonation affects the reduction potentials.[43,44] For example, plumbagin, menadione, and juglone (Fig. 8.6), redox-cycling quinones, are powerful inducers of MnSOD activity in *E. coli*. Diphenols/ semiquinones can also react with peroxyl radicals; indeed, both ubiquinol (in mitochondria and LDLs) and plastoquinol (in chloroplasts) have been suggested to act as antioxidants protecting against lipid peroxidation. Their semiquinone forms do not appear to generate $O_2^{\bullet-}$ at a significant rate during the normal functioning of mitochondria and chloroplasts.

8.6.2 Interaction with metals

Semiquinones ($SQ^{\bullet-}$) probably do not react directly with H_2O_2 to give $OH^{\bullet}$, but if metals are present reactions such as

$$SQ^{\bullet-} + Fe(\text{III}) \rightarrow Fe^{2+} + Q$$
$$Fe^{2+} + H_2O_2 \rightarrow Fe(\text{III}) + OH^{\bullet} + OH^-$$

$$\text{Net:} \quad SQ^{\bullet-} + H_2O_2 \xrightarrow{\text{Fe catalyst}} OH^{\bullet} + OH^- + Q$$

can occur. This is a **semiquinone-driven Fenton reaction**, analogous to $O_2^{\bullet-}$-driven Fenton chemistry. If the $SQ^{\bullet-}$ reduces O_2 to $O_2^{\bullet-}$ an additional set of reactions is

$$SQ^{\bullet-} + O_2 \rightarrow Q + O_2^{\bullet-}$$
$$O_2^{\bullet-} + Fe(\text{III}) \rightarrow Fe^{2+} + O_2$$

Diphenols can sometimes reduce transition metal ions, for example hydroquinone (Fig. 8.7) reduces Cu^{2+} to Cu^+.

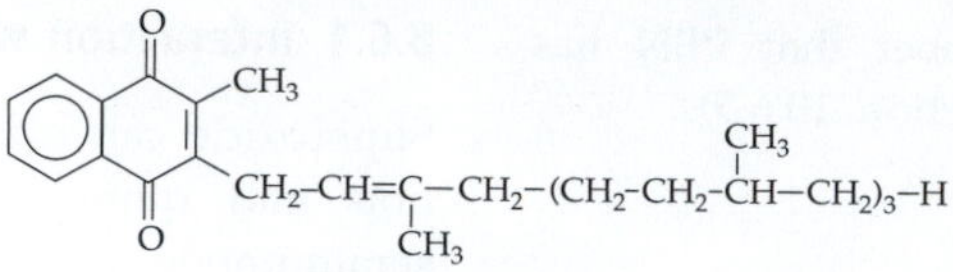

Vitamin K₁ in plants

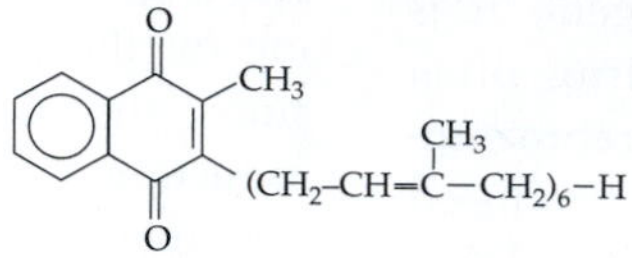

Vitamin K₂ in bacteria

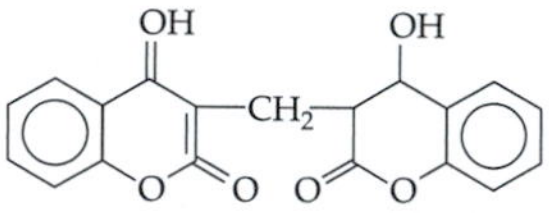

Dicoumarol
(Vitamin K antagonist)

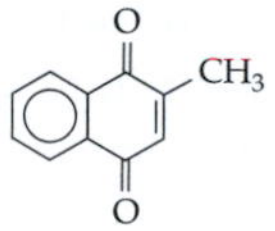

Menadione (vitamin K₃)

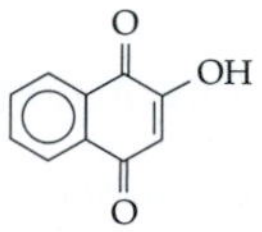

Lawsone

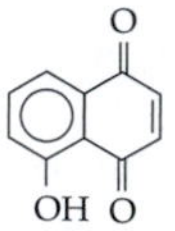

Juglone

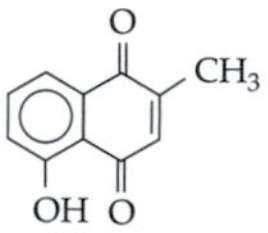

Plumbagin

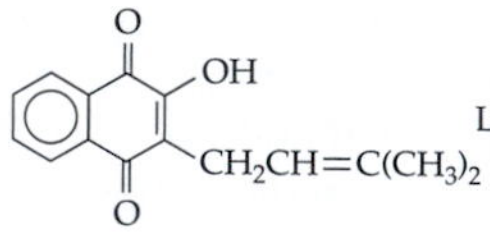

Lapachol

Figure 8.6 Some quinones. Vitamins K are cofactors required by enzymes that attach carboxyl groups to glutamate residues in some of the proteins involved in blood coagulation. Vitamins K₁ and K₂ were found to protect oligodendrocytes and neurons from death induced by severe GSH depletion; exactly how is uncertain (*J. Neurosci.* **23**, 5816, 2003). Different forms of vitamin K exist; the **phylloquinone** or K₁ form (n = 3 in the side-chain) derives from plants (also see Section 6.8.2) and the **menaquinone** series (n = 6–11 in the side-chain) from bacteria (including gut bacteria). **Dicoumarol** antagonizes vitamin K action and interferes with blood coagulation; it is found in sweet clover, which can cause haemorrhagic disease in animals. High doses of α-tocopherol might also antagonize vitamin K action (Section 3.20.2.5). **Menadione** is a synthetic compound lacking the isoprenoid side-chain, but still shows vitamin K activity in animal tests; hence the name 'vitamin K₃'. **Lawsone** is a coloured pigment found in henna, a paste made from leaves of *Lawsonia inermis* that has been used to dye hair since ancient times. **Juglone** is exuded by the roots of walnut (*Juglans regia*) trees, possibly to deter germination of other plant seeds in the vicinity of the tree. **Lapachol** is found in the wood of several trees and has been claimed to have antimalarial and anticancer activities.

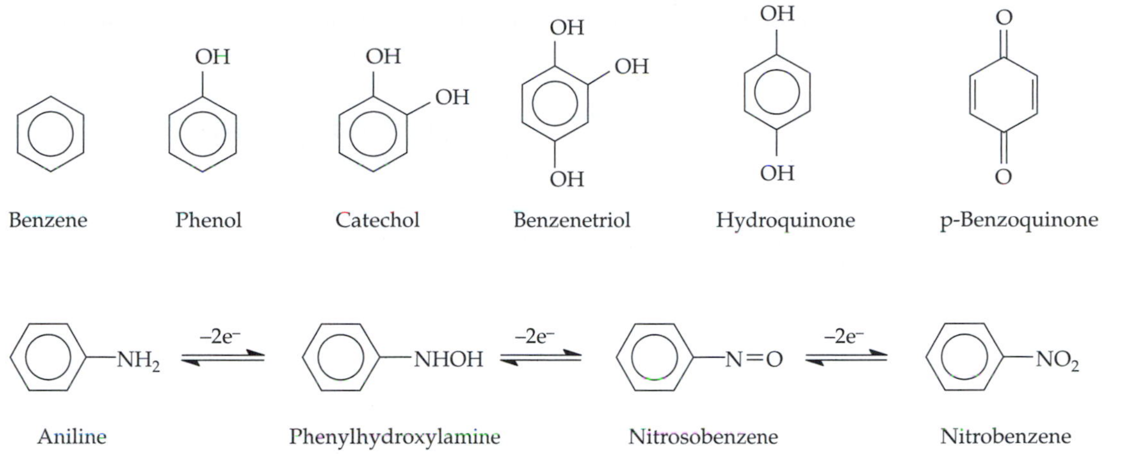

Figure 8.7 Benzene and its metabolites. Conversion of benzene to phenol and hydroquinone is catalysed by CYPs, largely in the liver. The bottom diagram (metabolism of aniline) is by courtesy of Professor Ron Mason.

8.6.3 Mechanisms of toxicity

Quinones can be toxic to aerobes by at least two mechanisms.[44] First, they or their semiquinones may react with GSH and protein –SH groups (ubiquinone and plastoquinone do not). Reaction with GSH can be non-enzymic and/or catalysed by GST enzymes, and GSH depletion may result. In addition, the conjugates with GSH are not always benign. Conjugates of hydroquinone (Fig. 8.7) with GSH cause kidney damage, for example. The conjugate is exported from the liver, metabolized by renal γ-glutamyltranspepti-dase (Section 3.9.3) and the resulting cysteine conjugate taken up by kidney cells to cause oxidative stress.[44]

Second, quinones may redox cycle, after reduction by cellular flavoproteins such as cytochrome P450 reductase

$$\text{Cellular reducing system}$$
$$Q \longrightarrow SQ^{\bullet-}$$
$$1e^- \text{ reduction}$$

$$SQ^{\bullet-} + O_2 \rightarrow Q + O_2^{\bullet-}$$

One example is menadione (Fig. 8.6), which can cause haemolysis, especially in erythrocytes deficient in G6PDH (Section 6.5). Reaction of menadione with oxyhaemoglobin causes oxidation and precipitation of the protein. A semiquinone is formed

$$Hb(Fe^{2+})O_2 + Q \rightleftharpoons Hb[Fe(III)] + O_2 + SQ^{\bullet-}$$
$$\text{methaemoglobin}$$

that can either re-reduce methaemoglobin or convert O_2 to $O_2^{\bullet-}$. Addition of SOD accelerates methaemo-globin formation, presumably by dismuting $O_2^{\bullet-}$ and thus altering the equilibrium (Section 2.5.3.5) to favour reaction of $SQ^{\bullet-}$ with O_2. In addition, menadione can add directly to the β93 cysteine –SH groups on haemoglobin[45] to form the adduct

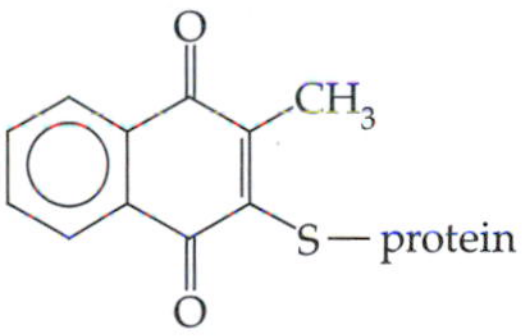

In hepatocytes, high concentrations of mena-dione deplete GSH, increase formation of $O_2^{\bullet-}$ and H_2O_2 and cause membrane blebbing, associated with increased intracellular free Ca^{2+} (Section 4.3.2). Menadione also causes DNA damage, but this seems largely due to the activation of Ca^{2+}-dependent nucleases rather than to oxidative damage, since rises in 8OHdG were not observed in menadione-treated hepatocytes despite extensive DNA strand breakage.[46]

8.6.4 Quinone reductase

Several enzymes in addition to NADPH-cyto-chrome P450 reductase can catalyse one-electron reduction of quinones into semiquinones and promote redox cycling, including glutathione reductase and thioredoxin reductase.[47] However, most tissues contain high activities of **quinone reductase (NAD(P)H: quinone oxidoreductase)** enzymes which catalyse a *two-electron* reduction of quinones into hydroquinones at the expense of NADH or NADPH.[48] The most important is **quinone reductase type 1 (QR1)**. Interestingly, its levels in human liver seem quite low as compared with other human tissues, whereas rat liver is a rich source of it.[49] Quinone reductase 1 contains FAD, is largely present in the cell cytosol and has also been called **DT diaphorase**. It can be inhibited by the anticoagulant **dicoumarol** (Fig. 8.6). This enzyme reduces not only quinones (including menadione, coenzyme Q and 'natural' vitamins K) but also some artificial electron acceptors such as tetrazolium salts.

What is QR for? It may help to maintain coenzyme Q in the reduced (ubiquinol) form.[48] Another role could be to decrease formation of $O_2^{\bullet-}$ *in vivo* by removing quinones, preventing their reduction to semiquinones by other enzyme systems. Hence QR1 is often regarded as a phase II detoxification system. Consistent with this, 'knockout' mice lacking QR1 show bone marrow abnormalities and elevated levels of oxidative DNA damage in liver and kidney, plus increased susceptibility to menadione toxicity.[50] Quinone reductase gene expression is under the control of the antioxidant response element and so QR1 levels are increased by several xenobiotics (Section 4.5.10).

8.6.5 Catechol oestrogens[44]

Oestrogens have been speculated to be antioxidants (Section 3.19), but this action is not established *in vivo*. Indeed, excessive exposure to oestrogens may promote cancer development. Several mechanisms are involved; one of them (of uncertain importance), may be the formation and oxidation of catechol metabolites. Oestrone and oestradiol (Fig. 3.23) can be converted by CYPs into 2-hydroxy and 4-hydroxycatechol derivatives which can oxidize to give quinones and semiquinones. These could both redox-cycle and form adducts with DNA bases, especially guanine.

Similar reactions may contribute to the effects of TCCD (Section 8.3.2).

8.6.6 Substituted dihydroxyphenylalanines and 'manganese madness'

Diphenols derived from phenylalanine (Fig. 8.8) play important physiological roles, but can also oxidize. For example, oxidation of the hormone **adrenalin**, the neurotransmitter **dopamine** and its precursor **L-DOPA**, and the hormone/ neurotransmitter **noradrenalin** produces $O_2^{\bullet-}$ and H_2O_2 and various quinones/ semiquinones.[51] Indeed, adrenalin oxidation can be used to assay SOD (Section 3.2.5). Oxidation of diphenols is accelerated by transition-metal ions, which can often also cause $OH^{\bullet}$ formation. Quinones and semiquinones can attack protein –SH groups and deplete GSH; such reactions may occur in the brains of patients with Parkinson's disease (PD) (Section 9.19). Indeed, treatment of animals or humans with excess manganese promotes rapid dopamine oxidation in the brain and can cause **manganese madness** (sometimes called **locura manganica**), a disease that has been observed in miners of manganese ores in parts of northern Chile, and less often in Australia and Taiwan. Locura manganica in its later stages superficially resembles PD clinically, although the most extensive brain damage is to the striatum and pallidum, and less to the substantia nigra, the main site of cell death in PD (Section 9.19). The symptoms of locura manganica are caused by lowered levels of L-DOPA/ dopamine, but ROS and semiquinones/ quinones may also contribute.[52] Similarly, large doses of adrenalin, noradrenalin or the synthetic catechol **isoproterenol** (Fig. 8.8) can produce an 'infarct-like' necrosis of heart muscle in animals, apparently involving oxidative damage.[51] Oxidation products of α-**methyl-DOPA**, a drug used to lower blood pressure in humans, have been suggested to contribute to the liver damage it can sometimes cause; α-methyldopamine may cause neurotoxicity in a similar way (Section 8.9 below).

Insects provide an interesting example of a *useful* role for dopamine autoxidation.[53] During formation of the hard exoskeleton, **N-acetyldopamine** and similar compounds undergo oxidation and reaction with proteins to toughen the structure.

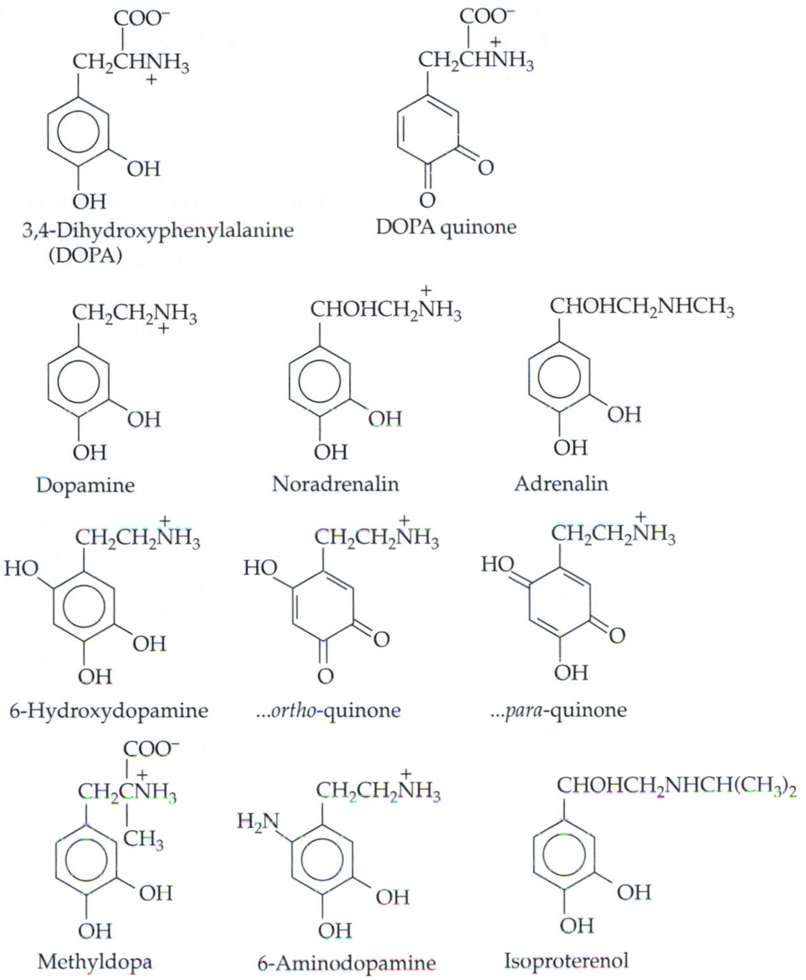

Figure 8.8 Derivatives of phenylalanine. Compounds with the catechol ring structure plus an amino group are often called **catecholamines**, for example dopamine and noradrenalin.

8.6.7 Neurotoxicity of 6-hydroxydopamine[54]

Oxidation of adrenalin, L-DOPA, dopamine and noradrenalin is probably slow *in vivo*, both because SOD is present to remove $O_2^{\bullet-}$ and break the 'chain reaction' of autoxidation and because concentrations of 'catalytic' transition metals are low. By contrast, **6-hydroxydopamine** (6-OHDA) and **6-aminodopamine** (Fig. 8.8) oxidize much faster, although traces of metal ions are still needed. Again, semiquinones and quinones are formed (Fig. 8.8 shows the two quinones that are produced

by 6-OHDA), together with H_2O_2, $O_2^{\bullet-}$ and $OH^{\bullet}$. Superoxide participates in the oxidation of further molecules of 6-OHDA and hence addition of SOD decreases the observed oxidation rate. Indeed, overexpression of a CuZnSOD gene protected isolated neurons against damage by 6-OHDA.[55]

When injected into the brains of animals (it cannot cross the blood–brain barrier so systemic injection does not work), 6-OHDA causes rapid and specific damage to catecholamine nerve terminals. Hence, it is widely used as a research tool to investigate the physiological roles of such terminals (Section 9.19.4). The selective action is probably due to the specific uptake of 6-OHDA by catecholamine neurons, followed by increased intraneuronal formation of ROS, semiquinones and quinones. This is supported by the observation that the brains of mice overexpressing MnSOD (but not EC-SOD) genes were less damaged by 6-OHDA.[56]

8.6.8 Benzene and its derivatives[44]

The aromatic hydrocarbon benzene, a widely used industrial solvent and fuel additive, can damage most tissues if ingested in sufficient quantity, including the liver and brain. However, the bone marrow is particularly vulnerable, and excess exposure to benzene is a risk factor for development of leukaemia. Levels of 8OHdG were reported to be elevated in DNA from blood lymphocytes of benzene-exposed workers.[57]

Benzene toxicity involves its conversion by CYPs (especially CYP2E1) into phenols (phenol, catechol, hydroquinone and 1,2,4-benzenetriol). These can undergo oxidation to quinones and semiquinones (Fig. 8.7), perhaps accelerated by the high levels of myeloperoxidase present in bone marrow. Adding CuZnSOD accelerates oxidation of hydroquinone to the more toxic benzoquinone, which is capable of forming DNA adducts; SOD removes $O_2^{\bullet-}$, so driving the equilibrium between the intermediate semiquinone radical and O_2 to the right.[43] Copper ions also promote hydroquinone oxidation. It has been suggested that formation of $ONOO^-$ contributes to benzene toxicity, by generating nitrobenzenes.[58]

Quinone reductase converts benzoquinone back to hydroquinone; indeed a polymorphism of the gene encoding QR1 which abolishes enzyme activity has been suggested as a risk factor for benzene carcinogenicity.

8.6.9 Toxic-oil syndrome and a new society[59]

In 1981, a new disease was reported in Spain, the **toxic-oil syndrome** or **Spanish cooking-oil syndrome**. At the height of the epidemic more than 20 000 people in central and north-west Spain were affected, of whom 11 000 required hospital-

ization and over 800 eventually died. The symptoms of the disease in its acute stage were respiratory distress, fever, headache, itching, nausea and, sometimes, muscular pains and neurological disorders. Lung damage caused most of the early deaths. When followed up later, about 10% of patients had developed muscular wasting and weakness, and another 49% had suffered some muscular or neurological impairment. Sufferers from the disease were found to have consumed 'olive oil' sold by door-to-door salesmen. Analysis showed that the oil in question had never seen an olive tree, and was basically oil obtained from seeds of the rape plant, *Brassica napus*.

Rapeseed oil imported into Spain was at that time treated with **aniline** (Fig. 8.7) to deter its consumption. Aniline is widely used in the manufacture of explosives, dyestuffs and other chemicals. Excess exposure produces haemolytic anaemia and damage to the spleen, accompanied by splenic fibrosis with increased lipid peroxidation and oxidative protein damage.[60] This is probably because some damaged erythrocytes are taken up by the spleen, which thus accumulates not only aniline and its metabolites but also excess iron. Damage to red blood cells by aniline appears to involve its metabolite **phenylhydroxylamine** (Fig. 8.7), which is oxidized by oxyhaemoglobin to give nitrosobenzene and methaemoglobin. Nitrosobenzene is then reduced by methaemoglobin reductase (or non-enzymically) back to phenylhydroxylamine, which oxidizes more oxyhaemoglobin in a cyclic manner. However, although aniline might have made some contribution to toxic-oil syndrome, the symptoms are different from those of aniline poisoning. It appears that attempts had been made to remove aniline from the rapeseed oil. During this 'purification', aniline-derived toxins were formed.

One good thing to come out of the toxic-oil affair was that it led to the setting up, largely through the efforts of Robin Willson and the late Trevor Slater, of the Society for Free Radical Research (SFRR) in the UK. From the seed they planted has grown a network of international societies with thousands of members: SFRR Europe, SFRR Africa, SFRR India, SFRR ASEAN, SFRR Asia, SFRR Australasia and SFRR America (The Society for Free Radical Biology and Medicine), plus four journals, *Free Radical Research* (official journal of SFRR Europe), *Redox Report, Antioxidants and Redox Signaling* and *Free Radical Biology and Medicine* (Official journal of the American society). Ironically, however, there is little evidence that free radicals and oxidative damage had anything to do with the toxicity of the adulterated oil.

8.7 Redox-cycling agents: toxins derived from Pseudomonas aeruginosa

Pseudomonas aeruginosa, a Gram-negative bacterium, can cause pneumonia in immunocompromised patients and often chronically infects the respiratory tract of patients with cystic fibrosis (Section 9.8). Many *P. aeruginosa* strains secrete **pyocyanin** (5-methyl-1-hydroxyphenazine), a redox-cycling agent with the structure

Production of $O_2^{\bullet-}$ by pyocyanin appears to account for its toxicity to *E. coli* (low levels raise MnSOD levels in this bacterium) and possibly to the lung in patients with *P. aeruginosa* infection.[61,62]

P. aeruginosa secretes an elastase that can cleave lactoferrin and transferrin to release iron, plus a siderophore (**pyochelin**) that allows iron uptake. Iron bound to pyochelin appears capable of catalysing $OH^{\bullet}$ formation from H_2O_2; hence the combination of pyochelin and pyocyanin is more cytotoxic than either agent alone.[62]

8.8 Alcohols

8.8.1 Ethanol

Many of us drink some ethanol (ethyl alcohol) in alcoholic drinks, and even in teetotallers traces are formed by gut bacteria and enter the blood. Ethanol is soluble both in water and in many organic solvents, and crosses cell membranes readily, including the blood–brain barrier. One beneficial effect that it has, apart from some social ones, is to partially protect experimental animals

against alloxan-induced diabetes (Section 8.5.1). It may do this (at the high concentrations used in the studies)[63] by scavenging $OH^{\bullet}$ to form the less-reactive hydroxyethyl radical:

$$CH_3CH_2OH + OH^{\bullet} \rightarrow CH_3\overset{\bullet}{C}HOH + H_2O$$

This reaction is used in spin-trapping experiments (Section 5.2.4). Indeed, the spin trap POBN (Section 5.2) has been used to detect this radical *in vivo* in ethanol-dosed rats.[64]

8.8.1.1 *Ethanol metabolism and CYP2E1*

In animals, most ethanol is metabolized in the liver by **alcohol dehydrogenase** (ADH) enzymes, to form the aldehyde **ethanal (acetaldehyde)**

$$CH_3CH_2OH + NAD^+ \rightarrow NADH + H^+ \\ + CH_3CHO$$

Ethanal is more toxic than ethanol and must be rapidly metabolized by **aldehyde dehydrogenases** in mitochondria

$$H_2O + CH_3CHO + NAD^+ \rightarrow NADH + H^+ \\ + CH_3COOH$$
$$\text{acetic (ethanoic) acid}$$

Polymorphisms of aldehyde dehydrogenase genes that produce an enzyme with less activity cause impaired tolerance of alcohol, sometimes manifested as a **flush reaction** on alcohol consumption.[65] High intakes of alcohol shift cellular $NAD^+/NADH$ ratios in favour of the reduced state in both cytosol and mitochondria; this may promote abnormal fat accumulation in the liver (Fig. 8.9).

Smaller amounts of ethanol can be oxidized by the peroxidatic action of catalase in peroxisomes (Section 3.7.4) and by certain CYPs. Many years ago, a **microsomal ethanol oxidizing system (MEOS)** was identified; it was observed that liver microsomes can oxidize ethanol (and some other alcohols, including butanol) and that rates of oxidation were increased in microsomes from animals chronically exposed to ethanol. We now know that repeated exposure to ethanol induces synthesis of **CYP2E1**, the **ethanol-inducible cytochrome P450**, in hepatocytes and Kupffer cells.[66] This CYP doesn't only oxidize ethanol to acetaldehyde; it acts on many other substrates, including acetone,

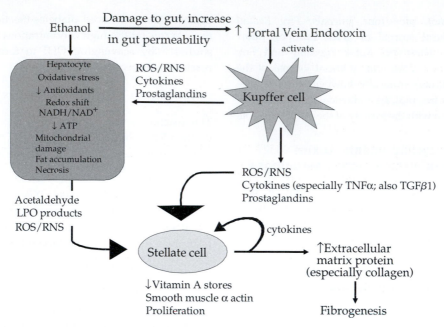

Figure 8.9 Effects of alcohol on liver cells. Chronic alcohol consumption triggers a series of events in hepatocytes, Kupffer cells and hepatic stellate cells that are believed to play important roles in the initiation and progression of alcohol-induced liver injury. Adapted from *Free Radic. Res.* **37**, 585, 2003, by courtesy of Dr SM Bailey and Taylor and Francis. Fat accumulation in response to ethanol is triggered by rises in the NADH/NAD$^+$ ratio, by interference with the DNA binding of **peroxisome proliferator-activated receptor-α (PPARα)**, a transcription factor which increases levels of enzymes involved in fatty acid transport and β-oxidation, and by stimulation of lipogenesis by activating **sterol regulatory element binding protein 1 (SREBP)**, a transcription factor that leads to higher activities of enzymes involved in cholesterol, fatty acid and triglyceride synthesis (*Am. J. Physiol.* **287**, G1, 2004). Similar events are involved in liver damage by inflammation generally (Section 9.12.3).

butanol, pentanol, aniline, paracetamol, benzene, pentane, halothane, isoflurane, chloroform, cocaine and CCl$_4$. Several xenobiotics that are metabolized by CYP2E1 to more reactive products can thus exert toxic effects at lower levels than usual in chronic alcohol consumers; examples are paracetamol (Section 8.10 below) and cocaine (Section 8.9 below). The CYP2E1 is present in various regions of the brain and levels can be increased by ethanol exposure (Section 9.16.5); it may be a more important route of alcohol metabolism there, since brain has only low levels of ADH.[67] Cytochrome P4502E1 is also elevated in diabetes and obesity, and its synthesis can be increased by several solvents other than ethanol, including acetone, benzene, CHCl$_3$ and dimethylsulphoxide.[66]

8.8.1.2 *Ethanol toxicity*
Ethanol is remarkably non-toxic at millimolar levels, and moderate intakes may be beneficial to the cardiovascular system, because they increase

plasma HDL levels and may promote NO$^•$ synthesis by the vascular endothelium. Other possible effects include antithrombotic and ischaemic preconditioning (Section 9.5.6).[68] There may be additional benefit from red wines because of their flavonoid content, although this has not been clearly established (Section 3.22.2); it may be the alcohol that exerts most or all of the cardioprotective effect.[68] Studies plotting cardiovascular disease incidence against alcohol intake often show a J-shaped curve: a small to moderate ethanol intake is good and excess (>35 drinks per week) increases incidence. Acceptable intakes have been quoted as 21 units per week in men and 14 in women (less in pregnant woman). One unit (10 g) of alcohol is contained in about 1 oz of whisky, one glass of wine or half a pint of beer. Of course, it must be realized that a pregnant woman who drinks is exposing the foetus to equivalent levels of alcohol, since alcohol crosses the placenta readily. Indeed, the **foetal alcohol syndrome** is characterized by growth retardation, damage to the nervous system (often accompanied by impaired cognitive function) and facial aberrations, such as eye abnormalities. In part, the ethanol may act by interfering with the normal function of glutamate in promoting synapse formation in the developing brain (Section 9.16.3).[69]

Prolonged intake of excess ethanol by humans damages many tissues, especially the liver. Alcohol-induced liver disease is characterized by fat accumulation, inflammation and necrotic death of hepatocytes and it can progress to fibrosis and cirrhosis (Fig. 8.9). Inflammation involves both hepatic resident macrophages (Kupffer cells) and lymphocytes and neutrophils recruited from the circulation. Production of TNFα by Kupffer cells plays an important role; indeed, in mice deficient in TNFα receptors, alcohol-induced liver injury is decreased.[66,70] Hepatic iron overload is common in patients with alcoholic liver diseases and the effects of alcohol are worsened if there is pre-existing iron overload, for example due to haemochromatosis.[71] Alcohol abuse is also a risk factor for pancreatitis (Section 9.12.1). Chronic alcoholism frequently causes cognitive impairment, possibly involving suppression of neurogenesis in the hippocampus.[72] In many countries, it is illegal to drive a motor vehicle with a blood ethanol concentration greater than 80 mg per 100 ml, corresponding to a concentration of approximately 17.4 mM. Some heavy drinkers reach levels of 300 mg per 100 ml of blood, or 65.2 mM.

8.8.1.3 *Does ethanol increase RS formation?*
These huge concentrations (by comparison with toxic levels of almost any other xenobiotic) have been shown in animals to affect antioxidant protective systems and cause oxidative damage. Injection of large doses of ethanol into rats decreased the SOD activity measurable in brain homogenates by about 25%, and an even greater decrease was produced by repeated injection. Similarly, exposure of neuronal or glial cells from rats, mice, hamsters, and chicks to 100 mM ethanol *in vitro* decreased SOD activity.[73] By contrast, some other scientists have reported *increases* in SOD activity in animals treated with ethanol for prolonged periods, possibly reflecting adaptation.

Both large doses of ethanol, and smaller doses given repeatedly, increase lipid peroxidation in the plasma and livers of animals and humans, as measured by rises in conjugated dienes and, more convincingly (Section 5.14.4.2), in ethane, phosphatidylcholine hydroperoxides, HNE and F_2-isoprostanes.[74,75] Large doses of ethanol decrease GSH levels in liver, neurons, and kidney of animals, which would tend to promote oxidative stress. Decreases in GSH levels in lung lining fluids in human alcoholics have also been observed.[76] Alcohol abuse interferes with methionine metabolism in the liver, slowing its conversion to *S*-adenosylmethionine by the **methionine adenosyltransferase (MAT)** enzyme and hence generating less cysteine further down the pathway. This contributes to the drop in GSH. Oxidative stress can further damage MAT, which has several cysteine residues essential to its function.[66] Mitochondrial from foetal brains showed increased HNE levels after the mothers had been dosed with ethanol, suggesting that oxidative damage might contribute to the foetal alcohol syndrome.[77] Finally, the ability of chronic ethanol consumption to decrease plasma testosterone levels in males has been suggested to involve increased oxidative damage in the pituitary gland.[78]

8.8.1.4 *How does it do that?*
One possibility is that increased mitochondrial $NADH/NAD^+$ ratios promote $O_2^{•-}$ formation (Fig. 8.9), somewhat analogous to the situation in diabetes (Section 9.4). Hydroxyethyl radicals generated during metabolism of ethanol by CYP2E1 can form adducts with proteins: antibodies against such adducts are present in blood from patients with alcoholic liver disease.[79] Another problem is that CYP2E1 is 'leakier' than other P450 isoforms; during its operation more $O_2^{•-}$ and H_2O_2 are released than for other CYPs (Fig. 1.10).[66]

Yet another source may be acetaldehyde. This is mainly metabolized by aldehyde dehydrogenases in liver, but some might be acted upon by **aldehyde oxidase**,[80] which produces $O_2^{•-}$ (Table 1.4). In addition CYP2E1 and XO can oxidize acetaldehyde, the latter producing $O_2^{•-}$ and H_2O_2. Indeed, the XO/dehydrogenase ratio can sometimes increase in the liver of ethanol-treated rodents.[80] However, the affinity of XO for ethanol is low, so that xanthine and hypoxanthine may well out-compete acetaldehyde as substrates *in vivo*. Acetaldehyde reacts reversibly with GSH (another contributor to falls in GSH concentration) and with protein –SH and NH$_2$ groups, for example on plasma albumin and in mitochondrial proteins. Some of these adducts might provoke an immune response. Indeed, protein adducts containing both acetaldehyde and MDA have been detected in animals and humans.[81] Acetaldehyde might even help convert dopamine and serotonin in the brain into neurotoxic products, such as **tetrahydroisoquinolines** and **tetrahydro-β-carbolines** (Section 9.19.3).[82] Acetaldehyde can be produced in the colon from ethanol by the action of colonic bacteria, and might contribute to colonic irritation resulting from excessive drinking.[83] Other potentially toxic products generated from ethanol include **fatty acid ethyl esters**, which have been suggested to be neurotoxic. Withdrawal of ethanol from neurons 'adapted' to its presence in culture can also, paradoxically, cause damage that may involve RS.[84]

8.8.1.5 *Do the RS explain ethanol toxicity?*

Excess ethanol exposure is accompanied by GSH depletion and elevated oxidative damage. Does this account for ethanol toxicity to humans? Some contribution seems likely, but how much is uncertain. Analysing the role of RS in tissue damage in human alcoholics can be made difficult by the fact that their diet is often inadequate, lacking enough α-tocopherol, selenium, B vitamins or PUFAs and sometimes too rich in saturated fats. Heavy drinkers are often cigarette smokers, compounding the pathology of two different toxic agents. The effects of ethanol in causing fatty liver may be due largely to altered NADH/NAD$^+$ ratios and changes in gene transcription (Fig. 8.9). However, mice lacking CuZnSOD show greater liver damage after alcohol administration, suggesting some role for ROS.[85] Indeed, liver fibrosis seems closely associated with lipid peroxidation. Fibrogenesis in the liver is mediated by **hepatic stellate cells**, which normally store vitamin A. After insult to the liver by ethanol, other toxins or viral infection, they can become activated to proliferate and produce collagen.[86] Both 4-HNE and F$_2$-isoprostanes appear to be powerful profibrogenic stimuli for stellate cells (Fig. 8.9).[86,87] **Non-alcoholic steatohepatitis**, liver damage associated with fatty infiltration of hepatocytes, is associated with obesity, and high-fat diets, and can lead to fibrosis. Again, ROS and HNE are involved.[88] Oxidative stress probably contributes to ethanol-induced cognitive impairment[72] and to the foetal alchohol syndrome (Section 8.8.1.3). Oxidative stress might help damage the intestinal mucosa and allow endotoxin to enter the circulation, potentiating inflammation (Fig. 8.9).[89]

To summarize, important sources of RS in alcohol-induced liver damage include mitochondria, CYP2E1, Kupffer cells and other phagocytes, possibly lymphocytes, TNFα, and endotoxin from the gut. Iron overload in the cirrhotic liver may aggravate oxidative injury, depending on the ability of the extra iron to catalyse free-radical damage. So would antioxidants help to ameliorate the toxicity of ethanol? Several studies have attempted to use them to treat liver damage/fibrosis. Some studies with high-dose α-tocopherol reported improvements, albeit only small ones (but remember that α-tocopherol is often ineffective at decreasing oxidative damage).[90] However, in rats on a high-fat diet plus ethanol, α-tocopherol made liver damage worse (Section 3.20.2.5). **Silymarin**, isolated from the milk thistle *Silybum marianum*, has been claimed to be beneficial against liver damage in humans in some (but not all) studies, and works well in animals.[87,91] Whether any benefit it has is due to antioxidant, or other, actions remains to be determined. Silymarin is a mixture of phenolic compounds, including **silybin**.

8.8.2 Allyl alcohol and acrolein

Alcohol dehydrogenase is not specific for ethanol; other substrates include methanol (CH_3OH), oxidized to **formaldehyde** (HCHO), and **allyl alcohol**, to acrolein. Acrolein we met already as a toxic unsaturated aldehyde produced during lipid peroxidation (Section 4.12.5.3). Indeed, feeding allyl alcohol to animals produces liver necrosis, preventable by supplying the alcohol dehydrogenase inhibitor **pyrazole**.[92] Acrolein is also found in automobile exhaust gases, overheated cooking oils, cigarette smoke (Section 8.12 below), and as a metabolite of **cyclophosphamide**, a drug used in cancer treatment. Acrolein reacts fast with thiols (largely by Michael addition to the double bond; Section 4.12.5.3), causing GSH depletion, and protein modification. High levels of acrolein also cause release of iron from cellular iron stores.[93]

8.9 Other recreational drugs

Some have called ethanol 'the world's most commonly used psychoactive drug', but there are many others. Like ethanol, **cocaine** (Fig. 8.10) can damage both adult and foetus.[94] It is metabolized in the adult liver, mainly by hydrolysis by esterases (detoxification), but about 10% can be acted upon by CYPs in various tissues to give **norcocaine** (the **N-oxidation pathway**), and **N-hydroxy-norcocaine**. The latter can form a nitroxide radical that may generate $O_2^{\bullet-}$ by redox cycling as well as being directly damaging to biomolecules, possibly by producing a nitrosonium ($\overset{+}{N} = O$) electrophile. These RS might contribute to damage; consistent with this (but far from establishing it) are observations that administration of the GSH precursor 2-oxothiazolidine-4-carboxylate (Section 10.6.9) or the spin trap PBN (Section 5.2.4) decreased embryo damage in pregnant mice given cocaine. The foetotoxicity of cocaine may involve not only direct damage, but also cocaine-induced vasoconstriction (itself possibly via ROS generation) that can subject the embryo to ischaemia–reperfusion.[95]

Other popular drugs are **methamphetamine** ('speed') and its derivatives, including **3,4-methylenedioxymethylamphetamine** (**MDMA**), sometimes called **ecstasy**. Ecstasy causes an abnormally large release of 5-hydroxytryptamine (5-HT) from neurons, followed by prolonged depletion of 5HT and damage to serotonergic nerve terminals and axons. The neurotoxicity of ecstasy is diminished in mice overexpressing CuZnSOD, suggesting that ROS are involved.[96] Indeed, $OH^{\bullet}$ formation has been detected in the brains of MDMA-treated animals,[97] using salicylate hydroxylation (Section 5.3.1). The hyperthermia caused by ecstasy may accelerate ROS production in the brain.

Ecstasy is demethylated by CYPs to 3,4-methylenedioxyamphetamine and then converted to **α-methyldopamine** (Fig. 8.10). Both may cause oxidative stress; nitrotyrosine formation and neuronal damage induced by methamphetamine were attenuated in nNOS-knockout mice,[98] suggesting a role for RNS. Administration of methamphetamine to pregnant mice increased levels of 8OHdG in the foetal liver and brain and led to impaired motor co-ordination after birth.[99] α-Methyldopamine readily oxidizes to generate ROS and quinones/semiquinones that bind to protein –SH groups and deplete GSH; their GSH conjugates may be precursors of other neurotoxic agents.[44]

What about cannabis? Smoking anything causes harm (Section 8.12 below). However, there are speculations that some constituents, such as the **cannabinoids**, could be antioxidants. For example, both Δ[9]-**tetrahydrocannabinol** and the non-psychoactive cannabinoid **cannabidiol** (Fig. 8.10) were reported to protect neurons against excitotoxicity (Section 9.16.4) and rats against brain damage induced by ethanol or by 6-hydroxydopamine, possibly by antioxidant actions, presumably due to the phenolic structures.[100,101]

8.10 Paracetamol (acetaminophen), a glutathione-depleting toxin[102]

Paracetamol (called **acetaminophen** in the USA) is a mild painkiller; unlike aspirin and other COX-1 inhibitors, it does not irritate the stomach. Paracetamol is safe in the recommended dosage, but overdoses (frequently in suicide attempts) damage the liver and kidneys. The liver damage caused by excess paracetamol is life threatening and often can only be dealt with by transplantation. Ethyl

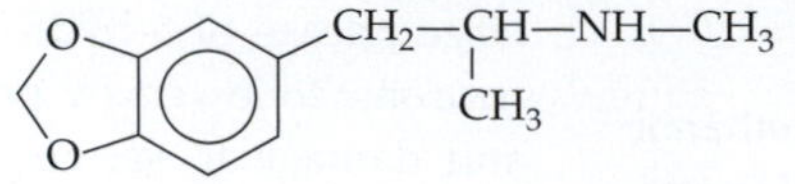

3,4-Methylenedioxymethamphetamine (MDMA)

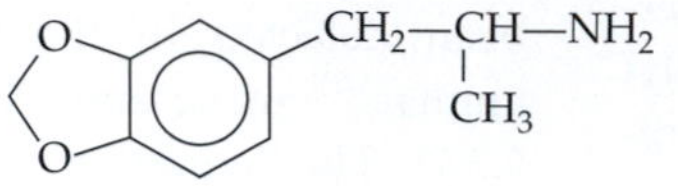

3,4-Methylenedioxyamphetamine

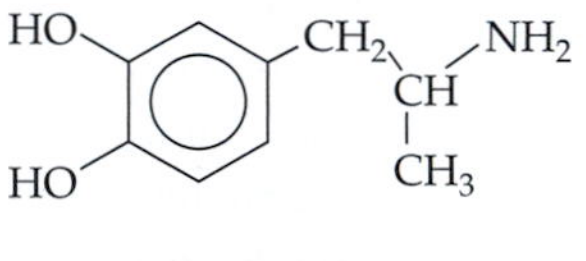

α-Methyldopamine

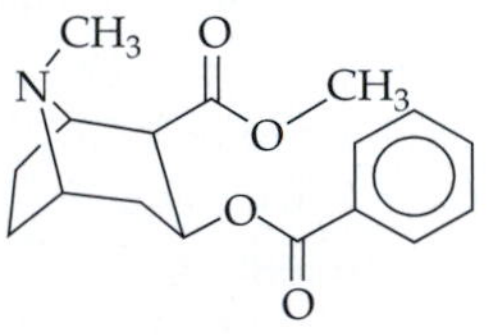

Cocaine 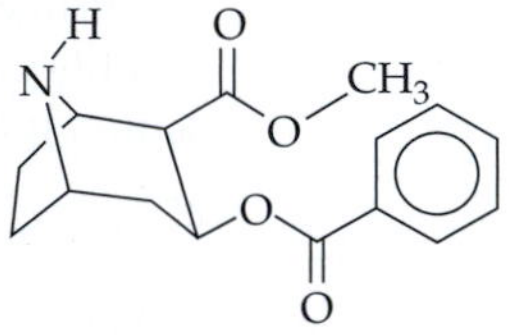   Norcocaine 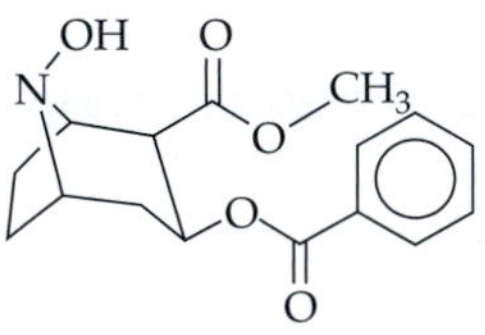   N-hydroxynorcocaine

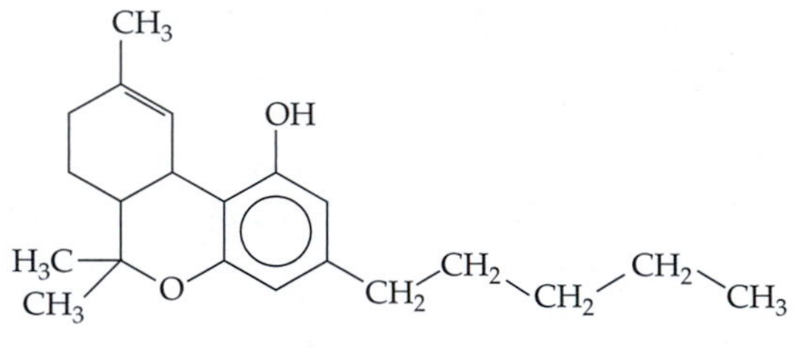

Δ⁹-Tetrahydrocannabinol (THC)

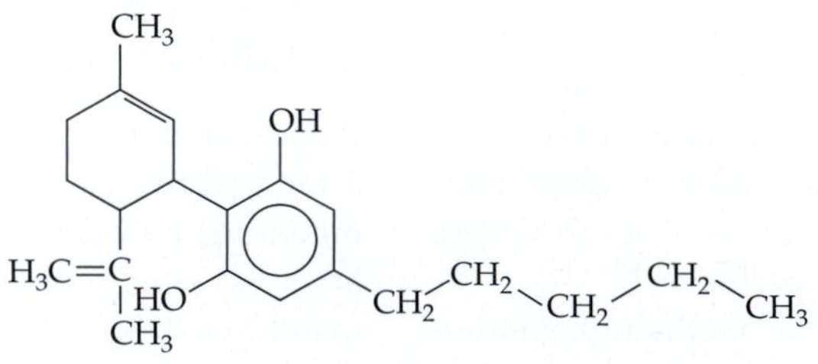

Cannabidiol (CBD)

Figure 8.10 Structures of some 'recreational drugs'.

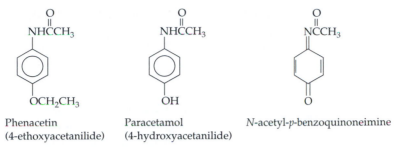

Phenacetin
(4-ethoxyacetanilide)

Paracetamol
(4-hydroxyacetanilide)

N-acetyl-*p*-benzoquinoneimine

Figure 8.11 Structures of phenacetin, paracetamol and the toxic quinoneimine.

paracetamol, **phenacetin**, is no longer marketed as a painkiller because of the risk of kidney damage.

Paracetamol is mostly metabolized by sulphation and glucuronidation, but is also a substrate for several CYPs, especially CYP2E1. Indeed, 'knockout' mice lacking CYP2E1 are less sensitive to paracetamol toxicity.[103] The action of CYPs on paracetamol produces a reactive **quinoneimine** (Fig. 8.11), which can bind to protein –SH groups as well as cause rapid depletion of GSH; the latter reaction occurs both spontaneously and is catalysed by GST enzymes. Conjugation with GSH and subsequent mercapturic acid formation (Section 3.9.5) help detoxify paracetamol, although the paracetamol–cysteine conjugate may be toxic to the kidney at high levels.[105] Paracetamol overdosage causes severe GSH depletion in the liver, allowing the quinoneimine to attack proteins, including PDI, glutamine synthetase, the Ca^{2+}-ATPase of the endoplasmic reticulum, the Ca^{2+} export system of the plasma membrane and mitochondrial proteins. Rises in intracellular free Ca^{2+} result, and contribute to hepatocyte death.[105] Activation of Kupffer cells and neutrophil recruitment make matters worse.

Sulphur-containing compounds, such as **N-acetylcysteine** or methionine, can protect the liver against paracetamol if administered early enough. They act by being metabolized to cysteine and maintaining intracellular GSH, and N-acetylcysteine may directly scavenge the quinoneimine as well. Alcoholics are more vulnerable to paracetamol because of decreased GSH and elevated CYP2EI. This does not occur when alcohol is in the body (since ethanol competes with paracetamol for metabolism by CYP2E1) but when alcohol is temporarily avoided yet the CYP2E1 is still present (e.g. taking paracetamol to treat the 'morning after the binge' symptoms).

Paracetamol-induced lipid peroxidation has been demonstrated in the livers of animals, but there is little evidence that peroxidation is a major contributor to paracetamol hepatotoxicity.[106] For example, only small increases in F_2-IPs were observed in the plasma of rats given hepatotoxic doses of paracetamol. More likely, the extensive GSH depletion and tissue injury caused by paracetamol lead to secondary lipid peroxidation and other free-radical reactions. Of course, rises in free Ca^{2+} can stimulate $NO^{\bullet}$, and hence $ONOO^{-}$, production, as well as activate the calpains that convert XDH to XO. Calpains released from damaged hepatocytes can injure other liver cells, and also cause systemic damage.[107] In addition, plasma of patients with paracetamol-induced liver failure contains 'catalytic' iron and copper ions[108] that might promote oxidative damage in plasma and other tissues.

The common environmental pollutant **naphthalene** targets the Clara cells of the lung, probably because they are rich in the CYP2F2 enzyme that catalyses its reaction with GSH. Depletion of GSH contributes to naphthalene cytotoxicity.[109]

8.11 Air pollutants[110]

There is much interest in the deleterious health effects of air pollution. To put this into perspective, remember that O_2 is a free-radical gas, whose appearance in the atmosphere has been called 'the worst case of air pollution ever to occur on Earth' (Section 1.1). We will now consider three other pollutants. First, a general principle; the damage

464 FREE RADICALS IN BIOLOGY AND MEDICINE

caused by inhaled gaseous toxins may be mediated not only by the toxin itself, but also by products of its reaction with constituents of the respiratory tract lining fluids. This is especially true for O_3, so we will consider it first.

8.11.1 Ozone, a non-radical reactive species

Ozone performs an essential 'antioxidant' role in the higher levels of the atmosphere by screening out UV light (Section 1.1), but it is a nuisance if formed at lower levels by photochemical reactions (Section 2.6.5). It readily damages plants, eyes and skin as well as the respiratory tract (Section 2.6.5, 6.9.3 and 6.12.1.4). Ozone adds across double bonds in lipids to generate ozonides, which can decompose to cytotoxic aldehydes (Fig. 2.17). It also attacks proteins (Section 2.6.5). In addition, O_3 can generate $^1O_2$ and $OH^\bullet$ (Section 2.6.5). Both lipids and proteins (e.g. in surfactant) may be targets of attack by O_3 in the respiratory tract. Millions of people worldwide are exposed to O_3 levels above the 1998 USA National Ambient Air Quality Standard (NAAQS) of 0.12 p.p.m. (120 p.p.b), more recently reduced to 0.08 p.p.m. Lung damage is both direct, and by inducing inflammation (Section 2.6.5). Ozone may also aggravate asthma in susceptible subjects (Section 6.3.3), including those with low dietary intake of antioxidants and/or those carrying the GSTM1 null allele (Section 3.9.5).[111]

Luckily, constituents of the respiratory tract lining fluids probably absorb most or all of the O_3 we breathe in. These fluids contain ascorbate, GSH and urate (Table 6.1), which act as O_3 scavengers.[110,112] In humans, nasal lining fluid is richer in urate than are the fluids lining the rest of the respiratory tract (Table 6.2). Since urate reacts fast with O_3 (and $NO_2^\bullet$), it may act to some extent as a nasal 'scrubber' of inhaled toxic gases.[112]

Ozone does not initiate lipid peroxidation, but free-radicals emanating from the products of its direct reactions with PUFAs (Fig. 2.17) might. Hence α-tocopherol could contribute to protection against O_3 toxicity. Indeed, several studies have claimed decreased O_3-induced lung damage in subjects supplemented with α-tocopherol and/or vitamin C, although others deny this.[110–113] A rise

in F_2-IPs was detected[114] in the lung lining fluids of guinea pigs exposed to 1 to 3 p.p.m. O_2 for 6 h, and F_2-IPs in breath condensate (Section 5.14.8) were increased in humans exposed to 0.4 p.p.m. O_3 for 2 h.[115] Any O_3 not scavenged by antioxidants in the lining fluids can react with lining fluid lipids, proteins and other constituents to form products (e.g. cytotoxic aldehydes) that may well be the main mediators of damage to the underlying cells.[110,116]

Repeated exposure of animals to O_3 can lead to adaptation (**tolerance**), that is further O_3 exposures produce less damage. Increased levels of ascorbate in lung lining fluids may contribute to adaptation in mice and rats,[117] as may rises in lung cell SOD, catalase, GPx and G6PDH activities. Consistent with this, adaptation of rats to O_3 renders them more resistant[118] to elevated O_2.

8.11.2 Nitrogen dioxide[110,119]

The toxic, brown, irritating gas nitrogen dioxide ($NO_2^\bullet$) is an intermediate in nitration by $ONOO^-$ (Section 2.6.1.1), but also occurs in the air around us. During combustion of organic material, nitrogen atoms react with O_2 to give oxides of nitrogen, including $NO^\bullet$ and $NO_2^\bullet$. The brown fumes of $NO_2^\bullet$ were first described in 1670 by the alchemist Clark, who called the vapours 'the flying dragon', but it was Priestley (the discoverer of O_2) who was the first to prepare pure $NO_2^\bullet$. Like $NO^\bullet$, $NO_2^\bullet$ is a free radical in which the unpaired electron is delocalized between the oxygen and nitrogen atoms, but $NO_2^\bullet$ is far more reactive than $NO^\bullet$. Nitric oxide can form $NO_2^\bullet$ by reaction with O_2 (Section 2.5.6.1) or with ozone. If sufficient levels of O_3 and $NO_2^\bullet$ are present in the atmosphere,[120] they can form **nitrate radical**, $NO_3^\bullet$, a powerfully oxidizing and nitrating species. Nitrate radical and $NO_2^\bullet$ can join together to give **dinitrogen pentoxide**, N_2O_5. Nitrate radical may account for the presence of nitrated proteins in pollen particles,[121] but there could also be a contribution from **peroxyacetyl nitrate**,

$$CH_3\overset{\overset{\displaystyle O}{\|}}{C}OONO_2$$

another constituent of polluted air.

In most large cities, the main source of $NO_2^\bullet$ in outdoor air is vehicle exhaust emissions. The NAAQS for $NO_2^\bullet$ in the USA is an annual average of 0.053 p.p.m., a figure regularly exceeded in several cities. In London in December 1991, air $NO_2^\bullet$ levels reached an all-time UK high of 0.42 p.p.m. Nitrogen dioxide is also found in indoor air (levels can exceed 1 p.p.m), being produced by gas cookers, wood-burning stoves, coal fires, kerosene heaters, and cigarette smoking (Section 8.12 below). Exposure to higher levels of $NO_2^\bullet$ can occur in acetylene welding, explosives manufacturing, military activities and in grain silos.

Healthy humans can tolerate short-term exposure to up to about 4 p.p.m. $NO_2^\bullet$ without obvious acute lung injury, but asthmatic subjects can be affected by levels <0.3 p.p.m. Levels above the NAAQS may predispose to respiratory illnesses, especially in children. In animals, levels of $NO_2^\bullet$ in the 1 p.p.m. range can increase susceptibility to infections with such organisms as *Staphylococcus aureus*, probably by interfering with the normal defence functions of alveolar macrophages. Indeed, alveolar macrophages obtained from humans exposed to 2 p.p.m. $NO_2^\bullet$ for 4 h whilst performing intermittent exercise had impaired phagocytic activity and decreased $O_2^{\bullet-}$ production.

Higher levels of $NO_2^\bullet$ (≥ 3–4 p.p.m.) cause demonstrable lung damage, both by direct injury to cells (especially to type I alveolar cells) and possibly also by inactivating α_1-antiproteinase and α_2-macroglobulin (Table 7.2), thus promoting elastase-dependent hydrolysis of lung elastin. Surfactant can be attacked by $NO_2^\bullet$ (Section 1.5.2), nitrating its proteins and impairing alveolar expansion and contraction.[122] Loss of alveolar structures, microscopically similar to emphysema, has been observed in animals exposed to high levels of $NO_2^\bullet$ (e.g. 20 p.p.m. for 30 days), but whether air pollution levels of $NO_2^\bullet$ are a risk factor for human emphysema is uncertain.

8.11.2.1 Nitrogen dioxide as a free radical[119,120,123,124]

Nitrogen dioxide dissolves in water to give nitric acid, a strong acid irritating to the respiratory tract, and a cause of damage to plants by 'acid rain' (Section 6.9.3); N_2O_5 also contributes to nitric acid formation

$$2\,NO_2^\bullet + H_2O \rightarrow HNO_3 + HNO_2$$
$$\text{nitric acid} \quad \text{nitrous acid}$$

$$HNO_3 \rightarrow H^+ + NO_3^-$$

$$HNO_2 \rightleftharpoons H^+ + NO_2^-$$

Nitrous acid, although a weak acid, can deaminate DNA bases (Section 4.8.2.10) and cause mutations. Reaction of $NO_2^\bullet$ with secondary or tertiary amines can generate carcinogenic nitrosamines. Overall, however, there is little evidence that $NO_2^\bullet$ at usual atmospheric levels is carcinogenic in animals. Nitrogen dioxide can initiate lipid peroxidation by abstracting hydrogen

$$LH + NO_2^\bullet \rightarrow L^\bullet + HNO_2$$

and by addition reactions

Both reactions generate carbon-centred radicals that combine with O_2 to give peroxyl radicals and propagate peroxidation. However, the former mechanism (H$^\bullet$-abstraction) is preferred[125] at low $NO_2^\bullet$ levels. Lipid peroxidation has been observed (e.g. as increased ethane exhalation) in the lungs of animals exposed to p.p.m. levels of $NO_2^\bullet$ and in human body fluids exposed to $NO_2^\bullet$.

8.11.2.2 Antioxidants[123,126] and $NO_2^\bullet$

Ascorbate reduces $NO_2^\bullet$ to NO_2^-, the reaction rate constant being quite high, about $3.5 \times 10^7\,M^{-1}s^{-1}$. Tocopherols can react directly with $NO_2^\bullet$ (especially γ-tocopherol; Section 3.20.2.7) as well as inhibit lipid peroxidation induced by $NO_2^\bullet$. Indeed, supplementation of humans with ascorbate and α-tocopherol prior to $NO_2^\bullet$ exposure has been reported as protective in several studies,[113] whereas α-tocopherol deficiency in rats, or ascorbate deficiency in guinea pigs, aggravated lung damage by $NO_2^\bullet$. Uric acid can also scavenge[110] $NO_2^\bullet$ ($k \sim 10^7\,M^{-1}s^{-1}$); levels of urate and ascorbate in lung lining fluids fell rapidly[127] in humans breathing 2 p.p.m. $NO_2^\bullet$. Urate is oxidized to urate radical, which can be recycled by ascorbate (Section

3.18.6). Oxidation of thiols by $NO_2^\bullet$ is slow unless they are in their ionized form

$$NO_2^\bullet + GS^- \rightarrow NO_2^- + GS^\bullet$$

Nevertheless, the amount of thiolate present at pH 7.4 allows GSH to scavenge $NO_2^\bullet$ with a rate constant[126] of about $2 \times 10^7 \, M^{-1}s^{-1}$.

Nitrogen dioxide can react with itself, the two unpaired electrons forming a covalent bond

$$NO_2^\bullet + NO_2^\bullet \rightleftharpoons N_2O_4$$
$$\text{Dinitrogen tetroxide}$$

Like $NO^\bullet$, $NO_2^\bullet$ reacts rapidly (rate constants $>10^9 \, M^{-1}s^{-1}$) with other free radicals, for example with $NO_3^\bullet$ to give N_2O_5, with $O_2^{\bullet-}$ to form **peroxynitrate** ($k \sim 5 \times 10^9 \, M^{-1}s^{-1}$)

$$NO_2^\bullet + O_2^{\bullet-} \rightarrow OONOO^-$$

and with alkoxyl and peroxyl radicals[123]

$$RO^\bullet + NO_2^\bullet \rightarrow ROONO$$

$$RO_2^\bullet + NO_2^\bullet \rightarrow RO_2ONO$$

Such reactions could modulate lipid peroxidation, and generate biologically active nitrated lipids (Section 2.6.1.3), but little attention has yet been paid to the possible importance of $OONOO^-$, ROONO and RO_2ONO *in vivo*.

8.11.3 Sulphur dioxide

Sulphur dioxide (SO_2), a colourless, choking gas formed by the combustion of fuels containing sulphur (e.g. low-grade coals), is another common air pollutant. Unlike O_3 and $NO_2^\bullet$, SO_2 is a reducing rather than an oxidizing agent. It contains no unpaired electrons, and thus is not a free radical. Sulphur dioxide dissolves in water to reversibly form sulphite and bisulphite ions, producing an acidic solution:

$$SO_2 + H_2O \rightleftharpoons H_2SO_3$$
$$\text{sulphurous acid}$$
$$H_2SO_3 \rightleftharpoons H^+ + HSO_3^-$$
$$\text{bisulphite ion}$$
$$HSO_3^- \rightleftharpoons H^+ + SO_3^{2-}$$
$$\text{sulphite ion}$$

In addition to inhalation of SO_2, humans are exposed to sulphite because it is used as a preservative in some drug preparations, wines (there can be millimolar levels in white wines),[128] and several foods, both as sulphites and metabisulphites (e.g. $Na_2S_2O_5$). Sulphite is also generated *in vivo* during the metabolism of methionine and cysteine. Usually it is oxidized to sulphate (SO_4^{2-}) by the mitochondrial molybdenum-containing enzyme **sulphite oxidase**, which uses cytochrome *c* as an electron acceptor, and is present in several tissues, liver having especially high levels.[129] High levels of SO_3^{2-} can cleave disulphide bridges, for example in albumin, by the **sulphitolysis** reaction

$$R-S-S-R + SO_3^{2-} \rightarrow RS-SO_3^- + RS^-$$

Whether this occurs *in vivo* is uncertain. Sulphites can also oxidize to generate ROS, which are involved in the toxicity of SO_2 to plants (Section 6.9.3). Indeed, the earliest use of SOD to investigate a reaction mechanism was a study of the role of $O_2^{\bullet-}$ in sulphite oxidation.[130]

Peroxidases, activated lymphocytes,[131] $ONOO^-$, and transition metal ions can bring about one-electron oxidation of SO_3^{2-} to sulphite radical (**sulphur trioxide anion radical**), $SO_3^{\bullet-}$, which can be spin trapped using DEPMPO (Section 5.2.4).[132] Sulphite stimulates the peroxidation of PUFA emulsions, microsomes and lipid extracts from rat lungs, possibly by the interaction of $SO_3^{\bullet-}$ (and/or species derived from it) with preformed lipid hydroperoxides and/or by abstraction of hydrogen atoms. In addition to $SO_3^{\bullet-}$, $SO_4^{\bullet-}$ (**sulphate radical**) and $SO_5^{\bullet-}$ (**peroxysulphate radical**) can form during sulphite oxidation.[133] Sulphate radical and $SO_5^{\bullet-}$ are highly reactive; $SO_4^{\bullet-}$ can oxidize the 'OH$^\bullet$scavengers' ethanol and formate, and $SO_3^{\bullet-}$ can oxidize methionine, tryptophan and β-carotene. Peroxysulphate radical is a peroxyl radical formed by reaction of $SO_3^{\bullet-}$ with O_2

$$SO_3^{\bullet-} + O_2 \rightarrow {}^-O_3SOO^\bullet \qquad k > 10^9 \, M^{-1}s^{-1}$$

It can react with more SO_3^{2-} to continue sulphite oxidation

$$SO_3^{2-} + {}^-O_3SOO^\bullet \rightarrow SO_4^{\bullet-} + SO_4^{2-}$$
$$k > 10^7\,M^{-1}s^{-1}$$

$$SO_4^{\bullet-} + SO_3^{2-} \rightarrow SO_4^{2-} + SO_3^{\bullet-}$$
$$k = 2.6 \times 10^8\,M^{-1}s^{-1}$$

Inhalation of excess SO_2 might thus lead to lung damage by radical reactions as well as by low pH. Humans and other animals often respond to inhaled SO_2 by bronchoconstriction; asthmatics may be more susceptible than healthy subjects.

Human inborn errors that result in inactive sulphite oxidase lead to death at a few months of age with multiple defects, including neurodegeneration. Accumulation of sulphite could lead to free radical formation in the brain, which might contribute. In addition, SO_3^{2-} at high levels can directly inhibit several important enzymes, such as glutamate dehydrogenase.[129]

8.12 Toxicity of mixtures: cigarette smoke and other 'toxic smokes'[134]

Although we have considered O_3, SO_2 and $NO_2^\bullet$ separately, we must remember that polluted air contains a mixture of toxins, and interactions between them can aggravate (or sometimes diminish) toxicity. One example is the reaction of O_3 and $NO_2^\bullet$ to form $NO_3^\bullet$ (Section 8.11.2).

One of the most complex mixtures is tobacco smoke. Smoking predisposes to emphysema, bronchitis, pneumonia, lung and several other cancers (including mouth, larynx, kidney, urinary tract, oesophagus, pancreas, liver, stomach, colon, cervix), atherosclerosis and many other diseases. It damages the vascular endothelium, facilitates platelet aggregation and blood coagulation and causes vasoconstriction. Maternal smoking can injure the foetus both by damaging the placenta and directly, for example nicotine can cross the placenta and impair lung development. On the other hand, tobacco users (smokers, tobacco chewers, snuff takers) are at lower risk of developing Parkinson's disease (Section 9.19.3), although, if it should develop, it progresses at the normal rate.[135] However, to put this 'advantage' into perspective, one can quote the 1989 US

Surgeon General's report: 'In 1985 [in the USA] smoking accounted for 87% of lung cancer deaths, 82% of deaths from chronic obstructive pulmonary disease, 21% of coronary heart disease deaths and 18% of stroke deaths'. The rest of the world has similar problems.

8.12.1 Chemistry of tobacco smoke

Cigarette smoke is a complex mixture of toxic agents, some of which are free radicals, others free-radical-generating agents, and yet others GSH-depleting compounds (Table 8.2). Smoke can be separated by filters into gas and particulate (sometimes called **tar**) phases, each with different chemistry. Overall, the gas phase is oxidizing and the particulate phase weakly reducing. Both contain free radicals.

One gram of tar contains about 10^{17} ESR-detectable radicals of several different types: many of them are stable, persisting for hours (Fig. 8.12). One prominent type is semiquinones, undergoing redox interconversions with quinones and hydroquinones to generate $O_2^{\bullet-}$ and H_2O_2. These ROS can be converted to $OH^\bullet$ by Fenton or Fenton-type chemistry; cigarette smoke contains a range of metals (Table 8.2) and it has been estimated that $>1\,\mu g$ of iron is inhaled per pack of cigarettes. In addition, 'catalytic' iron is available normally in the lower respiratory tract lining fluids (Section 6.3). Lung macrophages and respiratory tract lining fluids in smokers have elevated iron contents, and smoke may be capable of releasing iron from ferritin in these fluids. Cells damaged by cigarette smoke may also release iron.

Radicals in gas-phase cigarette smoke have much shorter lifetimes than those in the tar and are usually studied by spin trapping (e.g. Fig. 8.14). The gas phase contains over 10^{15} radicals per puff, including alkoxyl, peroxyl and, to a lesser extent, carbon-centred radicals. Up to 22 nmol of radicals per cigarette can be trapped. This is an underestimate; many cannot be detected because of inefficient trapping or fast decomposition of the spin adducts.[136] Smoke can be drawn as far as 180 cm down a glass tube without a significant decrease in radical concentration, which has frightening implications for what happens in the lungs. Since the

(a)

(b)

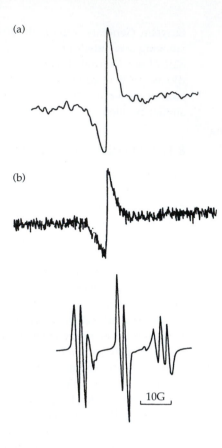

10G

Figure 8.12 Detection of radicals in cigarette smoke by electron spin resonance. (a) ESR signal from a glass-wool filter after smoke from four cigarettes has been drawn through it. The *g*-value is 2.002. (b) ESR signal from a glass-fibre filter after smoke from four cigarettes has been drawn through it. The *g*-value of the centre of the spectrum is 2.002. (c) ESR spectrum of the spin adduct formed by the trapping of radicals in cigarette smoke with PBN in benzene. Spectra by courtesy of Professor W. A. Pryor.

Table 8.2 Some constituents of cigarette smoke

Phase	Examples of constituents
Gas	Nitrogen, ammonia (NH_3), carbon monoxide (CO), CO_2, $NO^\bullet$, $NO_2^\bullet$, H_2S, methane, hydrogen cyanide (HCN), volatile aldehydes (e.g. ethanal, formaldehyde, acrolein, crotonaldehyde, $CH_3CH = CHCHO$), benzene, toluene, acetone, vinyl chloride, unsaturated hydrocarbons (e.g. butadiene, isoprene), methylamine, nitropropane (Section 3.13.4)
Particulate	Tar, nicotine, metals (e.g. cadmium, lead, aluminium, nickel, iron, manganese, chromium, arsenic), phenols/semiquinones/quinones, carcinogenic hydrocarbons (e.g. benzpyrene, benzanthracene, chrysene), other carcinogens (e.g. nitrosamines), fatty acids

'Cigarette smoke consists of tarry particles suspended in a complex mixture of both organic and inorganic gases and contains >4000 different known chemicals.' (*Am. Rev. Resp. Dis.* **136**, 1058, 1987). At least 69 of these are carcinogens, aided by several tumour promoters (*Chem. Res. Toxicol.* **14**, 767, 2001). The top of a burning cigarette reaches temperatures up to 900°C, facilitating homolytic bond cleavage to generate radicals.

radicals have short lifetimes, they must be constantly produced to maintain a steady-state level. Fresh cigarette smoke contains high concentrations of $NO^\bullet$ (~300–400 p.p.m.) and $NO_2^\bullet$, which react with unsaturated hydrocarbons in the smoke, such as isoprene. Nitrates are added to cigarettes to improve burning properties and these are a major source of the oxides of nitrogen. Radical-generating reactions include heat-induced homolytic fission of carbon–carbon bonds (Table 8.2) as well as the reactions

$$RH + NO_2^\bullet \rightarrow R^\bullet + HNO_2$$

$$R-CH=CH-R \ + \ NO_2^\bullet \longrightarrow \ R-CH-\overset{\bullet}{C}H-R$$
$$\underset{NO_2}{|}$$

$$R^\bullet + O_2 \rightarrow RO_2^\bullet$$

A steady-state level of radicals is quickly established. Reaction of oxides of nitrogen with $O_2^{\bullet-}$ generated from the tar phase might also occur

$$O_2^{\bullet-} + NO^\bullet \rightarrow ONOO^-$$
peroxynitrite

$$O_2^{\bullet-} + NO_2^\bullet \rightarrow OONOO^-$$
peroxynitrate

as well as

$$RO_2^\bullet + NO^\bullet \rightarrow ROONO$$

$$RO_2^\bullet + NO_2^\bullet \rightarrow ROONO_2$$

8.12.2 Mechanisms of damage by cigarette smoke[134]

Injury by cigarette smoke occurs by multiple mechanisms, including direct toxic effects of HCN, CO, aldehydes and carcinogens (Table 8.2). For example, HCN can inactivate peroxidase in the saliva of smokers.[137] Here we focus on the damage that involves RS.

1. Peroxyl radicals and RNS ($NO_2^\bullet$, $ONOO^-$, $OONOO^-$) cause direct damage, stimulating lipid peroxidation, oxidizing and nitrating proteins, lipids and DNA bases. Plasma, urine and (in some studies) breath condensate from cigarette smokers show elevated levels[138] of IPs. Urinary levels of etheno-guanine adducts (Section 4.12.5) are also elevated.[139] In several studies, levels of 8OHdG were found to be increased in the white blood cells, lung, sperm and urine of smokers,[134] and 8-nitroguanine excretion in urine is also elevated (Section 5.13.7), although levels of 3-nitrotyrosine in breath condensate (as measured by GC–MS with precautious to avoid artefactual nitration; Section 5.6.2.2) were not increased.[140]

2. Aldehydes (Table 8.2), especially acrolein, other unsaturated aldehydes, acetaldehyde and formaldehyde, can deplete GSH and modify protein –SH and –NH$_2$ groups. The 'total aldehydes' generated by smoking one cigarette, if completely dissolved in the lung lining fluid, would reach levels of 2 to 3 mM.

3. The hydroquinones/quinones in the tar phase may leach out into lung lining fluids, diffuse across cell membranes and undergo both extracellular and intracellular (e.g. in vascular endothelium)[141] redox cycling to generate semiquinones, $O_2^{\bullet-}$ and H_2O_2.

4. Cigarette smoke is proinflammatory and irritant and can activate alveolar macrophages to produce $O_2^{\bullet-}$, H_2O_2, and possibly $NO^\bullet$ (Fig. 7.12). It also promotes recruitment and retention of neutrophils in the lung; activation of neutrophils will additionally generate HOCl. In normal lungs there are about 50 to 70 phagocytes per alveolus, largely macrophages; in smokers macrophages increase two to four-fold and neutrophils 10-fold. The nicotine in cigarette smoke has been suggested to 'prime' neutrophils to produce an increased respiratory burst in response to stimuli.[142] However, too much smoking can depress phagocyte function and increase the risk of infection of the respiratory tract.

5. Both surfactant and α_1-antiproteinase can be inactivated by RS within cigarette smoke and/or generated by activated phagocytes, e.g. $NO_2^\bullet$, $ROONO_2$, $ONOO^-$ and HOCl. Smoking predisposes to the development of emphysema, in part via a localized inactivation of α_1-antiproteinase and other antiproteinases within the lung, allowing elastase released from neutrophils and macrophages to remain active. Lung lavage fluids from chronic smokers sometimes (but by no means always) show subnormal antiproteinase activity. Inappropriate apoptosis of lung cells by the ceramide pathway (Section 4.4.1.2)[143] may also be involved in emphysema. The term **chronic obstructive pulmonary disease (COPD)** is often used to encompass emphysema, excess mucus secretion and small airways inflammation. Cigarette smoking is the primary risk factor for COPD, although only a minority of smokers develop the full-blown syndrome.[138]

6. The carcinogenic action of such agents as benzpyrene may involve RS (Section 9.14).

7. Smoking is often associated with a poor diet, lacking plant-derived antioxidants and excessively rich in fat and ethanol, compounding the pro-oxidant effects of cigarette smoke.

8.12.3 How does the respiratory tract defend itself?[110,134]

The best defence against cigarette smoking is not to do it. However, the antioxidants in respiratory tract lining fluids do offer some protection (Tables 6.2 and 6.3). For example, GSH can help remove aldehydes, $RO_2^{\bullet}$, $OH^{\bullet}$, HOCl, $ONOO^-$ and $NO_2^{\bullet}$. Mucus may scavenge some HOCl, $RO_2^{\bullet}$, $OH^{\bullet}$ and RNS (Section 6.3.2), as well as binding particulates and removing them from the lung. As scavenging occurs, the mucus is degraded, but it is continuously replenished by the mucus-secreting cells of the trachea. Irritation of these cells by any mechanism (including smoking) causes increased mucus production (Section 8.12.4 below).

Ascorbate and urate react rapidly with $NO_2^{\bullet}$ and $RO_2^{\bullet}$, and ascorbate may also 'recycle' α-tocopherol; peroxidation of LDL is not observed in human plasma exposed to gas-phase cigarette smoke *in vitro* until ascorbate has been depleted.[144] Consumption of extra ascorbate by smokers decreased their F_2-IP levels.[145] Indeed, smokers 'turn over' ascorbate faster than non-smokers, and the recommended daily allowance of ascorbate in the UK and USA is set at a higher level for smokers. α-Tocopherol might be important in protecting against smoke-induced lipid peroxidation, but there is little evidence that α-tocopherol supplements lower F_2-IP levels in smokers.[146] Smokers show increased turnover of *RRR*-α-tocopherol, especially if their plasma vitamin C levels are low, and consuming extra vitamin C normalizes the turnover rate.[144] Smokers also have increased urinary excretion of the γ-tocopherol metabolite, γ-CEHC, and increased plasma levels of 5-nitro-γ-tocopherol (Section 3.20.2.7), suggesting accelerated turnover of γ-tocopherol as well.[147] This accelerated turnover was also decreased by ascorbate supplementation.[144]

Decreases in vitamin C and α-tocopherol, and increased lipid peroxidation, could conceivably contribute to accelerated atherosclerosis in smokers. In addition, smokers have decreased plasma HDL levels, which may relate to the ability of cigarette smoke (probably via aldehydes) to inhibit the enzyme **lecithin–cholesterol acyltransferase** (LCAT),[148] which catalyses the formation of cholesteryl esters in HDL. Smoking interferes with vascular endothelial $NO^{\bullet}$ synthesis and impairs vasodilation, by increasing endothelial ROS formation. This could involve increases in vascular NADPH oxidase and/or XO.[141]

How much of the increased cancer risk from smoking is due to carcinogens and how much to oxidative DNA damage is uncertain—probably the two are synergistic. Although ascorbate supplements decreased F_2-IPs in smokers, neither ascorbate, α-tocopherol nor β-carotene had any effect on urinary 8OHdG excretion,[134,149] implying that they would be unlikely to help much in preventing cancer. More worrying, high dietary levels of vitamin C and α-tocopherol *accelerated* the development of preneoplastic lesions in guinea pigs forced to breathe cigarette smoke.[150]

8.12.4 Adaptation[134,151]

Parts of the respiratory tract antioxidant defence system can adapt to cigarette smoke. Smoking stimulates mucus production; ROS in tobacco smoke can activate the transcription factor AP-1, leading to increased expression of the gene encoding mucin MUC5AC, a major airway mucin.[152] Activation of AP-1 also leads to increased levels of γ-glutamylcysteine synthetase, the rate-limiting enzyme of GSH synthesis.[153] Hence GSH levels in lung lining fluid and alveolar cells are often increased in smokers, although probably transiently depleted during the act of smoking. Genes encoding GPx2, GPx3, glutathione reductase, thioredoxin reductase, GST and G6PDH were also expressed more in the airway epithelium of smokers, whereas the *GPx3* gene was downregulated in emphysema.[151] Activities of DNA repair enzymes may also increase in smokers, although not always sufficiently to prevent rises in 8OHdG.[154] Susceptibility of smokers to lung cancer may in part depend on the relative activities of the CYPs that activate carcinogens, levels of detoxifying enzymes (such as quinone reductases and

GSTs), and the efficiency of DNA repair. All these enzymes are induced, to varying extents, by the 'xenobiotic exposure' of smoking.

8.12.5 Environmental tobacco smoke (ETS)

Exposure to ETS is unpleasant and irritating to many people, but does it cause harm? A growing body of evidence[155] suggests that the answer is 'yes, to some extent', and certain animal studies reveal that fresh 'sidestream' smoke may be more toxic than mainstream smoke. Humans exposed to ETS may have lower plasma ascorbate, higher urinary excretion of 8OHdG and elevated urinary or plasma F_2-IPs, and the IP levels were decreased by ascorbate supplementation.[155,156] More work is needed to ascertain whether oxidative damage plays a role in the alleged deleterious effects of ETS.

8.12.6 Other tobacco usage

Other uses of tobacco, which include snuff taking and tobacco chewing, are also associated with oral and upper digestive/respiratory tract cancer. The chewing of **betel quid**, sometimes with tobacco, is popular in certain parts of the world (e.g. Papua New Guinea, India and Taiwan) and has been associated with increased oral cancer, possibly related to the delivery of both carcinogenic nitrosamines and of RS to the mouth. Two major ingredients of betel quid, areca nut and catechu, oxidize at high pH (provided by the slaked lime, $Ca(OH)_2$, often added to the preparation chewed) to give $O_2^{\bullet-}$, H_2O_2 and $OH^\bullet$, especially as areca nut is rich in copper. Formation of $OH^\bullet$ has been demonstrated by adding phenylalanine to the betel quid and measuring formation of *ortho-* and *meta-* tyrosines (Section 5.3.1).[157]

8.12.7 Fire smoke[158]

Cooking smoke can contain cytotoxic agents, including aldehydes, that might contribute to lung cancer development (Section 4.12.5). Many people die in fires, most often as a result of smoke inhalation. This causes severe lung damage within minutes, often leading to death days or weeks later, for example by acute respiratory distress syndrome

(Section 9.7). Smoke from burning buildings includes contributions from wood, cellulose, paint, polystyrene, polythene, other plastics and rubber and has several chemical similarities to cigarette smoke: CO, aldehydes, oxides of nitrogen, ESR-detectable free radicals, HCN (from nitrogen-containing polymers such as nylon) and particulates are all present. In addition, the combustion of halogenated plastics (such as polyvinyl chloride) generates HCl, Cl_2 and phosgene.

One system often used to model smoke injury is the exposure of sheep to smoke from burning cotton. Reports have appeared that the resulting lung injury can be ameliorated with aerosols containing dimethylsulphoxide, α-tocopherol or desferrioxamine attached to a starch polymer.[159] In rabbits, the antioxidant U75412E (Section 10.6.8) offered some protection against acute lung damage after smoke inhalation.[160] The use of antioxidants in the treatment of smoke-exposed patients is an area worthy of further investigation, since so many people die from smoke exposure.

8.13 Diesel exhaust[120,136,161]

Diesel exhaust is rich in free radicals, including oxides of nitrogen, and diesel vehicles can emit 30 to 100 times more particulates than petrol-engined cars. The particles contain salts (mainly ammonium sulphate and nitrate) plus carbon particulates, to which are adsorbed carcinogenic hydrocarbons, nitro-aromatics and other toxins, including redox-active iron and polyphenols that can redox-cycle to generate ROS, and semiquinones/ quinones. Other metals often present include vanadium, copper, chromium, nickel and titanium. Those particles with an aerodynamic diameter of less than 2.5 microns (called **PM2.5 particles**) represent a particular threat because they penetrate deep into the lungs, settle there and generate ROS (including $OH^\bullet$). They can activate phagocytes, producing inflammation and more oxidative stress.[162] These particles are mutagenic and carcinogenic in cell and animal models, and several studies have shown increased lung levels of 8OHdG after exposing animals to diesel exhaust.[163]

The carcinogenic risk of diesel exhaust to humans is unclear, and, as for cigarette smoke, the lung can respond by upregulating defence enzymes. However, diesel exhaust particulates can aggravate asthma and COPD in humans, although more studies of the role of RS in this, and the prospects for effective antioxidant intervention, are required.[164] Highly redox-active *ultrafine* particulates (<0.15 microns) can cross membranes of lung cells, damage subcellular organelles such as mitochondria and even enter the bloodstream and be distributed to other tissues, including the brain. There is increasing worry about their potential to cause harm, especially given the current popularity of nanoparticles for industrial uses and as drug carriers.[162]

8.14 Toxicity of asbestos and similar particulates[165]

Silicon is the second most abundant element in the Earth's crust, often present as **silicon dioxide (silica)**, SiO_2, examples of which include sand and quartz. Many other minerals contain **silicate ion**, SiO_4^{2-}, examples being the various forms of **asbestos**. Excess exposure to silica dust causes acute and chronic lung damage (**silicosis**).

Inhalation of asbestos fibres for prolonged periods causes not only lung fibrosis but also two types of cancer, mesothelioma and bronchogenic carcinoma. Asbestos and several other silicates contain iron, some of which is in a form that can stimulate $OH^\bullet$ formation, lipid peroxidation, and oxidative DNA damage.[166,167] Iron is sometimes an integral part of the silicate crystal structure, for example in the **amosite**, $Fe_7^{2+}[Si_8O_{22}](OH)_2$, and **crocidolite**, $Na_2Fe_2^{3+}Fe_3^{2+}[Si_8O_{22}](OH)_2$, forms of asbestos. Alternatively, iron may be present on the surface, as with **chrysotile asbestos** $(Mg_3[Si_2O_5](OH)_4)$, where varying amounts of Mg^{2+} can be replaced by iron. Alveolar macrophages phagocytose asbestos fibres of the correct length and shape (e.g. longer than $8\,\mu m$ and less than $0.36\,\mu m$ diameter for rats), and the resulting macrophage-derived RS participate in iron-dependent radical reactions that contribute to fibrosis and cancer development. Indeed, mice lacking EC-SOD show more lung damage after intratracheal asbestos administration.[168] Macrophages also release elastase and proinflammatory cytokines and upregulate iNOS gene expression. Death of the macrophage frees the asbestos to be taken up by more macrophages in a vicious cycle (Fig. 8.13). Asbestos also causes death of alveolar type II cells.[167] Indeed, transfection of a gene encoding MnSOD into lung cells makes them more resistant to the toxic effects of crocidolite. Several papers show that workers exposed to asbestos excrete more 8OHdG.[169]

Redox reactions also participate in the deleterious effects of other dusts. An example is silicosis; quartz is more toxic to the lung when freshly ground, and both silicon radicals and Fenton chemistry may contribute.[165] When silica is fractured, breakage of the covalent bonds produces free radicals by homolytic cleavage ($SiO^\bullet$, $Si^\bullet$) as well as ions (Si^+, SiO^-) from heterolytic fission. Oxygen combines with some of these species to generate 'surface bound ROS', including $Si^+-O_2^{\bullet-}$, $SiO_2^\bullet$ and $SiO_3^\bullet$. These radicals decay with time, but traces are still present in aged dusts.[166] The damaging effects of welding fumes,[170] **oil fly ash** (a particulate air pollutant arising from combustion of fuel oil), **coal fly ash**, metal dusts, soot and fine coal particles may also involve metal-dependent oxidative damage. Coal and coal dusts contain stable carbon-centred radicals, up to 10^{19} per gram, immobilized in the carbon matrix; they can even be detected in the lungs of coal workers. Coals contain iron, the presence of which is one factor determining the ability of coal dusts to cause lung injury in miners.[171] Fine particles collected from air in the Stockholm city subway system were pro-oxidant to cells in culture[172] and contained a high proportion of **magnetite**, Fe_3O_4.

Fly ash from waste incinerators contains not only free radicals, metals and carcinogenic aromatic hydrocarbons, but also chlorinated toxins such as polychlorinated dibenzo-*p*-dioxins and polychlorinated dibenzofurans, which might contribute to oxidative damage (Section 8.3.2).

8.15 Toxicity of metals[173]

8.15.1 Cause or consequence?

The contribution of oxidative damage to the effects of 'catalytic' iron and copper has already been

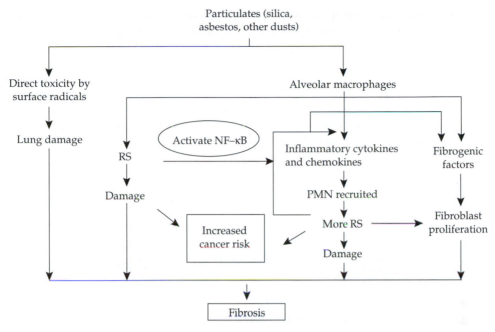

Figure 8.13 Mechanisms involved in the initiation and progression of lung damage by silicates. Reactive species are generated both directly from the mineral surface and during phagocytosis of particles. These ROS activate transcription factors in macrophages and increase production of chemokines, other cytokines, other RS and fibrogenic factors. Adapted from[165] by courtesy of Dr V. Castranova and Elsevier.

considered (Sections 3.15.5 and 4.8.2.2), as has the role of metals within asbestos, cigarette smoke, ashes, and other smokes and dusts (Section 8.14). Toxic particulates can contain a range of metals, for example oil fly ash can contain Fe, Ni, V, Cr, Mn and Cu.

Increased ROS generation has often been suggested to contribute to the toxicity of lead, cobalt, mercury, nickel, cadmium, molybdenum, vanadium, chromium and aluminium, as well as selenium and arsenic. For many of these elements, the evidence that oxidative stress is a primary cause of their toxicity is not convincing. Often, increased lipid peroxidation was demonstrated in cells exposed to metals in culture, or in tissues from animals poisoned by metals (often at absurdly high levels, irrelevant to human exposure). Such peroxidation may be a consequence of tissue injury and GSH depletion rather than an early contributor to metal toxicity.

Let us briefly review, for selected metals, the data available about the role of oxidative stress in the damage that they cause, beginning with those where the evidence is better than average.

8.15.2 Arsenic[174]

Arsenic, an element in group V of the Periodic Table, has two major oxidation states, As(III) and As(V). It is widespread in the environment, for example in soil, seawater and river water, fortunately usually at concentrations below 0.1 p.p.m. Sadly, higher arsenic levels occur in drinking water in some areas of Taiwan, Bangladesh, India and Argentina.

After its discovery in the Middle Ages, arsenic (usually as **arsenic trioxide**, As_2O_3) became one of the most popular poisons for disposing of rodents as well as unwanted rivals and spouses. A dose of 200 to 250 mg is usually lethal, but tolerance occurs upon repeated exposure to lower doses, possibly involving metallothionein induction. This has confounded poisoners throughout history. The trioxide has found a new use recently, as a treatment for acute promyelocytic leukaemia, and arsenicals have been used to kill trypanosomes (Section 3.12.1).

Arsenic in high doses is carcinogenic (e.g. high levels in drinking water can raise the incidence of skin and other cancers) and p.p.m. levels may predispose to atherosclerosis. **Arsenate** (AsO_4^{3-}) can be taken up by cells in mistake for phosphate and affects signal transduction systems. Some of it is reduced to **arsenite** (AsO_3^{3-}), which is more reactive and can bind to $-SH$ groups on GSH and cellular proteins. Indeed the antidote developed to one of the first toxic gases used in chemical warfare (the arsenical **lewisite**) is a dithiol, **British antilewisite** (2,3-dimercapto-1-propanol). Arsenite may also interfere with DNA repair mechanisms and methylation; indeed arsenic can itself form methyl- and dimethyl derivatives, which may act as tumour promoters. Studies on cells in culture show that arsenic treatment increases oxidative damage, by causing GSH depletion and possibly by increasing mitochondrial free radical production and activating NAD(P)H oxidase.[175] Hence antioxidants might be useful in treating arsenic poisoning. Consistent with a role for increased oxidative damage *in vivo*, arsenic-exposed subjects show elevated urinary 8OHdG excretion and increased levels of 8OHdG in tissues. Arsenic-related skin cancers showed higher 8OHdG levels than skin cancers of other origins.[176]

The ability of As_2O_3 to cause apoptosis in leukaemia cells involves RS production, and some antioxidants can delay arsenic-induced cell death.[174,175] Thus, patients being treated with arsenic should probably avoid taking antioxidants! Interestingly, the synthetic antioxidant Trolox *potentiated* As_2O_3 toxicity to tumour cells in culture.[177]

8.15.3 Nickel[178]

The transition element nickel has principal oxidation states of Ni^{2+} and Ni(III) and comprises about 0.01% of the Earth's crust. It is used by several organisms as an enzyme cofactor, for example in urea-hydrolysing enzymes (**ureases**) in plants and bacteria, and in bacterial NiSODs (Section 3.2.4). Inhalation of nickel-containing particulates (e.g. **nickel subsulphide**, Ni_3S_2 or the oxide, NiO) can lead to lung inflammation and fibrosis and even lung cancer, as has been seen in miners of nickel ores and refinery workers. Cells appear to phagocytose those particles, and some of the Ni^{2+} ends up in the nucleus.

Hydrated Ni^{2+} ions react slowly, if at all, with H_2O_2 to form $OH^{\bullet}$, nor are they efficient at decomposing organic peroxides. However, chelation of the Ni^{2+} to proteins and peptides (including the 'antioxidants' anserine and carnosine; Section 3.18.7) alters the reduction potential to facilitate $OH^{\bullet}$ generation and organic peroxide decomposition

$$Ni^{2+} - chelate + H_2O_2 \rightarrow Ni(III)chelate + OH^{\bullet}$$
$$(ROOH) \quad + OH^- \quad\quad (RO^{\bullet})$$

Nuclear protein–Ni^{2+} complexes can generate $OH^{\bullet}$; incubation of chromatin with Ni^{2+} and H_2O_2 leads to DNA base modifications characteristic of $OH^{\bullet}$ attack. These base modifications are also observed in DNA from the livers and kidneys of female rats injected with nickel. Toxic doses of nickel additionally induce lipid peroxidation and protein carbonyl formation in animals. Hence it is widely thought that oxidative DNA damage is involved in nickel genotoxicity, although the evidence is not conclusive. In addition, nickel can inhibit some DNA repair enzymes.[179]

8.15.4 Chromium[173,178]

Traces of chromium have been suggested (but not proven) to be essential in the diet of animals to facilitate glucose metabolism. Supplements of **chromium picolinate** are widely sold, but doubts have been raised about their safety.[173,180] Chromium has multiple oxidation states; Cr(VI), Cr(V), Cr(II) and Cr(III); the last is the most stable and it can bind to transferrin. Examples of each are sodium chromate (Na_2CrO_4) and dichromate $(Na_2Cr_2O_7)$, both Cr(VI) species, and the chlorides $CrCl_5$, $CrCl_3$ and $CrCl_2$. Chromium(V) reacts with H_2O_2 to form $OH^{\bullet}$

$$Cr(V) + H_2O_2 \rightarrow Cr(VI) + OH^- + OH^{\bullet}$$

and Cr(VI) can be reduced back to Cr(V) by ascorbate, GSH (forming $GS^{\bullet}$), $O_2^{\bullet-}$, and other cellular reducing systems. Ascorbate may first reduce Cr(VI) to Cr(IV), which then disproportionates to Cr(V) and Cr(III). Chromates apparently enter cells via the sulphate or phosphate transport systems. They are toxic, mutagenic and carcinogenic in humans and other animals; lung cancer is the most common cancer in workers exposed to excess Cr(VI), for example in the manufacture of chrome steel. It is possible (but not proven *in vivo*) that reduction to Cr(V) followed by OH$^\bullet$ generation causes DNA damage that contributes to carcinogenicity. Indeed, in the presence of ascorbate chromium(VI) can form 8OHdG in DNA, but then oxidizes the 8OHdG to spiroiminodihydantoin (Section 4.8.2.12).[181] Incubation of cells with Cr(VI) leads to the formation of ternary adducts in which Cr bridges DNA to either ascorbate, GSH or cysteine. The Cr(VI) is reduced and attaches to the phosphate groups on the DNA backbone. Another source of OH$^\bullet$ may be reaction of Cr^{2+} with H$_2$O$_2$, followed by re-reduction of Cr(III) to Cr^{2+} by cellular reductants

$$Cr^{2+} + H_2O_2 \rightarrow Cr(III) + OH^\bullet + OH^-$$

Chromium-induced oxidative stress may also contribute[182] to the toxicity of PM2.5 (Section 8.13).

8.15.5 Cobalt[178]

Cobalt is a transition metal with principal oxidation states of Co^{2+} and Co(III). It is widely used in the hard-metal industry, its salts as colouring agents for ceramics and glass, and the radioactive isotope cobalt-60 in radiotherapy. Cobalt is toxic (especially to the heart) and suspected to be carcinogenic in animals when given in large quantities. However, trace amounts are needed in the human diet as a constituent of vitamin B$_{12}$ (Section 7.2.4). Reaction of Co^{2+} with H$_2$O$_2$ produces a 'reactive species' that can degrade deoxyribose and hydroxylate phenol and salicylate (to 2,3- and 2,5-dihydroxybenzoates). The simplest explanation would be formation of OH$^\bullet$

$$Co^{2+} + H_2O_2 \rightarrow Co(III) + OH^\bullet + OH^-$$

but it has not yet proved possible to demonstrate this reaction *in vitro*.[183] Instead, an oxycobalt complex may form that can (among other reactions) oxidize CO$_2$/HCO$_3^-$ into CO$_3^{\bullet-}$ radical.[184] Nevertheless, incubation of chromatin with Co^{2+} and H$_2$O$_2$, or injection of Co^{2+} into rats, led to a pattern of oxidative DNA base damage characteristic of OH$^\bullet$ attack. As in the case of Ni^{2+}, it may be that Co^{2+} itself does not form OH$^\bullet$ from H$_2$O$_2$ but that certain Co^{2+} chelates with biomolecules can. In addition, cobalt may interfere with DNA repair.[179]

8.15.6 Cadmium[173]

Cadmium, most common oxidation state Cd^{2+}, is widely used in the manufacture of batteries, alloys and pigments, but is toxic (especially to the kidney) and carcinogenic. Usually toxicity arises from inhalation of Cd-containing fumes in factories. However, in Japan, **Itai-itai disease** (severe cadmium poisoning) occurred in humans when cadmium was discharged from a mine into a river used to supply drinking water. Apart from these cases, cigarette smoking is the major source of cadmium in adults. There are several suggestions (but not a great deal of hard data) that oxidative stress plays a role in cadmium toxicity. However, Cd^{2+} does not react with H$_2$O$_2$ to form OH$^\bullet$. Nevertheless, it does bind to –SH groups and can cause GSH depletion. Administration of cadmium to animals rapidly induces metallothionein synthesis (Section 3.16.1), but sadly Cd-containing metallothionein can be degraded in the kidney to reliberate Cd^{2+}, perhaps contributing to its renal toxicity. Like Co and Ni, Cd can interfere with DNA repair, especially mismatch repair.[179]

8.15.7 Mercury[173]

Mercury (common oxidation states Hg$^+$ and Hg^{2+}) is well known to be toxic to humans and other animals. This was dramatically illustrated in 1956 by **Minamata disease**, an outbreak of poisoning by methyl mercury (CH$_3$Hg) ingested from fish and shellfish from the Shiranui Sea around Kyushu Island, Japan. The marine life had been contaminated by mercury discharged in waste water from a chemical plant. Fish and shellfish died, as did local cats and many people: pathological findings included damage to the cortex, cerebellum and peripheral nerves. There was a significant increase in the birth of children with cerebral palsy. Organic mercurials such as CH_3Hg are lipophilic and cross the blood–brain barrier, whereas inorganic mercury salts in excess cause renal damage.

The mechanism of CH_3Hg neurotoxicity is unknown, but there are several suggestions that both oxidative stress (possibly as a result of mitochondrial damage) and increases in 'free' Ca^{2+} levels are involved. The Hg^{2+} ion binds avidly to –SH groups and can deplete GSH, which might contribute to renal damage. Low concentrations of Hg^{2+} ($\leq 10^{-9}$ M) were reported[185] to stimulate $O_2^{\bullet-}$ production by human neutrophils, although higher concentrations diminish it, by causing injury to the cells. Mercury(II) ions can displace Cu^+ ions from metallothionein *in vitro*, which might potentiate oxidative damage if it occurred *in vivo*. Excess exposure to mercury has been reported to lead to elevated urinary 8OHdG excretion in humans.[186]

8.15.8 Lead[187]

Humans can be exposed to lead from vehicle exhausts (although lead as a fuel additive has been phased out in many countries), lead-based paints (now banned in most countries), handling of lead-acid batteries and contamination of food and drinking water. Lead has two common oxidation states, Pb^{2+} and Pb(IV). Too much lead can cause hypertension, is neurotoxic and damages red blood cells, the immune system and the kidney. In children, blood lead concentrations in the micromolar range may be sufficient to impair development of the nervous system, in part by interfering with the action of NMDA receptors (described in Section 9.16.3). Mechanisms of lead toxicity include inhibition of δ-aminolaevulinic acid dehydratase (the first step in haem biosynthesis; Fig. 2.14), leading to accumulation of δ-aminolaevulinic acid. The Pb^{2+} ion can accelerate oxidation of oxyhaemoglobin to methaemoglobin (with increased formation of $O_2^{\bullet-}$). Lead(II) combines quickly with –SH groups on proteins and, at high concentrations, causes GSH depletion. Lead also alters Ca^{2+} homoeostasis, perhaps interfering with Ca^{2+}-dependent neurotransmitter release in the brain. Indeed, Pb^{2+} can enter cells by passing through Ca^{2+} channels. In rats, lead-induced hypertension

was ameliorated by feeding extra α-tocopherol in the diet, suggesting that ROS are involved.

8.15.9 Vanadium[188]

The transition element vanadium is widely used in industry and can contribute to the pro-oxidant effects of particulates (Section 8.14).[182] It exists in several oxidation states, for example V(V), V(IV), V(III) and V(II). Examples of each are (in decreasing order of oxidation state) sodium orthovanadate Na_3VO_4, the vanadyl ion VO^{2+}, and the vanadium chlorides, VCl_3 and VCl_2. Vanadium occurs in some peroxidase enzymes (Section 3.13.6) and traces have been suggested (but not proven) to be essential in animal diets, apparently to aid glucose metabolism. Vanadate inhibits ATPase enzymes, including the plasma membrane Na^+, K^+–ATPase. Indeed, commercial ATP samples can be contaminated with vanadium, as can preparations of albumin.[189] Vanadate inhibits phosphotyrosine phosphatases and thus potentiates phosphorylation of protein tyrosine residues in cells, and resultant signalling.[190]

Vanadate is reduced to V(IV) by ascorbate, GSH, other thiols and certain sugars. Vanadium (IV) can reduce O_2 to $O_2^{\bullet-}$

$$V(IV) + O_2 \rightleftharpoons O_2^{\bullet-} + V(V)$$

generate $OH^\bullet$ from H_2O_2

$$V(IV) + H_2O_2 \rightarrow V(V) + OH^- + OH^\bullet$$

and decompose lipid peroxides

$$LOOH + V(IV) \rightarrow V(V) + OH^- + LO^\bullet$$

In aqueous solution, vanadate catalyses the oxidation of NADH and NADPH by $O_2^{\bullet-}$ via a **peroxovanadyl** species

$$V(V) + O_2^{\bullet-} \rightleftharpoons V(IV) - OO^\bullet$$

$$V(IV) - OO^\bullet + NAD(P)H \rightleftharpoons$$
$$V(IV) - OOH + NAD(P)^\bullet$$

$$V(IV) - OOH + H^+ \rightleftharpoons V(V) + H_2O_2$$

$$NAD(P)^\bullet + O_2 \rightarrow NAD(P)^+ + O_2^{\bullet-}$$

Hence vanadium salts are capable of promoting oxidative damage. Indeed, scientists using them to inhibit phosphatases in studies of signal transduction must not ignore their potential to cause oxidative stress,[190] since ROS also inhibit phosphatases (Section 4.5.5.3).

It is possible that oxidative stress contributes to the toxic effects of excess vanadium, which have been observed in miners of vanadium ores and workers in some other industries.

8.15.10 Titanium[183]

Titanium is widely regarded as an inert metal, hence its frequent use in medical implants. Similarly, titanium dioxide (TiO_2) particles are often used as 'inert' controls when studying the effects of other particulates, although they can act as photosensitizers in some sun blocks (Section 6.12.2). A mixture of titanium(III) and H_2O_2 has been used for decades as a laboratory source of $OH^•$.

$$Ti(III) + H_2O_2 \rightarrow Ti(IV) + OH^• + OH^-$$

Reactive species have been hypothesized to be involved in the ability of titanium implants (e.g. hip replacements) to cause inflammation in surrounding tissues; at the interface of implant and bone, phagocyte activation can occur to produce RS, which can contribute to loosening of the implant.[191]

8.15.11 Aluminium[192]

Aluminium is the most abundant metal in the Earth's crust ($\sim 8\%$), and the third most abundant element (after oxygen and silicon). Animals are frequently exposed to it; it is slowly leached from aluminium cookware and cans, ingested from beverages such as tea and many processed foods, sprayed on skin as an 'antiperspirant', injected as a constituent of some vaccine preparations, and consumed in antacids containing the hydroxide $Al(OH)_3$. It contaminates solutions used for parenteral nutrition as well as many laboratory reagents, including ATP and albumin.[189]

Aluminium has a fixed oxidation number of 3, and aluminium salts can release the hydrated Al^{3+} ion, $Al(H_2O)_6^{3+}$, in aqueous solution. Only small amounts of Al^{3+} exist in aqueous solution except at low pH; aluminium salts at pH 7.4 rapidly hydrolyse and form sparingly soluble polyhydroxide species. The gastrointestinal tract does not readily take up aluminium. Nevertheless, high doses of $Al(OH)_3$ administered orally to rats or to humans (as antacids) do raise tissue and urine aluminium levels. The extent to which inhaled aluminium compounds (e.g. in deodorants) might enter sensory neurons of the olfactory epithelium and pass into the brain is uncertain. Some organic acids, such as citrate, bind Al^{3+} and accelerate its uptake from the gastrointestinal tract. Absorbed Al^{3+} can bind to transferrin, enter cells via the transferrin receptor, and be deposited in ferritin. Aluminium can be a major problem for plants, especially when mobilized from soils or sediments by exposure to low pH. Similarly, acidification of water and subsequent Al^{3+} release can kill fish by damaging their gills.

Aluminium's potential toxicity to humans was not appreciated until the early 1970s, soon after the development of haemodialysis procedures to treat patients with kidney disease. Many dialysis patients developed a neurological syndrome, **dialysis encephalopathy**, which was eventually shown to be caused by accumulation of high concentrations of aluminium (derived from Al-contaminated dialysis fluids) in the brain. Dialysis encephalopathy is accompanied by anaemia and bone demineralization, leading to increased risk of fracture.

Why is aluminium neurotoxic? There are several hypotheses. They include interference with Ca^{2+} uptake mechanisms, inactivation of G6PDH and inhibition of **dihydropteridine reductase**, an enzyme that catalyses NADPH-dependent reduction of dihydrobiopterin to tetrahydrobiopterin, a cofactor required for biosynthesis of tyrosine. Another idea is that Al imposes oxidative stress. Aluminium(III) ions do not usually stimulate free radical reactions, because of their fixed oxidation number. However, if peroxidation in liposomes, erythrocytes, synaptosomes, myelin, LDL, or microsomes is stimulated by adding Fe^{2+} ions, the presence of Al^{3+} increases the peroxidation rate.[193,194] It may be that Al^{3+}ions bind to membranes and cause a subtle rearrangement of membrane lipids that aids the propagation of lipid peroxidation.[193] Lead(II) can sometimes do the same.[193] Another suggestion is that aluminium forms a pro-oxidant complex with superoxide, $AlO_2^{\bullet 2+}$. The significance of these various mechanisms in producing encephalopathy is uncertain, although feeding a diet enriched in Al did increase F_2-IP levels in the brains of mice.[195]

8.15.12 Zinc

Zinc is essential to animals and may exert antioxidant properties under some circumstances (Table 2.5), but intakes far above the RDA can be toxic. In particular, excess Zn^{2+} in the brain can damage neurons. Levels of extracellular 'free' Zn^{2+} in brain are normally low, but appear to rise during excitotoxicity. It can then be taken up and accumulate in postsynaptic neurons, damaging them (Section 9.17.3.1). Zinc may also be rendered 'available' by other mechanisms, for example exposure of rat neurons to a $ONOO^-$-generating system caused a rise in Zn^{2+} levels, and apoptosis was decreased by Zn^{2+}-chelators.[196] Presumably $ONOO^-$ releases Zn^{2+} from transcription factors with 'zinc fingers', and/or from metallothioneins (Section 3.16.1).

In cell culture studies, antioxidants often protect against Zn^{2+}-induced toxicity. However, Zn^{2+} does not itself promote free radical reactions. Instead, it may damage mitochondria to increase ROS production. It can also increase the activity of NADPH oxidase in neurons.[197]

8.16 Antibiotics

Antibiotics are substances produced by living organisms that halt the growth of, and sometimes kill, fungi, bacteria or other microorganisms. Antiobiotics can be targets of oxidative damage, cause such damage or, in some cases, exert antioxidant effects.

As an example of the first, the polyene antifungal antibiotics (such as **amphotericin** and **candicidin**) bind to sterols in the membranes of fungal cells and cause membrane permeabilization. Their highly polyunsaturated structures (Fig. 8.14) make them prone to oxidize with the formation of peroxides, alkoxyl/ peroxyl radicals, and cytotoxic aldehydes. As a result, they can deteriorate on storage, by oxidation.[198] Indeed, it has been suggested that their toxic effects may sometimes involve products of oxidative damage.

8.16.1 Tetracyclines as pro- and antioxidatants

The **tetracyclines** (Fig. 8.14) act by inhibiting ribosome function in bacteria, but they are also sensitizers of singlet O_2 formation, as are the **quinolone** antibiotics such as **sparfloxacin, lomefloxacin, ciprofloxacin** and **ofloxacin**.[199] Tetracyclines chelate iron and copper ions, and the chelates with the last two metals can generate $OH^\bullet$ from H_2O_2 in vitro. This might sometimes be relevant in vivo. For example S. cerevisiae is usually resistant to tetracyclines, but mutants lacking CuZnSOD stop growth and show increased oxidative damage when exposed to these agents.[200] On the other hand, tetracyclines are powerful scavengers of HOCl and $ONOO^-$, and there are reports that they decrease ROS production by phagocytes (including microglia), suppress increases in iNOS, COX-2 and IL-1, and inhibit matrix metalloproteinases in animal models of stroke and neurodegenerative diseases. **Minocycline** (Fig. 8.14) seems especially effective and is being studied as a potential neuroprotective agent in stroke and neurodegenerative diseases such as ALS (Section 9.21.2) and Huntington's disease (Section 9.22.2).[201]

Hence it must never be assumed that an effect exerted by an antibiotic in vivo is necessarily mediated by antibacterial action. Pro-oxidant effects of antibiotics could aid the killing of bacteria (sometimes called a **phago-mimetic** effect)[202] whereas antioxidant effects could modulate inflammation.

Several antibiotics contain chlorine residues; these can be introduced by haloperoxidases (Section 3.3.16) or more-specific halogenating enzymes. In both cases, HOCl may be involved in the catalytic mechanism (Section 3.13.6).[203]

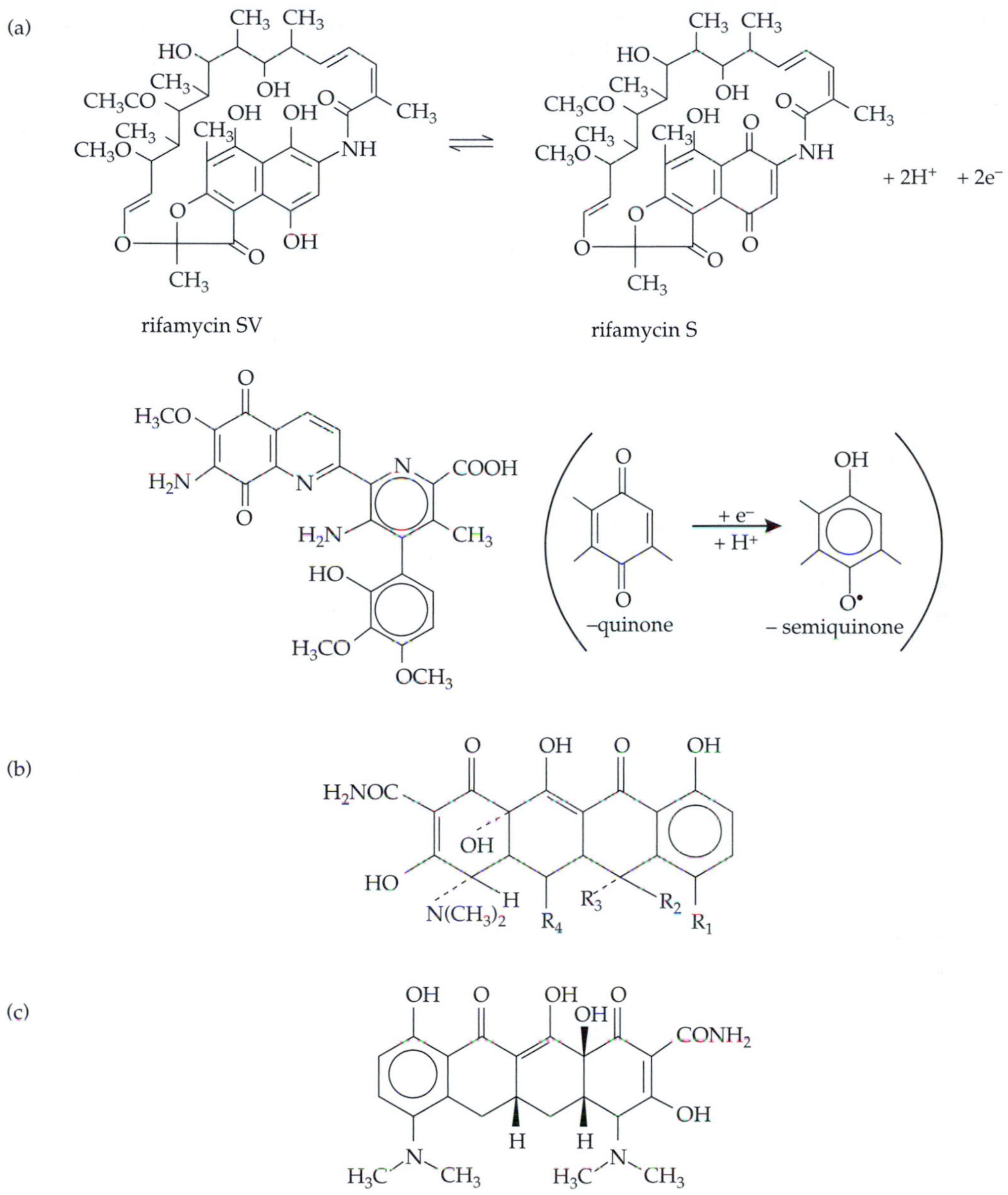

Figure 8.14 Structures of some antibiotics. (a) the diphenol rifamycin SV and the quinones rifamycin S and streptonigrin. (b) Tetracycline: $R_1 = H$, $R_2 = OH$, $R_3 = CH_3$, $R_4 = H$; oxytetracycline: $R_1 = H$, $R_2 = OH$, $R_3 = CH_3$, $R_4 = OH$; chlortetracycline: $R_1 = Cl$, $R_2 = OH$, $R_3 = CH_3$, $R_4 = H$; doxycycline: $R_1 = H$, $R_2 = H$, $R_3 = CH_3$, $R_4 = OH$. (c) Minocycline.

(d)

(e)

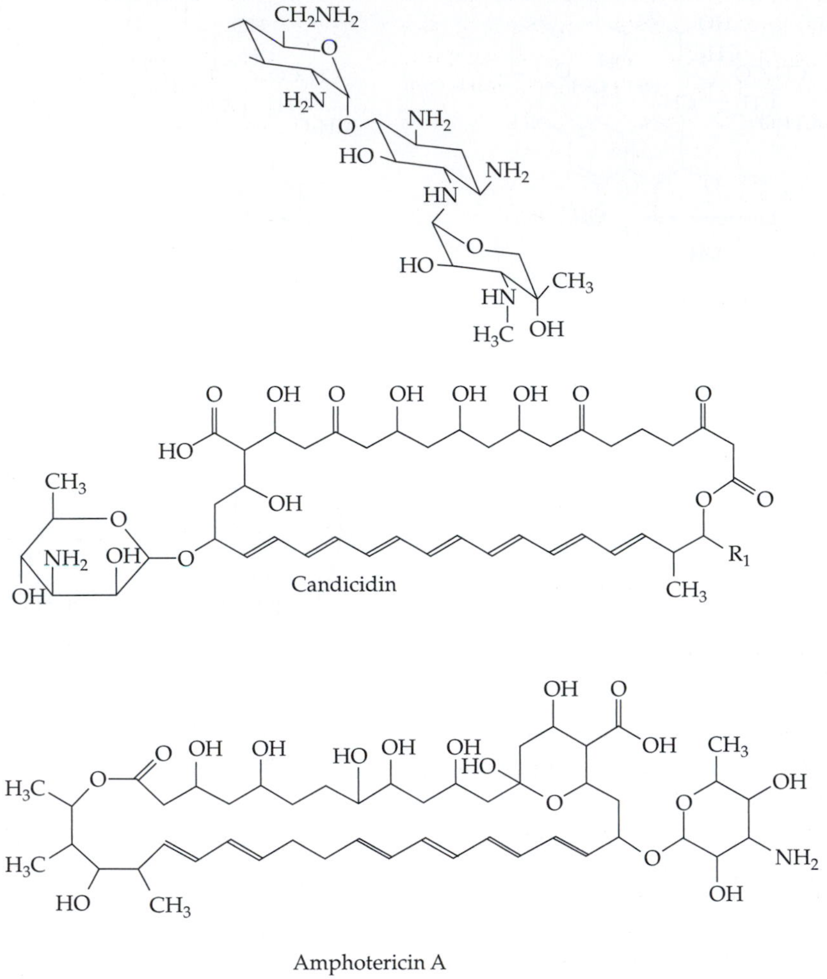

Candicidin

Amphotericin A

Figure 8.14 (d) Gentamicin C1a. (e) The polyene antibiotics.

8.16.2 Quinone antibiotics

Many anticancer antibiotics are quinones that redox cycle to produce $O_2^{\bullet-}$, semiquinones and H_2O_2 *in vivo* (Section 9.15). An example is **streptonigrin**, produced by *Streptomyces flocculus*. It was one of the first quinone antibiotics whose action *in vivo* was shown to involve ROS, but is now rarely used clinically because of side-effects. Its toxic action on *E. coli* requires O_2 and is decreased if SOD activity is raised.

Similarly, low levels of it can induce MnSOD. The quinone part of streptonigrin (Fig. 8.14) is reduced by bacterial enzymes to a semiquinone form that then reduces O_2 to $O_2^{\bullet-}$. Elevated intrabacterial iron levels enhance the bacteriocidal action of streptonigrin, presumably via $OH^\bullet$ formation.[204] For example, killing of the gonococcus by streptonigrin depended on the availability of iron to promote Fenton-type reactions.[205]

Rifamycin SV (Fig. 8.14), an antibiotic that has been used to treat tuberculosis, oxidizes in the presence of transition metal ions to give a quinone (**rifamycin S**), with intermediate formation of a semiquinone, and $O_2^{\bullet-}$

$$QH_2 + O_2 \overset{metal\ ions}{\rightleftharpoons} QH^{\bullet} + O_2^{\bullet-} + H^+$$
$$\text{rifamycin SV} \qquad \text{semiquinone}$$

$$QH^{\bullet} + O_2 \rightarrow Q + O_2^{\bullet-} + H^+$$

$$QH^{\bullet} + \text{metal ion} \rightarrow Q + H^+ + \text{reduced metal ion}$$

The bactericidal action of rifamycin SV may involve intracellular ROS generation, in addition to prevention of bacterial RNA synthesis.[206]

8.16.3 Aminoglycoside nephrotoxicity and ototoxicity

Reactive species may be involved in the side-effects produced by several antibiotics, including the anticancer ones (Section 9.15). Another example, aminoglycoside antibiotics such as **gentamicin** (Fig. 8.14) can damage the kidneys, accompanied by increased lipid peroxidation. Gentamicin binds iron ions to form a chelate that is a potent catalyst of lipid peroxidation, and damage to renal mitochondria by gentamicin may lead to iron ion release and formation of this chelate.[207] Indeed, desferrioxamine decreases gentamicin-induced kidney damage in rats. However, whether lipid peroxidation is an early, causative, stage in aminoglycoside-induced renal injury or a consequence of tissue injury is uncertain. For example, α-tocopherol administration to rats lowered gentamicin-induced lipid peroxidation in the kidney, but did not prevent the renal damage.[208] Iron chelators and α-tocopherol also decreased ear damage (**ototoxicity**) caused by high doses of gentamicin in guinea pigs. Ototoxicity of gentamicin appears more severe in malnourished animals, possibly due to lowered GSH levels.[209]

8.17 Noise and stress

Many people suffer from 'stress' of various kinds. One source of stress is excessive noise, and damage to the inner ear by this has been suggested to involve RS. Loud noise may cause direct mechanical damage to the cochlea, but in addition produces decreased blood flow followed by reperfusion injury, leading to formation of $O_2^{\bullet-}$ and $OH^{\bullet}$ radicals, and increased lipid peroxidation,[210] as measured by F_2-IPs.[209] Isoprostanes may worsen the problem by inducing vasoconstriction. Noise-induced hearing loss in animals can be decreased by desferrioxamine, the antioxidant edaravone (Section 10.6.7), lipid peroxidation inhibitors, the GPx mimetic Ebselen, or by raising GSH levels by supplying N-acetylcysteine or glutathione esters,[211] but not by CuZnSOD administration or over-expression (indeed, there are some reports that damage is worse if CuZnSOD is elevated[212]). Reactive species may also be involved in ear damage secondary to pneumococcal meningitis,[213] or caused by gentamicin (Section 8.16.3) or by the anticancer agent cisplatin.[214] Studies of mice with defects in balance showed that one of the genes involved encoded a $O_2^{\bullet-}$-generating NADPH oxidase, NOX3 (Section 7.10), levels of which are higher in the inner ear than in other tissues. Its metabolic role is uncertain, but cisplatin seems to stimulate $O_2^{\bullet-}$ production by it.[214]

Long-term 'stress' affects the functioning of the nervous, endocrine and immune systems and several papers have suggested a role for RS. In one animal model,[215] stress caused by immobilization (taping down all four limbs of a rat) is associated with increases in oxidative damage to lipids, proteins and DNA in the brain, possibly relating to increased $NO^{\bullet}$ production and mitochondrial dysfunction, together with ROS production by oxidation of dopamine and tetrahydrobiopterin.[216] How well this model relates to human stress is uncertain. Another model is sleep deprivation in animals, which may increase oxidative damage in the brain.[217] Some studies suggest that the level of stress/ depression in patients correlates with elevated levels of 8OHdG in white blood cells.[218] In another study, stressed mothers of chronically ill children showed an increased ratio of F_2-IPs to α-tocopherol, plus accelerated telomere loss in white blood cells.[219] Stress-induced ROS formation might worsen gastric damage caused by *H. pylori* infection.[220] Much more work needs to be done in this area to establish the exact contribution of RS to stress.

8.18 Nitro and azo compounds[221]

Several compounds containing nitro groups are used therapeutically, for example in cancer treatment (Section 8.19.3 below) and as vasodilators (e.g. nitroglycerine). Toxicity can occur from overdoses, or side-effects, of therapeutic nitro compounds, and from over-exposure to nitro compounds used in industry, such as 2-nitropropane (Section 3.13.4). The manufacture and use of explosives has provided many cases of toxicity of nitro compounds. Nitrated proteins are 'abnormal' and may provoke an immune response, for example when inhaled as constituents of pollens (Section 8.11.2).

8.18.1 Nitro radicals and redox cycling

The antibacterial drug **nitrofurantoin** (Fig. 8.15), sometimes used to treat urinary tract infections, can produce lung damage. Its toxicity both to bacteria and to lung may involve redox cycling. The drug is reduced (e.g. by NADPH–cytochrome P450 reductase in lung ER):

$$RNO_2 \xrightarrow[\text{electron}]{1e^-} RNO_2^{\bullet-}$$

followed by reoxidation of the nitro radical to produce $O_2^{\bullet-}$

$$RNO_2^{\bullet-} + O_2 \rightarrow RNO_2 + O_2^{\bullet-}$$

Nitrofurantoin is one of the agents that can induce haemolysis in patients with G6PDH deficiency (Section 6.4.5), again possibly by oxidative mechanisms.

Reduction of nitro compounds to $RNO_2^{\bullet-}$ can also be achieved by mitochondria, xanthine and aldehyde oxidases, and, in some cases, by

glutathione reductase. For example, reduction of trinitrotoluene by enzymes in the lens has been proposed to account for the propensity of this compound to produce cataract,[222] and nitrated metabolites may contribute to the toxicity of benzene (Section 8.6.8). Fish, crabs and mussels contain enzymes that can reduce nitro compounds, and oxidative stress may be involved in damage to aquatic organisms by nitro compounds in polluted waters.[223] Redox-cycling might account for the toxicity of nitrofurazone (Fig. 8.15) and its derivatives to *Trypanosoma cruzi* (Section 3.12.1). Some dinitrohalobenzenes (e.g. CDNB) interact with thioredoxin reductase to cause $O_2^{\bullet-}$ formation (Section 3.11).

3-Nitrotyrosine can also be converted to a nitro radical, capable of converting O_2 to $O_2^{\bullet-}$, by various reductase enzymes.[224] However, at the levels of 3-nitrotyrosine present *in vivo* (Sections 2.6.1.2 and 5.6.2), this is unlikely to contribute much to toxicity.

8.18.2 Further reduction of nitro radicals

In the absence of O_2, nitro radicals can undergo further reduction (e.g. by GSH), or disproportionation, to form nitroso (RNO) compounds

$$2RNO_2^{\bullet-} + 2H^+ \rightarrow R-N=O + RNO_2 + H_2O$$

$$RNO_2^{\bullet-} + GSH \rightarrow R-N=O + GS^\bullet + OH^-$$

Nitroso compounds might be further reduced to hydroxylamines (RNHOH) or even to amines, RNH_2. The extent of reduction, and which product is the ultimate toxin, depends upon the nitro compound administered and the organism studied.

$$RNO_2 \xrightarrow{1e^-} RNO_2^{\bullet-} \xrightarrow[H^+]{1e^-} RNO \xrightarrow[]{2e^-} R-NHOH \xrightarrow[H^+]{2e^-} RNH_2$$

One-electron reduction of nitroso compounds gives nitroxide radicals

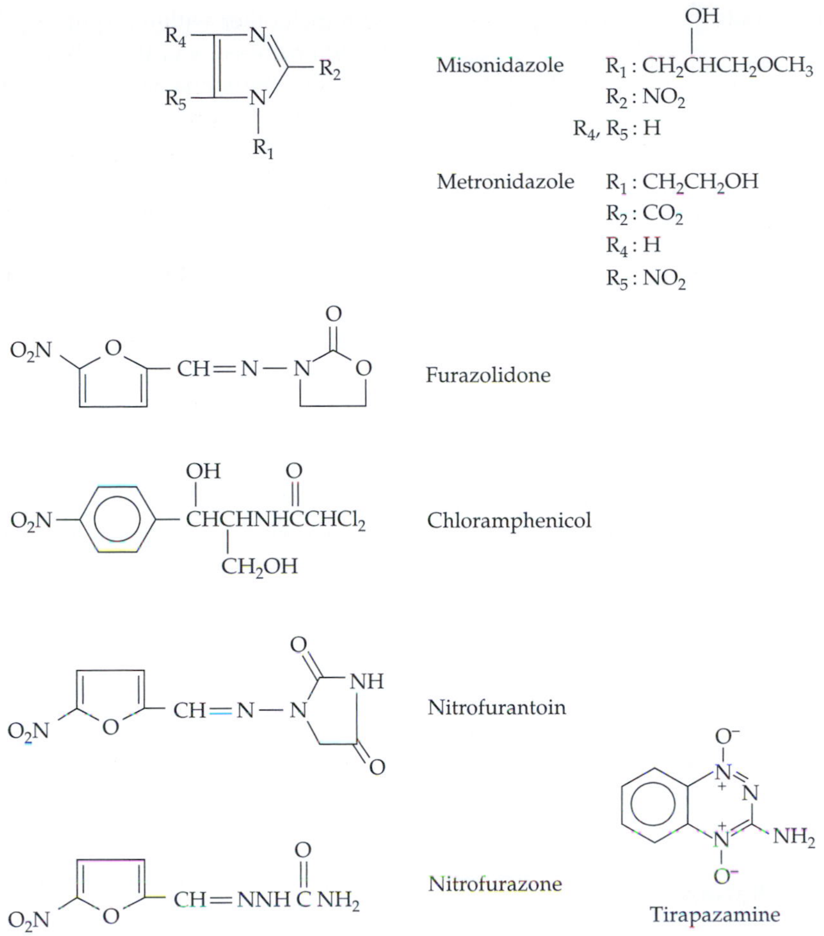

Figure 8.15 Some nitro compounds used in the treatment of disease. **Furazolidone** and **nitrofurazone** are antibacterial agents used in veterinary medicine: their toxicity to bacteria may involve RS. The antibiotic **chloramphenicol** acts against a range of bacteria, but its use is restricted since it can affect the bone marrow to sometimes produce severe and irreversible anaemia. Bone marrow damage may involve reduction of the nitro group to nitrosochloramphenicol as well as oxidation of the side-chain by CYPs to generate —NHCOCOCl species that form adducts with proteins.

$$RNO + e^- + H^+ \longrightarrow R-\overset{\displaystyle H}{\underset{\displaystyle |}{N}}-O^{\bullet}$$

as does one-electron oxidation of hydroxylamines

$$RNHOH \rightarrow e- + \quad R-\overset{\displaystyle H}{\underset{\displaystyle |}{N}}-O^{\bullet} +H^+$$

Vice versa, nitroxides can be reduced to hydroxylamines by ascorbate, thiols and various enzymes. Nitroxide radicals are also generated by addition of free radicals to nitrones and nitroso compounds; remember your spin trapping chemistry (Section

5.2). An amino cation radical ($RNH_2^{\bullet+}$) can be generated by one-electron oxidation of RNH_2, or one-electron reduction of RNHOH.

For many nitro compounds, the reduction products ($RNO_2^{\bullet-}$, RNO, etc.) are more cytotoxic than is $O_2^{\bullet-}$, so that the compounds cause more damage in the absence of O_2 than under aerobic conditions. For example, **metronidazole** (Flagyl®; Fig. 8.15) is used to treat infections caused by anaerobic bacteria and protozoa, such as the human intestinal parasites *Giardia lamblia* and *Entamoeba histolytica*.

8.18.3 Azo compounds[225]

Azo compounds contain the $-N=N-$ group. They can be reduced by NADPH–cytochrome P450 reductase, XO, and several other enzymes to generate an azo anion free radical, capable of reducing O_2 to $O_2^{\bullet-}$

$$R-N=N-R' \xrightarrow{1e^-} [R-N-N-R']^{\bullet-}$$
$$[R-N-N-R']^{\bullet-} + O_2 \rightarrow R-N=N-R' + O_2^{\bullet-}$$

Further reduction yields hydrazines, $R-NH-NH-R$, whose toxicity can also involve RS (Section 6.5.1).

Azo compounds are widely used in the pharmaceutical, food and cosmetic industries and as research tools (e.g. AAPH and AMVN; Section 4.11.8.2). Another example; **arsenazo III** has been used to measure Ca^{2+} movements because it changes colour when Ca^{2+} binds to it. However, arsenazo III can be reduced by cytosolic enzymes, mitochondria and microsomes, leading to $O_2^{\bullet-}$ generation by the above reactions. Oxidative stress alters Ca^{2+} homoeostasis (Section 4.3), so that this 'Ca^{2+} probe' can end up altering what it is trying to measure.

8.19 Ionizing radiation

If the energy of a photon exceeds the energy needed to displace an electron from a molecule, it may cause **ionization** of that molecule, knocking out the electron and leaving an ion $(X^{\bullet+})$ behind. Visible and UV light are insufficiently energetic to ionize most biomolecules, but γ-rays, X-rays, high-energy electrons (β-particles), high-energy neutrons, and α-particles (He^{2+} ions) can. These are often collectively called **ionizing radiation**. Oxidative damage and inappropriate reduction of metal clusters by 'stray' electrons are a problem during X-ray crystallography.[226]

When ionizing radiation passes through a biological system, energy is not deposited uniformly along its path but in small packages: these **spurs** have different sizes and may contain several excited molecules, ions and electrons. For example, in water exposed to γ-rays there is both ionization and excitation (Section 2.3.3.1) to form $H^\bullet$, $OH^\bullet$ and hydrated electrons. These products can recombine with each other within a spur (e.g. 2 $OH^\bullet$ forming H_2O_2) or diffuse into the bulk water. A significant part of the initial damage done to cells by ionizing radiation is due to $OH^\bullet$. DNA is a particularly important target, suffering double- and single-strand breaks, deoxyribose damage, base modification to form a multiplicity of products and cross-links with nuclear proteins. Double-strand breaks are especially important damaging agents because their repair can be error prone (Section 4.10.6). Also, radiation tends to produce 'clusters' of DNA damage; two or more adjacent lesions that interfere with repair of each other.[227] In patients undergoing radiotherapy, increased levels of 8OHdG in lymphocyte DNA and in urine have been observed.[228]

Radiation dose is measured in **Grays**, one gray being an absorbed dose of one joule per kilogram. A Gray is a large dose: humans exposed to 3 to 6 Grays of ionizing radiation have a 50% chance of dying within a few weeks from damage to the gastrointestinal system and bone marrow. At doses at or above 1 Gray, radiation sickness begins to occur, manifested as nausea, vomiting, fatigue, fever, diarrhoea and other symptoms. Subjects who survive are more prone to sterility, some forms of cancer and cataract, probably by formation of protein radicals that cross-link proteins and reduce lens transparency. There may be no 'safe dose' of ionizing radiation; even very low doses may increase cancer risk.[229]

8.19.1 The oxygen effect[230]

The damaging effects of ionizing radiation on cells are aggravated by the presence of O_2, by a factor (**the oxygen enhancement ratio**) of 2- to 3.5-fold (Fig. 1.12). This **oxygen effect** can involve several mechanisms. Attack of $OH^\bullet$ and other reactive radicals upon biomolecules often proceeds by $H^\bullet$ abstraction. The resulting radicals (designated $R^\bullet$ below) can sometimes be repaired by reaction with GSH or ascorbic acid, for example

$$R^\bullet + GSH \rightarrow RH + GS^\bullet$$

It was proposed many years ago by radiobiologists that O_2 'fixes' the damage by forming other radicals that cannot regenerate the original compound, for example

$$R^\bullet + O_2 \rightarrow RO_2^\bullet \text{ (peroxyl radical)}$$
$$RO_2^\bullet + GSH \rightarrow RO_2H + GS^\bullet$$
$$\text{(oxidized biomolecule)}$$

Indeed, GSH plays an important role in protecting against ionizing radiation, and treatment of organisms with buthionine sulphoximine (Section 3.9.3) to inhibit GSH synthesis increases radiosensitivity. Reduced glutathione, its precursors and other thiol compounds (such as **cysteamine**, $HSCH_2CH_2NH_2$ and mercaptopropionylglycine; Section 10.6.9), have been used as radioprotectors. GSH may be radioprotective not only by 'repair' reactions (shown above), but also by providing a substrate for GPx enzymes and possibly by scavenging OH$^\bullet$ radicals directly. In addition, it can react with $RO_2^\bullet$ radicals, preventing them from propagating chain reactions. However, the reactivity of the sulphur radicals produced should not be ignored (Section 2.5.5).

8.19.1.1 A role for superoxide?

If O_2 is present, the hydrated electrons formed by ionizing radiation can reduce it to $O_2^{\bullet-}$ (Section 2.3.3.1). In addition (although quantitatively less important), some peroxyl radicals formed by attack of OH$^\bullet$ on biomolecules can decompose to give $O_2^{\bullet-}$ (Section 2.5.4.1). Thus for α-hydroxyalkylperoxyl radicals formed from glucose

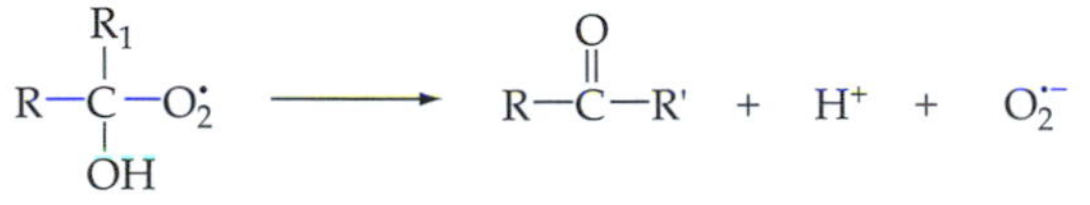

$$R-\underset{\underset{OH}{|}}{\overset{\overset{R_1}{|}}{C}}-O_2^\bullet \longrightarrow R-\overset{\overset{O}{\|}}{C}-R' + H^+ + O_2^{\bullet-}$$

Radiation can damage mitochondria, causing more electron leakage to O_2. Superoxide might aggravate injury by forming H_2O_2 and promoting metal ion release (Section 3.6.1). Indeed, tissue damage by radiation may lead to increased availability of transition metal ions *in vivo*; this has been demonstrated (as a rise in plasma non-transferrin-bound iron)[231] in patients exposed to radiation to ablate the bone marrow prior to transplantation with normal marrow. This iron may arise from dying cells, and/or by the action

of $O_2^{\bullet-}$ on metalloproteins. Some radioresistant bacteria repair DNA strand breaks exceptionally well, have high levels of SOD, or accumulate intracellular Mn^{2+} to scavenge $O_2^{\bullet-}$, whereas elevated intracellular iron levels aggravate bacterial radiation damage,[232] an effect also seen in animal cells. [233] Overexpression of MnSOD renders animal cells more resistant to radiation, and administration to mice of liposomes containing a plasmid encoding MnSOD (Section 10.6.3.1) decreases damage by radiation.[234]

Injection of CuZnSOD into mice has been reported to diminish mortality after X-irradiation, whereas injection of inactivated enzyme cannot. Its effects depend on the time and dose of SOD administered, and on the intensity of radiation used. The mechanism behind them remains to be established, but could be by diminishing the inflammatory response after radiation-induced tissue damage (which spreads damage to a range of tissues) rather than an effect on the primary radiation damage.[235] When interpreting some of the earlier studies, do bear in mind the possible contamination of SOD with endotoxin (Section 10.6.3). Irradiation activates transcription factors (partly by ROS production) and causes increased cytokine production, inflammation, increased expression of COX-2 and iNOS genes, ONOO$^-$ formation, fibrosis and often cell death by necrosis or apoptosis.[233] The ceramide pathway (Section 4.4.1.2) seems particularly important in apoptosis induced by ionizing radiation.[236]

How much, overall, might $O_2^{\bullet-}$ contribute to oxygen enhancement of radiation damage? Maybe a lot in animals. Not much in *E. coli*; mutants lacking FeSOD and MnSOD showed normal O_2 enhancement ratios.[237]

8.19.2 Antioxidants and radiotherapy

Should patients undergoing radiotherapy take antioxidants to protect against collateral damage to normal tissues? Or would they simply be protecting the tumour? In one study of head and neck cancer, patients were given α-tocopherol (400 units/day) and β-carotene (30 mg/day) during radiotherapy and for up to 3 years later. There was a tendency to have less severe acute adverse effects during therapy in the test group as compared with the placebo group. Unfortunately, the test group also showed a trend for cancer recurrence rates to be higher.[238] Hence, on the basis of current data, we see no case for patients to take such supplements.

8.19.3 Hypoxic-cell sensitizers[221,230]

The O_2 effect causes problems in the treatment of malignant tumours by radiotherapy. As tumours grow, areas within them become hypoxic, resist radiation treatment and serve as 'nuclei' for subsequent regrowth. There has therefore been interest in therapies combining increased O_2 exposure with radiation (Section 1.5.2) and in various drugs that, like O_2, make hypoxic cells more sensitive to ionizing radiation. Such drugs are collectively known as **hypoxic-cell sensitizers** (HCS). Another approach is to target HIFs, whose activation allows tumours to survive hypoxia (Section 1.3.2).

The first HCS to be identified was metronidazole (Fig. 8.15). Exposing animal cells in culture to metronidazole increased their susceptibility to ionizing radiation under anaerobic conditions, and experiments on tumour-bearing animals confirmed this effect *in vivo*, although high doses were required. Research continued to find better HCS, **misonidazole** (Fig. 8.15) being one candidate. It had little clinical success, however, and the focus shifted to finding drugs that are directly toxic to hypoxic cells. The antibiotic **mitomycin C** (Section 9.15.2) shows limited selectivity for hypoxic cells, but a more promising agent is **tirapazamine** (Fig. 8.15). It is being tested in head and neck cancer as a radiosensitizer, and also in combination with other chemotherapeutic agents such as *cis*-platin. Tirapazamine is reduced by several cellular systems to a free radical that reacts with O_2 to regenerate tirapazamine and produce $O_2^{\bullet-}$. If no O_2 is around, the reactive radical persists and damages DNA bases.

One reason for the 'oxygen effect' is prevention of the 'repair' of organic radicals. Metronidazole ($MN-NO_2$) and other HCS might act to prevent repair in a similar way, for example by forming a radical adduct

In addition, the products might injure hypoxic cells, either directly or after reduction to nitroso or other species.

8.19.4 Food irradiation[239]

Treatment of foodstuffs with ionizing radiation (high-energy electrons, γ-rays or X-rays) is an accepted method for sterilization, killing insects, or preventing germination and ripening. In many countries, laws govern the types of food that may be irradiated, and the dose of radiation used. Their enforcement requires methods to detect irradiated food and quantitate the radiation dose. The available techniques resemble those used to detect oxidative damage in living organisms (Chapter 5). For example, most irradiated spices and some other foodstuffs give more chemiluminescence when added to alkaline luminol solutions than do unirradiated control samples. Bone and calcified cuticle (e.g. in chickens, crustacea and some fish) develop long-lived ESR signals upon irradiation because the radicals are trapped in a solid matrix. Food scientists may measure end-products of lipid peroxidation (e.g. volatile hydrocarbons, peroxides, IPs, carbonyl compounds), DNA damage products (e.g. thymine glycol, 8OHdG), and oxidized amino-acid residues, (*ortho*-tyrosine, formylkynurenine, bityrosine, 2-oxohistidine). As yet, however, no single method to detect irradiation is applicable to all foods, just as there is no single 'best' method of detecting oxidative damage *in vivo*.

8.20 Summary and conclusion

For some toxins (e.g. ionizing radiation, paraquat and CCl_4), RS generation is the major, if not the only, mechanism by which they cause damage. For others, such as redox-cycling quinones and nitro compounds, it may be a significant contributor. For others, RS may play a minor role. Several toxins (e.g. metals, paracetamol) can deplete GSH and thus predispose the cell to secondary oxidative stress, which may (or may not) further contribute to the overall toxic effects. For yet others, RS may play no role whatsoever. As we said at the beginning, the demonstration of oxidative stress induced by a toxin, or the trapping of a toxin-derived RS, is not evidence that such species are important in the toxicity.

CHAPTER 9

Reactive species and disease: fact, fiction or filibuster?

Living matter has a dark side. It fights a lost battle against its own fragility and ends up scorched.

G. Schatz

9.1 Setting the scene

The biomedical literature is full of claims that free radicals and other reactive species (RS) are involved in human diseases (Table 9.1).[1,2] They have been implicated in over 150 disorders, ranging from rheumatoid arthritis and haemorrhagic shock through cardiomyopathy and cystic fibrosis to intestinal ischaemia, AIDS and even male-pattern baldness.[3] As early as 1984, we pointed out[4] that this wide range of disorders reveals that increased RS formation is not something unusual, and that it probably accompanies tissue injury in most, if not all, human diseases. Why? Simply because any form of tissue injury (even inserting a microelectrode) raises RS formation. Reasons for this are summarized in Fig. 9.1 and include liberation of 'catalytic' transition-metal ions and haem proteins, recruitment of phagocytes, damage to mitochondria causing increased leakage of electrons from the electron transport chain[5] and loss of antioxidants such as ascorbate, plasma thiols (e.g. the albumin–SH group)[6] and cellular GSH. An ancillary mechanism is that the antioxidant nutrient status of sick people may be compromised. Thus AIDS patients may absorb nutrients poorly,[7] and very sick patients may not eat at all. Patients in intensive care often show low plasma ascorbate[8]—would it be beneficial to correct this? Some studies suggest yes,[9] but more work remains to be done.

9.2 Does oxidative stress matter?

Yes it does. Some diseases are probably caused by oxidative stress. For example, many of the biological consequences of excess radiation exposure are due to oxidative damage (Section 8.19). The symptoms produced by chronic dietary deficiencies of selenium (Section 3.11.2) or of tocopherols (Section 3.20.2) might also be mediated by oxidative stress.

However, in most diseases, oxidative stress is a consequence and not a cause of the disease (Fig. 9.1). Tissue damage leads to formation of increased amounts of putative 'injury mediators', such as prostaglandins, leukotrienes, cytokines and, of course, RS. All of these have, at various times, been suggested to play important roles in tissue injury (Fig. 9.1).

If then, in most human diseases, more RS are produced as a consequence of tissue injury, do they make a significant contribution to the disease pathology, or is their formation of little or no consequence? Or is it even beneficial, for example in triggering rapid adaptive responses? The answer probably differs in different diseases (Fig. 9.2) and may even differ from patient to patient depending on his/her antioxidant defence status. For example, the outcome of stroke (Section 9.17.2 below) might be worse in subjects with low levels of antioxidants such as α-tocopherol in the brain. Tissue injury after trauma may be greater in subjects low in G6PDH activity (Section 6.4.3). In many diseases, RS may not

Table 9.1 Some of the clinical conditions in which the involvement of reactive species has been suggested

Category	Examples
Disorders affecting the immune system	Lupus, Hashimoto's thyroiditis, vascular inflammation, sarcoidosis, Grave's disease, AIDS
Ischaemia–reflow states	Stroke, myocardial infarction/arrythmias/angina/stunning, organ transplantation, inflamed rheumatoid joint, frostbite, Dupuytren's contracture, thalidomide-, phenytoin-, and cocaine-induced foetal damage, ischaemic preconditioning
Drug and toxin-induced reactions	See Chapter 8
Iron overload (tissue and plasma)	Idiopathic haemochromatosis, dietary iron overload (accidental poisoning, Bantu), thalassaemia and other chronic anaemias treated with multiple blood transfusions, nutritional deficiencies (kwashiorkor), alcoholism, multiorgan failure, cardiopulmonary bypass, fulminant hepatic failure, prematurity, alcohol-related iron overload, cancer chemotherapy/radiotherapy, lung transplant rejection (bronchiolitis obliterans)
Radiation injury	Consequences of nuclear explosions, accidental exposure, radiotherapy, background exposure (cosmic rays, radon)
Ageing	Disorders of premature ageing, ageing itself, age-related diseases, senescence
Red blood cells	Phenylhydrazine, primaquine and related drugs, lead poisoning, protoporphyrin photoxidation, malaria, sickle cell anaemia, favism, Fanconi's anaemia, haemolytic anaemia of prematurity, chemotherapy, G6PDH deficiency
Respiratory tract	Effects of cigarette smoke, other smoke inhalation, snuff inhalation, COPD, hyperoxia, broncho-pulmonary dysplasia, exposure to air pollutants (O_3, NO_2, SO_2, diesel exhaust), ARDS, mineral dust pneumoconiosis, asbestos carcinogenicity, bleomycin toxicity, paraquat toxicity, asthma, cystic fibrosis, allergic rhinitis, pulmonary hypertension, pulmonary sarcoidosis, lung transplant storage/rejection, idiopathic pulmonary fibrosis
Reproductive system	Defective placentation, sterility due to inflammation (both male and female), varicocele, hydatiform mole, pre-eclampsia; various problems of the newborn (premature or otherwise; see Chapter 6)
Heart and cardiovascular system	Alcohol cardiomyopathy, Keshan disease, atherosclerosis, anthracycline cardiotoxicity, cardiac iron overload, transplant storage/rejection, cardiac hypertrophy, eosinophilic endocarditis, tuberous sclerosis complex[a]
Kidney	Autoimmune nephrotic syndromes, glomerulonephritis, aminoglycoside nephrotoxicity, heavy metal nephrotoxicity (Pb, Cd, Hg), myoglobin/haemoglobin damage, haemodialysis, transplant storage/rejection, obstructive bladder disease, hyperoxaluria, cystinosis
Liver/gastrointestinal tract	Betel nut-related oral cancer, liver injury caused by endotoxin or halogenated hydrocarbons (e.g. CCl_4), exposure to diabetogenic agents, pancreatitis, hepatitis, oesophatitis, gastritis, gastric cancer related to *H. pylori*, NSAID-induced gastrointestinal tract lesions, oral iron poisoning, liver cancer related to parasites or viruses, Crohn's disease, ulcerative colitis, liver transplant storage/rejection, oral leukoplakia
Musculo-skeletal system	Osteoporosis, osteoarthritis, rheumatoid arthritis, gout, fibromyalgia, chronic fatigue syndrome, injury by exercise, inclusion body myositis
Brain/nervous system/related neuromuscular disorders	Hyperbaric oxygen, α-tocopherol deficiency, exposure to neurotoxins, Alzheimer's disease, mild cognitive impairment, autism, Parkinson's disease, Huntington's disease, stroke, neuronal ceroid lipofuscinoses, epilepsy, leprosy, allergic encephalomyelitis, aluminium overload, sequelae of traumatic injury, muscular dystrophy, tardive dyskinesia, Rett's syndrome, uraemia-induced encephalopathy, multiple sclerosis, amyotrophic lateral sclerosis, cerebral palsy, high altitude headache, Guam dementia; may also occur during preservation of foetal dopamine-producing cells for transplantation
Eye	Cataract, ocular haemorrhage, degenerative retinal damage/macular degeneration, retinopathy of prematurity, photic retinopathy, penetration of metal objects, other trauma, Eale's disease, pterygium, retinitis pigmentosa, uveitis, conjunctivitis
Skin	UV radiation, thermal injury, porphyria, hypericin and other photosensitizers, dermatitis, baldness, psoriasis, lichen sclerosus, leprosy, pseudoxanthoma elasticum, Smith–Lemli–Opitz syndrome[b]

Abbreviations: ARDS, acute respiratory distress syndrome; COPD, chronic obstructive pulmonary disease; NSAID, non-steroidal anti-inflammatory drug. Viral, bacterial and other parasitic infections can also cause oxidative stress.

[a] Affects brain, heart, skin and kidney (*Cancer Res.* **65**, 10881, 2005).

[b] Also affects the central nervous system.

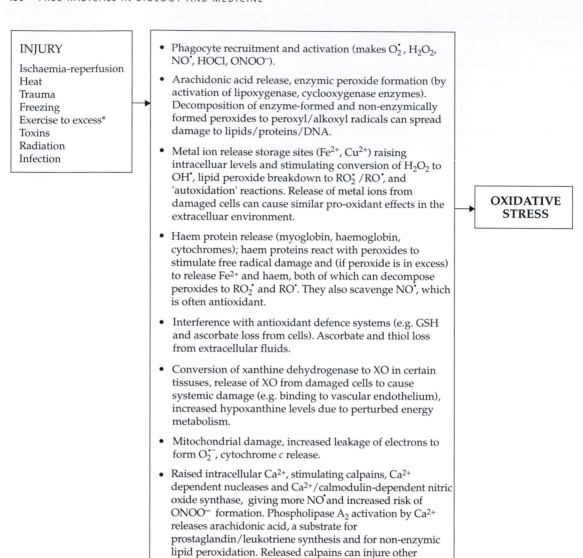

INJURY

Ischaemia-reperfusion
Heat
Trauma
Freezing
Exercise to excess*
Toxins
Radiation
Infection

- Phagocyte recruitment and activation (makes $O_2^{\bullet-}$, H_2O_2, $NO^{\bullet}$, HOCl, $ONOO^-$).

- Arachidonic acid release, enzymic peroxide formation (by activation of lipoxygenase, cyclooxygenase enzymes). Decomposition of enzyme-formed and non-enzymically formed peroxides to peroxyl/alkoxyl radicals can spread damage to lipids/proteins/DNA.

- Metal ion release storage sites (Fe^{2+}, Cu^{2+}) raising intracelluar levels and stimulating conversion of H_2O_2 to $OH^{\bullet}$, lipid peroxide breakdown to $RO_2^{\bullet}$/$RO^{\bullet}$, and 'autoxidation' reactions. Release of metal ions from damaged cells can cause similar pro-oxidant effects in the extracelluar environment.

- Haem protein release (myoglobin, haemoglobin, cytochromes); haem proteins react with peroxides to stimulate free radical damage and (if peroxide is in excess) to release Fe^{2+} and haem, both of which can decompose peroxides to $RO_2^{\bullet}$ and $RO^{\bullet}$. They also scavenge $NO^{\bullet}$, which is often antioxidant.

- Interference with antioxidant defence systems (e.g. GSH and ascorbate loss from cells). Ascorbate and thiol loss from extracellular fluids.

- Conversion of xanthine dehydrogenase to XO in certain tissues, release of XO from damaged cells to cause systemic damage (e.g. binding to vascular endothelium), increased hypoxanthine levels due to perturbed energy metabolism.

- Mitochondrial damage, increased leakage of electrons to form $O_2^{\bullet-}$, cytochrome c release.

- Raised intracellular Ca^{2+}, stimulating calpains, Ca^{2+} dependent nucleases and Ca^{2+}/calmodulin-dependent nitric oxide synthase, giving more $NO^{\bullet}$ and increased risk of $ONOO^-$ formation. Phospholipase A_2 activation by Ca^{2+} releases arachidonic acid, a substrate for prostaglandin/leukotriene synthesis and for non-enzymic lipid peroxidation. Released calpains can injure other cells/tissues.

OXIDATIVE STRESS

Figure 9.1 Some of the reasons why tissue injury causes oxidative stress. For example, merely placing a microdialysis probe in a muscle (Section 6.13.1) increased production of $OH^{\bullet}$ and $O_2^{\bullet-}$, and the system took at least 30 min for ROS production to return to 'normal' (*Free Rad. Biol. Med.* **39**, 1460, 2005). * To an extent that causes tissue damage/inflammation (Section 6.13).

be major players in tissue injury. For example, the increased lipid peroxidation demonstrated in the damaged muscles of patients with muscular dystrophy may be a consequence of the tissue damage, making little or no further contribution to damage. Hence antioxidants are not beneficial in this disease.[10] There is a plethora of papers measuring protein carbonyls, lipid peroxides etc. in samples from patients and showing elevations, with the assumption that such rises mean that oxidative damage is important. This is not to criticize the field unduly: exactly the same is true for the hundreds of papers that implicate $NO^{\bullet}$, prostaglandins, leukotrienes, cytokines etc. as major players just because

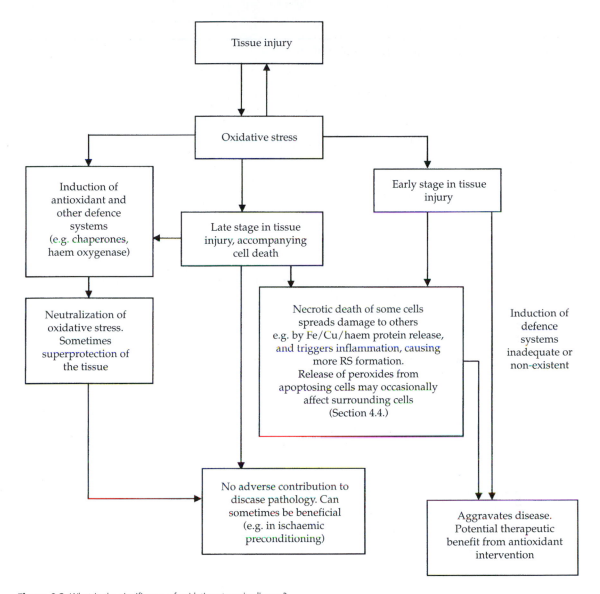

Figure 9.2 What is the significance of oxidative stress in disease?

the levels are up—the fact that there is more of something in a disease does not prove it is important.

Another factor to consider is how cells respond to oxidative stress (Fig. 9.2). In Section 4.2 we examined various types of response. Table 9.2 lists them again, with comments on how they are relevant to disease and how they can be both good and bad, depending on the circumstances.

9.2.1 Establishing importance

In order to show that RS are important in a particular disease, it is necessary to fulfil the criteria listed in Table 9.3, using appropriate traps and/or biomarkers (Fig. 9.3). Although oxidative stress may often be a secondary event, the appropriate use of such techniques has revealed that it does

Table 9.2 Cellular responses to oxidative stress in human diseases

Response (taken from Section 4.2)	Examples of possible effects	
	Good	**Bad**
Increased proliferation	Wound healing	Fibrosis
Upregulation of defences (chaperones, antioxidants, etc.)	Resistance to further injury (e.g. ischaemic preconditioning; Section 9.5.6 below), salvage of tissue	Persistence of abnormal cells (e.g. malignant cells, damaged cardiomyocytes with abnormal electrical activity predisposing to arrhythmias)
Upregulation of transcription factors (AP-1, NF-κB etc.; Section 4.5)	Phagocyte recruitment and activation, increased production of NO• and cytokines as defences against infection; increased synthesis of GSH or other antioxidants	Survival of unwanted cells Overproduction of NO•/cytokines/ROS (e.g. in chronic inflammation)
Necrotic cell death	Can 'trigger' the inflammatory response, signalling a problem and recruiting the resources to deal with it	Loss of essential cells (e.g. excitotoxicity in stroke; Section 9.17.2) Release of 'catalytic' metals etc. can aggravate damage and promote more inflammation
Apoptosis/senescence	Eliminates (or prevents division in the case of senescence) cells with excessive DNA damage, avoids malignancy	Loss of essential cells (e.g. in neurodegenerative disease) Release of peroxides from apoptosing cells (Fig. 9.2) Senescent cells can provide an 'environment' favouring malignancy (Section 10.3.5.1)

Table 9.3 Criteria for implicating reactive species (RS) as a significant mechanism of tissue injury in human disease

1. The RS (or the oxidative damage caused) should always be demonstrable at the site of injury.
2. The time-course of formation of the RS (or of the oxidative damage caused) must be consistent with the time-course of tissue injury, preceding or accompanying it.
3. Direct application of the RS over a relevant time course (point 2 above) to the tissue at concentrations within the range found *in vivo* should reproduce the tissue injury and oxidative damage observed.
4. Removing the RS or inhibiting its formation should diminish the tissue injury to an extent related to the degree of inhibition of the oxidative damage.

Point 4 is worth a further comment; the fact that an antioxidant diminishes tissue injury does not prove that RS are important, since many antioxidants exert additional biological effects (Section 10.6). One must measure the fall in oxidative damage and relate it to the protective effect. Vice versa, a number of drugs developed to target other mediators of injury may have antioxidant actions in addition (Section 10.6). Note that we could replace 'RS' in the above table by NO•, TNFα, IL-6 etc.; the same criteria have to be fulfilled to show the importance of any putative mediator of injury.

play a role in furthering tissue injury in several diseases. We have already considered the examples of porphyria (Section 2.6.4), α-tocopherol deficiency (Section 3.20.2), COPD (Section 8.12), hypertension (Section 7.10.3), drug-induced haemolytic disease (Section 6.5), cataract (Section 6.10), macular degeneration (Section 6.10.5) and malaria (Section 6.6.1). Other possible examples are retinopathy of prematurity (Section 1.5.3), Wilson's disease (Section 3.15.5.5) and haemochromatosis (Section 3.15.5.2).

Let us examine some other diseases in detail.

Antioxidant (AOX) depletion
Does not prove oxidative damage, only that the defence system is working

Total AOX potential, depletion of specific AOX, measurement of AOX-derived species, e.g. ascorbate radical, urate oxidation products)

Induction of AOX enzymes
Does not prove oxidative damage, only that the defence system is responding

Biomarkers of oxidative damege
Suggest that oxidative damage has occurred but rises in cell/tissue levels of biomarkers could reflect not only more damage but also less repair

Lipid

peroxides
cholesterol oxidation products
halogenated/nitrated lipids

MDA, HNE and other aldehydes
isoprostanes and related products

DNA

oxidized/nitrated/deaminated/chlorinated/brominated bases in cells and urine; aldehyde/DNA base adducts in cells and urine

Protein

–SH oxidation
carbonyl formation
aldehyde adducts
oxidized tyr, trp, his, met, lys, leu, ileu, val
nitrated/chlorinated/brominated tyrosine, trp, phe
protein peroxides/hydroxides

RS trapping
Spin traps
Aromatic probes (e.g. salicylate, phenylalanine), other detectors

RS formation does not equate to RS inportance. If RS are important and the traps are efficient, the traps should protect against tissue injury.

Figure 9.3 Some 'biomarkers' of oxidative stress or reactive species (RS) that can be used to study disease. There is a full discussion of biomarkers in Chapter 5; here we revisit the key points revisit to their application and to the interpretation of results.

9.3 Atherosclerosis

9.3.1 What is atherosclerosis?[11]

Cardiovascular disease is a major cause of death in the USA, Middle East, Europe, Singapore, India and increasingly in the rest of the world. Most heart attacks (**myocardial infarctions**) and many cases of localized cerebral ischaemia (**stroke**) are secondary to the condition of **atherosclerosis**, a disease of arteries that is characterized by a local thickening of the vessel wall that develops in the inner coat (**tunica intima**) (Fig. 9.4, Plate 16). The clinical effects of atherosclerosis are often evident in the coronary, carotid, femoral and iliac arteries and the aorta.

An early stage of atherosclerosis is the **fatty streak**. These are slightly raised, yellow, narrow, longitudinally lying areas. They are characterized by the presence of **foam cells** (Fig. 9.4), lipid-laden distorted cells that arise largely from macrophages, but sometimes from smooth muscle cells. Fatty streaks can develop into **fibrous plaques**, approximately round, raised lesions, usually off-white in colour and often a centimeter or so in diameter, slightly obstructing the vascular lumen. A typical fibrous plaque consists of a fibrous cap (composed mostly of smooth muscle cells and dense connective tissue containing collagen, elastin, proteoglycans and basement membranes) covering an area rich in macrophages, smooth

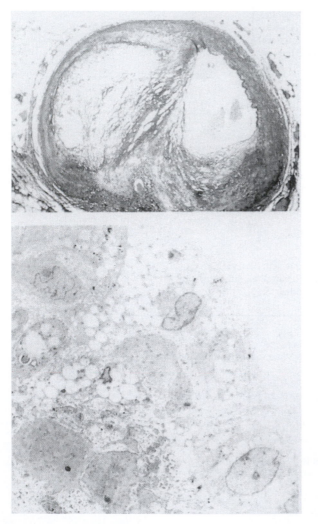

Figure 9.4 (see plate 16) Advanced atherosclerosis. Top: an atherosclerosed and thrombosed human coronary artery obtained during necropsy. Bottom: section through a lesion. Note the lipid-laden foam cells. By courtesy of Dr M.J. Mitchinson and the Upjohn Company.

muscle cells and T lymphocytes. Often there is a deeper necrotic core, which contains debris from dead cells, extracellular lipid deposits and cholesterol crystals. **Complicated plaques** are fibrous plaques that have been altered by necrosis, calcium deposition, bleeding and thrombosis.

Plaques can cause disease by limiting blood flow to a region of an organ such as the heart or brain. A stroke or myocardial infarction occurs when the lumen of an essential artery becomes completely occluded, usually by a thrombus forming at the site of a plaque. Thrombus formation is often triggered by plaque rupture, exposing noxious products such as tissue factor (Fig. 9.5a). Plaque disruption occurs most frequently where the fibrous cap is thinnest and most heavily infiltrated by foam cells;

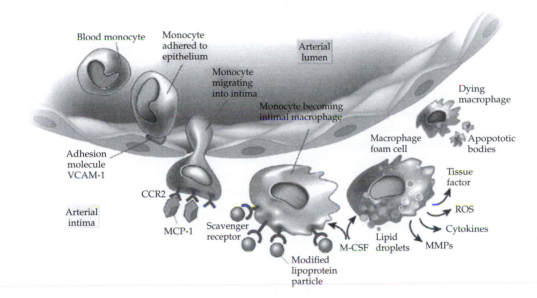

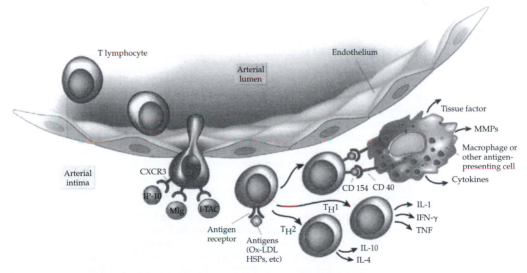

Figure 9.5 (a) Mononuclear phagocytes in atherogenesis. An outline of steps in the recruitment of mononuclear phagocytes to the nascent atherosclerotic plaque and their roles in the mature atheroma. The steps are depicted in an approximate time sequence proceeding from left to right. Normal arterial endothelium does not engage in prolonged contact with leukocytes, including the blood monocytes (Fig. 7.10).

macrophage-derived proteinases (e.g. collagenases, gelatinases, stromelysin, metalloelastase and matrilysin; Table 7.2) may be involved. Hence it is not only the presence of plaque that matters; its stability (tendency to rupture) is also a key factor.

9.3.2 Predictors of atherosclerosis[12]

Atherosclerosis is accelerated by homocysteine (Section 10.5.9), smoking (Section 8.12), diabetes (Section 9.4 below) and hypertension (Section 7.10.3), all conditions associated with oxidative stress and impairment of vascular endothelial function. Another important factor is inflammation; phagocyte recruitment occurs early in atherosclerosis development (Fig. 9.5) and inflammation also promotes thrombosis. Indeed, many authors now view atherosclerosis as a chronic inflammatory condition of the blood vessel wall. High blood levels of C-reactive protein (CRP) (Section 4.7.3) and of myeloperoxidase (MPO, Section 7.7.3) are associated with increased risk of cardiovascular events.[13,14] Indeed, CRP is present within plaque and may contribute to its development.[14]

Blood lipids also play a key role. In well-fed populations, atherosclerosis begins in the first decade of life. Fatty streaks can even be found in the foetus, to an extent increasing with maternal plasma cholesterol levels.[15] Section 3.20.2.6 explained the role of low-density lipoproteins (LDL) in fat metabolism; they are mostly produced from very-low-density lipoproteins (VLDL) in the circulation and are rich in cholesterol and its esters. LDL help to supply cholesterol, tocopherols and carotenoids to tissues by binding to cell surface receptors and being internalized.

In the disease **familial hypercholesterolaemia**, LDL receptors are defective or absent, so that blood LDL (and hence cholesterol) levels become very high. Atherosclerosis is accelerated, and myocardial infarctions can occur as early as 2 years of age. This observation focused attention on the role of cholesterol in promoting atherosclerosis. Indeed, later work showed that people with high blood LDL cholesterol develop atherosclerosis at an accelerated rate and that lowering elevated cholesterol levels (e.g. by blocking its synthesis by the liver using the **statin** family of drugs) decreases the incidence of myocardial infarction. One of the earliest responses induced by hypercholesterolaemia is increased levels of VCAM-1 in the endothelium, an adhesion molecule that promotes attachment of monocytes and lymphocytes (Fig. 9.5). Increased expression of genes encoding VCAM-1 may occur as a result of oxidized lipoprotein particles accumulating in the intima, acting to activate NF-κB and other

When endothelial cells undergo inflammatory activation, they increase their expression of adhesion molecules (Section 7.7.1). For monocyte recruitment, vascular cell adhesion molecule-1 (VCAM-1) has a major role. Once adherent to the activated endothelium, the monocyte moves between endothelial cells to penetrate into the tunica intima, the innermost layer of the arterial wall. This directed migration requires a chemoattractant gradient. Various chemokines participate, particularly interaction of monocyte chemoattractant protein-1 (MCP-1) with its receptor CCR2. Once resident in the intima, the monocyte acquires characteristics of the tissue macrophage. In the atheroma, the macrophage expresses scavenger receptors that bind internalized lipoprotein particles modified by oxidation (or glycation). These processes give rise to the foam cell, a hallmark of the arterial lesion (Fig. 9.4). Within the arterial intima, the macrophage is a key player in atherosclerosis and its complications. Foam cells secrete both RS and pro-inflammatory cytokines that amplify the local inflammatory response in the lesion. The activated mononuclear phagocyte has a key role in the thrombotic complications of atherosclerosis by producing matrix metalloproteinases (MMPs), which can degrade the extracellular matrix that lends strength to the plaque's fibrous cap. When the plaque ruptures as a consequence, it permits the blood to contact another macrophage product, the potent procoagulant protein **tissue factor**. Many macrophages congregate in a central core in the typical atherosclerotic plaque. Macrophages can die in this location, some by apoptosis, hence producing the 'necrotic core' of the atherosclerotic lesion. (b) The roles of T lymphocytes in atherogenesis. Similarly to monocytes, lymphocytes enter the intima facilitated by binding to adhesion molecules, including VCAM-1, in response to chemoattractants selective for lymphocytes. Known chemoattractants include a trio of interferon-γ (IFN-γ)-inducible chemokines of the CXC family including inducible protein-10 (IP-10), monokine induced by IFN-γ (Mig), and IFN-inducible T-cell α-chemoattractant (I-TAC). These chemokines bind to chemokine receptor CXCR3 expressed by T cells in the atherosclerotic lesion. Once resident in the arterial intima, the T cell may encounter antigens such as oxidized LDL (Ox-LDL) and heat-shock proteins (Hsps) of endogenous or microbial origin. Upon activation by engagement of the receptor with antigen, the T cell can produce cytokines that influence the behaviour of other cells present in the atheroma. Production of these mediators provides an amplification loop resulting from crosstalk between the cell of acquired immunity (the T lymphocyte) and the mononuclear phagocyte. Within the atheroma, as in other tissues, the helper T cells can polarize into those secreting generally proinflammatory cytokines (known as T_H1 cells) and those secreting predominantly anti-inflammatory cytokines (denoted T_H2 cells). Adapted from *Nature* **420**, 868, 2002 by courtesy of Dr Peter Libby and Elsevier.

transcription factors in the endothelial cell. In other words, LDL oxidation promotes monocyte recruitment, which then accelerates LDL oxidation (Section 9.3.4 below). As body cells receive the cholesterol they need, they down-regulate expression of LDL receptors, and LDL stays for a longer time in the circulation. In hypercholesterolaemia, LDL levels are higher and the LDL may be 'older' on average, perhaps facilitating its oxidation.[16]

Low-density lipoproteins enter the arterial wall both by transport in vesicles through endothelial cells, and by diffusion through the intercellular matrix. The amount entering depends on both the plasma LDL level and the arterial wall permeability, so that endothelial injury by any mechanism (including oxidative damage) facilitates LDL entry. Entered LDL bind to proteoglycans in the wall, promoting their retention. If they undergo oxidation/aggregation (see below), retention is further promoted. Smoking (probably at least partly via oxidative stress), and genetic predisposition to 'permeable' vessel walls, may also increase LDL penetration.

Other errors in fat metabolism also predispose to atherosclerosis, an example being **type III hyperlipoproteinaemia**. Plasma levels of cholesterol and triglyceride are markedly elevated. The disease is associated with defects in **apolipoprotein E** (apoE) or in receptors for it. Apolipoprotein E is a component of chylomicrons and VLDL and functions as a ligand for uptake of 'remnant particles', derived from VLDL and chylomicrons, by the liver (Section 3.20.2.6). In humans there are three common isoforms of apoE: apoE3, apoE2 and apoE4 (also see Section 9.20.2 below). They differ from each other by single amino-acid substitutions at residues 112 and 158 in the protein. The apoE2 form, with cysteine residues at both positions, is associated with impaired binding to the apoE receptors. Transgenic 'knockout' mice lacking apoE show accelerated atherosclerosis on a normal diet (even faster on a high-cholesterol diet), and are frequently used as a model of human atherosclerosis.

9.3.3 What initiates atherosclerosis?[11,12]

Atherosclerosis begins with impairment of the function of the vascular endothelium. In the average human adult, the vascular endothelium consists of over 10^{13} cells and weighs about 1 kg.[17] Damaging events include infection of the vessel wall (herpes viruses, cytomegalovirus and *Chlamydia* are among the agents implicated), and exposure to blood-borne toxins, including both xenobiotics (e.g. from cigarette smoke) and elevated levels of normal metabolites, such as glucose, LDL or homocysteine. Mechanical damage can also occur. For example, endothelial damage by turbulent blood flow at bifurcations in the arteries can be worsened by high blood pressure and sites of such 'flow stress' are particularly prone to atherosclerosis.[18] Flow stress is not always bad—it can increase levels of eNOS and antioxidant defence enzymes, a process that may be an adaptation triggered by ROS production (Table 4.7 points 12 and 13 and ref[18]) and can contribute to the cardiovascular benefits of regular exercise. It's the usual redox balance—some ROS are good, but too many, as in hypertension (Section 7.10.3), end up causing endothelial damage.

Endothelial injury allows more LDL to enter the vessel wall, and is soon followed by attachment of monocytes from the circulation, which enter the vessel wall and develop into macrophages. Monocyte recruitment is facilitated by increased expression of VCAM-1 and other adhesion molecules, and by **monocyte chemoattractant protein 1, MCP-1** (Fig. 9.5). Macrophages in the vessel wall secrete cytokines that can amplify a local inflammatory response, and matrix metalloproteinases that can damage the fibrous cap and weaken the plaque. Lymphocytes also enter the vessel wall by binding to adhesion molecules such as VCAM-1, being attracted by cytokines. Once there, lymphocytes can respond to antigens (e.g. from bacteria and viruses), to produce antibodies. They produce cytokines that 'cross-talk' with macrophages (Fig. 9.5b).

9.3.4 LDL oxidation and the foam cell[12]

The LDL entering the vessel wall undergoes oxidation (exactly how we will consider shortly). Macrophages possess some receptors for 'normal' LDL, but LDL that has undergone lipid peroxidation is recognized by different receptors. These were first identified as receptors that bound chemically acetylated LDL (the **acetyl-LDL receptors**), but are now usually called the **scavenger receptors**. Major ones are **scavenger receptors A (SRA**; at least five types) and **CD36**, a member of the **class B family** of scavenger receptors. The A and B class scavenger receptors recognize specific classes of lipid oxidation products. For example CD36 recognizes oxidized phosphatidylcholine residues that have a carbonyl residue on the fatty acid at position 2 of the glycerol backbone.[19] Uptake of oxidized LDL causes cholesteryl esters to accumulate in droplets in the macrophage cytoplasm, and eventually the foam cell results. A key factor promoting the transition of monocytes to macrophages and foam cells is **macrophage colony-stimulating factor, MCSF**, which increases SRA expression and cytokine production. Foam cells show increased expression of genes encoding MCP-1, matrix metalloproteinases, several cytokines and 15-lipoxygenase (Section 9.3.5.3 below).

Although uptake of oxidized LDL by macrophages might be regarded as a 'defence mechanism' to protect the vascular wall, it imposes an oxidative stress on the macrophage, for example causing it to synthesize more chaperones and to raise intracellular GSH levels.[20] Eventually, some foam cells succumb to the oxidation load, poisoning themselves with ingested oxidized lipids and dying by apoptosis or necrosis (Fig. 9.5), forming the 'necrotic core' of advanced atherosclerotic lesions.

Oxidized LDL is important not only because it can produce foam cells.[12] Depending on its degree of oxidation, LDL can be chemotactic for monocytes and T-cells, mitogenic for smooth muscle cells and macrophages, accelerate production of VCAM-1, MCP-1 and MCSF by endothelial and smooth muscle cells, and activate redox-sensitive transcription factors such as NF-κB. As with other ROS (Section 4.5.8), NF-κB shows a biphasic response; although low levels of oxidized LDL can lead to activation, high levels might suppress binding of the activated transcription factor to DNA.[21] Indeed, LDL in the early stages of oxidation (so-called **minimally modified LDL**) may be the most damaging; once it has oxidized further, it is recognized by the macrophage scavenger receptors, taken up by these cells and removed from contact with other cells in the vessel wall. For example, exposure of vascular endothelial cells in

culture to oxidized LDL increases expression of a $O_2^{\bullet-}$-producing NADPH oxidase, ICAM-1, VCAM-1 and cytokines via NF-κB. This is because endothelial cells can take up oxidized LDL via a receptor (**LOX-1; lectin-like oxidized LDL receptor-1**) different from the 'scavenger-receptors' on macrophages.[19,22,23] Indeed, activated NF-κB can be detected in smooth muscle cells, macrophages and endothelial cells within atherosclerotic lesions, but not usually in normal vessel wall.[22] Peroxides can accelerate cyclooxygenase- and lipoxygenase-catalysed reactions in endothelium, phagocytes, and in any platelets present, leading to enhanced formation of eicosanoids (Section 7.12.4). The expression of the endothelial receptor is increased by hypertension, diabetes and hypercholesterolaemia and levels are elevated in atherosclerotic lesions. Cyclooxygenase-2 (Section 7.12.23) is present in human atherosclerotic lesions, and PGE_2 may increase metalloproteinase expression in macrophages.[24] F_2-isoprostanes generated from arachidonic acid residues in LDL[25] could also contribute to dysfunction of the vessel wall, for example by promoting vasoconstriction or platelet aggregation (Section 4.12.3). By contrast, prostacyclin could help protect the endothelium.

Excess uptake of oxidized LDL by endothelial cells can injure or kill them (often by triggering apoptosis), so disrupting the endothelium. A counterbalancing factor may be the **peroxisome proliferator-activated receptor-γ (PPARγ)**, so-called because it is activated by peroxisome proliferator drugs (Section 9.14.2.1 below). This receptor is a transcription factor essential in animals for the development of adipose tissue and for correct glucose homoeostasis, and is the target of several drugs (the **thiazolidinediones**) that decrease tissue insulin resistance in type 2 diabetes. The receptor is highly expressed in foam cells in atherosclerotic lesions; ligands to PPARγ decrease atherosclerosis in LDL-receptor-deficient mice, suggesting that PPARγ activation has some antiatherosclerotic effect.[26] Constituents of oxidized LDL can activate this receptor, which would presumably be a beneficial effect *in vivo*.[27] Other members of the PPAR family, such as PPARα might also be involved.[26] Thus oxidized lipids might do good things and bad things in the vessel wall. Which is most important?

The **oxidative modification hypothesis** introduced by Steinberg et al[12] states that LDL oxidation is a key contributor to the development of atherosclerosis, i.e. that overall the oxidation products are bad. Before reviewing the evidence for and against this concept, let us ask how LDL might be oxidized in the vessel wall.

9.3.5 Mechanisms of LDL oxidation

Activated monocytes and macrophages produce $O_2^{\bullet-}$, H_2O_2, and possibly $NO^{\bullet}$. Other sources of ROS in the vessel wall include mitochondria, COX and lipoxygenase enzymes, NADPH oxidases (Section 7.10.3) and XO. The last binds readily to vascular endothelium and is present in human atherosclerotic lesions.[28] 'Uncoupled' eNOS (Table 1.4) can make ROS as well.

However, $O_2^{\bullet-}$, H_2O_2 or $NO^{\bullet}$ cannot oxidize LDL. Indeed, $NO^{\bullet}$ tends to inhibit LDL peroxidation, by scavenging peroxyl radicals (Section 2.5.6.2), and is generally thought to be antiatherosclerotic.[29] Nitric oxide also deters thrombosis, phagocyte adhesion to endothelium and NF-κB activation. Endothelial $NO^{\bullet}$ production in atherosclerotic lesions appears subnormal, perhaps due to its consumption by $O_2^{\bullet-}$ and to interference with eNOS activity by oxidized LDL.[30] Although iNOS is present in phagocytes and smooth muscle cells in atherosclerotic lesions, it is uncertain whether its overall effect is good (raising $NO^{\bullet}$ levels) or bad (raising $NO^{\bullet}$ to the extent that $ONOO^-$ is formed). For example, in the apo-E knockout mouse (Section 9.3.2), additional knockout of iNOS decreased the atherosclerosis produced by a high cholesterol diet, that is the $NO^{\bullet}$ seemed bad.[31] This is just one model of course, and mice are not men, although some men behave like them. Another factor to consider is that levels of the 'natural' NOS inhibitor ADMA (Section 2.5.6) can be elevated in atherosclerotic humans.[32]

9.3.5.1 *Metal ions*
Macrophages, vascular endothelial cells, smooth muscle cells and lymphocytes cause peroxidation of LDL when incubated with it *in vitro*. LDL oxidation by all these cell types *in vitro* requires traces of iron or copper ions, and is stimulated by certain thiol compounds. Is this an artefact of cell culture (Section 1.11) or physiologically relevant? Injury to vascular endothelium *in vivo* might liberate 'catalytic' metal ions (Fig. 9.1) and caeruloplasmin entering the vessel wall could conceivably degrade to release copper.[28] This protein breaks down at low pH and when exposed to proteinases or $ONOO^-$. Peroxides in LDL might release iron from haem proteins. Indeed, 'catalytic' metal ions have been detected in advanced human atherosclerotic lesions and can also be released by injury of normal vessel wall.[33] Administered copper ions are proatherosclerotic in some animal models.[34] Metal ions could accelerate lipid oxidation by promoting $OH^{\bullet}$ formation and/or by decomposing lipid peroxides to peroxyl and alkoxyl radicals; haem also facilitates peroxide decomposition. Even 'normal' circulating LDL may contain traces of peroxides (Section 9.3.8 below). In addition, the intact caeruloplasmin molecule might be able to oxidize LDL (Section 3.15.2). Thus rises in caeruloplasmin levels in the acute-phase response could contribute to the proatherogenic effects of inflammation. However, could free copper ions persist in the vessel wall? Albumin and many other proteins avidly bind copper ions and decrease their pro-oxidant effect (Section 3.16.3.5), as do negatively charged proteoglycans. Indeed, LDL bound to glycosaminoglycans are resistant[35] to oxidation by Cu^{2+}.

Haem oxygenase (HO-1) in lesions is a potential source of iron,[36] but haem is itself a powerful pro-oxidant for LDL,[37] so the overall effect of HO-1 could be antiatherosclerotic. Indeed, inhibition of HO-1 in rabbits accelerated atherosclerosis development,[38] although the CO produced by HO-1 might play some role in this (Section 3.17). Studies on developing atherosclerotic lesions in cholesterol-fed rabbits showed them to be enriched in iron (but *not* in copper), and decreasing this accumulation by using desferrioxamine (or venesection) delayed the appearance of atherosclerosis.[39] Several groups have attempted to correlate human body iron stores with extent of atherosclerosis, but the data are inconclusive (Section 10.4.10). This may be because stored iron (e.g. in ferritin, whose levels are generally increased in atherosclerotic lesions)[40] is generally not very pro-oxidant, if at all (Section 3.16.3.3); only 'catalytic' iron matters.

So where are we? Limited evidence suggests that haem and iron ions are proatherosclerotic *in vivo*, whereas evidence for a role of copper ions or caeruloplasmin is even more limited.

9.3.5.2 *Reactive nitrogen and chlorine species*[13]

Peroxynitrite readily oxidizes LDL.[41] Another role for RNS may be in the nitration of fibrinogen, a process which accelerates thrombus formation. Indeed, plasma levels of nitrated fibrinogen are increased in patients with coronary artery disease (Section 2.6.1). Hypochlorous acid produced by MPO can deplete antioxidants (especially ascorbate and thiols) and attack LDL directly. It oxidizes apoprotein B, especially on cysteine, forms chloramines from $-NH_2$ groups on LDL protein and lipid, and converts PUFA side-chains and cholesterol into chlorohydrins and chlorinated sterols (Section 7.7.3). Plasmalogens in LDL (Section 4.12.8) are particularly sensitive to oxidation by HOCl, generating chlorinated aldehydes, some of which might injure endothelial cells.[42] Myeloperoxidase can additionally oxidize LDL by converting tyrosine into tyrosyl radicals, which can initiate LDL peroxidation. Hypochlorous acid-treated LDL are recognized by macrophage scavenger receptors and promote platelet aggregation, perhaps contributing to thrombus formation after plaque rupture.[43] Myeloperoxidase binds tightly to the basement membranes of vascular endothelial cells and, in the presence of H_2O_2, can catalyse $NO^{\bullet}$ depletion, $NO_2^{\bullet}$ formation and protein nitration (Section 7.9.4). It has been claimed that subjects with a polymorphism in the promoter region of the MPO gene that leads to decreased activity show a lower incidence of heart disease.[13]

But hold on for a minute; LDL receptor-deficient mice that also lack MPO are *not* protected against atherosclerosis—in fact it is increased.[44] Knockout of EC-SOD failed to accelerate atherosclerosis in apoE-deficient mice, suggesting limited importance for $O_2^{\bullet-}$ and $ONOO^-$ in this model.[45] However, ROS, RNS and RCS do form in human atherosclerotic lesions, as evidenced by elevated levels of such biomarkers as bityrosine, 3-chlorotyrosine, 5-chlorouracil, chloro-aldehydes, 3-nitrotyrosine, *ortho*- and *meta*-tyrosine (putative biomarkers of $OH^{\bullet}$ generation; Section 5.3.1) and other amino acid oxidation products.[46,47] Nitrated γ-tocopherol has also been observed (Section 3.20.2.7). Nitrotyrosine could arise from $ONOO^-$ and/or from MPO-dependent reactions. One important target of nitration/chlorination in atherosclerosis may be apolipoprotein A-1 (Section 9.3.9 below).

9.3.5.3 *Lipoxygenases*[48]

Dual specificity 12/15-lipoxygenases (LOX) that can directly oxidize cholesterol and fatty acid side-chains in LDL have been detected in animal atherosclerotic lesions. Peroxide decomposition to radicals can then cause further (non-enzymic) peroxidation. Knockout of 12-/15- LOX in apo-E null mice decreased atherosclerosis on a high cholesterol diet, and inhibition of 15-LOX in rabbits by an (allegedly) specific inhibitor lacking antioxidant properties (**PD146176**), also decreased atherosclerosis.[49] The importance of LOX enzymes to human atherosclerosis is uncertain, and do remember that mice, rabbits and humans have different types of LOX (Section 7.12). Analysis of stereospecificity suggests that lipid oxidation products in human lesions do not arise enzymically,[50] although this does not rule out a 'seeding' role for lipoxygenases in LDL oxidation (i.e. they start it and it then continues non-enzymically). Lipoxygenases, especially 5-LOX (which has been detected in human atherosclerotic lesions), might also contribute to atherosclerosis by synthesizing leukotrienes that worsen the 'inflammatory state' of the vessel wall.

9.3.5.4 *Summing it up: which pro-oxidant(s) oxidize LDL in vivo?*

The extents of elevation of biomarkers of oxidative/ nitrative/ chlorinative damage in atherosclerotic lesions are variable between laboratories. We cannot say at the moment which species (metals, $ONOO^-$, other RNS, HOCl, LOX) is the most important initiator of LDL oxidation *in vivo*. In fact, given the complexity of lesions, they could all be important in different regions and/or at different stages of the lesion. Indeed, it is possible that no two lesions have exactly the same pattern of oxidative damage. For example, in diabetes-induced atherosclerosis, $OH^{\bullet}$ may be more important than HOCl or $ONOO^-$ (Section 9.4.6 below).

Remember also that the presence of LOX or bio-markers of oxidation, nitration and chlorination is not evidence that these processes are important. Nevertheless, it is intriguing that plasma 3-nitro-tyrosine levels are increased in subjects with coronary artery disease, and drop when patients are given statins to lower cholesterol.[51] It is further possible that atherosclerosis development in mice is more dependent on LOX and less so on MPO than in humans.[44] Indeed, MPO is much more abundant in human atherosclerotic lesions than in mouse ones. This means that murine models are of limited relevance to the human situation.

9.3.6 Other aspects of the involvement of RS in atherosclerosis

Reactive species have been proposed to play a role in the proatherogenic effects of homocysteine (Section 10.5.9). Matrix metalloproteinases can be activated by HOCl and other RS (Table 7.2), which could contribute to plaque rupture. Products of LDL oxidation are procoagulant[52] and may play some role in promoting calcification in advanced lesions.[53] Oxidation products of cholesterol (COPs) might be involved in atherosclerosis, since cholesterol is oxidized to multiple products in peroxidizing LDL. Indeed, cholesterol ester peroxides and hydroxides (the latter presumably reduction products of the peroxides) are present in advanced human lesions[54] and levels are elevated in the plasma of patients with coronary artery disease.[55] Some COPs are toxic to arterial smooth muscle cells, vascular endothelium and monocyte/macrophages in culture. The significance of this *in vivo* is uncertain, since mixtures of oxidation products resembling those found in lesions do not seem especially cytotoxic.[56]

9.3.7 Does evidence support the 'oxidative modification hypothesis' of atherosclerosis?

This hypothesis states that oxidation of LDL in vessel walls is a significant contributor to atherosclerosis development. Doubt has been cast on this concept recently by the failure of several intervention trials with antioxidants to affect the development of cardiovascular disease. However, this does not mean that the hypothesis is wrong (discussed in Section 10.5). Oxidation of LDL mostly occurs in the microenvironment of the blood vessel wall and not in the circulating blood. Nevertheless, several reports suggest that plasma LDL isolated from people with extensive atherosclerosis shows a mild degree of oxidation[52,57] and that the plasma level of oxLDL may predict cardiovascular events. Of course, some oxidized LDL might escape from the vessel wall back into the circulation. Consider also that the LDL from such patients might have lower antioxidant levels and tend to undergo more artefactual peroxidation during isolation (Section 9.3.8 below). Oxidized LDL is, in any case, rapidly cleared from the circulation, mostly by uptake by hepatic endothelial and Kupffer cells using scavenger receptors.[58]

What do we know? First, oxidized lipid is present in human and other animal atherosclerotic lesions; it has been detected as COPs, linoleic and arachidonic acid peroxides and hydroxides, F_2-IPs, and decomposition products of lipid peroxides (such as 4-HNE and MDA).[59] Lipid oxidation occurs despite the fact that the lesions contain α-tocopherol.[59] Increased oxidative protein and DNA damage, the latter usually measured as 8OHdG, is also observed in endothelial and smooth muscle cells and macrophages in atherosclerotic lesions,[60] but its significance is unclear. It may be another reflection of the fact that RS production and uptake of oxidized LDL place cells under oxidative stress.

Second, antibodies (some or all presumably produced by lymphocytes in the lesion; Fig. 9.5) that recognize oxidized LDL are found in plasma from patients with coronary artery disease. The antibodies recognize a range of epitopes, including aldehydes and specific oxidized lipids present in oxidized LDL.[61] The plasma antibody titre has been reported in some (but not all) studies to correlate with progression of atherosclerosis of the carotid arteries (as measured by ultrasound techniques).[62] Does production of such antibodies affects the progression of human atherosclerosis? The possibility that it could is suggested by animal experiments; immunization of mice or rabbits lacking LDL receptors with MDA-treated LDL led to high plasma antibody levels, and less atherosclerosis.[63] Similarly, antibodies recognizing oxidized mouse

LDL decreased atherosclerosis in LDL receptor-deficient mice.[61]

The third line of evidence often quoted to support the theory is that several antioxidants decrease the extent and/or progression rate of atherosclerosis in animals. One of the most effective is **probucol** (Fig. 9.6), but α-tocopherol, lazaroids (Section 10.6.8), flavonoids and flavonoid-rich plant extracts have sometimes worked in animals. Probucol was initially introduced as a drug to lower blood cholesterol levels, but it is also a chain-breaking antioxidant. Its major metabolite in rabbits, a *bis*-phenol (Fig. 9.6), is also an antioxidant. The antiatherogenic effect of probucol in rabbits is greater than expected from its cholesterol-lowering ability, an observation initially taken to suggest that its antioxidant activity might contribute. Similarly, butylated hydroxytoluene (BHT), has been shown to be antiatherosclerotic in some animal studies, despite the fact that high-dose BHT raises plasma lipid levels in animals.[64]

However, never assume that 'antioxidants' are working as such without measuring biomarkers of oxidative damage to prove it. Thus in rabbits, *bis*-phenol administration decreased lipid oxidation in the lesions but *not* the development of atherosclerosis, whereas probucol slowed both. Hence probucol's actions are not necessarily mediated by inhibiting lipid peroxidation.[65] Probucol may exert additional effects (e.g. HO-1 induction) dependent on its disulphur structure,[66] which is lacking in the *bis*-phenol metabolite. In apoE-knockout mice, a mixture of polyphenols extracted from red wine decreased atherosclerosis but *not* the levels of F_2-IPs in lesions or plasma, again suggestive of an antiatherosclerotic effect other than inhibiting lipid peroxidation.[67] In fact, a more effective 'antioxidant' approach may be

to lower elevated plasma cholesterol using statins.[12,13] Hypercholesterolaemic patients show elevated plasma F_2-IPs (even when corrected for their higher lipids). Levels drop after statin treatment, as do plasma levels of chloro-, nitro- and bityrosines.[13,51] Statins might also decrease the activity of endothelial NOX and the expression of adhesion molecules on the endothelial surface,[68] as well as increase eNOS levels.[30]

To summarize, the oxidation hypothesis, as originally formulated, is in doubt; if one can inhibit lipid oxidation but not lesion progression this argues against a key role of the former in the latter. Nevertheless, overexpression of catalase (but not CuZnSOD) in apoE-deficient mice substantially decreased the extent of atherosclerosis,[69] implying a role of H_2O_2. In addition, administration of α-tocopherol to apo-E deficient mice decreased *both* F_2-IP levels *and* the development of atherosclerosis,[70] whereas effects of α-tocopherol against atherosclerosis in other animals (including us!) have been much less clear-cut or absent. Relevant factors include the basal α-tocopherol content of the animals' diet, whether the α-tocopherol actually inhibited peroxidation in the test animal (it often does not) and finally whether its administration had an effect on plasma lipid levels, as observed in some studies. Of course, 'lack of importance of lipid oxidation', even if confirmed, does not equate to 'lack of importance of RS'; they do many things in atherosclerotic lesions.

9.3.8 Chemistry of LDL oxidation: is *in vitro* LDL oxidation a relevant model?

One prediction of the oxidation hypothesis is that the lower the resistance of LDL to oxidation, the greater the chance that it will become oxidized in the vessel

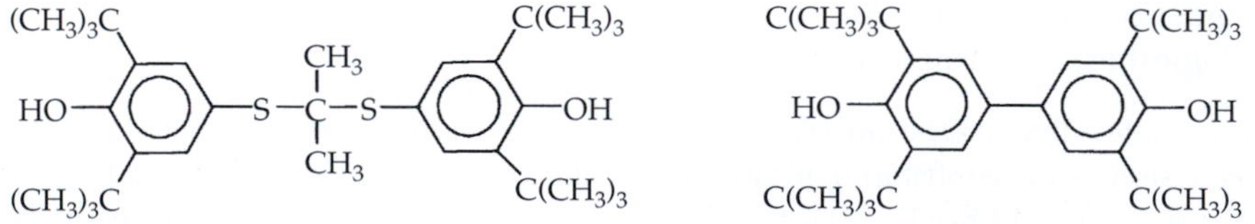

Figure 9.6 Structure of probucol, 4,4′–[(1–methylethylidene)–bis(thio)]bis–[2,6–bis(1,1–dimethylethyl)phenol], (*left*) and one of its metabolites, *bis*-phenol (*right*). The phenolic –OH groups confer chain breaking antioxidant activity. **AGI1067** is a succinate ester of probucol that has also been used as an antiatherosclerotic agent in humans (*Drugs Future* **28**, 421, 2003).

walls and contribute to the atherosclerosis. Hence it has become very popular to examine the sensitivity of LDL to oxidation *in vitro* and how this is altered by administration of antioxidants to animals or human volunteers prior to LDL isolation.[71] What do these studies tell us?

Most often, LDL is isolated from plasma by a process involving lengthy centrifugations. It is usually oxidized by incubation with Cu^{2+}, for example as copper(III) sulphate, $CuSO_4$. Many investigators measure the **lag phase** or **lag period**, the time taken before peroxidation of the Cu^{2+}-exposed LDL begins to accelerate. Other parameters measured include the slope of the 'acceleration' phase and levels of oxidation products (Fig. 9.7). Factors affecting LDL resistance to oxidation *in vivo* include:

1. Fatty acid composition; a greater proportion of saturated and monounsaturated fatty-acid side-chains increases oxidation resistance. For example, LDL isolated from humans or other animals fed on diets enriched in oleic acid were more resistant to oxidation *in vitro*. The reverse is true on feeding diets[73] containing a lot of PUFAs.

2. The concentration of Cu^{2+}. For Cu^{2+} concentrations in the μM range the lag phase decreases with

Cu^{2+} concentration up to a maximum. The 'active' Cu^{2+} is that which binds to histidine residues on apoprotein B.[74] At very low Cu^{2+} concentrations (up to 0.1 μM) the kinetics can change (Fig. 9.6) and the lag period may not be seen.[72]

3. The O_2 concentration.[75] Incubations are usually carried out under ambient O_2 (21%), whereas pO_2 in blood vessel walls may be as low as 2.5% O_2. At lower pO_2, the rate of LDL peroxidation is lower. Oxygen levels can fall rapidly in *in vitro* studies of LDL oxidation, but are rarely monitored.[76]

4. The content of antioxidants. Dietary supplementation with antioxidants that intercept lipid peroxyl radicals, such as α-tocopherol or probucol, usually increases the length of the lag phase in LDL subsequently isolated from the plasma.

5. The lipid peroxide content of the LDL particle. Copper ions appear to act largely or entirely by decomposing peroxides in the LDL to chain-propagating radicals[77]

$$LOOH + Cu^{2+} \rightarrow LO_2^{\bullet} + Cu^{+} + H^{+}$$

$$LOOH + Cu^{+} \rightarrow LO^{\bullet} + Cu^{2+} + OH^{-}$$

$$Cu^{2+} + LOOH \rightarrow LO^{\bullet} + Cu(III) + OH^{-}$$

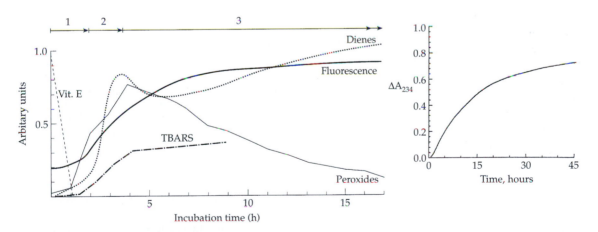

Figure 9.7 Sequence of events during copper ion-stimulated oxidation of LDL *in vitro*. Usually, α-tocopherol is first consumed and the 'peroxide pool' is filled, whereupon peroxidation accelerates. Peroxidation can be measured as formation of conjugated dienes at 234 nm, fluorescence at 430 nm with excitation at 360 nm, formation of lipid hydroperoxides, isoprostanes, COPs or production of thiobarbituric acid-reactive material (TBARS), although TBARS formation is not a good index of LDL oxidation. Period 1(top) is the lag phase, period 2 is the propagation phase. In phase 3, peroxides decompose to aldehydes and other products. Data provided by courtesy of the late Professor Dr Hermann Esterbauer. These kinetics are seen at μM Cu^{2+} concentrations, but they can be altered at lower Cu^{2+} levels[72]—see the Figure on the right. Here 0.03 μM Cu^{2+} was used; note the slower oxidation but the absence of a lag period.

Peroxide decomposition forms multiple carbonyl compounds, including MDA and HNE, which can modify apoB, as can $LO^\bullet$ and $LO_2^\bullet$ radicals. Modification of apoB can change the mobility of LDL on electrophoretic gels, sometimes used as an index of oxidation.

6. The assay used to measure LDL peroxidation. As expected from the complexity of peroxidation, different assays give different results (Fig. 9.7) and it is customary to use at least two different assay methods to measure LDL oxidation.

9.3.8.1 *The role of 'seeding peroxides'*

In general, the larger the peroxide content in LDL, the greater is the rate of Cu^{2+}-stimulated oxidation. Levels of peroxides in LDL isolated from different individuals vary a lot. Where do they come from? There are several possibilities:

1. Some may be artefactually introduced by *in vitro* peroxidation during the prolonged centrifugation procedures used to isolate LDL.
2. Some may arise from peroxides in dietary fats (Section 6.2). The extent of absorption of peroxidized lipids from the diet has been investigated in several laboratories, with conflicting answers. The gut is effective at detoxifying lipid peroxides (Section 6.2), but small amounts probably get through as a component of chylomicrons, especially if a diet rich in cooked fatty foods is consumed.[78] The major PUFA in oils used for human nutrition (e.g. sunflower and soya) is linoleate, which can be oxidized to 9- and 13-hydroperoxides. Arachidonate from meats gives a more complex mixture of peroxides, and even more complex mixtures result from peroxidation of dietary EPA and DHA.
3. Some peroxides can form in LDL *in vivo* due to its oxidation by RS and/or lipoxygenases, either as the LDL circulates in the blood or within the vessel wall, followed by its escape back into the circulation.
4. Cell membranes might transfer peroxides into LDL passing by them in the blood.[79]

9.3.8.2 *Antioxidants and LDL oxidation*[71]

An LDL particle is approximately spherical with a diameter of 19 to 25 nm and a relative molecular mass between 1.8 and 2.8 million. It contains, on average,

about 600 molecules of cholesterol, 1600 molecules of cholesterol ester (mostly cholesterol linoleate) and 170 molecules of triglyceride within a hydrophobic core (Table 9.4). In order to allow these insoluble lipids to travel in an aqueous solution (the blood plasma), the core is wrapped in a monolayer containing about 700 phospholipid molecules, mainly phosphatidylcholine, with their polar head groups oriented toward the aqueous phase. Apoprotein B is embedded in this outer layer. Antioxidants are present in both core and phospholipid coat, the most abundant being α-tocopherol (Table 9.4).

During the lag period, α-tocopherol is lost, as are several other constituents (Fig. 9.8). The length of the lag period depends on several factors, including the natural lag period of autocatalytic lipid peroxidation (Section 4.11), the 'seeding peroxide' content of LDL, and the inhibitory effect of α-tocopherol, plus some contribution from other antioxidants. Tocopherols react much faster with peroxyl radicals than do PUFAs (Section 3.20.2)

$$TocH + LO_2^\bullet \rightarrow Toc^\bullet + LO_2H$$

The tocopheryl radical ($Toc^\bullet$) has a weak capacity to abstract hydrogen from PUFAs, but is far less reactive than $LO_2^\bullet$ radicals. Indeed, if LDL is isolated from subjects who have consumed α-tocopherol supplements, the lag period after Cu^{2+} exposure of the LDL is significantly increased. For example, in subjects consuming *RRR*-α-tocopherol for 21 days, the oxidation resistance of LDL isolated from their plasma increased, on average, to 118%, 156%, 135% and 175% of control for doses of 150, 225, 800 or 1200 IU/day, respectively (1 IU = 0.67 mg *RRR*-α-tocopherol). Six days after the α-tocopherol supplements were stopped, LDL resistance to Cu^{2+}-mediated oxidation, and its α-tocopherol content, had returned to normal.

Tocopheryl radicals can be recycled to TocH if ascorbate is added to the LDL suspension

$$Toc^\bullet + ascorbate \rightarrow TocH + semidehydroascorbate$$

Added ascorbate delays the onset of LDL peroxidation even when it is started by adding Cu^{2+}, an apparent exception to the general rule that Cu^{2+}/ascorbate mixtures stimulate oxidative damage (Fig. 9.9). In fact, oxidative damage may be

Table 9.4 Composition of human low-density lipoprotein (LDL)[a]

Constituent	Mean amount (molecules/ LDL particle)	Constituent	Mean amount (molecules/ LDL particle)
Total lipids		*Antioxidants*	
Phospholipids	700	α-tocopherol	7–8(3–14)[b]
Phosphatidylcholine	450	γ-tocopherol	0.50
Triglycerides	170	Ubiquinol-10	0.10–0.30[c]
Free cholesterol	600		
Cholesterol ester	1600	*Putative antioxidants*	
		β-carotene	0.30
Fatty-acid esters		α-carotene	0.12
Palmitic	693	Lycopene	0.16
Palmitoleic	44	Lutein and zeaxanthin	0.04
Stearic	143	Phytofluene	0.05
Oleic	454		
Linoleic	1101		
Arachidonic	153		
Docosahexaenoic	29		
Total PUFAs	1282		

[a] Data abstracted from several publications of the late Professor Dr Hermann Esterbauer.[71] The figures must not be taken too literally, since the LDL composition in an given individual depends on diet. For example, consumption of large amounts of PUFAs increases their levels in LDL.
[b] Range in parentheses for subjects not consuming α-tocopherol supplements.
[c] Ubiquinol is easily oxidized during isolation, and the true value may be up to 0.5 molecules/LDL particle (Roland Stocker, personal communication, 1993).

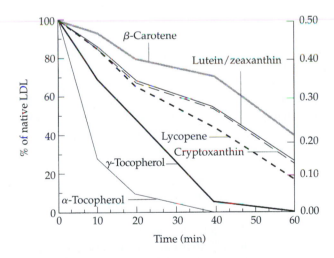

Figure 9.8 Sequence of loss of antioxidants during the lag phase of human LDL oxidation catalysed by Cu^{2+}. Data by courtesy of the late Professor Dr Hermann Esterbauer.

occurring, but not to the lipid. Incubation of LDL with Cu^{2+} and ascorbate led to conversion of histidine residues on apo-B to 2-oxohistidine, presumably by site-specific RS formation. Oxo-histidine binds Cu^{2+} less effectively, so that less Cu^{2+} remains associated with the LDL particle.[74] Ascorbate can also recycle probucol-derived phenoxyl radicals in LDL treated with probucol.[80]

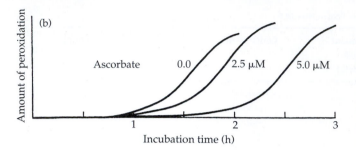

Figure 9.9 Effect of ascorbate on LDL peroxidation. After isolation from human plasma, LDL were exposed to Cu^{2+}. Ascorbate delayed the onset of peroxidation, the lag period rising with increasing concentrations. Diagram from *Free Radic. Res. Commun.* **6**, 67, 1989, by courtesy of the late Professor Dr Hermann Esterbauer and Harwood Academic Publishers.

The LDL contain ubiquinol (Table 9.4), another chain-breaking antioxidant (Section 3.18.5). When LDL is oxidized, ubiquinol disappears faster than tocopherols, probably because it recycles toco-pheryl radicals

$$CoQH_2 + Toc^\bullet \rightarrow CoQ^\bullet + TocH + H^+$$

However, the ubiquinol content of LDL is small (Table 9.2)—only ~10 to 50% of LDL particles contain it. Consumption of coenzyme Q_{10} supplements can raise the amount of ubiquinol-10 in LDL to a limited extent, but this was ineffective in decreasing atherosclerosis in a rat model.[81]

LDL contain several carotenoids, which are lost during the lag period (Fig. 9.8). The amounts present depend on diet, but in no case is there even approaching one molecule per LDL particle on average (Table 9.2), suggesting that any antioxidant effects would be limited at best. Indeed, raising the β-carotene content of LDL does not usually increase their resistance to oxidation *in vitro*,[75] and interest is now switching to the effects of supplements of lutein, lycopene, α-carotene and other carotenoids.

Flavonoids and other phenols can protect LDL against peroxidation *in vitro*, and it has been suggested that phenols in red wine, cocoa, nuts and chocolate might exert antiatherogenic effects. Indeed, administration of phenolic-rich plant extracts decreases atherosclerosis in several animal models. Of course, such phenols might act not only as chain-breaking antioxidants, but also as metal ion chelators and LOX inhibitors (Section 3.22.2)[82,83] Indeed, as mentioned earlier, red wine extract was antiatherosclerotic, but *not* by inhibiting lipid oxidation.[67] Whether flavonoids are significant antioxidants to LDL in humans is uncertain, given the low levels of unconjugated phenols present *in vivo* (Section 3.22.2).

9.3.8.3 *Pro-oxidant effects of antioxidants*[84]

In some *in vitro* systems, α-tocopherol can be made to exert pro-oxidant activity, acting to stimulate oxidative damage. Tocopherols are reducing agents, able to convert Fe(III) to Fe^{2+} or Cu^{2+} to Cu^+. Reaction of α-tocopherol with Cu^{2+} or Fe(III) generates the tocopheryl radical, which can react with PUFAs at a low rate (Section 3.20.2.5). Thus tocopherols accelerate metal-ion-dependent oxidative damage to LDL under certain circumstances, since Cu^+ and Fe^{2+} decompose peroxides more quickly than Fe(III) and Cu^{2+}. The relevance of these effects *in vivo* is uncertain, since α-tocopherol *in vivo* should always be present with coreductants (such as ascorbate and ubiquinol) which remove the α-tocopheryl radical.

Several other antioxidants can exert pro-oxidant effects in Cu^{2+}-induced LDL oxidation. This can happen with ascorbate (when oxidation has proceeded far enough to deplete α-tocopherol), urate, and some flavonoids.[85,86] They are probably acting by reducing Cu^{2+} to Cu^+, but again the physiological relevance is uncertain, since α-tocopherol is present in human lesions.

9.3.8.4 *Relevance of the model*

Although Cu^{2+}-dependent LDL oxidation *in vitro* is a widely used model, the evidence that Cu^{2+} ions participate in LDL oxidation *in vivo* is equivocal (Section 9.3.5.1). Whereas α-tocopherol must be depleted for rapid LDL oxidation to occur *in vitro* (Fig. 9.8), LDL oxidation products *coexist* with α-tocopherol in lesions. Thus α-tocopherol depletion is not necessary for oxidation to occur *in vivo*.[59] Indeed, α-tocopherol in LDL is not very effective in protecting them against damage by HOCl or ONOO⁻; ascorbate is better.[87] Hence some laboratories have examined oxidation and anti-oxidant depletion in isolated LDL exposed to HOCl, ONOO⁻, haem or haem proteins. For example, ONOO⁻ depletes α- and γ-tocopherols and carotenoids.[41] Others have used less physiologically-relevant systems, such as UV light or synthetic peroxyl radicals derived from AAPH, AMVN or related compounds (Section 4.11.8.2).

9.3.8.5 An artefact of eating?

One study[88] showed that consumption of olive oil, which is rich in antioxidant phenols such as hydroxytyrosol (Section 3.22), increased the lag time when subsequently isolated LDL were exposed to Cu^{2+}. However, the same effect was seen if the phenols were absent from the oil. In other words, the lag time of LDL oxidation might be increased by consumption of *any* food. How this occurs is uncertain, but if the data are reproducible it adds another question mark to the relevance of studies of *ex vivo* LDL oxidation.

When LDL were isolated from humans at different times of the year, the content of oxidized lipids present was different, causing variations[89] in the lag phase after exposure to Cu^{2+}. This seasonal effect must be considered when examining the effects of long-term dietary supplementations on LDL oxidizability.

9.3.9 The role of high-density lipoproteins

High-density lipoproteins (HDL) are anti-atherogenic; they remove excess cholesterol from cells (including macrophages and foam cells) within peripheral tissues, and transport it to the liver (**reverse cholesterol transport**). Like LDL, HDL have a hydrophobic core of triglycerides and cholesterol esters surrounded by a monolayer of phospholipids containing some cholesterol. Several proteins are embedded in the coat, the major ones being **apolipoproteins A1** (about 70% of total protein) and **-A2 (apo A1, apo A2)**. The beneficial cardiovascular effects of moderate intakes of ethanol and of PUFAs have been suggested to involve

rises in blood HDL levels (Sections 8.8.1 and 10.5.9). The enzyme **lecithin–cholesterol acyltransferase** (LCAT) esterifies free cholesterol entering HDL, facilitating storage in the core. Indeed, transgenic animals overexpressing the LCAT gene show higher plasma HDL levels and are more resistant to diet-induced atherosclerosis,[90] whereas 'knockouts' of LCAT raise tissue cholesterol levels. Inactivation of LCAT, for example by constituents of cigarette smoke (Section 8.12), might thus be proatherogenic.

The antiatherogenic actions of HDL do not stop at removing cholesterol. The HDL particles also exert anti-inflammatory properties and can remove peroxides from LDL.[91] Indeed, incubation of mildly oxidized LDL with HDL prevents some of the deleterious effects of the former. Peroxidized lipids can transfer from LDL to HDL, promoted by a cholesteryl ester transfer protein. They can then be degraded by two HDL enzymes, **platelet activating factor acetylhydrolase** (PAF acetylhydrolase) and **paraoxonase-1**, often abbreviated to **PON-1**. The related enzymes **paraoxonases-2** and **-3** may also contribute. The PAF acetylhydrolase enzyme is found in both HDL and LDL and helps remove PAF, a potent mediator of inflammation (Section 4.12). It can also hydrolyse peroxidized fatty acids arising from phospholipids during oxidation of LDL or HDL. Peroxidation of phospholipid-bound fatty acid followed by fragmentation to release an aldehyde leaves behind a substrate for PAF, which removes the oxidized 'residue' to give a lysophospholipid.

Paraoxonases are Ca^{2+}-dependent esterases, originally discovered by their ability to hydrolyse organophosphate and aromatic carboxylic acid esters. The former are widely used as insecticides and have been employed as nerve gases in chemical warfare. Examples are **sarin** (released by terrorists into the Tokyo subway system in 1995) and **soman**. The name 'paraoxonase' arises from the use of **paraoxon**, a toxic organophosphate, to assay the enzyme. The PON-1 enzyme hydrolyses phospholipid oxidation products (e.g. phospholipid-bound IPs and aldehydes) and cholesterol ester oxidation products derived from arachidonic or linoleic acid residues. Indeed, 'knockout' mice lacking PON-1 develop more atherosclerosis on a high-fat diet.[92]

You may be amused to know that ostrich HDL does not contain PON-1,[92] unlike the mammalian HDLs. The PON-1 gene has several polymorphisms, some of which influence activity. Two major forms of PON-1 exist: a high activity (towards paraoxon) form, and a low activity form in which arginine at position 192 is replaced by glutamine. Whether possession of a particular PON-1 phenotype affects atherosclerosis is unclear.[92]

Like LDL, HDL is subject to attack by LOX enzymes and RS, including $OH^\bullet$, HOCl and $ONOO^-$. Indeed, *in vitro*, HDL seem more easily oxidized than LDL, in part because of lower contents of α-tocopherol and other antioxidants.[93] Whereas normal HDL has anti-inflammatory properties, HDL isolated from patients with cardiovascular disease or diabetes may exert the opposite, that is proinflammatory effects.[48] This appears to relate to a high content of lipid peroxides and to the nitration and chlorination of tyrosine residues in apo-A1 by RS generated by MPO.[94] Indeed, nitration and chlorination of plasma HDL is increased in subjects with cardiovascular disease, and these modifications decrease the ability of HDL to remove cholesterol from macrophages.[91,94] This may be relevant *in vivo*, since the amounts of nitrated and chlorinated HDL are increased in human atherosclerotic lesions.[94,95]

9.3.10 Lipoprotein(a)[96]

This species is found only in humans and some other primates, and (oddly!) in the European hedgehog. It closely resembles LDL but contains an additional glycoprotein, **apo(a)**, linked to apoB by a disulphide bridge. There are over 30 different apo(a) isoforms. Increased plasma levels of lipoprotein(a) are an additional risk factor for atherosclerosis and it is present in atherosclerotic lesions. Like LDL, lipoprotein(a) can be oxidized to a form recognized by scavenger receptors, and it may also be able to collect and retain oxidized phospholipids from cells or other lipoproteins, possibly aggravating their pro-oxidant effect. The structure of apo(a) resembles that of **plasminogen**, the precursor of the enzyme plasmin that dissolves fibrin in blood clots. Thus another effect of apo(a) might be to antagonize plasminogen action and favour blood coagulation.

9.3.11 Unanswered questions

The evidence that lipid peroxidation occurs in atherosclerotic lesions is clear-cut. What remains unclear for humans is how important peroxidation is in lesion progression, how it is initiated, why some lesions develop and others do not, and how peroxidation might be modulated (if it all) by antioxidants. Indeed, how can peroxidation occur in vessel walls in the face of all the antioxidants that must diffuse into the wall from the plasma, and what contribution does caeruloplasmin make to LDL oxidation *in vivo*? There needs to be greater awareness that the different animal models used may have different mechanisms of atherosclerosis, and not all may be relevant to humans.

9.4 Diabetes

Diabetes mellitus (the Latin word *mellitus* means 'honey-sweet' and refers to the taste of diabetic urine) is a disease marked by elevated blood glucose (**hyperglycaemia**) and urinary glucose excretion. It is caused by faulty production of, or tissue response to, insulin. Insulin signalling is a key part of the regulation of metabolism, may involve ROS (Section 4.5) and is intimately linked to ageing (Section 10.3).

Complications of poorly controlled diabetes include systemic vascular disease (accelerated atherosclerosis), microvascular disease of the eye causing bleeding and retinal degeneration (**diabetic retinopathy**), cataract, kidney damage leading to renal failure and damage to peripheral nerves (**peripheral neuropathy**). Retina, kidney, renal glomeruli cells and neurons are freely permeable to glucose and are thus exposed to the full force of hyperglycaemia. By contrast, in the absence of insulin (or in failure to respond to it) muscle, adipose tissue and many other tissues do not take up glucose well, minimizing damage to them but contributing to elevated plasma glucose levels.

In the most common form of diabetes (**type 2 or non-insulin-dependent diabetes**) blood insulin levels are normal or elevated, yet tissue response to it is subnormal; there is said to be **peripheral resistance**. Liver also fails to respond to insulin, continuing to produce glucose despite the high plasma levels. Type 2 diabetes is seen most often in adults, and risk factors include obesity and lack of exercise, as well as poor diet. Sadly, in advanced countries, type 2 diabetes is increasingly appearing in children. As yet, however, most childhood diabetes is **Type 1**, in which insulin secretion is impaired or absent because of damage to the pancreatic islet cells that secrete this hormone.

The complications of diabetes correlate with the extent and time period of blood glucose elevation, so it is widely thought that excessive glucose is the major cause of tissue injury. In addition, blood LDL, VLDL and lipoprotein (a) levels are increased in diabetes, whereas HDL and PON-1 tend to be lowered. These changes contribute to pathology, especially the accelerated atherosclerosis.[92,97]

9.4.1 Can oxidative stress cause diabetes?

Some diabetogenic agents (e.g. alloxan) act by imposing severe oxidative stress on the β-cell (Section 8.5), but whether oxidative stress contributes to the origin of human diabetes is unclear. Exposing human islet cells to a mixture of IL-1β and IFNγ injured the cells, but overexpression of antioxidant enzymes did not protect.[98] There is a strong genetic predisposition to diabetes, which is clearest in the 1 to 2% of cases inherited in a simple autosomal dominant manner (**maturity onset diabetes of the young, MODY**).[99] Genes found to be defective in different MODY patients include those encoding the enzyme glucokinase (which converts glucose to glucose 6-phosphate) and the gene transcription factor HNF-1α (**hepatic nuclear factor-1α**). Inherited decreases in catalase activity have been suggested to predispose to diabetes (Section 3.7.8).

In some animals that develop diabetes spontaneously, such as the **non-obese-diabetic (NOD) mouse** and the **biobreeding (BB) rat**, there is an autoimmune attack on the β-cells, and RS (especially ONOO$^-$)[100] generated by attacking phagocytes are involved in islet cell killing. Indeed, α-tocopherol, SOD, the antioxidant EUK-8 (Section

10.6.4) and desferrioxamine have been reported to delay the onset of diabetes in NOD mice.[101,102] Type 1 diabetes in humans frequently involves autoimmune events (even insulin can act as an autoantigen) but the contribution of RS is unproven.[98] Nevertheless, antioxidants may find a role in helping to protect isolated human islets for use in transplantation from the oxidative stress of cell isolation procedures.[103,104]

9.4.2 Oxidative stress in diabetic patients

It may be unclear whether oxidative stress causes diabetes, but diabetes does cause oxidative stress. Plasma F_2-IPs and lipid peroxides (even if values are corrected for elevated plasma lipids) are usually found to be elevated in diabetics.[105] Rats rendered diabetic by streptozotocin treatment (Section 8.5.2) absorbed peroxides from oxidized fats in the diet to a greater extent than controls, suggestive of a diminished ability of the gut to detoxify food lipid peroxides.[78] However, this is unlikely to confound measurements of F_2-IPs since they do not appear to be absorbed from diet (Section 5.14.6). Diabetics excrete more 8OHdG in urine and have elevated levels of several DNA base oxidation products in their white cells.[106] What about antioxidants? There is disagreement as to whether plasma α-tocopherol levels in diabetic patients are low (one must correct for elevated lipids, and diabetics are often on low fat diets which could affect vitamin E uptake), but most researchers find that plasma vitamin C levels are subnormal and there are several reports of lowered GSH levels in various tissues.[107–109]

The significance of oxidative stress to diabetic pathology is uncertain but it probably contributes to the accelerated atherosclerosis, and possibly to renal damage, neuropathy, cataract, and retinopathy. Maternal diabetes increases the incidence of foetal abnormalities, and oxidative stress may contribute. Consistent with this, transgenic mouse embryos overexpressing the CuZnSOD gene showed fewer malformations than controls when exposed to hyperglycaemia caused by administration of streptozotocin to their mothers (Section 6.11.7). In rat embryos, the oxidative stress appeared to impair the expression of genes required for neural tube closure.[110]

9.4.3 How does the oxidative stress originate?

One possible source is elevated plasma lipids leading to increased lipid oxidation (e.g. by peroxisomal β-oxidation, which generates H_2O_2; Section 9.14.2.1). Elevated LDL itself promotes atherosclerosis. However, most attention has focused on glucose. Indeed incubation of many cell types (including neurons) with excess glucose causes increased ROS production, the key event being disruption of mitochondrial function[111] to release more $O_2^{\bullet-}$. This seems to occur because excess glucose metabolism generates too much NADH, overloads the electron transport chain and promotes electron leakage.[111] α-Ketoglutarate dehydrogenase can also generate ROS if NAD^+/NADH rations are too low (Section 1.10.5). Increased mitochondrial oxidation of fatty acids (producing NADH and $FADH_2$) can make things worse. Additional mechanisms may include stimulation of protein kinase C (PKC) activity, leading to activation of endothelial NOX. Activation of PKC can be achieved both by ROS (Section 4.5.5) and because hyperglycaemia promotes the synthesis[111] of the PKC activator DAG, diacylglycerol (Section 9.4.4 below). Catalysis of $O_2^{\bullet-}$-dependent NADH oxidation by cytosolic lactate dehydrogenase to generate ROS (Section 2.5.3.2), as well as facilitation of excessive cellular iron uptake by glucose,[112] might also contribute. Yet another factor, initially suggested by experiments on human aortic smooth muscle cells, may be that hyperglycaemia depresses ROS scavenging by the thioredoxin system. It appears to increase the levels of **thioredoxin-interacting protein (TiP)**, which binds to thioredoxin and blocks its redox-active cysteine residues (Section 3.11).[113] Indeed, diabetic (streptozotocin-treated) rats showed elevated levels of TiP and decreased thioredoxin in blood vessel walls.[113]

In diabetics, acute rises in plasma glucose are accompanied by rapid elevations in plasma F_2-IPs.[114] Even in healthy subjects, transient hyperglycaemia can increase plasma F_2-IP levels and decrease endothelial-dependent vascular relaxation,[115] a process markedly impaired in diabetics.

In type 2 diabetes, the islet cells themselves can be oxidatively damaged by hyperglycaemia, decreasing transcription of the genes encoding insulin and aggravating the diabetes.[116,117] Another mechanism may be the induction of uncoupling protein 2 (Section 1.10.6) in the islet mitochondria, causing falls in ATP that impair insulin secretion.[116] A further source of oxidative stress results from the reaction of sugars with $-NH_2$ groups.

9.4.4 Non-enzymatic glycation and glycoxidation[118]

Glucose in solution is a ring structure, in equilibrium with a small amount of an open-chain aldehyde form. Aldehydes can combine with $-NH_2$ groups, modifying DNA bases, proteins, and amino-lipids such as phosphatidylethanolamine, in a process referred to as **non-enzymic glycation** (Fig. 9.10). Glycation of proteins is the first step in the 'browning process', often called **Maillard browning**. It is named after Professor Louis Camille Maillard, who in 1912 began to elucidate the chemistry behind the colours formed upon heating mixtures of carbohydrates and amines. Indeed, the golden-brown colours (and some elements of the taste) of cooked foods are due to Maillard products. Maillard chemistry can generate pleasant aromas, such as those associated with roasted coffee. However, mutagenic heterocyclic amines can be formed by Maillard chemistry in meats and fish. Several phenolic antioxidants, including catechins, BHT and BHA, decrease formation of these mutagenic products. Whether dietary Maillard products can be absorbed and contribute to tissue damage is uncertain; a few studies suggest that they can.[119]

Glycation *in vivo* is slow and reversible at physiological glucose levels, tending mostly to affect proteins with a very slow turnover, for example collagen in some connective tissues, and lens crystallins (Section 6.10). Glycation is faster at elevated glucose, occurring in these and many other proteins in diabetic patients. Indeed, glycated haemoglobin levels are used as an index of how well blood glucose has been controlled over the previous month or so. Glycated haemoglobin (HbA_{1C}) contains a glucose Amadori product (Fig. 9.10) attached

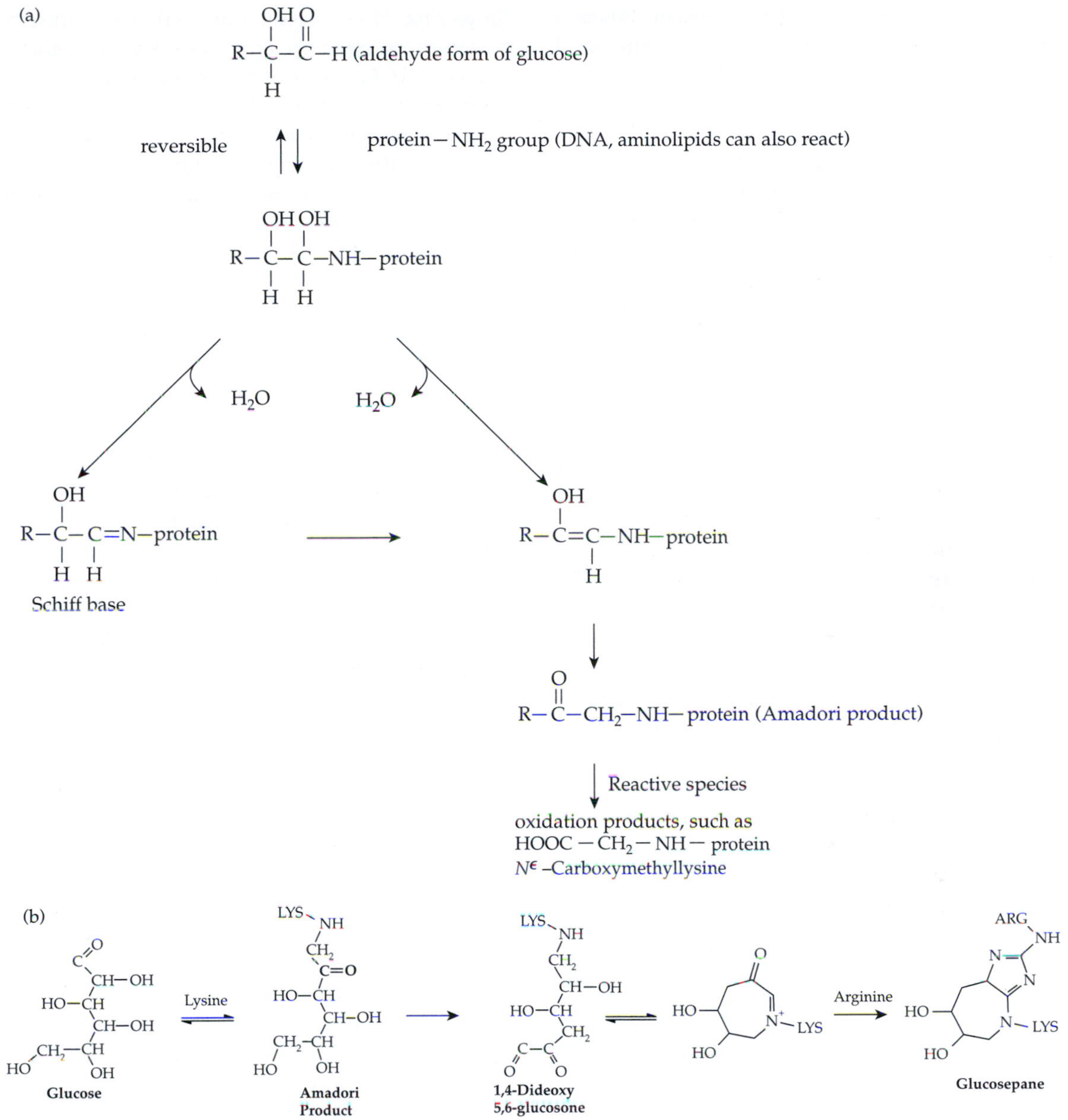

(a)

$$
\begin{array}{c}
\text{OH}\ \ \text{O} \\
\ \ |\ \ \ \ || \\
\text{R}-\text{C}-\text{C}-\text{H}\ \text{(aldehyde form of glucose)} \\
\ \ | \\
\ \ \text{H}
\end{array}
$$

reversible $\ \uparrow\downarrow\ $ protein$-$NH$_2$ group (DNA, aminolipids can also react)

$$
\begin{array}{c}
\text{OH}\ \text{OH} \\
\ |\ \ \ \ | \\
\text{R}-\text{C}-\text{C}-\text{NH}-\text{protein} \\
\ |\ \ \ \ | \\
\ \text{H}\ \ \text{H}
\end{array}
$$

H$_2$O   H$_2$O

$$
\begin{array}{c}
\text{OH} \\
\ | \\
\text{R}-\text{C}-\text{C}=\text{N}-\text{protein} \\
\ |\ \ \ | \\
\ \text{H}\ \ \text{H}
\end{array}
$$
Schiff base

$\longrightarrow$

$$
\begin{array}{c}
\text{OH} \\
\ | \\
\text{R}-\text{C}=\text{C}-\text{NH}-\text{protein} \\
\ \ \ \ \ \ | \\
\ \ \ \ \ \ \text{H}
\end{array}
$$

$$
\begin{array}{c}
\text{O} \\
|| \\
\text{R}-\text{C}-\text{CH}_2-\text{NH}-\text{protein (Amadori product)}
\end{array}
$$

Reactive species

oxidation products, such as
HOOC $-$ CH$_2$ $-$ NH $-$ protein
N^ϵ –Carboxymethyllysine

(b)

Figure 9.10 (a) Reaction of glucose with proteins (other monosaccharides can react similarly). The Schiff base and Amadori products can be attacked by RS to generate carbonyls, including glyoxal and dicarbonyls (Fig. 9.11). (b) Formation of a cross-linked arginine/lysine complex (**glucosepane**) by glucose. From *J. Biol. Chem.* **280**, 12310, 2005 by courtesy of the American Society for Biochemistry and Molecular Biology and Professor Vincent Monnier. Glucosepane is a major constituent of glycation products in cataractous human lenses (*J. Biol. Chem.* **277**, 24907, 2002).

to the N-terminal valine of the β-chain. Whereas haptoglobin can prevent pro-oxidant effects of normal haemoglobin (Section 3.16.3.4), it is less good (especially the Hp2–2 form) at doing so for glycated haemoglobin.[120] Indeed, diabetics with Hp2–2 haemoglobin were reported to suffer more cardiovascular disease.[120] Glucose also glycates CuZnSOD in the erythrocyte, decreasing its activity; this may account for the lower SOD activity reported in the blood of some diabetics.[108] Both CuZnSOD and caeruloplasmin can fragment after glycation, to release pro-oxidant copper ions.[121]

Glycation products can be oxidized by several RS, including OH$^\bullet$ and ONOO$^-$, to give **advanced glycation end-products** (AGEs; Figs 9.10 and 9.11). Indeed, ROS have been described as 'fixatives of glycation'. Accumulation of AGE on proteins is accompanied by browning (the animal equivalent of the browning of cooked foods), increased fluorescence and cross-linking. Formation of AGEd proteins is usually irreversible (unless the protein is degraded), occurs over periods of months to years, and can inhibit the function of enzymes and transcription factors. Accumulation of AGEs in collagen decreases the elasticity of connective tissue

(impairing blood vessel function) and damages basement membranes of the kidney. In diabetic patients, AGEs are present in many tissues, on circulating LDLs, and in atherosclerotic lesions. Chemical structures found in AGEs include **carboxymethyllysine** and **pentosidine**, a fluorescent cross-link between lysine and arginine residues in AGE-modified proteins (Fig. 9.11). Another important product involving lysine and arginine cross-linking is **glucosepane** (Fig. 9.10).

Glucose is not the only contributor to AGEing. Increased ROS production in diabetes decreases the activity of the glycolytic enzyme glyceraldehyde-3-phosphate dehydrogenase (G3PDH),[111] allowing triose phosphates to accumulate for ready conversion into DAG. Inactivation of G3PDH seems to involve[111] its ADP-ribosylation by PARP-1 (Section 4.2.4). Some of the triose phosphates can convert to **methylglyoxal,** which participates in AGE formation.[108] Methylglyoxal is also produced by attack of RS upon Schiff bases, and both glyoxal and methylglyoxal are produced during lipid peroxidation. The glyoxalase system (Section 3.9.1) is important in controlling such events *in vivo*, but will be compromised if GSH levels are low.[108]

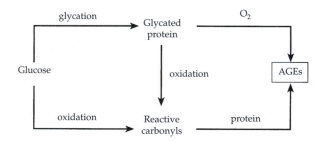

Carboxymethyl-lysine

Pentosidine

Figure 9.11 Glycoxidation reactions. The combination of glycation and oxidation can result in the formation of advanced glycation end-products (AGEs) whose increased accumulation is associated with tissue injury in diabetes. Glucose can be oxidized before binding to proteins, or glycated proteins can themselves oxidize, releasing ROS. **N$^\varepsilon$-Carboxymethyl-lysine** (Fig. 9.10) and **pentosidine** have been identified as glycoxidation-derived constituents of AGEs, but there are many others, e.g. 2-ammonio-6-(3-oxidopyridinium-1-yl) hexanoate, a lysine derivative, is found in aged human lenses and levels are elevated in cataract (*J. Biol. Chem.* **279**, 6487, 2004).

Another way of making AGEs is to first oxidize the glucose and then allow the oxidation products to react with protein. Monosaccharides can oxidize, catalysed by traces of iron and copper ions, to produce $O_2^{\bullet-}$, H_2O_2, $OH^{\bullet}$ and toxic carbonyls which can damage proteins (Figs 9.10 and 9.11).

Oxidative stress thus contributes to AGE formation (Fig. 9.11) and the word **glycoxidation** is often used to describe the pathways involved. Once formed, AGEd proteins cause more oxidative stress. Glycation of proteins in the electron transport chain can impair normal electron flow and promote 'leakage' to form $O_2^{\bullet-}$.

Binding of glucose to the amino groups on both apoB and on lipids in LDL facilitates LDL oxidation. In addition, AGEd proteins are toxic to many cell types.[118] For example, exposure of endothelial cells to AGEs activates NF-κB, increases adhesion molecule (including VCAM-1) production and NOX activity, and may decrease GSH levels. This occurs in addition to the direct deleterious effects of high glucose on vascular endothelium. Proteins bearing AGE have been implicated in the excessive proliferation of blood vessels that occurs in diabetic retinopathy. Several cell types, including monocyte/macrophages and endothelial cells, recognize AGEs using cell-surface receptors, **RAGE** (receptors for AGE), that are distinct from the scavenger receptors. The RAGE receptors are expressed in atherosclerotic lesions, especially in diabetics,[122] are involved in monocyte migration and activation in response to AGEs, and appear to recognize carboxymethyllysine (Fig. 9.11). In addition, several scavenger receptors, including SR-A, CD36 and LOX-1 recognize AGEd proteins.[19,58] Normally, RAGE may enable macrophages to recognize and engulf glycosylated cells, for example AGE-modified erythrocytes. RAGE receptors bind several other ligands, including β-amyloid and HMGB1, a promoter of inflammation released from necrotic cells (Section 4.4).[118]

9.4.4.1 *Reversing AGEing?*
Aminoguanidine

$$H_2N-NH-\overset{\overset{+}{N}H_2}{\underset{\|}{C}}-NH_2$$

a hydrazine compound that reacts with dicarbonyls, is in clinical trials in diabetic patients; its ability to prevent AGE formation may retard the development of kidney, eye, blood vessel and nerve damage.[123] **Pyridoxamine**

a compound related to vitamin B_6 (**pyridoxine**) has a similar effect.[124] Other agents, such as **ALT-711**, have been described that appear to dissolve AGE structures and can decrease the AGE content of tissues.[123]

9.4.5 Other mechanisms of glucose toxicity: aldose reductase[111]

Aldose reductase, an enzyme found in several mammalian tissues (including lens and retina), has been proposed to contribute to the development of diabetic cataract. It converts glucose to the polyalcohol **sorbitol** by reducing the aldehyde group

$$RCHO + NADPH + H^+ \rightarrow RCH_2OH + NADP^+$$

The hyperglycaemia, combined with inhibition of G3PDH, raises intracellular glucose levels and accelerates enzyme action. Inhibitors of aldose reductase can delay the onset of diabetic complications in animals, but have not given convincing results in humans. Why abnormal activity of aldose reductase should be toxic is unknown; one suggestion is an excessive osmotic stress in the lens, as sorbitol accumulates to high concentrations. However, cataracts from human diabetics do not appear to contain osmotically active concentrations of sorbitol and so the importance of this mechanism is unclear. Sorbitol can be oxidized by NAD^+-dependent enzymes to fructose, further raising NADH levels. In addition, high aldose reductase activity may drain away NADPH (needed by thioredoxin and glutathione reductases), so making tissues more vulnerable to oxidative damage.

9.4.6 How important is oxidative stress in diabetes?

Elevated lipid peroxidation can be demonstrated in early diabetes. Hence it is not merely a consequence of tissue injury from diabetic complications.[125] Similarly, in one study, patients with higher urinary excretion of 8OHdG later developed more severe nephropathy.[126] Type 2 diabetes is often preceded by the **metabolic syndrome**, a cluster of metabolic abnormalities (low HDL, hypertension, high triglycerides, mild hyperglycaemia due to insulin resistance) usually associated with abdominal obesity. Plasma F_2-IPs are already elevated at this stage[127,128] and ROS may contribute to the insulin resistance.[128A] Abdominal obesity (a risk factor for type 2 diabetes) is also associated with increased F_2-IP levels in both human and obesity-prone rats, perhaps because abdominal adipose tissue and hepatocytes in fatty livers release cytokines that provoke an inflammatory state.[105] In the **Zucker diabetic fat (ZDF) rat**, a model of the metabolic syndrome, development of renal damage was delayed by the antioxidant ebselen (Section 10.6.10).[129] Oxidative stress probably contributes, via LDL oxidation and AGE/RAGE interactions, to the accelerated progression of atherosclerosis in diabetics. Measurements of protein modification products in atherosclerotic lesions from diabetic monkeys suggested that $OH^\bullet$ rather than $ONOO^-$ was important; levels of o-tyrosine, m-tyrosine and bityrosine were raised but 3-nitrotyrosine was not.[130] Oxidative stress may also contribute to neuropathy, for example by decreasing nerve GSH levels.[107]

Interestingly, however, mice overexpressing GPx1 developed hyperglycaemia and elevated blood insulin,[131] the suggested explanation being that ROS are a second messenger of insulin action (Section 4.5.5).

9.4.6.1 Do antioxidant supplements help diabetic patients?

Intervention trials with high-dose α-tocopherol gave little or no evidence of benefit in diabetes,[132] although it is unclear to what extent lipid peroxidation was decreased by the interventions (probably little, if at all). Lipoic acid (Section 3.18.4) has been suggested, but not proven, to decrease the severity of diabetic neuropathy by maintaining GSH levels and/or by its direct antioxidant properties.[107,109] However, lipoic acid administration improved endothelial function in subjects with metabolic syndrome, but did not decrease their plasma F_2-IP levels, suggestive of benefit by non-antioxidant mechanisms.[133] By contrast, **irbesartan** (an agent that blocks the angiotensin receptor; angiotensin II is associated with increased ROS production [Section 7.10.3]) did decrease IP levels as well as improving vascular effects; the effects of lipoic acid and irbesartan were additive, again suggesting that benefits of lipoate are not antioxidant-related.[133]

Since ascorbate levels are subnormal in diabetics, would they benefit from ascorbate supplementation? Ascorbate has antioxidant properties, but it can also glycate proteins. One epidemiological study suggested that high ascorbate intake in subjects who had been diabetic for many years was associated with *increased* risk of complications.[134] More work is needed before clear-cut conclusions can be drawn. Oxidative stress in diabetes results mainly from hyperglycaemia, and is probably best controlled by carefully monitoring and controlling plasma glucose levels and keeping LDL levels down.

9.5 Ischaemia–reperfusion

We have already considered the roles of hypoxia–reperfusion in birth and in sickle-cell anaemia (Section 6.11.8 and 6.4.4). Let's now examine some other examples of this phenomenon. Damage to the heart or brain by deprivation of O_2 (**ischaemia**) is a major cause of death worldwide. Rupture of an atherosclerotic lesion, followed by thrombosis and the blockage of an essential coronary or cerebral artery, are the usual cause (Section 9.4). Removal of the blood supply to a tissue also halts the supply of nutrients and the removal of metabolic waste products. Severe restriction of blood flow, leading to O_2 concentrations lower than normal (**hypoxia**), but not complete O_2 deprivation, results if the blocked artery is the major, but not the only, source of blood to the tissue. The terms hypoxia and ischaemia tend to be used interchangeably (albeit this is incorrect!) in the literature.

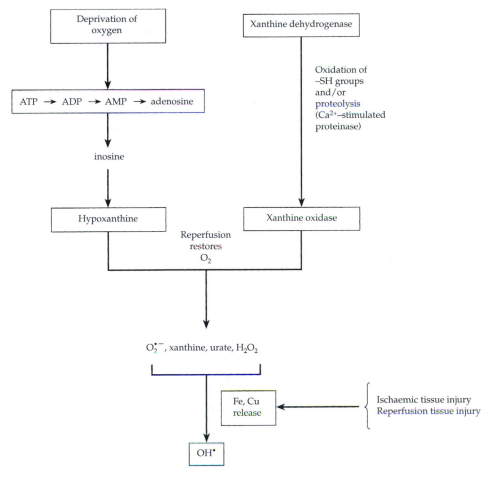

Figure 9.12 A suggested mechanism for tissue injury upon reoxygenation of ischaemic or hypoxic tissues. Modified from J.M. McCord *Fed. Proc.* **46**, 2402, 1987. The enzyme that converts adenosine to inosine is **adenosine deaminase**. Adenosine is a vasodilator, decreases phagocyte RS production, modulates the activity of numerous other cell types and may help to protect cells against some of the consequences of ischaemia–reperfusion (Sections 7.9.2 and 9.5.6).

Tissues made hypoxic or ischaemic survive for a variable time, depending on what tissue it is and the species it is from. Thus skeletal muscle is fairly resistant to ischaemic injury, whereas the brain is far more sensitive. Many tissues can adapt to cope with some degree of hypoxia (Section 1.3.2). However, any mammalian tissue made ischaemic for a sufficient period will be irreversibly injured. Tissues respond to O_2 deprivation in several ways.[135] Early responses usually include increased rates of glycogen degradation and glycolysis, leading to lactate production and acidosis. Levels of ATP eventually fall and the cells' normal ion gradients are disrupted (Section 4.3). The

AMP formed is degraded, hypoxanthine accumulates (Fig. 9.12) and intracellular Ca^{2+} levels rise, activating Ca^{2+}-stimulated proteinases and phospholipases (providing fatty acid substrates for eicosanoid synthesis) and nitric oxide synthases (if present). Of course, O_2 is a substrate for COX and NOS enzymes and so complete O_2 deprivation will block $NO^\bullet$ and eicosanoid formation.

9.5.1 Reoxygenation injury[135]

If the period of O_2 deprivation is not long enough to injure the tissue irreversibly, much can be salvaged by reperfusing it with blood, reintroducing O_2 and nutrients. In this situation, reperfusion is beneficial. However, it was shown in the early 1980s that reintroduction of O_2 to an ischaemic tissue can cause an additional insult to the tissue (**reoxygenation injury**) that is, in part, mediated by a burst of ROS production. The relative importance of reoxygenation (often called **reperfusion**) injury depends on the time of ischaemia. If this is sufficiently long, the tissue is irreversibly injured and will die, so reoxygenation injury adds little or nothing to the damage, at least to that tissue. Nevertheless, reperfusion of a dead or dying tissue can release toxic agents into the circulation, including xanthine oxidase (XO),[136] biologically active oxidized lipids (e.g. IPs, PAF-like products [Section 4.12]) and 'catalytic' transition-metal ions, causing problems to other body tissues. These may contribute to **multiple organ dysfunction syndrome (MODS)**, a leading cause of death in very sick patients. This syndrome can result from several events, including major trauma, overwhelming infection, and gut, liver or skeletal muscle ischaemia/reoxygenation. In particular, damage to the gut can allow bacteria and bacterial products (e.g. endotoxin) into the circulation, and some groups have called the gut 'the motor of multiorgan failure'. The syndrome is characterized by a release of 'stress hormones', such as catecholamines and cortisol, and by a systemic inflammation (**systemic inflammatory response syndrome, SIRS**) with overproduction of cytokines, complement activation and mitochondrial dysfunction with falls in ATP. Some studies have suggested limited benefit of *N*-acetylcysteine in decreasing the incidence of MODS, but most have not.[137,138]

However, if the period of ischaemia is short, the reoxygenation injury component may become important and the amount of tissue damage can be decreased by including antioxidants in the reoxygenation fluid. What length of time is 'short' depends on the tissue and the degree of O_2 deprivation. There can also be a 'burst' of NO$^•$ and eicosanoid production when O_2 is restored.

9.5.2 A role for xanthine oxidase?

Almost all the xanthine-oxidizing activity in healthy animal tissues is the dehydrogenase (XDH), which transfers electrons not to O_2, but to NAD$^+$, as it oxidizes xanthine or hypoxanthine into uric acid. When tissues are damaged, some XDH can be converted to XO (Fig. 9.12) by oxidation of –SH groups or by limited proteolysis. Proteolytic cleavage of surface-exposed loops in the protein causes a conformational change around the FAD binding site that blocks access to NAD$^+$ and allows electrons to pass to O_2. Oxidation of –SH groups may form a disulphide bond that leads to similar changes.[136] Depletion of ATP in hypoxic tissue causes hypoxanthine accumulation. This hypoxanthine can be oxidized by XO when the tissue is reoxygenated, causing rapid generation of $O_2^{•-}$ and H_2O_2. Released transition-metal ions can then promote OH$^•$ formation (Fig. 9.12).

Xanthine oxidase can also contribute to systemic injury for example in MODS. It binds readily to vascular glycosaminoglycans to form ROS injurious to vascular endothelium. Even if XDH is released from damaged tissues, it is rapidly converted to XO in plasma.[136]

9.5.3 Intestinal ischaemia–reoxygenation[135,139]

Intestinal ischaemia–reperfusion injury in humans is associated with high morbidity and mortality; interruptions to the blood supply of the gut can occur in haemorrhagic or septic shock (Section 9.5.7 below), thrombosis, strangulated hernias and torsions of the intestine. Apart from the brain, the gut is the most sensitive body organ; ischaemia readily damages the gut lining, especially the cells at the tips of the villi, and reperfusion aggravates damage. Even a brief period of gut ischaemia can allow bacteria and bacterial products such as endotoxin to enter the body and contribute to MODS (Section 9.5.1).

Indeed, the earliest evidence supporting the scheme in Fig. 9.12 came from studies upon intestine. Partial occlusion of the artery supplying blood to a segment of cat small intestine, followed by reperfusion, causes histologically observable damage to the tissue and increases intestinal vascular permeability. Intravenous administration of SOD, or oral administration of allopurinol (to inhibit XO), to the cats before perfusion, decreased damage, and infusion of hypoxanthine plus XO into the arterial supply of a segment of normal cat intestine mimicked the damage, an effect that was decreased by SOD, $OH^•$ scavengers or desferrioxamine. Iron ions able to catalyse $OH^•$ production could be released by cell necrosis, proteolytic digestion of metalloproteins, release of iron from ferritin or iron–sulphur proteins[140] by $O_2^{•-}$, and/or breakdown of haemoglobin (e.g. by H_2O_2) liberated as a result of bleeding upon tissue reperfusion. Intestinal ischaemia in cats results in accumulation of hypoxanthine, which disappears quickly on reperfusion, and both lipid peroxidation and GSSG formation can be measured in the reperfused intestine. It has also been reported that SOD or desferrioxamine administration diminish the mortality consequent upon bowel ischaemia in rats.

Rat, human and cat intestines are rich in XDH activity. Although allopurinol is not specific as an inhibitor of XDH and XO, other evidence for the involvement of this enzyme has been obtained. **Pterinaldehyde** (2-amino-4-hydroxypteridine-6-carboxaldehyde), a powerful XO inhibitor that often contaminates commercial preparations of the vitamin folic acid (Fig. 1.16), also offered protection. Feeding animals a diet rich in tungsten decreases tissue XDH activity; intestinal segments from rats pretreated in this way showed less reoxygenation injury after hypoxia than segments from normal rats. The tungsten works by being incorporated into XO instead of molybdenum, producing an inactive enzyme.[141]

The model in Fig. 9.12 thus explains many aspects of intestinal ischaemia–reoxygenation in some animals, although its importance to human gut has been questioned because the XDH to XO conversion seems very slow.[142] Indeed, XO is not the only source of ROS in reoxygenated intestine (or other tissues) and it may not be the major source in humans.[136] Mitochondria damaged by ischaemia may 'leak' more electrons than usual from their electron transport chain, forming more $O_2^{•-}$ (especially from complex I) when O_2 is restored.[5] Excess intramitochondrial $O_2^{•-}$ can interfere with energy metabolism by inactivating enzymes such as aconitase, simultaneously releasing iron.[140] Reactive species can arise from phagocytes entering (or already present within) reoxygenated intestine. Reperfused

tissues can release leukotriene B_4, PAF and other chemoattractants for neutrophils, and increase levels of adhesion molecules by signalling pathways that involve ROS. Adhesion molecule expression can also increase in hypoxia, by HIF-related mechanisms (Section 7.7.1.1). Neutrophils then adhere to endothelium and may activate to generate products ($O_2^{•-}$, H_2O_2, HOCl, chloramines, eicosanoids, elastase) that worsen injury. Indeed, neutrophil depletion of animals, or pretreatment of them with antibodies that prevent neutrophil adherence to endothelium, has diminished reoxygenation injury to intestine and other tissues in some animal studies.

Intestinal ischaemia can lead to acceleration of heart rate and increased blood pressure. Apparently, ROS produced by reoxygenation can stimulate sensory nerve endings in the viscera to produce cardiovascular responses.[143]

9.5.4 Cardiac ischaemia–reoxygenation

9.5.4.1 *The phenomenon*
The model in Fig. 9.12 soon attracted the attention of cardiologists, since myocardial infarction (essentially ischaemic/hypoxic injury to heart muscle) is a major cause of death, and thrombolytic therapy is widely used to dissolve blood clots and promote reperfusion. Heart muscle can survive up to 60 to 90 min of ischaemia, depending on the animal. The healthy animal heart needs about 8 to 15 ml O_2 per 100 g tissue every minute when the body is at rest, and this can rise to over 70 ml during vigorous exercise.

After short periods of ischaemia or hypoxia, reoxygenation of isolated perfused hearts has been shown to produce additional tissue damage that is diminished by adding MnSOD, CuZnSOD, catalase, spin traps such as PBN, scavengers of $OH^•$ radical such as dimethylsulphoxide or mannitol, desferrioxamine or allopurinol to the reperfusion fluids. In addition, hearts isolated from transgenic animals overexpressing catalase, MnSOD or GPx1 show less reperfusion injury[144] whereas hearts from animals lacking various antioxidant enzymes, or G6PDH, show more.[145,146] One point worth making—studies showing protection by mannitol should not assume that it is acting as an $OH^•$ scavenger.[147] For example, mannitol and glucose react with OH$^{\bullet}$ equally fast, but mannitol protects better than glucose against ischaemia–reperfusion in isolated rat heart. Deleterious cell volume changes can occur in response to ischaemia and/or ROS, and mannitol may help prevent these by exerting osmotic effects.

The manifestations of cardiac reoxygenation injury vary according to species and experimental protocol. For example, reoxygenation of isolated rat hearts after brief ischaemia can produce irregular contractions (**arrhythmias**).[147] Reoxygenation after 15 to 20 min ischaemia can result in delayed return of contractile function (**myocardial stunning**) in pig, rabbit and dog hearts.[148] The **stunned myocardium** does not contract, but is not irreversibly injured and will eventually recover normal function (hours to days later). The molecular mechanism of stunning is unclear; its rapid onset and the protective effects of thiol compounds in some studies have led to suggestions that OH$^{\bullet}$ oxidizes –SH groups on membrane ion-transport systems that are essential for maintaining membrane potential and keeping intracellular Ca^{2+} low. Normal heart function depends on periodic 'waves' of electrical activity to stimulate the heart muscle to contract in an ordered sequence, so it is easy to envisage how disruptions of membrane ion transport could provoke stunning or arrhythmias. Calcium overload can activate calpains (Section 4.3.2) and cause proteolytic damage to myofibrils; the time taken to repair this damage may contribute to the delayed recovery of function.[148]

9.5.4.2 *Importance of the model used*
Many studies showing protective effects of antioxidants have used hearts isolated from mice, rats, rabbits, dogs or pigs and perfused with buffer. These studies are easy to control and standardize. Problems include contamination of buffers with transition-metal ions, and the absence of the range of antioxidants and metabolites normally present in blood. Hence it is easy to overestimate the potential physiological significance of protective effects when an antioxidant is added to a buffer that (unlike blood) has no basal antioxidant activity. Alternatively, studies can be performed with organs *in situ*. For example, in 'open-chest' anaesthetized dogs (the chest is opened, a coronary artery partially or completely occluded, and the blockage removed after various periods) several studies showed that pretreatment of animals with SOD plus catalase, or allopurinol, decreased the amount of tissue death (size of the **infarction**) produced by prolonged (≥ 60 min) occlusion, followed by reoxygenation. This model has also been used to show the involvement of OH$^{\bullet}$ in myocardial stunning resulting from shorter (10–15 mins) ischaemia followed by reoxygenation (Fig. 5.6).[148]

The extent of protection by antioxidants has varied widely in different experiments, especially in studies of infarct size, the most controversial area. At least three reasons account for this.

1. The importance of reoxygenation injury as a fraction of total tissue damage declines as the ischaemic period increases. In experiments with prolonged ischaemia, so much tissue injury may be done by O_2 deprivation that reperfusion injury adds little and antioxidants are unlikely to offer much protection. In dog heart, for example, coronary occlusion for less than about 20 min can lead to stunning on reperfusion, but rarely any infarct. Occlusion for more than 4 h followed by reperfusion gives an infarct about the same size as that resulting from permanent occlusion (i.e. damage is maximum and cannot be further increased).[148] In this model, antioxidants are protective against stunning, but do not usually alter infarct size after prolonged occlusion.

2. In 'whole-animal' studies (e.g. using open-chest pigs or dogs), the extent of O_2-deprivation during arterial occlusion can vary considerably because of collateral vessels. Thus 'ischaemia' is often hypoxia, to variable extents. If flow does not cease completely, not only does some O_2 enter the 'ischaemic' tissue, but also some metabolic products, such as H^+, are removed and acidosis is less severe.

3. Some of the antioxidants used show bell-shaped dose–response curves. For example, in studies upon arrhythmias in isolated rat hearts after a brief period of ischaemia, there is an optimal concentration of SOD for protection, and higher or lower concentrations give smaller protective effects.[147] Similar effects are observed if release of enzymes from damaged cells is measured (Fig. 9.13). The reasons remain to be established. For example, a

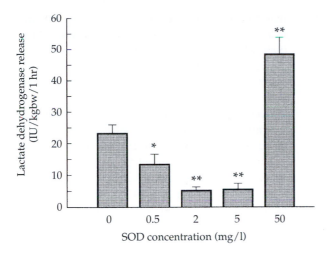

Figure 9.13 Effect of human recombinant MnSOD on lactate dehydrogenase release in isolated rabbit hearts subjected to 1 h of ischaemia followed by 1 h of reperfusion. Means and standard errors are shown (*, $P < 0.05$; **, $P < 0.01$). While MnSOD lowered enzyme release at lower doses, it *increased* the release at the highest dose. From *Free Rad. Biol. Med.* **9**, 465, 1990 by courtesy of Professor Joe McCord and Elsevier.

deleterious effect of impurities in some of the antioxidants studied might become significant at very high antioxidant concentrations, and if SOD is contaminated with endotoxin (Section 10.6.3), pretreatment of animals with it can alter endogenous antioxidant levels.

Other studies have used 'conscious' dog, rabbit or pig models in an attempt to eliminate possible confounding effects of anaesthesia, surgical trauma and mechanical ventilation.[148] Probes that record myocardial function and a hydraulic coronary 'balloon occluder' are implanted into an anaesthetized animal, which is then allowed to recover. Switching on the occluder in the awake animal for a short period, followed by reperfusion, produces myocardial stunning which can be attenuated by thiol compounds and desferrioxamine. Spin adducts from preadministered PBN can also be detected in coronary venous blood after hypoxia–reperfusion. Both the extent of the stunning and the amounts of PBN adducts detected are lower in 'conscious' than in 'open-chest' dogs, but the stunning phenomenon is still evident.[148] In conscious rabbits, overexpression of EC-SOD decreased infarction after ischaemia–reperfusion.[149]

9.5.4.3 *The relevance of xanthine oxidase*[136]
Multiple reports that antioxidants and allopurinol protect against cardiac ischaemia–reoxygenation injury in various animals support the relevance of the model in Fig. 9.12. Indeed, the adenosine deaminase inhibitor **erythro-9-(2-hydroxyl-3-nonyl) adenine**, which should block formation of hypoxanthine, also decreased ROS formation in the isolated reperfused rat heart.[150]

However, all is not clear-cut. Rat and dog heart contain XDH, but its rate of proteolytic conversion to XO during ischaemia is slow (e.g. in rat heart one study reported that about 20% of enzyme is present as oxidase to start with and it takes about 4 h of ischaemia for this to increase to 30%). Of course, the basal level of XO could still lead to extra ROS generation because of increased hypoxanthine. Unfortunately, rabbit, pig and human hearts have been reported not to contain *any* XO. If so, how can one explain the protective effects of allopurinol reported by several groups? It might prevent the depletion of purine nucleotides that can be used as substrates for resynthesis of ATP on reoxygenation.[151]

Of course, other sources of RS, such as mitochondria[5,152] may also be important. Mitochondria are more 'leaky' after a period of ischaemia. Also, if ischaemia is incomplete (i.e. limited O_2 is still present), the electron transport chain will be highly reduced and electron leakage could conceivably be favoured. Indeed, a mitochondrially targeted antioxidant was able to protect rat hearts against reperfusion injury (Section 10.6.11). Some $O_2^{\bullet-}$ might arise from cytochromes P450 in the heart, although their levels are generally low.[153]

Phagocytes may be an important source of ROS. Neutrophils play little role in the arrhythmias and stunning seen after brief ischaemia followed by reperfusion,[147,148] but they are important after longer ischaemic periods.[154] Thus depleting animals of neutrophils, or injecting them with antibodies that prevent neutrophil adherence to endothelium, before performing ischaemia–reperfusion has decreased infarct size in some studies.[155] Activation of complement during ischaemia–reperfusion can provoke neutrophils to release more ROS.[156] Neutrophil adherence to vascular endothelium is promoted by ROS and may contribute to the **no-reflow phenomenon**, the inability to reperfuse areas of previously ischaemic tissue, often thought to be due to plugging of capillaries by swelling of endothelial cells and neutrophil accumulation. Thus, as for gut, postischaemic cardiac injury involves inflammation. The vasoconstrictive effect of IPs formed during oxidative damage (Section 4.12.3) might also contribute.[157]

9.5.4.4 *The relevance of transition metals*

If $OH^\bullet$ is formed in the reoxygenated heart by Fenton chemistry (Fig. 9.12), then a source of transition-metal ions must be identified (not neglecting the contamination of buffers by them in studies with isolated hearts). Their importance is suggested by the generally protective effects of iron chelators (such as desferrioxamine) on ischaemia–reoxygenation-induced damage even *in vivo*[148] and the fact that hearts isolated from iron-overloaded animals are more susceptible to reoxygenation injury.[158] Remember, however, that desferrioxamine can do things other than chelating iron; it can scavenge ROS directly and also lead to activation of HIF (Section 10.7.1).

Iron and copper[159] might become more available as a result of cell injury, bleeding, or the action of $O_2^{\bullet-}$ on iron-containing proteins (Section 9.5.3). In heart, another source of RS could be myoglobin. Exposure of myoglobin to excess H_2O_2 causes liberation of haem and iron ions.[160] Myoglobin-H_2O_2 mixtures also exert pro-oxidant effects by ferryl formation (Section 3.15.3).

9.5.4.5 *Nitric oxide: good or bad?*[161]

The role of $NO^\bullet$ and $ONOO^-$ in ischaemia–reperfusion injury is unclear. Many papers imply that $NO^\bullet$ is good, yet several say it is bad. Nitric oxide will increase blood flow, scavenge $O_2^{\bullet-}$ (helpful only so long as the $ONOO^-$ produced can be removed), depress neutrophil adherence to endothelium, remove ferryl myoglobin by reacting with it and deter platelet aggregation. Nitric oxide also seems to play a key role in preconditioning (Section 9.5.6 below). By contrast, $ONOO^-$ can inactivate Ca^{2+} pumps in the heart, impairing contractility. Indeed, increased protein nitration was observed in failing human hearts.[162] Chronic high blood pressure or other 'overload stresses' can cause hypertrophy of the ventricles and sometimes eventual heart failure. Several papers (including some human studies)[163] suggest that proproliferative effects of excess ROS production (from mitochondria, NOS, and NOX enzymes) contribute to the abnormal remodelling of the ventricular wall.[164]

9.5.4.6 *Clinical relevance*

Since oxidative stress is involved in the common risk factors for coronary heart disease (diabetes, hypertension, cigarette smoking, obesity, hypercholesterolaemia), it is not surprising to find that patients with heart disease show elevated IP levels.[165,166] The protective effects of antioxidants against ischaemia–reperfusion in isolated hearts and various animal models cannot be doubted, with the caveat that their ability to influence infarct size after prolonged ischaemia is debatable. However, are these actions of antioxidants clinically relevant?

In many human myocardial infarctions, occlusion of a coronary artery may be maintained for so long that ischaemic injury is the sole cause of tissue death, reoxygenation injury being irrelevant. However, the early use of agents (such as **streptokinase** or **tissue plasminogen activator**) to dissolve thrombi is now commonplace, and thrombolysis sometimes occurs spontaneously. Several studies have shown that thrombolysis in humans is accompanied by increased oxidative damage.[166] Combined use of an antioxidant and a thrombolytic agent might thus be predicted to give enhanced benefit, although results of clinical trials using human recombinant CuZnSOD have been disappointing (maybe the wrong dose [Fig. 9.13], the wrong antioxidant or its inability to reach the site of ROS production perhaps; Section 10.6.11).[167] Thrombolysis is generally a slow process, rather than an abrupt reoxygenation, perhaps mitigating ROS formation.

9.5.4.7 *Cardiopulmonary bypass*

In open-heart surgery, patients are usually placed 'on bypass', the blood being diverted from the heart through an oxygenation system. Several studies suggest that reoxygenation injury contributes to the 'stunning-like' myocardial dysfunction sometimes seen after the heart is reperfused.[165] In addition, prolonged use of oxygenators can lead to damage to erythrocytes, complement activation, phagocyte adherence to endothelium, and release of 'catalytic' iron and copper ions.[168] The last problem can be especially significant in babies, since their plasma transferrin saturation tends to be greater than adults (Section 6.11.8.6).[169] There is now an increasing tendency, when possible, to perform surgery on the beating heart ('off pump'), to minimize such problems.[168,170]

9.5.5 Angioplasty, restenosis and bypass grafting

Another relevant area is the reopening of partially atherosclerosed arteries by **angioplasty**. In balloon angioplasty, a coronary artery is completely occluded when the balloon is inflated to 'squash' the atherosclerotic lesions. Abrupt reperfusion occurs upon balloon deflation, when blood flows through the 'cleared' artery. Usually the short duration of the occlusion (1–2 min) precludes significant reoxygenation injury to the heart, although elevations in blood F_2-IP levels may occur in patients and some studies suggest that allopurinol prevents this.[171] Coronary artery constriction, attenuated by SOD administration, was observed in dogs after balloon angioplasty.[172] Presumably, excess $O_2^{\bullet -}$ generation resulting from reoxygenation of the vascular endothelium transiently decreased net $NO^{\bullet}$ production. The 'squashing' of the atherosclerotic lesions may liberate transition metal ions and oxidized LDL into the circulation.[173]

A more important problem is the high incidence (>50% of cases) of **restenosis** after angioplasty. This involves endothelial damage caused by the balloon, and by any stents placed to keep the vessel open, leading to accelerated atherosclerosis marked by excessive proliferation of smooth muscle cells and fibroblasts. High doses of probucol decrease the severity of restenosis somewhat.[174,175] This might involve a contribution from probucol's antioxidant effects, but its other actions in inhibiting cell proliferation and promoting repair of damage to the endothelium seem more important. Restenosis is associated with increases in NOX, and consequent production of $O_2^{\bullet -}$, in the vessel wall, especially in smooth muscle cells and fibroblasts. Hence $O_2^{\bullet -}$ may contribute to their proliferation (Section 4.2.1).[174] Indeed, a peptide inhibitor that blocks NOX activity decreased restenosis in a rat model,[176] and restenosis in rabbits was decreased by raising EC-SOD levels in the arterial wall.[177] The contribution of lipid peroxidation to restenosis is uncertain, for example in rabbits coenzyme Q supplementation decreased lipid oxidation but did not delay restenosis after balloon-injury of the aorta.[178]

An alternative treatment for coronary atherosclerosis is bypass grafting. Again, one problem is accelerated atherosclerosis in the grafted vessels, involving increased levels of NOX.[179] Endothelial injury, perhaps caused by hypoxia (e.g. during the preparation and placement of the vessel), followed by reoxygenation, might contribute.[180] Short-term animal studies suggest that antioxidants (e.g. desferrioxamine–manganese and lazaroids; Section 10.6.8) might exert protective effects.[181,182]

9.5.6 Ischaemic preconditioning[135,161,183]

Short periods (a few minutes) of myocardial ischaemia can produce tissue changes that result in decreased sensitivity to a subsequent ischaemic insult. Similar phenomena are seen in other tissues, including brain, gut, muscle and skin. There are two phases of protection: a transient one that occurs within minutes but disappears within about 2 h, and a delayed phase that takes hours to appear but can then last for days. For example, if dog hearts are preconditioned by several 5-min periods of coronary artery occlusion, a subsequent 40-min reocclusion results in infarcts up to 75% smaller than in controls. The effects of preconditioning can also be observed against stunning and arrhythmias, and may have clinical relevance in **angina pectoris**. In this disease, atherosclerosis decreases blood supply through the coronary arteries. Exercise can cause the heart's O_2 requirements to exceed its blood supply, causing acute chest pain. Repetitive brief ischaemia in angina patients may, paradoxically, help protect against myocardial infarction.

The mechanism of preconditioning is intensively debated. Adenosine released from ischaemic myocytes is involved (legend to Fig. 9.12) in the early phase. It binds to receptors, stimulates phospholipase activity, raises DAG levels, activates protein kinase C and promotes its translocation to the plasma membrane (Section 4.5.5). During subsequent ischaemia, the PKC already on the membrane can be rapidly activated by DAG. Its activation causes phosphorylation and activation of ATP-sensitive potassium channels in plasma membrane and mitochondria, which seems to exert tissue-protective effects. For example, opening of the mitochondrial inner membrane ATP-dependent K^+ channel, which allows K^+ to enter the matrix, modulates mitochondrial ROS production (some studies show ROS production to be decreased, but others that more ROS are made and trigger signalling pathways involved in cytoprotection).[184] Once the PKC has left the membrane and gone back to its normal location, the protective effect disappears. Reactive species produced during reperfusion can activate PKC (Section 4.5.5), and, in cases where this is important, the preconditioning is abolished by antioxidants.[185]

Delayed preconditioning involves NO• (from eNOS and, in part, produced by increased expression of the gene encoding iNOS), probably again via activation of PKC and other kinases. Another factor contributing to delayed preconditioning may be rises in the levels of defences such as MnSOD and Hsps and increases in proteasome activity (to facilitate removal of damaged proteins that might impair contractility).[186] Pre-exposure to ethanol can also protect the heart and intestine against ischaemia–reperfusion, by causing ROS-dependent PKC activation.[187] Some anaesthetics, such as **isoflurane**, are cardioprotective; in a rat model, the delayed cardioprotection observed after exposure to this agent involved ROS and RNS.[188]

9.5.7 Shock-related ischaemia–reoxygenation[135]

Severe bleeding can cause a rapid fall in blood pressure. This places many tissues at risk, since it results in hypoperfusion with blood and hence hypoxia. When blood volume is restored, a 'shock' syndrome (**haemorrhagic shock**) can result, to which RS contribute. Stomach, gut, kidney and pancreas are among the organs that can be affected. Pretreatment of animals with allopurinol or SOD before haemorrhagic shock has been reported to minimize damage to various tissues.[189] Allopurinol and desferrioxamine increased survival in dogs subjected to severe haemorrhagic shock.[190]

Shock can also be induced by severe infection.[191] Septic shock is characterized by abnormally low blood pressure and inadequate perfusion of many organs. There is marked overproduction of $O_2^{\bullet-}$ (from activated phagocytes, other NOX, mitochondria, and possibly XO) and of NO•, largely involving iNOS gene expression in various organs in response to cytokines. Hence $ONOO^-$ production also occurs. Mitochondrial ATP production is impaired, in part by NO•. Treatment of septic shock includes antibiotics and administration of adrenalin or noradrenalin to maintain blood pressure. However, response to these catecholamines is often limited, and it has been suggested that this is due to their oxidation[191] by $O_2^{\bullet-}$. Mimetics of SOD, SOD itself and several other antioxidants have been tested in human sepsis patients, with variable results;[191,192] they may work best in the most severe cases (where deleterious effects of ROS outweigh beneficial ones e.g. antibacterial effects).[193]

9.5.8 The eye

The retina may become hypoxic as a result of atherosclerosis of ocular blood vessels (especially in diabetes), damage to the retinal pigment epithelium or by vascular occlusion by sickled red blood cells in patients with sickle-cell anaemia. Rises in intraocular pressure (e.g. in glaucoma) can also decrease blood flow and cause oxidative damage (Fig. 6.19). In animals, it has been shown that reperfusion of ischaemic retina leads to ROS production; for example, OH• was identified[194] by the salicylate method (Section 5.3.1).

9.5.9 Plants[195]

Plants can suffer hypoxia–reoxygenation, for example if the roots of a plant (or the whole plant) are flooded, which restricts the access of O_2. The plant responds by halting the synthesis of most proteins, but up-regulates the synthesis of others, the **anaerobic polypeptides**, one of which is alcohol dehydrogenase.

Many plants appear, morphologically, to survive flooding only to die on subsequent emergence, a classical reperfusion injury. Reactive species can be involved. For example, lipid peroxidation after flooding was higher in rhizomes of the flooding-sensitive plant *Iris germanica* than in rhizomes of the tolerant *Iris pseudacorus*. The latter species increases CuZnSOD activity during anoxia, but the former does not.

9.5.10 Chemical ischaemia–reperfusion: carbon monoxide poisoning[196]

Carbon monoxide, CO, is a colourless, odourless, tasteless gas produced by incomplete combustion of carbon-containing materials. It occurs in wood smoke, car exhausts, polluted air and cigarette smoke (Section 8.12), and is generated *in vivo* by haem oxygenase (Section 3.17) and as a minor end-product of lipid peroxidation.

Low levels of CO are useful *in vivo* (Section 3.17) and may even contribute to the ability of HO-1 to protect tissues against ischaemia–reperfusion (Section 9.6.1 below). However, high CO levels are poisonous. Coma can occur at carboxyhaemoglobin levels of >40% (levels in healthy non-smoking subjects are usually $\leq 0.7\%$) and lower levels can adversely affect the activity of organs especially sensitive to hypoxia, such as the heart and brain. Toxicity of CO results from its avid binding to haem proteins, especially haemoglobin (where it out-competes O_2 for binding by a factor of about 220, and the resulting **carboxyhaemoglobin** dissociates only slowly). Cytochrome oxidase can also be inhibited and mitochondrial ROS production from the 'backed up' electron transport chain thereby increased.

Treatment of CO poisoning is to remove the patient from the CO source and administer pure (or even hyperbaric) O_2. It is thus likely that tissue ischaemia–reoxygenation occurs. Patients often appear to recover from CO poisoning only to display delayed neurological effects, to which RS might contribute. Indeed, increased production of RS (including $OH^\bullet$ and $ONOO^-$) and lipid peroxidation have been reported in the brains of animals after CO exposure.[197]

9.5.11 Freezing injury

Cold-induced vasoconstriction in the skin is an important mechanism to reduce heat loss—low temperature enhances the response of receptors on smooth muscle cells to noradrenalin, facilitating blood vessel contraction. It has been suggested that increased mitochondrial generation of ROS plays a role in the signalling pathway increasing receptor sensitivity.[198]

However, severe and prolonged chilling of tissues causes hypoxia, and rewarming may create a reoxygenation injury. Thus it has been hypothesized that RS contribute to frostbite injury, although there is little evidence that antioxidants such as SOD would be protective in humans.[199]

Several vertebrates naturally tolerate freezing, for example the North American red-sided garter snake *Thamnophis sirtalis parietalis* can be frozen for several hours at $-2.5°C$, with about 50% of the body water as ice. It can also endure ischaemia (under N_2 gas) for up to 2 days. One survival strategy may be a rapid increase in antioxidant defences at the onset of freezing or anoxia.[200] A comparable strategy may be used by the ground squirrel *Citellus citellus*, in which an increase in tissue antioxidant defences is observed just before the onset of hibernation, presumably to minimize oxidative stress on reawakening.[201]

9.5.12 Sleep apnoea

Many humans suffer from this problem; their airways become obstructed during sleep, creating hypoxia that then (hopefully!) wakes them up, whereupon normal breathing resumes and pO_2 rises (reoxygenation). Their problems include not only fatigue due to interrupted sleep, but also an increased risk of hypertension, myocardial infarction and neuronal death in the brain. It has been suggested that ROS may be involved in these events,[202] for example by increases in the activity of NOX enzymes, although more data are needed to establish this in humans. Hypoxia due to living at high altitudes has also been suggested to increase oxidative damge (e.g. as elevated 8OHdG excretion), particularly during exercise.[203]

9.6 Organ preservation, transplantation and reattachment of severed tissues

9.6.1 Heart and kidney

The preservation of organs for transplantation, and the transplant surgery itself, can involve reperfusion injury. One aspect is **cold hypoxia**, the organ becoming hypoxic when stored at low temperature in a preservation fluid. Another is **warm hypoxia**, when the organ is inside the body and warming up, but unperfused as its blood vessel connections are being made. Once the organ is plumbed in, the body may mount an inflammatory/immune attack upon it. If severe, this can cause eventual rejection, a process to which phagocyte-derived RS may contribute. Indeed, one study suggested that the level of alkanes in expired air, a putative marker of lipid peroxidation (Section 5.14.8), can be used to identify patients rejecting their heart transplants.[204]

Newly transplanted hearts may suffer atherosclerosis of the coronary vessels, a process to which the host inflammatory-immune response contributes. One study of 40 patients indicated that supplementation with 500 mg vitamin C plus 400 units of α-tocopherol for 1 year decreased atherosclerosis in heart transplant recipients.[205] Increasing the levels of CuZnSOD or HO-1 in transplanted hearts decreased atherosclerosis and rejection in animals; CO accounts for at least part of the protective effect of HO-1, for example by promoting vasodilation, deterring phagocyte infiltration and decreasing thrombosis (Section 3.17). Bilirubin might sometimes contribute, for example in rats given bilirubin or biliverdin there was less restenosis after balloon injury.[206]

As for kidney transplants, several groups have reported that pretreatment of whole animals or isolated kidneys with SOD, catalase, allopurinol or desferrioxamine decreases reperfusion injury.

Rodent kidney contains XDH, although its irreversible (proteolytic) conversion to XO in ischaemic tissues occurs only slowly (half-life of about 6 h). There is much less XO in dog or human kidney. Hence the model in Fig. 9.12 is unlikely to account for reperfusion injury in kidney; ROS from sources other than XO may be important. Indeed, in transplanted human kidneys subjected to 25 to 28 h of cold hypoxia, SOD infusion into the renal artery at implantation produced significant improvement in short-term renal function; the difference was less marked with storage times below 25 h.[207] Similar data have been published using allopurinol. However, the clinical impact of such therapy on renal transplant surgery has been minor; the priority is to obtain the freshest kidneys possible and improve the preservation fluids, which often already contain allopurinol (Section 9.6.2 below). One interesting model perhaps worth further study is the ringed seal, *Phoca hispida*. During prolonged diving, blood flow is redistributed to the heart and nervous system, and the kidney is severely vasoconstricted. The seal kidney, both *in vivo* and as an isolated organ, is much more tolerant of ischaemia–reperfusion than other animal kidneys. Whether this is due to elevated antioxidant defences or other reasons remains to be estblished.[208]

Transplanted kidneys are frequently infiltrated by host phagocytic cells, and the RS they produce might contribute to transplant rejection, for example by facilitating fibrosis (Table 9.2). Indeed, enhanced immunostaining for nitrotyrosine has been measured in 'rejected' human kidney transplants. One of the nitrated targets is MnSOD (Section 7.9.4); exposure of this enzyme to $ONOO^-$ inactivates it. Is this an early or late event? It's hard to tell in humans, but in a rat model, increased mitochondrial nitrated MnSOD was seen prior to renal dysfunction.[209] Patients awaiting new kidneys are maintained by dialysis, a process that may cause oxidative stress (Section 7.10.5).

9.6.2 Liver

Hypoxia–reperfusion can occur in transplanted livers. During cold preservation, liver endothelial cells and hepatocytes can be sensitized to injury by several mechanisms, including rises in their low molecular mass iron pool,[210] accelerating damage by any ROS generated after the new liver is perfused. For example, human transplant recipients have been reported to exhale more ethane (Section 5.14.8) at the time of organ reperfusion[211] and liver GSH levels drop rapidly at that time.[212] Patients also showed increased urinary F_2-IPs.[213]

Liver contains XDH, but this is only slowly converted to XO during ischaemia, although both enzymes can be released into the blood from damaged liver and contribute to extrahepatic damage. In human liver, XDH is present in hepatocytes and bile duct epithelial cells, where it concentrates at the luminal surface. Indeed, the enzyme appears to be excreted into bile.[214] Other sources of oxidative stress in reperfused livers include more $O_2^{\bullet-}$ from damaged mitochondria, adherence of circulating neutrophils to the vascular endothelium, and activation of both these neutrophils and the macrophages (**Kupffer cells**) present in the liver itself.[215] Indeed, raising the levels of MnSOD in mouse liver mitochondria decreased both liver damage and the extent of activation of AP1 and NFκB after hypoxia–reoxygenation, indicative of a role for mitochondrial ROS.[216]

The role of Kupffer cells can be investigated by selectively killing them using **gadolinium chloride**, GdC1$_3$. Endothelial damage at early stages of liver reoxygenation may involve activation of Kupffer cells, whereas neutrophils (and, in some animals, XO) may contribute to later damage. Transplanted livers usually come from accident victims, who have sometimes been drinking heavily, and so their function might be compromised by ethanol (Section 8.8).

9.6.3 Limbs, digits and sex organs

Limb ischaemia or hypoxia can result from severe atherosclerosis (especially in diabetics with poor control of blood glucose, who may suffer gangrene of the extremities), thrombosis, arterial injury resulting in rapid blood loss, and (to a controlled extent) in the use of tourniquets to provide a 'bloodless field' in orthopaedic surgery. Modern surgical techniques for reattachment of severed digits, limbs and even penises can result in the reoxygenation of tissue that has been hypoxic for hours. Another problem is **intermittent claudication**, caused by narrowing or obstruction of leg arteries. Sufficient blood may reach the muscles at rest, but exercise leads to ischaemia and severe muscle pain in the calves.

Skeletal muscle is more resistant to ischaemic injury than most tissues. However, after some hours of ischaemia, an ischaemia–reperfusion injury to muscle can be demonstrated,[217] and is greater in mice lacking EC-SOD.[218] For example, experiments with rat hindlimbs have demonstrated OH$^{\bullet}$ formation during ischaemia–reperfusion using salicylate hydroxylation, observed the presence of lipid-derived radicals that could be trapped by PBN in both muscle and blood, and shown some protective effects of SOD plus catalase against the injury.[219] Levels of XO in pig or human muscle are lower than in rat,[220] although allopurinol has been claimed to be beneficial in decreasing lower limb swelling after leg artery bypass surgery.[221] In patients with claudication, OH$^{\bullet}$ formation was demonstrated (by aromatic hydroxylation) during the rest period after exercise.[222] In another study, surgical vessel reconstruction to improve blood flow was observed to decrease urinary F_2-IPs in patients, measured on the second postoperative day.[223]

Limbs and digits are not just muscle of course; the vascular endothelium may be far more sensitive to damage by ischaemia–reperfusion than the muscle. This can lead to a 'no reflow' situation as neutrophils adhere to damaged endothelium, and thrombosis occurs. Reperfusion of large areas of damaged muscle (e.g. crushed legs) can cause systemic injury to which both complement activation and ROS appear to contribute, for example by release into the bloodstream of XO, myoglobin and transition-metal ions.[224]

Dupuytren's contracture,[225] a disease in which tendons in the hand shorten abnormally and pull the fingers into a closed position, has been suggested to involve ischaemia–reoxygenation. Elevated levels of hypoxanthine and XO occur in the palmar fascia.

9.6.4 Organ preservation fluids[226]

As mentioned above, antioxidants are frequently added to organ preservation fluids. Examples are mannitol (although its major action may be as an osmotic agent that delays cell swelling), GSH and allopurinol. For example the **University of Wisconsin preservation fluid** has millimolar levels of added GSH. However, by the time the fluid is used, this is largely or completely oxidized to GSSG.[227] The fluid also contains high K^+ levels, 1 mM allopurinol, **lactobionic acid** (a weak Ca^{2+} and iron chelator), 5 mM adenosine (which may suppress phagocyte ROS production), the trisaccharide sugar raffinose and hydroxyethyl starch. The last two decrease cell swelling. Organs can be preserved for hours by flushing with this solution and storing at 0 to 5 °C. Some researchers have advocated supplementing this and other organ preservation fluids with desferrioxamine,[210] other thiols (e.g. bucillamine), PARP-1 inhibitors or a chimeric MnSOD that binds to vascular endothelium (Section 10.6.3).[228]

9.6.5 Other examples

Oxidative damage may contribute to the death of islet cell grafts implanted to treat diabetes, (Section 9.4.1),[102,229] of neurons injected to treat Parkinson's disease (Section 9.19 below), of myoblasts used to repair damaged hearts[230] and in adverse reactions to skin grafts. For example, there are reports that the 'survival time' of skin flaps is increased by SOD, desferrioxamine or allopurinol.[231]

9.7 Lung damage, shock and ARDS[6]

Ischaemia–reoxygenation can occur during the preservation of lungs for transplantation; RS may contribute, although few of them probably come from XO since its activity in human lung is low.[232] Reoxygenation injury can also occur when collapsed lungs are re-expanded, and if pulmonary vessels are blocked by thrombi that then dissolve. For example, reperfusion of isolated animal lungs after ischaemia leads to increased production of $O_2^{\bullet-}$ and H_2O_2, in part by activation of an a NOX enzyme in the pulmonary endothelium.[233] Thus addition of antioxidants (e.g. dimethylthiourea) to lung preservation fluids has been advocated, and supplying catalase (in a modified form that binds to pulmonary endothelium) to the rat lung during cold storage decreases injury after transplantation and improves graft function.[234] Upregulation of

HO-1 also protects the lung, CO being the major protective agent.[235]

A major problem for transplanted human lungs is inflammation, neutrophil infiltration, infection and fibrosis. Indeed, **obliterative bronchiolitis**, a fibroproliferative disease that blocks up the airways and interferes with lung function, is a major cause of long-term morbidity and mortality after lung transplantation. Iron accumulation in transplanted lungs and ROS formation may play a role in its pathology.[236] Lung transplant recipients were reported to have low antioxidant levels in plasma and lung lining fluids for at least 1 year post-surgery,[237] perhaps indicative of their consumption by ongoing RS production.

Lung damage can also result from events elsewhere in the body, such as injury to the gut resulting in sepsis and MODS (Section 9.5.1). Indeed, ischaemia–reperfusion damage to the liver of rats led to nitration and inactivation of MnSOD in the lung.[238] The lung damage associated with MODS varies from mild to very severe, the latter producing the **acute** (sometimes called **adult**, although this term is less popular now because children can suffer the condition) **respiratory distress syndrome (ARDS)**. The ARDS syndrome is defined as severe hypoxia resistant to O_2 administration, caused by pulmonary oedema. It can arise as a complication of haemorrhagic or endotoxic shock (Section 9.5.7), aspiration of stomach contents into the lung, cardiopulmonary bypass or severe tissue damage, for example caused by burns (Section 6.12.3) or accidents. The ARDS syndrome kills thousands of patients worldwide. It leads to death in about 50% of cases, and even today mortality has decreased only modestly from when ARDS was first described in 1967. Bronchopulmonary dysplasia in babies (Section 6.11.8) resembles ARDS.

The ARDS syndrome is marked by a dramatic appearance of neutrophils and neutrophil-derived products in the lung, involving upregulation of adhesion molecules on lung endothelial cells, production of cytokines by alveolar macrophages and other phagocytes, and activation of the complement system. It is widely thought that RS from activated phagocytes are important mediators of lung injury. Indeed, the acute lung injury produced in rats after severe skin burns or injection of cobra-venom factor (both causing complement activation and neutrophil infiltration into lung) can be minimized by treating the animals with SOD, catalase, desferrioxamine or apolactoferrin, and worsened by infusion of iron(III) salts, implying that iron-dependent formation of $OH^\bullet$ is involved.[239] Activated neutrophils produce HOCl and secrete elastase; lung elastic fibres can be degraded if α_1-antiproteinase is inactivated by HOCl or $ONOO^-$. However, neutrophils should not automatically be assumed to be the 'bête noir' in ARDS. They also have beneficial effects; combating pulmonary infection and releasing lactoferrin, which can inhibit iron-dependent oxidative damage (Section 7.7.2). Alveolar macrophages are another source of RS, elastase, other proteinases and cytokines in ARDS, and additional RS can come from mitochondria and XO. Although normal human lung contains little XO, circulating enzyme from other injured body tissues can readily bind and remain within the lung.[232]

9.7.1 Oxidative stress in ARDS: does it occur and does it matter?[6]

So are RS important in ARDS? Oxidative stress certainly occurs (Table 9.5), but attempts to target it as a therapeutic strategy have been disappointing. Oxidative stress can result from ARDS itself, the condition that triggered ARDS (Table 9.5, legend) and from the elevated O_2 administered to patients to maintain blood pO_2. It has even been suggested that the routine clinical practice of administering O_2 could be bad because it interferes with tissue-protective responses to hypoxia.[240] Lung previously injured, for example by aspiration of gastric contents or infection, may be more susceptible to O_2-induced damage. In addition, it has been suggested that prolonged mechanical ventilation induces oxidative damage in the diaphragm and lung, that may facilitate inflammation.[241] But clinically there is often no choice, the O_2 is needed. Reactive species could damage alveolar surfactant (e.g. $ONOO^-$ nitrates surfactant proteins) and α_1-antiproteinase as well as impairing their synthesis by alveolar type II cells.

Reactive species are intimately linked to cytokines (Section 4.7), the levels of many of which are elevated in ARDS and in septic patients at high risk of ARDS. Special attention has been paid to TNFα, which increases cellular ROS and produces proinflammatory mediators. Yet, TNFα also induces antioxidant defences, especially MnSOD (Section 4.7.1). This cytokine itself is not therefore necessarily bad; it seems more the *balance* of proinflammatory (including TNFα) and anti-inflammatory (e.g. IL-10) cytokines that influences outcome in ARDS, and in sepsis. Indeed, therapies directed at neutralizing TNFα have not proved effective in ARDS. Similarly, the antioxidant properties of N-acetylcysteine *in vitro*, together with the observed depletion of thiols in ARDS patients (Table 9.5), led to clinical trials of this substance, which have (sadly) demonstrated that thiol supplementation is of little benefit to most patients, although N-acetylcysteine did offer some benefit in another condition, idiopathic pulmonary fibrosis (Section 10.6.9.2). The complexity of ARDS and the large number of mediators of tissue injury involved (complement, RS, cytokines, proteinases, prostaglandins, leukotrienes) make it perhaps unlikely that any single intervention will have a major clinical benefit. Remember also that RS are sometimes good things, helping to damp down inflammation (Section 7.9.5) and modulate MMP activity (Table 7.2). In addition, ARDS is a blanket term for several closely related conditions provoked by different stimuli, and it is likely that the role played by RS differs in each. Thus ARDS can even develop in neutropaenic patients, that is it can occur without significant neutrophil infiltration into the lung.

9.8 Cystic fibrosis[243]

Cystic fibrosis (CF), one of the commonest inherited human diseases (incidence about 1 in 2500 in Caucasians), is due to an abnormality in a protein encoded by a gene on chromosome 7. Several mutations are known, but the most common is a three-base-pair deletion that eliminates a phenylalanine residue at position 508, giving a misfolded protein that stays in the ER and never reaches the plasma membrane. This protein (the **cystic fibrosis transmembrane conductance regulator**, CFTR) couples ATP hydrolysis with Cl^- transport across epithelial surfaces. It probably has other physiological functions as well, such as transport of other

Table 9.5 Evidence for oxidative stress in ARDS[6]

Observation	Comments
Oxidized α_1-antiproteinase found in lung lavage fluid	Essential methionine residue oxidized, presumably inactivated by HOCl, ONOO$^-$, chloramines etc. (*Am. J. Physiol.* **278**, L961,2000).
Elevated H_2O_2 levels in exhaled air	Elevated H_2O_2 in urine from ARDS patients reported (*Chest* **105**, 232, 1994).
Elevated F_2-isoprostanes in breath condensate	*Chest* **114**, 1653, 1998. Isoprostanes may not only be biomarkers of lipid peroxidation but may have pathological effects, since some are powerful constrictors of airway smooth muscle (*Am. J. Resp. Crit. Care Med.* **166**, S25, 2002). Other evidence of lipid peroxidation includes increased plasma HNE (*Crit. Care Med.* **24**, 241, 1996).
Diminished levels of ascorbate in body fluids[a]	Ascorbate can be oxidized by RS and the DHA taken up by activated neutrophils. Nutrition in very sick people is also compromised. Some studies suggest that the risk of developing ARDS in surgical patients might be diminished by administering ascorbate and α-tocopherol.[138]
Reports of decreased α-tocopherol	Data conflicting: it is essential to standardize α-tocopherol levels against lipid before comparison as lipid levels in body fluids change in ARDS, e.g. cholesterol levels can fall sharply.
Oxidation/ chlorination of proteins in plasma and lung lining fluid Nitrotyrosine (NT) formation	Loss of –SH groups, increased levels of protein carbonyls and of chloro-and *ortho*-tyrosine (*Am. J. Resp. Care Med.* **142**, A28, 1994; *Free Radic. Res.* 20, 289, 1994). Immunostaining of lungs from ARDS patients revealed nitrotyrosine, scarcely detectable in normal lung (*J. Clin. Invest.* **94**, 2407, 1994). Plasma NT also increased; plasma proteins modified by nitration include caeruloplasmin, transferrin, and α_1-antiproteinase (*Am. J. Physiol.* **278**, L961, 2000). Some circulating antibodies reported to recognize nitrated proteins.
[b]Presence of 'catalytic' iron in plasma (BDI)	Patients with impaired liver function and multiple organ failure show increased transferrin saturation and 'catalytic' iron in plasma. Patients without such complications show increased transferrin saturation but not usually to an extent leading to BDI. Lung lining fluid transferrin levels rise in ARDS due to increased leakage from plasma, and can bind BDI.
Upregulation of haem oxygenase in the lung	Often quoted as a evidence of oxidative stress (Section 3.17). May contribute to the changes in iron metabolism (*Crit. Care Med.* **32**, 1130, 2004).
Diminished caeruloplasmin 'ferroxidase' activity	Plasma caeruloplasmin protein levels often elevated (acute phase response), also in lung lining fluid (increased leakage from plasma) but ferroxidase activity per unit protein is decreased. Could be due to increased release of proteinases, since caeruloplasmin is sensitive to proteolytic damage, and/or to damage by ONOO$^-$ (*Am. J. Physiol.* **278**, L961, 2000).
Loss of plasma –SH groups	Normal levels $\approx 500\,\mu M$; fall to $\sim 300\,\mu M$ in ARDS.
Decreased GSH levels in lung fluids	Levels in alveolar lining fluid are $\sim 20\,\mu M$, much lower than normal. Levels of GSSG elevated (*Am. Rev. Resp. Dis.* **148**, 1174, 1993).
Increased xanthine oxidase	Xanthine oxidase may be released from other injured tissues to cause damage to lung by binding to cell surfaces. Levels of plasma hypoxanthine increase, indicative of hypoxia (*Am. J. Resp. Care Med.* **155**, 479, 1997).
Increased activity of angiotensin II	Could promote ROS production (Section 7.10.3). See *Nature* **436**, 112, 2005.

[a] Often $<5\,\mu M$ in plasma; normal values were $\sim 50\,\mu M$ in the same studies.
[b] BDI, bleomycin-detectable iron.
Please remember that the oxidative stress measured could be due not only to the ARDS, but also to its causes (trauma, sepsis, etc.) and to O_2 administration.

anions (e.g. ATP) and GSH. Indeed, GSH levels in lung lining fluids are subnormal in CF patients.[244]

The defect in CF impairs the movement of water and electrolytes across various epithelial surfaces, most notably in the respiratory tract, but also in the liver, bile ducts, pancreas, gastrointestinal tract and skin (the sweat excretion system). In the respiratory tract there is decreased Cl^- secretion and increased Na^+ absorption, resulting in inadequate hydration of the respiratory tract mucus. This makes it stickier and difficult to clear, and predisposes the CF patient to chronic lung infection. This infection, and the ensuing inflammatory-immune responses, lead to progressive lung destruction. Oxidative stress contributes to this injury, but, as with ARDS, its significance is uncertain (Table 9.6). For example, both ROS and elastase can increase mucus production (ref [245] and Section 8.12.4). The commonest pathogen chronically infecting the lung is *Pseudomonas aeruginosa*, an organism rich in catalase (Section 3.7.1)

that releases siderophores and redox-cycling agents which aggravate oxidative damage to the lung (Section 8.7). It also produces an enzyme that can cleave transferrin and lactoferrin to release iron (Section 8.7) but can secrete an extracellular polysaccharide (**alginate**) to protect itself against ROS. Indeed, some of the antibiotics administered to CF patients may confer benefit by antioxidant as well as antibacterial actions (Section 8.16). *P. aeruginosa* can also infect the lungs of ARDS and immuno-compromised patients. Elevated lung ROS levels can damage the bacterial DNA, paradoxically sometimes helping *P. aeruginosa* to mutate faster and acquire resistance to antibiotics.[247]

9.8.1 Cystic fibrosis and carotenoids

Cystic fibrosis patients have low plasma levels of β-carotene (often ~0.04 µM as opposed to normal levels of around 0.2 µM), lutein, zeaxanthin,

Table 9.6 Evidence consistent with increased oxidative stress in plasma and cystic fibrosis

Elevated F_2-isoprostanes in exhaled air[246]
Elevated levels of plasma lipid peroxidation products (measured by GPx assay or by HPLC)
Increased susceptibility of lipoproteins to peroxidation
Increased susceptibility of erythrocytes to peroxide-induced hemolysis
Elevated breath pentane levels
Increases in myeloperoxidase in sputum
Increased phagocyte-derived 'long-lived oxidants' in sputum
Increased 'catalytic' iron in sputum and respiratory tract lining fluids
Evidence of protein oxidation, chlorination, and nitration in sputum
Increased plasma protein and bronchoalveolar lavage fluid carbonyls (*Am. J. Clin. Nutr.* **80**, 374, 2004; *Chest* **129**, 431, 2006)
Decreased GSH levels in bronchoalveolar lavage fluid, some suggestions that inhaled GSH may be helpful (*Chest* **127** 308, 2005; *Free Rad. Biol. Med.* **39**, 463, 2005)
Increased amounts of pro-oxidant cytokines (e.g. TNFα)
Increased neutrophil and monocyte numbers in lung
Decreases in plasma selenium (and plasma and erythrocyte GPx levels)
Decreases in plasma ascorbate and α-tocopherol (in some but not all studies)[a]
Decreased plasma β-carotene
Increased oxidative damage to DNA (assayed by urinary 8OHdG)
Elevated dityrosine levels in plasma and bronchoalveolar lavage fluids
Inactivation of α_1-antiproteinase
Decreased plasma TRAP (Section 5.17) values
Increased levels of HO-1 and ferritin in the lung (*Am. J. Resp. Care Med.* **170**, 633, 2004)
Increased CO in exhaled air, presumably from the HO-1 but possibly some from lipid peroxidation (*Thorax* **55**, 138, 2000)

For references not cited above, see *Adv. Pharmacol.* **38**, 491, 1996 and *Thorax* **49**, 738, 1994.

[a] Important to standardize to plasma lipids when expressing α-tocopherol levels.

lycopene and α-carotene. Carotenoid levels in the macula of the eye are also subnormal (Section 6.10.4). The decreases cannot easily be explained by lower carotenoid intake or disordered fat absorption and (at least for β-carotene) are greater in more severe disease. Is there increased turnover of carotenoids? If so, is it due to their acting as antioxidants? Some studies suggest yes; for example administration of β-carotene to children with CF was reported to decrease plasma TBARS (measured using HPLC) from $\sim$90 nM to $\sim$70 nM (close to the values found in normal children).[248] However, carotenoids have other biological actions (Section 3.21). It would be good to measure products of carotenoid oxidation in CF patients (to establish their putative antioxidant activity), and also to carry out studies of carotenoid turnover in CF. In another study, supplementation with a mixture of α-tocopherol, vitamin C, selenium and retinol did not decrease plasma F_2-IPs, nor did it improve lung function in CF patients.[246]

9.9 Chronic inflammatory diseases: more examples

The acute inflammatory response is essential in helping to eliminate dangerous pathogens. Inflammation is normally self-limiting and its benefit outweighs any tissue damage caused (Section 7.9). However, anything causing abnormally large and/or prolonged activation of the immune system has the potential to cause severe injury. Thus infection by organisms that the host finds hard to eliminate (Section 7.9.6) can cause problems; we have just seen this for *P. aeruginosa* in CF (Section 9.8). Other examples include leprosy and tuberculosis. Persistent inflammation also contributes to asthma (Section 6.3), atherosclerosis (Section 9.3), diabetes (Section 9.4), ischaemia–reperfusion (Section 9.5), psoriasis (Section 6.12), graft rejection (Section 9.5), Alzheimer's disease (Section 9.20 below) and MODS/ARDS (Sections 9.5 and 9.6). Yet another example is **gout**, where severe inflammation is triggered by precipitation of sodium urate crystals within joints. Gout is treated with allopurinol.

Perhaps the most striking consequences of abnormal phagocyte/lymphocyte action are seen in the **autoimmune diseases**. The body has mechanisms to deter formation of antibodies against its own components. Failure of these allows formation of **autoantibodies** that can bind to normal biomolecules, and provoke attack by the immune system. Sometimes, only one tissue is affected. For example, in **Hashimoto's thyroiditis** infiltration of the thyroid gland by lymphocytes and phagocytes is accompanied by tissue damage and fibrosis, and the presence of circulating antibodies against such thyroid constituents as thyroglobulin (Section 7.5.1). In **myasthenia gravis**, a neuromuscular disorder characterized by weakness and fatigue of voluntary muscles, antibodies against the neurotransmitter acetylcholine are present.

Small amounts of autoantibodies are sometimes demonstrable in 'normal' subjects, and their incidence increases with age. One mechanism for this may be oxidative damage to tissues, creating new antigens by oxidation of amino acid residues and/or by the binding of end-products of lipid peroxidation such as HNE.[249] Indeed, 'senescent antigen' is used by macrophages to recognize worn-out erythrocytes (Section 6.4). It has even been reported[250] that exposure to a $O_2^{\bullet-}$-generating system (hypoxanthine plus XO) or to $ONOO^-$ causes DNA to become antigenic when injected into animals, the former possibly because of $O_2^{\bullet-}$-dependent generation of $OH^{\bullet}$. Both $OH^{\bullet}$ and $ONOO^-$ can attack the DNA to generate novel antigens.

In some other autoimmune diseases, such as **systemic lupus erythematosus** (SLE), **scleroderma** (a connective tissue disease characterized by fibrosis of the skin and often the internal organs), and **autoimmune vasculitis**, lesions are widespread and autoantibodies are present against many tissues. For example, antineutrophil antibodies seem important in several vascular autoimmune diseases, such as **Wegener's granulomatosis**. Myeloperoxidase is one important antigen recognized.[251] Lupus mainly affects young women, and produces a variety of lesions involving the skin, kidneys, muscles, joints, heart and blood vessels. Patients are light-sensitive and in about 40% of cases develop a characteristic 'butterfly' rash across the cheeks and nose when exposed to sunlight. Among the wide range of autoantibodies produced are some directed against CuZnSOD,[252] DNA, RNA, erythrocytes, subcellular organelles and plasma proteins. The kidney lesions in lupus are probably due to deposition of immune complexes on the basement membranes of glomeruli, followed by complement activation. It has been speculated[250] that some of the anti-DNA antibodies arise from oxidative damage to DNA or nucleoproteins. In addition, oxidized mitochondrial DNA may be proinflammatory.[253] Antibodies directed against phospholipids are present in patients with lupus and some other autoimmune diseases and in some females with repeated failures of pregnancy. Some of them cross-react with oxidized LDL and it is possible that they are directed against products of lipid peroxidation *in vivo*. Most of these antibodies require a phospholipid-binding protein found in plasma, **$β_2$-glycoprotein I** (sometimes called **apolipoprotein H**) to allow them to recognize phospholipids.[254] This protein can also be oxidatively damaged, and oxidized forms may also be proimmunogenic.[254] Patients with antiphospholipid antibodies (and other lupus patients) indeed show elevated lipid peroxidation, measured as F_2-IPs,[255] and increased circulating oxidized LDL. The serum of lupus patients has been reported to contain **clastogenic factors**, agents that induce chromosome damage when added to cells in culture, an effect prevented by inclusion of SOD in the culture medium.[256] More work is needed to elucidate their molecular nature.

Several drugs can induce a condition resembling lupus, including **hydralazine, isoniazid, chlorpromazine, procainamide** and (much less frequently) penicillamine, α-methyl-DOPA, and diphenylhydantoin (Chapter 8). Metabolites of, or products formed by attack of RS upon, these drugs may bind to proteins to give products that behave as 'foreign antigens' (Section 9.10.6.2 below).[257]

9.9.1 Are RS important mediators of autoimmune diseases?

It seems likely that RS play some role in tissue damage in the autoimmune diseases, although how much is not clear. For example, scleroderma and lupus patients show elevated urinary IPs, indicative of increased lipid peroxidation.[255,258] Serum proteins from lupus patients have elevated levels of

carbonyls, nitrotyrosine and methionine sulphoxide.[259] Skin fibroblasts from scleroderma patients showed increased NOX activity and released more $O_2^{•-}$ in culture,[260] perhaps relevant to their excessive proliferation *in vivo* (Sections 4.2.1). Lupus patients have been suggested to have defects in the repair of 8OHdG in DNA.[261]

However, increased production of RS does not prove their importance as mediators of tissue injury. Autoimmune diseases generally have active and quiescent phases, which makes evaluation of medical treatment difficult. This should be borne in mind when assessing the effectiveness of any therapy, including the use of antioxidants, in any study other than a fully randomized double-blind controlled clinical trial over a long period. Too many claims of benefit from, for example SOD, are based on short-term 'open' studies of small numbers of patients.[262] Nevertheless, injection of SOD or other antioxidants can decrease inflammation in animal models, such as several models of renal injury (Section 7.10.5). For example, SOD bound to a high-molecular-mass polymer such as **Ficoll** decreases inflammation induced by injecting **carrageenan**, an irritating substance derived from seaweed, into the feet of rats. Both SOD and catalase showed inhibitory effects against inflammation induced by the implantation of carrageenan-soaked sponges beneath the skin of rats. Nitric oxide, probably via $ONOO^-$, also contributes to this model of inflammation.[263] Injection of a low-molecular mass SOD mimetic, M40403 (Section 10.6.4) decreased inflammation, nitrotyrosine formation and pain in rats injected in a hindpaw with carrageenan.[263]

9.9.1.1 *Artefacts to watch for: contamination of commercial antioxidants and oxidation on sample storage*

One criticism that can be levelled at many of the above experiments with antioxidant proteins is the lack of controls. Controls with inactivated SOD and catalase should be performed to rule out 'non-specific' anti-inflammatory effects of proteins, or of contaminants within the enzyme preparations. These can include bacterial endotoxin[264] and **thymol**, an antioxidant preservative in commercial catalase solutions. Endotoxin contamination of

SOD could easily explain some of its reported anti-inflammatory effects.

Another artefact can affect measurements of oxidative damage in patient material. Body fluids can undergo lipid peroxidation on prolonged storage (even at $-70\,°C$) or mishandling (e.g. repeated freeze–thawing), in part because of release of copper ions from caeruloplasmin.[265] Several studies identifying 'cytotoxic factors' in the plasma of patients with various diseases have been led astray by the artefactual generation of peroxidation products. One cannot necessarily allow for this by using controls of normal body fluids stored for the same time. Plasma contains powerful antioxidants that limit lipid peroxidation; depletion of these protective mechanisms and rises in caeruloplasmin occur during many diseases, so that the fluid are less stable on storage than those from healthy subjects. Hence studies of oxidative damage should, whenever possible, be carried out on freshly drawn or properly stored samples. For example, plasma or serum samples stored for later analysis of isoprostanes must have antioxidants such as BHT added.

9.9.1.2 *Periodontal disease: a missed opportunity?*[266]

Inflammation of the gums is a major cause of tooth loss worldwide, and appears to be due to an inflammatory/immune response to dental plaque accumulation around the gum margin. Given that increased oxidative damage can be demonstrated in this region[267] (although more work is needed with modern techniques) and that topical application of antioxidants should be easy, it is surprising to the authors that more work has not been done in this area, although one study did show that the antioxidant M40403 decreased inflammation in a rat model of periodontal disease (Table 10.2). A similar comment can be applied to chronic skin inflammations such as acne. In both acne and periodontal disease, increased 'catalytic' iron may be involved (Section 6.12 and references[267,268]).

9.10 Rheumatoid arthritis[269]

Joint inflammation often accompanies autoimmune diseases, such as SLE, and is a complication of iron overload in idiopathic haemochromatosis (Section 3.15.5), but some of the severest cases are due to rheumatoid arthritis (RA). This disease is characterized by chronic joint inflammation, especially in the hands and legs, and is more frequent in females. Indeed, RA has many features of an autoimmune disease and there is genetic predisposition to it, but the cause of most cases is unknown. T-lymphocytes play a key role, which has led to the proposal that RA is a persistent, cell-mediated immune response to an unknown antigen. The blood plasma and joint fluid of RA patients often contain autoantibodies directed against **immunoglobulin G** (IgG), mostly against the Fc region of this protein. Something must cause IgG to become antigenic in RA; this may be because the carbohydrate side-chains are different and/or because IgG is damaged by RS generated during the inflammation.[270]

9.10.1 The normal joint

In normal synovial joints, articular cartilage covers the bone ends and both are enclosed by a thin and fibrous synovial membrane, made up of lining cells that face the joint cavity, plus overlying fatty and fibrous material. The lining cells (**synoviocytes**) are of at least two types: type A cells are essentially macrophages and type B cells are secretory, fibroblast-type cells. The synovial lining synthesizes **hyaluronic acid** (Fig. 9.14) and secretes it into the synovial fluid (SF), where it is largely responsible for the viscosity of the fluid. The synovial lining also acts as a barrier to the free movement of proteins from plasma into the synovial fluid. The macrophage-like cells may function to engulf debris produced as a result of 'wear and tear' in the joint. The volume of SF in healthy synovial joints is small, for example only about 0.5 ml in human knee joints. It lubricates the joint, supplies nutrients to, and removes waste from, the cartilage.

Articular cartilage is a dense tissue containing cells (**chondrocytes**) embedded in a matrix of collagen fibres and proteoglycans (mostly **aggrecan**). Cartilage does not contain blood vessels and receives O_2 by diffusion from the bone and SF, so that cartilage O_2 levels are low. One important nutrient it requires is ascorbate, needed for collagen synthesis (Section 3.20). Chondrocytes take up ascorbate in a Na^+-dependent process (using SVCT2) and concentrate it to millimolar intracellular

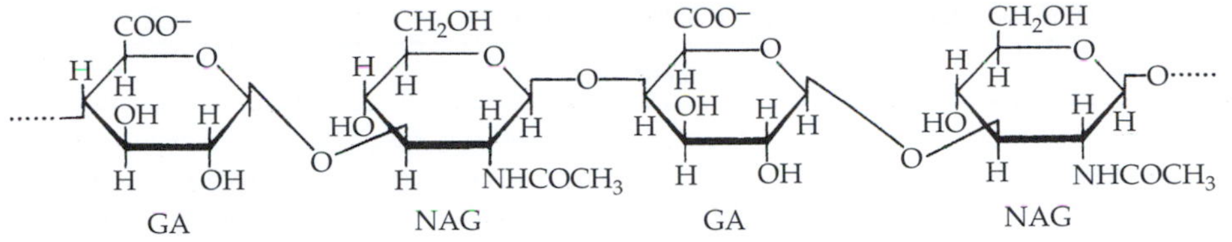

Figure 9.14 Structure of hyaluronic acid. Hyaluronic acid is a long polymer formed by joining together alternately two different sugars: glucuronic acid (GA) and *N*-acetylglucosamine (NAG). The negative charge on the carboxyl groups of GA at physiological pH causes them to repel each other, so that the molecule extends out in solution. Hence solutions of hyaluronic acid are extremely viscous.

levels.[271] They can also take up DHA, using glucose transporters.[271] Chondrocytes contain the usual complement of antioxidants, including peroxiredoxins, and cartilage has a high level of EC-SOD in the matrix.[272]

9.10.2 The RA joint[269]

The onset of RA is usually slow, appearing as pain, stiffness and swelling of the joints. The synovial lining thickens and folds, there is growth of new blood vessels, infiltration of lymphocytes, increased numbers of macrophages and proliferation of fibroblasts. The permeability of the synovial lining rises, allowing more proteins to enter the joint from the plasma. Iron deposits form within the synovial cells, much being located in ferritin and haemosiderin. The progression of RA is variable; in some subjects it is mild and self-limiting, but in it others leads to destruction of the articular cartilage, bone erosion, and impairment of joint function. Severe RA is also associated with accelerated atherosclerosis and cardiovascular disease. How do these events happen?

Bone is normally remodelled as required by a balance of opposing reactions; digestion by **osteoclasts** (a macrophage-type cell), deposition of new matrix by **osteoblasts** and then calcification of this matrix. This balance is altered to favour net bone loss in severe RA. Why? Partly because of increased osteoclast activity due to the expression of the **RANKL (receptor activator of NF-κB ligand) protein** on T-cells and synoviocytes in the rheumatoid joint. This ligand attaches to the **RANK (receptor activator of NF-κB)** receptor on osteoclasts, promoting their maturation and activation. Reactive species may be involved in the intracellular

signalling. In addition, osteoblasts are readily damaged by RS (Section 9.10.3 below), including H_2O_2, oxidized lipids and $ONOO^-$. By contrast, low concentrations of ROS or oxidized lipids *accelerate*[273,274] bone resorption by osteoclasts; these cells even make ROS, using an NADPH oxidase, NOX4 (Section 7.10.7).[275] In other words, a pro-oxidant environment favours bone loss.

Cartilage destruction appears largely mediated by increased activity of matrix metalloproteinases (Table 7.2), aided by inactivation of antiproteinases. Macrophage elastase (**matrix metalloproteinase-12**) may be especially important.[276] In addition, chondrocytes can be damaged[277] by $ONOO^-$ and other RS; H_2O_2 readily inhibits cartilage proteoglycan synthesis,[278] for example by interfering with ATP synthesis, in part by inhibiting G3PDH in chondrocytes. Indeed, intra-articular injection of H_2O_2-generating systems causes severe joint damage in animals.[279] The low ascorbate concentrations in RA SF (Table 9.7) might hinder collagen resynthesis, adding to the problem.

Damage in the RA joint usually occurs from the periphery (where the synovial lining meets the articular cartilage) by the growth of the inflamed synovial lining over, and into, the cartilage. This 'overgrowing' tissue is called **pannus**; the word comes from the Latin for 'cloth', the pannus being said to resemble a reddish cloth spreading over the cartilage. Pannus is often vascularized and contains iron deposits, and most cells in pannus are large and mononuclear, many having fibroblastic features. Most of the macrophages arise from blood monocytes attracted by chemotactic factors produced in the joint. The cytokine TNFα secreted by activated macrophages induces activation of NF-κB in synoviocytes, leading to increased production of

Table 9.7 Evidence revealing increased oxidative damage in rheumatoid disease

Observation	Comment
Increased lipid peroxidation products in serum and synovial fluid (SF)	Elevated F_2-isoprostanes (*Ann. Rheum. Dis.* **60**, 627, 2001) and increased levels of 4-HNE. In addition, decreased α-tocopherol (per unit lipid) in SF is consistent with lipid peroxidation, as are reports of 'foam cells' containing oxidized LDL in rheumatoid synovium. LDL isolated from RA SF showed altered electrophoretic mobility consistent with oxidation (*Free Rad. Biol. Med.* **22**, 705, 1997). High doses of α-tocopherol were reported to diminish pain but not other parameters of inflammation in RA patients (*Ann. Rheum. Dis.* **56**, 649, 1997).
Depletion of ascorbate in serum and SF	Presumably results from oxidation of ascorbate during its antioxidant action. Activated neutrophils take up DHA rapidly.
Decreased GSH in synovial T-lymphocytes	May result from oxidative stress or activation (*J. Immunol.* **158**, 1458, 1997). Synovial T-lymphocytes frequently stain positive for H_2O_2 production in the RA joint (*Arth. Rheum.* **52**, 2003, 2005).
Increased exhalation of pentane	Putative end-product of lipid peroxidation (Section 5.14.8).
Increased concentrations of urate oxidation products	Products measured appear to be end-products of RS attack upon urate (Section 5.12).
Activation of NF-κB in rheumatoid synovia	Probably mediated by TNFα and other cytokines, possibly by ROS as second messengers (Section 4.5.8) (*Arth. Rheum.* **39**, 583, 1996; *Arth. Rheum.* **40**, 226, 1997).
Increase in formation of 2,3-DHB from salicylate	2,3-DHB appears to be a product of attack of OH$^\bullet$ upon salicylate in patients taking high-dose aspirin (Section 5.3).
Hyaluronic acid degradation Formation of 'fluorescent' proteins	Pattern of degradation is suggestive of OH$^\bullet$ production (*Biochem. J.* **273**, 459, 1991). Fluorescence probably caused by oxidative damage to proteins. Nitrated and chlorinated IgG found in RA SF (*J. Immunol.* **165**, 6532, 2000).
Increased steady-state levels (in cellular DNA) and increased urinary excretion of 8OHdG	Indicative of oxidative DNA damage. Oxidized mitochondrial DNA was detected in plasma and synovial fluid of >50% of RA patients (*Arth. Res. Ther.* 5, R234, 2003).
Increased levels of protein carbonyls in synovial fluid	Indicative of oxidative protein damage, but could also result from binding of HNE and other aldehydes to proteins (Section 5.15.3).
Nitrotyrosine	3-Nitrotyrosine detected in SF and tissues of RA patients, but not clear if levels are elevated compared with control or OA patients (our unpublished data; also see ref[272] and *Arth. Rheum.* **46**, 2341, 2002; *J. Rheumatol.* **30**, 1173, 2003). Serum levels of nitrated peptides derived from collagen were reported to be elevated in both OA and RA (*Osteoarth. Cartilage* **13**, 258, 2005). Overall contribution of ONOO$^-$ to RA is unclear.
Increased inactivation of antiproteinases	Synovial fluid α_2-macroglobulin shows increased chlorination and oxidation (as carbonyls) and inactivation in RA (*Arch. Biochem. Biophys.* **391**, 119, 2001). This protein is known to be inactivated by HOCl (Section 2.6.3). Increased levels of oxidized α_1-antiproteinase also detected in plasma (*Clin. Chim. Acta* **317**, 125, 2002).
Glycation	N^ϵ-carboxymethyllysine levels increased in synovial tissue, indicative of glycoxidation (Section 9.4). Elevation also seen in OA patients (*Ann. Rheum. Dis.* **61**, 488, 2002).

Abbreviations: 2,3-DHB, 2,3-dihydroxybenzoate; HNE, hydroxynonenal; LDL, low-density lipoprotein: 8OHdG, 8-hydroxy-2′-deoxyguanosine; OA, osteoarthritis. For references not cited, see *Ann. Rheum. Dis.* **54**, 505, 1995.

IL-1, IL-8, iNOS, COX-2, monocyte chemoattractant protein-1 (MCP-1) and TNFα itself, among other products. Both IL-1 and TNFα promote bone resorption. In addition TNFα and other cytokines increase expression of adhesion molecules to facilitate phagocyte recruitment. The actions of TNFα seem very important in RA, since the drugs **infliximab** (**Remicade**®) and **etanercept** (both TNFα binding agents) are effective in decreasing symptoms, and often inducing remission, in RA patients. Their use has to be circumspect, because they can increase susceptibility to infection.[280]

The SF of the inflamed rheumatoid joint swarms with neutrophils. Some are activated, and the SF thus contains increased quantities of their products, including lysozyme, lactoferrin and prostaglandins. Neutrophils are also present at the interface of cartilage and pannus.[281] The volume of SF is increased in the swollen inflamed rheumatoid joint, but its viscosity is lower than normal, because the hyaluronic acid present has a lower average molecular mass than normal. The cartilage wear particles, produced by increased friction in the joints, might activate phagocytes and make matters worse.

9.10.3 Does increased oxidative damage occur in RA?

Yes (Table 9.7). One advantage of studying RA is that it is easy to sample from the knee joint, since aspiration of SF is a therapeutic procedure sometimes employed to reduce swelling and pain. Interest in the role of oxidative damage in RA stems from the seminal work of McCord, who noted the decreased viscosity of SF in RA patients and showed that a similar decrease could be produced by exposing SF, or solutions of hyaluronic acid, to a system generating $O_2^{\bullet-}$ (xanthine/XO). Later work by the authors showed that hyaluronate degradation is not caused by $O_2^{\bullet-}$, but by $OH^{\bullet}$ generated by $O_2^{\bullet-}$-driven Fenton chemistry. The required iron was probably contaminating the reagents. Nevertheless, the chemical pattern of damage to hyaluronate in RA synovial fluids (as demonstrated using nuclear magnetic resonance) is consistent with $OH^{\bullet}$ attack,[282] although hyaluronate can also be degraded by HOCl and may additionally be secreted as abnormally short chains by the dysfunctional synovium in RA. Aspiration of RA SF into solutions of phenylalanine or salicylate produces patterns of aromatic hydroxylation[283] consistent with $OH^{\bullet}$ production.

How might $OH^{\bullet}$ arise in the joint? One possibility is reaction of $O_2^{\bullet-}$ with HOCl (Section 2.6.3). Another is from $ONOO^-$ (Section 2.6.1), although the importance of $ONOO^-$ in RA (as judged by nitrotyrosine production) is unclear (Table 9.7). A third is Fenton-type chemistry; indeed 'catalytic' iron (but not copper) can be measured in about 40% of synovial fluids aspirated from inflamed RA knee joints.[284] This iron could arise from necrotic cells,

by H_2O_2-mediated degradation of haemoglobin (liberated by microbleeding in the RA joint), and by the action of $O_2^{\bullet-}$ on synovial fluid ferritin. Indeed, iron release occurs when SF is exposed to $O_2^{\bullet-}$, especially at acidic pH.[285] Haem oxygenase might also play a role perhaps.[285A]

9.10.4 What is the origin of the oxidative stress?

9.10.4.1 *Immune cells, bone and cartilage*
One obvious source is activated macrophages and neutrophils, releasing $O_2^{\bullet-}$, H_2O_2, proteinases, HOCl (neutrophils only), eicosanoids and $NO^{\bullet}$ (by induction of iNOS). Several RS (e.g. $OH^{\bullet}$, HOCl, $ONOO^-$) might alter the antigenic behaviour of immunoglobulin G and other proteins, producing fluorescent aggregates that might activate phagocytic cells, provoke antibody formation, and be proinflammatory.[270,286] So might hyaluronic acid degradation products, some of which can activate macrophages.[287] Hypochlorous acid, $ONOO^-$ and $O_2^{\bullet-}$ react with ascorbate, which may help to explain its low levels in RA body fluids (Table 9.7). Hypochlorous acid and $ONOO^-$ inactivate α_1-antiproteinase, α_2-macroglobulin (Table 7.2), and other proteins (**tissue inhibitors of metalloproteinases, TIMPs**) that normally antagonize the action of matrix metalloproteinases.[288] Fibroblasts[260] and osteoclasts[273] in the RA joint can release $O_2^{\bullet-}$ and $NO^{\bullet}$, and osteoblasts and chondrocytes may make $NO^{\bullet}$. Synovial fluid T-lymphocytes from RA patients seem highly active in ROS production (Table 9.7). Human SF, like plasma, contains little catalase, GPx or GSH and only traces of SOD activity (largely as EC-SOD), so is not good at quenching RS.

9.10.4.2 *Hypoxia–reoxygenation*
The K_m for O_2 of the NADPH oxidase of rat neutrophils is within the range of physiological O_2 concentrations in body fluids.[289] If the same is true of human phagocytes, then local O_2 concentrations at sites of inflammation might modulate ROS production. Indeed, it has been proposed that the inflamed rheumatoid joint, upon movement and rest, undergoes hypoxia–reperfusion.[290] Tensing an inflamed rheumatoid knee joint can generate intra-articular pressures above capillary perfusion

pressure, resulting in sharp drops in O_2 concentration. Upon relaxing the joint, the O_2 level gradually returns to normal and ROS may be generated. Some may come from XO, which has been identified in synovial membranes. Indeed, hypoxanthine concentrations are elevated in SF from RA patients.[290]

9.10.5 Does oxidative damage matter in RA?

Increased oxidative damage occurs in RA (Table 9.7) but how far does it contribute to the chronicity of the inflammation and the cartilage and bone destruction? It seems likely that it could; we have already seen that iron overload or intra-articular injections of H_2O_2-generating systems damage joints.[279] A further illustration of the potential proinflammatory action of ROS may be provided by **alkaptonuria**, a disease caused by an inborn defect in **homogentisate oxidase**, an enzyme involved in the degradation of tyrosine.[291] Alkaptonuric patients accumulate homogentisic acid, show pigmentation of cartilage and connective tissue and may gradually develop severe inflammatory arthritis, presumably due to oxidation of homogentisic acid to generate ROS and quinones/semiquinones. Polymerization of the latter may account for the pigmentation observed.

However, there is little direct evidence that RS are important in RA. Early studies claiming that intra-articular injections of SOD are beneficial were unconvincing[262] and this line of research does not appear to have been pursued in humans, although interest in other therapeutic uses of SODs continues (Section 10.6.3). Reactive species could even be beneficial! When mice lacking neutrophil NADPH oxidase were subjected to intra-articular injection of zymosan (an irritant-induced inflammation) or pretreated with an antibody against lysozyme followed by intra-articular injection of a modified lysozyme (an immune-complex-mediated inflammation), they showed an *aggravated* inflammatory response. There was more cartilage and bone erosion, and *enhanced* synovial expression of TNFα, IL1α, RANKL and some matrix metalloproteinases.[292] Consistent with this, increased severity of collagen-induced arthritis and autoimmunity, as well as some spontaneous severe arthritis (in females), were found in rats and mice with mutations in the *Ncf1* gene; these animals

have decreased phagocyte ROS production because the gene encodes $p47^{phox}$ (Section 7.7.2).[293] Hence in these animal models *less* ROS equates to *more* inflammation. Since rats and mice are not humans, studies on chronic granulomatous disease patients (Section 7.7) might throw light on the clinical relevance of ROS, but at the moment the answer to the question posed at the beginning of this section is 'on a balance of probabilities, RS are not key contributors'. As in atherosclerosis (Sections 4.12.2 and 9.3.4), some oxidized lipids may be beneficial, for example by antagonizing vascular leakage at sites of inflammation,[294] and RS may help damp down lymphocyte proliferation and inactivate cytokines (Section 7.9.5).

9.10.6 Drugs for the treatment of RA: antioxidant, pro-oxidant or neither?

Cyclooxygenase (COX) inhibitors, blocking prostaglandin production and hence decreasing pain and swelling, are still commonly used in the day-to-day treatment of RA, although interest is now switching to the control of lymphocyte proliferation by such agents as **methotrexate** and to the use of anti-TNFα agents and molecules that decrease the activity of NF-κB.[269,280] The first COX inhibitor to be synthesized was **aspirin**, a drug with a long history which still springs surprises on us today. Even the ancient Egyptians were aware of the analgesic effects of an extract of willow leaves. In 1763, the Reverend Edmund Stone of Oxford, England, read a report to the Royal Society on the antifever action of willow bark and in 1876 the Scottish physician MacLagan reported its effectiveness in arthritis. The active component was later extracted and shown to be salicylate and in 1899 the Bayer Company in Germany introduced acetylsalicylate (aspirin). Aspirin ingested by humans is quickly hydrolysed to salicylate by esterases in the digestive tract and liver (Section 8.1).

Several other **non-steroidal anti-inflammatory drugs (NSAIDs)** have been developed as COX inhibitors; they include diclofenac sodium, indomethacin, ibuprofen, phenylbutazone, piroxicam and mefenamic acid. Major side-effects of COX inhibitors are gastrointestinal disturbances and renal injury. None of these drugs decreases cartilage damage or bone erosion in RA, and some may enhance it, perhaps by encouraging IL-1 formation by macrophages in the pannus or (in the case of salicylate) by inhibiting synthesis of cartilage proteoglycans. Selective inhibitors of COX-2, an enzyme present in various cells in the RA joint as a result of cytokine action, have also been examined. A popular agent is **celecoxib** (Fig. 9.15). In principle, a COX-2 inhibitor should not produce the typical side-effects of a COX-1 inhibitor. However, as COX-2 inhibitors have become more widely used they also turn out to have side-effects.

Some thiol compounds have been used to treat RA; they include **penicillamine** (often given as its disulphide, which is reduced to penicillamine *in vivo*; Fig. 9.15), **bucillamine** and gold–thiol complexes such as **aurothiomalate** and **aurothioglucose**. Several drugs developed for other diseases have found use in RA, such as the antimalarials **chloroquine** and **hydroxychloroquine**, the antibiotic **rifamycin**, and **sulphasalazine** (Fig. 9.15). Sulphasalazine consists of **5-aminosalicylic acid** linked by an azo (–N=N–) bond to **sulphapyridine**. *In vitro*, millimolar levels inhibit both lipoxygenase activity and prostaglandin biosynthesis, although it is not clear if this accounts for the clinical actions of sulphasalazine. In RA, the effective agent seems to be sulphasalazine itself or sulphapyridine, rather than 5-aminosalicylate.

9.10.6.1 Anti-inflammatory drugs as antioxidants?[295]

Anti-inflammatory drugs can affect oxidative damage in several ways:

1. Any drug that inhibits inflammation (by any mechanism) will lead to decreased production of RS, e.g. by reducing phagocyte numbers. **Corticosteroids** decrease phospholipase A_2 activity, decreasing arachidonic acid release and hence diminishing eicosanoid formation. They also decrease levels of IL-1, TNFα and iNOS. Naturally occurring corticosteroids include cortisol, and synthetic ones include **prednisolone** and **dexamethasone**. Steroids are effective drugs in RA, but side-effects limit prolonged use of high doses.

2. Drugs might scavenge RS. Most, if not all, anti-inflammatory drugs react quickly with $OH^•$ (rate constants 5×10^9 to $1 \times 10^{10} M^{-1} s^{-1}$). This is

predictable from their structures (Fig. 9.15), since aromatic and thiol compounds react fast with $OH^•$. Is it important *in vivo*? Millimolar or higher drug levels would be required to compete with biomolecules for any $OH^•$ generated, and most drugs achieve nowhere near such concentrations *in vivo*. One exception is aspirin; in aspirin-treated RA patients salicylate concentrations in plasma and synovial fluid do reach millimolar. Indeed, levels of 2,3-dihydroxybenzoate, a product of $OH^•$ attack on salicylate, are elevated in plasma from aspirin-treated RA patients.[295] *In vitro*, many drugs react with HOCl and ONOOH, but in few cases is the reaction fast enough for scavenging to be feasible at the drug concentrations present *in vivo*. Feasible (which doesn't mean that they actually do it *in vivo*!) HOCl and ONOOH scavengers include penicillamine and gold sodium thiomalate. Salicylate also reacts with ONOOH, undergoing hydroxylation and nitration (Section 5.3.1).

3. Drugs may chelate transition metal ions needed for $OH^•$ generation and lipid peroxidation. Little information is available on whether this could happen at therapeutic drug levels, but it is feasible for salicylate.

4. Drugs might depress activation of NF-$κ$B in synovial cells, thus decreasing inflammation by lowering levels of COX-2, iNOS, cytokines etc. Indeed, much research is now directed towards novel agents that minimize NF-$κ$B activation.[269] Salicylate is a weak inhibitor of i$κ$B kinase $β$ (Section 4.5.8).[296]

5. Drugs might decrease production of ROS by phagocytes. There have been several claims, but few convincing demonstrations, that NSAID levels at sites of inflammation can do this. One agent that does decrease neutrophil $O_2^{•-}$ production is **tetomilast** (Section 10.8.2).

9.10.6.2 As pro-oxidants?[257,295]

The gold-containing compound **auranofin**, S-triethylphosphinegold(I)-2,3,4,6-tetra-O-acetyl-1-thio-$β$-D-glucopyranoside, sometimes used in RA, was reported to inhibit thioredoxin reductase and stimulate mitochondrial ROS production at levels achievable *in vivo*. Aurothiomalate has similar effects (at higher concentrations) and also inhibits

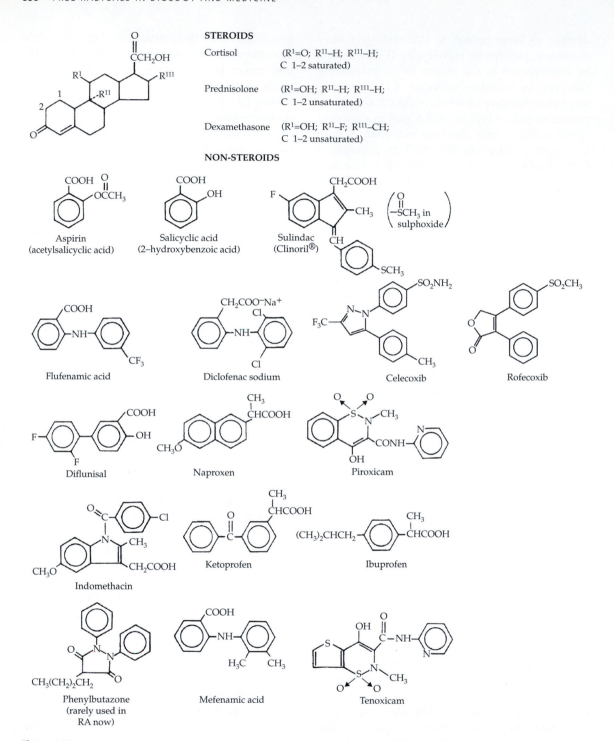

Figure 9.15

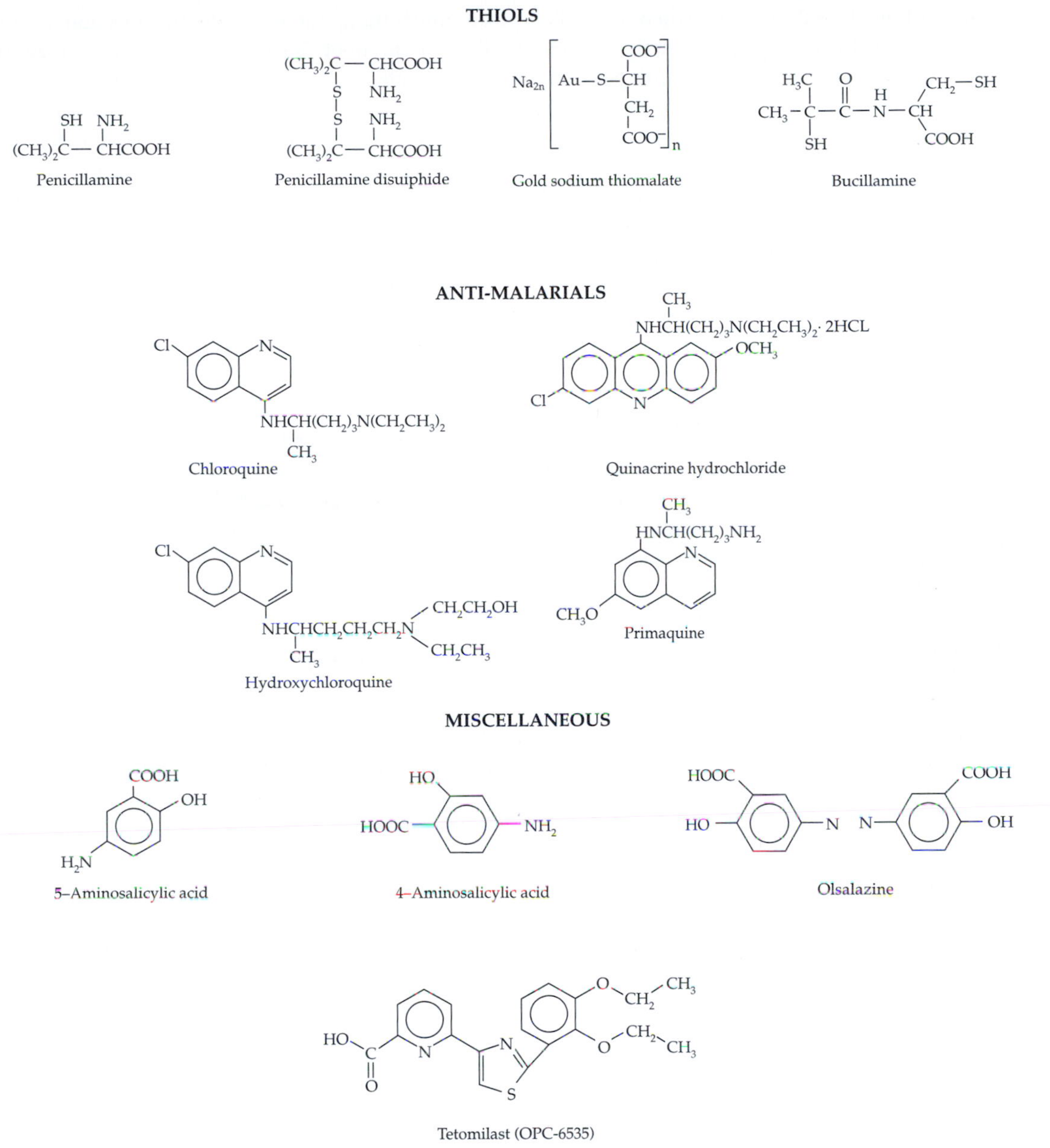

Figure 9.15 Structures of some drugs used in the treatment of inflammatory diseases. Sulindac is a pro-drug (a sulphoxide) that must be reduced to the CH_3SO- form to be active, probably by methionine sulphoxide reductases (*Biochim. Biophys. Acta* **1703**, 203, 2005).

GPx.[297] Some drugs used in the treatment of RA might themselves be converted into RS. For example, *in vitro* studies show that radicals derived from penicillamine, indomethacin, phenylbutazone, diclofenac, some fenamic acids and the aminosalicylate component of sulphasalazine can inactivate α_1-antiproteinase, oxidize ascorbic acid and accelerate lipid peroxidation. Such radicals might form *in vivo* when drugs are oxidized by MPO (e.g. diclofenac, indomethacin, phenylbutazone), the peroxidase action of COX (e.g. phenylbutazone) or by direct reaction of the drug with RS (e.g. aminosalicylate, penicillamine). For example, thiyl ($RS^{\bullet}$) and more reactive ($RSO_2^{\bullet}$ and $RSO^{\bullet}$)

radicals (Section 2.5.5.2) formed when penicillamine reacts with RS could combine with proteins, alter their antigenicity, and account for penicillamine's ability to cause autoimmunity in RA. The importance of these various reactions *in vivo* is unclear as yet.

Several drugs not used in the treatment of RA may also generate RS *in vivo* as a contribution to their side-effects. One is phenytoin (Section 6.11.7). Another is **clozapine**, an antipsychotic that can damage the bone marrow; its oxidation to a toxic product by MPO may be involved.[257]

9.10.7 Iron and rheumatoid arthritis

Rheumatoid arthritis is accompanied by changes in body iron metabolism. A rapid fall in the 'total iron' content of plasma at the onset of disease (Table 9.8) is followed by a drop in haemoglobin and increased deposition of iron in the synovial membranes. The drop in blood iron is due to the inflammation.[298] It is an example of the **anaemia of chronic disease**, also seen in chronic infections and in patients with cancer. Attempts to reverse this 'anaemia' by giving oral iron salts to RA patients are usually ineffective; it is not due to iron deficiency, but to increased synthesis of hepcidin by the liver in response to such cytokines as IL-6. Hepcidin decreases uptake of iron from the gut and favours its retention in macrophages in the spleen, so that plasma levels fall (Section 3.15.5).

Indeed, oral iron treatment can even worsen the symptoms of RA, as can intravenous iron administration, for example by injection of iron dextran to treat 'severe anaemia'. Although the side-effects are often attributed to the dextran, it may be the iron that is at fault.[299] Exacerbations of joint inflammation in RA patients given iron dextran occurred at the same time as plasma transferrin became saturated with iron and 'catalytic' iron was present in body fluids. Consistent with this, iron-overloaded haemochromatosis patients frequently show joint inflammation (Section 3.15.5), and bleeding into the joints of haemophiliac patients is associated with inflammation. Indeed, injection of blood into the joints of animals can trigger inflammation.[300] However the use of iron-chelating agents such as desferrioxamine as potential anti-inflammatory agents in animal models of RA gave inconclusive results, and preliminary studies in humans revealed little benefit and several side effects.[301]

9.11 Inflammatory bowel disease[302]

Reactive species may be involved in tissue injury in the inflammatory bowel diseases (IBDs) such as **Crohn's disease** and **ulcerative colitis**. The former is a recurrent inflammation and ulceration of the whole digestive tract, although it is often most severe in the lower part of the ileum, and in the colon and rectum. In ulcerative colitis, the ulceration and inflammation affect the colon and rectum only. In both conditions, autoantibodies to bowel components can be found in plasma. Patients suffer

Table 9.8 Protein and iron concentrations (mean ± SD) in plasma and synovial fluid from rheumatoid patients

	Plasma		Synovial fluid from rheumatoid knee-joint (n = 9)
	Normal control (n = 8)	Rheumatoid (n = 8)	
Total non-haem iron (μM)	17.9 ± 6.7	7.5 ± 5.7	8.9 ± 4.1
Transferrin (g/l)	2.92 ± 0.38	2.76 ± 4.2	1.67 ± 0.31
% Transferrin saturation with iron	29.9 ± 10.2	16.1 ± 12.8	26.3 ± 11.7
Albumin (g/l)	50.3 ± 44	36.3 ± 7.9[a]	17.2 ± 6.3
Caeruloplasmin (g/l)	0.259 ± 0.079	0.469 ± 0.085[a]	0.256 ± 0.077

Data abstracted from *Biochim. Biophys. Acta* **869**, 119, 1986.

[a] Changes characteristic of the acute phase response (Section 4.7.3).

severe diarrhoea, pain, fever, weight loss and are at increased risk of developing colorectal cancer. The origin of these diseases may involve an abnormal immune response to the gut flora.

As in the case of RA, the tissue injury and inflammation associated with IBDs involves the extensive recruitment and activation of neutrophils, monocytes, and lymphocytes and the overproduction of cytokines (e.g. TNFα), eicosanoids, proteinases and RS, including HOCl and $ONOO^-$. Hydrogen peroxide, HOCl and chloramines are capable of increasing the permeability of the gut wall and promoting electrolyte secretion, perhaps contributing to the diarrhoea. Bleeding is common in the inflamed gut and may provide a source of iron for $OH^{\bullet}$ generation. In addition, faeces often contain 'catalytic' iron unabsorbed from the diet (Section 6.2). Immunocytochemical evidence for formation of nitrotyrosine has been obtained in several animal models of IBD and in biopsies from patients with ulcerative colitis and Crohn's disease. Actin is one of the proteins nitrated.[303] Intrarectal administration of bolus $ONOO^-$ to animals provokes a severe inflammation, consistent with a contribution to injury in IBDs.[304] However, increased $NO^{\bullet}$ production in IBD patients must not be assumed to be all bad, since $NO^{\bullet}$ may depress phagocyte recruitment, for example by decreasing synthesis of adhesion molecules.[302]

Is the increased production of RS in IBD a major contributor to tissue injury? The answer is unclear as yet, but it is interesting to note that transgenic mice lacking both GPx1 and GPx2 (the two major GPx types that metabolize peroxides in colonic epithelium)[305] show spontaneous colonic inflammation and cancer development.[306] In a mouse model of IBD, levels of GSH dropped in the colon prior to onset of inflammation; prevention of this by administering N-acetylcysteine slowed inflammation.[302] Patients with Crohn's disease show elevated plasma IP levels; in one study these were decreased by administration of vitamin C plus α-tocopherol, but it is not clear if there was clinical benefit.[307] The increased risk of cancer in ulcerative colitis may involve DNA damage by RS; indeed, levels of 8OHdG and of etheno-DNA adducts in the inflamed colon are elevated.[308]

Nevertheless, be cautious. A popular animal model of IBD is to administer dextran sodium sulphate in the diet: this sulphated polysaccharide induces chronic colon inflammation.[304] When this was done to mice lacking phagocyte NADPH oxidase (knockout of p47^{phox}), the inflammation was *unchanged*. However, in one[302] (but not another)[309] study in mice overexpressing CuZnSOD the inflammation was *more* severe, hinting that $O_2^{\bullet-}$ might be neutral or beneficial, reminiscent of recent studies in animal models of RA (Section 9.10.5).

9.11.1 The salazines

One popular treatment for IBD is sulphasalazine (Fig. 9.15); the active constituent is 5-aminosalicylate (**mesalazine** or **mesalamine**) generated by hydrolysis of sulphasalazine by colonic bacteria. Indeed, both this and other aminosalicylates, such as **4-aminosalicylate**, are used to treat IBD.

Aminosalicylates are powerful scavengers of $OH^{\bullet}$, $ONOO^-$ and HOCl *in vitro* and may be able to decrease NF-κB activation *in vivo*.[302] Since they accumulate in the bowel to millimolar levels during therapy, scavenging of RS is feasible.[310] Evidence consistent with this is provided by the isolation from faeces of IBD patients of what appear to be ROS-generated oxidation products of 5-aminosalicylate.[311] However, it is also possible that oxidation products of aminosalicylates (e.g. iminoquinones and quinones) could cause damage, for example by attacking proteins.[312]

9.12 Inflammation of other parts of the gastrointestinal tract

9.12.1 Pancreas[313]

Pancreatitis is an inflammatory disease causing intense pain and destruction of pancreatic tissue. It can be provoked by several factors, including excess alcohol (Section 8.8.1.2), pancreatic-duct obstruction by gallstones or by a period of ischaemia, for example after haemorrhagic shock. Cytokines, NF-κB activation, adhesion molecules, phagocytes and iNOS are again involved, and severe pancreatitis can trigger ARDS. Some studies have shown that the injury induced by fatty-acid infusion, ischaemia or partial duct obstruction in isolated perfused no pancreas can be diminished by including SOD and catalase in the perfusing medium. Conflicting results have been obtained as to whether SOD and catalase are effective against pancreatitis in whole animals,[313,314] although there is increased lipid peroxidation in the inflamed tissue.[315] Indeed, F_2-IP levels are increased in bile from patients with pancreatitis and there are more etheno–DNA adducts in the inflamed tissue.[316] Whether or not RS contribute significantly to this disease is an important issue, since current treatments for pancreatitis are inadequate. Double-blind trials suggested that supplementation with a mixture of ascorbate, selenium, β-carotene, α-tocopherol and methionine can decrease the severe pain associated with chronic pancreatitis[317] but little other evidence of clinical benefit of antioxidants is available in the literature.

9.12.2 Oesophagus and stomach

Reactive species have been suggested to be involved in inflammation of the oesphagus (e.g. after reflux of acid from the stomach due to weakness of the sphincter) and in gastric damage secondary to haemorrhagic shock or inflammation. They may also contribute to gastric injury in chronic infection by *Helicobacter pylori*. This organism infects the stomachs of much of the world's population and, in a minority of cases, causes inflammation (with neutrophil, lymphocyte and monocyte infiltration), predisposition to ulcer formation, and elevated risk of gastric cancer. Similar *Helicobacter* species are found in the stomachs of other animals. Levels of 8OHdG, 8-nitroguanine (Section 5.13.7), and lipid peroxidation are elevated in the gastric mucosa of infected patients, and GSH levels are subnormal, as are ascorbate levels in the gastric fluid.[318] The phagocyte infiltration and RS formation may be attempts to eradicate the bacterium, but sadly they are not successful (indeed, *H. pylori* turns them against the host; Section 7.9.6). *H. pylori* is resistant to ROS, in part due to its high content of catalases, peroxiredoxins, iron-binding proteins and methionine sulphoxide reductase.[319,320] It contains the enzyme urease, which releases CO_2 that can combine with $ONOO^-$,

decreasing $ONOO^-$'s bactericidal action (Section 2.6.1.1).[321]

So are RS damaging in *H. pylori* infection? Host DNA is oxidatively damaged, including the *p53* gene (Section 5.13.8). This organism can be eradicated by antibiotic treatment, but additional supplements of vitamin C and α-tocopherol did not appear to add clinical benefit.[322] Indeed, in mice lacking phagocyte NADPH oxidase, gastric damage by *H. pylori* was *more* severe. This was not due to an increase in bacterial numbers but rather to tissue injury by neutrophil granule components.[323] Yet more evidence to reinforce the growing view that RS sometimes act to down-regulate inflammation (Section 7.9.5).

9.12.3 Liver

Inflammation of the liver (**hepatitis**) is a major clinical problem. Causes include alcohol abuse (Section 8.8), infection with viruses such as hepatitis C or parasites such as *Opisthorchis* (Section 9.13.6 below) and, less commonly, exposure to toxins such as chlorinated hydrocarbons (Section 8.2). Sources of RS include infiltrating neutrophils, activation of Kupffer cells, and possibly NADPH oxidase enzymes in hepatocytes. Iron accumulation often occurs in damaged liver, and may contribute to injury.[324] Hepatitis is a risk factor for the development of liver cancer (Section 9.13.6 below). Indeed, increased levels of 8OHdG and 8-nitroguanine are present in inflamed human liver[325] and patients infected with hepatitis B excrete more etheno-DNA adducts in urine.[316] Mice lacking CuZnSOD also show elevated 8OHdG in liver and are at increased risk of hepatoma.[326] Plasma F_2-IPs are elevated in hepatitis patients[327] and studies have examined the effects of administering α-tocopherol. Sadly, clinical improvements have generally been minimal or absent.[328] Of course, the vitamin E may not have decreased the oxidative damage (Section 3.20.2.8).

Inflammation of the bile ducts (e.g. as a result of immunological attack) can interfere with normal drainage of the bile, leading to liver damage by the retained bile constituents, and eventual liver fibrosis. Both the initial ductal inflammation and the subsequent liver damage (including the fibrosis;

Fig. 8.9) have been suggested to involve RS. For example, bile salts can activate NOX enzymes under certain conditions.[316,329] Chronic inflammation of the gall bladder is a risk factor for cancer development there, and levels of 8OHdG are elevated in the inflamed tissue.[330]

9.13 Oxidative stress and cancer: a complex relationship

9.13.1 The cell cycle[331]

Most cells in an adult, multicellular organism are not dividing and must receive mitogenic signals (e.g. platelet-derived growth factor (PDGF), epidermal growth factor (EGF), insulin-like growth factor 1 (IGF-1), transforming growth factor β (TGF-β), fibroblast growth factor (FGF), nerve growth factors (NGFs), erythropoietin, IL-2, or IL-3) to start the process. Some growth factors act on a range of cells (e.g. PDGF, FGF, EGF, IGF-1, TGF-β) whereas others are more selective; for example, IL-2 acts on T-lymphocytes, NGFs on neurons, and erythropoietin on bone marrow erythrocyte precursor cells. Cells will only respond if they express receptors for the growth factor, binding to which activates intracellular signalling mechanisms that lead to changes in gene expression (Section 4.5.5). In adult humans, most neurons and skeletal muscle cells do not normally divide at all, hepatocytes perhaps once a year or so, whereas some epithelial cells in the gut may divide twice daily as the gut lining is constantly renewed. In culture, many cells supplied with serum as a source of growth factors will grow until a confluent monolayer is obtained—in general, when cells touch each other, proliferation is inhibited. Both adhesion molecules and gap junctional proteins (e.g. **connexins**) are involved in this **contact inhibition**.

To produce a pair of genetically identical daughter cells, the DNA must first be accurately replicated. Cell division begins with **mitosis** (**M phase**), the process of nuclear division. The nuclear envelope breaks down, chromatin condenses into visible chromosomes, and the cellular microtubules form a **mitotic spindle** on which the chromosomes eventually separate. In **anaphase** the chromosomes move to the poles of the spindle and reform intact nuclei, and the cell then divides in

two. In most cells M phase is short (often 60 min or less) by comparison with **interphase**, the gap between M phases.

Replication of nuclear DNA occurs in the **S phase** (S for 'synthesis') of interphase. Cells in S phase can be recognized experimentally because they take up DNA precursors, for example tritium-labelled thymidine or **bromodeoxyuridine**, a thymidine analogue that can be recognized in the nucleus by antibody staining techniques (Section 5.13). The interval between completion of mitosis and the start of a new round of DNA synthesis is the **G1 phase**; the **G2 phase** is the gap between finishing DNA synthesis and the onset of mitosis. The G1 and G2 phases provide time for cell growth and synthesis of other components, and for repairing any errors made in DNA replication. Cells in G1, if not yet committed to DNA replication, can halt their progress around the cell cycle and are then said to be in a resting, **G0**, state. Withdrawal of growth factors from proliferating cells sends them into G0.

Control of the cell cycle needs many proteins; an essential group is the **cyclin-dependent protein kinases** (**cdk**), whose ability to phosphorylate their targets is regulated by another important protein class, the **cyclins**. Different cyclin/cdk complexes are assembled and activated at different points in the cell cycle. Ubiquitin and the proteasome (Section 4.14.2) play key regulatory roles by degrading cyclins. Also important are **checkpoints**; the cell must have fulfilled certain criteria (e.g. DNA replication completed, a certain minimum size), before moving on to the next stage. For animal cells, one major checkpoint is in G1. A feedback control is essential to delay mitosis until DNA replication is complete in S phase. Damage to DNA also generates a signal to delay mitosis, until repair is (hopefully!) complete. The checkpoint mechanisms not only halt replication but are also involved in promoting repair of DNA damage.

Proteins involved in the G1 checkpoint include ATR and ATM (Section 4.10.6). The latter recognizes double-strand breaks, whereas ATR is activated by UV-radiation and unreplicated DNA (stalled DNA replication). Both switch on checkpoint kinases that can activate p53 by phosphorylation (Section 9.13.4 below). The p53 protein is also involved in the **G2**

checkpoint, which deters cells from starting mitosis if they experience DNA damage in G2, or if they enter G2 with some unrepaired DNA damage from the G1 phase. The movement of cells from G1 to S can also be blocked by lack of nutrients or oxidative stress. The latter effect is partly mediated by DNA damage induced by RS, but also involves **FOXO transcription factors** (Section 4.5.5.2). If nutrients are missing, FOXOs accumulate in the nucleus. Similarly, oxidative stress provokes FOXO activation by acetylation. The active FOXOs leads to increases in the levels of cytostatic and proapoptotic factors.

9.13.2 Tumours

A multicellular organism is essentially a clone of cells which collaborate, regulating their own proliferation in the interests of the whole organism. There are about 10^{16} cell divisions per lifetime in the human body, and about 10^{12} in the mouse. The 'spontaneous' mutation rate due to errors made by DNA polymerases has been estimated as 10^{-6} per gene per cell division. Hence each gene might have undergone 10^{10} mutations in the human (10^6 in mouse) lifespan. Mechanisms to repair damage and eliminate mutated cells are thus essential.

A **tumour** may be defined as an abnormal lump or mass of tissue, the growth of which exceeds, and is unco-ordinated with, that of the normal tissue, i.e. normal intercellular collaboration has broken down. Most tumours form discrete masses, but in the **leukaemias** (tumours of myeloid or lymphoid cells) the tumour cells spread through the bone marrow or lymphoid tissues, and circulate in the blood. Tumours vary widely in their growth rates. The most important classification is that of **benign** or **malignant**. Benign tumours remain at the site of origin. When growing in a solid tissue, they usually become enclosed in a layer of fibrous material, the capsule, formed by the surrounding tissues. Benign tumours rarely kill, unless they press on a vital structure or secrete abnormal amounts of hormones.

Most fatal tumours are **malignant**, or **cancerous**. Unlike benign tumours, the cells of malignant tumours invade locally, and often also pass through the bloodstream and/or lymphatic system to form secondary tumours (**metastases**) at other sites. This involves release of the cell from the matrix, prevention of the apoptosis that usually occurs when cells detach from their normal environment (**anoikis**; Section 4.4.1), and migration through the tissue and vessel walls to enter the circulation. Rates of growth and metastasis differ from tumour to tumour, for example basal cell cancer of the skin epidermis (which arises from keratinocyte precursors) rarely metastasizes, whereas melanoma (which arises from pigment cells) frequently does. Rapidly growing malignant tumours usually lose their histological resemblance to their tissue of origin. Cancers are classified according to the tissues from which they arose, for example **carcinomas** arise from epithelial cells and **sarcomas** from connective tissue or muscle.

9.13.3 Carcinogenesis

The process of conversion of a normal cell to the malignant state is called **carcinogenesis**, and agents that induce it are **carcinogens**. Carcinogenesis is a complex, multistage process; essentially, an abnormal cell is generated and then gives rise to a larger number of increasingly abnormal cells as a result of a series of mutations, cell divisions and changes in the pattern of gene expression.

Factors predisposing to malignancy are both inherited and environmental. For example, breast cancer risk is affected by genetic predisposition (e.g. in the genes, *BRCA1* and *BRCA2*; Section 4.10), both involved in cell cycle checkpoints. Cancer incidence is affected by diet; for example, a high-calorie (especially fat-rich) diet is thought to be a risk factor for breast and colon cancer, whereas diets rich in fruits and vegetables are protective against several types of cancer (Section 10.5). Some people are more sensitive to environmental or self-administered (e.g. cigarette smoke) carcinogens than are others, in part due to differences in the relative levels of their phase I and phase II xenobiotic metabolizing enzymes (Sections 8.1 and 10.5). The environment of the tumour is also important; for example are inflammatory cells present (inflammation can promote tumour development [Section 9.13.6 below] but also damage malignant cells), is intercellular communication taking place, what is the level of growth factors and hormones that influence cell growth and proliferation, and can the tumour get an adequate blood supply?

The development of cancer in animals takes years and involves progressive tissue and cellular changes (Table 9.9 and Fig. 9.16). Take **cervical cancer** as an example. Normal cell proliferation in the cervix occurs in the basal layer of epithelial cells. New cells move upwards, differentiate, become keratinized, and eventually slough off the surface. Cervical screening frequently reveals **dysplasia**; dividing cells occur outside the basal layer and some disordered cell arrangement is visible. Dysplasia may persist harmlessly or disappear, but sometimes it progresses to **carcinoma** *in situ*; the whole epithelium appears disordered and contains proliferating cells, many of abnormal shape and size. Carcinoma *in situ* may again persist without problems, but in some cases it gives rise (over several more years) to a malignant **cervical carcinoma**, whose cells break out of the epithelium by crossing the basement membrane to invade the underlying connective tissue.

Studies of the action of carcinogens in mouse skin (painting the skin with carcinogenic hydrocarbons such as **benzpyrene** or **dimethylbenzanthracene**; Section 9.14 below) were the first to reveal that two distinct stages of carcinogenesis can be defined, and later work identified a third stage (Table 9.9). This three-stage model applies (with reservations) to many cancers.

9.13.3.1 *Initiation*

Initiation is caused by DNA alteration, for example reaction of carcinogens with DNA. The major protections against initiation are limiting exposure to carcinogens, efficiency of carcinogen detoxification by phase I/II enzymes, DNA repair, elimination (e.g. by apoptosis) of cells with damaged DNA or sending such cells into senescence (Section 10.3.5).

Successful initiation requires not only DNA modification but also at least one round of DNA replication and cell proliferation to allow the mutation to be 'fixed' in the DNA before repair can remove it, so that it becomes irreversible. The cell proliferation may be occurring normally in a dividing tissue, could be stimulated by the initiator, or might occur secondarily because of the need to replace some cells killed by the carcinogen. Of course, if all the initiated cells are killed the problem disappears. Most human cancers are carcinomas, in part because epithelial cells often proliferate rapidly in the healthy animal and they are frequently exposed to carcinogens, for example in inhaled air or from diet.

9.13.3.2 *Tumour promoters*

Initiation can be followed by **promotion**. Tumour promoters cause expression of the latent phenotype of initiated cells (Table 9.9) by **selection** and **clonal expansion**, promoting cell proliferation and/or

Table 9.9 The stage of carcinogenesis

Stage	Description
Initiation	Characterized by irreversible genetic changes. Examples of initiators include chemicals that react directly with DNA (can be endogenous, such as RS, or xenobiotic) and ionizing radiation. Single initiated cells are not morphologically recognizable; may have subtle phenotypic changes after multiplication.
Promotion	Usually reversible process of gene activation; often the result of action of xenobiotics or endogenous substances; involves entire tissue (initiated and non-initiated cells); may produce a benign tumour from initiated cells. May have several stages (early reversible, and late irreversible).
Progression	Conversion of benign to malignant tumours, usually accompanied by faster growth, invasiveness, metastasis, increased genetic instability. May be associated with further irreversible genetic change. Examples include progression of benign papillomas to squamous cell carcinoma in mouse skin, benign colon polyps to adenocarcinoma, and focal benign hepatic nodules to hepatoma.

Adapted from Table 1 in *Blood* **76**, 655, 1990 by courtesy of Prof. S.A. Weitzman and the publishers. Considering the number of cell divisions and errors in DNA replication over the human lifespan, it is perhaps remarkable that only about one-third of humans develop cancer. This is because cells can die, halt proliferation or senesce at every stage (Fig. 9.16).

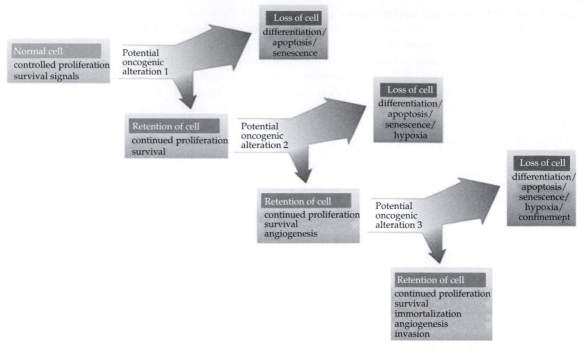

Figure 9.16 Development of cancer is more complex than the straightforward linear accumulation of oncogenic mutations. Potentially oncogenic proliferative signals are coupled to a variety of growth-inhibitory processes, such as the induction of apoptosis, differentiation or senescence, each of which restricts subsequent clonal expansion and neoplastic evolution. Tumour progression occurs only where these growth-inhibitory mechanisms fail to work or are thwarted by compensatory mutations. From *Nature* **411**, 342, 2001 by courtesy of Elsevier and Drs G.I. Evans and K. H. Vousden.

decreasing apoptosis. Many carcinogens, in large doses, are both initiators and promoters. However, a dose of a carcinogen too small to induce a tumour can lead to cancer if supplied together with certain non-carcinogens, the so-called **tumour promoters**. For example, **croton oil**, a non-carcinogen, promotes the development of cancer by subcarcinogenic doses of the hydrocarbon methylcholanthrene, but only if the oil is given with, or after, the methylcholanthrene. Croton oil comes from seeds of the plant *Croton tiglium*. Fractionation of the oil showed that the most powerful tumour promoter present is **phorbol myristate acetate** (PMA, Fig. 9.17), a compound frequently used to induce the respiratory burst in phagocytic cells (Section 7.7). Many tumour promoters, including PMA, are potent inducers of inflammation, but no single mechanism explains the action of all the different promoting agents. Another promoter is **2,3,7,8-tetrachlorodibenzo-*p*-dioxin**, TCDD (Section 8.3).

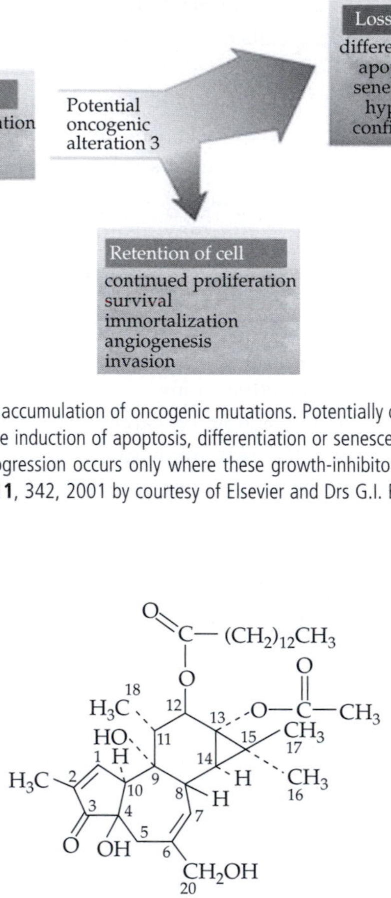

Figure 9.17 Structure of phorbol myristate acetate (PMA). The full chemical name of this compound is 12-*O*-tetradecanoylphorbol-13-acetate.

During promotion, the altered DNA of the initiated cell is revealed by changes in the expression of genes that regulate cell differentiation and growth. Tumour promoters can produce reversible changes in cell proliferation and phenotypic expression

(Table 9.9). Removal of the promoter often results in the tissue returning approximately to normal, although it will still be initiated.

9.13.3.3 *Progression*

The final stage of carcinogenesis is the development of a premalignant lesion into a malignant one. This **tumour progression** involves additional changes in DNA. For example, colorectal cancers are common age-related cancers worldwide; they arise from the epithelium lining the colon and rectum. Often they are preceded by a benign tumour, an **adenoma**, called a **polyp**. Malignant (**transformed**) cells in culture lose contact inhibition and can proliferate without attachment to a substratum. Often there is down-regulation of connexin synthesis and hence of communication through gap junctions. They grow so well that many studies of cell and molecular biology are performed upon malignant cells in culture, perhaps not always a good model of normal physiology (Section 1.11).

9.13.4 Genes and cancer

No single gene defect directly causes cancer in humans. Changes in three types of genes are usually involved, **oncogenes**, **tumour-suppressor genes** and **stability genes**.[332]

9.13.4.1 *Oncogenes*

Oncogenes were first discovered by virologists. Several viruses induce tumours in animals, for example the **Rous sarcoma virus** causes sarcomas in chickens. From many of these viruses **oncogenes** have been identified, specific genes that can transform animal cells in culture into a malignant state when the virus infects them. Rous sarcoma virus contains the oncogene *src*. It was soon found that normal mammalian cells contain genes (**proto-oncogenes**) that resemble the viral oncogenes. Thus the normal cellular analogue of the viral *src* (**v-*src***) gene is *c-src* (sometimes just written as *src*).

Proto-oncogenes are frequently related to cell growth, in that often they encode growth factors, growth factor receptors, proteins involved in transferring the growth 'signal' from receptors to the nucleus (e.g. protein kinases) or proteins involved in the control of the cell cycle or cell death (Table 9.10). Many oncogenes have been identified by means other than the use of viruses, for example by direct identification in malignant tumours or

Table 9.10 Some oncogenes originally identified in transforming viruses

Oncogene	Function of gene product	Source of virus	Virus-induced tumour
src	Tyrosine kinase	Chicken	Sarcoma
abl	Tyrosine kinase, involved in suppressing apoptosis (Section 4.5.5)	Mouse, cat	Leukaemia, sarcoma
erb-B	Tyrosine kinase: epidermal growth factor receptor	Chicken	Erythroleukaemia, fibrosarcoma
fos, jun	Fos and Jun proteins associate to form AP-1 (Section 4.5.9)	Mouse, chicken	Osteosarcoma, fibrosarcoma
raf	Protein kinase (serine/threonine) actived by Ras	Mouse, chicken	Sarcoma
myc	Transcription factor; normally acts in nucleus as signal for cell proliferation, collaborates with *max* gene	Chicken	Sarcoma, myelocytoma, carcinoma
H-*ras*, K-*ras*	GTP-binding proteins; cycle between active (GTP-bound) and inactive (GDP-bound) states; hydrolysis of GTP stops activity (Section 4.5.5)	Rat	Sarcoma, erythroleukaemia
v-rel	Gene-regulatory protein related to NF-κB (Section 4.5.8)	Chicken	Lymphoma in spleen and liver
sis	Platelet-derived growth factor B-chain	Monkey	Sarcoma

Most human cancers are not related to viral infection, but some are, e.g. **Burkitt's lymphoma** (Epstein–Barr virus) and **adult T-cell leukaemia/lymphoma** (human T-cell leukaemia virus type I, HTLV-I). Sometimes viruses can induce cancer by provoking inflammation (Section 9.13.5 below). In general, viral infection alone does not produce cancer—many other events are involved. Thus <5% of adults infected with HTLV-I develop leukaemia. DNA tumour viruses often also encode proteins that inactivate tumour suppressor genes.

analysis of chromosomal abnormalities. Examples are *lck*, *neu*, N-*ras* and *bcl*-2; the last is involved in suppressing apoptosis (Section 4.4). In essence, oncogenes are activated proto-oncogenes, such that the gene is always expressed, or at least expressed under conditions where the wild-type gene is not. Activation can be by mutation of the proto-oncogene, gene amplification, or chromosomal rearrangements that place the gene in a region of the chromosome being transcribed. For example, the oncogene *erbB* (Table 9.10) is a mutated form of the EGF receptor that 'sends a signal' all the time.

Mutated proto-oncogenes are found in most human and other animal tumours. For example, *Ras* mutations are common in human cancers. *Ras* oncogene protein products have diminished ability to hydrolyse GTP. The GTP-bound configuration is active in signal transduction and the GDP-conformation inactive (Section 4.5.5), so that loss of GTPase promotes excessive signalling.

9.13.4.2 *Tumour suppressor genes*

A mutation in an oncogene has been compared[332] to a car with a stuck accelerator—the car moves even if you take your foot off it (foot equals growth signal!). However, the car will still stop if the brake is pressed. A mutation in a **tumour-suppressor gene** is analogous to a faulty brake—it no longer works to halt proliferation of an abnormal cell. Whereas mutations creating oncogenes tend to be dominant, since they create proliferation signals, mutations in suppressor genes are usually recessive, that is both copies of the gene must be inactivated. Often, there is a point mutation in one allele, and the other disappears later by loss of part or whole of a chromosome. Sometimes tumour suppressor genes are 'silenced' rather than mutated or lost, for example by methylation of promoter regions.

The most important tumour suppressor gene is *p53*, so-called because the relative molecular mass of its protein product is 53 000. The p53 protein, sometimes called 'the guardian of the genome', is a transcription factor that acts to stop cell division. It is activated by phosphorylation in response to DNA damage,[333] for example by RS (especially H_2O_2) and by a wide range of chemotherapeutic drugs (which may sometimes involve RS; Section 9.15 below). It is also activated (sometimes again via ROS!) if the cell senses abnormal growth signals due to oncogene activation. Active p53 protein increases transcription of other genes, including *p21* (encoding a cyclin kinase inhibitor), *GADD45* (growth arrest on DNA damage) and *mdm2*, which encodes a protein involved in p53 destruction. Thus p53 regulates its own level. Levels of phosphorylated p53 rise in cells subjected to stresses that result in DNA damage (e.g. radiation, hyperoxia), and this halts DNA replication until DNA damage is repaired. Stimulation of p53 can also trigger senescence (Section 10.3.5) or apoptosis in some cell types under certain conditions, for example by promoting the synthesis of proapoptotic proteins such as bax (Section 4.4.1). Mice lacking p53 rapidly develop cancers.

The actions of p53 are intimately linked with ROS (Fig. 9.18). First, the normal low cellular levels of p53 are involved in maintaining the cellular antioxidant defence network, promoting the transcription of genes encoding MnSOD, GPx1 and proteins that regenerate oxidized peroxiredoxins, among others.[333] Second, ROS can increase p53 activity, for example in cells with active *ras* oncogene (Section 10.3.5). Third, higher levels of p53 can cause ROS *production* by the p66shc protein (Section 10.4.1) and by other mechanisms, and this ROS contributes to its cytostatic and proapoptotic effect.

If both p53 genes are inactivated, cells can enter the cell cycle with damaged DNA. Mutations of p53 are very common lesions in human cancers. Although p53 protein is most often inactivated by mutation of its gene, its activity can also be diminished by changes in genes encoding proteins that interact with p53. One such protein is **MDM2** (encoded by the *mdm2* gene mentioned above), which helps to ubiquitinate p53 for degradation by the proteasome. If levels of this rise, p53 levels will fall. Indeed, levels of p53 in a cell are a balance between production and destruction.

The P53 protein is stabilized and activated as a transcription factor by phosphorylation (e.g. by ATM), as mentioned above, but this is not all. Another mode of regulation is by **acetylation**, which further increases p53 activity. Deacetylases involved in ageing (Section 10.3.4) reverse this and favour cell survival under stress.

In addition to p53, other tumour suppressor genes exist. One is *APC*. The disease **familial**

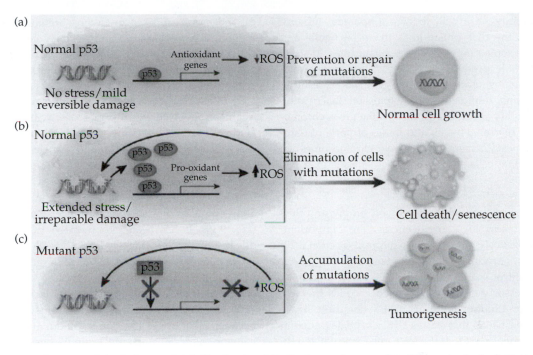

Figure 9.18 The p53 protein has both pro- and antioxidant functions. (a) In the absence of stress or after mild stress, low levels of p53 drive the expression of several antioxidant genes that decrease ROS levels. P53 can also facilitate DNA repair. (b) Greater activation of p53 after severe or extended stress leads to the formation of ROS by several mechanisms, resulting in elevated ROS levels and cell senescence or death. Both of these mechanisms contribute to tumor suppression. (c) Loss of p53 function increases intracellular levels of ROS, which damage DNA and increase the mutation rate. The inability to activate p53-induced apoptosis in response to these oncogenic alterations ultimately results in the development of cancer. The p53 protein can also be inactivated by oxidation of its cysteine residues (Section 9.13.5.3). Adapted from *Nature Medicine* **11**, 1278, 2005 by courtesy of Elsevier and Drs Karim Bensaad and Karen Vousden.

adenomatous polyposis coli, in which polyp development occurs early in life and colon cancer almost invariably develops, is associated with a defect in *APC*.

9.13.4.3 *Stability genes*

Stability genes keep DNA 'normal', by repairing damage to it (Section 4.10) or otherwise ensuring that cell division and chromosomal segregation proceed accurately.[332] When stability genes malfunction, mutations in other genes occur more often and the risk of creating an oncogene or inactivating a suppressor gene is increased. Usually, both alleles of the stability gene must be mutated for maximum effect. For example, defects in DNA repair predispose to cancer development. In **xeroderma pigmentosum**, an inborn recessive defect in the ability to repair UV-induced lesions in DNA (Section 4.10.8.2), there is a high risk of skin cancer on exposure to sunlight. Patients with **Fanconi's anaemia**, a disorder caused by mutations in several genes (Section 9.13.7 below) show an elevated level of 8OHdG in DNA and an increased incidence of malignancies. Elevated cancer risk is also seen in **Werner's syndrome** (Section 10.3.3) and in **ataxia telangiectasia**, caused by mutation in the *ATM* gene encoding the ATM protein involved in cell-cycle checkpoints (Section 9.13.1). Cells from ataxia telangiectasia patients lack checkpoint control; for example after irradiation they proceed into S phase without repairing DNA.

Mutations in proto-oncogenes, tumour suppressor or stability genes sometimes occur in the germline, giving a hereditary predisposition to cancer. Cancer is not guaranteed to develop, but the risk is increased because the cells have a 'head start' on the normal cell (one gene class defective, only two to go). Mutations may also occur 'randomly' in a cell, to give a sporadic tumour. Often, the first mutation is in an oncogene and causes some degree of clonal expansion that starts the whole process (Table 9.9). Subsequent mutations in any or all of the three gene classes result in additional rounds of clonal expansion. Inactivation of stability genes contributes to the gross chromosomal rearrangements and losses of parts of chromosomes (or sometimes whole chromosomes) in malignant cells.

9.13.4.4 *Angiogenesis and cancer*

A growing tumour needs a blood supply, and thus genes affecting angiogenesis are important. Angiogenesis in response to hypoxia (Section 8.19) involves production of such agents as VEGF, under the control of HIF (Section 1.3.2). Another tumour suppressor gene is **VHL**, which encodes the **von Hippel–Lindau protein**, an E3 ubiquitin ligase (Section 4.14.2) that causes HIF1α to be degraded in the presence of O_2. If the *VHL* gene is mutated, HIF is stabilized and VEGF production accelerated. Germline mutations in *VHL* increase the risk of cancer, especially in kidney, and are associated with abnormal angiogenesis.[334] By contrast, p53 stimulates the expression of genes encoding some antiangiogenic factors.[333]

9.13.5 Reactive species and carcinogenesis

So much for the molecular biology of cancer, but what's it got to do with RS? A few moments thought will reveal that RS could be involved in all aspects of carcinogenesis; they can be proproliferative (Section 4.2.1), induce senescence (Section 4.2.3), increase p53 activity, cause apoptosis, facilitate apoptosis triggered by other agents, suppress apoptosis (Section 4.4.1), cause DNA damage (Section 4.8), activate FOXOs (Section 9.13.1) and recruit phagocytes (Section 7.7). Which of these actions is the most important *in vivo*? We have no clear idea, and there may be no single answer (Section 9.13.6 below).

Let us first review what RS can do.

9.13.5.1 *DNA damage*

Exposure to ionizing radiation has long been known to favour cancer development. Radiation-induced carcinogenesis appears to involve initiation, promotion, activation of proto-oncogenes, and inactivation of stability- and tumour-suppressor genes. Some genetic damage by radiation occurs by direct absorption of energy by DNA, but much is mediated by OH$^\bullet$ (Section 8.19). In other words, OH$^\bullet$ might be involved in all stages of carcinogenesis. Hydroxyl radical attack upon DNA generates several mutagenic purine, pyrimidine and deoxyribose oxidation products (Section 4.9).

The incidence of most cancers rises with the fourth or fifth power of age in animals, e.g. about 35% of humans have cancer by age 85 (Fig. 9.19). It has been hypothesized that this is due to a lifetime of attack by ROS.[335] Is endogenous RS production and DNA damage large enough to account for this? The 'steady-state' levels of oxidative base lesions in DNA in normal cells vary according to the measurement method and between laboratories (Section 5.13), but an average value for all lesions may be around 1 per 10^5 DNA bases, or more. Enough to cause cancer? By comparison with the levels of adducts of known carcinogens that are detected in carcinogen-exposed cells, it could be.[336] For example, levels of benzpyrene adducts in DNA from cancers taken from smokers range from 0.062 to 0.53 per 10^5 bases. In rat liver the levels of carcinogen-DNA adducts associated with a 50% incidence of hepatoma ranged from 0.053 to 2.083 per 10^5 bases for a range of carcinogens. In mouse liver the respective figures were 0.812 to 5.543 adducts per 10^5 bases for several carcinogens. Of course, one can always debate the relative mutagenicity of xenobiotic carcinogen adducts versus ROS-derived DNA lesions. However, many of the latter are significantly mutagenic (Section 4.9.1), they are formed in our DNA since conception, and the levels present could have even more impact if damage is located in specific genes relevant to cancer (Section 5.13.8). Reactive chlorine, bromine, sulphur and nitrogen species can also attack DNA, to give mutagenic lesions (Section 4.9.1). Indeed, as early as 1984 it was shown that exposure of mouse fibroblasts to ROS leads to malignant transformation.[337,338] Incubation of plasmids bearing proto-oncogenes (e.g. K-*ras*) with ROS followed by their transfection into cells could also cause transformation.[339]

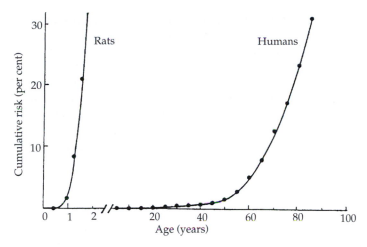

Figure 9.19 The cumulative risk of cancer as a function of age in humans. Note the sharp rise in cancer incidence in older people. Apart from a few rare cancers (e.g. testicular cancer, leukaemias), cancer is generally a disease of old age. The same phenomenon occurs, usually on a shorter time-scale, in other mammals such as mice and rats (From *Free Radic. Res. Commun.* **7**, 122, 1989, by courtesy of Professor Bruce Ames and Harwood Academic Press). At first sight the rates seems high, but the enormous number of mutations that occur over a lifetime caused by polymerase errors, spontaneous deamination and depurination of DNA, plus the actions of RS and exogenous carcinogens, makes one admire the high efficiency of protective mechanisms (Fig. 9.16) in ensuring that the majority of us do *not* develop cancer.

Several organic peroxides (e.g. **benzoyl peroxide**) are tumour promoters in mouse skin; their conversion into free radicals is thought to be involved.[340] Section 4.10.8.1 reviews some animal studies consistent with the concept that unrepaired oxidative DNA damage can lead to cancer, and arguments about its relevance are further developed in Section 9.13.6 below.

9.13.5.2 *Increased oxidative DNA damage in cancer?*

Many studies have shown increased levels of 8OHdG in human and other animal tumours.[341] In some cases, mass spectrometry has been used to suggest that a range of oxidative DNA base damage products is elevated, indicative of damage by OH$^\bullet$. Several authors suggest that malignant tumours are in a 'pro-oxidant' state, generating more ROS (e.g. from increased mitochondrial $O_2^{\bullet-}$ formation [Section 9.13.7 below] and by NOX enzymes)[342,343] that might contribute to genetic instability. Another source in some tumours might be **proline oxidase**, an H_2O_2-generating mitochondrial enzyme that converts proline to pyrroline-5-carboxylate.[344] In principle, decreases in DNA repair might also explain rises in base damage products, but, paradoxically, a few studies

report increased activities of DNA repair enzymes in human cancers.[345] It seems that rates of oxidative DNA damage are increased in malignancy and repair does not keep up. The p53 protein is intimately involved in these events (Fig. 9.18). First, if p53 is inactivated ROS levels rise because some genes encoding antioxidant enzymes are no longer properly transcribed (Section 9.13.4.2). Second, if levels of active p53 are high, it can increase ROS generation, for example by increasing levels of proline oxidase[344] and by mechanisms involving p66shc (Section 10.4.1). Third, ROS can inactivate p53 directly (Section 9.13.5.3 below).

Do the various mutations detected in malignant tumours arise by oxidative DNA damage? Maybe, but we can't be sure. Most attention has focused on 8OHdG, since it is mutagenic and is produced in DNA in significant amounts by several RS (Section 4.8.2). The G $\rightarrow$ T transversions often seen in cancer-related genes such as *p53* could result from the mutagenic effect of 8OHdG. However, they could also be generated by certain carcinogens and by errors in the replication of DNA containing abasic sites. Oxidative damage could account for C $\rightarrow$ T and G $\rightarrow$ A transitions frequently seen in various cancer-related genes, but again these changes are not specific for attack by RS. For example, $C \rightarrow T$ can result from deamination of 5-methylcytosine to thymine. By contrast, tandem mutations provide good evidence for UV-induced DNA damage to p53 in skin cancers (Section 6.12.1). It is interesting to note that oxidative DNA damage is elevated even in cancers induced by carcinogens whose mechanism of action does not involve RS (Section 9.14.2 below).

Reactive species need not damage DNA directly to facilitate cancer development. Oxidative damage to lipids and to proteins (e.g. DNA repair enzymes) could also contribute (Fig. 9.20).

9.13.5.3 Redox regulation

Low levels of ROS stimulate cell proliferation. For example, NIH-3T3 fibroblasts in culture transfected with a *ras* oncogene generated excess $O_2^{\bullet-}$ by the action of an NADPH oxidase, and this $O_2^{\bullet-}$ contributed to abnormal proliferation.[346] Several transcription factors are subject to redox regulation, especially NF-κB and AP-1 (Section 4.5), but also p21 and p53. The p53 protein has ten cysteine residues, some of which are involved in binding a zinc ion required for activity. Oxidation of p53 inhibits its action as a transcription factor. For example, p53 can be oxidized and nitrated by $ONOO^-$, and nitrated p53 was detected in human glioblastoma, a highly malignant brain cancer.[347] Oxidized cysteines on p53 can be re-reduced by Ref-1 (Section 4.10.3) and the thioredoxin system.[348] Oxidative inactivation of p53 will in turn raise cellular ROS levels (Section 9.13.5.2).

9.13.5.4 Intercellular communication[349]

Communication through gap junctions is generally decreased in tumour cells, which may facilitate proliferation. Several tumour promoters, and oxidative stress (Section 3.9.1), decrease gap-junctional communication.

9.13.5.5 Suppressing apoptosis

Certain tumour cell lines in culture appear to use ROS to deter apoptosis, by mechanisms involving suppression of caspase activity and changes in intracellular pH (Section 4.4.1.2). This could be one advantage of the 'pro-oxidant' state of some tumours.[350] Several ROS can inhibit PTEN,

favouring cell survival by stimulating the Akt pathway (Section 4.5.5.3).

9.13.5.6 Metastasis

Reactive species might contribute to metastasis.[351] Consistent with this, human metastatic prostate cancer showed higher levels of 8OHdG, HNE and 3-nitrotyrosine than did primary cancer.[352] Facilitation of metastasis may involve changes in cell surface morphology, cell mobility, and increased vascular permeability. In addition, degradation of extracellular matrix involves matrix metalloproteinases, some of which are secreted in latent forms (by both tumour cells and phagocytes) that can be activated by RS (Table 7.2). These enzymes can also liberate growth factors bound to matrix constituents (Section 7.7.1.1). For example, levels of stromelysin-1 (MMP3) are increased in many breast tumours. Exposure of mouse mammary epithelial cells to this enzyme increased their ROS production, causing oxidative DNA damage and genomic instability.[353] In addition, ROS might help suppress anoikis (Section 9.13.2).[351] Would, therefore, a judicious use of antioxidants have an antimetastatic effect? Maybe (Section 10.6.3).

9.13.5.7 Cachexia

Advanced malignant disease is accompanied by body wasting, including loss of muscle mass. Cytokines, especially TNFα, play an important role, in part by inducing oxidative stress (Section 4.7.1). Indeed, levels of lipid peroxidation, protein oxidation and 3-nitrotyrosine were increased in the wasted muscles of mice with hepatoma.[354]

9.13.5.8 Physiological relevance?

One should be cautious when examining mechanisms in tumour cells grown in culture, since they have adapted to the culture process and may use signalling mechanisms not employed *in vivo* (Sections 1.11 and 4.5.12). However, the potential carcinogenic effect of ROS is supported by the increased cancer rates in mice lacking CuZn-SOD,[326] GPx1 and 2 (Section 3.8)[306] and peroxiredoxins (Section 3.11), and by the finding in several tumours of NOX enzymes, in particular NOX1 (Section 7.10.1). This protein is normally present in colon, prostate, uterus and vascular smooth

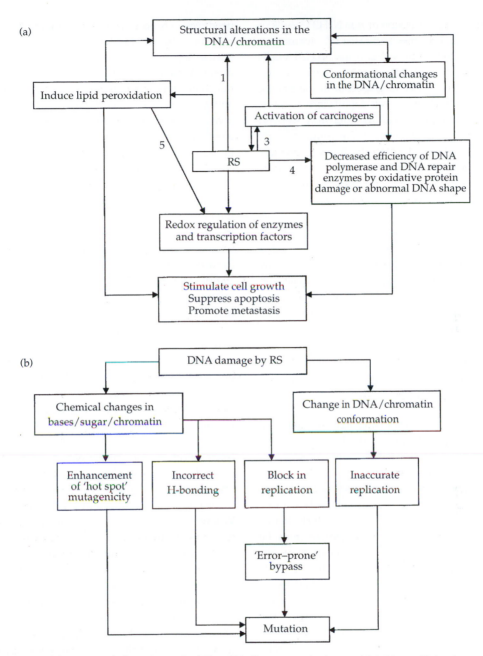

Figure 9.20 Some of the ways in which reactive species (RS) could facilitate cancer development. (a) 1. Direct oxidative damage to DNA. 2. Aldehyde end-products of lipid peroxidation (e.g. MDA and HNE) form mutagenic adducts with DNA bases. For example, M_1-dG (Section 4.12.5.3) is present in colonic mucosa (*Cancer Epidemiol. Biomark. Prevent.* **11**, 207, 2002). Radicals ($RO^\bullet$ and $RO_2^\bullet$) formed during peroxidation might also attack DNA. 3. Reactive species can activate carcinogens, and some then generate more RS. 4. They could damage proteins, e.g. DNA repair enzymes and polymerases (increasing the error rate of replication). 5. Hydroxynonenal can be proproliferative and is a powerful redox modulator (Section 4.12.5.3). (b) How structural changes in the DNA can cause mutations.

muscle, and overexpression of it in NIH3T3 cells or prostate cancer cell lines increased $O_2^{\bullet-}$ formation. Cell proliferation increased and the N1H3T3 cells developed some features of malignancy (Section 7.10.1).[342] But is NOX1 increased in human colon cancer? It's not clear as yet; reports are variable (some say it *decreases*) and its level may depend on the differentiation state of the tumour.[355] By contrast, NOX1 is elevated in human prostate cancers.[343] Some human prostate cancers contain mutations in mtDNA that may increase mitochondrial ROS production.[356] Mitochondria could be important, since mice heterozygous for the *Sod2* gene, with 50% of normal mitochondrial MnSOD levels, showed elevated 8OHdG in nuclear DNA of all tissues, and increased risk of developing lymphomas, adenocarcinomas and pituitary adenomas.[357] Finally, enzymes such as prolyl and lysyl oxidases in some tumours generate ROS that could sometimes contribute to cell survival, proliferation and metastasis.

9.13.6 Chronic inflammation and cancer: a close link but is it due to RS?

Reactive species can promote cancer. But they can also inhibit cell proliferation, kill cells or drive them into senescence (Sections 7.10.1 and 10.3.5). For example, DNA damage induced by RS is one trigger of p53 activation, and p53 binding to DNA may facilitate repair of oxidized bases, but only up to a point (Fig. 9.18).[333] So what is the net effect? In one tissue under one set of circumstances RS may be procarcinogenic, whereas a small change of circumstances may make them have the opposite effect. Thus when people ask 'are antioxidants good for cancer?', the answer can be 'maybe–it depends on the cancer, stage, tissue and environment.' For example, we saw that mice lacking CuZnSOD have increased rates of liver cancer development.[326] Why only liver? We don't know.

One well-known fact is that chronic inflammation is a risk factor for cancer. Examples include the effects of asbestos (Section 8.14), inflammatory bowel disease (Section 9.11), pancreatitis, oesophagitis, bile duct inflammation (Section 9.12.3), *H. pylori* infection (Section 9.12.2) and infection with the parasite *Schistosoma haematobium*, which

produces chronic bladder inflammation with increased risk of bladder cancer. In both Asia and Africa, hepatocellular carcinoma is commoner than in the West and is often associated with chronic infection and inflammation caused by hepatitis B and C viruses, or liver flukes of the *Opisthorchis* genus. Indeed, a transgenic mouse strain expressing a hepatitis B virus protein in the liver (provoking an immune response) showed chronic hepatitis and elevated liver 8OHdG levels, which preceded the development of hepatoma.[358] Where it has been measured (usually as 8OHdG), most or all of these inflammatory conditions in humans are accompanied by increased oxidative (and nitrative; Section 9.13.6.1 below) DNA damage.[341] Methodological caution is needed in such studies, since a biopsy sample may include not only tumour cells but also inflammatory cells, which may be activated to damage their own DNA and raise bulk 8OHdG levels in the whole tissue sample. Nevertheless, the authors feel that the available evidence overall supports increased oxidative DNA damage in inflammation-related cancer. Mice with disrupted *GPx1* and *GPx2* genes show increased intestinal cancer (Section 3.8), but *only* if gut bacteria are present to trigger inflammation.[306]

Just as inflammation can cause cancer, a tumour often induces an inflammatory response. For example, it may secrete cytokines that recruit phagocytes and lymphocytes. Many tumours are infiltrated by monocyte-derived macrophages. Whether this response is good (helping to suppress tumour growth) or bad (facilitating more mutations in the tumour cells and promoting metastasis by secreting proteolytic enzymes) is uncertain and may differ from tumour to tumour. Studies in animals have suggested that progression to malignancy involves activation of NF-κB, which suppresses apoptosis.[359] Thus in a colitis model in mice, knockout of the I$\kappa\kappa\beta$ gene, whose product is needed for NF-κB activation in intestinal epithelium, did *not* decrease the severity of inflammation, but tumour incidence was decreased by 80%. Interestingly, knockout of the NF-κB system in macrophages also decreased tumour incidence (by 50%), implying that (in this system at least) the host inflammatory response was procarcinogenic. However, anticytokine therapy (e.g. anti-TNFα) has had little clinical effect in human cancers.[359] NF-κB activation may also play a role in metastasis.[359]

One apparent exception to the general rule that 'chronic inflammation increases cancer risk' is RA. In RA, there is increased oxidative damage to DNA, lipids and proteins (Table 9.7) but no clear evidence that RA patients develop cancers at an increased rate, at least not at the most intense site of oxidative stress, the inflamed joint. One hypothesis is that this is because of the nature of the synovial cells. Synovium seems to be a hostile environment for tumour development, although it has been argued that the excessive synovial cell proliferation in RA resembles neoplastic transformation and might be related to the growth-promoting properties of ROS.[269,360] Several NSAIDs used to treat RA have anticancer effects, decreasing the incidence of colorectal and some other cancers by inhibiting COX-2.[359] Diabetes is associated with some inflammation and is accompanied by increased oxidative DNA damage (Section 9.4), but again the evidence of any increased cancer risk is weak, although the risk of colorectal cancer might be slightly elevated.[361]

So where then does oxidative damage fit in? The increased risk of cancer development, correlated with elevated 8OHdG levels, in animals lacking CuZnSOD or MnSOD, overexpressing a hepatitis B protein, or missing certain DNA repair enzymes (Section 4.10.8) supports a link between the increased oxidative DNA damage seen in cancers and the origin of the cancer. However, a rise in 8OHdG *alone* is insufficient to lead to cancer, since its levels are elevated in RA and in some DNA repair enzyme knockouts in mice, without rises in cancer incidence. It is also unclear where oxidative DNA damage fits into the sequence of events that results in cancer; studies on prostate suggested that it was elevated in benign prostatic hypertrophy[362] whereas studies on colon cancer found 8OHdG elevated in carcinoma but not adenoma.[363] Levels of 8OHdG are often elevated in premalignant lesions in tissues treated with carcinogens (Section 9.14.2 below).

9.13.6.1 *A role for reactive nitrogen and chlorine species?*
We should not forget the RCS and RNS; N_2O_3, HNO_2, HOCl, HOBr and ONOO$^-$ can damage DNA (and oxidize 8OHdG!) to mutagenic products (Section 4.8.2.12). Thus we might have a clearer picture if we measured a range of DNA oxidation, halogenation and deamination products.

Nitric oxide and other RNS might play multiple roles in cancer but, as for ROS, their overall role is unclear. They can promote DNA damage and inhibit caspases, delaying apoptosis. They can inhibit cytochrome oxidase and slow mitochondrial ATP formation (Section 2.5.6), impairing cell proliferation and slowing tumour growth. Indeed, that might be the 'purpose' of NO$^\bullet$ production by macrophages around a tumour. Some of the antiproliferative effects of RNS involve activation of p53, indirectly (via DNA damage) and directly by promoting its phosphorylation,[364] although too many RNS could oxidize and inactivate p53 (Section 9.13.5.3). Often, iNOS induction occurs as part of the inflammatory response associated with tumours, and formation of nitrating species such as ONOO$^-$, as evidenced by the presence of nitrotyrosine, is measurable. Nitric oxide can generate NO_2^- (Section 2.5.6), which at the low pH found in hypoxic areas of tumours, might form HNO_2 and N_2O_3. Reactive nitrogen species have been suggested (but not yet proven) to be especially important in causing DNA damage (measured as 8-nitroguanine [8-NG] formation) in chronic inflammation induced by the *Opisthorchis* parasites.[365] Levels of 8-NG are also elevated in the stomach of humans infected with *H. pylori* and in the colon of mice with IBD.[365]

9.13.7 Changes in antioxidant defences in cancer[352,366]

Mitochondria from several malignant animal tumours, and from many tumour cells in culture, show low MnSOD activity. Transfection of the MnSOD gene into cells can suppress the malignant phenotype in some (but not all) cell lines. Some authors suggest that elevated MnSOD generates more H_2O_2, which causes inhibition of proliferation, sometimes via p53 activation. Consistent with this, overexpression of catalase can often prevent the effects of excess MnSOD in cell lines. Low activities of CuZnSOD, catalase and GPx are also often reported in transformed cell lines.

One must be careful when extrapolating from cultured cells to *in vivo*, so what do direct measurements on malignant tissue show? Results are variable, but in general there is no clear pattern of marked decreases in MnSOD or other antioxidant enzymes in freshly obtained human cancerous tissue. Indeed, levels of MnSOD are sometimes (e.g. in mesothelioma, neuroblastoma, melanoma, stomach, ovarian, and breast cancer) elevated, perhaps as a response to increased oxidative stress.[363,367] Indeed, some investigators propose that high MnSOD activity is associated with increased tumour invasion, metastasis and a poor prognosis, possibly because a cellular redox imbalance induced by MnSOD overexpression increases levels of matrix metalloproteinases.[363,367] Probably what is important *in vivo* is not the level of any one enzyme, but the balance of RS production, antioxidant defence, and the repair systems, including the ratio of SOD to H_2O_2-consuming enzymes. The activity of the peroxiredoxin/thioredoxin system may also be increased in some malignant cells,[366] as is that of putative antioxidant protein DJ-1 (Section 9.19.5 below).

In fact, it is often difficult to interpret data on antioxidant enzyme levels in biopsy specimens given their heterogeneity, a problem already mentioned for 8OHdG (Section 9.13.6). In addition, areas within a tumour mass can be hypoxic (Section 8.19.3) which may decrease antioxidant levels. For example,[368] in rat breast cancer, SOD levels were found to be about $54\,\mu g/g$ tissue at the centre of the tumour, but $117\,\mu g/g$ at the edge. Exposure of the tumour-bearing rats to elevated O_2 concentrations raised both values, to 162 and $286\,\mu g/g$, respectively. It is also important to measure enzyme *activity* and not just gene expression or protein level. Increased mRNA does not always equate to more enzyme, and inactivated enzymes (e.g. nitrated MnSOD) can show up in protein measurements.

The increased risk of cancer in Down's syndrome (Section 3.14.2), Bloom's syndrome, ataxia telangiectasia and Faconi's anaemia has prompted investigations of cellular antioxidant defences in these conditions, although in none of the last three does the primary gene defect directly affect antioxidant defence. Nevertheless, mice lacking the ATM protein show increased oxidative damage

accompanied by *rises* in thioredoxin, MnSOD, CuZnSOD, and GSH in some tissues.[369] Cells from Fanconi patients are hypersensitive to O_2 and to ROS-generating agents in culture, and these patients show elevated leukocyte 8OHdG levels.[370] Indeed, several mutated genes that can lead to Fanconi's anaemia are involved in redox reactions. For example, one of them (*FANCC*) regulates microsomal electron transport, and another (*FANCG*) controls the expression of CYP2E1 (Section 8.8.1.1). Yet others play a role in redox-dependent cell signalling, for example through Akt kinase (Section 4.5.5), whereas *FANCD1* is involved in cell cycle checkpoints and DNA repair, and is now known to be identical with BRCA2.

Levels of lipid peroxidation are decreased in some cancers and tumour cell lines,[371] but again this does not seem to be a general feature of human malignant tumours.[352,363,367]

9.13.8 Transition metals and cancer

Malignant disease, like chronic inflammation (Section 9.10.7), produces changes in body iron and copper distribution. In most cases, plasma iron falls and caeruloplasmin rises. These 'acute-phase response' changes are induced by cytokines from the tumour and/or host inflammatory cells. One suggestion[372] is that they are a host's attempt to withhold iron from the tumour and slow down its cell division. In general, tumours do contain less 'total iron' and have less iron in ferritin than do normal cells. This is not always the case, however, since human breast tumours appear to accumulate iron.[373] In some cancers, including Hodgkin's disease, breast cancer and leukaemia, the concentrations of ferritin in the blood are significantly increased.[373,374] In cancer patients, chemotherapy or radiotherapy can produce sharp rises in 'total blood iron' and plasma transferrin saturation, the latter often approaching or reaching 100%. Indeed, non-transferrin-bound iron is sometimes present (Section 4.3.3).[375]

Can iron contribute to cancer? Iron-dependent oxidative DNA damage is widely thought to account for the increased risk of hepatoma in iron-overloaded haemochromatosis patients (Section 3.15.5). However, attempts to demonstrate increased levels of 8OHdG and other base oxidation products in liver DNA from patients have been unsuccessful (ref[376] and authors' unpublished data), although elevations in etheno–DNA adducts, probably arising via lipid peroxidation, have been reported.[376] Nevertheless, several iron chelates are carcinogenic in animals,[377] including asbestos (Section 8.14). Indeed, the first report of iron carcinogenicity was in 1959, when multiple injections of iron dextran into rats were shown to lead to tumours at the site of inoculation. Injection of **ferric nitrilotriacetate** into rats or mice causes increased lipid peroxidation, oxidative DNA damage (measured as 8OHdG in tissue and urine) and, eventually, renal cancers.[377] The DNA damage is not random, for example the *ras* oncogenes or *p53* are not affected. Instead, two other tumour suppressor genes, *p15* and *p16*, are among the targets of oxidative damage.[377] By contrast, p53 mutations *are* detected in the livers of haemochromotosis patients. Iron may also promote local invasion and metastasis, and it can aggravate the carcinogenicity of other compounds, for example hexachlorobenzene or polychlorinated biphenyls in mice (Section 8.3). There are suggestions that high body iron stores predispose humans to develop cancer (discussed further in Section 10.5.10).

There is also interest in copper. For example, the LEC rat develops hepatitis and hepatoma, associated with increased copper accumulation in the liver (Section 3.15.5.5). Copper-induced DNA damage might be involved, since LEC rats show elevated 8OHdG in several tissues.[378]

9.14 Carcinogens: oxygen and others

The O_2 that surrounds us is essential to life yet probably carcinogenic. Oxygen is not a direct carcinogen; it must first be metabolized (to ROS). The same is true of many of the molecules that are more usually regarded as carcinogens. They are metabolized to **electrophiles**, molecules that seek areas of high electron density, such as the purine and pyrimidine bases of DNA. In 1775, the English surgeon Percival Pott reported that the incidence of cancer of the scrotum in chimney sweeps was correlated with deposition of soot and tar in the scrotal creases. Later work showed that repeated application of coal tar to the skin of animals produces malignant tumours at the application site. Aromatic hydrocarbons such as **benz[α]pyrene** (Fig. 9.21), abbreviated elsewhere in this book to benzpyrene, were isolated from coal tar and shown to be carcinogenic. Carcinogenic hydrocarbons are present in combusted organic matter, for example soot, vehicle exhaust particulates and cigarette tar (Sections 8.12 and 8.13). In the late 1800s, the German physician Rehn noticed an association between exposure of dye workers to aromatic amines such as **benzidine** (Fig. 9.21) and the development of bladder cancer. Not until the 1930s was it shown that some aromatic amines cause this cancer.

Many naturally occurring and man-made chemicals are carcinogenic; Table 9.11 lists a few. About one-third of cancer cases in Europe and North America originate from exposure to carcinogens in tobacco products.[379]

9.14.1 Carcinogen metabolism

Many carcinogens, for example benzpyrene, are **complete carcinogens**, both initiators and promoters of carcinogenesis. Others are initiators only (**incomplete carcinogens**) and produce malignant transformation only if a promoter is present. Low doses of a complete carcinogen , too small to produce cancer, can be made to do so by a tumour promoter. The biological effects of a carcinogen depend on the dose, the animal species used, sometimes the gender of the animal and the mode of carcinogen administration.

Most carcinogens act by attacking DNA. The resulting carcinogen–DNA adducts can lead to mutations that activate proto-oncogenes, inactivate tumour suppressor genes, or cause genetic instability. Some carcinogens, such as **N-methyl-N'-nitrosoguanidine** (Fig. 9.21), modify DNA directly, for example by methylating guanine. Most have to be converted *in vivo* into their active form, the **ultimate carcinogen**. Conversion of a **procarcinogen** to the ultimate carcinogen can proceed in one or more steps. If more than one step is required, the intermediates are called **proximate carcinogens**. The necessary metabolism is sometimes carried out by

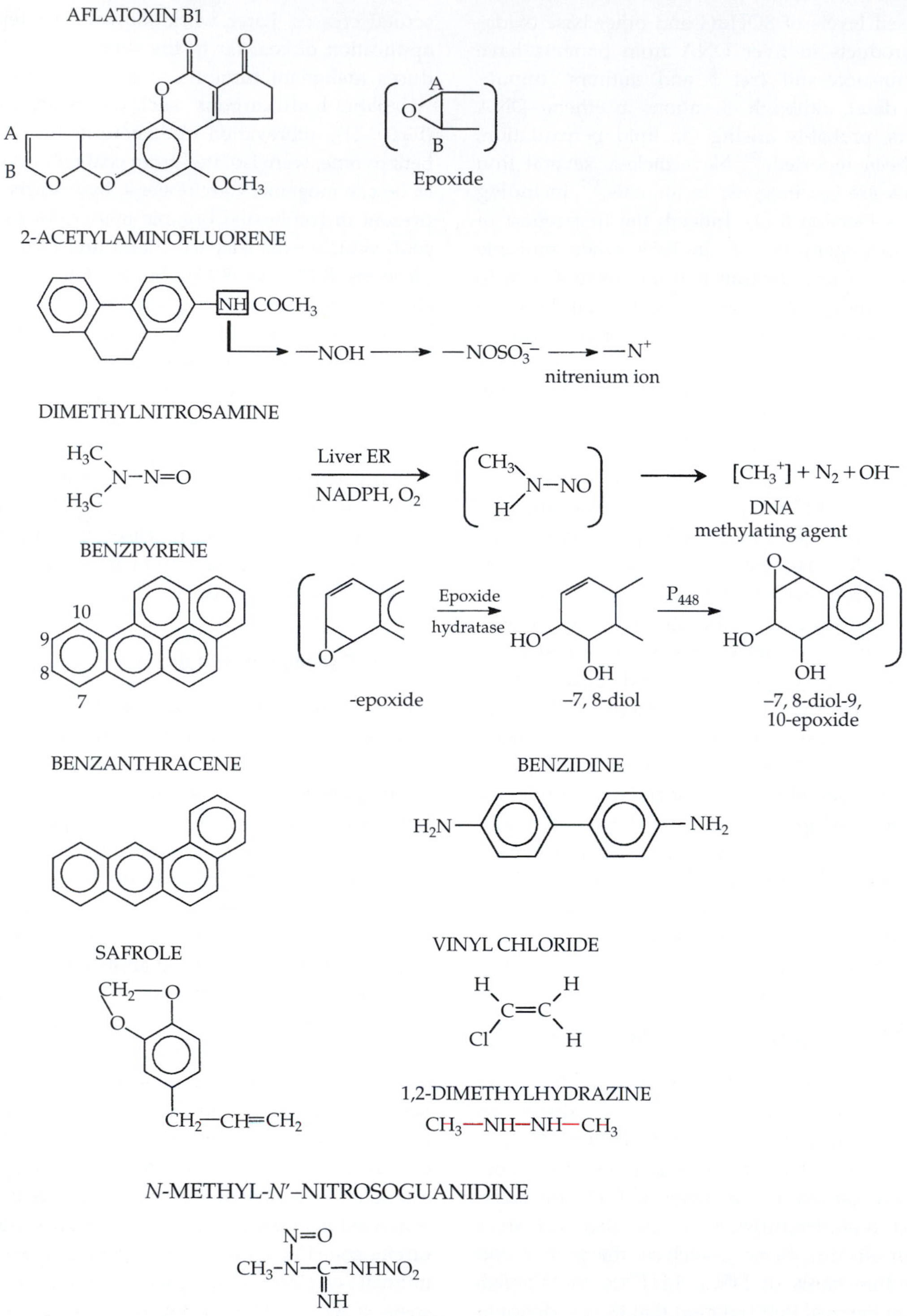

AFLATOXIN B1

A
B

OCH₃

Epoxide

2-ACETYLAMINOFLUORENE

NH COCH₃

—NOH ⟶ —NOSO₃⁻ ⟶ —N⁺

nitrenium ion

DIMETHYLNITROSAMINE

H_3C
$\quad$ N—N=O
H_3C

$\xrightarrow[\text{NADPH, O}_2]{\text{Liver ER}}$

CH_3
$\quad$ N—NO
H

$\longrightarrow$ $[CH_3^+] + N_2 + OH^-$

DNA
methylating agent

BENZPYRENE

10
9
8
7

-epoxide

$\xrightarrow[\text{hydratase}]{\text{Epoxide}}$

HO

OH

−7, 8-diol

$\xrightarrow{P_{448}}$

O

HO

OH

−7, 8-diol-9,
10-epoxide

BENZANTHRACENE

BENZIDINE

H_2N— —NH_2

SAFROLE

CH_2—O
$\quad$ O

CH_2—CH=CH₂

VINYL CHLORIDE

H$\quad$H
$\quad$C=C
Cl$\quad$H

1,2-DIMETHYLHYDRAZINE

CH_3—NH—NH—CH_3

N-METHYL-*N'*–NITROSOGUANIDINE

N=O
CH_3—N—C—$NHNO_2$
$\quad\quad\quad$ ‖
$\quad\quad\quad$ NH

Figure 9.21

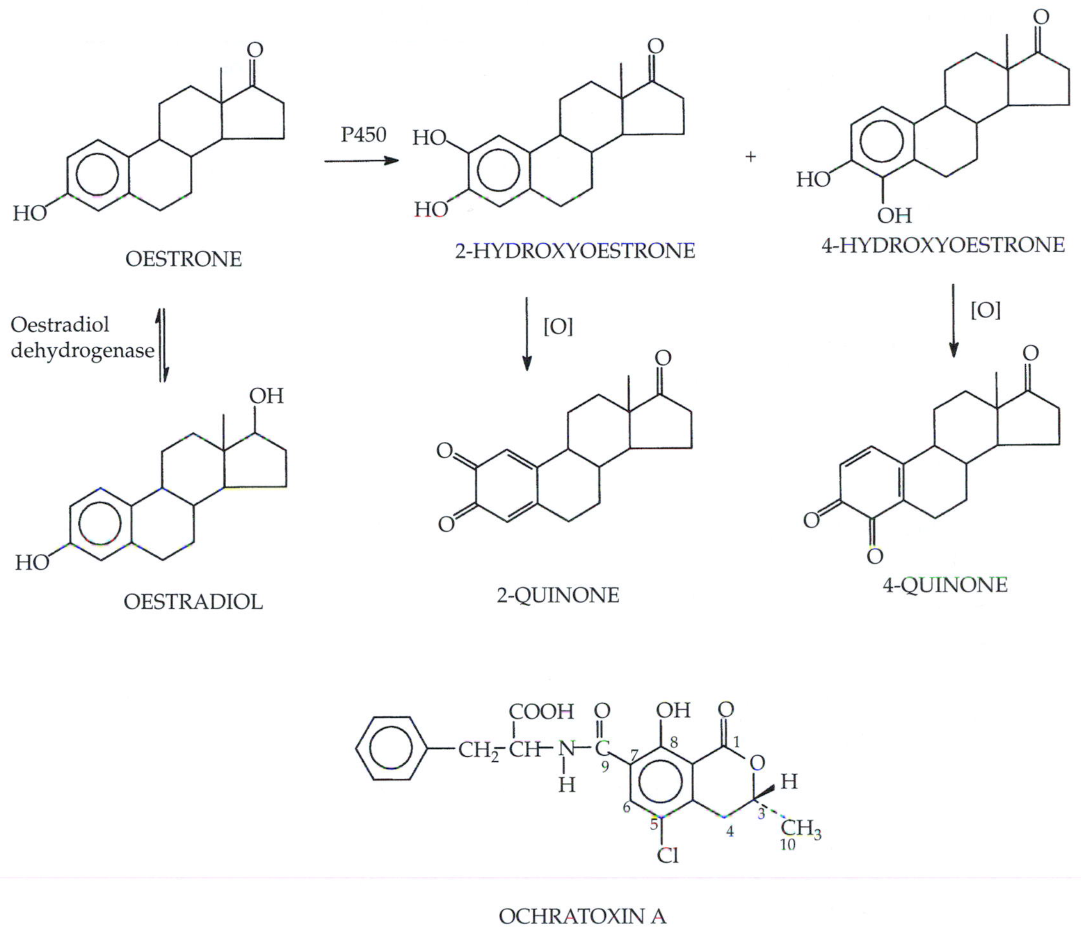

Figure 9.21 The structure and metabolism of some carcinogens.

gut bacteria, for example the hydrolysis of cycasin (Table 9.11) to the proximate carcinogen **methyla-zoxymethanol**, which then decomposes to a DNA-damaging product.[380] More often, enzymes in the body tissues are involved. Individual variations in carcinogen metabolism are in part genetically determined, depending on the levels of the various CYPs and phase II enzymes, as well as on rates of repair of DNA–carcinogen adducts. The first example of metabolic activation to be discovered was the conversion of the aromatic amine derivative **2-acetylaminofluorene** (Fig. 9.21) to an N-hydro-xylated product by CYPs. This type of metabolism is common to several aromatic amines, including het-erocyclic amines formed in cooked foods (Table 9.11).

The N–OH product can undergo several reactions, including sulphation to give an N–O–sulphate ester. Loss of sulphate produces a reactive **nitrenium ion**, which combines with guanine residues in DNA.

Benzpyrene also needs metabolic activation; the ultimate carcinogen is a **7,8-diol-9,10-epoxide** (Fig. 9.21). Cytochromes P-450 (especially CYP1A1 and 1A2) convert benzpyrene into a 7,8-epoxide. This is acted upon by the enzyme **epoxide hydra-tase** to form a diol, which is a substrate for further epoxidation. The resulting 7,8-diol-9,10-epoxide combines with guanine in DNA and cause $G \rightarrow T$ transversion mutations. Epoxidation can occur at other positions on the ring, although the products are less carcinogenic. Phenobarbital, an inducer of

Table 9.11 Example of chemical carcinogens

Chemical	Source	Site of cancer
A. Industrial chemicals		
Aromatic amines		Bladder
Asbestos[a]		Bronchus, pleura
Tars, oils		Skin, lungs
Diethylstilboestrol		Vagina
Arsenic[a]		Skin, bronchus
Benzene[a]		Bone marrow
Vinyl chloride		Liver
Aromatic hydrocarbons[f]		Lung
B. Naturally occurring chemicals		
Cycasin	Cycads	Liver, kidney, intestine (rats)
Ptaquiloside[b]	Bracken	Bladder, intestine (rats, cows)
Ochratoxin A[c]	Fungi (several *Aspergillus* and *Penicillium* spp.)	Liver, kidney[b]
Nitrosamines and others	Betel quid[a]	Mouth
Safrole	Oil of sassafras	Liver (rats)
Aflatoxins[d]	The fungus *Aspergillus flavus*	Liver (several species)
Agaritine[e]	The fungus *Agaricus bisporus*	Skin (in mouse models)
Heterocyclic amines	Family of products generated during cooking of meat.	Liver, GI tract, mammary gland, lung (*Nutr. Rev.* **62**, 427, 2004)

[a] The carcinogenicity of these molecules is discussed in Chapter 8. Arsenic is also employed in chemotherapy (Section 8.15.2).

[b] The purification and structure of ptaquiloside can be found in *Tetrahedron Lett.* **24**, 4117 and 5371, 1983.

[c] Presence in food has been implicated in the fatal renal disease **Balkan endemic nephropathy**, although its contribution is uncertain (*Chem. Res. Toxicol.* **18**, 1091, 2005).

[d] Several are known; the most active is aflatoxin B1.

[e] Agaritine in *A. bisporus* is metabolized to a phenylhydrazine, from which diazonium salts and various carbon-centred radicals can be generated (*Chem. Biol. Interac.* **94**, 21, 1995).

[f] Aromatic hydrocarbons can also be generated by charring of meats during cooking.

CYPs, accelerates carcinogenesis due to benzpyrene. **Aflatoxin B1**, a powerful hepatocarcinogen, is also metabolized to an epoxide, which binds to guanine (Fig. 9.21). Epoxides can be detoxified by glutathione S-transferases, being converted into derivatives which are excreted (Section 3.9.5).

9.14.1.1 *Carcinogens can make RS*

In a few cases, the DNA-attacking agent derived from a carcinogen may be a RS. Some authors have suggested that it is a phenoxyl radical of ochratoxin A (Fig. 9.21) that attacks guanine, but this is controversial.[381] Reactive species may contribute to carcinogenesis induced by the administration of high doses of oestrogens to rodents. Oestrogens can be converted into catechols by CYPs (Fig. 9.21).

Catechols can then oxidize in the presence of metal ions (e.g. copper) or oxidase enzymes to form semiquinones and quinones that can modify DNA bases and redox-cycle to generate ROS.[382] Excess oestradiol has additionally been suggested to increase mitochondrial ROS production,[383] although it may have the opposite effect at physiological levels (Section 3.19).

Reactive species might also modulate DNA damage by other carcinogens. First, they can alter the activities of detoxification enzymes (Section 4.5.10). Second, prostaglandin synthetase, MPO, and lactoperoxidase can oxidize several procarcinogens *in vitro* to yield RS. For example, COX and peroxidases can convert benzpyrene into 6-hydroxybenzpyrene, which rapidly oxidizes into a mixture of quinones, with production of $O_2^{\bullet-}$. Benzpyrene 7,8-diol (Fig. 9.21) need not always undergo epoxidation; it can be reduced by aldo-keto reductase enzymes to a catechol, which can oxidize to give ROS, quinones, and semiquinones, all capable of attacking DNA.[384] Other substrates for the peroxidase action of COX include benzidine, 2-aminofluorene, and 2-naphthylamine. Lactoperoxidase can oxidize a range of products, including aromatic amines. Oxidizing lipids have been reported[385] to convert benzpyrene into mutagenic products (including 6-hydroxybenzpyrene), and to form diol epoxides from benzpyrene-7,8-diol, probably by the action of peroxyl radicals. Oxidizing sulphite ions can produce diol epoxides from the 7,8-diol, perhaps by the action of $^{\bullet}O_2SO_3^-$ radical (Section 8.11.3). Indeed, SO_2 has been claimed to promote the development of lung cancer in animals treated with benzpyrene.[386]

However, the contributions of these various reactions to cancer development is unclear as yet, although it has been suggested that polymorphisms affecting MPO activity influence DNA-carcinogen adduct formation in smokers.[387] One such polymorphism is at position 463 in the promoter region; the presence of A produces less MPO gene transcription than if G is present. Some papers suggest that the 463A allele decreases the risk of smoking-induced tumours, although data are controversial. Such effects could relate to MPO-dependent metabolism of carcinogens, but might also of course involve modulation of the inflammatory processes associated with cancer.

9.14.2 Carcinogens and oxidative DNA damage

Damage to DNA by most carcinogens does not involve RS. Yet, rises in 8OHdG (and in other base oxidation products, when measured) in the neoplastic, and often the preneoplastic, lesions are common in carcinogen-treated tissue (Table 9.12). There are some negative reports, but the timing of measurements and poor methods of measuring 8OHdG might account for this. Thus the balance of evidence supports the view that oxidative DNA damage is involved in carcinogenesis, whatever carcinogen started the process.

9.14.2.1 *Peroxisome proliferators*[388]

Reactive species have been implicated in the actions of **peroxisome proliferators**. Several compounds, including trichloroethylene, some drugs that lower blood lipid levels (e.g. **clofibrate**, **ciprofibrate**, **nafenopin**, **gemfibrozil**), plasticizers (e.g. di-(2-ethylhexyl)phthalate), and phenoxyacetic acid herbicides (e.g. 2,4-dichlorophenoxyacetic acid), produce liver enlargement in animals, accompanied by increases in the number of hepatic peroxisomes. Peroxisomes not only increase in number, but their balance of enzyme activities changes. Thus the activity of the peroxisomal system for β-oxidation of fatty acids (which generates H_2O_2) often increases more than that of catalase. These agents sometimes also cause proliferation of hepatic ER and its associated CYPs, perhaps additional sources of $O_2^{\bullet-}$ and H_2O_2.

Some peroxisome proliferators increase the incidence of malignant tumours in rodent (but not human) liver, but neither they nor their metabolites react directly with DNA; the term **non-genotoxic** (or **epigenetic**) **carcinogen** is often used for agents of this type, whereas a **genotoxic carcinogen** is one where it (or its metabolites) damage DNA directly. How do peroxisome proliferators work? One idea is that the excess H_2O_2 in peroxisomes (e.g. due to increased oxidation of fatty acids) is not fully metabolized by the limited catalase activity present, leaks out of these organelles, reaches the nucleus, and causes oxidative DNA damage. Indeed, perfusion of lauric acid, a substrate for peroxisomal β-oxidation, into livers of fasted rats produced only small increases in the efflux of GSSG (Section 3.8.4), presumably because catalase degraded the H_2O_2. However, if the rats had been pretreated with nafenopin, lauric acid infusion did increase GSSG efflux, consistent with escape of H_2O_2 from peroxisomes. Of course more GSSG means that H_2O_2 is being metabolized by GPx, which is not evidence that H_2O_2 reaches the nucleus. So does oxidative DNA damage increase? Some, but not all, studies say yes. However, such increases are observed with several carcinogens (Table 9.12) and so their significance must not be over-interpreted. Clofibrate also increases mitochondrial ROS production and 8OHdG levels in mtDNA in mice.[389] Overall, in a court of law, RS would be acquitted of causing

Table 9.12 Some of the carcinogens shown to increase levels of 8-hydroxy-2′-deoxyguanosine in DNA *in vivo*

Agent	Species	Tissue/body fluid	Effect on [8OHdG]	Comment
γ-Radiation	Several	Several	Increases	Complete carcinogen; other base damage products also raised, pattern indicative of OH• attack on DNA
Potassium bromate	Rat	Renal tumours	Levels rise ~24 h after injection (*Japan J. Cancer Res.* **82**, 161, 1991)	
2-Nitropropane	Rat	Liver	Levels rise ~75% 6 h after injection (*Cancer Lett.* **91**, 139, 1995)	Hepatocarcinogenic; 8-aminoguanine also produced (*Chem. Res. Toxicol.* **6**, 269, 1993)
Ferric NTA	Rat	Kidney	Levels increase prior to renal cancer	Section 9.13.8
Benzene	Mouse	Bone marrow	5 × rise 1 h after administration (*Cancer Res.* **53**, 1023, 1993)	Leukaemogenic agent (Section 8.6.8)
Benzpyrene	Rat	Liver/kidney	3.5 × rise in liver, 2 × rise in kidney following oral treatment (*Cancer Lett.* **113**, 205, 1997)	
NNK[a]	Mouse	Lung	~2 × rise (*Carcinogenesis* **13**, 1269, 1992)	Induces lung cancer
Arochlor[b] + iron	Mouse	Hepatoma	3–5 × rise (*Carcinogenesis* **13**, 247, 1992)	
4-Hydroxyamino-quinoline-N-oxide	Rat	Pancreas	Significant rises (*Cancer Lett.* **83**, 97, 1994)	Powerful carcinogen in rats
Cigarette smoke	Human	Blood/urine	Elevated in blood cells and urine, also elevated in lung cancer patients who ceased smoking (*Int. J. Cancer* **114**, 153, 2005)	Section 8.12.1
Nickel (Ni^{2+}) ions	Rat	Kidney	8OHdG and other base products rapidly elevated; pattern characteristic of OH• (*Chem. Res. Toxicol.* **5**, 811, 1992)	Induces kidney tumours
Polycyclic aromatic hydrocarbons	Human	White blood cells	Levels of 8OHdG elevated in workers exposed to these agents industrially (*Carcinogenesis* **23**, 273, 2002), also urinary 8OHdG excretion increased (*Occup. Env. Med.* **61**, 692, 2004)	

Agent	Species	Organ	8OHdG	Comments
Hydrogen peroxide	Trout	Liver	Increased	Dietary H_2O_2 enhances liver carcinogenesis by N-methyl-N'-nitro-N-nitrosoguanidine; H_2O_2-enhancing effect reported to be correlated with elevated levels of 8OHdG (*Carcinogenesis* **13**, 1639, 1992)
2-Fluoroenylacetamide	Rat	Liver	Elevated	Elevations in 8OHdG and several other base-oxidation products observed (*Chem. Biol. Interac.* **94**, 135, 1995)
Transgenic mice expressing HBV large envelope protein in liver[c]	Mouse	Hepatoma	Rises early in life and continues to rise as liver damage progresses (*Proc. Natl. Acad. Sci. USA* **91**, 12808, 1994)	
Aflatoxin	Rat	Liver	Single i.p. injection raised liver 8OHdG (*Carcinogenesis* **16**, 419, 1995)	Hepatocarcinogen
Dimethylbenzanthracene	Mouse	Skin	Elevated up to 15 ×	Higher 8OHdG levels correlate with shorter time to first appearance of papillomas (*Proc. Natl. Acad. Sci. USA* **92**, 5900, 1995)
Acrylonitrile	Rat	Brain	Elevated ~2-fold (*Arch. Toxicol.* **72**, 429, 1998)	Acrylonitrile associated with tumours in several organs, including brain
Arsenic	Human	Skin	Levels of 8OHdG elevated (*J. Invest. Dermatol.* **113**, 26, 1999)	Arsenic is pro-oxidant and carcinogenic (Section 8.15.2) but can also be used in chemotherapy (Section 9.15 below)

[a] 4-(Methylnitrosamine)-1-(3-pyridyl)-1-butanone, a 'tobacco-specific' nitrosamine.

[b] A polychlorinated biphenyl.

[c] Animal model for hepatitis B virus (HBV) infection.

peroxisome proliferator-induced cancer on the basis of 'not proved beyond reasonable doubt.' Of course, acquittal does not equate to innocence.

9.14.3 Reactive nitrogen species and cancer

Nitrous acid and $ONOO^-$ can be produced in tumours (Section 9.13.6.1) and damage DNA. Reaction of secondary or tertiary amines with HNO_2/N_2O_3 produces **N-nitrosamines** (in the case of a secondary amine, for example, N–H is replaced by N–N=O). Nitrosamines are formed in the stomach from dietary amines (Section 9.12.2), and can be generated at sites of inflammation when RNS from activated phagocytes react with amines. Nitrosamines are found in human faeces (levels increase on a high-meat diet)[390] and tobacco smoke is a rich source of nitrosamines, some of which are 'tobacco specific'. At least one of these (Table 9.12) is a powerful carcinogen, especially for lung. Nitrosamines require metabolic activation (involving CYPs) to agents that attack guanine (Fig. 9.21). Ascorbate,[391] and possibly various plant phenols (such as flavonoids)[392], may be scavengers of nitrosamines *in vivo*. One 'bioassay' for such reactions *in vivo* is to feed nitrate plus the amino acid proline; proline is converted into the non-carcinogenic **nitrosoproline**, which is excreted in urine. For example, both ascorbate and, to a lesser extent, α-tocopherol decreased nitrosoproline excretion in humans given NO_3^- and proline.[391]

9.15 Cancer chemotherapy

Cancer treatment by radiotherapy or chemotherapy aims to kill malignant cells with as little damage as possible to normal cells. In malignant tumours, an abnormally large proportion of cells is dividing and so most chemotherapeutic agents are designed to interfere with cell division. The first reported use of chemotherapy was in 1942, when the DNA-modifying agent **nitrogen mustard** was used in a patient with lymphoma. One class of chemotherapeutic agents is the alkylating agents; they or their metabolites bind to DNA, and modify it, interfering with replication and transcription. The nitrosourea **carmustine** (BCNU) also

inhibits glutathione reductase (Section 3.8.3). **Cytosine arabinoside** contains an arabinose sugar instead of ribose, and its incorporation into DNA interferes with replication. **Cisplatin** (*cis*-diamminedichloroplatinum(II); Fig. 9.22) probably acts by cross-linking guanine residues in DNA, whereas **vincristine**, **vinblastine** and **taxol (paclitaxel)** interfere with mitotic spindle formation. DNA damage or stalled DNA replication will activate p53 and halt proliferation; thus the effects of DNA-damaging drugs are often diminished in cancers where p53 is lost.

Other anticancer drugs interfere with metabolic reactions. **Methotrexate** inhibits the enzyme dihydrofolate reductase and prevents transfer of methyl groups in several biosynthetic reactions, including synthesis of thymine for DNA. **5-Fluorouracil** is an analogue of thymine and prevents DNA synthesis by inhibiting thymidylate synthetase. **Hydroxyurea** inhibits ribonucleoside diphosphate reductase (Section 7.2.2). Hormone antagonists such as **tamoxifen** have been developed to treat cancers whose growth depends on steroid hormones.

Many other anticancer agents are produced by living organisms. They include the **anthracyclines,** other quinone-containing drugs (such as mitomycins and streptonigrin), some metal-chelators (such as tallysomycin and the bleomycins), and aureolic-acid-based antibiotics (such as mithramycin, chromomycins and olivomycins). Another promising class of anticancer drugs is the **proteasome inhibitors**, which block the cell cycle by interfering with both NF-κB activation and the ubiquitin-dependent degradation of cyclins (Section 4.14.2). Drugs based on indoleacetic acid are also under development (Fig. 3.20).

Of course, any normal cells undergoing rapid division (e.g. in the intestinal epithelium, hair follicles, gonads and bone marrow) will be damaged by most of these drugs. These and other side-effects limit the doses of most chemotherapeutic agents that can be used.

9.15.1 Oxidative stress and chemotherapy

Reactive species are often suggested to be involved in the mechanisms of action of, and/or in the side-effects produced by, anticancer drugs, for example

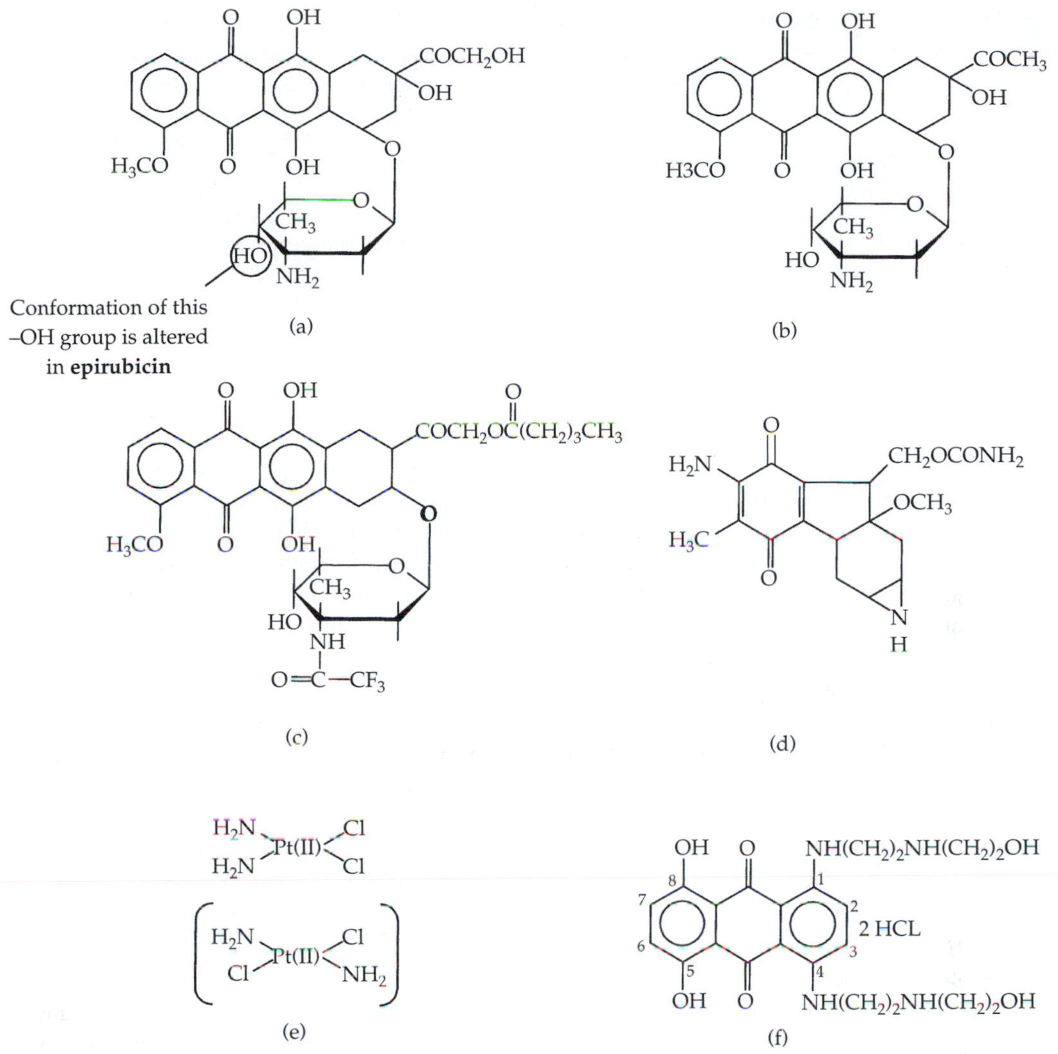

Figure 9.22 Structures of some antitumour drugs. (a) Adriamycin; (b) daunomycin; (c) AD32; (d) mitomycin C; (e) *cis*-diamminedichloroplatinum(II); the *trans*-isomer (below, in brackets) is not an effective antitumour drug; (f) mitoxantrone.

in kidney damage by cisplatin[393] and the neuro-toxicity of cytosine arabinoside.[394] The effects of taxol may involve ROS and RNS as well as directly interfering with mitosis.[395] If malignant cells are already under oxidative stress as a feature of malignancy (Section 9.13.5.2), adding more ROS might 'push them over the edge' and cause cell death (Fig. 9.23). Indeed, some groups have attempted to target H_2O_2-generating enzymes such

as XO or D-amino acid oxidase to tumours in animals.[396] If more ROS production were to occur in normal cells, however, there would be the potential for damaging side-effects and malignant transformation. Indeed, all the anticancer DNA damaging agents are potentially mutagenic and carcinogenic. For example, arsenic trioxide, As_2O_3, is effective in treating acute promyelocytic leukaemia,[397] but its pro-oxidant effects may account for

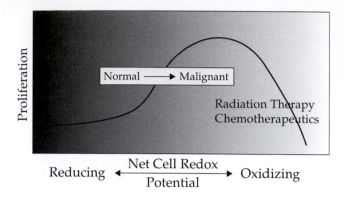

Figure 9.23 Impact of cell redox potential on cell proliferation. Small shifts in the redox potential toward oxidation can have large effects on increasing the proliferative capacity of malignant cells. This is in contrast to the highly oxidizing environment created by radiation therapy or some chemotherapeutic drugs that are strongly cytostatic/cytotoxic. From *Free Rad. Biol. Med.* **36**, 718, 2004 by courtesy of Drs VL Kinnula, JD Crapo and Elsevier. It has even been speculated that high-dose ascorbate could be pro-oxidant to tumour cells *in vivo* by generating H_2O_2 (*Proc. Natl. Acad. Sci. USA* **102**, 13604, 2005). The p53 protein also influences the redox state of the cell (Fig. 9.18).

its carcinogenicity (Section 8.15.2). Another interesting agent is **2-methoxyestradiol**, which appears to decrease CuZnSOD activity in cells (not apparently by direct inhibition[398]). It was reported to be selectively toxic to chronic lymphocytic leukaemia cells that already showed high basal ROS levels, and of low toxicity to normal lymphocytes.

Let us explore some ROS-generating anticancer agents in more detail.

9.15.2 The anthracyclines and other quinones[399]

Several antitumour antibiotics are quinones (Fig. 9.22). Hence redox cycling and/or reaction of semiquinones with –SH groups (Section 8.6) might participate in their anticancer activity. Generation of $O_2^{\bullet-}$ and H_2O_2 by redox cycling could produce DNA damage if they led to generation of $OH^\bullet$ close to DNA. Reduction of Fe(III) to Fe^{2+}, which facilitates $OH^\bullet$ generation, could be achieved by $O_2^{\bullet-}$, and by semiquinones ($SQ^{\bullet-}$).

$$(A) \quad SQ^{\bullet-} + O_2 \rightarrow Q + O_2^{\bullet-}$$

$$O_2^{\bullet-} + Fe(III)\text{-chelate} \rightarrow O_2$$
$$+ Fe^{2+}\text{-chelate}$$

$$(B) \quad SQ^{\bullet-} + Fe(III)\text{-chelate}$$
$$\rightarrow Fe^{2+}\text{-chelate} + Q$$

The balance between pathways A and B will depend on the reaction rate constants and the concentrations of O_2 and Fe(III)–chelate. In general, route B is only favoured at low O_2 concentrations.

The first antitumour antibiotic whose action *in vivo* was proposed to involve ROS was **streptonigrin** (Section 8.6), although it is no longer used clinically. Another is **mitomycin C** (Fig. 9.22). This drug, isolated from *Streptomyces caespitosus*, is used, in combination with other agents, in the treatment of several cancers. *In vitro*, it can be reduced by microsomal or nuclear electron-transport chains in the presence of NADPH. Reduction forms a semiquinone that can react with O_2 to form $O_2^{\bullet-}$. NADPH-cytochrome P450 reductase converts mitomycin C under hypoxic conditions into products that attack DNA directly, and cross-link the strands. Usually the cytotoxicity of mitomycin C is greater under hypoxic conditions, suggesting that its reductive activation and DNA cross-linking is more important in damaging its target cells than is redox cycling. The action of mitomycin C against large 'solid' tumours, which often contain hypoxic areas (Section 8.18), is consistent with this conclusion. Mitomycin C can additionally be reduced by quinone reductase (Section 4.5.10); two-electron reduction by this enzyme again forms a DNA-damaging product.

The role of ROS has been given greatest attention for the anthracyclines, tetracyclic antibiotics produced by various *Streptomyces* strains. The four-ring structure is attached to a carbohydrate, removal of which usually causes loss of antitumour activity. Anthracyclines are widely used in the treatment of leukaemias, breast cancer, Hodgkin's disease, and sarcomas. The best known are **daunorubicin** (sometimes called **daunomycin**) and doxorubicin (often called **adriamycin**). Both are products of *Streptomyces peucetius*. In both, the attached sugar is **daunosamine** (Fig. 9.22).

Like all antitumour drugs, the anthracyclines produce side-effects, the most serious being heart damage. Acute cardiotoxicity can occur within minutes of drug administration, revealed as arrhythmias and electrocardiographic changes. More serious than this is a chronic irreversible congestive heart failure, which becomes a significant problem once a certain amount of anthracycline has been administered. This cardiotoxicity limits the total amounts of doxorubicin and daunorubicin that can safely be given to cancer patients. One partial solution has been to use **epirubicin** (Fig. 9.22), which exerts equal anticancer activity but is metabolized faster, allowing larger doses to be given.

How anthracyclines work is not entirely clear, and multiple mechanisms are probably involved. Once they have entered the nucleus (a process which may involve their binding to the proteasome, followed by movement of the complex into the nucleus and its dissociation), doxorubicin and daunorubicin can intercalate between DNA bases, interfering with DNA replication and RNA transcription. Probably their major anticancer action is to affect **topoisomerase II**, an ATP-dependent enzyme involved in unwinding DNA for replication; it passes an intact double helix through a transient double-stranded break in the DNA backbone. Anthracyclines stop the enzyme from resealing these breaks. Other mechanisms of action may include partial inhibition of proteasome function, and interference with ion transport. Indeed, the doxorubicin derivative **AD32** (*N*-trifluoroacetyladriamycin-14-valerate, **valrubicin**; Fig. 9.22) will not bind to DNA, and yet is still an antitumour agent.

What about ROS? Reduction of the quinone moiety can be achieved by NADPH-cytochrome P450 reductase, XO, eNOS, the electron transport chain of the nuclear envelope, and the mitochondrial NADH-dehydrogenase complex (simultaneously interfering with normal electron transport). Damage could then be caused by semiquinones and/or by ROS. However, intercalation of anthracyclines into DNA prevents their reduction by enzymes (because of inaccessibility), and so it seems unlikely that ROS contribute much to the DNA damage (probably much less than topoisomerase inhibition does). Of course, some H_2O_2 formed elsewhere in the cell by redox cycling might diffuse into the nucleus and contribute to DNA damage.

9.15.2.1 *Mechanisms of cardiotoxicity: redox cycling and others*[399]

Changes in Ca^{2+} handling may contribute to the cardiotoxic effects of adriamycin. **Doxorubicinol**, a major metabolite of doxorubicin formed by NADPH-dependent reduction of the side-chain keto group to –CHOH by a **carbonyl reductase** enzyme, is a much more powerful inhibitor of membrane-associated ion pumps than is doxorubicin. It especially interferes with cardiac Ca^{2+} metabolism.

Whereas ROS may not contribute much to their DNA-damaging effects, they seem to be more important in the cardiotoxicity of anthracyclines, especially as several newer anthracycline analogues with less cardiotoxicity (such as **mitoxantrone**, which also acts on topoisomerase II) appear to undergo less redox cycling *in vitro*. The anthracycline semiquinone can oxidize to lose its sugar, giving a therapeutically inactive **aglycone** which can still, nevertheless, redox-cycle and may partition into mitochondria, facilitating local ROS generation, cytochrome c release, and apoptosis of cardiac myocytes. Indeed, doxorubicin cardiotoxicity in mice is accompanied by cardiac protein nitration and inactivation of creatine kinase, consistent with $ONOO^-$ production (Section 2.6.1).[400]

Why should heart be a target of damage? One possibility could be its modest levels of antioxidant defences. Indeed, transgenic mice overexpressing catalase, metallothionein or mitochondrial MnSOD in the heart are resistant to the acute cardiotoxicity of adriamycin. Treatments of animals with ascorbate, ubiquinone, PBN, α-tocopherol, probucol or *N*-acetylcysteine have often shown protective effects against the acute toxicity of doxorubicin. In general, however, they are less effective against chronic cardiotoxicity, a more serious clinical problem. Of course, some of these scavengers (e.g. thiols) might react directly with semiquinones.

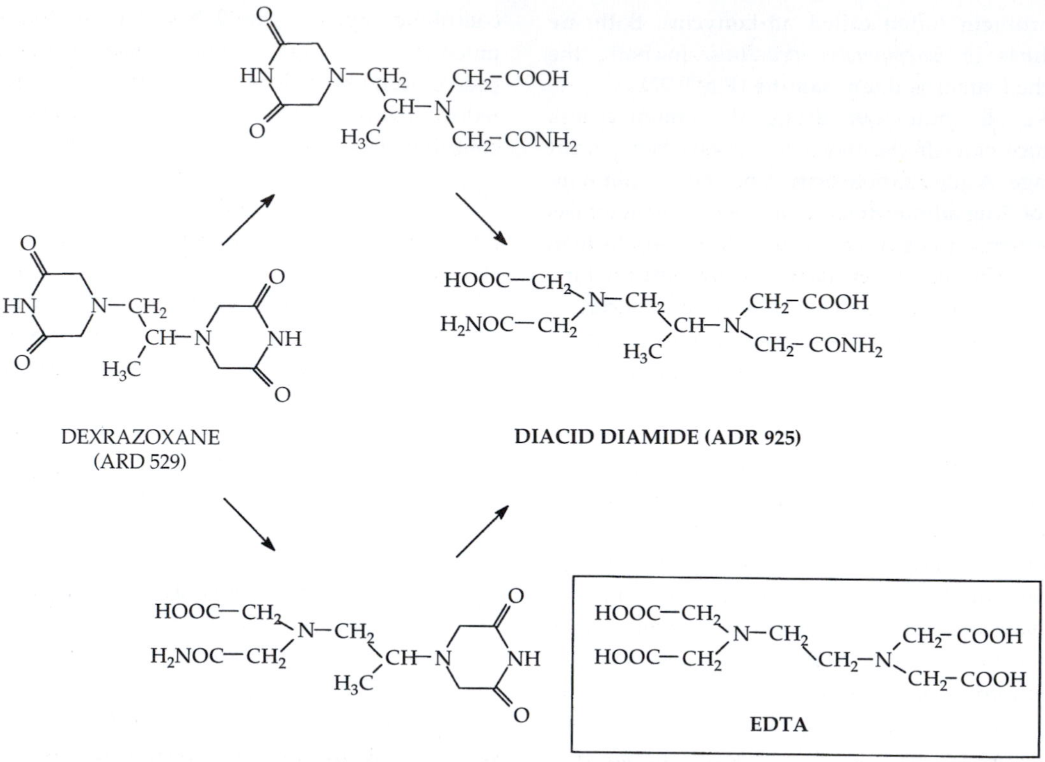

Figure 9.24 Two-step hydrolysis of dexrazoxane to an EDTA-like diacid diamide. From[399] by courtesy of Dr G. Minotti and the American Society for Pharmacology and Experimental Therapeutics.

9.15.2.2 *Iron and anthracyclines*[399,401]

The compound **ICRF-187** (or **dexrazoxane**) has cardioprotective actions in humans and other animals and allows higher doses of anthracyclines to be used. Dexrazoxane undergoes two enzyme-catalysed (or, more slowly, non-enzymic) hydrolysis steps to form a diacid diamide (**ADR 925**) that resembles EDTA (Fig. 9.24). Although ICRF-187 can inhibit topoisomerase II, evidence suggests that it acts mainly by iron chelation. Hence iron must contribute to anthracycline cardiotoxicity. Indeed, doxorubicin and daunorubicin can chelate several metal ions, including Fe^{2+}, Fe(III) and Cu^{2+}. Chelates of doxorubicin with Fe^{2+} can oxidize in air to generate $O_2^{\bullet-}$ and $OH^\bullet$. Doxorubicin forms a stable complex with Fe(III), in which three doxorubicin molecules associate with each Fe(III). The Fe(III) is slowly reduced to Fe^{2+}, which can then reoxidize, forming $O_2^{\bullet-}$ and $OH^\bullet$. In addition, thiol compounds such as cysteine or GSH can reduce the doxorubicin–Fe(III) complex, leading to increased formation of $O_2^{\bullet-}$ and H_2O_2. A combination of doxorubicin and iron, **quelamycin**, was once tested for anticancer activity but found to be highly toxic to heart and other tissues. The levels of several DNA base oxidation products in blood cells are increased in patients given epirubicin or doxorubicin, consistent with $OH^\bullet$ formation *in vivo*.[402]

Where might the 'catalytic' iron in the heart come from? Superoxide can release iron from aconitase and ferritin (Section 3.6). Cancer chemotherapy can cause 'non-transferrin-bound' iron to appear in plasma, for uptake by cardiac cells (Section 3.15.5.4).[375] The origin of this iron is uncertain, but it may be released from damaged cancerous (and normal) cells. Increasing the number of transferrin receptors by converting aconitase to IRP-1, leading to increased iron uptake into cardiac cells and decreased ferritin synthesis (Section 3.15.1.5), is another possibility.[403]

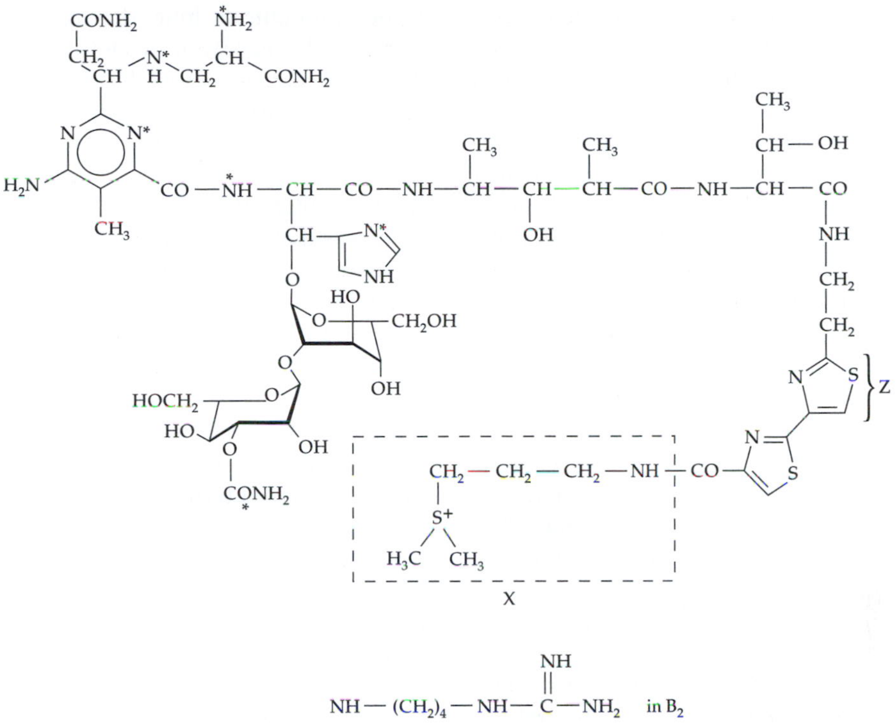

Figure 9.25 Structure of bleomycin A_2. In bleomycin B_2 the substituent shown replaces the terminal group (X) of bleomycin A_2. The asterisks denote the atoms that interact with transition-metal ions. The **phleomycin** antibiotics differ from the bleomycins in the absence of one of the double bonds in the ring marked Z. Bleomycin is usually supplied by the manufacturers as a sulphate salt.

Ferrylmyoglobin (Section 3.15.3) can oxidize doxorubicin to several products, including **3-methoxyphthalic acid,**

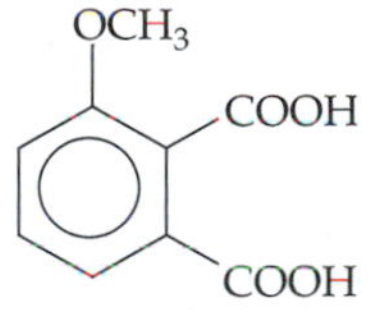

which has been detected in the hearts of doxorubicin-treated mice.[404] Since this product appears non-cardiotoxic, myoglobin may help to protect the heart against damage by anthracyclines. Myeloperoxidase can also oxidize anthracyclines to this and other products.[405]

9.15.3 Bleomycin[406]

Bleomycin is the collective name given to a family of glycopeptide antibiotics produced by *Streptomyces*

verticillus. The clinical preparation usually used, **Blenoxane**, is a mixture of bleomycins that differ slightly in structure, although bleomycins A_2 and (to a lesser extent), B_2 are the major components (Fig. 9.25). Bleomycins are active against several human cancers, including Hodgkin's disease and cancer of the head, neck or testis.

Bleomycins bind to DNA, especially adjacent to guanine residues, and cause single-strand, and some double-strand, breaks; triggering apoptosis, or halting the cell cycle. Breakdown of the deoxyribose by bleomycin forms, among other products, **base propenals** (base–CH=CH–CHO), which further decompose to release MDA. Since MDA reacts with TBA to give a pink chromogen, the TBA assay can be used to follow DNA breakdown by bleomycin (Section 4.3.3.1).

Bleomycins are powerful chelators of transition-metal ions by donation of electrons from nitrogen and from a carbonyl group (Fig. 9.25). Indeed, transition metal ions are needed for bleomycin to degrade DNA. *In vitro*, complexes of bleomycins with Fe^{2+}, Cu^+, Co^{2+}, Mn^{2+} and vanadium(IV) can damage DNA, but iron ions are probably the most important *in vivo*.

An Fe^{2+}-bleomycin complex capable of degrading DNA (in the presence of O_2) can be generated by adding Fe^{2+} salts to bleomycin or by reducing a Fe(III)–bleomycin complex, e.g. by ascorbate, GSH, $O_2^{\bullet-}$ or the nuclear electron transport chain. Ferric–bleomycin will also degrade DNA if H_2O_2 is added; O_2 is not then required. In all cases, the DNA-degrading intermediate appears to be an oxo–iron, probably Fe(V)=O, species. If bleomycin is incubated with Fe^{2+} under air in the absence of DNA the bleomycin destroys itself; it is protected by addition of DNA, which then becomes the target of attack. Catalase, SOD or other antioxidants offer little or no protection to DNA against damage by bleomycin. Indeed, ascorbate, propyl gallate and some other phenolic antioxidants make the damage worse *in vitro* by reducing Fe(III)–bleomycin back to the Fe^{2+} state.[407] DNA degradation can be inhibited by preventing iron binding to the bleomycin, for example with EDTA, DETAPAC, desferrioxamine or ICRF-187.

9.15.3.1 *Side-effects of bleomycin*
A major side-effect of bleomycin is lung inflammation and fibrosis. Matrilysin (matrix metalloproteinase 7) is involved in the neutrophil recruitment (Section 7.7.1). Activation of phospholipase A_2 (bleomycin toxicity is attenuated in mice lacking this enzyme)[408] and overproduction of TGFβ by pulmonary macrophages and alveolar type II cells are also important. The TGFβ1, 2 and 3 cytokines normally play important physiological roles in helping to repair tissue damage, for example in wounds, and are powerful chemoattractants for fibroblasts. Too many of them will promote fibrosis. Lung damage by bleomycin may involve RS, since microsomal fractions from rat lungs can reduce Fe(III)–bleomycin in the presence of NADPH, forming Fe^{2+}–bleomycin and hence ROS, which could contribute to fibroblast proliferation (Section 4.2.1). Consistent with this, mice lacking EC-SOD show more lung inflammation and fibrosis after bleomycin administration, whereas overexpression of EC-SOD is protective.[409]

Bleomycin-induced lung damage in animals is increased by exposure to elevated O_2. The lung may be a target because it has low activities of **bleomycin hydrolase**, a cysteine proteinase which breaks down bleomycin into an inactive form. This hydrolase is present in most body tissues and its level in malignant tumours is one factor that affects their sensitivity to bleomycin.[410]

Another relevant factor is the availability of iron within the tissue. Thus intravenous injection of bleomycin into rats produces no lung injury, yet simultaneous tracheal installation of ferric ions leads to marked bleomycin-dependent lung damage.[411] However, attempts to use desferrioxamine to prevent bleomycin-induced lung fibrosis in animals have given negative or marginally positive results,[411] perhaps because desferrioxamine does not penetrate easily into lung cells. The chelator ICRF-187 (Section 9.15.2) has been claimed to be protective in some animal studies, but not others. Intraperitoneal administration of nicotinamide decreased bleomycin-induced lung damage in hamsters,[412] possibly by acting as a precursor of NAD^+ and preventing 'lethal NAD^+ depletion' due to PARP activation (Section 4.2.4). Carbon monoxide was reported to decrease lung fibrosis in bleomycin-treated mice.[413]

The toxicity of bleomycin to bacteria (remember it's an antibiotic!) might also involve ROS, since strains of *E. coli* K12 with increased SOD and catalase activities, due to previous exposure to paraquat, are more resistant to bleomycin.[414]

9.15.4 Should cancer patients consume antioxidants?

If, on the whole, RS are bad things in cancer, then antioxidants should have an anticancer effect. Indeed they do, in some animal models. For example, increased dietary intake of α-tocopherol decreased liver tumour formation in transgenic mice overexpressing c-*myc* and *TGF*α genes[415] (remember however that α-tocopherol has biological effects unrelated to antioxidant activity; Section 3.20.2.9). In a transgenic mouse model of prostate cancer, administration of a mixture of vitamin E, selenium and lycopene (Section 3.20.2.9) slowed cancer development.[416] Antioxidants might also be beneficial in chemotherapy[417] if some of the side-effects are caused by RS.

Few good clinical trials have been conducted to date to address these issues. Those that have been done provide little evidence of benefit from antioxidant supplementation in cancer patients,[417–419] although such studies rarely provide evidence to show that the supplements did decrease oxidative damage, and so are inconclusive. Indeed, in patients undergoing radiotherapy there is a suggestion of harm from antioxidants (Section 8.19.2). Whether antioxidants have value in preventing cancer development is also uncertain (Section 10.5). One apparent exception is some older studies on **oral leukoplakia**, a precancerous mouth lesion that can develop after excessive exposure to tobacco and alcohol and may progress to cancer. It was reported in 1993 that some of the lesions regress after oral administration of α-tocopherol or β-carotene.[420] More work is needed to confirm this.

9.16 Oxidative stress and disorders of the nervous system: setting the scene[421,422]

9.16.1 Introduction to the brain

All aerobic cells suffer oxidative damage, yet the mammalian brain is often said to be especially sensitive. One reason is its high O_2 consumption; in adult humans, the brain accounts for only a few percent of body weight, but about 20% of basal O_2 consumption (Fig. 1.9). Hence it processes a lot of O_2 per unit tissue mass. The discrepancy is even more striking in young children—much smaller bodies but not proportionately smaller brains. The other reasons we will examine shortly (Section 9.16.5 below), but first let us make some general comments to set the scene. Figure 9.26 outlines the structure of the brain, covering the parts dealt with in this Chapter.

The adult brain contains about 10^{11} to 10^{12} nerve cells (**neurons**), which are supported and protected by at least twice as many **glial cells** (**glia** is derived from the Greek for 'glue'). The neuron, the basic working unit of the brain, is a specialized cell evolved to transmit information to other nerve cells (or to muscle or gland cells).

Neurons consist of a cell body, **dendrites** (short, branched extensions from the cell body), an **axon** that transmits electrical signals (by the opening and closing of specific ion channels) and a **nerve terminal** (Fig. 9.27). The neuronal cytoskeleton helps maintain the axon structure and facilitates transport of materials between the cell body and the nerve terminal, which can be a considerable distance away (axon lengths vary from mm to metres [in long motor neurons]). Hence damage to cytoskeletal proteins (e.g. by oxidation or nitration) leads to neuronal dysfunction, sometimes to an extent that causes axonal degeneration and neuronal death. Neurons with long axons must maintain large areas of membrane, and transport a range of materials (vesicles, proteins, etc.) from the cell body down the axon to the terminal (**anterograde transport**). All parts of the neuron contain mitochondria (presumably locally generating ATP) but the major site of protein synthesis is the cell body. Materials also move in the opposite direction (**retrograde transport**). Transport of some materials occurs quickly (50–200 mm/day) and that of others more slowly (0.1–3.0 mm/day). If an axon is severed, the segment beyond the cut will degenerate; this is an active process of self-destruction involving the proteasome. The nerve terminal forms part of a **synapse**, the communication mechanism between neurons. Synapses can be **excitatory** or **inhibitory**; the former release neurotransmitters that decrease the membrane potential of the target cell and make it more likely to fire an action potential, whereas an inhibitory neurotransmitter does the opposite. Neurons do not normally divide, and until fairly recently it was thought that the number of neurons before birth. The discovery of **adult neuronal stem cells** has transformed this view, but it is unclear how many new neurons they generate in the adult brain. Neurogenesis seems most important in the hippocampus.

There are several types of glial cell, including **microglia, astrocytes** and **oligodendrocytes**. The last synthesize and maintain the myelin sheath which insulates most axons (Fig. 9.27). Astrocytes co-operate in the metabolism of (Section 9.16.2 below) and help protect (Section 9.16.6 below) neurons, and are involved in the blood–brain

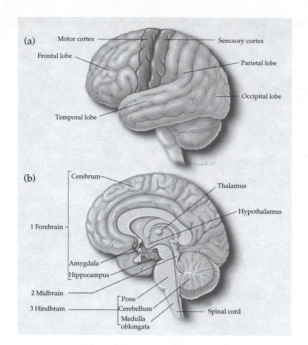

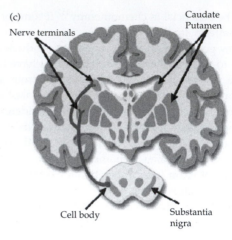

Figure 9.26 The brain. (a) **Cerebral cortex**. This is divided into four sections: the **occipital**, **temporal**, **parietal** and **frontal** lobes. Functions such as vision, hearing and speech, are distributed in selected regions (some are associated with more than one function). (b) **Major internal structures.** The forebrain (1) is credited with the highest intellectual functions—thinking, planning and problem-solving. The hippocampus is involved in memory. The thalamus serves as a relay station for information coming into the brain. Neurons in the hypothalamus serve as relay stations for internal regulatory systems by monitoring information coming in from the autonomic nervous system and controlling the body through those nerves and the pituitary gland. On the upper surface of the midbrain (2) are two pairs of small hills, **colliculi**, collections of cells that relay sensory information from sense organs to the brain. The hindbrain (3) consists of the pons and **medulla oblongata**, which help control respiration and heart rhythms, and the **cerebellum**, which helps control movement as well as cognitive processes that require precise timing. Parts a and b reproduced from[421] by permission of the Society for Neuroscience, USA. (c) A section through the human brain to show the **caudate** and **putamen**, which constitute the **striatum**. A section through the midbrain shows the **substantia nigra (SN)**. Dopaminergic neurons whose cell bodies are located in the SN send projections that terminate, and release dopamine, in the striatum. With degeneration of the dopaminergic pathway less dopamine is released in the striatum. Striatal dopamine deficiency results in complex changes in the brain's motor circuitry that lead to the motor deficits characteristic of Parkinson's disease (Section 9.19). From *Bioessays* **24**, 308, 2002 by courtesy of Dr R. Betarbet and Wiley.

barrier. They are also present around synapses and nodes of Ranvier (Fig. 9.27).[423]

The endothelium of the small blood vessels in the brain is, in general, much less permeable to molecules than other vascular endothelia, although essential molecules (such as glucose and ascorbate) and most lipid-soluble molecules (such as ethanol, other organic solvents and anaesthetics) can still penetrate. Many other molecules are excluded from the brain by this so-called **blood–brain barrier**. The blood–brain barrier also involves the capillary basement membrane, cells called **pericytes** present in this membrane, and the end-feet of astrocytes ensheathing the blood vessels.[424]

9.16.2 Energy metabolism

Neurons use most of the O_2 they take up in mitochondria, to make the ATP needed to maintain ion gradients (high intracellular K^+, low Na^+, very low 'free' Ca^{2+}). Sodium influx is needed to propagate action potentials; Na^+ must then be pumped out of the neurone using Na^+, K^+-ATPases. The human brain uses glucose for energy production, relying on glycolysis and the Krebs cycle, and needs about 4×10^{21} ATP molecules every minute. It can also utilize lactate from the circulation, which must first be converted to pyruvate using NAD^+ and lactate dehydrogenase (Fig. 1.7).[425]

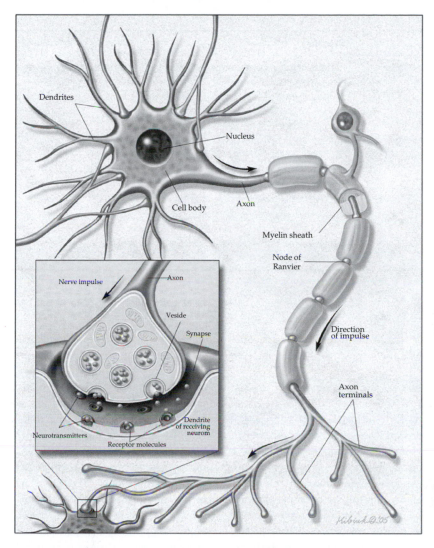

Figure 9.27 Neurons: a neuron fires by transmitting electrical signals (**action potentials**) along its axon. When signals reach the end of the axon, they trigger the release of **neurotransmitters** that are normally stored in pouches called **vesicles**. Neurotransmitters bind to receptors on the surfaces of adjacent neurons. The point of virtual contact is known as the **synapse**. The **nodes of Ranvier** accelerate transmission of the action potential. Adapted from[421] by permission of the Society for Neuroscience, USA.

Lactate is also released as an end-product of glycolysis in astrocytes, and taken up by neurons; it may be their major metabolic fuel *in vivo*. The brain is rapidly affected by interruptions of the glucose supply, since little glycogen is stored there (e.g. injection of excess insulin produces **hypoglycaemic coma**). Its heavy reliance on oxidative phosphorylation makes the brain also vulnerable to interruptions of O_2 supply. Similarly, inhibitors of mitochondrial ATP synthesis readily cause neuronal death (Table 9.13).[426] Examples include cyanide, **3-nitropropionic acid** (an inhibitor of mitochondrial succinate dehydrogenase) and **rotenone** (an inhibitor of complex I). 3-Nitropropionic acid is produced by some fungi, exposure to which has caused neurotoxicity in animals (e.g.

Table 9.13 Some neurotoxic agents whose action may involve oxidative stress

Type of agent	Examples	Relevant sections of this book
Inhibitors of energy metabolism	Cyanide, carbon monoxide, iodoacetate, rotenone, antimycin A, nitropropionic acid, malonic acid, MPP$^+$	This chapter
Excitotoxic agents	Kainate, quinolinate, domoic acid, β-N-oxalylamino-L-alanine	This chapter and Fig. 7.3
Metals	Copper, lead, mercury, tin, aluminium, manganese, iron	This chapter and Section 8.15
Organic solvents	Ethanol, toluene, n-hexane, pyridine	Sections 8.2, 8.8, 9.16.5, 9.19.3
Agents affecting antioxidant defences	Buthionine sulphoximine (GSH depletion), aminotriazole (catalase inhibitor), chloropropionic acid (GSH depletion), mercaptosuccinate (GPx inhibition)	Sections 3.9, 9.16.5
Free radical generators	6-hydroxydopamine, paraquat, sulphite, CCl$_4$	Sections 8.6, 8.11.3, 9.19.3
Other agents	Cocaine, methamphetamine, ecstasy, heroin, haloperidol, morphine, chlorpromazine, phenytoin	Section 8.9
Ammonia	Elevated level (e.g. in inborn disorders of the urea cycle, or in liver failure) is highly neurotoxic; oxidative stress may be involved (*Metab. Brain Dis.* **19**, 313, 2004)	–

cattle in the USA) and humans (in subjects in China who ate sugar-cane infected with such a fungus).[426,427]

Neurons also use energy in secretion; arrival of an action potential at the nerve terminal opens ion channels to allow Ca^{2+} influx, leading to release of neurotransmitter into the synapse by exocytosis. Each subgroup of neurons is associated with a particular neurotransmitter or group of neurotransmitters. The released neurotransmitter binds to receptors on the target neuron, for example there are multiple types of receptor for the neurotransmitter **dopamine**. Other neurotransmitters include **acetylcholine, serotonin, noradrenalin, γ-aminobutyrate (GABA), glycine** and **glutamate**. Acetylcholine is also released by neurons connected to voluntary muscle, for example in promoting vasoconstriction. Glutamate is stored in synaptic vesicles in neurons. After release, it is taken up by both neurons and astrocytes; the latter convert it into **glutamine** (the side-chain –COOH becomes –CONH$_2$) by the ATP-dependent enzyme **glutamine synthetase**. Glutamine is then released and taken up by neurons for hydrolysis into glutamate.[423]

The inability of most neurons to divide renders the brain sensitive to loss of function if neurons die. Fortunately, many parts of the brain have considerable redundancy and plasticity. Neurons in culture are prone to injury, often leading to necrosis or apoptosis, if treated with toxins that interfere with energy metabolism, exposed to RS such as ONOO$^-$ or H$_2$O$_2$, or if 'growth factors' (better called **neurotrophic factors**) are withdrawn from the culture medium. During development of the nervous system, a range of neurotrophic factors regulates proliferation of different neurons; they include nerve growth factor (NGF), brain-derived neurotrophic factor (BDNF), ciliary neurotrophic factor, neurotrophins 3, 4 and 5, and fibroblast growth factor. For example, BDNF seems to promote hippocampal-dependent memory; some humans carry a variant form in which a valine at position 66 is replaced by methionine. It has been claimed to be associated with poorer memory.[428] All of these factors are capable of protecting neurons in culture against various types of injury. Thus they are not only 'growth factors' but also 'support factors'. Often they act, in part, by increasing levels of neuronal antioxidants.

9.16.3 Glutamate, calcium and nitric oxide

Most of the excitatory synapses in the brain use glutamate as a neurotransmitter, whereas glycine and GABA are inhibitory neurotransmitters. Glutamate binds to **NMDA, AMPA** and **KA** receptors. They are named after **agonists**, molecules used in the laboratory to activate such receptors, **N-methyl-D-aspartate**, **α-amino-3-hydroxy-5-methyl-4-isoxazole-4-propionate** and **kainic acid**. The excitatory action of glutamate plays key roles in learning, memory and brain development and some of the neurotoxicity of Pb^{2+} is due to its ability to impair the functioning of NMDA receptors (Section 8.15.8).

Binding of glutamate to these various receptors opens cation channels and depolarizes the membrane of the target neuron (e.g. binding to AMPA receptors allows in Na^+), increasing the likelihood that the second neuron will fire an action potential. The NMDA receptor requires both membrane depolarization and glutamate binding before it opens to allow Ca^{2+} and Na^+ into the cell (the fall in potential displaces Mg^{2+}, which blocks the 'resting' channel). Glutamate also binds to receptors coupled to GTP-binding proteins (Section 4.5.5), the so-called **metabotropic** glutamate receptors. Binding of glutamate to all types of its receptors leads, directly or indirectly, to rises in intracellular free Ca^{2+}. Calcium is an important signalling molecule in neurons, which therefore expend a lot of ATP in maintaining low intracellular Ca^{2+} using transporters in the ER, plasma membrane, and mitochondria (Section 4.3.2).

Nitric oxide is used as an intercellular messenger by neurons in the peripheral nervous system (e.g. in regulation of penile erection and gut function) and by 1 to 2% of neurons in the brain (somewhat more in cerebellum). They contain **nNOS** (neuronal NOS), which is Ca^{2+}/calmodulin-regulated (Section 2.5.6.6).[429] Nitric oxide plays a role in development of **synaptic plasticity**—the strengthening or weakening of synaptic connections between neurons depending on how often they are used. This process is very important in long-term memory. Transgenic 'knockout' mice lacking nNOS show enlargement of the stomach, behavioural changes, and are more resistant to the toxicities of malonate (a succinate dehydrogenase inhibitor), the neurotoxin MPTP (Section 9.19.2 below), and to ischaemia–reperfusion damage to the brain. Indeed, injection of 3-nitropropionate (Section 9.16.2) or of malonate into the brains of rats or mice leads to neuronal death in which $NO^\bullet$ and $ONOO^-$ appear

to be involved. **7-Nitroindazole** is a nNOS inhibitor used in neurological research, but it can also inhibit monoamine oxidase and is hence not specific.[430]

The endothelial cells of brain blood vessels contain eNOS, which has an important vasodilatory role in regulating cerebral blood flow.

9.16.4 Excitotoxicity

The term **excitotoxin** was coined in the 1970s when the ability of high levels of glutamate or aspartate to kill neurons was observed. Similar neurotoxicity can be produced by NMDA, AMPA, kainic acid or **domoic acid** (a neurotoxin which binds to kainate receptors). Domoic acid is produced by the seaweed *Digenea domoi*; eating mussels contaminated with this toxin induces acute gastrointestinal symptoms followed by neurological damage. Kainic acid was also first described as a product of a seaweed, *Digenea simplex*. High levels of quinolinic acid, a product of the kynurenine pathway, in the brain can also cause excitotoxicity by binding to NMDA receptors (Fig. 7.3).

Concentrations of glutamate in brain extracellular fluids are normally low (<1 µM). The death of cells or collapse of normal ionic gradients (e.g. due to severe energy depletion) in neurons can cause massive glutamate release. It binds to receptors on adjacent neurons, leading to excessive and prolonged increases in intracellular free Ca^{2+} and Na^+ within them. Neurons treated with excess glutamate or other excitotoxins swell rapidly and die, usually by necrosis. Rises in Ca^{2+} interfere with mitochondrial function, cause overproduction of $NO^\bullet$ (in NOS-positive neurons, although the $NO^\bullet$ can then diffuse over a wide area in the brain) and increase ROS generation, in some animals (but probably not humans) by promoting conversion of XDH to XO by Ca^{2+}-stimulated proteinases. Peroxynitrite can be formed, and in some cases mitochondrial MnSOD is nitrated and inactivated.[431] Rises in Ca^{2+} stimulate phospholipases, increasing concentrations of free fatty acids and hence eicosanoid production.[432] Hence studies of neurons or neuron-like cells in culture in different laboratories have shown variable protective effects against excitotoxic damage upon adding inhibitors of NOS or of XO, or by a variety of antioxidants, including overexpression of CuZnSOD. Interestingly, nNOS-containing neurons are fairly resistant to excitotoxicity, but can sometimes respond to excess glutamate or NMDA by releasing enough NO$^\bullet$ to injure adjacent neurons. The mechanisms underlying resistance are uncertain, but one of them may be a high level of MnSOD.[433]

9.16.5 Why should the brain be prone to oxidative stress?[422]

It is often said that brain and nervous tissue are prone to oxidative stress (Section 9.16.1). Neurons seem more susceptible than glia. Oxidative stress can also occur in the cells comprising the blood–brain barrier, and increase its permeability. Why is brain more sensitive, apart from its high O_2 uptake? Several reasons.

1. The high Ca^{2+} traffic across neuronal membranes; interference with Ca^{2+} sequestration by oxidative stress and/or disruption of energy metabolism produces especially rapid rises in intracellular free Ca^{2+}, activating nNOS, phospholipase A_2 and calpains (Section 4.3.2). Some neurons and glia contain the TRPM2 cation channels, which rapidly allow Ca^{2+} in when ROS such as H_2O_2 are present (Section 4.3.2.2).[434]

2. The presence of excitotoxic amino acids (Section 9.16.4). Excitotoxicity increases $O_2^{\bullet-}$ and NO$^\bullet$ formation. Oxidative stress can damage neurons and promote the release of glutamate, generating a 'vicious cycle' of events. Other relevant events may be the ability of several RS (including ONOO$^-$) to decrease glutamate uptake by glial cells and to inactivate glutamine synthetase. Indeed, this enzyme is inactivated in Alzheimer's disease (Section 9.20 below).

3. Neuronal mitochondria generate $O_2^{\bullet-}$ (mostly from complex I; Section 1.10.4). Levels of 8OHdG, mutations, and deletions increase with age in brain mitochondrial DNA (Section 10.4).

4. Several neurotransmitters (not glycine or glutamate) are autoxidizable molecules. Dopamine, its precursor L-DOPA, serotonin and noradrenalin react with O_2 to generate $O_2^{\bullet-}$, H_2O_2 and quinones/semiquinones that can deplete GSH and bind to protein –SH groups (Section 8.6.6). Superoxide can

react with noradrenalin (Section 2.5.3), dopamine and serotonin[435] to initiate their oxidation, which then continues with production of more ROS, quinones, etc. Dopamine–GSH conjugates are degraded by peptidase enzymes to produce dopamine–cysteine conjugates (e.g. **5S-cysteinyldopamine**), which can be detected in several brain regions, and levels are elevated in Parkinson's disease (Section 9.19 below).

5. Autoxidation of neurotransmitters is accelerated not only by $O_2^{\bullet-}$ but also by transition metal ions, such as manganese (Section 8.6.6) and iron. Iron is found throughout the brain; important iron-containing proteins include cytochromes, ferritin, aconitases, non-haem-iron proteins in the mitochondrial electron transport chain, CYPs and the tyrosine and tryptophan hydroxylase enzymes, which catalyse the first steps in the synthesis of dopamine and serotonin respectively.[436] There are about 60 mg of non-haem iron in the 'average' adult human brain. Several brain areas (e.g. substantia nigra, caudate nucleus, putamen, globus pallidus) have a high iron content, which can be detected by magnetic resonance imaging.[437] Much iron in healthy brain is in ferritin, with some in haemosiderin. Oligodendrocytes express receptors for ferritin and appear to obtain most of their iron from it.[436] In adults, iron crosses the blood–brain barrier inefficiently, for example in haemochromatosis (Section 3.15.5.2) the peripheral iron overload is scarcely reflected in the brain. The iron content of the brain is low at birth but rapidly increases in early life to reach a maximum at about 30 years. If insufficient dietary iron is available to babies and children there may be permanent impairments of brain function. Transferrin delivers most of the required iron across the blood–brain barrier, utilizing receptors located on the brain microvasculature.[436]

However, there is a problem; damage to brain readily releases iron (and copper) ions in forms capable of catalysing such free radical reactions as OH$^\bullet$ formation from H_2O_2, lipid peroxidation (Fig. 9.28) and autoxidation of neurotransmitters. Injection of iron salts into the brains of animals can produce epilepsy-like convulsions, dopamine depletion and death of neurons accompanied by

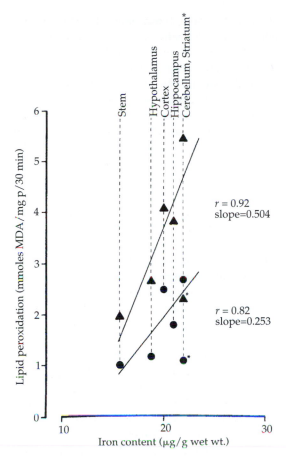

Figure 9.28 Peroxidation of brain homogenates. Regions of rat brain were homogenized and the iron content and rates of TBARS (Section 5.14.9) formation measured (no iron or ascorbate was added). Iron levels in striatum and cerebellum were the same (striatum values are designated by *). Lines were fitted by the least-square method. The closed circles represent values obtained from homogenates incubated under air and the triangles are the values obtained under 100% O₂. Iron content and rate of peroxidation are well-correlated. Data adapted from *Neurochem. Res.* **10**, 397, 1995 by courtesy of Professor Robert Floyd and the publishers.

lipid peroxidation, oxidative damage and OH$^\bullet$ generation (as detected by aromatic hydroxylation). 'Catalytic' iron released by brain damage can persist because the **cerebrospinal fluid (CSF)** that surrounds the brain and spinal cord has little or no iron-binding capacity. 'Total iron' values in CSF from normal humans have been reported as 0.29 to 1.12 μM. The transferrin content is $\sim$0.24 μM. Since one mole of transferrin binds two moles of iron

ions, these data suggest that CSF transferrin is often at, or close to, iron saturation.

6. Neuronal membrane lipids contain a lot of highly polyunsaturated fatty acid side-chains, especially docosahexaenoic ($C_{22:6}$) acid (DHA) residues. Homogenization of brain tissue causes rapid lipid peroxidation (Fig. 9.28), which can be largely inhibited by iron-chelating agents such as desferrioxamine. In addition, products of lipid peroxidation can injure the brain. 4-Hydroxynonenal (Section 4.12.5.3) is especially cytotoxic to neurons (increasing Ca^{2+} levels, inactivating glutamate transporters and damaging neurofilament proteins)[438,439] and can inactivate α-ketoglutarate dehydrogenase ($\alpha\kappa$GDH), a key enzyme of the tricarboxylic acid cycle.[440] 4-Oxo-2-nonenal may be equally or more toxic.[438] Isoprostanes may act as vasoconstrictive agents in brain[441] and can damage developing oligodendrocytes in premature babies (Section 6.11.8.2). Cyclopentenone IPs and prostaglandins (Section 4.12.3) may also be highly neurotoxic.[442]

7. Brain metabolism generates a lot of H_2O_2, not only via SOD but also by other enzymes. Especially important are **monoamine oxidases**,[443] flavoprotein enzymes located in the outer mitochondrial membranes of neurons and glia. They catalyse the reaction

$$monoamine + O_2 + H_2O \rightarrow aldehyde + H_2O_2 + NH_3$$
$$(RCH_2NH_2) \qquad\qquad (RCHO)$$

For example, dopamine is oxidized to 3,4-dihydroxyphenylacetaldehyde, which an aldehyde dehydrogenase then converts to DOPAC (3,4-dihydroxyphenylacetic acid). Monoamine oxidases exist in two forms (**MAO-A** and **-B**). The former preferentially oxidizes hydroxylated amines such as serotonin and noradrenalin, whereas MAO-B prefers to act on non-hydroxylated amines. Both can oxidize dopamine. The ammonia generated is disposed of by several mechanisms, including its use in conversion of glutamate to glutamine by glutamine synthetase. **Clorgyline** is a drug that inhibits MAO-A, **selegiline** is selective for MAO-B and **pargyline** inhibits both.

8. Antioxidant defences are modest (Section 9.16.7 below). In particular, catalase levels are low in most brain regions (Table 3.7); levels are a bit higher in hypothalamus and substantia nigra than in cortex or cerebellum. Brain catalase is located in small peroxisomes (**microperoxisomes**) and its activity in rat or mouse brain is rapidly inhibited if aminotriazole is administered to the animals, showing that brain generates H_2O_2 *in vivo* and that at least some of it reaches catalase.[443] The catalase probably cannot deal with H_2O_2 generated in other subcellular compartments.

9. Some glia are **microglia**, resident macrophage-type cells that arise from monocytes entering the brain during embryonic development. Normally, they help clear cellular debris (including apoptotic cells) and protect neurons.[444] However, microglia can become activated to produce $O_2^{\bullet-}$, H_2O_2, and cytokines such as IL-1, IL-6 and TNFα. In turn, such cytokines can prime microglia to generate more ROS upon activation and to produce iNOS and NO$^\bullet$. Cytokines can additionally be produced by activated astrocytes, which may again respond to them by iNOS induction. Thus microglia and astrocytes are major players in inflammatory processes in the brain.

10. Cytochromes P450 are present in some brain regions.[445] For example, CYP46 (Section 9.20.1 below) metabolises cholesterol. In rats, CYP2E1 is present in hippocampus, substantia nigra and blood–brain barrier, and CYP2D6 is present in several human brain regions.[445] Since CYP2E1 can produce more ROS than other CYPs (Section 8.8.1), it is another potential source of oxidative stress (although the magnitude of this may be small because brain P450 levels are low compared with those in, for example, the liver). However, CYP2E1 metabolizes ethanol, acetone, halothane, related anaesthetics, and organic solvents such as CCl_4 and $CHCl_3$ and may be inducible in human brain by ethanol and smoking.[446] Thus it could contribute to solvent neurotoxicity. Brain CYP2D6 levels are also elevated in human alcoholics; this isoform metabolizes many drugs that act on the nervous system, for example tricyclic antidepressants and MAO inhibitors.[445]

11. Reactive species, both directly (e.g. by down-regulating the synthesis of proteins involved in tight junctions between cells) and/or by activation of matrix metalloproteinases, can contribute to

'opening up' the blood–brain barrier, allowing neurotoxins and inflammatory cells to enter the brain.[448]

12. Like many other cells, neurons contain PARP-1, which responds to DNA damage, can lead to 'lethal NAD^+ depletion' (Section 4.2.4), and is involved in opening TRPM2 channels (Section 4.3.2.2). Overall, however, NAD^+ may be neuroprotective; NAD^+ added to neurons can slow axonal degeneration, an effect that seems to require the enzyme SIRT1 (Section 10.3.4).[449] This enzyme may contribute to the neuroprotective effects of caloric restriction in some animal models of AD.[449]

13. Loss of trophic support can lead to oxidative stress and apoptosis in neurons, in part by excess activation of neuronal NOX enzymes. Production of ROS by these enzymes may play important roles in brain development[450] but their overactivation in the developed brain can lead to inappropriate neuronal death.[451]

9.16.6 Antioxidant defences in the brain[422]

9.16.6.1 *Keeping oxygen low*

One important defence may be to keep brain pO_2 as low as possible consistent with normal function. Low O_2 decreases autoxidation reactions, mitochondrial $O_2^{\bullet-}$ production and oxidase activities. Of course, keeping pO_2 low has a disadvantage; it renders the brain highly sensitive to interruptions of the O_2 supply. The presence of neuroglobin (Section 1.3.1) in neurons, but not glia, has been hypothesized to assist correct O_2 delivery to mitochondria;[452] this protein seems less pro-oxidant in the presence of H_2O_2 than haemoglobin or myoglobin (Section 3.15.3).

9.16.6.2 *Superoxide dismutases and peroxide-removing enzymes*

All parts of the nervous system contain CuZnSOD, MnSOD, GSH (at millimolar levels), GPx enzymes and the thioredoxin/peroxiredoxin system.[453] The brain also contains glutathione S-transferases; isoforms differ between neurons and glia. Mitochondrial MnSOD is essential; mice lacking it suffer neurodegeneration after birth (Section 3.4.2), marked by cell death (especially in the cortex and brainstem) and severe motor disturbances.[454] No such problems are seen in mice lacking CuZnSOD, whereas mice overexpressing CuZnSOD are more resistant to ischaemia–reperfusion and to certain neurotoxins (Box 3.1). Indeed, neurons from transgenic mice overexpressing CuZnSOD survive longer after transplantation into other animals, and overexpression of CuZnSOD in normal neurons delays the ROS-dependent apoptosis that is triggered by removal of growth factors (Section 9.16.5), or by addition of H_2O_2. By contrast, decreasing CuZnSOD levels promotes apoptosis under these conditions.

Nevertheless, overexpression of CuZnSOD may contribute to the pathology of Down's syndrome (Section 3.14.2). Further evidence consistent with the view that not only too little but also too much CuZnSOD can be deleterious in the nervous system comes from the observation that not only mice overexpressing EC-SOD, but also mice lacking EC-SOD, show impairments of brain function. This occurs in part (but not entirely[455]) because $NO^\bullet$ and $O_2^{\bullet-}$ are involved in the regulation of cerebral blood flow: too much $O_2^{\bullet-}$ risks hypoxia and too little can promote $NO^\bullet$-dependent vasodilation that delivers too much O_2 to the brain.[456]

Mice lacking GPx1 show no evidence of brain abnormalities at 2 to 3 months of age, but the damage caused by administration of mitochondrial toxins (malonate, MPTP, nitropropionic acid) is worse. It thus seems that lack of GPx1 can be compensated for (e.g. by the peroxiredoxin system) under normal conditions, but not when mitochondria are damaged.[457] Brain is a 'privileged organ' with respect to selenium, efficiently retaining it and maintaining GPx1 and thioredoxin reductase activities even under conditions of severe dietary deficiency. Selenoprotein P is important in delivering selenium to the brain (Section 3.11.2); mice lacking this protein die with severe degeneration of motor neurons unless their diet is enriched with selenium.[458]

9.16.6.3 Glutathione

It is generally thought that neuronal GSH levels are lower than in glia, and that glia may assist neurons by efficiently degrading extracellular H_2O_2. Astrocytes may release GSH, which is degraded by

γ-GGT (Section 3.9.3) on their cell surface to produce cys–gly, which can be further degraded by an enzyme present on the neuronal membrane and the cysteine taken up for coversion to GSH.[459] In general, glia appear less susceptible to RS (including $ONOO^-$) than are neurons and more able to accelerate GSH synthesis under stress. However, many of these conclusions are based on studies of isolated cells, and the isolation process is itself a 'stress' that could increase glial GSH levels. For example, in a study on rat brain using antibodies to detect total glutathione, levels appeared *higher* in neurons than glia. Injection of kainate depleted levels in neurons whilst raising those in astrocytes.[460]

Severe depletion of GSH in mice by administration of buthionine sulphoximine (Section 3.9.3), causes neuronal damage and mitochondrial degeneration, perhaps indicative of the special importance of the mitochondrial GSH pool. Paradoxically, excess cysteine can also be neurotoxic.[461] Cysteine seems to be weakly excitotoxic and can act synergistically with glutamate. In addition, cysteine readily oxidizes to form $O_2^{\bullet-}$, H_2O_2, and thiyl radicals (Section 2.5.5), although the contribution of this to its neurotoxicity is unknown. Overproduction of H_2S from cysteine may be another mechanism of injury.[461] Another interesting observation is that, in mice, activities of glutathione reductase and glyoxalase-1 seem somehow linked to level of anxiety.[462]

The pentose phosphate pathway enzymes are needed in neurons and glia to provide NADPH for glutathione and thioredoxin reductases.

9.16.6.4 Ascorbate[422,463,464]

All animal species examined to date have high ascorbate levels in the brain. Ascorbate concentrations in human CSF are higher than in plasma (Section 3.20.1), whereas neurons and glia have active transport systems that concentrate ascorbate even more, to millimolar intracellular levels. Neurons readily take up ascorbate, whereas astrocytes take up dehydroascorbate (DHA) and convert it to ascorbate intracellularly. Indeed, it has been proposed that neurons may release DHA for 'recycling' by astrocytes. Ascorbate levels in CSF and brain are maintained high even when there are falls in plasma levels, suggestive of ascorbate's importance there. Key roles include involvement in dopamine hydroxylation, collagen synthesis and formation of the myelin sheath.[463] Indeed, mice lacking the SVCT2 ascorbate transporter (Section 3.20.1) show severely decreased ascorbate levels in brain (and other tissues), indicating that this may be the most important transporter for brain ascorbate uptake. These mice die within a few minutes of birth with respiratory failure and brain haemorrhage,[465] indicating that ascorbate is essential in the lung and brain to cope with 'birth hyperoxia' (Section 6.11.8). However, brain catecholamine levels were normal, suggesting that impairment of dopamine-β-hydroxylase activity was not the mechanism involved.[465] Weak blood vessels due to lack of collagen? Or oxidative stress perhaps? Time will tell, hopefully.

However, if iron or copper are available, for example in damaged brain, ascorbate could conceivably *stimulate* oxidative damage. Haemoglobin toxicity (Section 9.17 below) may involve its pro-oxidant actions in the presence of peroxides and also its release of haem and iron ions on decomposition. Unlike ascorbate's pro-oxidant effect with 'free' iron ions, ascorbate inhibits oxidative damage caused by haem protein/peroxide mixtures (Section 3.20). Hence its net effects at sites of tissue injury are hard to predict. For example, administration of DHA to mice decreased neuronal damage in a stroke model,[466] suggesting that overall (at least in this model) ascorbate is beneficial.

9.16.6.5 Chain-breaking antioxidants: vitamin E
Tocopherols are important in the brain, especially α-tocopherol; analysis of brain tissue shows little or no tocotrienols or β-, γ- or δ-tocopherols to be present, although they can be detected in CSF. Also, feeding tocotrienols to pregnant mice caused them to appear in both maternal and foetal brain.[467] Much brain α-tocopherol is derived from HDL (Section 3.20.2). Severe and prolonged deprivation of α-tocopherol, as occurs in fat malabsorption syndrome or ataxia with isolated vitamin E deficiency (AVED), produces neurological damage probably associated with increased oxidative stress (Section 3.20.2).[468] α-Tocopherol-deficient diets take a long time to lower brain α-tocopherol levels; for

example, it is necessary to feed rats such a diet for a year in order to decrease brain levels to <3% of control. A study in dogs suggested that peripheral nerves respond faster to dietary α-tocopherol repletion or depletion than the brain.[469] Similarly, it takes many weeks to increase the α-tocopherol content of brain in adult mammals supplemented with this vitamin.[468]

Hence brain α-tocopherol levels seem tightly regulated. This point is highly relevant when assessing the therapeutic effects of α-tocopherol supplementation in clinical trials; large doses need to be given for long periods to raise brain levels significantly. Levels of α-tocopherol appear normal in the brains of centenarians, patients with Alzheimer's or Parkinson's diseases, or in foetuses with Down's syndrome.[468] High doses of α-tocopherol have been reported in some studies to improve cognitive function in aged rodents[470] and in Alzheimer's patients (Section 9.20 below), although the extent of the benefit is uncertain. Again, we caution that effects of α-tocopherol are not necessarily related to its antioxidant ability (Section 3.20.2.9).

9.16.6.6 Coenzyme Q[422]
Defects in the ability to synthesize ubiquinone cause encephalopathy, and oral administration of coenzyme Q to rats was reported to increase its levels in the brain and to protect against striatal lesions induced by malonate or 3-nitropropionic acid. Coenzyme Q also protects against MPTP toxicity in mice (Section 9.19.2 below) and may have some therapeutic benefit in Huntington's disease (Section 9.22.2 below) and Freidreich's ataxia (Section 9.22.1 below). Neuroprotective effects could involve its electron transport action in mitochondria and/or the antioxidant action of ubiquinol ($CoQH_2$). In one study, the learning ability of old mice was improved by feeding a mixture of coenzyme Q and α-tocopherol, but not by either agent alone.[471]

9.16.6.7 Carotenoids and flavonoids[422]
Little information is available on the levels of carotenoids and flavonoids in brain. No carotenoids were detectable in human brain stem or in rat brain, even after dietary supplementation.

Nevertheless, there is evidence that some phenolics can cross the blood–brain barrier, with several animal studies claiming that monophenols such as ferulic acid and flavonoids such as epigallocatechin gallate, hesperitin and naringenin can enter.[472] In such studies, it is essential to wash out residual compounds from the vascular system before extracting the tissue for analysis. Some (but not all) reports suggest a protective effect of orally administered *Ginkgo biloba* extracts against the development of dementia. Such effects (if real) are often attributed to the flavonoids present, which include myricetin and quercetin. Mice whose diets were supplemented with *Ginkgo* did show changes in neuronal gene expression, suggesting that something had entered the brain.

9.16.6.8 *Metal-binding and related protective proteins*[422]

Although largely synthesized in the liver, caeruloplasmin is additionally made in brain. The brain form, largely present in astrocytes, is not secreted but instead anchored to glycosylphosphatidylinositol on the membrane (Section 3.15.2). Acaeruloplasminaemia is associated with degeneration of the retina and basal ganglia and elevated lipid peroxidation (Section 3.15.2). Prion protein may also be involved in brain copper metabolism (Section 9.22.3 below).

Haptoglobin is present in CSF, and may help to bind haemoglobin released as a result of bleeding. It has been hypothesized that low haptoglobin levels may predispose to epilepsy, but more data are needed to confirm this.

Brain also contains metallothioneins, including a 'brain-specific' metallothionein-III isoform. Transgenic mice lacking metallothioneins I and -II (but oddly, not mice lacking metallothionein-III!) showed impaired repair of brain damage after cortical injury (Section 3.16.1). Metallothioneins are major stores of intracellular zinc and alterations in zinc metabolism may contribute to the pathology of neurodegenerative diseases (Section 9.17.2.1 below).

Haem oxygenase is widespread in the brain; both constitutive (HO-2) and inducible (HO-1) forms have been detected. Indeed, its product CO may be a neurotransmitter. The levels of HO-1 increase after ischaemia–reperfusion, subarachnoid haemorrhage and in Alzheimer's disease.

9.16.6.9 *Repair of oxidative damage*[422]

Brain contains the ubiquitin–proteasome system to degrade abnormal (including oxidatively damaged) proteins. DNA repair enzymes are present in nucleus and mitochondria[473] and are important. For example, inhibition of uracil-DNA glycosylase in cultured rat hippocampal neurons increased levels of DNA damage and led to p53-dependent apoptosis,[474] and the brains of mice lacking Ku70 (Section 4.10.6) showed increased oxidative DNA damage and cell death.[475] Indeed, the disease **spinocerebellar ataxia with axonal neuropathy-1** may result from defects in the repair of single-strand breaks induced by ROS or other agents.[476]

Methionine sulphoxide reductases (MsrA and B; Section 4.14.1) are also found in brain. Mice lacking MsrA show a peculiar neurological phenotype, 'tip-toe walking'.[458]

9.16.6.10 *Histidine-containing dipeptides*[422]

Carnosine, homocarnosine and related compounds are present at high levels in brain and have been postulated to exert antioxidant effects, for example by chelating transition metal ions and binding cytotoxic aldehydes produced during lipid peroxidation (Section 3.18.7).

9.16.6.11 *Defence of the blood–brain barrier*[477]

Another important aspect in the maintenance of normal brain function is the antioxidant defence of the capillary endothelial cells that contribute part of the blood–brain barrier. Rat microvessels are rich in GSH, GPx, glutathione reductase, and catalase when compared with the rest of the brain. Glutathione appears important in maintaining the integrity of the blood–brain barrier, and GSH depletion can help to open up the barrier.

9.16.6.12 *Plasmalogens*

These have been suggested to exert antioxidant properties (Section 4.12.8). Such a role is feasible in the brain, since plasmalogens form a major proportion of phospholipids in the adult human brain, often esterified with DHA.[478] However, their contribution to antioxidant defence there is unclear as yet.

9.17 Oxidative stress in brain ischaemia, inflammation and trauma

9.17.1 Inflammation: a common feature

Inflammation is a key player in most, if not all, human disorders, and the nervous system is no exception. Systemic inflammation can predispose to atherosclerosis and stroke, and stroke is rapidly followed by inflammation. Inflammation in the brain can involve activation of microglia to produce RS and cytokines, and/or entry of peripheral inflammatory cells via increased levels of adhesion molecules on the blood–brain barrier triggered by its exposure to cytokines or RS.[424] For example, injection of endotoxin into the brains of mice provoked rises in both F_2- and F_4-IPs.[479] Endotoxin does not usually cross the blood–brain barrier, but can do so if it is damaged (e.g. by traumatic injury) or 'opened up' (e.g. by cytokine exposure). Animal studies have shown that administration of antioxidants (e.g. *N*-acetylcysteine, spin traps, uric acid) can protect against brain damage resulting from bacterial **meningitis**, inflammation of the membrane that covers the brain. Oxidative and nitrative damage may occur first to the blood–brain barrier (helping to damage it) and then spread into the brain.[424,480] Thus, in human meningitis, HNE and nitrotyrosine were detected in blood vessels in the subarachnoid space. Nitrotyrosine and allantoin (Section 5.12) levels rose in the CSF, and ascorbate fell.[481]

9.17.2 Multiple sclerosis[482]

Inflammation plays a key role in multiple sclerosis (MS), and there are repeated suggestions that RS contribute to the injury observed. The symptoms of MS are due to impaired nerve conduction caused by damage to the myelin sheath, apparently by an inflammatory reaction involving lymphocytes, glial cells and macrophages recruited (initially as monocytes) from the circulation by increased levels of adhesion molecules on vascular endothelial cells. Multiple sclerosis is an autoimmune disease; sug-gested autoantigens include $\alpha\beta$ crystallin (a small heat shock protein found in oligodendrocytes and astrocytes in MS lesions), oxidized lipids, the enzyme transaldolase (part of the pentose phosphate pathway) and several myelin proteins, including **myelin basic protein, myelin-associated basic glycoprotein** and **myelin oligodendrocyte glycoprotein (MOG)**. Several myelin proteins cause **autoimmune encephalomyelitis** (inflammation and demyelination of the central nervous system) when injected into animals. In these animal models and in MS itself there is increased iNOS and cytokine production, higher levels of matrix metalloproteinases, increased oxidative damage and more nitrotyrosine. In the animal models, some protection by *N*-acetylcysteine amide (Section 10.6.9.2), catalase, BHA, EUK-8 (Section 10.6.4), epigallocatechin gallate, lipoic acid or urate has been claimed[482,483]; the latter was suggested to act by scavenging ONOO⁻ since it decreased nitrotyrosine levels.[483] By contrast, flavonoids increased damage in one mouse model,[484] and whether antioxidants have a role in the treatment of human MS is an open question. Indeed, rats lacking the *Ncf1* gene showed not only more aggressive collagen-induced arthritis (Section 9.10.5) but also more severe encephalomyelitis after injection of MOG.[292] This implies that the phagocyte ROS production could have, overall, an *anti-inflammatory* effect under certain circumstances. However, in other circumstances, ROS make things worse (e.g. references [466,485]).

9.17.3 Brain ischaemia[486]

There are essentially two types of brain ischaemia/hypoxia (as for other tissues, these terms tend to be used interchangeably by neuroscientists). **Global ischaemia** occurs when O_2 supply to the whole brain fails or is severely limited. It occurs after asphyxia, myocardial infarction, haemorrhagic shock or poisoning by CO. It can also occur during birth; hypoxic injury to the neonatal brain can produce acute damage and long-term dysfunction (Section 6.11.8). Cerebral blood flow in adult humans is about 50 ml per 100 g of brain per min; flows below 18 ml will lead to injury, and O_2 supply must be re-established within minutes to prevent neuronal damage.

Local (sometimes called **focal**) **ischaemia** results from failure of the blood supply to part of the brain, for example by rupture of a blood vessel (**haemorrhagic stroke**) or the more common (~85%) **thrombotic stroke** due to thrombus formation in an atherosclerosed vessel. The former has the additional problem that, as with any bleeding into the brain, intracranial pressure rises because of the rigid skull and more brain damage is done. Haemoglobin is also neurotoxic. For example, bleeding into the brain due to trauma or rupture of a blood vessel is sometimes followed by **cerebral vasospasm** and thus a secondary ischaemia.[487] In local ischaemia, cells in the centre of the ischaemic zone are damaged most rapidly, but cells in the surrounding area (often called the **ischaemic penumbra**) that receive some O_2 (but not enough) from other blood vessels are also at risk. Animal models have been developed to mimic both types of ischaemia. For example, ligation of the carotid and vertebral arteries gives global ischaemia whereas ligation of the midcerebral artery is a popular focal model. Stroke is the third most frequent cause of medically related deaths and the second leading cause of neurological morbidity (after Alzheimer's disease) in the USA and Europe. It is the fourth most common cause of death in Singapore. Actions that help to prevent stroke include treatment of hypertension and hypercholesterolaemia, and a diet rich in fruits and vegetables (Section 10.5).

Global brain ischaemia for short periods damages only certain groups of neurons, as is observed in individuals resuscitated too long after a cardiac arrest. Most sensitive are the so-called **pyramidal neurons** in the CA1 region of the hippocampus. Other groups of neurons here and elsewhere (e.g. in layers 3, 5 and 6 of the cerebral cortex and in parts of the striatum, hypothalamus and cerebellum) have intermediate sensitivities. By contrast, the majority of neurons can tolerate 30 min or more of ischaemia (at least in animal studies). Death of susceptible neurons does not occur immediately but 1 to 5 days after reoxygenation. However, cerebral ischaemia lasting more than about 60 min produces tissue infarction in which all cells within the severely ischaemic region die. Ischaemia–reperfusion also damages the blood–brain barrier.

The brain displays ischaemic preconditioning; in various animal models, brief ischaemia can decrease injury resulting from subsequent, more prolonged ischaemia. Administration of low (controlled!) doses of 3-nitropropionic acid can also induce tolerance against subsequent ischaemia. Suggested mechanisms of ischaemic preconditioning in brain include adenosine release, increased synthesis of neurotrophic factors and Hsps, and modulation of K^+ channels (Section 9.5.6).[488]

9.17.3.1 *Mediators of damage*[486]

The best way of treating brain ischaemia is to restore blood supply as soon as possible. In thrombotic stroke, rapid but cautious administration of thrombolytic agents is often beneficial, but is clearly not suitable for haemorrhagic stroke. Even then, reoxygenation injury might occur and cause further damage, especially in the ischaemic penumbra. Hence there has been much interest in attempts to develop therapies to prevent neuronal death. The most important event in ischaemic injury appears to be failure of ATP synthesis, leading to release of glutamate from neurons by reversed operation of a membrane transporter that normally takes glutamate into neurons.[489] The resulting excitotoxicity (Section 9.16.4) raises Ca^{2+} and Na^+ levels in other neurons, ATP levels fall there as well, and the damage perpetuates. Cell swelling in the injured brain due to abnormal ion composition contributes to tissue oedema. Other relevant events include acidosis, release of haem and 'catalytic' iron from necrotic cells, and activation of phospholipases A_2 and C. Phospholipase activation causes rapid rises in arachidonic acid levels and excessive formation of eicosanoids, since COX-2 is normally present in brain (Fig. 9.29). Neuronal NOS is Ca^{2+}-dependent, so $NO^\bullet$ production may rise excessively. Of course, eicosanoids, $NO^\bullet$ or $O_2^{\bullet-}$ cannot form in an ischaemic tissue since O_2 is required to produce them, but in fact pO_2 rarely falls to zero, and they can certainly form after reperfusion. Rises in Ca^{2+} activate calpains—one target of digestion by these proteinases may be the Na^+/Ca^{2+} exchange system, hindering cells from exporting Ca^{2+} and slowing

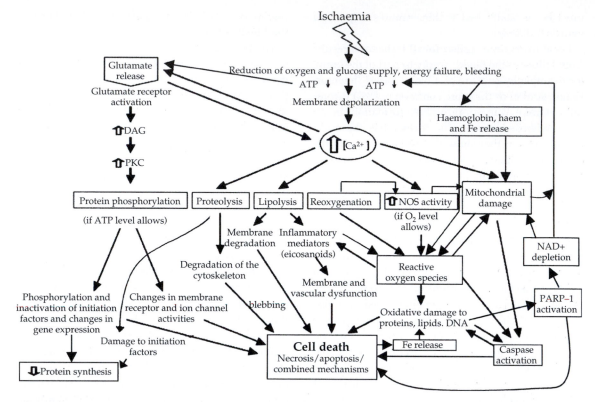

Figure 9.29 Mechanisms of cell injury in stroke. During ischaemia, less O_2 and glucose reach the affected area and ATP levels fall. This and the depolarization of membranes leads to increased intracellular free Ca^{2+} and release of glutamate. Glutamate receptors are then activated and a further increase in Ca^{2+} occurs, to damaging levels, with excessive Ca^{2+}-dependent proteolysis and lipolysis. There is also a marked depression in protein synthesis rates. Although reoxygenation is required for recovery, it results in the generation of RS. Together with increased NOS activity and mitochondrial damage, this can lead to caspase activation, the release of inflammatory mediators, and oxidative damage, ultimately leading to its cell death. DAG, diacylglycerol; PKC, protein kinase C. Cell death can involve necrosis, apoptosis and often features of both. Extensively modified from[486] by courtesy of Dr P.J. Crack and the publishers.

the restoration of correct ion gradients during reperfusion.[489] Ischaemia–reperfusion in mouse cortex produces rises in several DNA base oxidation products, a pattern indicative of attack by OH$^\bullet$ (Section 4.8.2.1).[490] DNA damage may contribute to cell death, since mice lacking uracil-DNA glycosylase show larger infarcts after brain ischaemia.[491] So might end-products of lipid peroxidation such as HNE, oxononenal, and products of the isoprostane pathway (Section 9.16.5). That RS do play a role in ischaemia–reperfusion injury is indicated by observations that transgenic mice overexpressing MnSOD, CuZnSOD, GPx1 or thioredoxin are usually more resistant to cerebral ischaemia–reperfusion and traumatic injury. Antioxidants decrease oxidative lipid, DNA and protein damage and may help to protect mitochondria (e.g. by preventing $O_2^{\bullet-}$ from inactivating aconitase) and thus maintain ATP levels and prevent ion gradient derangements and glutamate release.[492]

Where do RS come from? Likely sources include increased electron leakage from the mitochondrial electron transport chain, XO (in some animals, probably not humans)[493] and faster oxidation of neurotransmitters catalysed by released transition-metal ions. Brain ischaemia in mice led to increased levels of the mRNA that encodes uncoupling protein-2 in microglia in the peri-infarct area; this protein regulates ROS production in mitochondria (Section 1.10.6) and raising its level could be an attempt at defence by slowing mitochondrial $O_2^{\bullet-}$ production.[494]

Another proposed mediator of injury is Zn^{2+}, a neurotoxin at high levels (Section 8.15.12). Excitoxicity has been suggested to cause sufficient Zn^{2+} release from stores in synaptic vesicles to reach toxic extracellular levels in brain. Metallothionein is another possible source (Section 9.16.6.8); it can release Zn^{2+} if attacked by RS (Section 3.16.1).

As well as their role in post-stroke inflammation, microglia may play an earlier role. Ischaemia–reperfusion led to elevated levels of microglia CD36 (a scavenger receptor, Section 9.3.4) in mouse brain; mice lacking CD36 showed less ROS production and smaller infarcts.[495]

9.17.3.2 *Therapeutic interventions?*

One possible treatment is to lower brain temperature, which slows down falls in ATP, deleterious changes in ion gradients, and lipid peroxidation.[496] It has shown some benefit in decreasing neurological damage in patients resuscitated after cardiac arrest, but is difficult to apply to stroke patients and has several side-effects.[497]

Multiple agents have been shown to decrease neuronal loss after ischaemia in animal models, including Ca^{2+} blockers, inhibitors of nNOS, XO or phospholipase A_2, agents that prevent binding of glutamate to its receptors, and antioxidants such as PEG-SOD,[a] SOD mimetics, ebselen, some plant phenols, N-acetylcysteine, desferrioxamine, dehydroascorbate, lazaroids (Section 10.6.8), edaravone, PBN or related compounds such as NXY-O59 (Section 10.6.5), and proteasome inhibitors. The last is somewhat paradoxical because these agents can be neurotoxic (Section 9.18 below); possibly they dampen inflammation by decreasing activation of NF-κB.[498] The success of these various interventions depends on the dose and animal model used, the extent and duration of hypoxia, the length of follow-up of the animals (some agents delay neuronal death rather than preventing it, an effect easily missed in a short-term study), the baseline levels of brain antioxidants (e.g. α-tocopherol-deficient animals suffer more damage after ischaemia–reperfusion),[499] and other parameters of experimental design.

[a] CuZnSOD conjugated to the polymer polyethylene glycol.

The fact that this wide variety of interventions can work in animals suggests that cell death is not due to a single event, but to multiple events acting in parallel and/or synergistically (Fig. 9.29). Suggestions as to why some neurons are more vulnerable than others include their levels of various glutamate receptors, basal levels of oxidative stress, ability to take up Zn^{2+} and propensity to suffer proteasomal dysfunction and/or to undergo rises in intracellular free Ca^{2+} (e.g. whether TRPM2 is present) and mitochondrial damage.[500] The ability to activate signal pathways that promote neuronal survival, such as the PI3-K/Akt pathway (Section 4.5.5) may also be important.[486]

Sadly, none of the agents mentioned above has yet given convincing clinical benefit in human stroke patients, although NXY-059 seems promising. Unlike the highly controlled animal models, human patients vary in their degree of hypoxia, the time at which they appear in hospital with problems and the time taken to diagnose a stroke. Hence they can be at widely different points along the 'cytotoxic chain of events', and it would be naïve to expect a single agent to benefit the majority of subjects. There may also be a 'gender effect', a trend to better outcome in females than males, which has been speculated to be due to better antioxidant protection in the former (Section 3.20). For example, in one study CSF F_2-IP levels were higher after traumatic brain injury in male than in female patients.[501]

The inflammatory-immune response is intended to help repair tissue injury, but an excess response could lead to further damage involving phagocyte-derived RS.[502] The potential for injury is revealed by studies showing that ischaemic injury to the brain is decreased in mice lacking the A_{2A} adenosine receptor on neutrophils. This receptor stimulates neutrophil cytokine production, implying that recruitment of neutrophils by adenosine can worsen damage.[503] However, in other circumstances adenosine is beneficial (Section 9.5.6). Interestingly, mice deficient in receptors for TNFα (a cytokine often picked as the 'bad guy' during inflammation) show *increased* neuronal damage after focal cerebral ischaemia or injection of the excitotoxin kainic acid.[504] Similarly, increased production of NO$^{\bullet}$ is not necessarily bad; it can decrease levels of adhesion molecules, improve blood flow (by vasodilation) and inhibit lipid peroxidation, for example.

Ischaemia–reperfusion also affects the blood–brain barrier, causing increased leakiness and raising levels of adhesion molecules, attracting lymphocytes and neutrophils.[424] Reactive species can damage the barrier directly (e.g. causing swelling of astrocytes and damage to endothelial tight junctions), and by activating metalloproteinases (Section 9.16.5).

9.17.4 Traumatic injury

Traumatic injury to the brain or spinal cord involves both direct tissue damage (crushing, tearing, bruising) and secondary damage involving many of the events relevant to stroke, such as release of transition metal ions, Zn^{2+} and haemoglobin, increased $NO^\bullet$ production, protein nitration, phospholipase and calpain activation, release of fatty acids and rises in glutamate.[432] For example, damage to the rat spinal cord caused extracellular iron release accompanied by $OH^\bullet$ formation, as detected by salicylate hydroxylation (Section 5.3.1).[505] Blood vessels ruptured by the trauma leak blood, and the parts of the brain they normally feed will become hypoxic. Bleeding and oedema (due both to cell swelling resulting from abnormal ionic composition and to fluid leakage) raise intracranial pressure and further decrease blood flow. The vasospasm that can occur several days after intracranial bleeding seems to involve oxidative damage, e.g. by $OH^\bullet$ production[506] and by end-products of lipid peroxidation such as IPs. For example, F_2-IP levels were higher in the CSF of patients with subarachonoid haemorrhage who suffered vasospasm that in these who did not.[507] Binding of $NO^\bullet$ by haemoglobin is also involved. During the first 5 days after an intracranial bleed, the erythrocytes in the CSF slowly haemolyse and glial cells gather at the site to take up the iron and eventually store it as ferritin or haemosiderin. Much haemoglobin is converted to bilirubin by HO but part undergoes non-enzymic oxidation and degradation.[487] Injury or ischaemia increase HO-1 levels, especially in glia. HO-2, constitutively expressed in brain, also plays a role.[508]

Is HO good or bad? Degradation of haem removes one potential pro-oxidant but causes release of another, iron ions. Transgenic mice overexpressing HO-1 were less sensitive to ischaemic brain injury, apparently due to increased ferritin synthesis secondary to the increased HO.[508] Bilirubin produced by haem degradation might have some antioxidant activities, but its degradation can produce vasoconstricting compounds (Section 3.18.1). By contrast, when haemoglobin was injected into the striatum of mice, *less* oxidative damage was seen if the mice lacked HO-2.[509] The usual redox balance!

Soon after trauma, inflammatory/immune responses begin, involving cytokines, activation of transcription factors (e.g. NF-κB), activation of microglia, and recruitment of circulating phagocytes. Traumatic injury can directly damage the blood–brain barrier, allowing entry into the brain of agents that do not normally cross. The inflammatory-immune response after injury may be good, bad or, more likely, both (as in the case of stroke).

Many agents tested for the treatment of stroke have also been examined in models of traumatic injury. For example, PEG-CuZnSOD appears to be beneficial when administered to rats after percussive brain injury. It probably enters the brain only because the blood–brain barrier is damaged. Indeed, increasing EC-SOD levels decreased the severity of vasospasm in a rabbit model of subarachnoid haemorrhage.[510]

9.18 Oxidative stress and neurodegenerative diseases: some general concepts[422,426,437,511–514]

The various **neurodegenerative diseases** (diseases in which neurons degenerate and die) have different symptoms, affect different parts of the brain, and have different causes. Before examining the most common ones individually, it is worth emphasizing what they have in common; impaired mitochondrial function, increased oxidative damage, defects in the ubiquitin–proteasome system, the presence of abnormal, aggregated proteins, changes in iron metabolism (Table 9.14) and some involvement of excitotoxicity and of

Table 9.14 Common features of the major neurodegenerative diseases

	Parkinson's disease	Alzheimer's disease	Amyotrophic lateral sclerosis	Freidreich's ataxia	Huntington's disease	Prion diseases
Mitochondrial dysfunction	Complex I ↓, αKGDH[a] ↓	Complex IV ↓ (some studies), αKGDH[a] ↓, Pyruvate dehydrogenase ↓	Complex I and IV ↓ (varying reports)	Frataxin is a mitochondrial Fe–S protein; levels of complexes I, II, III and aconitase decreased	Complexes II, III ↓, αKGDH[a], aconitase ↓	Reported in brains of scrapie-infected mice
Proteasome dysfunction	Specific genetic defects in this pathway cause inherited PD. Proteasome proteolytic activities subnormal in sporadic PD	Proteasome proteolytic activities subnormal	Proteasome activity may be decreased by aggregates of mutant SODs in FALS[a] (e.g. *Neurobiol. Dis.* **18**, 509, 2005)	No data	Aggregates (see below) include proteasome subunits and may impair proteasome function	Accumulation of ubiquitinated proteins observed in animal models and CJD brain suggestive of proteasome dysfunction[515]
Abnormal protein aggregates	Lewy body	Amyloid plaques, neurofibrillary trangles	A range of aggregates described, often containing ubiquitin, neurofilaments, dorfin[b] etc. in motor cortex and spinal motor neurons CuZnSOD is a major component of aggregates in FALS[a] caused by SOD1 mutations	Frataxin aggregates in nucleus	Aggregates containing huntingtin, ubiquitin, heat-shock proteins and proteasome subunits	Abnormal protein aggregates (Section 9.22.3)
Changes in iron metabolism	More iron in substantia nigra (Table 9.16)	Iron in plaques	Iron deposition in dying motor neurons	'Catalytic' Fe levels might be elevated due to abnormal frataxin, although this has not been shown experimentally (*J. Biol. Chem.* **280**, 6701, 2005; *Hum. Mol. Genet.* **14**, 463, 2005) Iron deposits in heart	Iron deposited in lesions (*J. Neural Trans.* **111**, 1455, 2004)	Iron levels reported as raised in affected areas (*Brain Res.* **884**, 98, 2000)
Oxidative and nitrative damage	See Section 9.19	Section 9.20	Section 9.21	Section 9.22.1	Section 9.22.2	Section 9.22.3

[a] αKGDH, α-ketoglutarate dehydrogenase; FALS familial amyotrophic lateral sclerosis; CJD Creutzfeldt–Jakob disease.

[b] Dorfin is an E3 ubiquitin ligase (*J. Biol. Chem.* **277**, 36793, 2002), also found in Lewy bodies.

inflammation. Oxidative damage is manifested as increases in lipid peroxidation end-products (e.g. HNE, F_2-IPs), DNA (and often RNA) base oxidation (usually measured as 8OHdG or 8OHG) and protein damage. The protein aggregates frequently contain proteins that are nitrated, bear carbonyl residues, have attached aldehydes such as HNE or acrolein and, sometimes, carry AGE-products (Section 9.4.4).

It seems likely that all these events constitute a vicious cycle, and any one of them could initiate neuronal cell death, rapidly recruiting the others to its evil purpose (Fig. 9.30). Thus damage to mitochondria (e.g. by neurotoxins that target them or by abnormal proteins such as mutant CuZnSODs or hyperphosphorylated tau; Sections 9.20 and 9.21 below) generates more ROS and causes oxidative damage that modifies proteins. In AD, decreases in energy production may raise β-secretase activity and cause more $A\beta$ generation (Section 9.20 below). Oxidized and nitrated proteins are usually removed

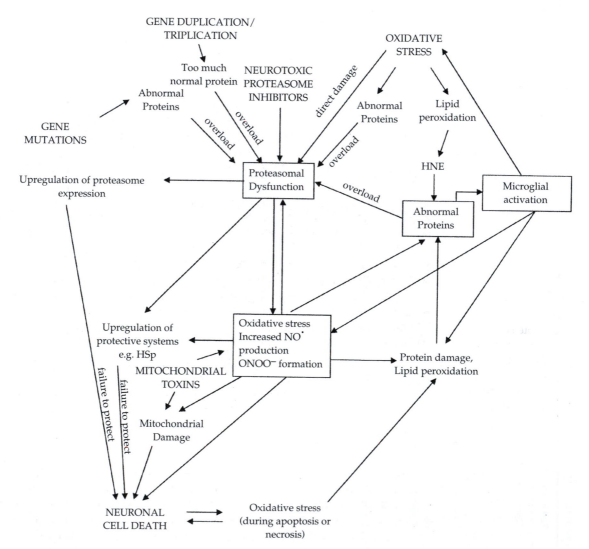

Figure 9.30 Interplay of mitochondria, oxidative damage and the proteasome in neurodegeneration. Low-level proteasome inhibition can cause transient neuroprotection (e.g. by induction of heat-shock proteins, Hsp).[511]

Table 9.15 Processes generating abnormal proteins in neurodegenerative diseases

---

Overexpression of a normal gene, causing too much normal protein to accumulate (e.g. triplication of the synuclein gene in some rare familial cases of PD)

Gene mutations, producing an abnormal protein

Aberrant splicing of mRNA, producing an abnormal protein

Faulty post-translational modification, producing an abnormal protein

Oxidation of amino acid residues by reactive oxygen species

Nitration and/or oxidation of amino acid residues by reactive nitrogen species

Halogenation and/or oxidation of amino acid residues by reactive chlorine or bromine species

Glycation/glycoxidation

Spontaneous deamination or deamidation

Modification by end-products of lipid peroxidation such as HNE, other aldehydes and isoketals

Modification by end-products of the eicosanoid pathway, e.g. cyclopentenone prostaglandins, levuglandins

Modification by quinones or semiquinones produced by oxidation of neurotransmitters or their precursors (L-DOPA, dopamine, serotonin, noradrenalin)

---

by the proteasome (Section 4.14.2). Inhibition of the proteasome allows abnormal proteins to accumulate and produces oxidative stress; exactly how is unclear—potential mechanisms include increased mitochondrial ROS production[516] or rises in nNOS producing[511] more NO•. Abnormal proteins resulting from gene mutations could overload the proteasome (Table 9.15); its activity tends to decrease with age in the brain (Section 10.4.5), making neurons more vulnerable in older people. Protein aggregates may stimulate RS formation, for example by activating microglia. Finally, RS-producing agents could initiate neurodegeneration, since RS damage mitochondria, cause rises in Ca^{2+}, and may inhibit proteasome function directly (e.g. by oxidative or nitrative inactivation of proteasome subunits) or indirectly (e.g. by interfering with ubiquitination, or overloading the proteasome by creating more oxidatively modified proteins). In particular, HNE and isoketals (Section 4.12.3) can inactivate proteasome hydrolytic activities, and proteins modified by these agents are poor substrates for the proteasome and 'clog it up'.

Where does iron fit into the story? A common view (e.g. for PD and ALS) is that its deposition is a late stage in tissue injury, with the implication that it is unimportant. However, the pathology of subarachnoid haemorrhage and caeruloplasmin deficiency in humans clearly shows the potential of haem and/or iron to cause neuronal damage (Section 9.17.3). So does that of mice lacking IRP2

(Section 3.15.1.5). A (rare) inborn error in the gene encoding ferritin L-chains is associated with abundant iron deposition in the basal ganglia accompanied by neurodegeneration.[437] Similarly, a juvenile-onset autosomal recessive severe movement disorder known as **Hallevorden–Spatz syndrome** is associated with iron deposition in the globus pallidus and substantia nigra. The defective gene encodes **pantothenate kinase**, an enzyme involved in the biosynthesis of coenzyme A. The faulty enzyme leads to cysteine accumulation, and it has been hypothesized that a pro-oxidant mixture of iron and cysteine (Section 2.5.5) contributes to neurodegeneration.[517] The iron content of most brain areas increases with age, and iron, copper and other metals promote the aggregation of several proteins including α-synucleins (Section 9.19 below) and β-amyloid (Section 9.20 below). Iron chelation could protect against the neurotoxicity of a proteasome inhibitor (Section 9.19.3 below).

How do neurons die in these various diseases? Sometimes largely by necrosis, for example in excitotoxicity. Sometimes probably by apoptosis. As more studies are done, however, the role of 'intermediate' types of cell death, with features of both, is becoming more prominent. Some studies suggest that in mature neurons one action of oxidative stress (at a certain level) is to upregulate expression of genes encoding cell cycle proteins, as if the neuron were about to enter the cell cycle. Most neurons cannot divide, however, and apoptosis results.[518] This cell cycle activation seems to be associated with a response to elevated levels of DNA damage.[474,518]

There is intense debate about whether inclusion bodies or other protein aggregates (Table 9.14) are toxic to neurons. In general, it may be the early stages of aggregate formation (e.g. of huntingtin or β-amyloid) that are toxic rather than the final insoluble complexes; in fact, formation of the latter may be beneficial if it helps convert toxic oligomers to an insoluble form.[519] Some cells handle aggregated proteins by using microtubules to move them all to a single site in the cell, the **aggresome**, which can then be dealt with by uptake into lysosomes. This mechanism seems to fail in the neurodegenerative diseases.

9.19 Parkinson's disease[514,520]

Parkinson's disease (PD) was first described in 1817, by the English physician James Parkinson, as the 'shaking palsy', but his essay on the topic was ignored for almost half a century and it was not until the 1900s that the disease was named after him. The disease usually appears in middle to old age (rarely before 50), often as a rhythmic tremor in a foot or hand, especially when the limb is at rest. As the disease develops, patients have increasing problems in controlling movement. Movement is slow (**bradykinesia**), tremor becomes more prominent, initiation of movement is difficult (**akinesia**) and there is muscle rigidity. The disease is slowly progressive and can be detected in up to 5% of people aged over 85. Parkinson's disease is the most common movement disorder and second most common neurodegenerative disease, after Alzheimer's disease (AD).

Parkinson's disease destroys neurons in the **substantia nigra (SN) pars compacta** (Fig. 9.26) in the upper part of the brainstem; the word 'nigra' reflects the fact that these neurons are rich in granules containing the black pigment **neuromelanin**.[521] Cells also die in another part of the brain in PD, the **locus coeruleus**, leading to lowered noradrenalin levels. Neuromelanin arises from dopamine oxidation to quinones and semiquinones, followed by cross-linking. Like other melanins,

neuromelanin is redox-active and binds metal ions. It contains residues derived from cysteinyl dopamine and appears to be a 'mixed-type melanin', containing some cysteine sulphurs (unlike eumelanins), but not as much as in phaeomelanins (Section 3.18.9). About 20% of neuromelanin granule content is lipid, mostly **dolichol**.[522]

Parkinson's disease is associated with the appearance of **Lewy bodies** in the residual neurons in the SN and several other brain regions. Lewy bodies are electron-dense inclusion bodies, with an especially dense core from which filaments radiate. They are found in about 10% of 'normal' persons above the age of 60, in another disorder, **dementia with Lewy bodies**, and in about 15% of AD patients. Hence they are not specific to PD. A major constituent of Lewy bodies is **α-synuclein**, a protein of unknown function abundant in presynaptic nerve terminals throughout the brain. Other proteins present include ubiquitin and neurofilaments. Synuclein and/or other proteins in Lewy bodies are oxidized, nitrated and contain HNE. α-Synuclein has four tyrosine residues and is rapidly nitrated by $ONOO^-$; indeed, nitration might be one factor that facilitates its aggregation,[512] although some studies suggest that nitration might be antiaggregatory. Remember that $ONOO^-$ does many things to proteins other than nitration (Section 2.6.1), which might help explain variable results.

9.19.1 Genetics or environment?

Almost all cases of PD are **sporadic**, that is they appear without obvious genetic cause. However, identification of rare inherited variants (at least eight types to date) has given insight into disease pathology. For example, in 1997 two groups of patients with autosomal dominant PD were found to have mutations in α-synuclein, an observation that led to the discovery of this protein in the Lewy body. These mutant α-synucleins have a much greater tendency to polymerize and aggregate than wild-type synuclein.

Some of the rare juvenile (appearing before age 20) or early onset (before age 40–50) PD cases are caused by recessive mutations in **parkin**, an enzyme involved in ubiquitination, and found in Lewy bodies. Parkin is an E3 ligase (Fig. 9.31)

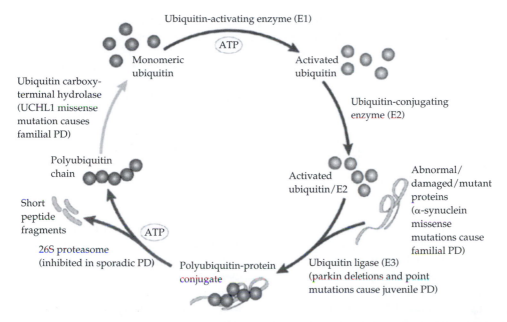

Figure 9.31 (see plate 17) Defects in the ubiquitin–proteasome system in Parkinson's disease. Blue section shows the normal ATP-dependent identification and labelling of unwanted proteins with ubiquitin molecules (ubiquitination) as a signal for ATP-dependent degradation by the 26S proteasome complex (proteolysis; red section). Green section shows recovery and recycling of ubiquitin molecules that are released from proteins. Also depicted are ways in which potential defects in the system cause PD. The UCHL1 enzyme, one of the most abundant proteins in brain (up to 2% of total brain protein) releases free ubiquitin and allows the cycle to continue.[514] A variety of deletion and point mutations in the parkin gene can lead to PD. From *Nature Rev. Neurosci.* **2**, 589, 2001 by courtesy of Prof. Peter Jenner and *Nature* publishers.

whose substrates include α/β tubulin, glycosylated α-synuclein, and a range of other proteins. If parkin is defective one might guess that its substrates would accumulate and contribute to protein aggregation and neurotoxicity. Surprisingly, patients with parkin defects sometimes do not show Lewy bodies. Nevertheless, further attention was drawn to the ubiquitin–proteasome system by the discovery of PD-causing mutations in the gene encoding **ubiquitin carboxy-terminal hydrolase L1, UCHL1** (Fig. 9.31, Plate 17). These mutations interfere with normal protein turnover. However, it was soon discovered that both UCHL1[523] and proteasome activities in the SN are low even in sporadic PD. Levels of the α-subunits and the PA700 proteasome activator are both decreased in SN.[524]

9.19.2 Treatment

As Fig. 9.26c shows, the substantia nigra sends nerve fibres to the **striatum** (meaning 'striped'); the terminals of these fibres secrete dopamine as a neurotransmitter. Striatal neurons relay the message to the cortex, helping to control movement. The progressive death of nigral cells mean that less dopamine is available. Hence PD patients benefit from therapy with L-DOPA. Dopamine cannot cross the blood–brain barrier, but L-DOPA can and is decarboxylated to dopamine in the brain. It is administered together with an inhibitor of DOPA decarboxylase that does not cross the blood–brain barrier (e.g. **benserazide, carbidopa**) so that it is only decarboxylated in the CNS. The combination of L-DOPA and carbidopa is called **Sinemet®; Madopar®** is L-DOPA plus benserazide. Another treatment (still experimental) is to graft dopamine-producing cells into the brain.

Treatment with L-DOPA can produce distressing side-effects and its efficacy diminishes with time. Dopamine can oxidize *in vivo* (Section 9.19.4 below) and metabolism of excess dopamine by MAO might produce damaging levels of H_2O_2 and

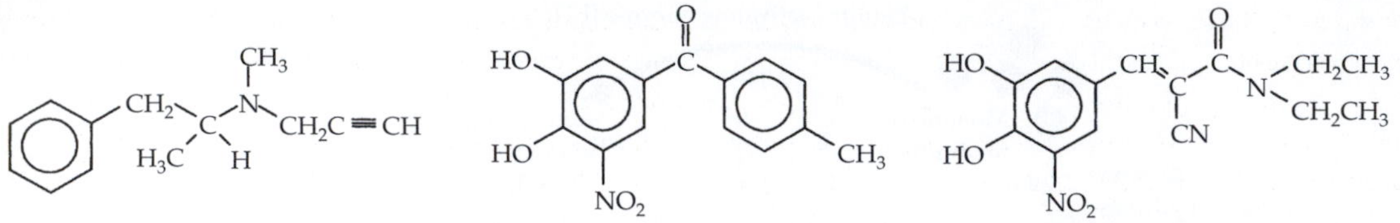

Figure 9.32 The structures of deprenyl (selegiline), tolcapone and entecapone. Deprenyl has no direct antioxidant ability whereas tolcapone and entecapone are catechols and thus capable of scavenging ROS and binding metal ions. However, their semiquinone/ quinone oxidation products could conceivably be toxic (*Chem. Res. Tox.* **16**, 123, 2003).

contribute to further neuronal death, although the evidence for this *in vivo* is equivocal.[525,526] Several alternative or additional therapies exist. One is to block dopamine metabolism, for example by inhibiting its methylation using inhibitors of catechol-*O*-methyltransferase (COMT) such as **entecapone** or **tolcapone**, or by inhibiting MAO. Thus selegiline (**deprenyl**) is an inhibitor of MAO-B, which should both preserve dopamine and decrease H_2O_2 production. L-Deprenyl (Fig. 9.32) is rapidly metabolized to (−)methamphetamine. Prolonged administration of deprenyl to animals has been reported to increase levels of CuZnSOD in the SN and, to a lesser extent, in other brain areas. Hence it could be neuroprotective by mechanisms additional to MAO-B inhibition.[527] Consistent with this, L-deprenyl has been reported to protect neurons against damage by several toxins and to raise neuronal GSH levels. Its metabolite **desmethylselegiline** is also neuroprotective *in vitro* even though it is only a weak inhibitor of MAO-B.[527] Some COMT inhibitors have antioxidant properties *in vitro*, as can be predicted from their phenolic structures (Fig. 9.32). Whether these properties are important *in vivo* is uncertain. Yet another therapeutic approach is to use agents that directly stimulate dopamine receptors, such as **bromocriptine, pramipexole, ropinirole** and **pergolide**. Some of these have been suggested to act additionally by raising neuronal antioxidant defences.[528,529]

9.19.3 Toxins and PD

One important clue about possible causes of sporadic PD came from studies of drug abusers. In 1982, clinicians at hospitals in California were surprised by a sudden influx of young patients with severe parkinsonian symptoms. They were found to have used 'synthetic heroin' from a drug pusher, but sadly it was contaminated with **1-methyl-4-phenyl-1,2,3,6-tetrahydropyridine (MPTP)**.[530] A report published in 1979 was then unearthed describing a 23-year-old graduate student who developed PD after trying to synthesize the drug Demerol, which became contaminated with MPTP as a by-product of the synthesis. Ironically, MPTP had been synthesized, tested (and fortunately discarded!) as an *anti*-PD drug by a major pharmaceutical company in the late 1950s.

Unfortunately, MPTP can cross the human blood–brain barrier and be oxidized by MAO-B, which is largely located in glial mitochondria. Oxidation of MPTP in astrocytes produces $MPDP^+$, which then forms MPP^+ (Fig. 9.33). This is recognized by the dopamine transporter **DAT**, and so MPP^+ released by glia is taken up by SN neurons, a process that may be accelerated by MPP^+ binding to neuromelanin after uptake. Neurons in the SN are killed, producing dopamine depletion, a rapid onset of parkinsonian symptoms and formation of inclusion bodies containing α-synuclein. How are neurons killed? α-Synuclein plays a role; mice lacking it develop normally, but are less sensitive to MPTP. Primarily, however, MPP^+ accumulates in mitochondria and is a powerful inhibitor of mitochondrial complex I (NADH dehydrogenase); neuronal cell death can result from interference with ATP production.[514] Secondary consequences include rises in ROS production from the electron transport chain, and

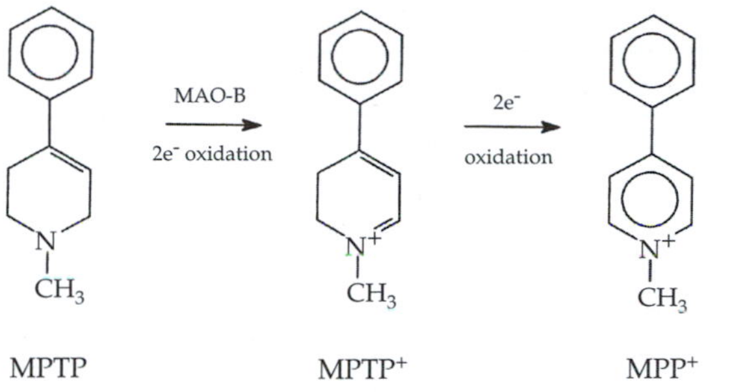

Figure 9.33 MPTP metabolism. It is oxidized to MPDP$^+$ (1-methyl-4-phenyl-2,3-dihydropyridine ion) which forms MPP$^+$, the 1-methyl-4-phenylpyridinium ion. Inhibitors of monamine oxidase, such as pargyline or deprenyl, diminish damage by MPTP. How MPDP$^+$ is converted into MPP$^+$ is not completely clear. Mitochondrial ubiquinone might oxidize it, simultaneously forming ubiquinol (*FEBS Lett.* **461**, 196, 1999).

elevations of Ca^{2+} leading to increased production of NO$^\bullet$ and ONOO$^-$; MPTP-treated mice show elevated brain nitrotyrosine levels.[531] Glial activation associated with neuronal death may also contribute to NO$^\bullet$ and other ROS production, and a role for MPO in nitration has been suggested (Table 9.16). Indeed, nNOS inhibitors, or knockouts of MPO or nNOS, decrease MPTP neurotoxicity in animals. Mice overexpressing MnSOD or CuZnSOD are also less sensitive to MPTP. Iron accumulation, and elevations in COX-2, can also be involved in MPP$^+$-induced cell death. For example, when MPP$^+$ was added to cultured cerebellar granule cells, ROS were produced. This led to aconitase inactivation, which in turn triggered production of more transferrin receptors (Section 3.16.1.5) that raised cellular iron content.[532]

There is some resemblance between MPTP (Fig. 9.33), paraquat (Section 8.4) and several other industrial chemicals. This raised the possibility that PD is caused by toxin(s) in the environment, and several (inconclusive) epidemiological studies attempted to link PD incidence to pesticide exposure, drinking well water or living in rural areas.[533] In addition some (but not all) animal studies suggest that chronic exposure of animals to paraquat by i.p. injection can cause selective degeneration of the SN accompanied by oxidative damage and protein nitration,[534] although paraquat is a poor complex I inhibitor. Paraquat enters the brain (at least in rats) using a 'neutral' amino acid transporter in the blood–brain barrier that normally carries L-valine and L-phenylalanine. Thus, preadministration of these amino acids could protect against the effects of paraquat.[535] Paraquat's effects in causing neurodegeneration and oxidative damage may be aggravated if it is coadministered with other toxins, such as the fungicide **maneb**.[536]

However, PD is found throughout the world, suggesting that if a single toxin is responsible, it must be present universally. It seems more likely to the authors that several toxins can damage SN and predispose to PD in later life. One is hexane, an organic solvent used in adhesives, varnishes and fuels. Hexane is metabolized to produce hexanol, hexanone, hexanediols and **2,5-hexanedione**, a neurotoxin.[537] Another is a toxin found in the **yellow star thistle**, consumption of which can cause a PD-like syndrome in horses.[538] Yet others include **deguelin** and **annonacin**, complex I inhibitors found in certain plants.[539,540] Indeed, complex I inhibitors (including rotenone) may be (worryingly!) common in nature. Injection of the proteasome inhibitor lactacystin into mouse or rat SN can produce neurodegeneration, movement disorders and protein aggregates.[541] Desferrioxamine gave some protection, suggesting an involvement of iron.[541] Proteasome inhibitors occur naturally and, if some could enter the brain after consumption in the diet, PD might result. In addition, investigators have tried to identify compounds, formed endogenously in the brain, that might mimic the action of MPTP. One such group is the **tetrahydroisoquinolines** (e.g. **N-methyl-(R)Salsolinol**[542]) formed from L-DOPA, another is the **tetrahydro-β-carbolines**.[514,543] Both can produce parkinsonian symptoms in animals after long-term treatment and both are found at low levels in certain foods (e.g. cheese, chocolate powder and wine; also see Section 8.8.1.4). Their importance is unclear.

Ironically, despite its many deleterious effects (Section 8.12), tobacco usage lessens the risk of developing PD (even when corrections are made for earlier death in smokers). Preferred explanations include raising brain GSH levels, an effect of nicotine in stimulating dopamine release by dopamine neurons, and chemicals in tobacco that

Table 9.16 Evidence consistent with oxidative stress in Parkinson's disease

Observation	Comments
Direct evidence (measurement of increased oxidative damage or other biomarkers of RS production)	
Increased lipid peroxidation	Measured in SN as HNE-protein adducts in Lewy bodies, and increased peroxides (by HPLC/chemiluminescence assays), also rises in isofurans (see paragraph below). No changes in SN α-tocopherol levels reported or any beneficial effect of administering α-tocopherol in PD.
Increased oxidative DNA damage	Rises in 8OHdG reported in mitochondrial and 'total DNA'; little or no rise in other DNA base oxidation or deamination products, suggesting rise is not due to OH$^\bullet$ or ONOO$^-$ attack on DNA. Levels of FapyGuanine decreased and total damage to guanine unchanged in SN suggestive of a change to a more oxidizing environment (Section 4.10). This is also suggested by a rise in isofurans but not F$_2$-isoprostanes (*J. Neurochem.* **85**, 645, 2003) (Section 5.14.6). Could there be a local rise in O$_2$ due to defective mitochondrial function? Increased oxidative damage to RNA also reported, and an increase in 8OHdGTPase (Section 4.10.2) in the mitochondria of SN neurons.
Increased protein damage	Rises in protein carbonyls observed in SN but also in several other brain regions, including those unaffected in PD. Possibly related to the presence of Lewy bodies in several brain areas. SOD1 is reported to be oxidized in PD brain (carbonyls, −SH group oxidation), but not present in Lewy bodies (*J. Biol. Chem.* **280**, 11648, 2005). Damage to complex I proteins may be oxidative (*J. Neurosci* **26**, 5256, 2006).
Increased nitrotyrosine	Lewy bodies in SN stain with antibodies against nitrotyrosine. This could be due to ONOO$^-$ and/or to MPO, since MPO is detected in human PD brain and in the brains of mice treated with MPTP, and knockout of MPO decreases MPTP toxicity to mice (*J. Neurosci.* **25**, 6594, 2005).
Increased levels of dopamine oxidation products	Levels of cysteinyl–DOPA and –dopamine increased in SN (*J. Neurochem.* **71**, 2112, 1998).
Indirect evidence (evidence suggestive of effects of, or response to, oxidative stress)	
Fall in GSH, no marked rise in GSSG	GSH decreases about 40% in SN, not in other brain regions.
Increased iron content	SN zona compacta (but not other brain regions) has higher iron levels in PD, apparently with unaltered ferritin. Uncertain whether this extra iron is 'catalytic' for free radical reactions. No increase in Cu or Mn detected but Zn may increase. Source of excess Fe unknown but increased expression of receptors for lactoferrin has been reported on neurons and microvessels in SN. Lactoferrin may also be made by activated microglia (*Mol. Brain Res.* **96**, 103, 2001).
Changes in SOD	Total SOD activity elevated but unclear if CuZnSOD, MnSOD or both rise. Oddly, levels of mRNA for CuZnSOD reported to *fall* (*Brain Res.* **968**, 206, 2003). Some SOD1 may be oxidized and inactivated (see above).
Changes in enzymes of GSH metabolism	Small decreases in catalase and GPx reported in SN and other brain regions by some (not all) researchers. Levels of mRNA for GPx1 reported as subnormal (*Brain Res.* **968**, 206, 2003). γ-Glutamyl transpeptidase (involved in degradation and recycling of GSH) elevated. No marked changes in glutathione reductase or γ-glutamylcysteine synthetase (the rate-limiting enzyme in GSH synthesis).
Other evidence consistent with the concept	
Defects in mitochondrial function	Decreased complex I activity in SN, also in some peripheral tissues (e.g. in platelets and skeletal muscle). Coenzyme Q$_{10}$ levels reported as decreased in platelet mitochondria in PD.
Increased glycoxidation	Formation of AGE requires both glycation and oxidation.
More haem oxygenase I	Occurs in neurons (associated with Lewy bodies) and astrocytes. Could be triggered by several stress mechanisms.
Activation of NF-κB	Could be explained by oxidative stress.
More COX-2	Found in Parkinsonian SN and MPTP-treated mice. COX-2 suggested to participate in dopamine oxidation (*Proc. Natl. Acad. Sci.* **100**, 5473, 2003).

For references see [422,426,520,524] unless cited in the text.

AGE, advanced glycation end-products; SN, substantia nigra.

inhibit MAO, but none is supported by strong evidence as yet.[543,544]

9.19.4 Oxidative stress and mitochondrial defects in PD[422,426,520,524,545]

Comparison of brain tissue from patients who died with PD with normal control tissue reveals increased oxidative damage and defective mitochondrial function (Table 9.16). Decreases in complex I activity have been found in the SN (probably in both neurons and glia) but not in other brain regions. Since the decreases are specific to complex I (activities of the other mitochondrial electron-transport complexes seem unaltered), they are unlikely to be related to cell death, gliosis or loss of mitochondria, and may involve oxidative damage to complex I (Table 9.16).

Mutations in mitochondrial DNA (mtDNA) cause several diseases that affect the basal ganglia, including Leigh disease, Leber's disease with dystonia and MELAS (Section 1.10.5). Although there is little evidence that PD involves mtDNA mutations, these observations do show how mitochondrial dysfunction could lead to neurodegeneration. Damaged mitochondria may generate more ROS than usual, and ROS can further inhibit complex I. Hence it is possible that oxidative stress and mitochondrial defects contribute to a 'vicious cycle' in PD (Fig. 9.30). Some studies suggest that high-dose coenzyme Q has modest clinical benefit in PD, perhaps by protecting mitochondria.[545] Falls in ATP could interfere with ubiquitination and proteasome function (Fig. 9.31), further impairing this system. Another contributor to neuronal cell death could be production of $O_2^{\bullet-}$, $NO^{\bullet}$ and cytokines by activated glial cells in the SN, although its overall importance is unclear.[546] Nevertheless, protein nitration is observed in Lewy bodies. Activation of microglia might sometimes be provoked by neuromelanin released by dying neurons.[521]

Dopamine and L-DOPA can oxidize *in vitro* to generate semiquinones, quinones, $O_2^{\bullet-}$, and H_2O_2, a process facilitated by transition-metal ions. Does this happen *in vivo*? Probably; levels of products formed by conjugation of these quinones and semiquinones with GSH followed by cleavage of the glutathione side-chain, are elevated in SN in PD (Table 9.16). Dopamine oxidation by MAO produces not only H_2O_2 but also dihydroxyphenylacetaldehyde, which is potentially neurotoxic if not rapidly metabolized.[547] The effects of 6-hydroxydopamine (Section 8.6.7), show the potential of oxidation to cause neuronal death. Damage by 6-hydroxydopamine is potentiated by iron injection or depletion of GSH (e.g. by intracerebral administration of buthionine sulphoximine) and decreased to some extent by pretreating animals with α-tocopherol or desferrioxamine. 6-Hydroxydopamine-induced lesions in the rat striatum show increased iron levels, and 6-hydroxydopamine has also been reported to inhibit mitochondrial complex I.[514] Indeed, in PD, where most of the dopaminergic neurons have been lost, a rise in dopamine turnover in the remaining cells would be expected in the face of decreased GSH (Table 9.16).

9.19.4.1 *Early or late?*

One important question is whether the changes in mitochondria and oxidative damage in PD occur early in neurodegeneration and contribute to it, are a consequence of neurodegeneration, or an effect of treatment (patients who die with PD will often have taken L-DOPA for years). Another point to consider when pondering the data in Table 9.16 is that one is comparing a healthy SN with SN in which >80% of the neurons have died and been replaced by other cell types, including microglia.

One way of attempting to distinguish cause from consequence is to perform animal experiments. For example, injection of buthionine sulphoximine into the brains of rats decreased GSH levels by up to 70% but did not alter SOD levels or mitochondrial complex I activity, nor did it cause nigrostriatal degeneration.[524] However, these were short-term experiments. Mice lacking a neuronal cysteine transporter had decreased brain GSH levels and developed behavioural abnormalities and brain atrophy, but only when 11 months of age or older. The atrophy was accompanied by increased levels of HNE and 3-nitrotyrosine.[548]

6-Hydroxydopamine and MPTP have provided valuable (although imperfect) tools for understanding PD. Rodents have high levels of MAO-B in the blood–brain barrier and thus are far less sensitive than primates to systemically administered

MPTP (it is oxidized in the barrier to MPP^+, which cannot cross into the brain), but MPP^+ or MPTP can be injected directly into their brains to cause damage to the SN. Alternatively, primates can be studied; treatment of monkeys with MPTP led to iron deposition in the substantia nigra (as a late event) but acute treatment did not decrease GSH or complex I activity. Genetic studies have also given valuable insights. Overexpression, in the nigrostriatal areas of rats or monkeys, of the mutant synucleins associated with some cases of familial PD causes neurodegeneration and formation of synuclein-containing inclusions.[549] Overexpression of the wild-type gene had the same effect; indeed triplication of the gene encoding α-synuclein (resulting from a chromosome abnormality) is a rare cause of familial PD. Hence too much normal α-synuclein, and any of the mutant α-synucleins, is bad. Cells transfected with mutant α-synucleins are more sensitive to apoptosis induced by a range of toxins, including H_2O_2, iron and HNE, and show increased levels of oxidative damage and protein aggregate formation. Cell data on the effects of overexpression of normal α-synuclein are conflicting: in some studies it protected the cells against toxins, but in others it did not.[550] There is variation between different cell lines, and probably also with the degree of overexpression achieved: high level overexpression of any protein might disturb neuronal metabolism (Fig. 9.30).

Another approach to distinguish cause from consequence in PD is based on the observation that abnormal numbers of Lewy bodies and some neurodegeneration are occasionally present in the SN of subjects who died with no observable PD symptoms (Table 9.17). Some neurologists propose that these individuals were in the presymptomatic stages of PD (and thus would not have been treated with L-DOPA). Others dispute this; it is impossible to be sure because this so-called **incidental Lewy body disease** (ILBD) is only diagnosed postmortem, so one cannot follow up the subjects to see if PD develops later. However, if one accepts the former interpretation, one can ask which parameters of damage are still detected.[524] The answers (Table 9.17) suggest that GSH depletion is an early event in PD development and could facilitate slow neurodegeneration,[548] whereas iron accumulation may occur later. A later accumulation of iron does not necessary equate to its unimportance, e.g. mice overexpressing ferritin L-chains in the SN showed less damage after MPTP treatment.[551]

Other data have been obtained with complex I inhibitors. Let us consider them now.

9.19.5 What does it all mean?

In some studies, treatment of rats or monkeys with low-dose rotenone over long periods produces PD-like symptoms and neurodegeneration accompanied by oxidative damage, nitrotyrosine formation, and generation of inclusion bodies containing α-synuclein.[552] Unlike MPP^+, rotenone does not concentrate in dopamine neurons, yet it can still induce fairly selective damage to the SN, killing some cells and impairing dopamine release from others.[552] It follows that SN neurons may be especially sensitive to complex I inhibition, so that any toxin affecting complex I might cause PD-like neurodegeneration. Such toxins may be widespread in

Table 9.17 Oxidative stress in substantia nigra of 'incidental Lewy body' cases: a comparison with overt Parkinson's disease[524]

Parameter	Comments
Features shared by ILBD and PD Decreased GSH, no rise in GSSG. Increased level of Bcl-2.	~40–50% fall in GSH for both. Suggests fall is not due to L-DOPA treatment or gliosis. Bcl-2 rise is perhaps a response to stress?
Changes observed in PD but not in ILBD Decreased mitochondrial complex I (but *trend* to lower values in ILBD), increased iron or zinc levels, changes in ferritin, raised protein carbonyls.	Could be that small rises are difficult to detect, but implication is that these events are later stages in the disease pathology.

Abbreviations: ILBD, incidental Lewy body decrease.

the environment; even rotenone in some places.[553] However, the ILBD data (Table 9.17) question an early role for complex I defects. Perhaps they are misleading us. Indeed, another clue pointing to a key role for mitochondria is provided by the observation that early-onset PD can be caused by mutations in the nuclear gene encoding a mitochondrial protein, **PINK1**, a protein kinase that is somehow able to protect cells against apoptosis induced by proteasome inhibition.[520]

However, PD need not always start with mitochondrial defects. The studies with 6-hydroxydopamine show that oxidative stress can cause neurodegeneration. Dopamine oxidation products (which are known to accumulate in PD) can both damage mitochondria and inactivate the proteasome. The effects of mutations in the ubiquitin–proteasome system, together with the finding that UCHL1 activities are decreased even in sporadic PD,[523] suggest that all the events shown in Fig. 9.30 are important. Indeed, this fall in UCHL1 activity involves oxidative damage, since the protein shows elevated levels of carbonyls and methionine sulphoxide.[523] Mice lacking UCHL1 (the *GAD mouse*) show widespread neurodegeneration, formation of protein aggregates and increased oxidative damage.[554] Decreases in complex I activity may also involve oxidative damage.

Another clue comes from the **DJ-1 protein**– several mutations in the gene encoding this cause autosomal recessive PD. It has been speculated that DJ-1 may have several functions, including accelerating GSH synthesis and acting directly as an antioxidant (it has an easily oxidizable –SH residue) that translocates to mitochondria under conditions of oxidative stress.[520,555] Abnormal DJ-1 proteins may aggregate and overwhelm the proteasome (Fig 9.30). Interestingly *DJ-1* is an oncogene, and elevated expression is detected in breast, lung and prostate cancers.

9.20 Alzheimer's disease[422,556]

9.20.1 Definition and pathology

Dementia is defined by the World Health Organization as 'an acquired global impairment of higher cognitive functions, including memory, the ability to deal with daily life, the performance of sensorimotor and social functions, language communication, and control of emotional reactions, without marked reduction of consciousness'. Six percent or more of people aged 65 and above in the world suffer from dementia, and in the West most of these have **Alzheimer's disease** (AD). The incidence of AD in the USA may be as high as 30% in those aged 85 or over, but it seems less common in Singapore. In AD, several brain regions involved in learning and memory, such as the basal forebrain and hippocampus, suffer synaptic damage and eventual major neuronal loss. Full-blown AD is often preceded by **mild cognitive impairment (MCI)**, in which memory function for age is abnormally poor, but the subject is otherwise normal. Other forms of dementia include dementia with Lewy bodies, and **vascular dementia**, caused by impaired blood supply to the brain due to atherosclerosis. As we shall see (Section 9.20.3) the distinction between different types of dementia is not clear-cut. For example, vascular problems contribute to AD.

Two pathological features of AD, first reported by the German psychiatrist Alois Alzheimer in 1906, are the presence of **neurofibrillary tangles** and **senile plaques** in the brain (Fig. 9.34). Tangles are fibrous masses inside affected neurons. They consist of pairs of filaments, each about 10 nm in diameter, twisted around each other (**paired helical filaments**). They contain several proteins, the major one being **tau** (τ) phosphorylated to an abnormally high extent and with attached ubiquitin. Tau normally functions to promote correct microtubule assembly and facilitate axonal transport.

Senile plaques (sometimes called **neuritic plaques**) are extracellular localized areas of degenerating and frequently swollen axons, neurites, and glia surrounding a core of aggregated β-**amyloid peptides (Aβ)** with a β-sheet conformation. Many of the neurites contain paired helical filaments. Plaques are most common in the amygdala, hippocampus and cerebral cortex, but occur elsewhere. Also present in AD are diffuse deposits of Aβ, often called 'diffuse' or 'preamyloid' plaques, not accompanied by neurites or glia. Amyloid is additionally deposited in blood vessel walls in the AD brain. Neurofibrillary tangles and plaques are found in young adults with Down's syndrome

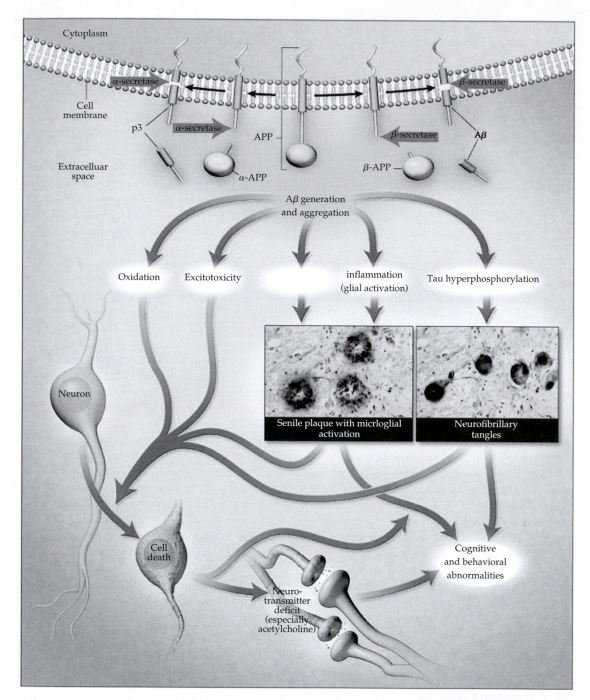

Figure 9.34 Pathogenesis of Alzheimer's disease (AD). The amyloid cascade progresses from the generation of the β-amyloid peptides (Aβ) from the amyloid precursor protein (APP), through multiple secondary steps to eventual neuronal death. The APP is made in the ER and passes through the Golgi apparatus to reach the plasma membrane, undergoing glycosylation and other modifications during its passage. At the cell surface, APP is attacked by **α-secretase**, which cleaves in the middle of the Aβ sequence, destroying that sequence and releasing soluble **APPα** into the extracellular environment. This molecule appears neuroprotective and lower levels of it in AD may facilitate neuronal damage. In healthy brain, this is the major route of APP cleavage. Uncleared APP can be recycled by endocytosis and either completely degraded or returned to the cell surface.

(Section 3.14.2) and, to a much more limited extent, in the normally ageing brain. However, in the AD brain soluble Aβ is at least five times higher than in controls, and precipitated Aβ may be 100 times higher.

β-Amyloid (Aβ) is a family of peptides produced by cleavage of larger proteins (**amyloid precursor proteins, APPs**); APPs are transmembrane proteins, present in most cells, with a short intracellular C terminus and a longer extracellular N terminus. In humans they are encoded by a gene on chromosome 21 and form a set of proteins varying from 695 to 770 amino acid residues long; APP695 is abundant in neurons. They are secreted by many cell types and several functions have been ascribed to them; in neurons, they may facilitate survival and growth during brain development, as well as neuronal responses to excitatory neurotransmitters. The normal turnover of APP involves proteolytic processing (by **α-secretase**) to release the N-terminal sequence and leave a fragment in the membrane. By contrast, release of Aβ involves **γ-** and **β-secretase** enzymes (Fig. 9.34). Cholesterol is intimately involved in APP cleavage. Indeed, inhibiting cholesterol synthesis using statins seems to decrease the risk of AD, perhaps by lowering Aβ formation by decreasing β- and γ-secretase action.[557] The brain is rich in unesterified cholesterol, almost all of which is synthesized there. Myelin contains most of the cholesterol; much of the rest is present in the plasma membranes of glia and neurons. Cholesterol level is maintained constant in the brain by a balance of synthesis and turnover. The latter involves CYP46A1 converting cholesterol to **24(S)-hydroxycholesterol**, which exits through the blood–brain barrier and is cleared by the liver.

The Aβ peptides can be 39 to 43 amino acids long, depending on where APP is cleaved; $A\beta_{1-40}$ is the commonest. Aβ-Peptides made in the laboratory are initially soluble in water and non-toxic to neurons. They become toxic on incubation, a process related to their aggregation, which probably involves traces of transition metal ions in laboratory reagents and cell culture media (Section 9.20.3 below). As well as Aβ, senile plaques contain many other proteins. They include $α_1$-antichymotrypsin, ubiquitin, acetylcholinesterase, proteoglycans and serum amyloid P. Of special interest there is **apolipoprotein E** (Section 9.3.2). In brain, apoE is made by astrocytes (little comes from plasma) and synthesis increases after traumatic injury and in several neurodegenerative diseases. It may play a key role in brain lipid metabolism and appears essential for neuronal and glial development.

9.20.2 Genetics of AD[556]

Genetics strongly influences the chance of developing AD. Other risk factors are also important, and may synergize with genetic predispositions. They include a low dietary intake of folic acid,[558] low education level, high plasma cholesterol (Section 9.20.1) or homocysteine[558] and repeated minor brain trauma, an example being **dementia pugilistica** ('punch-drunk syndrome') in boxers. Experiments on mice suggest that diets rich in DHA might be protective, especially as DHA levels decrease in the AD brain.[559]

In a few cases, a particular genetic trait almost guarantees that AD will develop. Such **familial AD**, with early onset and rapid progression, can be caused by several mutations. Some are in the gene on chromosome 21 that encodes APP, in regions within or close to that encoding the Aβ sequence. Transgenic mice overexpressing one of these mutant APP proteins (APP_{695}; Lys670 → Asn; Met^{671} → Leu, a dual mutation first identified in a large Swedish family with early onset AD), seem normal at birth but by 9 to 10 months of age behavioural deficits appear and are accompanied by brain amyloid plaques. These mice have proved to be a useful model of AD. In Down's syndrome the presence of

---

β-Secretase, a membrane-bound aspartyl proteinase, cleaves APP at the N-terminus of the Aβ sequence. The truncated N-terminus is released, whereas the cell-associated C-terminus can be cleaved by **γ-secretase** to give Aβ (lengths from 39–43 amino acids), or degraded completely. The γ-secretase complex contains at least four proteins, including **presenilin**, also an aspartyl proteinase. γ-Secretase acts on several other cell proteins, which may hinder attempts to use it as a therapeutic target in AD. The APP mutants in familial AD enhance its cleavage by this pathway and stimulate Aβ formation. Modified from *N. Engl. J. Med.* **351**, 56, 2004 by courtesy of Dr J.L. Cummings and the Massachusetts Medical Society. Levels of β-secretase may increase in neurons with mitochondrial defects (*J. Neurosci.* **25**, 10874, 2005).

three copies of chromosome 21 may account for the early appearance of AD-type pathology. Early onset AD can also result from mutations in the genes encoding **presenilins** (**PS1** and **PS2**), transmembrane proteins involved in secretase action (Fig. 9.34) and cellular Ca^{2+} metabolism.

The gene encoding apoE is located on chromosome 19 and has three alleles (Section 9.3.2). The most common isoform, apoE3, is a 299 amino acid protein with one cysteine residue, at position 112. Apoprotein E2 and apoE4 differ in that the former has an extra cysteine (replacing an arginine) at 158 whereas the latter has lost the cysteine at 112, which is replaced by arginine. Since apoE4 lacks cysteine, it cannot form disulphide bonds with itself (to form homodimers) or with other proteins. Possession of the apoE4 allele is a risk factor for development of AD, perhaps because the apoE4 protein facilitates plaque formation (or microglial activation by plaques: Section 9.20.3 below) more than the other forms. It could also modulate cholesterol metabolism, which in turn affects $A\beta$ production. By contrast, the apoE2 form is negatively associated with AD.

9.20.3 Mechanisms of neurodegeneration[422,556]

Most neuroscientists believe that the $A\beta$ peptides are the culprits causing neurodegeneration. Structures formed in the early stages of $A\beta$ aggregation cause damage to synapses and are generally neurotoxic. The form with 42 amino acids, $A\beta_{1-42}$, is the worst and is the major $A\beta$ present in plaques, despite the fact that much more $A\beta_{1-40}$ is made *in vivo*. Once released, further modifications can occur to $A\beta_{1-42}$, including loss of amino acids from the N terminus, which may increase its neurotoxicity.[560] The final aggregated $A\beta$ in plaques may no longer be directly neurotoxic (i.e. plaque formation can be argued as neuroprotective because it has precipitated the toxic 'early aggregates' out of solution). However, the plaque may cause further injury by provoking an inflammatory response of microglia. Which mechanism predominates? This question is relevant in attempts to use antibodies against $A\beta$ to solubilize plaques and clear $A\beta$ in animals and humans,[561] a strategy which has given variable results. If soluble $A\beta$ is neurotoxic, the antibodies must sequester it safely or else damage will be increased. If the intact plaque is neurotoxic, the antibodies should always be beneficial. Amyloid β is also deposited in vessel walls in AD and may lead to endothelial dysfunction, for example by increasing the levels of NOX enzymes, so forming ROS that antagonize NO•, generate $ONOO^-$, interfere with the expression of genes that control normal vessel function, and aggravate dementia by impairing blood flow.[562] Indeed, endothelial function was better in APP-overexpressing mice that also overexpressed CuZnSOD.[562]

Why should 'partially-aggregated' $A\beta$ be neurotoxic? This has been variously attributed to increased intracellular free Ca^{2+} (perhaps by opening TRPM2 channels,[434] or by forming 'cation channels' by insertion of the peptides into the plasma membrane), inhibition of mitochondrial function (hyperphosphorylated tau may also damage mitochondria), aconitase inactivation, decreasing the expression of proteins essential for synaptic function, and RS generation, leading to lipid peroxidation and cholesterol oxidation. All of these are linked events, of course. Indeed, the effects of $A\beta_{1-42}$ (or the 25–35 fragment of it) on neurons in culture are prevented by many antioxidants. The $A\beta_{25-35}$ fragment aggregates and develops neurotoxicity exceptionally rapidly and is thus often used in experiments, although it is not found *in vivo*.

How can $A\beta$ lead to RS production? First, it can make RS itself. The methionine residue at position 35 is essential for ROS generation by $A\beta_{1-42}$, and copper ions promote the reaction. Bound copper interacts with met35 to oxidize it to a radical[563]

$$metS + Cu^{2+} \rightarrow Cu^+ + metS^{\bullet+}$$

and eventually to the sulphoxide. Copper can also oxidize tyrosine residues on $A\beta$, and tyrosine radicals then cross-link $A\beta$ by bityrosine formation. Mixtures of $A\beta$ and Cu^+ can cause oxidation of ascorbate, L-DOPA, dopamine or cholesterol, accompanied by H_2O_2 production and conversion of histidine in $A\beta$ to 2-oxohistidine. One of the physiological roles of APP may be to bind copper and regulate neuronal copper metabolism, since APP-knockout mice show increased copper in liver and brain.[563]Cholesterol is oxidized to **4-cholesten-3-one**, levels of which are increased in the AD brain.[564]

Second, Aβ may stimulate ROS production by brain cells. It can activate NADPH oxidase in astrocytes, producing RS that damage neurons.[565] Mitochondria may also be targets; Aβ can associate with a mitochondrial enzyme that catalyses oxidation of several alcohols and of 3-hydroxyacylcoenzyme A. What this enzyme (called **ABAD**, the **Aβ-binding alcohol dehydrogenase**) does *in vivo* is uncertain, but its levels rise in AD.[566] Coexpression of Aβ and ABAD in cells causes mitochondrial ROS production, cytotoxicity and lipid peroxidation; overexpression of ABAD in APP-transgenic mice worsened the neurological defects.[566]

So Aβ neurotoxicity *in vitro* involves oxidative stress and mitochondrial dysfunction. Is this relevant *in vivo*? Most certainly;[422,556] mitochondrial defects reported in AD include decreased activities of pyruvate and α-ketoglutarate dehydrogenases,[545] and of cytochrome oxidase, key enzymes in ATP production.[566] Mice transgenic for a mutant APP also showed lowered αKGDH. As for oxidative stress, strong evidence supports its role in AD, stronger than for any other neurodegenerative disease. Rises in 8OHdG and other DNA base oxidation products in both nuclear and mitochondrial DNA,[567] 8OHG (indicative of RNA oxidation), protein carbonyls, glutamic and aminoadipic semialdehydes (Section 5.15.3), methionine sulphoxide, nitrotyrosine, acrolein, 4-HNE, HO-1 and IPs in brain tissue have been reported, although α-tocopherol levels seem normal in the affected brain regions. Plaques and paired helical filaments contain oxidized, glycated and nitrated proteins, and CSF from AD patients was also reported to contain elevated levels of oxidized, nitrated and glycated proteins.[568] One oxidized protein associated with plaques is CuZnSOD.[569] Plaques contain copper and iron in forms capable of facilitating oxidative damage;[563,570] indeed, traces of such metals may be essential for Aβ aggregation to occur *in vivo* (as they are for aggregation *in vitro*). Thus metal chelating agents such as the drug **clioquinol** (5-chloro-7-iodo-8-hydroxyquinoline) may have therapeutic benefit,[563]

although concern has been expressed that clioquinol itself might be somewhat neurotoxic.[571] Zinc is also present in plaques; although Zn^{2+} is not redox-active, it may facilitate Aβ aggregation. Zinc ions can be released from damaged neurons (Section 9.17.2.1). However, Zn^{2+} can compete with Cu^{2+} for binding to Aβ and decrease its neurotoxicity, although a high Zn/Cu ratio is required since Aβ preferentially binds copper.

Microglial activation by plaques would increase RS and cytokine production, consistent with the presence of microglia and various complement components in plaques. Of course, microglia may not be all bad; their activation may be an attempt to remove Aβ, for example by the secretion of proteinases. Levels of iNOS, 12/15-lipoxygenase and COX-2 are all increased in AD. Is inflammation important? Regular consumption of certain NSAIDs, such as indomethacin or ibuprofen (but not aspirin), seems to decrease the chance of developing AD. Too many prostaglandins could damage neurons by forming levuglandins, for example.[572] However, NSAIDS might additionally affect APP processing and hence decrease Aβ production,[557] so be cautious in assuming that their effect is anti-inflammatory. The RAGE receptor is found on microglia, vascular endothelial cells and neurons and might contribute to activation of the first and damage to the last two, since in AD AGEd proteins occur in plaques and tangles.[566] Indeed, type 2 diabetes is a risk factor for AD; high glucose promotes AGE formation and high insulin may raise Aβ levels by interfering with its degradation.[573] In addition, hypercholesterolaemia may facilitate oxidative damage in the brain.[574] A recent paper used probes of RS to dramatically demonstrate the pro-oxidant effects of Aβ plaques in mice (Fig. 5.15).

Chlorotyrosine levels are elevated in the AD brain, and immunostaining for MPO detects this enzyme in some microglia, plaques and neurons. By contrast, MPO is low or absent in the normal brain,[575] although present in PD brain (Table 9.16). Why MPO appears in these diseases is unknown.

9.20.4 Cause or consequence?

Why do we think that oxidative damage is important in AD? First, lipid peroxidation, measured as

F_2-IPs in brain tissue or CSF, is already elevated in patients with MCI. Neuroprostane levels are also increased in the AD brain, and levels tend to rise further as dementia progresses.[576] Brain protein carbonyls and HNE levels are also elevated in MCI, and oxidative DNA and RNA damage are also.[577] By contrast, the balance of evidence suggests that plasma or urinary IP levels are not elevated in AD, i.e. the higher levels in the CNS are not reflected systemically.[576] High doses of α-tocopherol (2000 units per day) were reported to produce a significant delay in the progression of AD in humans, although, sadly, the same dose did not affect the progression of patients with MCI to AD.[578] Given that α-tocopherol enters the brain only slowly, is not efficient at decreasing lipid peroxidation in humans, and is not depleted in AD brain, its apparent effect in AD gives hope that antioxidants designed to target the brain could have a significant therapeutic impact. A small study on humans with mild probable AD suggested that a combination of α-tocopherol and vitamin C decreases CSF F_2-IPs more effectively than α-tocopherol alone.[579]

Second, the oxidative protein damage observed in AD is not random, but highly selective and affects enzymes involved in protein turnover, energy metabolism and control of excitotoxicity. Proteomics[580] has revealed that heavily oxidized proteins in affected regions of the human AD brain include UCHL1 (also oxidized in PD),[523] creatine kinase, glutamine synthetase, CuZnSOD[569] and α-enolase. In earlier studies (Section 10.4.5), 'total' protein carbonyl levels in various regions of the brain in old mice were correlated with impairment of cognitive and motor functions,[422] which is not surprising given the key metabolic roles of the above enzymes. Similarly, only certain proteins become heavily nitrated in the AD brain, including α-enolase, β-actin and triosephosphate isomerase. Remarkably, mRNA oxidation in AD is also selective; only certain mRNAs contain 8OHG and others are unaffected.[581] Even protein modification by HNE is not random: a glial glutamate uptake transporter is one of the specific proteins attacked. Another is tau; HNE inhibits dephosphorylation of the protein. These data indicate that damage by RS in AD is highly targeted, and require specific molecular mechanisms to explain them.

Third, studies on transgenic animals reveal that oxidative damage is an early and important event, for example in mice overexpressing mutant human APP, brain IP formation preceded plaque deposition[582] and inhibition of F_2-IP formation by α-tocopherol administration delayed plaque formation and cognitive impairment.[583] α-Tocopherol works better against neurodegeneration and atherosclerosis (Section 9.3.7) in transgenic mice than it does in humans, unfortunately. In mice expressing different human apoE alleles, brain levels of F_2-IPs paralleled changes in Aβ levels.[584] In *C. elegans* overexpressing Aβ$_{1-42}$, rises in protein carbonyls preceded plaque formation, whereas a modified Aβ$_{1-42}$ lacking the methionine residue did not cause carbonyl formation.[585] In mice overexpressing APP, deposition of Aβ was paralleled by rises in HNE, pentosidine, iron and HO-1 as well as inactivation of UCHL1. Finally, APP-overexpressing mice with lowered MnSOD activity showed faster plaque development.[586]

Fourth, the association of AD with high plasma homocysteine levels, and its negative association with regular exercise, are explicable by the effects of these parameters on oxidative damage (Section 10.5.11).

The proteasome is also defective in AD, showing lowered hydrolytic activities. One reason may be the presence of **UBB^{+1}**, a mutant ubiquitin carrying a 19-amino acid C-terminal extension that is found in affected neurons in AD and Down's syndrome, apparently generated by errors during transcription. This mutant ubiquitin cannot attach itself to an expanding polyubiquitin chain, and also appears to inhibit the proteasome.[587] In addition, HNE-modified and other abnormal proteins (including HNE-Aβ and hyperphosphorylated tau) in AD may clog up the proteasome.[588]

To summarize, we believe that AD arises because of accumulation of Aβ, which happens in the aged brain due to impaired clearance and possibly increased formation. Mutations increasing Aβ formation (and possibly some affecting clearance) speed up AD onset. The Aβ is neurotoxic by several mechanisms, RS formation being one of the most important. Of course, in stating this, we are neglecting the importance of tau. Another area we have not touched upon is possible defects in the various mechanisms by which Aβ is exported from the brain.

9.20.5 An old red herring: aluminium in AD

Interest in the role of aluminium arose from reports that the cores of senile plaques are enriched in aluminium and silicon. Unfortunately, this turned out to be an artefact caused by contamination of the plaques (which bind metals avidly) by aluminium in laboratory reagents.[570] Aluminium causes encephalopathy (Section 8.15.11), but not AD-type pathology, and no increased incidence of AD has been observed in workers exposed to high aluminium levels. However, feeding aluminium to APP-overexpressing mice (but not normal mice) accelerated plaque deposition and raised the levels of F_2-IPs and Aβ, effects prevented by α-tocopherol supplementation.[589] *In vitro*, aluminium can accelerate iron-dependent lipid peroxidation (Section 8.15.11) and so it has the *potential* to worsen AD if it gets into the brain.

9.20.6 Other amyloid diseases[589A]

Amyloid β deposits are found in several other conditions, including in the drusen in macular degeneration (Section 6.10.1.1),[590] and in the muscles in **sporadic inclusion body myositis**, a degenerative muscle disease seen in some old people.[591] What is called 'amyloid' is also deposited in several other diseases, including tuberculosis, syphilis, rheumatoid arthritis and multiple myeloma. In fact, the term 'amyloid' is rather non-specific, being used to refer to any tissue deposit of rigid, proteinaceous material. The name means 'starch-like', a misnomer since it is protein, not carbohydrate. Amyloids show whitish birefringence in unstained sections and a green birefringence under polarized light after staining with Congo Red. Amyloid proteins usually adopt β-pleated sheet conformations (as in AD). Several different proteins can form amyloid (including the enzyme lysozyme and certain immunoglobulins) and even oxidized LDL can form amyloid-like structures.[592] Sometimes amyloids are useful, for example a β-sheet conformation of the

protein **Pme117** forms a scaffold to aid the synthesis of melanin in melanosomes (Section 3.18.9).[593]

Amyloid deposits form when soluble proteins undergo structural changes that cause them to aggregate. Several rare, inherited types of severe amyloid deposition have been described,[594] such as **familial Mediterranean fever**, found principally in Mediterranean Jews and Armenians. This disease is eventually fatal, often because of damage to the kidneys by the amyloid deposits. Another is **familial amyloid polyneuropathy**, caused by proaggregatory mutations in the gene encoding the protein **transthyretin** (which transports thyroxine in plasma). The cytotoxicity of this and other types of amyloid may involve oxidative damage, as indicated by rises in HNE and carbonyls.[595] However, the few studies conducted to date suggest that antioxidants have little therapeutic benefit.[594,596]

9.21 Amyotrophic lateral sclerosis (ALS)[422,512,597]

Amyotrophic lateral sclerosis is a degeneration of motor neurons in the motor cortex, brainstem and spinal cord. Motor neuron dysfunction is accompanied by neurofilament abnormalities and ubiquitin-positive inclusion bodies (Table 9.14); neuronal death accompanied by glial proliferation follows. 'Amyotrophic' refers to the muscle wasting associated with the disease. Synonyms for ALS include **Lou Gehrig's disease** (after the New York Yankees baseball player who ended his distinguished career in 1938 because he developed ALS), **Charcot's disease** (after the French neurologist who first reported it in 1874) and, by common usage, **motor neuron disease** (MND). Strictly, however, ALS refers to one form of MND, since some other diseases target motor neurons.

The mean age of onset of ALS is 57 years; it begins as painless muscle weakness and impaired muscle tone, leading to atrophy. Problems with speech and swallowing follow. The disease is chronic and progressive, often leading to death within a few years of its appearance, usually of pneumonia or respiratory failure secondary to muscle paralysis. Males are affected twice as often as females and the average incidence in the USA is about 1 to 2 per 100 000. Ninety percent or more of ALS cases are sporadic, $\leq 10\%$ are inherited. The latter (**familial**) forms of ALS have an earlier mean age of onset and men and women seem equally at risk (unlike sporadic ALS).

9.21.1 Familial ALS (FALS) and superoxide dismutase[512,598]

Several different mutations cause FALS (e.g. some are in genes encoding proteins involved in axonal transport), but about 20% of FALS cases (i.e. 2% of all ALS cases) have defects in the gene on chromosome 21 that encodes CuZnSOD. More than 105 mutations in this gene have been identified in different patients, almost all autosomal dominant. A list may be found at *www.alsod.org*. The altered amino acid residues in the mutant CuZnSOD proteins are rarely located at the active site, but instead at amino-acid residues that play a role in enzyme stability, dimer interaction, or affecting access to the active site. Most mutants have decreased enzyme activity, but rarely does it fall below 40% of normal, and some are fully active. For example, a Gly → Ala mutation at position 93 decreases SOD activity by about 64%.

Transgenic rats or mice overexpressing genes encoding some of these mutant CuZnSODs (e.g. Gly93 → Ala or Gly85 → Arg) develop motor neuron degeneration, the pathology and mode of progression of which resemble human ALS. By contrast, overexpression of normal human CuZnSOD in mice results in some pathological changes (including limited neuromuscular impairment; Section 3.4.2) but little neurodegeneration. Since rodents expressing mutant CuZnSODs also express their own CuZnSOD, the ALS syndrome they develop cannot be due to a lack of $O_2^{\bullet-}$ dismutating activity. The greater the expression of the mutant transgene, the more quickly the mice develop disease. Hence the mutant CuZnSODs must have acquired a toxic property. This concept is supported by cell culture studies; raising the CuZnSOD content of cells delays apoptosis induced by withdrawal of growth factors from the culture medium and increases resistance to several neurotoxins. However, mutant SODs render the cell more sensitive to serum withdrawal, HNE or H_2O_2.[599] But what is this cytotoxic property of mutant SODs and why should it be confined to motor neurons, since the mutant enzyme in the patients is present in other tissues as well? The simple answer is that we don't know, although some clues have emerged.

The mutant CuZnSODs are generally less stable *in vitro* than normal CuZnSOD and tend to aggregate, forming fibrils that could be toxic (although this has not been clearly demonstrated). They might misfold after release from the ribosome, or denature more quickly than normal *in vivo* to release Zn^{2+} and potentially pro-oxidant copper ions. They also appear more susceptible to breakdown when H_2O_2 is added, a process involving $OH^{\bullet}$ generation (Section 3.2.1.6). Zinc may be easily lost from some (but by no means all) of the abnormal CuZnSODs, exposing the active site copper. Indeed, some of the mutant enzymes catalyse H_2O_2-dependent peroxidase-type reactions (e.g. oxidizing ascorbate and thiols) and form nitrating species from peroxynitrite at an increased rate (the zinc-depleted enzyme is especially good at this). The abnormal SODs may bind to neurofilaments, directing oxidative damage and nitration to neurofilament proteins. Since CuZnSOD is present not only in cytosol but also in the mitochondrial intermembrane space, a toxic protein could lead to mitochondrial dysfunction, which has indeed been described in ALS (Table 9.14). Mitochondrial degeneration is especially obvious in the transgenic mouse models, and appears to precede symptoms. However, some authors have presented data suggesting that SOD without metals can be neurotoxic, casting doubt on the importance of metal-dependent redox reactions.

So why motor neurons? Many of them contain a lot of CuZnSOD, because of their size; large motor neurons may have axons more than 1 m in length. Transport of CuZnSOD from the cell body to the end of the axon appears to be by the slow mechanism (Section 9.16.1) and it is possible that denaturation, aggregation or association with neurofilaments occur during its travels. Slow transport through long motor neurons may take 1 to 2 years to reach the nerve terminus. Neurofilament aggregation is a marked feature of ALS and presumably impairs delivery of essential molecules and organelles down the axon. In transgenic mice, decreased axonal transport rates were demonstrable well before neurodegeneration.[600] Abnormal SODs are degraded by the proteasome and might 'clog it up', causing decreased activity. Another suggested factor is that mutant SODs bind to and damage mitochondria in motor neurons but not other cells.[601]

However, when gene expression in mice is targeted so that mutant SODs form only in motor neurons, or all neurons, or only in astrocytes, no degeneration is evident. It follows that the presence of a mutant SOD in a motor neuron is a necessary but *not* a sufficient cause of death. It must also be present in other cell types around the neurons (in FALS, of course, it is present in all cell types). Indeed, removing the mutant gene from microglia markedly extended the lifespan of transgenic mice.[602,603] Why should expression in several cell types be needed? Neurons do not work in isolation; they depend on glia. For example, astrocytes with mutant CuZnSOD may have defects in glutamate uptake; failure to clear extracellular glutamate will promote excitotoxicity. Motor neurons may be especially sensitive to excitotoxicity, since they express high levels of AMPA receptors and may not be good at buffering high intracellular Ca^{2+} levels.[604]

The various SOD mutations are associated with different rates of disease progression in FALS. One set of mutations (e.g. Ala4 → Val) is linked to rapidly progressive disease (death in about 1 year), another set (e.g. Gly93 → Ala) with average disease duration (2–5 years) and yet another set (e.g. Leu126 → Ser and His46 → Arg) with 'benign' progression (10 years survival or more). It will be interesting to compare the cytotoxicity of the proteins encoded by these various mutants.

9.21.2 Oxidative damage and excitotoxicity in ALS[422,512,597,598]

Increased oxidative damage occurs in ALS, but its importance to the disease pathology is unclear. No changes in CuZnSOD, MnSOD or catalase activities have been found in sporadic ALS, but 8OHdG, protein carbonyls, HNE, glycoxidation products and 3-nitrotyrosine are elevated in ALS spinal cord (although reports of elevated *free* nitrotyrosine levels in CSF were probably arte-

facts.[605]). In mutant SOD-1 transgenic mice, nitrated proteins found in the spinal cord included enolase, ATP synthase and actin; nitration was observed before appearance of symptoms.[606] Oxidized proteins (bearing carbonyls) included CuZnSOD and UCHL1.[607] Motor neurons do not normally contain much NOS, but may develop iNOS when injured, and $NO^\bullet$ could originate from astrocytes or microglia. Increases in the levels of COX-2, iron and zinc in the ALS spinal cord have been demonstrated and levels of toxic cyclopentenone prostaglandins (Section 7.12) may also rise.[579] Levels of 8OHdG in CSF, plasma, and urine are elevated in ALS, and increase further as the disease progresses.[608]

Mice transgenic for mutant SODs are a popular tool to examine potential therapies for ALS. RNA interference to decrease expression of the gene encoding the mutant enzyme delays disease onset and slows progression.[609] Inhibitors of nNOS or PARP-1 had little or no effect on the course of disease in transgenic mice, nor did restriction of energy intake. By contrast, administration of coenzyme Q_{10}, polyamine-modified or putrescine-modified catalase, creatine (which raises creatine phosphate levels), the antibiotic minocycline (Section 8.16.1), the copper chelators trientine and penicillamine, the antioxidants carboxyfullerene (Section 10.6.7), EUK-8, EUK-134 and AEOL 10150 (Section 10.6.4), the spin trap DMPO (Section 5.2.4), α-tocopherol, lipoic acid, COX inhibitors, the lipoxygenase inhibitor NDGA and N-acetylcysteine have been reported to extend lifespan in this model and/or to delay onset of the disease to a limited extent. These data are consistent with roles for copper, oxidative damage, eicosanoids and defective energy metabolism in the neuronal damage. The drug **riluzole**, which inhibits glutamate release at presynaptic terminals, also extends lifespan in these mice, as does the antibiotic **ceftriaxone**, which may act by promoting the uptake of glutamate by astrocytes.[610] Both excitotoxicity and oxidative damage (interrelated phenomena, of course) could thus contribute to ALS pathology. Indeed, riluzole is used in the treatment of ALS and extends patient survival slightly. However, no clear evidence for beneficial effects of α-tocopherol, selegiline, N-acetylcysteine or an antioxidant cocktail has been obtained in humans, nor did administration of 500 mg of α-tocopherol per day for 18 months improve outcome for patients on riluzole therapy.[611]

Overexpression of the *bcl*-2 gene, which encodes an antiapoptotic protein (Section 4.4) prolongs lifespan in transgenic mice, as well as in cell transfected with mutant CuZnSOD enzymes, suggesting that apoptosis is an important cell death mechanism *in vivo*.[599]

9.22 Other neurodegenerative diseases

9.22.1 Friedreich's ataxia[612,613]

Friedreich's ataxia (FA), the most common hereditary ataxia,[b] has an incidence of about 1 in 50 000. Onset is usually after age 15. The disease primarily affects neurons with long axons, which die back from the periphery. In the past, some cases of AVED (which responds dramatically to α-tocopherol; Section 3.20.2) were mistaken for FA (which does not). Friedreich's ataxia is caused by mutations in a gene on chromosome 9 that encodes a protein (**frataxin**) involved in mitochondrial iron metabolism. The mutations usually involve expansion of a trinucleotide (GAA) repeat sequence in intron 1, the overall effect of which is to decrease transcription of the gene. Low frataxin hinders the formation of Fe/S clusters in aconitase and in complexes I, II and III. It has also been speculated (but not proven) to raise the intramitochondrial level of iron 'catalytic' for free radical reactions. Frataxin levels in the cerebellum and spinal cord are normally higher than in the cortex, which may help to explain the pathology. The heart is rich in frataxin and premature death of FA patients often involves cardiac problems. The antioxidant **idebenone** (Section 10.6.7) has limited therapeutic benefit in FA, consistent with a role for oxidative damage. Indeed, it decreased the elevated urinary levels of 8OHdG reported in FA patients.[612] Mixtures of coenzyme Q and α-tocopherol are also reported as helpful.[613] However, they improve cardiac function more than they do the neurological symptoms.

[b] This term is defined in Section 3.20.2.6.

9.22.2 Huntington's disease[427]

Huntington's disease (HD; sometimes called **Huntington's chorea**) is an autosomal dominantly inherited disease characterized by psychiatric disorders, dementia and involuntary twitchings, writhings and other movements. It is named after the physician George Huntington, who described it in 1872 in the only paper he ever published. Chorea relates to the Latin *choreus* and the Greek *choros*, having to do with dancing (referring to the abnormal movements). It is caused by a fairly selective degeneration of striatal neurons, accompanied by astrocytosis, leading to atrophy of the caudate nucleus and putamen. The disease does not usually appear before age 30 and can last for 20 years or more, with progressively worsening symptoms. Huntington graphically described this as 'the hapless sufferer is but a quivering wreck of his former self'. The prevalence in the USA and Europe has been estimated as 4 to 10 per 100 000.

HD is caused by a defect in a gene on chromosome 4, which encodes the protein **huntingtin**. Its function is unclear, although it could be involved in the transport of the neurotrophic factor BDNF along microtubules,[614] among other processes. The gene encoding huntingtin is expressed in many tissues, especially neurons, testis, lung and ovary. Within the normal gene, the trinucleotide CAG occurs in sequences repeated 9 to 39 (mean 19) times and encodes a string of glutamine residues starting at position 18 in the protein. In HD the repeat frequency is greater (range 36–121, mean 43) and, correspondingly, the polyglutamine sequence is longer. Repeat lengths of ≥ 40 make it likely that a subject with even one copy of the abnormal gene will develop HD. Repeat lengths tend to increase from generation to generation so that the disease can become more severe in succeeding generations (**genetic anticipation**). Very high (>50) repeat lengths can lead to early disease onset (sometimes before age 30). The abnormal huntingtin gains a toxic function, related to too many glutamine repeats. Increased numbers of CAG repeats have been identified in different genes in at least eight other neurodegenerative diseases, including **spinocerebellar ataxia types 1,2,3,7 and 17** and **spinal-bulbar muscular atrophy**. In the last, there is an excessive number of CAG repeats within the coding region of the androgen-receptor gene. Affected males have a syndrome resembling a motor neuron disease, as well as impaired response to androgen.

Why does having extra glutamines make huntingtin neurotoxic? The defective protein shows an abnormal propensity to aggregate and form inclusion bodies that contain ubiquitin and proteasome components and impair the function of the proteasome; aggregation may be the origin of its toxicity.[513] As in the case of Aβ (Section 9.20), it may not be the final huntingtin aggregates that are toxic, but early stages of aggregation.[519]

Does oxidative damage contribute to HD? The evidence that it does is less abundant than for AD or PD,[422] although rises in striatal 8OHdG have been reported in some studies,[615] as have increased levels of F$_2$-IPs in patients' CSF (but not in their plasma or urine).[579] Rises in 8OHdG, increased lipid peroxidation, nitrotyrosine formation and mitochondrial dysfunction were reported in a transgenic mouse model of HD; mice expressing the relevant part of the mutant human gene develop progressive neurodegeneration from about 6 weeks of age.[615] The antioxidants lipoic acid or **BN82451** (Section 10.6.7) increased survival and motor performance and slowed neuronal death in the animals, as did coenzyme Q, clioquinol, cystamine and minocycline.[615,616]

Defects in energy metabolism can be detected in HD patients by imaging techniques, and falls in complex II, III and aconitase activities are reported in post-mortem material, possibly because the abnormal huntingtin associates with and damages mitochondria. Indeed, injection of complex II inhibitors, such as nitropropionic acid or malonate, into animals causes striatal damage resembling that in HD, and complex II inhibition is well known to increase mitochondrial ROS production.[427] Creatine administration increased brain ATP levels and improved survival in the transgenic mouse model.[617] There may be some benefit of high-dose coenzyme Q in HD patients.[545]

9.22.3 Prion diseases[618]

Scrapie, a neurodegenerative disease of goats and sheep, was first described some 250 years ago as presenting with excitability, ataxia, itching and eventual paralysis and death. Its transmissibility was accidentally demonstrated in 1937, when a flock of sheep was inoculated with an extract of brain tissue from an animal that turned out to harbour the disease, and many of the sheep went on to develop it. In the 1950s, Australian administrators exploring new territories in Papua New Guinea discovered a previously unknown tribe (the **Foré**) in which death from the disease **kuru** ('to shiver', in their tribal language) was often observed, especially in women and children. The lesions of kuru and scrapie in the brain look similar, and kuru was soon shown to involve an agent that could be transmitted to monkeys. The high kuru incidence was attributed to cannibalism; women and children eating the brains of infected subjects. The men were more likely to eat the flesh, thus developing kuru less often. In the 1920s, Creutzfeldt and Jakob described the human neurodegenerative disease named after them as **Creutzfeldt–Jakob disease** (CJD), which usually occurs sporadically in late middle age.

Few readers will be unaware of the epidemic of **bovine spongiform encephalopathy** (BSE) in cattle in the UK, especially as eating tissue from cattle infected by this 'mad cow disease' seems responsible for the occurrence of a small number of atypical cases of CJD (**variant CJD, vCJD**) in young people. More than 75 cases of CJD had previously occurred in children given growth hormone prepared from human pituitary glands obtained at autopsy; this practice has been abandoned since some of the glands must have come from cadavers with unrecognized disease. Other cases occurred in patients who received grafts of meningeal tissue, derived from donors with unsuspected disease, during neurosurgery. The vCJD cases have clinical features closer to those of the growth hormone cases, and kuru, and less similar to sporadic CJD. Spaces created in the brain by neuronal death create a sponge-like appearance, hence the name **transmissible spongiform encephalopathies** often given to these diseases. There is marked astrogliosis.

Scrapie, BSE, CJD and kuru are all thought to be caused by **prions** (proteinaceous infectious particles). Prion, a glycoprotein with 231 amino acids, is found in all mammals in many tissues, with levels highest in the brain. The problem arises when normal prion protein (**PrP^c**) becomes converted to an abnormal form (**PrP^{Sc}**), which differs not in amino acid sequence, but only in conformation, having adopted an abnormal β-sheet structure. The abnormal protein cannot be degraded and accumulates, leading to neuronal dysfunction and death, and can precipitate to give PrP-amyloid plaques that may provoke glial activation.

In 'sporadic' cases of CJD in elderly people, this transformation is probably a rare, random event. However, several (also rare) inherited mutations in the PrP^c gene that favour PrP^{Sc} formation, and cause autosomal dominant prion disease, have been described. Contact with PrP^{Sc} can also trigger the disease; if it gains access to a normal tissue, it alters the conformation of PrP^c to generate more PrP^{Sc}. That is probably what happened in BSE, vCJD, kuru and the growth hormone and surgical cases. Indeed, 'knockout' mice lacking PrP^c cannot be infected with scrapie, unlike normal mice. They show various abnormalities (in some studies), indicating an important role for PrP^c *in vivo*. One possibility is that it helps bind copper and prevent its pro-oxidant effects in the brain.[619] Indeed, mice lacking it showed increased brain protein carbonyls and MDA[619] and greater brain infarcts after ischaemic injury,[620] perhaps related to decreased CuZnSOD.[621]

Fragments of PrP^c (e.g. residues 121–231 or 106–126) are toxic to neurons in culture. As with Aβ, this may involve formation of membrane ion channels and/or oxidative stress, in part due to redox reactions of the peptide with copper or iron.[622] Neurodegeneration in scrapie-infected mouse brain is accompanied by increased levels of iron, HO-1, HNE, F$_2$-IPs and nitrotyrosine[623,624] and could be slowed by administering penicillamine.[625] Levels of F$_2$-IPs in CSF, and of HNE in brain are elevated in human CJD patients.[514,624]

9.22.4 Neuronal ceroid lipofuscinoses[626]

The neuronal ceroid lipofuscinoses (NCL) are autosomal, recessively inherited, fatal disorders that occur worldwide in about 1 per 100 000 live births, but more frequently in Scandinavia. Some patients develop symptoms during infancy (**infantile NCL**), others in early childhood (**late infantile NCL**),

others in late childhood (**juvenile NDL**) and yet others after adolescence (**adult NCL**). Juvenile NCL has sometimes been called **Batten's disease** and the adult form, **Kuf's disease**. There are also several variant types. The onset of NCL is marked by behavioural abnormalities which worsen to include disturbances of vision and speech, and muscular and mental deterioration, associated with seizures. In the terminal stages the brain is severely damaged and patients assume a contracted position. Similar diseases occur in dogs, cattle and sheep.

At least eight different genes are involved in NCL. Infantile NCL is caused by an inherited defect in a lysosomal proteinase (**palmitoyl protein thioesterase**), which removes fatty acids such as palmitate esterified to cysteine residues in lipoproteins. Late-infantile NCL is also caused by a lysosomal defect (in **tripeptidyl peptidase**). Other forms of NCL are caused by defects in lysosomal membrane proteins, some of which remain to be identified.

Attention was focused on NCL by free radical researchers because the disease is accompanied by accumulation of fluorescent pigments resembling the 'age pigment' ceroid (Section 10.4.6) in the brain (especially in cortex and cerebellum) and elsewhere. However, the original assumption that 'age pigment' is largely peroxidized lipid was mistaken, and there is no clear evidence of increased oxidative damage or defects in antioxidant protection in NCL (nor, to be fair, has it been studied systematically). The pigments are located within 'storage bodies' originating from lysosomes. In adult, juvenile and late infantile (but not infantile) NCL most of the protein within these bodies is **subunit c**, a hydrophobic component of mitochondrial ATP synthase. Lysosomes normally engulf cytoplasmic components by autophagy, and degrade them. In NCLs, engulfment continues but degradation (especially of subunit c) is impaired, so that abnormal lysosomes accumulate.

Hence involvement of oxidative damage in NCL must, at best, be indirect. There have been anecdotal reports that patients with NCL respond to treatment with antioxidants, but double-blind controlled clinical trials have not been reported. However, glial cell activation is a common feature of NCLs, so a contribution of RS is feasible. Autophagy is essential to normal neuronal function.[626A]

9.22.5 Tardive dyskinesia[627]

Tardive dyskinesia is a disorder characterized by abnormal involuntary movements of muscles in the face and limbs. Its cause is unknown, although long-term treatment of patients with antipsychotic drugs is a risk factor. It has been proposed that drug-related oxidative stress is involved in its development and that α-tocopherol administration is beneficial to patients, but insufficient data have been published to reach clear-cut conclusions. The condition is tending to disappear anyway as better antipsychotic agents come into use.

9.22.6 Cycads, flying foxes, Guam and lathyrism: now all history?[628]

In the first half of the last century, the native Chamorro Indians of Guam and Rota, islands in the western Pacific, showed a markedly-elevated incidence of neurodegenerative disorders with features of both ALS and PD with dementia (**ALS–parkinsonism–dementia complex**). The disparate symptoms seemed to be different manifestations of the same disease, called *lytico-bodig* by the locals. The incidence has been declining since the 1950s, as the Chamorros adopt an increasingly 'US-style' life, and is now rare in anyone born after 1960. It has been proposed that a neurotoxin present in extracts from nuts of the false sago palm (*Cycas circinalis*), formerly a common part of the Chamorro diet but now consumed less often, caused these diseases. This neurotoxin may be the amino acid, *β*-*N*-**methylamino-L-alanine** (α-amino-β-methyl aminopropionic acid) (Fig. 9.35). It can kill neurons by an excitotoxic mechanism, binding to NMDA receptors. It is additionally speculated that Chamorros acquired more of this toxin because they liked to eat the meat of the flying fox, a fruit bat

that feeds on cycads. This mammal is now almost extinct. The toxin is also produced by some strains of cyanobacteria, and it has been speculated to contribute to the occurrence of sporadic AD in other parts of the world.[629] Yet another proposal is that Chamorros were exposed to excess rotenone, because they used extracts of plants containing it to paralyse fish to catch and eat (a procedure now, fortunately, illegal there).[552]

The disease **lathyrism**, which manifests as paralysis of the legs, has been observed in many poor countries (especially India and Ethiopia). It is related to consumption of seeds of *Lathyrus sativus*, the chickling pea. *L. sativus* seeds contain a neurotoxin, *β*-*N*-**oxalyl-α,β-diaminopropionic acid** (*β*-*N*-**oxalylamino-L-alanine**) (Fig. 9.35) which activates AMPA receptors. Prolonged consumption of *L. sativus*, especially when the diet is poor in other nutrients, leads to death of motor neurons, probably by an excitotoxic mechanism. Sadly, this disease is not history: it still occurs.[630] Excitotoxicity, of course, implies oxidative stress, and a poor intake of antioxidant nutrients may make matters worse.

9.23 Oxidative stress and viral infections[632,633]

Oxidative damage can contribute to the damage done by bacterial infections, for example in meningitis (Section 9.17). The same is true for viruses. The immune response of the host, aided by increased production of such cytokines as TNFα, can generate large amounts of RS in a (usually successful) attempt to eliminate the virus. For example, NO• inhibits replication of many viruses in cells in culture, either directly and/or by damaging the infected host cell and preventing the

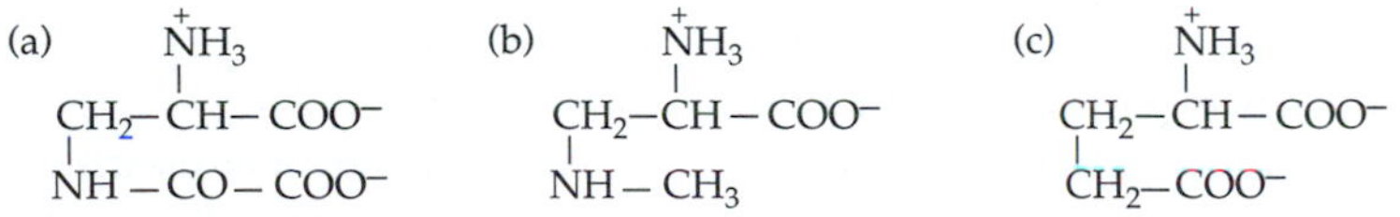

Figure 9.35 Structures of some plant neurotoxins. (a) *β*-*N*-Oxalylamino-L-alanine; (b) *β*-*N*-methylamino-L-alanine. Compound (a) is associated with lathyrism in several parts of the world; compound (b) with the increased incidence of ALS–PD–dementia syndromes in the Chamorro Indians. (c) The structure of the excitatory amino acid glutamate, for comparison.

virus from using it to replicate. Reactive oxygen species, and RNS derived from $NO^\bullet$ (HNO_2, $ONOO^-$, N_2O_3), can cause mutations in the viral genome. Too many of these will inactivate the virus, but another possibility is that they could promote mutations and facilitate viral evolution– another example of the Janus nature of RS.

Mobilization of the host defence system involves activation of NF-κB in the immune system, but this can be subverted by viruses for their own advantage, since viral gene promoters often contain NF-κB-binding sequences that promote transcription of viral genes. The persistent activation of NF-κB by some viruses (including those that cause **acquired immunodeficiency syndrome (AIDS)**, hepatitis B and C, and influenza) may also help suppress apoptosis of the host cell. A striking example is HTLV-1, which causes adult T-cell leukaemia (Table 9.10). The viral **tax** protein activates NF-κB and other transcription factors involved in causing malignancy. The hepatitis B virus **HBx** protein acts similarly and its presence increases the risk of hepatocellular carcinoma.[631]

With some infections, as with chronic inflammations, an overexuberant immune response can damage the host more than the infecting agent. As an example, infection of laboratory mice with an influenza virus produced significant mortality that could be decreased by administering SOD (linked to a polymer to prolong its lifetime in the circulation) or allopurinol. Mortality was due to lung damage, and involved XO, $NO^\bullet$, $ONOO^-$ and activated macrophages.[632] Increased levels of 8-nitroguanine were detected in the lung. Infection of the brains of mice with herpes simplex type I virus caused increased formation of 8OHdG and HNE, associated with inflammation.[633] Viral infections of vascular endothelium may contribute to atherosclerosis (Section 9.3.3), and selenium deficiency in mice allows a usually benign coxsackievirus to cause heart damage (Section 3.11.2).

However, most attention has been paid to the **human immunodeficiency viruses (HIV)**, the causative agents of AIDS. These pathogens, HIV-1 and -2, belong to a family of retroviruses whose other members infect monkeys. The former is more pathogenic to humans than HIV-2. The HIV viral particles contain a **capsid** enclosing the single-stranded RNA genome plus three viral enzymes: proteinase, reverse transcriptase and integrase. Reverse transcriptase copies viral RNA into DNA, which integrase incorporates into the host genome. The viral genome contains two genes that encode regulatory proteins, *Tat* and *Rev*. Tat (**transactivator of transcription**) protein activates gene transcription from the viral promoter as well as NF-κB in the host cell, whereas Rev facilitates export of viral mRNA from the cell nucleus. The capsid is surrounded by a matrix protein which in turn is covered by an envelope consisting of a lipid bilayer that contains the proteins **gp120** (outer envelope protein) and **gp41** (transmembrane).

Infection with HIV results from intimate exposure to the blood or other body fluids of an infected person. It usually results in a brief illness associated with a period of rapid viral replication. The virus mostly infects $CD4^+$ lymphocytes; T-helper lymphocytes expressing the cell-surface antigen **CD4**. Such lymphocytes are essential to the functioning of the immune system and those present in mucosal surfaces are an early target of destruction by HIV. The $CD4^+$ glycoprotein is recognized by the HIV-1 envelope protein complex (via gp120) to allow the virus to bind to host cells. Other receptors are needed for virus to enter; normally they bind chemokines such as MIP-1α, MIP-1β and RANTES (Table 4.8). Soon, the viral load falls and the patient becomes asymptomatic. This low apparent viral load results from an equilibrium between production of new virus and destruction of infected $CD4^+$ T-lymphocytes. As many as 2×10^9 of these cells, about 5% of the total body pool of $CD4^+$ cells, are destroyed and replaced per day. Over many years, $CD4^+$ cell numbers tend to fall as the ability of the immune system to replace them fails. When they fall below the minimum needed for normal immune function, patients develop 'opportunistic' infections with organisms normally easily eliminated (e.g. *Pneumocystis carinii* pneumonia), and full-blown AIDS appears.

Therapeutic agents used in triple combinations are effective in controlling HIV infection, although they do have side-effects. They include inhibitors of reverse transcriptase (e.g. **azidodeoxythymidine (AZT)**, **dideoxyinosine** (ddI) and **dideoxycytidine** (ddC)), and inhibitors of the proteinase enzyme used by the virus to cleave newly synthesized proteins into the forms needed for viral assembly. Examples of proteinase inhibitors are **ritonavir, indinavir** and **saquinavir**.

9.23.1 Reactive species, antioxidants and HIV

The presence of HIV in the brain can lead to neuronal death and glial proliferation, resulting in cognitive and motor defects. The most severe form of this is called **AIDS dementia complex**. Neurological damage by HIV involves immune activation of astrocytes and macrophages, leading to increased production of TNFα, IL-1β, other cytokines, iNOS, ROS, and eicosanoids, with formation of HNE and nitrotyrosine.[634] As well as these products, gp120 protein is toxic to neurons; the toxicity requires external glutamate and Ca$^+$ and is blocked by agents that antagonize glutamate receptors. Hence an excitotoxic mechanism involving RS may contribute to neuronal death.[634,635] Tat protein can be similarly toxic. With the advent of triple therapy, AIDS dementia complex is decreasing in frequency, fortunately. The brain damage that can sometimes be done by other viruses, such as measles virus and herpes simplex type I, also involves ROS and cytokines.[634]

9.23.1.1 Changes in glutathione?

The first suggestions that oxidative stress might be important in HIV infection came from measurements of GSH. Plasma and lung lining fluids from HIV-infected patients were reported to show decreased levels of GSH, cysteine and cystine. Monocyte and lymphocyte levels of GSH were also claimed to be subnormal. The size of the reported falls varied between laboratories, with particular disagreement about whether or not there is a fall in lymphocyte, plasma or lung lining fluid GSH in asymptomatic HIV-positive patients rather than in those with AIDS.[636] In Rhesus macaque monkeys, plasma, cysteine and intracellular GSH levels also fall 2 weeks after infection with simian immunodeficiency virus.[637] However, administration of *N*-acetylcysteine to raise GSH levels does not seem to confer much, if any, clinical benefit in humans,[638]

nor did administration of an antioxidant cocktail.[639] This may not be surprising, since there is little evidence for increased oxidative damage in asymptomatic HIV-infected subjects.[640] Indeed, high doses of α-tocopherol may be contra-indicated, since they can increase P450 levels and affect antiretroviral drug metabolism (Section 3.20.2.7).

The falls in GSH are most striking in patients with AIDS, where malnutrition due both to poor appetite and to impaired intestinal absorption of nutrients could contribute. Probably for these reasons, plasma concentrations of several vitamins and minerals, including zinc, magnesium, selenium, vitamin B$_{12}$, β-carotene and other carotenoids, are low in some AIDS patients. Hence correct nutrition is an important part of therapy.

9.23.2 Redox regulation of viral expression[641]

Studies on HIV-infected lymphocyte cell lines in culture reveal that imposing oxidative stress (e.g. by H$_2$O$_2$ or UV light) sometimes increases HIV gene expression (often via NF-κB), whereas antioxidants diminish it. In human (but not chimpanzee!) T-lymphocytes, expression of the HIV tat protein decreases GSH levels and expression of the gene encoding MnSOD, and increases ROS production. The Tat protein contains multiple cysteine residues and is thus susceptible to oxidation; oxidized Tat will not promote viral gene expression. Thus a limited degree of oxidative stress could conceivably encourage HIV production (via NF-κB activation), whereas high levels of oxidative stress might deter it by oxidizing Tat and NF-κB, and triggering lymphocyte apoptosis. Hence, as usual, the redox balance is all important.[642] Levels of thioredoxin, and its redox state, also influence the behaviour of infected cells.[641] In addition, activation of NF-κB in the host cells is not all bad; it leads to increased synthesis of several cytokines, including RANTES, a chemokine that can block HIV infection of cells.

Inhibition of viral replication by antioxidants in cultured cells is also observed for other viruses, including herpes simplex type I, respiratory syncytial virus (RSV), cytomegalovirus, murine Sindbis virus, hepatitis B virus and Epstein–Barr virus (EBV). Whether this could happen *in vivo*

Table 9.18 How important is oxidative stress in human disease?

Condition	Is oxidative stress a primary cause?	If oxidative stress is secondary, does it contribute significantly to disease pathology?	Is there evidence that antioxidants have, or will have, therapeutic benefit?
Radiation-induced damage	Yes	Yes[a]	Yes (Section 8.19.2)
α-Tocopherol deficiency[b]	Probably	–	Yes (Section 3.20.2)
Selenium deficiency	Very likely (animals); likely (humans)	–	Yes (Section 3.11.2)
Atherosclerosis	Sometimes[c]	Maybe	Limited for humans
Hypertension	Sometimes	Sometimes	Some
Diabetes	Possibly sometimes	Yes (phagocyte attack on islets; toxicity of glucose)	Limited
Rheumatoid arthritis	No[d]	Uncertain, phagocyte RS production may even be protective	No
Autoimmune diseases	Probably no[d]	Uncertain, phagocyte ROS production may even be protective	Limited
Inflammatory bowel disease	Probably no[d]	Probably, although phagocyte ROS production could sometimes be protective	A little
ARDS	Generally no[e]	Possibly	No
Cystic fibrosis	No	Possibly some	Limited
Cancer	Some cases, yes[f]	Probably	Limited, e.g. protective against side-effects of chemotherapy
Stroke/Traumatic CNS Injury	No	Sometimes	Limited
Parkinson's disease	Possibly	Probably	No
Alzheimer's disease	Probably no	Probably	Some
ALS	No	Hard to decide as yet	No
Neuronal ceroid lipofuscinoses	No	No data	No good data
Multiple sclerosis	No	Possibly	No
Drug side-effects	In a few cases	In a few cases	Limited
Huntington's disease	No	Possibly	Some
Freidreich's ataxia	No	Probably	Some
HIV infection/AIDS	No	Possibly	No

[a] Secondary production of RS by inflammation.
[b] Humans and other animals.
[c] Reactive species can damage vascular endothelium to start the process.
[d] Although oxidatively-modified proteins/DNA can be antigenic.
[e] But may contribute to phagocyte recruitment.
[f] Chronic inflammation-related, may contribute to mechanisms of carcinogen action.

is uncertain. Respiratory syncytial virus, for example, activates the NADPH oxidase of alveolar epithelial cells, elevates ROS generation and inactivates protein phosphatases, increasing net protein phosphorylation.[643] Patients with infectious mononucleosis caused by EBV develop a wide range of antibodies because of the extensive B-cell activation caused by the disease. One of them is directed against MnSOD and inhibits the enzyme activity.[644]

9.23.3 Side-effects of therapy

The first drug used to treat AIDS was AZT; it is still used as part of drug combinations. Treatment with AZT was associated with mitochondrial damage in about 20% of patients, in part by inhibiting the mitochondrial DNA polymerase (**pol-γ**).[645] Rises in mitochondrial 8OHdG levels in AZT-treated animals, and increased urinary 8OHdG excretion in patients, have been reported. Excretion of 8OHdG in AZT-treated patients can be decreased by oral supplements of α-tocopherol plus vitamin C.[645] Indeed, oxidative stress may be more associated with anti-HIV therapy than with actions of the virus.[646] For example, one side-effect of triple therapy is to cause abnormalities in lipid metabolism, such as peripheral fat wasting (**lipoatrophy**). Patients with this condition were reported to have elevated plasma F_2-IPs when compared to others not showing this side-effect.[647]

9.24 Conclusion

In reviewing current understanding of the relationship between oxidative stress and human disease, it is important to keep in mind the criteria listed at the start of this Chapter. Table 9.18 is an attempt to assess how far these criteria are met by the various diseases we have considered. Compare it with the table in the last edition of this book (Table 9.17); not a lot has changed!

CHAPTER 10

Ageing, nutrition, disease and therapy: a role for antioxidants?

With the passage of the years, phagocytic cells become incontinent, rampage through our tissues, gnaw at our vitals and cause the catastrophe that we recognize as ageing.

E. Metchnikoff

10.1 Introduction

Increased oxidative damage occurs in most if not all, diseases (Chapter 9). In some, it contributes to tissue injury, so that therapeutic intervention with antioxidants should be beneficial, provided that the agents used actually do decrease the oxidative damage. Additionally, diet-derived antioxidants are often thought to be important disease-preventing agents. Chapter 10 examines both these issues.

The incidence of many diseases, including cardiovascular and neurodegenerative diseases, osteoporosis, and osteoarthritis increases with age.[1] Let us therefore first examine whether oxidative damage is involved in ageing itself.

10.2 An introduction to theories of ageing

'Ageing' is a word hard to define precisely. In general terms, it can be described as a progressive decline in the efficiency of physiological processes (not necessarily all at the same rate) after the reproductive phase of life. The ability of cells and organisms to recover from an insult, such as traumatic injury (or oxidative stress) decreases with age, and the risk of disease increases. For example, muscle atrophies with age, and is slower to regenerate after injury. One of the many problems in studying ageing experimentally is the difficulty of separating ageing from age-related

disease (indeed, it may be impossible). Most old animals (including humans) have overt, or subclinical (e.g. atherosclerosis, β-amyloid plaques) diseases that can influence parameters of oxidative damage.

10.2.1 General principles

As an organism ages, its chance of death increases, so that all individuals of a given species are dead by some age, characteristic of that species. The maximum lifespan achieved to date in humans is 122 years; the French lady Jeanne Calment was born on February 21 1875 and died in August 1997. The longest-lived male to date was Shigechiyo Izumi, a Japanese, who died at age 120.

In many countries today (and, until recently, in all countries), few individuals reach their potential lifespan because of infectious diseases and/or poor nutrition. In advanced countries, such deaths are now rare. Those few people who die under the age of 35 usually do so from accidents, a limited range of infectious diseases such as AIDS, or suicide. By contrast, old people usually die of cancer, cardiovascular diseases, stroke or pneumonia, the last relating to an inability to tolerate infection, tissue injury or prolonged confinement in bed. In Chapter 9, we commented on the age-dependency of the neurodegenerative diseases. The overall incidence of cancer also rises with age (Fig. 9.19); for most cancers the

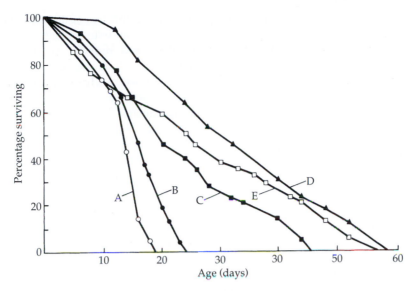

Figure 10.1 Effect of activity on the lifespan of the housefly, *Musca domestica*. Fifty normal flies (A) or dewinged flies (B) were placed in a large cage. In group C, each fly was placed alone in a large cage; the insects are disturbed less often and so fly less. In other groups, normal flies (D) or dewinged flies (E) were placed in small bottles, one per bottle, to prevent flying. Data by courtesy of Prof. Raj Sohal (also see[2] and *J. Gerontol* **61A**, 136, 2006). Mitochondrial respiratory activity declines with age in flies, and mitochondrial ROS production may increase (*Biochem. J.* **390**, 501, 2005).

incidence increases approximately proportionally to the fourth or fifth power of age.[1] This is seen both in short-lived species such as rats and mice and in humans (about 30% have cancer at the age of 85). Thus the average lifespan (or **mean lifespan**) of humans in 'advanced' societies is greater than that of less-developed ones, but the potential lifespan is probably the same.

10.2.2 What features of ageing must theories explain?

Whatever theory is proposed to explain ageing, it must account for several phenomena, one of which is the link to metabolic rate. Cold-blooded animals, such as insects and reptiles, live longer at lower temperatures. For example, the mean lifespan of *Drosophila* is 120 days at 10°C, but only 14 days at 30°C. Similarly, the nematode worm *C. elegans* lives longer (and moves more slowly) if the temperature is reduced. Insects consume much more O_2 when flying than at rest. Prevention of houseflies from flying by removing their wings, or by confining them in small bottles, increases lifespan (Fig. 10.1).[2] For most animal species, there is an inverse correlation between basal metabolic rates and

lifespan. In general, larger animals live longer and consume less O_2 per unit body mass than do smaller ones. Certain animals live longer than predicted by this correlation, including pigeons, canaries, bats, naked mole rats and humans. Some of these anomalies are discussed in Section 10.4.1 below.

10.2.2.1 *Caloric restriction (CR)*[3]

Another striking effect on lifespan is provided by **caloric restriction** (eating fewer calories whilst maintaining intake of essential vitamins and minerals), sometimes referred to as 'undernutrition without malnutrition'. It produces highly significant increases in lifespan in several species, including insects, worms, mice, fish, dogs, cows and rats. Thus the 'average' mouse in the 'average' laboratory lives about 28 months. Feeding it 53, 31 or 25% of its normal caloric intake extends lifespan to an average of 33, 45 or 47 months (as ever, be wary of extrapolation; it will not live forever if you don't feed it at all).[4] Caloric restriction delays the appearance of cancers (both spontaneous ones and those induced by administered carcinogens), slows age-related declines in the immune system and brain function, and increases the physical activity of animals. It even attenuates the development of Aβ plaques in APP-transgenic mice, apparently by increasing α-secretase activity (Fig. 9.34), and enhances tissue sensitivity to insulin, accompanied by falls in plasma insulin.[5] A few studies have produced increases in lifespan by restricting the intake of one specific component (such as methionine)[6] rather than total food intake–more research in this area is required.

10.2.2.2 Obesity, oxidative stress and CR in primates
Of course, laboratory animals are kept under conditions unrepresentative of nature. Their physical activity is decreased by caging, and food is supplied *ad libitum*. However, many humans live essentially the same way (little exercise, a lot of food)[7] and obesity is a major health problem in many parts of the world. Obesity shortens lifespan, increases the risk of many diseases and is associated with oxidative stress (usually measured as plasma and/or urinary F_2-IPs). For example, in a large cohort of subjects in Framingham, USA, the main determinants of urinary F_2-IP levels were smoking, diabetes and obesity.[8] Adipose tissue (particularly abdominal fat) is not only a storage depot for triglyceride but also a producer of proinflammatory cytokines such as TNFα and IL-6.[9] High-fat diets have been shown to increase levels of oxidative damage in animal studies, possibly (in part) because adipose tissue itself makes RS. Thus in obese mice NOX enzymes are active in the fat cells.[10] Losing weight causes F_2-IP levels to drop in humans. Hence oxidative stress and a proinflammatory state contribute to the link between obesity and disease. High-fat diets can also aggravate the deleterious effects of smoking and excess ethanol consumption.

So would humans benefit from CR? Those who over-eat do benefit from eating less, and certain epidemiological studies suggest that some degree of CR would be beneficial. However, too little food (≤ 1400 kcal/day) is also associated with increased mortality,[11] although often such a diet may lack sufficient vitamins and minerals, unlike 'laboratory' CR. Nevertheless, the potential for benefit is shown by experiments on CR in Rhesus monkeys that began in 1987 at the National Institutes of Aging (NIA) in the USA. Half eat *ad libitum* and the rest receive 30% less of the same diet.[12] Data so far are consistent with rodent studies, in that CR-monkeys and rodents are smaller, mature later, have lower blood glucose and insulin levels and slightly lower body temperatures, yet increased daytime activity. The NIA is also supporting studies in humans.[13]

Another dramatic example of the effect of diet on lifespan can be seen with the queen honeybee (*Apis mellifera*). The queen can live for as long as 6 years and produces hundreds of eggs each day whereas worker bees live for only a few weeks or months. The difference in lifespan relates to the exclusive feeding of the queen with royal jelly, a secretion produced by worker bees.[14]

10.3 What theories of ageing exist?[15–18]

Theories proposed to explain ageing fall into three general groups. There are **genetic theories**, in which gene-controlled, programmed 'biological clocks' such as telomeres (Section 10.3.5 below) regulate growth, maturity and old age, **neuroendocrine theories**, and **damage-accumulation theories** (Table 10.1). In fact, this distinction is silly, because all these mechanisms are important and interrelated.

10.3.1 Do genes influence ageing? The story of C. elegans

Yes they do; a database exists that characterizes over 200 genes linked in some way to human ageing (*genomics.senescence.info*). Most evidence for a role of genes has come from studies on *C. elegans*, *Drosophila* and yeast, although there are some animal and human data.

C. elegans normally lives for about 20 to 25 days when food (bacteria such as *E. coli*) is abundant. At 20°C, it develops from embryo to sexual maturity in about 3 to 4 days, lays most of its eggs in the next 3 to 4 days, and then survives for the rest of its lifespan with deteriorating function, for example muscle loss accompanied by slowing movement.[19] *C. elegans* is a hermaphrodite and reproduces primarily by self-fertilization, first producing sperm, and later eggs for the sperm to fertilize.

Table 10.1 Some theories of ageing

Theory	Summary of theory as originally proposed
Free radical	Random deleterious effects of free radicals produced during normal aerobic metabolism.
Cross-linkage	Random cross-links of DNA and proteins disrupt function.
Error catastrophe	Cumulative random errors in protein synthesis, affecting protein function and gene transcription.
Glycation	Glycation of proteins and other molecules leads to AGE formation and disruption of cell function.
Longevity determinants	Ageing is caused by the products of cellular metabolism, and the rate of ageing is governed by protection against these damaging products. Overlaps with free radical theory.
Membrane hypothesis	Membrane damage leads to decreased elimination of waste products, decreased protein synthesis and loss of water from the cytoplasm leading to decreased enzymic activities.
Inflammatory hypothesis	NF-κB and AP-1 activities rise in tissues as they age and cause formation of more cytokines, COX, prostaglandins (and RS) that damage tissues (*Antiox. Redox Signal.* **8**, 572, 2006).
Neuroendocrine	Changes in neural function and hormones cause age-related physiological changes by interfering with co-operation between organs and impairing the response to external stimuli. Some theories also incorporate changes in the immune system produced by neuroendocrine alterations; thus as one ages the immune system because less good at dealing with infectious agents but more likely to cause autoimmunity.

Multiple **damage-accumulation theories** have been proposed, but are similar in that they assume some progressive accumulation of damage because repair and maintenance are always less than those required for 'indefinite' survival. Evolution has little 'interest' in maintaining the body in the postreproductive years.[7] Faulty macromolecules can accumulate both by generating more of them (e.g. by more errors in gene transcription or mRNA translation, and/or by damaging macromolecules more) and/or by failure of systems that repair or degrade them. Some of these theories overlap with the genetic theories of ageing. A popular idea in its time was the **error—catastrophe theory**, introduced in 1963. It proposed that errors in transcription of RNA and its translation into protein eventually lead to accumulation of altered non-functional proteins in old cells, reaching levels that ultimately lead to an 'error catastrophe' of failure to function. Sadly, although some altered non-functional or less active enzymes have been isolated from aged cells, there is no evidence for accumulation of altered proteins to very high ('catastrophic') concentrations in any tissues from old animals, and only limited evidence that the fidelity of transcription or translation decreases with age. A similar criticism can be made about the 'membrane hypothesis'; membranes are not falling apart in cells from old animals.

When threatened (e.g. by food restriction or over-crowding), *C. elegans* halts its regular life cycle and forms a developmentally arrested, reproductively immature, long-lived form, the **dauer larva**. This is stress-resistant and can survive for a long time until conditions improve, whereupon it resumes development into the adult. Because of the short lifespan and well-characterized structure and genetics of *C. elegans*, many scientists have looked for genes that influence lifespan in this worm. They have reaped a rich harvest.[18,20] For example, mutations of the ***age-1*** gene slow muscle degeneration and can extend life expectancy by 40 to 100%; they do not affect reproduction, and movement is normal. This is an important control; in cold-blooded animals increased metabolic activity often shortens lifespan. Any change that alters O_2 consumption (e.g. by increasing or decreasing activity) or food intake (promoting over-feeding or CR) could produce indirect effects on lifespan,

which might be mistaken for identification of an 'ageing gene'.

Mutations in the ***daf-2*** gene also increase lifespan; the DAF-2 protein resembles the mammalian receptors that allow cells to respond to insulin or insulin-like growth factors (IGFs) (Figs 10.2 and 10.3). The *Daf2* gene product is involved in dauer formation;[21] harsh environmental conditions act, in part, by decreasing insulin/IGF signalling, whereas when food is restored ligands are released from secretory cells in the nervous system to activate the pathway.[18] Ligand binding to DAF-2 activates a kinase cascade in which the protein encoded by *age-1* is required. The end-result is to phosphorylate a transcription factor, **DAF-16**, which is then sequestered in the cytoplasm in an inactive form (Fig. 10.3). The DAF-16 protein is a member of the family of forkhead transcription factors of class O (FOXO) (Section 4.5.5.2), which are stopped from working upon phosphorylation because they are

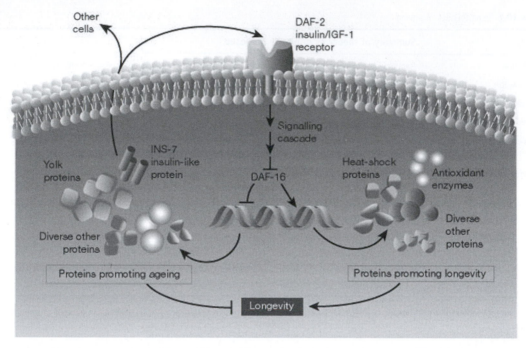

Figure 10.2 Ageing versus long life: the molecules involved. The transcription factor DAF-16 controls the expression of a battery of genes that affect lifespan. Prolongevity genes include those that encode antioxidant enzymes, or heat-shock proteins that can restore misfolded proteins to their correct conformations.[18] Genes that promote ageing include some that encode yolk proteins, consistent with a link between ageing and reproduction. Another pro-ageing protein is the insulin-like **INS-7**, which, by binding to the insulin/IGF-1 receptor (**DAF-2**), may repress DAF-16 on the same and other cells. This suggests the presence of a positive feedback loop that regulates DAF-2 activity.[18] Many other proteins are involved, but their mechanistic links to ageing are as yet unclear. Arrows indicate activation; T-bars indicate inhibition. From *Nature* **424**, 259, 2003 by courtesy of Elsevier and Drs David Gems and Joshua McElwee.

excluded from the nucleus. Left unphosphorylated as a result of mutations in *age-1* or *daf-2*, DAF-16 protein enters the nucleus and causes the transcription of genes that promote longevity and resistance to stresses, including heat and oxidative stress (Fig. 10.2). Genes whose expression is increased by active DAF-16 include those encoding antioxidant defences (Section 10.4.1 below), antimicrobial proteins (*C. elegans* feeds on bacteria, but they can also damage its gut), heat-shock proteins (Hsps) and members of the ubiquitin–proteasome system. By contrast, DAF-16 decreases expression of genes encoding some other proteins, including **INS-7** (Fig. 10.2).

Another *C. elegans* gene whose mutation confers increased lifespan and stress resistance is *clk-1* (*clk* for 'clock'), which encodes a mitochondrial protein involved in the synthesis of coenzyme Q. These mutants lack the normal *C. elegans* CoQ_9 (Fig. 1.8)

and must obtain CoQ from the diet (*E. coli* contains CoQ_8). The mutation impairs[22] electron transfer from complex I to complex III, but does not seem to affect metabolic activity much. The CoQ_9 precursor that accumulates (**demethoxyubiquinone**) may even be a better antioxidant than CoQ_9.[3]

C. elegans mutations that shorten lifespan have also been described,[18] but one must be careful here; any mutation that makes an animal sick might shorten its lifespan, and need not be affecting ageing *per se*. The gene *mev-1* encodes a subunit of cytochrome *b* in complex II of the electron transport chain, whereas *ctl-1* codes for a cytosolic catalase. Mutations in either of these may aggravate oxidative damage, the first by increasing mitochondrial ROS production and the second by decreasing an antioxidant defence. Mutants in *mev-1* show shortened lifespan, whereas *ctl-1* mutations are reported to shorten lifespan in some studies[17] but not

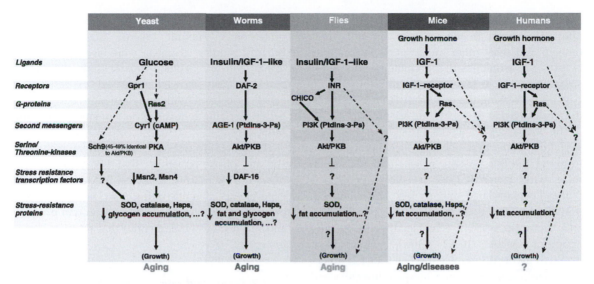

Figure 10.3 Conserved regulation of longevity. In yeast, worms and flies, the partially conserved glucose or insulin/IGF-I-like pathways decrease antioxidant enzymes and heat shock proteins, reduce the accumulation of glycogen or fat, and increase growth and mortality. Mutations that reduce the activity of these pathways extend longevity. In yeast and worms, the induction of stress-resistance genes is required for longevity extension. In mice, IGF-I activates signal transduction pathways analogous to the longevity regulatory pathways in lower eukaryotes and increases mortality. However, the intracellular mediators of life-span extension in GH- or IGF-I-deficient mice have not been identified. In humans, mutations or diseases that result in plasma GH or IGF-I deficiencies cause dwarfism, obesity and other adverse effects, but their effect on longevity is unclear. From *Science* **299**, 1342, 2003 by courtesy of the publishers and Dr Valter D. Longo. For details of the PI3 and Akt pathways consult Section 4.5.5.

others.[23] Knockout of peroxisomal catalase in *C. elegans* causes a drastic shortening of lifespan.[23]

10.3.1.1 *What about animals?*

Just as an insulin-like signalling pathway affects longevity in *C. elegans*, hormones and receptors may do the same in flies and mammals (Fig. 10.3). Indeed, CR in animals decreases insulin and IGF-1 levels. Unlike *C. elegans*, which has one gene (*daf-2*) encoding an insulin/IGF-like receptor, animals have separate receptors for insulin and IGF-1, affecting various aspects of metabolism.[24] Binding of IGF-1 to its receptors is involved in the actions of several molecules controlling energy metabolism, including growth hormone, insulin, IGF-2, leptin and adrenal steroid hormones. It also plays a key role in maintaining muscle mass. Completely inactivating the IGF-1 receptor is lethal in mice, but heterozygous knockouts seem normal and indeed live up to 30% longer, especially females.[25] Mice with a targeted disruption of the gene encoding insulin receptors in adipose tissue (but not in liver; loss of the gene there causes diabetes) have lifespan extended by about 18% (further

evidence that fat is linked to ageing). Several other mutations decreasing hormone production can increase lifespan; some **dwarf mouse strains** show abnormal development of the pituitary gland, have low levels of growth hormone, which in turn leads to low levels of IGF (growth hormone normally increases IGF-1 production), and live longer. One is the **Ames dwarf mouse**, which lives about 3 years and has a defect in a pituitary transcription factor that controls the secretion of growth hormone and insulin.[26] Over-expressing the gene encoding the protein **klotho** (which is involved in maintaining correct cellular Ca^{2+} signalling by controlling the activity of Ca^{2+} channels) in mice can increase lifespan, apparently by hindering insulin and IGF-1 signalling.[27]

Animals have FOXOs resembling DAF-16. The FOXO members **FOXO1**, **FOXO3a** and **FOXO4** are regulated by hormones and growth factors via the PI kinase–Akt pathway (Fig. 10.3; Section 4.5.5.2); when unphosphorylated they enter the nucleus and modulate the expression of genes affecting apoptosis, cell cycle arrest, differentiation, gluconeogenesis, fat breakdown, DNA repair and antioxidant defence (exactly which genes are affected depends on the cell type, the cell environment and what other transcription factors may be present). Mutations that promote insulin/IGF-1 signalling seem to favour cancer development, in part by decreasing the actions of FOXOs in inhibiting cell division or promoting apoptosis.[18]

The IGF receptor works through at least two signalling pathways, one of which involves two forms of the Shc protein, **p66shc** and **p52shc**. In mice with fewer IGF-1R receptors, p66Shc is underphosphorylated and so less active. Indeed, mutating *p66Shc* extends mouse lifespan by 30% and promotes resistance to oxidative stress and apoptosis (Section 10.4.1 below).[28] By contrast, overactivity of p53 in mice (Section 9.13.4.2) makes them age faster (shortened lifespan, hunchbacked spine, thinning of the skin, loss of muscle mass, poor wound healing and osteoporosis), possibly related to the role of this protein in cell senescence (Section 10.3.5 below).[29] Indeed, p53-mediated apoptosis requires p66shc (Section 10.4.1 below). These mice are however, less likely to develop cancer (given the role of *p53* as a tumour-suppressor gene) and do not show all features of ageing; brain amyloid deposits, cataracts or intestinal atrophy do not develop.[29]

Microarray analysis has been used by various groups to try to understand what happens during ageing. Genes whose expression is increased with age in mouse heart include those involved in carbohydrate metabolism, the cell cycle and synthesis of the extracellular matrix, whereas genes involved in fat metabolism showed less expression.[30] The ageing hypothalamus showed increased expression of genes encoding cell cycle regulatory proteins, proteins in the mitochondrial electron transport chain, chaperones, metallothionein and CuZn-SOD.[31] However, these changes were not generally seen in the mouse cortex.[31] Nevertheless, in both regions, there was decreased expression of genes encoding apoE, ion transport systems such as Na^+/K^+-ATPase and Ca^{2+}-ATPase and proteins involved in synaptic transmission.[31] In rat hippocampus, ageing seems associated with increased expression of genes involved in inflammation, cholesterol metabolism and iron metabolism (among others), whereas genes encoding proteins

involved in synaptic plasticity, chaperones and a proteasome subunit were downregulated.[32] Broadly similar changes were seen in human frontal cortex.[33] Skeletal muscle from old Rhesus monkeys also showed increased expression of genes associated with inflammation and less of genes encoding mitochondrial enzymes, including MnSOD.[34]

These data do not add up to a clear picture as yet, and please remember that any changes identified on microarray must be followed up with experiments demonstrating that increased gene expression gives rise to increased protein product, and (even more fundamental) that that product is important.

10.3.2 Genes and human longevity

Ageing might involve deleterious effects of the expression of genes in late life that confer benefit in early life, especially if they enhance reproductive success (e.g. keeping you alive to reproduce). An ability to rapidly store fat in the body when food is available is remarkably useful if food is periodically in short supply, as happened during human evolution. It's a nuisance in many countries now that food is free-flowing.[7] Genes that keep you alive when young so that you can reproduce and pass them on to the next generation will be selected for, whatever they do during the postreproductive years. The mutant gene responsible for Huntington's disease (Section 9.22.2) has been hypothesized to be selected for in this way;[35] young adults possessing it may be more fertile. Similar advantages may come from thalassaemia (Section 3.15.5.3) and idiopathic haemochromatosis (Section 3.15.5.2); the first helping to prevent early death from malaria and the second allowing iron to accumulate in the body when the diet is rich in it, which may favour survival of mother and baby during pregnancy if the food supply is erratic. A vigorous inflammatory response to kill pathogens is beneficial, even if overexuberant inflammation gives you cancer and cardiovascular diseases later in life.[7]

This concept is taken to extremes by the Pacific salmon.[16] It grows, reproduces once and then deteriorates fast and dies–it virtually 'falls apart'.

Since the chances of a Pacific salmon surviving to reproduce again are small, evolution did not favour 'holding back resources' for survival after reproduction. To quote[16] 'the rapid deterioration of Pacific salmon after mating is a natural byproduct of a life history that has been geared by natural selection to stake everything on a single bout of reproduction. As soon as the signal to reproduce is triggered, a massive effort is made to mobilize all available resources to maximize reproductive success, even if this leaves the adult so severely depleted or damaged that death ensues'.

10.3.3 Premature human ageing[36]

The human **progeroid** ('premature ageing') syndromes (**Hutchinson–Gilford syndrome** and **Werner's syndrome**) provide striking evidence that some genes have major effects on ageing (or what looks like ageing). Hutchinson–Gilford syndrome (sometimes called **progeria**) is a rare, dominantly inherited disease (one in every 4–8 million births). Newborns appear normal but at about 1 year old, severe growth retardation is observed. Loss of hair and subcutaneous fat make the skin appear old (Fig. 10.4) and pigmented 'age spots' are present. The subjects have an average weight of ~11 to 14 kg and a height of around 100 cm as teenagers. They have normal to above average intelligence but sadly many die by about 12 years, often due to heart failure or stroke consequential to accelerated atherosclerosis. The defective gene normally encodes (by alternative splicing of mRNA) two structural proteins in the nucleus, **lamin A** and **lamin C**. Their loss eventually causes nuclei to collapse, and there is impaired repair of DNA damage. Mice deficient in lamin A, or in the proteinase involved in its formation, similarly show 'premature ageing'. Excessive activation of p53 (Section 10.3.1.1) triggered by the nuclear abnormalities,[37] may also contribute. Defects in lamin may also occur randomly and spontaneously during normal ageing.[37A]

Werner's syndrome is a rare, autosomal-recessive mutation in a gene on chromosome 8. Affected individuals seem normal during childhood but stop growing during their teens. Greying and whitening of the hair occur at an early age, and the skin appears old with a scaly appearance. Patients develop

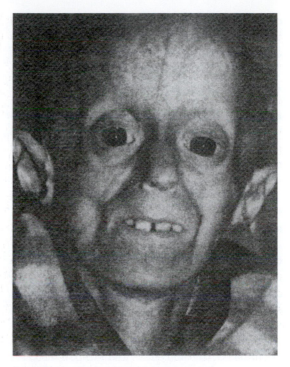

Figure 10.4 A 12-year-old girl with progeria.

early cataracts, tumours, bone demineralization and diabetes and show muscle atrophy, poor wound healing, poor gonad development and accelerated atherosclerosis. They usually die in their 40s from atherosclerosis-related conditions or cancer. The defective gene encodes an enzyme with helicase and exonuclease activities that is essential for genome stability and unwinding of the DNA double helix to allow transcription, replication and repair of damage, including oxidative damage.[38] Mice carrying mutations in the **XPD** gene, which encodes a helicase (Section 4.10.8), also show signs of premature ageing. Mutations in *XPD* in humans can cause **trichothiodystrophy**, characterized by some (but not all, e.g. no increased cancer incidence) features of premature ageing. Different mutations in the same gene can result in xeroderma pigmentosum (Section 4.10.8.2). Patients with **Cockayne syndrome** (Section 4.10.8.2) also show some features of accelerated ageing; the affected gene again encodes a helicase.

However, the progeroid syndromes are not fully representative of 'accelerated human ageing'. Features of normal ageing absent in progeria include increased frequency of cancer, cataracts and bone demineralization. Similarly, Werner's syndrome has been called a 'caricature of ageing', although there is an increased risk of cancer and cataract development.

10.3.4 Mechanisms of caloric restriction[3,18]

How does CR work? Important clues have come from studies with the yeast *S. cerevisiae*. It produces progeny by budding, leaving 'old' material (including oxidized proteins)[39] in the mother cell. Eventually the mother cells become senescent, usually after about 20 to 25 divisions. To quote Nemoto and Finkel from *Nature* **429**, 149 (2004), 'the middle-aged yeast cell is slower, fatter and less interested in reproduction', rather like many middle-aged humans. When glucose is plentiful, yeast cells bud rapidly, and then senesce. If glucose is restricted, cell division slows, stress resistance mechanisms are upregulated, lifespan extends and reproduction slows or ceases. The response to glucose involves protein kinases (Fig. 10.3); if genes encoding them are mutated, division slows and lifespan increases even when glucose is plentiful. This increase can be blocked by further mutations that impair either NAD^+ production or the activity of an **NAD^+-dependent histone deacetylase enzyme** called **Sir2 (silent information regulator 2)**. It catalyses cleavage of nicotinamide from the ribose ring of NAD^+ and attaches the acetyl group from the protein to the rest, forming *O*-acetyl-ADP-ribose. Despite its name, Sir2 is not specific for histones and can remove acetyl groups from other proteins. Overexpression of the *Sir2* gene decreases yeast senescence even when glucose is plentiful, whereas inactivation of it accelerates senescence. *C. elegans* has a gene resembling *Sir2*, which encodes a component of the DAF pathway, before DAF-16. Indeed, overexpression of *Sir2* in *C. elegans* increases lifespan, an effect reversed by knocking out *daf-16*. What about animals? Present there as well, for example **SIRT1** is a human deacetylase enzyme that closely resembles the yeast and *C. elegans* proteins—it is one of at least seven human enzymes of this type. It may have several metabolic roles, including regulating liver glucose metabolism. Indeed, Sir2-like proteins (**sirtuins**) with deactylase activity seem to be present in all organisms, from *E. coli* to humans. The phenolic

compound **resveratrol** (Fig. 3.33) activates Sir2 and SIRT1 and can increase the lifespan of yeast, *Drosophila* and *C. elegans*.[40] Would drinking wine increase human lifespan? Sadly, probably not; human plasma levels of resveratrol are low in wine drinkers since there is rapid metabolism by sulphation and conjugation with glucuronic acid.[41] But console yourself; moderate wine intake may be good for you in other ways (Sections 3.22 and 8.8).

The Sir2 and SIRT1 enzymes act on several substrates, including p53, deacetylation of which decreases its proapoptotic activity (Section 9.13.4.2). For example, in PC12 cells,[42] withdrawal of nutrients activates FOXO3a that then promotes increased expression of SIRT1. The activity of animal FOXOs can be modulated by acetylation that is reversed by sirtuins, and sometimes this deacetylation can over-ride the nuclear exclusion effects of phosphorylation. The overall effect of SIRT1 may be to increase the ability of FOXOs and p53 to induce cell cycle arrest and raise antioxidant defences, but decrease their proapoptotic effects.[43] Sirtuins are involved in the neuroprotective effects of CR in some animals (Section 9.16.5), and possibly also in the increased physical activity of CR animals.

By what mechanism does CR affect the sirtuins? Nicotinamide and NADH inhibit them. In yeast, CR relieves this by decreasing NADH levels (due to less glucose metabolism; Fig. 1.7) and/or by increasing the levels of an enzyme (**Pnc1**) that hydrolyses nicotinamide to nicotinic acid, which can then be used to make more NAD^+.

Caloric restriction in rats increases tissue levels of SIRT-1 and eNOS; rises in the latter may be involved in raising SIRT1 and promoting mitochondrial biogenesis in CR animals.[45] One effect of raising SIRT-1 levels is to cause fat mobilization from adipose tissue, by antagonizing the action of PPAR-γ (Section 9.3).[46] Indeed, agonists of PPAR receptors can 'mimic' caloric restriction in some systems.[47] In *Drosophila*, CR elevates levels of Sir2, an effect essential to produce the age-enhancing effect.[48] However in *C. elegans* Sir2 does not seem involved in the effect of CR; although the increased lifespan produced by overexpressing *Sir2* requires *daf-16*, the effects of CR are still seen if *daf-16* is knocked out.[18]

10.3.5 Telomeres and cellular senescence[38,49]

Telomeres are found at the ends of chromosomes in eukaryotic cells. In most eukaryotes, they contain multiple (several thousand in humans) DNA base repeat sequences (TTAGGG in humans) that are generated by an RNA-containing enzyme, **telomerase**. The RNA provides a template for the addition of the repeat sequences to DNA. Telomerase activity is regulated by **telomere repeat binding proteins** (TRBP) that decrease telomerase activity when the correct length has been obtained. Why are telomeres needed? DNA polymerases use the information in one DNA strand to make another. However, they need a primer (usually RNA) to start off the new strand; it attaches at the 5′ end of the DNA sequence being copied (Section 4.8.1). Without telomeres, there would be a loss of DNA at each round of replication; the primer is removed from the new strand and the sequence of bases in the DNA to which it was bound will not be present in the new DNA strand. Up to 200 base pairs are lost from telomeres at each chromosomal division. Telomeres also protect the chromosome ends from damage or fusion, helping to maintain genomic stability. Mice lacking telomerase eventually become sterile and show some features of premature ageing.

It was reported in 1961 that mammalian primary cells undergo only a certain number of cell divisions when cultured in the laboratory. For example, fibroblasts taken from a human foetus will divide only about 50 times. This was called the **Hayflick limit**, after the pioneer in ageing biology who first described it. When it is reached, the cells no longer respond to mitogens despite the fact that receptors for them can still be present (although levels of these receptors may sometimes fall) and are said to be in **senescence** (a terminal G_0 state of non-division). Senescent human cells have, on average, lost about half of their telomeric length and show accumulation of oxidized and ubiquitinated proteins and decreased proteasome activity.[50] Hence telomere shortening has been suggested to be a 'molecular clock' of the ageing process. Short telomeres have been proposed to trigger senescence by signalling cell cycle checkpoints involving p53 and sometimes p16. Senescence is also accelerated (probably not via actions on telomeres) in cells overexpressing oncogenes, as one mechanism deterring cancer development (Fig. 9.16). For example, the *ras* oncogenes may accelerate ROS production that can increase p53 levels and trigger senescence (although under different circumstances ROS can be proproliferative (Sections 9.13.5.3 and 9.13.6).

Telomerase is absent from most somatic cells (exceptions include germline cells, bone marrow stem cells and the cells derived from them). By contrast, it is present in many malignant tumours, suggesting that telomere elongation is involved in inappropriate cell replication and tumour growth. If cultured cells are exposed to certain viruses (e.g. Epstein–Barr virus, human papilloma virus), many cells will die, but 'immortal' cells that continue to grow are soon selected; most such cells have telomerase and do not undergo telomere shortening. Thus inactivation of telomerase is one approach to cancer therapy. Genes affecting telomere length or the rate of telomere loss could obviously influence the ageing process at the cellular level. Cells from patients with progeria or Werner's syndrome, for example, have pronounced shortening of telomeres.

10.3.5.1 *An artefact of cell culture?*[51,52]

Is senescence of cells grown in the laboratory relevant *in vivo* or is it purely an artefact of cell culture? Cell culture imposes oxidative stress (Section 1.11); indeed, growing cells at low pO_2 increases the number of cell divisions and delays senescence, which is well-known to be one consequence of oxidative stress (Section 4.2.3). Oxidative stress causes DNA damage and can accelerate the loss of telomeres, as well as protein damage (indeed, increasing proteasome activity can delay senescence).[50] It follows that telomeres are not a fixed 'molecular clock' of ageing–they respond to stress also. Indeed, in mouse embryonic fibroblasts in culture, oxidative stress appears more important than telomere loss as a cause of senescence. For human fibroblasts, both are probably involved. For example, decreasing CuZnSOD activity in human fibroblasts in culture by RNA interference led to senescence[51] involving activation of p53, whereas overexpression of SOD delayed senescence and telomere shortening.[54] Accelerated telomere shortening in cells from patients with ataxia telangiectasia

(Section 4.10.8.2) also appears to involve oxidative stress.[55] The G-rich nature of telomeres may make them sites of oxidative damage, since G is the DNA base most sensitive to attack by RS (Section 4.8.2). Oxidative damage to G can also weaken the association of TRBP with the telomeric DNA.[56]

The older an animal from which cells are taken, the fewer cell divisions occur in culture, suggesting some relationship of senescence to ageing. Consistent with this, overexpression of telomerase in *C. elegans* increases lifespan, an effect that requires DAF-16. However, most cells in *C. elegans* and other animals are not undergoing division anyway and so are hard to identify as senescent or not. Possibly the extra telomerase is working by promoting stress resistance. Increased levels of a **β-galactosidase** enzyme (and to some extent elevated p16 levels) are thought to be markers of senescence. In some (but not all) studies β-galactosidase has been detected in human skin, to an extent increasing with age. It has also been reported in certain cells within atherosclerotic lesions, venous ulcers, tissues around liver cancers, arthritic joints and pre-malignant tissues from both human and mouse (Fig. 9.17).[49,52] Introduction of telomerase into some cell lines in culture can delay senescence and decrease β-galactosidase expression, although one must be careful to check that antioxidant defences do not also change. Why β-galactosidase appears, and what it does, is uncertain.

It is worth noting that senescent cells are not necessarily harmless. For example, senescent fibroblasts secrete abnormally high levels of matrix metalloproteinases, growth factors and cytokines. This might contribute to tissue damage/local inflammation, creating an environment that favours the spread of malignant cells and promotes cancer.[38]

10.4 Oxidative damage: a common link between all the theories of ageing?

10.4.1 Introduction to the free radical theory of ageing

An important concept[18] emerging from studies on *C. elegans*, flies and rodents is that insulin/IGF1 affects lifespan through mechanisms involving protein kinases and FOXOs. The effects on lifespan may be 'by-products' of the ability of these pathways to modulate resistance to stress. Do RS and antioxidants contribute? Let us see.

The **free-radical theory of ageing** was introduced in 1956 by Denham Harman, who proposed that ageing results from random deleterious damage to tissues by free radicals. In subsequent papers, he focused on mitochondria as both free-radical generators and targets of damage, and Miquel *et al.* proposed a mitochondrial theory of ageing (progressive damage to mitochondrial DNA, for example by ROS, leading to mitochondrial dysfunction that affects the whole cell). We now know that many RS are not free radicals, so that Harman's theory should perhaps be renamed the **oxidative damage theory of ageing** or **the RS theory of ageing**.

Harman's theory has some immediately attractive features in relation to explanations of ageing:

1. Reactive species are produced during normal metabolism, sometimes accidentally and sometimes for useful purposes. Antioxidant defences do not remove them completely, so that ongoing oxidative damage to DNA, lipids and proteins is detectable in aerobes (Table 4.1). Indeed, calculations are consistent with a role for oxidative DNA damage in the age-related development of cancer (Section 9.13.5.1).

2. Production of RS can be envisaged as the consequence of genes selected because they confer benefit in early life, for example by facilitating signal transduction. When humans first crowded together in cities, infectious disease became a major threat. Phagocyte production of RS is beneficial in the short term by decreasing the risk of death from infections before or during the reproductive years. Evolution doesn't care if overexuberant RS production gives you cancer decades later.[7]

3. The theory explains the relation between metabolic rate, O_2 consumption and lifespan. If a fixed percentage of the O_2 consumed forms ROS, then the more O_2 consumed per unit mass of tissue, the more ROS will be made. Indeed, urinary excretion of 8OHdG and other DNA base damage products was reported to correlate with metabolic rate and lifespan in different mammals[57] and prevention of flight activity in houseflies (Fig. 10.1) decreased levels of oxidative damage to mitochondrial proteins.[2] Cooling-down cold blooded animals or stopping flies from flying presumably decreases ROS production.

But suppose that the percentage of O_2 that forms ROS is not fixed, but variable. Then there will be anomalies, but we can often learn a lot from 'exceptions to the rule'. One such anomaly is discussed in paragraph (5) below. Another is the 'rat/bird paradox'. Total O_2 consumption at rest is higher in pigeon and canary than in rat, but they have different mean lifespans: (rat 3 years, pigeon 35 years, canary 24 years). It turns out that mitochondria from avian tissues generate less ROS *in vitro* than rat mitochondria, providing a possible explanation of the difference.[58] Even in the same species, individuals vary. A positive association between **metabolic intensity** (food intake per gram of body mass) and lifespan was observed in mice, but no relationship of lifespan to the actual body mass. Mice with the highest metabolic intensity had greater O_2 consumption, but the inner membranes of their skeletal muscle mitochondria had greater proton conductance,[59] presumably leading to less ROS formation (Section 1.10.6).

4. Mitochondria are well-established as a major source of ROS in eukaryotic cells, although the expression of uncoupling proteins that regulate ROS formation (Section 1.10.6) is an important variable.[59] Several studies suggest that the electron transport chain gets leakier with age[60] and produces more ROS. If so, this can impact on nuclear gene transcription (Section 4.5.7). Levels of mitochondrial H_2O_2-producing enzymes, such as monoamine oxidase, may increase with age in certain tissues. Indeed, treatment of rats with the MAO inhibitor deprenyl (Section 9.19) was reported to increase lifespan and raise brain CuZn-SOD levels.[61] Many studies have reported increased oxidation of mtDNA as compared with nuclear DNA, and that mtDNA 8OHdG levels increase with age. However, methodological problems in 8OHdG analysis in mtDNA have left the issue of the correctness of these data open (Sections 1.10.5 and 5.13.4). Similar assay problems with SOD make it unclear as to whether or not mitochondrial SOD activities fall with age.[62]

Certainly, mtDNA accumulates defects with age, but these may not be caused by oxidative stress.

Hence whether RS-related mitochondrial defects are a cause of ageing seems uncertain. Mitochondria within the same tissue in old animals can be heterogeneous in their levels of oxidative damage and respiratory chain activities.[60,63] Thus in aged rat heart, only mitochondria between the myofibrils have impaired complex III and IV activities and increased ROS production, whereas mitochondria just beneath the plasma membrane were unaffected.[60] Mitochondria possess several copies of their mtDNA and are degraded after a few weeks by sequestration into lysosomes, diminishing the risk that they will fail completely.[64] Nevertheless, studies in mice show the potential of mtDNA defects to produce an ageing phenotype. For example, when mitochondrial DNA polymerase is mutated to remove its error-correcting function, so that point mutations and deletions accumulate, the mice show some features of accelerated ageing (shortened lifespan, reduced subcutaneous fat, hair loss, osteoporosis, curvature of the spine, decreased fertility), although oxidative DNA damage did not seem to contribute much.[65] Similar mutations have been found in a few human cases of **progressive external ophthalmoplegia**; patients show paralysis of the eye muscles and various other tissue defects, as well as increased levels of mtDNA mutations.[65] Mitochondrial dysfunction is especially evident during ageing in flies (Fig. 10.1).

5. Caloric restriction in rodents and monkeys (in so far as the latter have been studied) often decreases levels of oxidative damage to DNA, lipids and proteins and attenuates age-related declines in repair systems, such as DNA repair and the proteasome (Section 10.4.4 below).[66] It decreases plasma levels of glucose, IGF1 and insulin. Plasma ascorbate levels can fall, perhaps because ascorbate is made from glucose and this substrate may be less available.[67]

How does CR work? Lots of ways (Section 10.3.4), but decreases in oxidative damage may contribute. It seems to decrease mitochondrial ROS generation and levels of oxidative damage to mtDNA[66] One study on rat liver mitochondria suggested that this involved increased proton leaks across the inner membrane, an effect reversed by infusing insulin into the animals.[68] However another group, while confirming decreased ROS production in CR animals, did not detect a rise in proton leak.[69] Caloric restriction of yeast also decreased mitochondrial ROS generation, although it raised mitochondrial respiration rates.[70]

6. The long-lived *age-1* and *daf-2* mutants of *C. elegans* have elevated antioxidant defences (cytosolic and peroxisomal catalases, CuZnSOD, MnSOD) and increased resistance to agents inducing oxidative stress, such as paraquat. By contrast, *mev-1* mutants make more ROS and lifespan is shortened. Active DAF-16 promotes the transcription of genes encoding catalases, CuZnSOD and MnSOD. Do these changes contribute to the increased longevity? Yes, since antisense RNAs directed against the relevant genes prevented rises in enzyme activity and decreased the lifespan of *daf-2* mutants.[18,19] Mild heat shock also activates DAF-16, which is in turn required for the synthesis of some Hsps. Indeed, the lifespan of *C. elegans* and flies is extended by transient heat shock. This is an example of **hormesis**—a low level of a stress leads to subsequent protection against bigger insults.[18] By contrast, in *clk-1* mutants ROS production in mitochondria appears to be decreased rather than antioxidant defences raised.[3] Similarly, in animals, deacetylation of FOXOs by SIRT-1, or impaired phosphorylation of them, increases their transcriptional activity and can raise cellular levels of antioxidants such as MnSOD.

7. Mutating *p66shc* in mice not only extends lifespan but also promotes resistance to oxidative stress (Section 10.3.1.1); these mice show lower F_2-IP, 8OHdG and 3-nitrotyrosine levels and are resistant to atherosclerosis induced by a high-fat diet.[71] Normally p66Shc suppresses FOXO activity by promoting phosphorylation. If p66shc no longer works, FOXO causes transcription of antioxidant defence enzymes. Indeed, p66Shc is required for oxidative stress-activated p53 to induce apoptosis; cells from mice lacking it are resistant to apoptosis induced by ischaemia, withdrawal of growth factors or paraquat.[71] It has been proposed that p66shc is a redox protein that interacts with the mitochondrial

electron transport chain to generate ROS.[71] Hence ROS can act both upstream and downstream of p53 (Section 9.13.4.2).

8. Ames dwarf mice show low levels of oxidative DNA damage and protein carbonyls in liver and appear to be resistant to oxidative stress. Increased activities of CuZnSOD and catalase in several tissues have been reported.[26]

Calculations by Cutler *et al.*[72] suggest that longer-lived species have better antioxidant protection in relation to rates of O_2 uptake than shorter-lived species. Thus the SOD activity of human liver, expressed per unit metabolic rate, seems higher than that of other primates and much higher than that of other mammals. Since SODs appear to have similar structure and function in all animals, Cutler *et al.*[72] suggested that a change in gene regulation has allowed synthesis of higher *relative* cellular SOD concentrations in humans, contributing to longevity (humans live much longer than other primates). In other words, at least some of the genes encoding antioxidants may be 'longevity-determining' genes (Table 10.2). However, changes in SOD alone might not be enough to increase lifespan (Section 10.4.2 below) and application of similar analyses to other antioxidants did not identify a clear-cut pattern; GPx and GSH were not positively correlated with lifespan—in fact, correlations tended to be negative. Perhaps the peroxiredoxins (Section 3.11) should be examined. Or perhaps the secret of longevity is to make fewer ROS—then you don't need as many antioxidants!

9. Differences in RS production and antioxidant defence may help explain the relationship of gender to lifespan (Section 3.20).

So how might RS affect lifespan? They could:

1. cause oxidative damage to important molecules;
2. promote apoptosis or senescence that impair tissue renewal; senescent cells might also contribute to tissue damage (Section 10.3.5);
3. generate inappropriate cellular signalling (Section 10.4.7 below), perhaps even activation of the insulin pathway (Section 4.5.12);
4. cause, or contribute to, age-related diseases.

Table 10.2 Genetic changes that could affect oxidative damage

System/ factor affected by genetic change	Examples
Antioxidant defence enzymes	SOD, catalase, GPx, peroxiredoxins, haem oxygenases
Low-molecular-mass antioxidants	Enzymes synthesizing and catabolizing GSH, ascorbate (non-primates), urate (non-primates), carnosine, bilirubin, biliverdin, etc.
Repair systems	Proteasome, Lon proteinase, other proteinases, DNA repair, PHGPx, enzymes that metabolize cytotoxic aldehydes (e.g. GSTs), chaperones
Availability of transition-metal ions 'catalytic' for free-radical reactions	Transferrin, ferritin, caeruloplasmin, metallothionein, haemopexin, haptoglobin, Fe^{2+} transporters, Cu^{2+}-ATPases, lactoferrin, haem oxygenases
Targets of oxidative damage	Alterations in conformation of proteins, DNA, chromatin, membranes, lipoproteins, etc. that make it easier or harder for RS to attack sensitive targets; changes in DNA methylation, histone acetylation, etc.
Uptake or processing of dietary antioxidants	Vitamins C and E, rate and type of carotenoid cleavage in gut, flavonoid uptake and metabolism
Reactive species production	Types of cytochrome P450, 'leak rates' from mitochondrial electron transport, levels of NOX and other oxidases producing $O_2^{\bullet-}$ and/or H_2O_2, myeloperoxidase, other peroxidases
Rate at which oxidatively damaged cells die	P53, *bcl*-2, *bax*, other genes affecting cell cycle and apoptosis/ necrosis/ senescence

10.4.2 Testing the theory: altering antioxidant levels[73]

Attempts have been made to test the free radical theory of ageing by examining the effect of antioxidants on the longevity of various organisms. Thiol compounds (such as glutathione and mercaptoethylamine), chain-breaking lipid soluble antioxidants such as BHT, α-tocopherol and **Santoquin** (ethoxyquin; Table 10.13, below) and SOD mimetics (Section 10.6.4 below) have often been used. Thus, in the laboratory, α-tocopherol prolongs the lifespan of *Drosophila*, *C. elegans* and the rotifer *Philodina*, the SOD mimetics EUK-134 and EUK-8 extend the lifespan of *C. elegans* (in some but not all studies)[74] but not of houseflies,[75] and the nitrone LPBNAH (Section 10.6.5 below) made *Philodina* live longer.[76] Interestingly, *C. elegans* lifespan was increased by *removing* coenzyme Q from the diet of adult worms, and it was hypothesized that *E. coli* CoQ$_8$ might even be pro-oxidant.[77] By contrast, feeding CoQ$_{10}$ increased lifespan.[77]

Sadly, the effects of administered antioxidants on the lifespan of mammals are small or zero, for example lipoic acid or coenzyme Q had no effect on lifespan in mice.[30] High-dose α-tocopherol has no

effect on lifespan in rodents,[78] although it has sometimes been reported to diminish the decline in immune response with age.[79] Early claims that antioxidants such as mercaptoethylamine and Santoquin raise the lifespan of mice by up to 18% have been challenged. It appears that some of the control animals did not live as long as they should have done; perhaps their diet was bad or they were stressed, so that they died earlier. Thus the antioxidants might have acted to diminish oxidative damage produced by poor diet or environmental stress rather than increasing 'real' lifespan. We have no idea what is the *optimal* diet for small organisms such as *Philodina*. The antioxidant (e.g. α-tocopherol) content of laboratory animal diets is another important variable, and has tended to increase over the past three decades. In some older studies, effects of antioxidants were probably corrections of dietary deficiencies that shortened lifespan rather than real effects on lifespan in an optimally nourished animal.

Another problem is that these studies *assumed* that antioxidants would decrease oxidative damage in healthy animals, without testing it. Sadly, they often do not, rendering a lack of effect inconclusive. In addition, any agent that does work might do so by other mechanisms, for example resveratrol via the sirtuin pathway (Section 10.3.4) and PBN as an anti-inflammatory agent (Section 10.6.5 below). Excessive dosing of animals with an antioxidant might decrease the rate of synthesis or uptake of 'natural' antioxidants, so that the total 'tissue antioxidant potential' remains unaltered. For example, feeding female rats a diet rich in BHT decreased liver α-tocopherol content.[80] Similarly, inhibiting SOD or catalase in houseflies using aminotriazole or diethyldithiocarbamate led to compensatory changes in other antioxidants.[81] In mice, lipoic acid administration decreased the expression of genes encoding chaperones, whilst coenzyme Q downregulated genes encoding peroxiredoxin 5 as well.[30] However, a combination of lipoic acid and N-acetylcarnitine was reported to decrease 8OHdG levels and improve cognitive function in old rats.[82] This mixture is sold as a health supplement, *Juvenon*®. Only time will tell if it has value to humans.

10.4.2.1 *Transgenic organisms: the picture gets blurred*[75,83]

A better approach might be to genetically manipulate antioxidant defences and examine the effects on lifespan; such an approach confirmed that antioxidant enzymes are important in the life extension of *daf-2* mutants of *C. elegans* (Section 10.4.1) What about animals? 'Knockout' mice lacking MnSOD do not live long enough for ageing rates to be examined, but mice lacking CuZnSOD and GPx1 may become useful models. However, rodents overexpressing SOD do not live longer, nor do mice heterozygous for defects in MnSOD have shorter lifespans despite increased levels of 8OHdG and more cancer development.[84] It is, of course, essential when interpreting any such data to check that genetic alterations do not lead to secondary changes in other antioxidant defences, or to behavioural changes (e.g. impaired appetite) that can influence lifespan, for example by inducing CR. It must also be shown that the manipulation did decrease oxidative damage, for example overexpressing SOD to too great an extent may have the opposite effect! (Section 3.14.2). The subcellular location of the antioxidant can be important; overexpression of catalase in the mito-

chondria of heart and skeletal muscle increased lifespan in mice, but not if the catalase was targeted to the nucleus or peroxisomes.[85] The mitochondria showed less 8OHdG and seemed better-preserved structurally during ageing. The tissue distribution can also be important, as we see below.

Much transgenic work has been carried out on *Drosophila*, but results are variable and can differ from mammals. For example, increased expression of MnSOD and catalase in *Drosophila* mitochondria *shortened* lifespan.[85] In one set of studies, global overexpression of CuZnSOD by 32 to 42% had little effect on lifespan and the ability to withstand oxidative stress, although selective overexpression in motor neurons, (which normally have low CuZnSOD levels in *Drosophila*) did appear to increase longevity. Similarly, overexpressing γ-glutamylcysteine synthetase (γ-GCS) to increase GSH levels in neurons raised lifespan more than global expression.[86] Global overexpression of catalase alone did not affect lifespan in *Drosophila*. However, when genes for SOD and catalase were both globally overexpressed, lifespan of *Drosophila* increased by up to one third.[75] The normal age-related loss of function was decreased, and the flies showed lower levels of protein carbonyls and 8OHdG, and increased resistance to DNA damage by ionizing radiation. They were more active than control flies and their calculated 'lifetime O_2 consumption per unit body mass' had increased. By contrast, *Drosophila* lacking CuZnSOD show decreased lifespan. Overexpression of methionine sulphoxide reductase or MnSOD has increased *Drosophila* longevity in some studies.

The extent of overexpression (more is not necessarily better) and its tissue and subcellular location are critical variables in explaining different experimental results. Another is the lifespan of the control flies—the most dramatic effects are usually found when this is relatively short, whereas, when it is longer, effects of overexpressing antioxidants tend to disappear.[75] This is reminiscent of the early studies with antioxidants in rodents discussed above—one wonders why control flies in different laboratories live for variable times. Thus we cannot yet reach a firm conclusion from transgenic experiments upon flies or rodents.

10.4.3 'Rapidly-ageing' mice

Several such animals have been used to study oxidative damage. Examples include the **OXYS rat** (bred in Russia) and the **senescence accelerated mice**. They have shortened lifespan, appear to age rapidly and show increased oxidative damage to DNA, lipids and proteins. Various antioxidants can decrease oxidative damage and slow neurocognitive decline in these animals.[87,88] However, are they demonstrating 'real ageing' or are they just sick animals? We don't know yet.

10.4.4 Does antioxidant protection fail with age?

Generally, the answer is no, but with exceptions.[58] There are no marked falls in antioxidant defence with age in human or other mammalian tissues and some increases have been reported, for example α-tocopherol: PUFA ratios rise with age in rat tissues and some human cells (e.g. erythrocytes)[89] and SOD activities can rise in some tissues of ageing animals whilst falling in others.[90] However, the ability to increase antioxidant defence enzymes under stress may be more affected by age. For example, in liver of old rats Nrf2 (Section 4.5.10) levels were subnormal, which impairs activation of the ARE system.[91] However, the reverse seemed to be true in memory T-lymphocytes from old mice.[92] Of course, if RS production increases and antioxidants do not (or not enough), damage can still occur. Mitochondrial ROS production may rise (see above); another factor may be increases in potentially pro-oxidant enzymes with age, such as XO,[93] monoamine oxidase (Section 10.4.1), urate oxidase[94] (not in primates), NOX enzymes, and MPO.[95]

Several reports indicate that GSH/GSSG ratios, especially in mitochondria, are lower in at least some tissues from old *Drosophila* and rodents, and more protein–SSG adducts are present in the tissues. Murine T-lymphocytes are one exception![92] Falls in GSH could be due to increased consumption of this thiol and/or to decreased γ-GCS activity, perhaps in part[91] relating to impaired Nrf2. Caloric restriction appears to attenuate these changes,[96] and Ames dwarf mice have increased γ-GCS activity.[26] Brain tissue from old rats showed increased expression of Hsps, correlated with falls in GSH;[97] indeed rises in Hsps have been reported in several old organisms. In elderly humans, blood GSH levels and GSH/GSSG ratios seem to fall,[98] but it is hard to know what this signifies—is it less release by the liver and/or faster clearance (Section 3.9.3)? Carnosine (Section 3.18.7) levels are reported to decline with age in human and rat skeletal muscles.[99] Elderly subjects seem to require more vitamin C in their diets to maintain the same plasma levels, possibly due to a fall in SVCT1 levels.[100] Ascorbate levels in lymphocytes may also fall with age, correlated with drops in GSH (Section 3.20.1.2).

10.4.5 Does oxidative damage increase with age?

Measurements of biomarkers in humans and other animals suggest that, in general, oxidative damage does not increase enormously with age. Nevertheless, there are some changes. Rhesus monkeys showed higher levels of HNE-modified proteins in skeletal muscle with age, an effect attenuated by CR.[101] Nitrated proteins do not increase with age in Rhesus monkey muscle or rat brain,[102] but they do in the heart of rats; these nitrated proteins include aldolase, α-enolase, creatine kinase, MnSOD, the Ca^{2+}-ATPase of the sarcoplasmic reticulum and GAPDH.[103,104] *C. elegans* accumulates protein carbonyls with age; the rate is decreased in *age-1* and *daf-2* mutants, but increased in *mev-1* mutants or if *daf-16* is knocked out.[105] One target of oxidative damage (why we don't know) is **vitellogenin-6**, a yolk protein produced during egg laying.

Older rats have been claimed to exhale more ethane and pentane than younger ones and to show higher F_2-IP levels in plasma, liver and kidney.[106] However, increases in F_4- or F_2-IPs and HNE were not obvious in normal brain from old rats or humans.[107] Levels of protein carbonyls, MDA, HNE and 8OHdG in the brains and other tissues of Mongolian gerbils, rodents and humans show a trend (sometimes not that clear-cut if one examines the data carefully) to rise with age and, in the aged mouse brain, carbonyl levels correlate with loss of cognitive function.[82,108] Protein carbonyl levels in fibroblasts cultured from patients with progeria or

Werner's syndrome are strikingly elevated.[108] There is an accumulation of AGE products as years advance in such human proteins as collagen and crystallins, which have a slow turnover rate; their formation involves both oxidation and glycation (Section 9.4.4).

10.4.5.1 *Be cautious with global biomarkers*

If oxidative damage is focused on only certain molecular targets and/or organelles (e.g. mitochondria), large changes in oxidative damage or antioxidant levels at those sites could be 'swamped out' by lack of change elsewhere if the whole cell or tissue is assayed with 'global' biomarkers such as 8OHdG or carbonyls. For example in ageing human brain, rises in 8OHdG were particularly marked in the promoters of several genes whose expression is decreased, such as some involved in synaptic transmission and long-term potentiation.[33] In houseflies, oxidative damage to only two mitochondrial proteins, aconitase and adenine nucleotide translocase, accumulates with age.[2] Heavy oxidative damage to only a few proteins is seen in stressed *S. cerevisiae* cells[39] and in the brains of SAMP8 mice[88] and human AD patients (Section 9.20). Age-dependent selective increases in cardiolipin oxidation in rat heart mitochondria have been reported (Section 4.11.2.1). In rat liver, the protein **carbonic anhydrase III** seems to undergo exceptionally rapid oxidative modification with age, and falls in aconitase with age have also been observed in mitochondria from some rodent tissues. Carbonic anhydrase III is a peculiar protein; its carbonic anhydrase activity is low and knockout of the gene produces no phenotype in mice. It also undergoes glutathionylation (Section 3.9.6) with age and is oxidized even faster in the livers of mice lacking CuZnSOD.[109]

Levels of oxidative damage are a balance between damage rates and speed of repair (or replacement) of damaged molecules. Hence rises in damage levels could involve failure of repair systems with age. Indeed, both Lon proteinase (Section 4.14.2) and proteasome activities decline with age in some animal tissues, especially brain.[110,111] In mice, the decline in Lon in liver was associated with increased levels of oxidized mitochondrial proteins, including aconitase.[112] As for DNA, a positive correlation between the efficiency of DNA-repair enzymes (including PARP-1) and species longevity has been claimed, and DNA repair activity has been reported to decline in old animals in several, but not all, studies.[113] Methionine sulphoxide reductase (Section 4.13.1) may also be important; overexpression of Msr-A in *Drosophila* significantly extended lifespan,[75] whereas mice lacking it died earlier.

Overall therefore, the balance of evidence supports a rise in oxidative damage with age, although there are some contradictory data. Damage in the promoters of essential genes, or directly inhibiting important proteins, may be the key events. As an interesting aside, Stadman and Levine[114] found increased protein carbonyls with age in rats. Ten years later, they could not repeat this using the same rats, from the same supplier, fed on the same diet. One clue, the new batch of rats was living about 30% longer.

10.4.6 Lipofuscin and ceroid; fluorescent 'red herrings'?[115]

One of the earliest pieces of evidence put forward to support the free-radical theory of ageing was the presence in old tissues of **age pigments**, initially thought to be accumulated end-products of lipid peroxidation. The first description of the intracellular pigment **lipofuscin** was made in 1842 by Hannover, who described it in neurons. Lipofuscin was later found to accumulate, in amounts increasing with age, in many tissues of humans and other animals, including rats, *C. elegans*, *Drosophila* and houseflies. It is also found in several fungi. In general, the most metabolically active tissues show most lipofuscin deposition. In houseflies, the lipofuscin content of muscles increases with flight activity; flies that are more active live for shorter times and accumulate it faster. There is little lipofuscin in human heart up to the second decade of life, but it then accumulates at a rate of about 0.3% of the total heart volume in each further decade of life. On the other hand, lipofuscin appears earlier in some tissues, such as the spinal cord. Large motor neurons of human centenarians may be more than 70% occupied by 'age pigments'.

Lipofuscin varies in colour from red, through yellow, to dark-brown, and occurs intracellularly as granules 1 to 5 μm in diameter bounded by a single membrane. Both the number and size of granules increase with age. Many different lipids are present in the pigments, including triglyceride, phospholipids and cholesterol, and an equally wide variety of proteins. For example, AGE-modified proteins are frequently found, lipofuscin within the retinal pigment epithelium contains large amounts of retinal derivatives (Section 6.10), and much of the lipofuscin protein in most NCL patients is a mitochondrial protein, subunit c (Section 9.22.4). Lipofuscin granules are rich in metal ions such as zinc, copper and, especially, iron. They seem to be the end-product of lysosomal catabolism of unwanted cellular components (**autophagy**), such as damaged mitochondria. Oxidation may be accelerated in the lysosomal environment by low pH and the presence of transition metal ions. Extraction of lipofuscin granules with organic solvents solubilizes part of them, and the resulting solution has fluorescence characteristics similar to those of the conjugated Schiff bases, dihydropyridine dicarbaldehydes, and aldehyde polymers formed during lipid peroxidation (Section 5.14.10). However, these extracted fluorophores display blue fluorescence, whereas microscopists observe green to yellow fluorescence from lipofuscin *in situ*. Hydroxynonenal does not appear to be involved in lipofuscin fluorescence, but conjugates of MDA with protein thiol groups might be.[116]

Another pigment that superficially resembles lipofuscin is **ceroid**, a term introduced in 1942. Like lipofuscin, ceroid originates from uptake of material into lysosomes. The ceroid content of animal tissues rises if they are fed on diets deficient in α-tocopherol or rich in PUFAs. Such feeding can induce (e.g. in pigs and minks) a 'yellow fat disease' that can be prevented by feeding more α-tocopherol, or other antioxidants (Section 3.20.2). Macrophages in culture accumulate ceroid when they are exposed to lipids rich in PUFAs, and ceroid within macrophages as well as extracellular ceroid (presumably released from dead cells) are present in human atherosclerotic lesions.

Lipofuscin and ceroid deposition are promoted by several abnormalities of fat metabolism, including abetalipoproteinaemia (Section 3.20.2). Presumably more lipid than usual is degraded within lysosomes in such diseases. Accumulation of intracellular age pigments is not evidence that lipid peroxidation is important in disease pathology, since peroxidation probably occurs within the lysosome and these pigments are presumably safe so long as they stay there.

10.4.7 Oxidative stress, oxidative damage and signal transduction

One important feature of ageing is decreased response to stimuli. For example, hepatocytes from old rats showed less ERK activation (by phosphorylation) when exposed to EGF or to low (pro-proliferative) levels of H_2O_2 than did hepatocytes from young animals, whereas higher levels of H_2O_2 were more damaging to these older cells.[117] Thus loss of signal transduction capacity with age (even though cells may still have their surface receptors for mitogens, cytokines, etc.) may sometimes involve losses of protein kinase activities. Its overall effect might be to diminish the useful roles of ROS, for example in promoting increased Hsp levels in response to stress. By contrast, basal levels of Hsps tend to go up with age (Section 10.4.4), possibly in an attempt to deal with abnormal proteins. In contrast, too many ROS in the wrong place could facilitate inappropriate signalling (e.g. through the insulin pathway), or unwanted activation of NF-κB and AP-1, generating cytokines that trigger a mild chronic inflammation. Inflammation contributes to most diseases; is it also a general feature of ageing? This may be so in the brain and perhaps elsewhere (Table 10.1).[32,118]

10.4.8 The oxidative damage theory of ageing: summing it up

Harman's theory, expanded in the light of modern knowledge, is gaining credence because it fits with the genetic studies in *C. elegans*, *Drosophila* and mice and forms a link between most or all of the other suggested theories (Table 10.2). Many longevity-determining genes could be, directly or indirectly, linked to oxidative damage (Table 10.2).

But do RS *cause* ageing? We cannot confidently say yes for humans on present data, although data for *C. elegans* seem convincing. Remember that as tissues deteriorate with age, more oxidative damage is a likely consequence of disorganization and cell death (Section 9.2); rises in parameters of oxidative damage with age do not prove a cause–consequence relationship. A second important question is mechanism. *C. elegans* is genetically uniform and kept in a defined environment in the laboratory; despite this there are wide variations in individual longevity, consistent with an element of randomness (of free radical damage perhaps) in ageing. Yet oxidative damage often affects specific molecular targets (Section 10.4.5.1).

More food for thought, an adult *C. elegans* has no dividing cells and so can never be a close model for human ageing,[20] which involve not only damage to postmitotic cells (e.g. most neurons) but also impaired proliferation in tissues where cell division continues.[20] More research is needed. However, current data suggest that human centenarians generally do not show insulin resistance and their cells cope better with stressors.[118] But do they die 'old but healthy'? No, one study showed that most die of age-related diseases, especially cardiovascular, although deaths from cancer seemed rare. [119]

10.5 Nutrition, health and oxidative damage

That food and health are intimately linked is an old concept; in 400 BC the physician Hippocrates wrote, 'let food be your medicine and medicine be your food' (he liked giving apples and dates to his patients!). Indeed, it is widely thought that diet-derived antioxidants play a role in the prevention of human disease. This view arose largely from epidemiological studies showing inverse correlations of blood antioxidant levels (or dietary antioxidant intakes) with the risk of developing (or, in some studies, dying from) various diseases. However, attempts to validate a cause–consequence relationship by intervention studies (feeding antioxidants and observing effects on disease outcome) have produced confusion rather than enlightenment. Also, should an antioxidant be found to prevent a disease, it must not be automatically assumed that it does so by an antioxidant mechanism. For example, flavonoids in red wine, chocolate and cocoa have been speculated to be cardioprotective, but flavonoids exert many biological effects (Section 3.22.2.1), and the jury is still out on whether or not beneficial effects of moderate wine drinking are due only to the alcohol (Section 8.8). In addition, many other nutrients affect oxidative damage (Table 10.3).

10.5.1 Learning from epidemiology[120]

Epidemiology is the science that explores the distribution and determinants of disease in populations. Its methods were first applied to epidemic diseases such as smallpox and cholera, hence the name. One early example was the discovery that cholera incidence is related to consumption of water from specific (contaminated) sources.

Epidemiological studies may be descriptive (e.g. correlating the incidence of a disease to a particular habit or diet) or experimental (e.g. taking a dietary supplement and examining what happens). Many countries conduct regular surveys of food consumption patterns, nutritional status indicators and incidence of various diseases. Epidemiologists use these data in attempts to relate disease incidence to diet in different countries (**cross-cultural studies**), within regions of the same country, or over time (**longitudinal studies**)—looking for changes in disease incidence and attempting to relate them to changes in diet. For example, one can compare the incidence of myocardial infarction (Fig. 10.5) or stomach cancer between different countries, and can also observe what happens to incidence rates when people move between countries. In **cohort studies**, subjects are identified on the basis of their exposure to the factor of interest and followed to examine their disease status. Cohort studies are often **prospective**, healthy subjects being followed forwards in time. For example plasma antioxidant levels or dietary intake might be measured at the start of the study and subsequent disease appearance in the subjects examined. In **case–control studies** subjects are recruited on the basis of the presence or absence of a particular disease. Controls are randomly selected and

Table 10.3 Some links between diet and oxidative damage

Type of link	Constituent	Needed for
Direct	Antioxidant nutrients	(e.g. vitamin E, other plant-derived phenols such as flavonoids, carotenoids, vitamin C)
Indirect	Fe	Catalase, FeSOD, prevention of hypoxia (O_2 transport by haemoglobin, O_2 storage by myoglobin), nitric oxide synthase ($NO^\bullet$ often has antioxidant properties). Both Fe deficiency (can increase electron leakage from the mitochondrial electron transport chain) and Fe overload can promote oxidative damage.
	Mn	MnSOD. Excess Mn is neurotoxic by promoting RS formation from dopamine (Section 8.6.6).
	Cu	CuZnSOD, caeruloplasmin, normal iron metabolism. Both Cu deficiency and overload cause oxidative stress, each involving increased mitochondrial ROS production (*Toxicology* **189**, 147, 2003).
	Zn	CuZnSOD, metallothionein, glyoxalase II, membrane stabilization, displacement of iron, component of some transcription factors. High Zn^{2+} levels induce apoptosis in neurons (Section 8.15.12).
	Mg	Cofactor for multiple enzymes (e.g. in pentose phosphate pathway). No specific link to antioxidant defence but magnesium deficiency in animals causes inflammation and increases oxidative damage in several tissues (e.g. *Cardiovasc. Res.* **31**, 677, 1996). Magnesium deprivation caused GSH depletion and oxidative death in murine cortical cultures (*Brain Res.* **890**, 177, 2001).
	Amino acids/proteins	Synthesis of antioxidant defence enzymes, metal binding proteins, albumin (as 'sacrificial antioxidant'), GSH, e.g. dietary protein intake can affect rates of synthesis of GSH (*Am. J. Clin. Nutr.* **80**, 107, 2004).
	Riboflavin	Glutathione reductase (has FAD cofactor). Essential for correct mitochondrial electron transport and fatty acid oxidation.
	Thiamine	Key component of pyruvate and α-ketoglutarate dehydrogenases. Used in **transketolase**, an enzyme in the pentose phosphate pathway which supplies NADPH for glutathione and thioredoxin systems. Thiamine deficiency causes neuronal damage accompanied by oxidative stress (*J. Neuropath. Exp. Neurol.* **58**, 946, 1999) and accumulation of methylglyoxal (*FEBS Lett.* **579**, 5596, 2005).
	Selenium	GPx, thioredoxin reductases, methionine sulphoxide reductases, selenoprotein P, other selenoproteins.
	Nicotinamide	NAD^+, $NADP^+$, NADPH, NADH: energy metabolism, repair of DNA, PARP (Section 4.2.4), glutathione and thioredoxin reductases, aldehyde reductases, maintaining catalase function, regulates sirtuins (Section 10.3.4).
	Folic acid	Minimizes levels of plasma homocysteine—a risk factor for cardiovascular disease (Section 10.5.9 below).
	Inducers of antioxidant defences	Agents that increase expression of genes coding antioxidant and/or other defence systems (Table 10.7; Fig. 10.6).

matched for other criteria (e.g. age, sex and smoking status) as far as possible. Associations between the disease and a dietary factor are usually expressed as an **odds ratio** (or **relative risk**). Table 10.4 shows an example.

Nested case–control studies are case–control studies using patients from ('nested in') a cohort study, who develop a particular disease. Exposures measured as part of the cohort study are compared between patients and controls from within the same cohort. For example, the **Honolulu heart study** examined 8006 Hawaiian men whose α-tocopherol intake was assessed at enrollment, and followed them to see who developed coronary heart disease. A nested case–control study of 84 of these subjects who developed Parkinson's disease (PD) showed that, by comparison with 336 age-matched controls from the same cohort, there

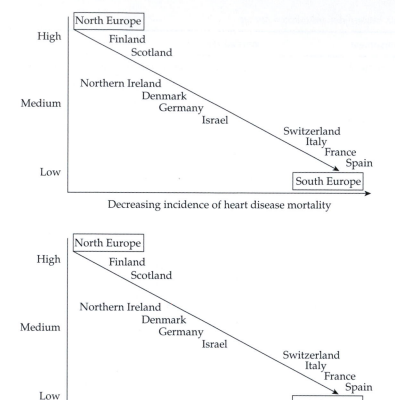

Figure 10.5 A cross-cultural study: mortality due to heart disease (above) and plasma α-tocopherol levels (below) in different European countries. Diagram adapted from *Am. J. Clin. Nutr.* **53**, 3265, 1991 by courtesy of the publishers and Dr Fred Gey.

appeared to be no relationship of dietary α-tocopherol intake to the risk of developing PD.[121]

10.5.2 Epidemiology and antioxidants[120,122–124]

Many epidemiological studies have examined antioxidants, but let us look first at some of the early ones that suggested the importance of antioxidants as disease-preventing agents. There are marked differences in cardiovascular disease incidence in different European countries: in general, the incidence is high in the north (e.g. Finland and Scotland) and low in the south (e.g. southern Italy). If populations are standardized to correct for known risk factors (e.g. plasma cholesterol, smoking), there is an inverse correlation between coronary events and lipid-standardized plasma α-tocopherol (Fig. 10.5). Data from this and other studies allowed calculation of plasma antioxidant levels apparently associated with low risk of cardiovascular disease (Table 10.4). Similarly, the **Zutphen elderly study**[125] (Section 3.22.2) examined risk factors for chronic disease in old men and found a decreased risk of mortality from heart disease in subjects with elevated flavonoid intake, even after correction for intakes of vitamin C, α-tocopherol and β-carotene (Table 10.4). No clear effects of flavonoid intake on cancer risk were observed in this (or later) studies.[126]

The **Nurses' Health Study**, a prospective cohort study, began in 1976 in the USA with 121 700 female nurses. In 1980, 87 245 nurses aged 34 to 59, free of obvious cardiovascular disease, completed dietary questionnaires that attempted to assess their consumption of a range of antioxidants. At 8 years follow-up, 437 non-fatal heart attacks had occurred

Table 10.4 Relationship between risk of coronary heart disease (CHD) and plasma concentrations/intakes of certain antioxidants

Antioxidant	Concentration (μM) associated with		
	Moderate risk of CHD[a]	Small risk of CHD[a]	
Carotene (mostly β-carotene)	<0.3	>0.4–0.6	
α-Tocopherol	<24	>27–28	
α-Tocopherol; cholesterol ratio (μmol/mmol)	<4.1	>4.8–5.6	
Ascorbate	<24	>35–60	
	Daily flavonoid intake (mg)[b]		
	0–19	19.1–29.9	>29.9
Mortality from CHD	20.4	14.5	9.9
Relative risk after correction for intake of total energy, saturated fats, blood pressure, physical activity, weight, smoking, total and HDL cholesterol	1.00	0.58	0.47

[a] Moderate risk of CHD, >250 deaths/10[6]; small risk, <130 deaths/10[6]. Data are abstracted from Gey, KF (*Bibl. Nutr. Diet.* **51**, 84, 1994 and *J. Nutr. Biochem.* **6**, 206, 1995) and are based on data from a range of studies. Similarly, in elderly subjects (70–75 years) there was an inverse correlation between plasma α-plus β-carotene and mortality from cancer and cardiovascular disease (*Am. J. Clin. Nutr.* **82**, 879, 2005).
[b] From Hertog, MGL *et al. Lancet* **349**, 699, 1997.

as well as 115 deaths from coronary disease. Those nurses in the top 20% of dietary α-tocopherol intake (as calculated from the questionnaire) showed 23 to 50% less heart disease after adjustment of the data to correct for age and smoking. Women who took α-tocopherol supplements for short periods had little apparent benefit, but those who took them for more than 2 years had a relative risk of major coronary heart disease of 0.38 to 0.91 after adjustment for age, smoking, other risk factors and intake of other antioxidant nutrients. There was no relation to vitamin C intake, although this was above 60 mg/day even in the lowest quintile and so is inconclusive (see Table 10.4 and the comment in Table 10.5). In another study on 34 486 postmenopausal women, the incidence of death from coronary heart disease decreased with calculated α-tocopherol intake from food, although no relation to vitamin C intake was observed.

In 1986, the **Health Professionals Study** began; 39 910 US males (dentists, veterinary surgeons, pharmacists, opticians, osteopaths, and podiatrists) 40 to 75 years old and free of obvious coronary disease, completed questionnaires designed to assess their intake of vitamin C, β-carotene and α-tocopherol. During 4 years of follow-up, 667 cases of coronary disease were observed. After controlling for age and other risk factors, a lower risk for coronary disease was observed among men with calculated high α-tocopherol intakes. For men consuming more than 60 International Units per day the relative risk was 0.49 to 0.83 compared with those taking less than 7.5 units per day. As compared with men who did not use α-tocopherol supplements, men who consumed at least 100 units per day for at least 2 years had a relative risk of 0.47 to 0.84 for coronary disease. By contrast, β-carotene intake was not associated with a lower risk among those who had never smoked, but among smokers, high β-carotene intake did appear associated with lower risk. A high intake of vitamin C was not associated with a lower risk of coronary disease but again this was, on the whole, a well-nourished population.

However, in a European multicentre study (EURAMIC; European Community Multicentre Study on Antioxidants, Myocardial Infarction and Breast Cancer), α-tocopherol and β-carotene concentrations in human fat were measured. There was no difference in α-tocopherol levels between people who had had heart attacks and controls. Fat α-tocopherol levels were used as a (putatively) more accurate measure of α-tocopherol status than dietary questionnaires. Low β-carotene levels were associated with a higher incidence of myocardial infarction, but only in patients who smoked.[127]

10.5.3 Problems of interpretation

The studies reviewed above suggested the importance of antioxidants, yet they relied on measurements of diet and disease incidence, neither of which is easy to quantitate accurately. The quality of medical records and disease classifications varies between countries. Dietary intake is commonly measured using 24-h dietary recalls, keeping diaries of food intake over several days or food-frequency questionnaires. Food-composition tables can then be used to calculate nutrient intake. All these methods have their problems, as one can easily imagine, added to which there is considerable interindividual variation in the uptake of dietary α-tocopherol and carotenoids from the gut by humans. Food-composition tables may be inaccurate; the composition of a food may vary between countries and regions and depends on how long it is stored. Bias in recording can alter risk estimates (e.g. if obese people systematically under-record their food intake whereas non-obese people do not). Also, diets change with time, a problem in longitudinal studies. Too many of these uncertainties in assessment of diet, or disease incidence, will obscure any relationship.

Some studies measured 'biomarkers' of body antioxidant levels, for example white cell ascorbate, plasma β-carotene or levels of α-tocopherol in adipose tissue or erythrocytes. More studies are needed on the relation between dietary intake and such parameters. For example, concentrations of α-tocopherol and vitamin C in plasma change quickly after alterations in dietary intake whereas α-tocopherol levels in adipose tissue do not. We already mentioned that the same intake of vitamin C produces lower plasma levels in elderly subjects than in younger ones (Section 10.4.4). Unfortunately, plasma concentrations of α-tocopherol

correlate poorly with LDL α-tocopherol content, and correlations between plasma and adipose tissue levels are similarly weak.[128]

However, the major problem with interpreting the studies is that *correlation does not prove a cause–consequence relationship*. For example, cross-cultural studies show a relation between cardiovascular disease rates and the number of television sets or telephones per thousand members of the population. This is (presumably!) not a cause-and-effect relationship but due to the fact that TV sets and telephones (and the consumption of dietary supplements!) are markers of increasing 'prosperity', itself usually associated with more cardiovascular disease. Several criteria are used to assess the strength of a correlation and its likelihood to be a cause–consequence relationship (Table 10.5).

It is widely agreed by nutritionists that diets rich in vegetables and fruits are associated with lowered incidence of cardiovascular disease, diabetes, stroke and certain types of cancer, especially lung and oral (but not breast and maybe not colorectal) cancers (Table 10.6). β-Carotene is a common constituent of plants. In humans, the higher the plasma β-carotene, the lower the risk (on a population basis) of developing some forms of cancer (Table 10.4). But does β-carotene itself protect against cancer? Or is it simply a marker for diet? Thus eating more plants might raise plasma β-carotene levels, but it could be anything (or any combination of things) in the plants that is the protective agent.[129] Plants contain a huge range of potentially-protective agents (Table 10.7). A fruit- and vegetable-rich diet is often low in fat, and high fat intake is a risk factor for some cancers. Such a diet may lower plasma cholesterol, ameliorating this risk factor for cardiovascular and Alzheimer's (Section 9.20) diseases. Fruits and vegetables are good sources of folic acid. Multiple toxins have also been identified in plants (Table 10.8); toxins at low doses may, ironically, be protective if they induce defence mechanisms. Oltipraz and sulphoraphane (Table 10.7), (Fig. 10.6) may help increase levels of phase II enzymes by creating mild oxidative stress, for example.[130]

Similarly, suppose that a group of subjects consumes large amounts of vitamin C and α-tocopherol and also shows lower incidence of heart disease than average. Does this mean that these

Table 10.5 Commonly used criteria for inferring causation from epidemiological data: a critique

Proposed criterion	Comment
Biological plausibility, i.e. there are physiological reasons for expecting the correlation. For example, LDL oxidation is involved in atherosclerosis and *in vitro* is inhibited by α-tocopherol, so one would expect α-tocopherol to have an antiatherosclerotic effect.	Runs the risks of ignoring phenomena which, at the time, have no obvious explanation yet for which the statistical evidence is equally strong. Also runs the risk of assuming what you are supposed to be trying to prove.
Strength of the correlation; strong relation observed consistently in several studies conducted by different countries.	Difficulties in collecting reliable data tend to obscure relationships. Thus if the correlation is very clear-cut it is difficult to explain it away, e.g. that between cigarette smoking and lung cancer. In 1854 Dr John Snow was so convinced by the strength of the correlation between cholera and drinking water from a particular well that he removed the pump handle (an intervention trial which stopped the epidemic).
The effect is **dose-responsive**, e.g. the lower the intake of a given nutrient the higher the incidence of a particular disease. Often subjects are divided into **tertiles** (groups of 33.3%), **quartiles** (25%), or **quintiles** (20%) of intake, blood levels, etc.	A negative result can occur if there is a correlation only over a given range of intakes. For example, 60 mg of vitamin C per day may be enough to give maximum protective effect against cardiovascular disease (Table 10.4). A study of vitamin C intake versus such disease in a country with a well-nourished population (average vitamin C intake well above 60 mg/day) will not show a relationship.
Trends in the population over time match changes in disease incidence.	An example is the alteration of lung cancer incidence with changes in smoking habits in several countries.

None of these criteria can prove causation.

Table 10.6 Epidemiological studies of the relationship between fruit and vegetable intake and cancer prevention

Site	Fruit (F) or Vegetable (V)	Relative risk	95% Confidence limits	Number of studies
Strong inverse correlations				
Oral/pharynx	F	**0.45**[*]	0.38−0.53	10
Pancreas	F	**0.80**[*]	0.69−0.83	7
Lung cancer	F	**0.77**[*]	0.71−0.84	16
Lung cancer	V	**0.80**[*]	0.73−0.88	14
Stomach	F	**0.85**[*]	0.77−0.95	11
Weak or no inverse correlations				
Bladder cancer	F	0.87	0.72−1.04	5
Colorectal cancer	F	1.00	0.96−1.05	19
Stomach cancer	V	0.94	0.84−1.06	7
Breast cancer	V	0.94	0.83−1.07	6
Colorectal cancer	V	0.97	0.87−1.08	16
Prostate cancer	V	0.95	0.84−1.08	6

The data and figures used are extracted from IARC Handbook of Cancer Prevention, Vol. 8, Fruit and Vegetables, IARC Press, Lyon, 2003, with permission from IARC Press. In general, case−control studies have given better evidence for protective effects than cohort studies; the above table takes both into account. Other agencies have ranked the risks somewhat differently (*Nutr. Rev.* **63**, 303, 2005) and we are sure that debate will continue for some time yet.

Table 10.7 Potential anticancer effects of dietary constituents

Class	Examples
Antioxidant effects in stomach/small intestine/ colon	Vitamin C reacting with nitrosamines in stomach. γ-Tocopherols, carotenoids and flavonoids scavenge RS in the GI tract (Section 6.2).
Agents interfering with metabolic activation or promoting metabolic deactivation, of carcinogens	Inhibitors of P450 (e.g. constituents of grapefruit juice, garlic, parsley, chilis and several herbal medicines),[a] although some compounds found in plants upregulate CYPs (*Carcinogenesis* **21**, 1157, 2000). An example is **glucoraphanin**, the precursor of sulphoraphane in broccoli (*Carcinogenesis* **25**, 61, 2004). Many compounds such as 1,2-dithiole-3-thiones (e.g. **Oltipraz**), sulphoraphane,[b] other isothiocyanates, rosemary extract) induce 'phase II' enzymes via the ARE and also raise GSH levels (Section 4.5.10). This can happen in cells of the GI tract (Section 6.2.1) or in other body tissues after uptake of the compounds.
Lipoxygenase/COX inhibitors	Resveratrol, flavonoids, other phenolic compounds. Can inhibit these enzymes in GI tract cells and perhaps in other body tissues if there is sufficient uptake.
Inhibitors of cell proliferation	Resveratrol, several flavonoids including green tea phenolics, curcumin. Several suggestions (not well supported) that green (and to a lesser extent, black) tea consumption has an anticancer effect (*N. Engl. J. Med.* **344**, 632, 2001). Catechins reported to block folate mechanism (*Cancer Res.* **65**, 2059, 2005).
Antagonists of oestrogen's action in promoting growth of certain tumours	Isoflavonoids, indole-3-carbinol, lignans.
Inhibitors of metastasis	Flavonoids, e.g. by inhibiting matrix metalloproteinases (*Mol. Pharmacol.* **65**, 15, 2004). Carotenoids may encourage cell–cell communication in transformed cells (Section 3.21).
Inhibitors of angiogenesis	Genistein (an isoflavonoid), epigallocatechin gallate (*Mol. Pharmacol.* **65**, 15, 2004).
Fibre	Increased speed of movement of faeces through colon; dilutes carcinogens and/or slows their formation.
Stimulation of immune response	Carotenoids, e.g. β-carotene, although data are variable.
Caloric restriction/low fat intake	High fat diets, high plasma cholesterol, and obesity promote oxidative damage. Diets rich in fruits and vegetables often have decreased fat and calorie content and tend to lower plasma cholesterol.
Selenium	Content in plants variable; related to soil content. Has anticancer effect in several animal studies, apparently by inducing protective enzymes and possibly by modulating GPx activity (loss of GPx1 and GPx2 in mice increases cancer of the GI tract; Section 3.11).
Phytoalexins	Resveratrol (grapes, wines). Antioxidant, anti-inflammatory, induce phase II enzymes.
Iron chelators	It has been speculated that high body iron stores are a risk factor for cardiovascular disease and cancer. Phytates, other organic phosphates, flavonoids may decrease iron uptake.
Down-regulators of transcription factors (e.g. NF-κB)	Capsaicin (found in *Capsicum* peppers; *J. Immunol.* **157**, 4412, 1996). Caffeic acid phenethyl ester (*Proc. Natl. Acad. Sci. USA* **93**, 9090, 1996), resveratrol, sulphoraphane.
Telomerase inhibitors	Catechins (*BBRC* **249**, 391, 1998, *Cancer Res.* **63**, 824, 2003).
Proteasome inhibitors	Epigallocatechin gallate, genistein, other phenols, curcumin (*J. Biol. Chem.* **216** 13322, 2001; *Biochem. Pharmacol.* **66** 965, 2003; *J. Biol. Chem.* **279**, 11680, 2004).
Receptor binding	Several flavonoids, as well as lutein and curcumin, can bind to the aryl hydrocarbon receptor and decrease the toxicity of dioxin (Section 8.3) to cells (*FEBS Lett.* **476**, 213, 2000; *J. Agr. Fd. Chem.* 52, 2499, 2004).

[a] Compounds in grapefruit juice (e.g. **bergamottin**) and Seville oranges inhibit CYP3A4 in the gut and can increase the oral bioavailability of several drugs (*Nature Med.* **7**, 29, 2001; *Drug Metab. Rev.* **1**, 41, 2005). For a review on resveratrol see *FASEB J.* **17**, 1975, 2003.

[b] Sulphoraphane, 1-isothiocyanato-4-(methylsulphinyl)butane, is present in broccoli and is a powerful inducer of quinone reductase and other phase II enzymes but not of CYPs. Oltipraz is found in cruciferous vegetables. Dithiolthiones have been reported to induce haem oxygenase and ferritin when administered to rats (*Carcinogenesis* **17**, 2291, 1996). Structures are shown in Fig. 10.6.

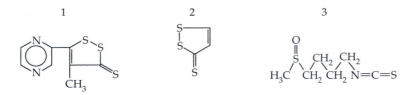

Figure 10.6 Structures of some of the compounds mentioned in Table 10.7: (1) oltipraz; (2) 1,2-dithiole-3-thione; (3) sulphoraphane.

Table 10.8 Examples of toxins found in plants

Type	Main food sources	Potential toxic effect
Thiosulphinates	Onions, garlic, other *Allium* species	Haemolysis; reported in cows, sheep, cats and horses consuming garlic or onions. Decompose on heating to a range of mono-, di-, tri- and tetrasulphides that can generate ROS and sulphur radicals on interaction with haemoglobin. Low doses may be beneficial by inducing phase II enzymes (*Free Rad. Biol. Med.* **34**, 1200, 2003).
Proteinase inhibitors	Legumes (e.g. soybeans)	Impaired food utilization
Cyanogens	Peas, beans, linseed, flax, cassava	Cyanide poisoning
Allergens	Potentially all food proteins, especially nuts and grains	Allergic response, anaphylactic shock
Carcinogens		
Aflatoxin	*Aspergillus flavus*	Carcinogenic
Safrole	Sassafras	
Sesamol	Black pepper, sesame seed	
Some flavonoids and other phenolic compounds (at high levels)		
Cycasin, other toxins	Cycads	Carcinogenic (Section 9.14); can be neurotoxic (Section 9.22.6).
Carminic acid	A major component of cochineal[a]	Close structural similarities to doxorubicin and can undergo redox cycling *in vitro* (*Food Addit. Contam.* **3**, 289, 1986).
Favism	–	Section 6.5
Alkaloids	Widely distributed	Hepatotoxic, cause lung damage, sometimes carcinogenic
Neurotoxins	Widely distributed	Section 9.16
Excitotoxins		
Complex I and II inhibitors		
Lathyrogens		
Nitrates/nitrites	Spinach, other leafy vegetables	Nitration and deamination reactions (e.g. by HNO_2 in the stomach)
α-Amanitin	*Amanita phalloides* toadstool	Salivation, vomiting, convulsions, death
Atractyloside	Thistle *Atractylis gummifera*	Inhibits mitochondrial adenine nucleotide translocator to block ATP release to cytosol
Gossypol	Cottonseed	Section 6.11.4
Psoralens	Celery, parsnips	Skin photosensitivity (Section 6.12)
Food reductones	Coffee, soy sauce	Oxidize to generate H_2O_2, e.g. hydroxyhydroquinone in coffee (*J. Agr. Fd. Chem.* **49**, 4950, 2001).

Adapted from Pariza, MW (1996) In *Present Knowledge in Nutrition*, 7th edn (Ziegler, EE *et al.*, eds), Chapter 57 (IRL Press, Washington DC). Note the overlap between 'protective agents' (Table 10.7) and toxins; low levels of toxins might be beneficial by inducing defence systems. Glucoraphanin/sulphoraphane is one example (Table 10.7). Indeed, the famous physician Paracelsus (1493–1541) wrote, 'All substances are poisons: there is none which is not a poison. The right dose differentiates a poison and a remedy.'

[a] A red food colourant obtained from the insect *Napalea coccinellifera*.

vitamins prevent heart disease? Not necessarily, since consumers of vitamin pills might be more interested in their health than average, such that they exercise more and eat better. Poor people suffer more disease than richer people, and poor people may not care about or even be able to afford vitamin supplements. In the UK and probably elsewhere, the lowest social classes have the lowest plasma vitamin C and α-tocopherol levels and poverty is strongly linked to disease incidence.[131]

10.5.4 The gold standard of intervention trials: hope unfulfilled[129,131,132]

The best way around the 'cause–consequence' conundrum is to conduct **intervention trials**. One could, for example, supplement a group of subjects with an antioxidant and compare their fates with a matched placebo group. The use of a placebo, ideally completely indistinguishable from the test compound, allows both subjects and investigators to be unaware of who is receiving what (**double-blinding**).

Intervention trials are the 'gold standard' of epidemiology; in principle they will give a clear answer. However, they are expensive and problems can occur if subjects do not comply with the regime (ideally, compliance should be monitored, for example by measuring blood levels of the administered substance), or if baseline parameters drift with time. For example, suppose that over a 5-year study testing the effects of vitamin C supplements on the incidence of cardiovascular disease, average dietary intakes of vitamin C in the population increase, for example due to its addition to more foods or to a general drift in the population towards eating more vitamin C-rich foods because of encouragement by public health agencies. This will minimize differences between those receiving vitamin C supplements or placebo.

Sadly, the intervention trials with antioxidants have yielded a morass of confusing data. Let us examine some in detail and see what went wrong.

10.5.5 The need for biomarkers

One major problem is that any beneficial effects of antioxidants such as ascorbate (Tables 10.4 and 10.5) may be exerted only over a certain range of intake. If most or all of the study population is already getting that amount from the diet, the trial may mistakenly conclude that the antioxidant is useless. A related error is that almost all studies assumed that feeding antioxidants would decrease oxidative damage, without measuring such damage to prove that it did decrease.[129] Yet we now know that 'antioxidants' often do not decrease oxidative damage *in vivo*. For example, several studies show little effect of flavonoids on oxidative damage (Section 3.22.2), only low intakes of vitamin C are associated with rises in 8OHdG (Section 3.20.1.1), and high-dose α-tocopherol is poorly effective at decreasing plasma F_2-IPs in healthy humans (Section 3.20.2.1). Studies in Denmark showed that urinary excretion of 8OHdG was decreased about 28% by feeding male (but not female) subjects Brussels sprouts,[133] but not by supplementing them with β-carotene, vitamin C, α-tocopherol or coenzyme Q_{10}.[134] This study was one of the first to show that food constituents able to decrease oxidative DNA damage need not be the 'classical' nutritional antioxidants. Some other studies have shown effects of antioxidant-rich foods in decreasing oxidative damage levels *in vivo*, but several have not[129,135] or have given mixed messages. For example giving smokers 250 g of blueberries each day for 3 weeks decreased plasma lipid peroxides[136] but not F_2-IPs. We believe that, whenever possible, epidemiological studies of the protective effects of antioxidants against human disease should be accompanied by measurement of biomarkers of oxidative damage, to check that an antioxidant effect was actually achieved. It may be only these 'normal' individuals who, for genetic or other reasons, show elevated levels of oxidative stress who respond.[129,132]

The use of biomarkers can be criticized. First, there is little evidence that the commonly used biomarkers of oxidative damage are correlated with later development of disease, although suggestive data for a predictive effect of F_2-IPs are accumulating. However, if they are not built into intervention trials, we will never know if they predict or not. Second, there are methodological issues. However, we feel that urinary 8OHdG and plasma/urinary IPs (IPs measured by mass spectrometry), are now good enough for general use

(Sections 5.13.6 and 5.14.6). The use of biomarkers might help government agencies in setting recommended dietary allowances (RDAs) for the antioxidant nutrients.[129]

10.5.6 Some intervention trials: a state of CHAOS

10.5.6.1 *Cardiovascular studies*
In the **CHAOS (Cambridge Heart Antioxidant)**[137] study, 2002 patients with coronary atherosclerosis were randomized to receive supplementary α-tocopherol or placebo and followed for 510 days. α-Tocopherol supplementation decreased the incidence of non-fatal myocardial infarctions by almost 50% but did not decrease (indeed it tended to increase) that of fatal ones. Sadly, almost all subsequent trials have failed to confirm these effects. Let us look at some examples.

The **GISSI study** in Italy examined 11 324 patients who had survived a recent myocardial infarction. It found that 1 g of (n-3) polyunsaturated fatty acids per day (as fish oil), but not 300 units of DL-α-tocopherol, decreased the risk of a second cardiac event. The **HOPE (Heart Outcomes Prevention Evaluation)** study was also 'hopeless'; 400 units of α-tocopherol daily failed to decrease cardiovascular events in 9541 subjects at high risk because of pre-existing cardiovascular disease or diabetes, nor did it decrease other complications in the diabetics.[138] The UK **Medical Research Council/British Heart Foundation (MRC/BHF)** study[139] examined 20 536 adults with arterial disease or diabetes; a mixture of α-tocopherol, vitamin C and β-carotene had no benefit. We think it safe to conclude that most or all patients with extensive atherosclerosis do not benefit from α-tocopherol. Some studies also suggest that high doses (400 units/day or more) may be deleterious (also see Section 8.19.2).[138,140] Vitamin C supplementation also shows limited, if any, evidence of benefit.[141]

However, this is not the same as saying that α-tocopherol cannot prevent the *development* of atherosclerosis. Some trials have addressed this point and appear more encouraging, but far from uniformly so.[142] In the **ASAP (Antioxidant Supplementation in Atherosclerosis Prevention)** study, a combination of slow-release vitamin C and

α-tocopherol decreased the progression of carotid atherosclerosis in 256 men, but not 264 women, a point to which we return in Section 10.5.7. A small trial (40 patients) showed an inhibition of atherosclerosis development in the new hearts of transplant patients by administration of vitamin C and α-tocopherol (Section 9.6.1). However, the **WAVE (Women's Angiographic Vitamin and Estrogen Trial)**[143] study showed no benefit of an α-tocopherol/vitamin C combination on coronary atherosclerosis, nor did 600 units of α-tocopherol daily for 10 years decrease heart disease in 39 876 healthy women.[144] Even worse, subjects on a combination of α-tocopherol, vitamin C, β-carotene, selenium, niacin and simvastatin (an inhibitor of cholesterol biosynthesis) showed a 0.7% progression in coronary artery stenosis; giving just niacin and simvastatin produced 0.4% regression. Hence the antioxidant supplement diminished the positive effect of the niacin/simvastatin.[145]

10.5.6.2 *The Linxian study*[146]
The county of Linxian in China has a high death rate from cancer of the oesophagus and stomach. In a trial of vitamin supplementation, 29 584 subjects (mostly non-smokers) aged 40 to 68 were given various supplements, or placebo. It was found that a daily supplement containing 50 µg selenium, 15 mg β-carotene and 30 mg α-tocopherol produced about 21% falls in death from stomach cancer, 13% for all cancers and about 9% fewer deaths overall after 5 years, whereas supplementation with a mixture containing 120 mg vitamin C (plus 30 µg of molybdenum!) did not. Although the effect on cancer mortality is convincing, it is uncertain which component(s) of the supplement was responsible (it may have been the selenium). Other studies examining the effects of selenium supplements on cancer incidence have given variable results but have not ruled out an anticancer effect, especially for prostate cancer.[147,148] By contrast, other intervention trials with β-carotene, α-tocopherol and vitamin C, alone or in combination, against cancer of the digestive tract or breast have given disappointing results. There is no evidence of benefit, and in seven out of 14 studies recently reviewed there was a suggestion of increased mortality.[147] The HOPE study, for

example showed no effect of α-tocopherol on overall cancer incidence.[138]

10.5.6.3 *The Finnish study (α-tocopherol/β-carotene [ATBC] cancer prevention study) and CARET*[146,149]

This study should have been a wake-up call to the enthusiastic and uncritical promoters of high-dose supplements. Unfortunately, it has not deterred them from 'pushing' flavonoids, herbal extracts, carotenoids other than β-carotene, and the like.[150] The study began in Finland in 1985 and examined 29 133 male smokers (age range 50–69 years, mean age 57 years) who had smoked (on average) 20 cigarettes a day for 36 to 37 years. Some received 20 mg of β-carotene per day, others 50 mg of DL-α-tocopherol, some both, and some placebo. They were followed for 5 to 8 years and the incidence of lung cancer noted. α-Tocopherol had no significant effect on lung cancer, but (as in CHAOS) tended to decrease the incidence of another non-fatal (but not fatal) myocardial infarction in subjects who has already suffered one. However, after 3 years, subjects receiving β-carotene showed a significantly greater incidence of lung cancer than controls (relative risk 1.16), an increased risk of myocardial infarction and an 8% increase in total mortality. On the bright side, there was a decreased risk of prostate cancers (sadly, an effect not confirmed in all subsequent studies with α-tocopherol[144]).

Epidemiological studies show that high plasma β-carotene levels are associated with lower risk of lung cancer (Table 10.4). The ATBC study suggests that β-carotene itself is not the protective agent, and may simply be a 'marker' of a diet rich in fruits and vegetables. Indeed, even in this study, subjects with a high intake of β-carotene *from diet* were less likely to develop lung cancer, whatever they were supplemented with.[151] Many subjects who have smoked for 36 to 37 years are well on the way to developing various pathologies, including lung cancer, and it seems unlikely to the authors that β-carotene or α-tocopherol could reverse this. Hence a logical result of this trial would be 'no effect', especially as β-carotene supplements are in any case ineffective in decreasing oxidative DNA damage in humans.[129,134] Indeed, the **Physician's Health Study** in the USA examined the effect of 50 mg β-carotene or 325 mg aspirin versus placebo in 22 071 male physicians. There was no significant effect (good or bad) of β-carotene on cardiovascular disease or cancer, but only 11% of the participants were current smokers.[152,153] In the **Women's Health Study**,[144] 50 mg β-carotene for 2 years (this part of the trial was terminated early) also had no effect on cancer incidence, but again only 13% were smokers. Nor did β-carotene affect cancer risk in the **skin cancer prevention study**.[153]

Why then did β-carotene increase lung cancer in the ATBC study? Suggested explanations include:

1. A random statistical 'fluke'. This seems unlikely because the data are supported by the β-**Carotene and Retinol Efficacy Trial** (CARET).[154] This was a double-blind trial of supplemental β-carotene plus retinyl palmitate in 18 314 asbestos workers and smokers. It was terminated 2 years early because lung cancer incidence appeared increased by up to 28% in the supplemented subjects. Of course, it could have been either retinol and/or β-carotene that was responsible. Since supplementation of the subjects ceased, the excess risk has tended to disappear.[153]

2. β-Carotene at high doses could be toxic or could interact with cigarette smoke to produce toxic products, or exert a proproliferative effect on promoted cells. Data consistent with this have been obtained in rats[155] and ferrets.[153,156]

3. The β-carotene may have been contaminated with breakdown products that accelerate proliferation of promoted cells, since this and other carotenoids are unstable (Section 3.21.3.2).

4. The β-carotene could have interfered with uptake of other carotenoids (putatively more protective) from the diet. Data from CARET seem consistent with this; individuals on placebo who consumed more fruits and vegetables had a lower risk of lung cancer but this effect was *not* seen in the supplemented subjects.[154]

In any case, the data show that the best way of protecting against smoke-induced pathology is to give up smoking rather than to keep smoking and take supplements. If you must smoke, do not consume β-carotene supplements but do eat lots of fruits and vegetables.

10.5.7 Some rays of hope and a gender bias

The **SUVIMAX (Supplementation en Vitamines et Mineraux Antioxidants)**[157] study examined 7876 French women aged 35 to 60 and 5141 men aged 45 to 60 (all apparently healthy) over seven or more years. They were given either a placebo, or a pill containing 120 mg vitamin C, 30 mg α-tocopherol, 6 mg β-carotene, 100 µg of selenium and 20 mg of zinc every day. These low doses of nutrients had no significant effect on cancer or cardiovascular disease for the group as a whole, nor did they lower blood lipids (in fact there was a tendency to raise them). However, for men only, there was a protective effect (relative risk 0.69) on cancer incidence at several sites (e.g. skin, lung, digestive tract) and on all cause mortality (relative risk 0.63), but no protection against cardiovascular disease. A similar gender effect was seen in the ASAP trial (Section 10.5.6.1). Why do women benefit less? They may have higher endogenous antioxidant defences (Section 3.20) and also eat better and have higher plasma antioxidant levels.[157] Pregnant women at risk of pre-eclampsia may sometimes benefit from antioxidants (Section 6.11.6); perhaps they start from a lower level.

Overall, SUVIMAX and ASAP imply that you do not need high doses of supplements to gain benefit. It may be that in a large population, even in advanced countries such as France and the UK, and more so in rural China, the bottom quintile or quartile is so badly nourished that they are close to antioxidant nutrient deficiency, and supplements combining small doses of multiple nutrients may be the best way of correcting that. Indeed, in the Linxian study (Section 10.5.6.2) the population was generally poorly nourished. The lowest quintile of plasma ascorbate in 1214 elderly subjects examined[158] in the UK was <17 µM. This segment of the population may be the only one that benefits, explaining why trials on well-nourished health professionals have been negative. To confuse things a bit more, in the **Stockholm Heart Epidemiology Program (SHEEP)**, consumption of a low-dose multivitamin supplement was associated with a lower risk of myocardial infarction for *both* men and women.[159] Some studies have shown antioxidant supplements to be associated with lower risk of infection in elderly subjects, whereas high-dose α-tocopherol supplements seem in general to be ineffective, with *suggestions* of harm in some studies. Any effect overall is likely to be small.[160,161]

The authors are not convinced by the suggestions that high does of α-tocopherol are harmful, although why bother taking them if they do no good? By what mechanisms could they be harmful? Some argue that the other tocopherols, especially γ-tocopherol, have benefit (Section 3.20.2.7) and high doses of α-tocopherol decrease plasma levels of γ-tocopherol.

10.5.8 Lycopene, other carotenoids and human disease

Epidemiological studies have drawn attention to the possible protective roles of other carotenoids. Several have focused upon lycopene (Section 3.21.3.3). A high lycopene intake was suggested to protect against cardiovascular disease, but the data are inconclusive.[141,152] A greater mass of data suggests that high lycopene intakes or plasma levels are inversely associated with risk of prostate cancers, and intervention studies are underway to look for a casual relationship.[162] But be careful with lycopene supplements; this carotenoid is very unstable and its oxidation products may do the opposite of what is intended (Section 3.21.3.2).

10.5.9 Other dietary factors and oxidative damage

The PUFA content of the diet affects cardiovascular disease; (n-3) PUFAs such as linolenic acid and EPA decrease LDL levels and tendency to thrombosis. In animals, dietary fish oil or (n-3) supplements have been shown to decrease both the vulnerability of the heart to arrhythmias after ischaemia–reperfusion and the production of eicosanoids and cytokines by activated phagocytes. Overall therefore, the cardiovascular effects of PUFAs appear to be beneficial, although not all studies have been positive.[163] In the GISSI study (n-3) PUFA supplements were protective, decreasing sudden cardiac death (Section 10.5.6.1).

Animal studies suggest that high intakes of PUFAs may increase dietary requirements for α-

tocopherol (Section 3.20.2). The vitamin E content of various vegetable and fish oils varies widely, a point to be considered in nutritional studies. High intakes of PUFAs may not be needed for health benefits; only 1 g/day was used in the GISSI study and eating fish twice a week might give the same benefit as high-dose supplements.[163] Docosahexaenoic acid is very important to brain function[164] and brain development in babies (Section 6.11.8.6)[165] and supplements of it have been suggested as beneficial in AD. Although EPA and DHA are highly peroxidizable *in vitro*, there is no evidence that this happens *in vivo* (Section 4.11.4 and [165]).

Elevated plasma levels (above 15 μM) of the thiol **homocysteine**

$$\overset{+}{\underset{|}{NH_3}}$$
$$HSCH_2CH_2CH-COO^-$$

are a risk factor for stroke, AD (Section 9.20.2), and cardiovascular disease.[159,166] Homocysteine arises from the essential amino acid **methionine**. Homocysteine levels depend on the activity of several enzymes which require vitamins B_6, B_{12} and folic acid (Fig. 10.7), such that inadequate intake of any of

these vitamins can elevate plasma homocysteine. Mutations in the genes encoding these enzymes can also lead to increases in homocysteine; one of the most common is a polymorphism in the gene encoding methylenetetrahydrofolate reductase that decreases enzyme activity, and has the overall effect of raising the folic acid intake required to maintain normal plasma homocysteine levels. It has been suggested (although by no means proved) that homocysteine damages vascular endothelium and predisposes to atherosclerosis by causing oxidative stress, raising F_2-IP levels and decreasing cellular GPx1 activity.[166] If so, the effects of inadequate intake of these B-vitamins illustrate how oxidative stress can result from deficiencies in nutrients that are not generally regarded as antioxidants. Similarly, magnesium or thiamine deficiency can lead to oxidative stress (Table 10.3). Low intakes of folate are associated with increased incidence of colorectal cancer, AD and of neural tube defects in unborn babies. Folate is required for the synthesis of thymine (the CH_3-group in thymine is provided by folate metabolism)[167] and low intake may cause DNA damage by allowing mistaken incorporation of uracil instead of thymine.

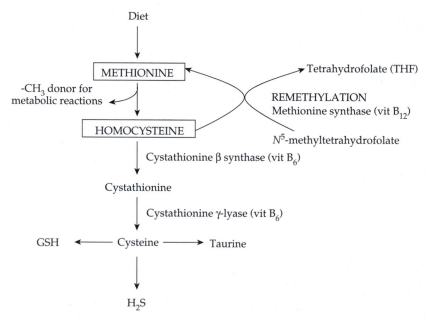

Figure 10.7 Folate metabolism and homocysteine formation. This diagram is considerably simplified; several intermediate steps are omitted. **Methylenetetrahydrofolate reductase** is involved in the regeneration of N^5-methylTHF from THF.

10.5.10 Iron, ageing and disease: another gender gap

Inhibiting, or overexpressing, antioxidant enzymes in flies has, at best, only moderate effects on lifespan (Section 10.4.2.1). One manipulation that did shorten lifespan was to feed the insects extra iron; indeed, iron accumulates in flies with age,[81] as it does in tissues of other animals and even in senescent yeast.[168] Iron has always been a paradox; essential for life yet pro-oxidant in the wrong molecular form. Excess or 'mal-placed' iron is intimately involved in many diseases, especially neurodegenerative disorders (Table 9.14).

Women suffer fewer heart attacks than men until after the menopause, one suggestion being that menstrual bleeding keeps body iron stores low. Another factor may be less RS production and greater antioxidant defences in females (Section 3.19). There have been several attempts to correlate body iron stores (usually assessed as plasma ferritin levels) with the incidence of cancer and cardiovascular disease, but data are inconclusive[169] and risks may be greatest if both iron and blood lipids are elevated.[170] Iron does play a role in the early stages of atherosclerosis (at least in rabbits; Section 9.3.5),[171] but measuring total tissue iron can be misleading, for at least two reasons. First, elevated body iron stores may indicate high consumption of haem iron-rich foods, especially cooked meats. Such a fat-rich diet is itself a risk factor for disease.[172] Second, most body iron is in ferritin and other proteins, relatively safe in terms of its pro-oxidant capacity. Indeed, desferrioxamine is poorly effective at decreasing iron in vessel walls, whereas creating iron overload in rabbits by injecting iron dextran did not raise iron in blood vessels.[171] This can explain why desferrioxamine decreases atherosclerosis in rabbits only after prolonged treatment and why iron overload does not necessarily accelerate atherosclerosis; the iron has to be in the correct place and in a pro-oxidant form.[171] Nevertheless, the increased iron content of older tissues may allow release of more pro-oxidant iron upon tissue damage, so that oxidative damage secondary to tissue injury can be aggravated.[173]

10.5.11 Antioxidants, epidemiology and neurodegenerative disease

Several studies suggest an inverse relationship between antioxidant intake and incidence of neurodegenerative problems. For example, in the **Shibata study** a cohort of Japanese subjects aged 40 years or older had their plasma vitamin C measured in 1977 and were followed until 1997. Low plasma vitamin C was found to be a risk factor for stroke.[174] Similarly, high vitamin C intake was associated with lowered stroke risk (especially in smokers) in the **Rotterdam study**, a study of 7983 subjects aged 55 or over.[175] However, in the Health Professionals Study, dietary intakes of α-tocopherol, vitamin C or β-carotene were not related to stroke incidence; indeed high-dose α-tocopherol seemed to marginally raise the risk of haemorrhagic stroke.[176,177] The basal levels of antioxidants in the various subjects studied may determine the effects of antioxidant supplements; in well-nourished populations they do not on the whole seem beneficial against stroke.[176–178]

What about PD or dementia? Few data support a role for dietary antioxidants in preventing PD,[121] but the potential importance of diet and lifestyle in AD is illustrated by the observation that CR decreased brain protein oxidative damage (measured as carbonyls) in mice within a few weeks, and this was associated with improved sensorimotor co-ordination.[179] Carbonyl levels were also decreased in rat brain after a programme of regular exercise,[180] and epidemiological studies suggest that regular exercise is a negative risk factor for AD development.[181] What about vitamin C and α-tocopherol? Several (but not all) epidemiological studies report that their intakes are negatively correlated with risk of AD development.[182] This was seen in the Rotterdam study, for example (the effect was clearest in these subjects who smoked). They are supported by a range of studies showing that high dose vitamin C and/or α-tocopherol improve memory in elderly subjects. The balance of published data is suggestive of a modest benefit,[182] although α-tocopherol did not help in MCI (Section 9.20.4).

Be cautious when judging the data, however. It is difficult to alter levels of α-tocopherol and vitamin C in the brain by changing plasma levels

(Sections 9.16.6.4 and 9.16.6.5). Also, supplements could affect memory by improving vascular function or (in the case of high-dose α-tocopherol) be mildly anti-inflammatory. Third, even if they enter the brain their effects on oxidative damage there might be limited. For example, α-tocopherol supplementation in old mice increased its levels in the brain, but did not decrease neuroprostanes, although F_2-IP levels fell.[183] Remember also that cognitive impairment may lead to changes in diet, nor can people with cognitive impairment be relied upon to complete dietary questionnaires accurately.

Studies with animals have also been positive, although not uniformly so. Feeding rats, mice or dogs with α-tocopherol ameliorated age-related declines in cognitive function.[182,184] Supplementation of the diet of rats with spinach, strawberries or blueberries (the last were the most effective) appeared to improve neuronal function,[185] and there is increasing evidence that polyphenols can enter the brain.[185,186] One possibly relevant observation is that feeding berry extracts to mice increases expression of the gene encoding γ-GCS in the brain.[187] Indeed, a (flavonoid-rich) extract of the plant *Ginkgo biloba* is widely thought to be beneficial in improving cognitive function; some (but not all) clinical trials in the elderly support this view, although the benefit (if any) is small.[188] Given the rising incidence of AD as populations age, we need to pay much more attention to whether changes in diet could delay its onset or ameliorate its symptoms.

10.5.12 What does it all mean? Some dietary advice

For healthy subjects, these seem to be little benefit from consuming high-dose supplements of single antioxidants. Indeed, high intakes of β-carotene may decrease body levels of other carotenoids, and high-dose α-tocopherol that of other tocopherols; some of these other carotenoids and tocopherols may be important to human health (but have not been proved to be so). Maintaining a good intake of fruits and vegetables, eating fish periodically, avoiding too much red meat, avoiding obesity, exercising moderately (Section 6.13.2), treating hyperhomocysteinaemia, hypertension or hypercholesterolaemia and taking a daily multivitamin/

mineral pill containing the RDA of all the nutrients required in the human diet (except possibly iron in the case of men) may be the best ways of minimizing oxidative damage. Indeed, F_2-IP levels are more affected by plasma cholesterol levels and obesity than they are by taking antioxidants (Section 10.2.2 and [189]). Don't smoke, but if you are already a tobacco addict, then all the above dietary advice, especially the fruits and vegetables, becomes even more important. Smokers should avoid high-dose β-carotene, and possibly high-dose α-tocopherol as well,[190] but should take more vitamin C and B vitamins (we suggest 500 mg of C daily and twice the RDA of the B vitamins). Those whose religion (if any) allows may gain added benefit by drinking alcohol in moderation (Section 8.8). Too much alcohol is not good for you, especially if combined with a bad (high fat, low fruits and vegetables) diet; if you over-indulge regularly you may benefit from increasing your intake of the B vitamins.

10.6 Antioxidants and the treatment of disease

In Section 10.5, we considered the role of antioxidants in disease prevention. A good 'tissue antioxidant status' may also help us resist the sequelae of trauma, since tissue injury leads to increased oxidative stress (Section 9.2). Thus, the extent of tissue damage after stroke (Section 9.17.3.2) or Aβ deposition may be lower in patients who have high antioxidant levels in the brain. Open-heart surgery, organ transplantation, and stays in the intensive care unit can lead to falls in plasma and/or tissue antioxidant levels.[191] Pretreatment of kidney transplant recipients with a mixture of vitamins (including vitamin C and α-tocopherol) led to better early graft function.[192] Although this study does not prove that it was the antioxidants rather than the other vitamins that were protective, studies of smaller numbers of subjects do suggest benefit from antioxidants.[193] By analogy, research in the livestock industry has shown that supplementation of pigs or cattle with α-tocopherol improves the resistance of the meat to spoilage.[194] It might do the same for our meat.

10.6.1 Therapeutic antioxidants[188,195]

There has been much interest in the therapeutic use of antioxidants. This may involve the use of naturally occurring antioxidants (with or without structural modifications) or completely synthetic molecules (Table 10.9). In addition, some drugs already used clinically may exert part or all of their effects by antioxidant mechanisms (Table 10.9), one example being aminosalicylates in the treatment of inflammatory bowel disease (Section 9.11.1) and another being various antibiotics (Section 8.16).

Any antioxidant proposed for therapeutic use must be non-toxic, but other questions should be addressed as well. They include

1. What biomolecule(s) is the antioxidant designed to protect? Is that biomolecule an important target of injury? For example, there is no point in inhibiting lipid peroxidation if the critical injury is to DNA or proteins.
2. How does the antioxidant work—by scavenging RS, preventing their formation, increasing endogenous defence systems or aiding repair of damage?
3. If it acts by scavenging, can the resulting antioxidant-derived radicals cause damage (Table 10.8)? They might be directly damaging, and/or reduce O_2 to $O_2^{\bullet-}$. It is advantageous if antioxidant derived radicals do not react with O_2 and can be 'recycled' to reform the antioxidant, for example by ascorbate or GSH.
4. Some RS have useful roles *in vivo*. Could the antioxidant interfere with them?

Suppose that clinical trials show that the antioxidant is beneficial. What does this tell us? It could mean that RS make a significant contribution to disease pathology, and/or that the antioxidant has beneficial pharmacological effects unrelated to its antioxidant action. We will see examples of this later. It is thus important to accompany clinical testing of a putative 'antioxidant drug' with measurements of oxidative damage biomarkers, to show that any benefit is related to antioxidant activity.

10.6.2 Approaches to antioxidant characterization[196]

A first step in evaluating putative therapeutic antioxidants is to establish what they are capable

Table 10.9 Some antioxidants available for therapeutic use

Category of compound	Example
Naturally occurring	SOD (CuZnSOD, MnSOD, EC-SOD; recombinant or purified), SOR, tocopherols, tocotrienols, coenzyme Q, lipoic acid, vitamin C, adenosine, transferrin, lactoferrin, cysteine, GSH, histidine-containing dipeptides, pyridoxamine, carotenoids, flavonoids, other plant phenolics, desferrioxamine, other 'natural' iron chelators, melatonin, coelenterazine, antibiotics
Synthetic	Thiols (e.g. mercaptopropionylglycine, *N*-acetylcysteine), synthetic metal-ion chelators (e.g. ICRF-187, Exjade, hydroxypyridones), fullerenes, xanthine oxidase inhibitors, inhibitors of $O_2^{\bullet-}$ generation by phagocytes, lipid-soluble chain-breaking antioxidants, inhibitors of phagocyte adhesion, GSH donors, SOD/catalase mimetics, derivatives of vitamins E or C, coelenterazine derivatives, modified antibiotics
Already in clinical use and might have antioxidant activity *in vivo* (but were not developed as antioxidants)	Penicillamine,[a] bucillamine,[a] aminosalicyates[a] (alone or as components of sulphasalazine), apomorphine,[a] selegiline, flupirtine, omeprazole, 4-hydroxytamoxifen,[a] ACE inhibitors (e.g. quinapril, ramipril, captopril) or angiotensin II receptor antagonists (e.g. losartan), ketoconazole, tetracyclines, probucol, propofol, some β-blockers (e.g. carvedilol, metoprolol),[a] cimetidine, some Ca^{2+} channel blockers,[b] phenylbutazone,[a] nitecapone,[a] entecapone,[a] idebenone, troglitazone,[a] tacrolimus

[a] Compounds which react with RS to form products with the potential to cause damage.

[b] Several β-blockers/Ca^{2+} blockers inhibit peroxidation *in vitro*; it is uncertain if they do so *in vivo* at the therapeutic levels normally achieved.

of doing. A battery of *in vitro* antioxidant characterization methods has been developed (Table 10.10). Two important (but often forgotten) points are that:

1. A compound should be tested at concentrations that are achievable *in vivo*.
2. In assaying antioxidants, one should employ biologically relevant RS, and think carefully about what targets of damage to use. For example, in 'screening' peroxynitrite scavengers, the authors use at least two types of assay, including ability to prevent $ONOO^-$-dependent tyrosine nitration as well as inactivation of α_1-antiproteinase (α_1-AP) on addition of $ONOO^-$. Because the assays do not measure the same aspects of peroxynitrite reactivity, 'scavengers' do not always behave in the same way. For example, uric acid inhibits $ONOO^-$-dependent tyrosine nitration but not α_1-AP inactivation.[197] α-Antiproteinase is inactivated by a wide range of RS and is useful for detecting damaging antioxidant-derived radicals.

The results of *in vitro* tests can be used to evaluate the likelihood that a compound exerts direct antioxidant effects *in vivo*. Thus if your compound needs mM levels to act as a good RS scavenger *in vitro* but is only present at micromolar levels *in vivo*, throw it away. Most (or all) putative antioxidants react fast with $OH^\bullet$ *in vitro* and are often suggested for use *in vivo* on this basis. However, it is unlikely that they can work as $OH^\bullet$ scavengers *in vivo* since most will never be present at levels remotely approaching those of endogenous molecules that react at diffusion-controlled rates with $OH^\bullet$, such as 0.5 mM albumin in plasma (rate constant $>10^{10} M^{-1}s^{-1}$) and 4.5 mM plasma glucose ($\sim 10^9 M^{-1}s^{-1}$). The authors are underwhelmed when told 'compound X is a good $OH^\bullet$ scavenger, so it's a promising antioxidant'. Our (usually politely unspoken) thought is 'tell us something that isn't a good $OH^\bullet$ scavenger, it may be useful as a control substance'.

Even an excellent antioxidant *in vitro* will not necessarily work *in vivo*. For example, it could be rapidly excreted, metabolized to inactive products or not reach the correct site. In addition, some compounds that have limited (or zero) direct antioxidant activity may exert antioxidant actions *in vivo* by being metabolized to better antioxidants, inhibiting generation of RS and/or by increasing endogenous antioxidant defences. Selegiline (Section 9.19.2) and melatonin (Section 3.18.3) may be examples of the latter. Some agents (e.g. carnosine) may bind cytotoxic end-products of lipid peroxidation. For example **pyridoxamine**, a metabolite of vitamin B_6, reacted rapidly with dicarbonyls when administered to rats at high doses, and the adducts were excreted in the urine.[198]

Let us look at some examples of putative therapeutic antioxidants.

10.6.3 Superoxide dismutases and catalases

Antioxidants enzymes available for therapeutic use include recombinant human SODs (CuZnSOD, MnSOD and EC-SOD). Indeed, transgenic mice that secrete human EC-SOD in milk have been obtained.[199] But if SODs are injected into animals, they have short plasma half-lives. To avoid this problem, a variety of 'longer-lived' SOD conjugates are available,[200] including polyethylene glycol (PEG)-SOD, Ficoll–SOD, lecithinized SOD, polyamine-conjugated SOD, cationized SOD, genetically engineered SOD polymers, SOD conjugated to fragments of (or the entire) HIV–tat protein (which facilitates their uptake into cells),[201] pyran–SOD, hyaluronic acid–SOD, hexamethylenediamine–SOD and albumin–SOD complexes. Several catalase conjugates[202–204] have also been made. For example, some animal studies show that intravenous administration of PEG–SOD and PEG–catalase decreases ischaemia–reperfusion injury to the brain or spinal cord; injury to the blood–brain barrier may allow them to enter the damaged tissue. Careful controls are needed because PEG itself can be neuroprotective.[205] Dismutases with heparin-binding domains have been developed which (like EC-SOD) can bind to endothelial cells. An interesting example is to fuse MnSOD with the heparin-binding domain of EC-SOD.[206] The involvement of ROS in cancer metastasis (Section 9.13.5.6) has prompted studies of the effects of antioxidant enzymes. Thus galactosylated or PEG-modified catalase decreased metastasis in mice.[203]

Many older papers reported anti-inflammatory effects of SOD, and some of catalase, in various

Table 10.10 Some assays used for screening putative antioxidants *in vitro*

Species screened	Assays	Comments
Superoxide	Superoxide is generated (e.g. by xanthine/xanthine oxidase) or added (e.g. as KO_2) and allowed to react with a detector molecule. The inhibition of the reaction is measured. Pulse radiolysis can be used to directly observe reactions with $O_2^{\bullet-}$.	Sections 2.3.3.1, 2.5.3 and 5.4
Hydrogen peroxide	Reaction with H_2O_2 is measured.	Multiple methods available (Section 5.8).
Singlet O_2	Scavenging/quenching of $^1O_2$ is measured.	Section 5.9
Nitric oxide	$NO^{\bullet}$ is generated. The reaction is followed directly, or as inhibition of the reaction of $NO^{\bullet}$ with a target molecule.	Section 5.5
Hydroxyl radical	$OH^{\bullet}$ is generated and allowed to react with a target (e.g. deoxyribose or a spin trap). Inhibition is measured. Pulse radiolysis can be used to directly observe reactions with $OH^{\bullet}$.	Sections 2.3.3.1, 5.2 and 5.3
Inhibition of Fenton chemistry	Effects on iron/H_2O_2-dependent damage to target molecules are measured.	Antioxidants that affect $OH^{\bullet}$-dependent damage can act by scavenging $OH^{\bullet}$ and/or by blocking $OH^{\bullet}$ formation, by removing its precursors ($O_2^{\bullet-}$, H_2O_2, HOCl, etc.) and/or by chelating metals.
Peroxyl radical	Reaction with a model peroxyl radical, e.g. AAPH-derived radicals or trichloromethylperoxyl ($CCl_3O_2^{\bullet}$) is measured, or the effects on lipid peroxidation are examined directly.	Peroxyl radical scavenging ability does not necessarily parallel ability to inhibit lipid peroxidation in membranes or lipoproteins: other factors (e.g. lipophilicity and interaction with any endogenous antioxidants) are important. For example, dihydrolipoic acid does not inhibit iron/ascorbate-dependent peroxidation in liposomes, but it recycles α-tocopherol radical in microsomes to inhibit peroxidation. Hence we recommend direct testing on biological membranes or lipoproteins. Nevertheless, studies with model peroxyl radicals are useful in optimizing antioxidant activity in the design of chain-breaking antioxidants.
Peroxynitrite	Nitration of tyrosine, inactivation of α_1-antiproteinase, oxidations of ABTS, pyrogallol, DCFDA or dihydrorhodamine123.	Peroxynitrite has complex chemistry; many antioxidants react with its decomposition products (e.g. $NO_2^{\bullet}$) or direct with ONOOH; few scavenge $ONOO^-$ directly (Section 2.6.1). Some of the metalloporphyins (Section 10.6.4 below) are an exception.
Hypochlorous acid	Oxidation of thionitrobenzoate; inactivation of α_1-antiproteinase (Section 5.7).	Some molecules (e.g. taurine) react with HOCl to generate products that also inactivate α_1-antiproteinase.
Total antioxidant activity	See Table 5.16.	Different methods give different answers.
Cell-based studies	Various 'probes' of cellular RS can be used (Section 5.11).	The antioxidant must be able to enter the cell. Watch out for effects in cell culture media (Section 1.11).

Whatever assay is used, one must check for any effects of the putative antioxidant on the assay system. For example, does it interfere with generation of RS (e.g. inhibiting XO) or react with the end-product detected (e.g. ascorbate reducing DMPO-$OH^{\bullet}$ to an ESR-silent species; Fig. 5.3)?

animals. Results tended to be variable both within (e.g. different enzymes of equal activity not having the same anti-inflammatory effect) and between laboratories. One factor that may account for many of these problems is the frequent contamination of SOD and catalase preparations with endotoxin.[207] Treatment of animals with traces of this substance increases endogenous antioxidant enzymes and is protective against subsequent insults (Section 3.4.5). The authors have been unable to find any report in a good journal of a double-blind controlled clinical trial showing a positive effect of SOD in a chronic inflammatory or autoimmune disease in humans, although brief reports of uncontrolled studies continue to be published.

Nevertheless, interest continues in the possible protective role of instilled recombinant human CuZnSOD, liposome-encapsulated SOD (with or without catalase), or catalase alone in protecting the lung against damage. For example, catalase targeted to the pulmonary endothelium improved outcome after lung transplantation in rats. Targeting was achieved by conjugating the catalase to an antibody recognizing PECAM-1 or, in some studies, ICAM-1 (Section 7.7.1).[202] A few human studies with SOD have shown promise; administration of recombinant human CuZnSOD to premature babies decreased inflammation somewhat and there were signs of improvement in clinical outcome in later life. Critically-ill babies treated with the SOD at birth had a decreased incidence of pulmonary illnesses (asthma, infections) when assessed at 1 year of age.[208]

Many bacteria contain superoxide reductase (SOR) enzymes (Section 3.3) which remove $O_2^{\bullet-}$ but do not make H_2O_2. The *Pyrococcus furiosus* SOR is very stable and able to function in eukaryotic cells, so might conceivably be useful.[209]

10.6.3.1 *Viral vectors*

An alternative approach is to deliver not the antioxidant enzymes but the genes encoding them, for example using viral vectors. Thus in one study genes encoding MnSOD or CuZnSOD attached to an adenoviral vector were injected into rats 3 days before bile duct ligation. The activity of both enzymes increased in the liver, but the MnSOD gene offered more protection against liver damage than that encoding CuZnSOD.[210] There are also

reports of radioprotective effects of SOD genes (Section 8.19.2). Therapy with eNOS or MnSOD genes improved wound healing in diabetic mice (Section 6.12.3) and adenoviral delivery of the 1-cys peroxiredoxin gene to the lungs of mice protected against injury by 100% O_2.[211] Of course, this method is difficult to use in acute situations, and questions persist about the safety of viral vectors.

10.6.4 SOD/catalase mimetics[212]

Several low-molecular-mass compounds that react with $O_2^{\bullet-}$ and/or H_2O_2 have been described (Fig. 10.8; Table 10.11). Most contain transition-metal ions. Examples include a complex of manganese ions with desferrioxamine, and copper ions chelated to amino acids or to anti-inflammatory drugs. However, many of the 'SOD-mimetic' copper chelates described in the early literature probably dissociate to release copper ions *in vivo* (Table 10.11) and there is now less interest in their use. Research now focuses around iron or manganese porphyrins such as FeTMPyP, AEOL 10150 (Table 10.11) and other manganese complexes such as EUK-8, EUK-134 and M40403 (Fig. 10.8) that catalyse the removal of $O_2^{\bullet-}$. Unlike the 'sheltered' catalytic site of SOD, the metal centres are more 'open' to undergo redox reactions with a wider range of biomolecules, although the extent of this is modulated by the ligands around the metal. However, these compounds have the advantage that they can penetrate readily into cells. The manganese in SC–55858, SC–54417, M40401 and M40403 is held by five co-ordination points and is only available for one-electron transfers. Thus these compounds can transfer an electron to and from $O_2^{\bullet-}$, catalysing its dismutation, but will not react with H_2O_2 or $ONOO^-$. However, they can, of course, undergo one-electron transfers with other cellular redox-active agents and enzymes (e.g. NADPH-cytochrome P450 reductase). *Hence do not regard any of these compounds as specific scavengers of $O_2^{\bullet-}$ in vivo*. In the EUK series (named after the company **Eukarion** that is developing them) the tetra-co-ordinated manganese can react with $O_2^{\bullet-}$, H_2O_2 and $ONOO^-$, as can that in the porphyrin AEOL10150 (the AEOL series is named after **Aeolus pharmaceuticals**). The compound

Table 10.11 Some SOD mimetics containing transition metals

Compound	Comments	References
Mn^{2+}–polyphosphate, –lactate, –succinate and –malate	Slowly catalyse $O_2^{\bullet-}$ dismutation; in the absence of chelating agents, Mn^{2+} is a poor catalyst. Manganese chelates are important catalysts of $O_2^{\bullet-}$ dismutation in some bacteria.	Section 3.5.2
Desferal–Mn(IV) and related Mn complexes	A green complex formed by reaction of desferrioxamine with manganese dioxide, MnO_2; 1 μM is equivalent to 1 unit of SOD in the cytochrome c assay. Has antioxidant effects in bacteria. Shown in various animal models to protect against vascular injury, e.g. in endotoxic shock.	*Drug. Dev. Res.* **25**, 139, 1992; *Arch. Biochem. Biophys.* **310**, 341, 1994; *Eur. J. Pharmacol.* **304**, 81, 1996; *J. Biol. Chem.* **271**, 26149, 1996; *Cardiovasc. Drug Ther.* **10**, 331, 1996; *Transplantation* **62**, 1664, 1996; *Proc. Natl. Acad. Sci. USA* **93**, 2312, 1996; *J. Am. Chem. Soc.* **118**, 4567, 1996; *Adv. Pharmacol.* **38**, 247, 1996; *Arch. Biochem. Biophys.* **288**, 215, 1991
Copper complexes	$Cu^{2+}_{(aq)}$ and some chelates of it catalyse $O_2^{\bullet-}$ dismutation at low pH equally or more rapidly than equimolar amounts of CuZnSOD. Cu^{2+} is less effective at physiological pH or when bound to proteins such as albumin. Some copper–amino-acid complexes (e.g. with lysine or with histidine) are still good catalysts at pH 7.4, as are complexes of copper with 3,5-diisopropyl salicylate or indomethacin. Many of these copper complexes are unstable, however, and problems can be caused due to the release of Cu^{2+} ions (e.g. as catalysts of $O_2^{\bullet-}$ dismutation or $OH^{\bullet}$ formation). EDTA decreases or abolishes reaction of $O_2^{\bullet-}$ with copper salts but has no effect on CuZnSOD. Several complexes, e.g. $Cu(II)_2(3,5\text{-diisopropyl salicylate})_4$ may be able to inhibit other enzyme systems, including NOS and cytochromes P450.	*Biochem. Biophys. Res. Commun.* **81**, 576, 1978; *Arch. Biochem. Biophys.* **203**, 830, 1980; *Biochim. Biophys. Acta* **745**, 37, 1983; *J. Med. Chem.* **27**, 1747, 1984; *Arch. Biochem. Biophys.* **315**, 185, 1994; *J. Inorg. Biochem.* **60**, 133, 1995
Metalloporphyins	Examples are Fe or MnTMPyP, MnTBAP and AEOLs 10150 and 10113 (Fig. 10.8). Have a modified protoporphyin structure.	Section 10.6.4 and reference[212]
Other manganese complexes	(Modified EDTA-type structures with aromatic rings). EUK-series, M40403, M40401, SC-55858, SC-54417	Section 10.6.4 and reference[212]

Table 10.12 Redox-active catalytic antioxidants are effective in animal models of diseases

Model system	Species used	Antioxidant(s) found to be protective
Lung		
Bleomycin fibrosis	Mice	AEOL10201
Radiation fibrosis	Rats	AEOL10113
Cigarette smoke injury	Rats	AEOL10150
Antigen-induced asthma	Mice	AEOL10113
	Guinea pigs	M40403
Haemorrhage-induced injury	SOD3 knock-out mice	AEOL10150
Bronchopulmonary dysplasia	Baboon	AEOL10150
Carrageenan-induced inflammation	Rats	M40403
Cardiovascular		
Splanchnic artery occlusion	Rats	AEOL10217
Heart ischaemia–reperfusion	Rats	M40403
		EUK8
Haemorrhagic shock	Rats	EUK8
		EUK134
Nitrate tolerance	Rats	AEOL10201
Interleukin-2-induced hypotension	Mice	M40403
Endotoxin-induced shock	Rats	M40401
		EUK8
Hypoxic pulmonary vasoconstriction	Mice	EUK8
Stenosis after balloon injury	Rats	M40401
Central nervous system		
Kainate injury	SOD2 knockout mice	AEOL10201
Cerebral vasoconstriction	Amyloid overproducing transgenic mice	AEOL10201
	Rats	AEOL10201
Corrects neurobehavioural defect in ATM-knockout	Mice	EUK139
ALS	Mutant CuZnSOD transgenic mice	EUK8
		EUK134
		AEOL 10150
Spinal cord injury	Rats	AEOL10201
Paraquat-induced neurodegeneration	Mice	EUK134
		EUK189
Spongiform encephalopathy	SOD2 knockout mice	EUK8
		EUK134
Ischaemia–reperfusion	Rats	AEOL10113
	Mice	AEOL10150
	Gerbils	M40401
Phencyclidine injury	Rats	M40401
Hyperalgesia	Rats	M40403
Age-induced cognitive impairment	Mice	EUK189
		EUK207
Meningitis-induced hearing loss	Rats	AEOL10150
Liver		
Acetaminophen injury	Mice	AEOL10201
Fas-induced injury	Mice	AEOL10201
Ischaemia–reperfusion	Rats	AEOL10150

Table 10.12 (cont.)

Gastrointestinal		
Acetic acid-induced colitis	Rats	AEOL11201
Trinitrobenzene sulphonic acid-induced colitis	Rats	M40403
Cerulein-induced pancreatitis	Mice	M40401
Renal		
Gentamicin injury	Rats	M40403
Endotoxin	Mice	AEOL10113
Ischaemia–reperfusion	Rats	EUK134
Endocrine		
Diabetes	NOD mice	AEOL10113
		EUK8
Joints		
Collagen-induced arthritis	Rats	M40403
Other		
Peridontitis	Rats	M40403

Abbreviations: ATM, ataxia telangiectasia mutated; NOD, non-obese diabetic.

Adapted from *Drug Discovery Today* **9**, 559, 2004 by courtesy of the publishers and Dr Brian J. Day. Also see *Free Rad. Biol. Med.* **36**, 938, 2004. The compound AEOL10201 is MnTBAP, AEOL10110 is MnTM-4-PyP, AEOL10112 is MnTM-2-PyP, AEOL10113 is MnTE-2-PyP and AEOL10150 is MnTDE-1,3-IP (which has undergone clinical trials for ALS).

FeTMPyP also reacts with $ONOO^-$. Indeed, several of these compounds react faster with $ONOO^-$ than CO_2 does. For example, MnTMPyP reacts quickly with $ONOO^-$ (rate constant 4.3×10^6 at $37\,°C$), and with carbonate radical.[213] The manganese is converted to an oxo–Mn(IV) complex, which can be reduced by GSH, ascorbate, $O_2^{•-}$ or urate. Reaction of these compounds with $O_2^{•-}$ usually involves a mechanism similar to that of MnSOD

$$Mn(III) + O_2^{•-} \rightarrow Mn^{2+} + O_2$$

$$Mn^{2+} + O_2^{•-} + 2H^+ \rightarrow Mn(III) + H_2O_2$$

whereas reaction with H_2O_2 probably forms an oxo–Mn(IV) complex.

'SOD mimetics' have been shown to protect against oxidative damage in a wide range of cell and animal model systems (Table 10.12) and EUK-8 and -134 increased the lifespan of *C. elegans* in some studies (Section 10.4.2). However, they may also exert other effects *in vivo*, for example slowing Ca^{2+} influx, and FeTBAP and MnTBAP increased levels of HO-1 in cell cultures.[214] We await with interest the results of their application to humans.

10.6.5 Spin traps/nitroxides[215]

Spin traps are used to detect free radicals *in vivo* and *in vitro* (Section 5.2). If a spin trap intercepts a biologically damaging radical *in vivo*, then it ought to protect against injury. If it does not, any or all of the following explanations apply:

1. the radicals trapped are not important contributors to damage;
2. not enough radical is trapped for significant protection;
3. the trap, its metabolites and/or products of its reaction with free radicals cause damage themselves.

The idea of using spin traps as therapeutic antioxidants arose from studies showing that α-phenyl-*tert*-butylnitrone (PBN) could protect rats against death from shock induced by gut ischaemia–reperfusion or endotoxin injection. Later work showed that PBN can protect against myocardial ischaemia–reoxygenation injury and heart transplant rejection in animals. It was also found to protect against cerebral ischaemia/reperfusion in gerbils, and it was noticed in the control animals that PBN administration to old gerbils decreased levels of brain protein carbonyls and appeared to improve cognitive function.

However, things are not so simple. *In vitro* characterization of PBN shows it to be a poor chain-breaking antioxidant or inhibitor of lipid peroxidation,[216] so its mechanism of action may not be as a radical scavenger. Several traps, including PBN, can have other metabolic effects, including metabolism to generate NO• (Section 5.2). The traps PBN, POBN and DMPO bind to CYPs and inhibit some of their oxidase activities.[217] After injection into animals, PBN is rapidly taken up by all tissues (including the brain); concentrations in gerbil brain are estimated to approach 0.5 mM after injection of 150 mg PBN/kg body weight. Rather than being a directly acting antioxidant, PBN may protect by decreasing the expression of genes encoding iNOS, COX-2 and proinflammatory cytokines, whilst stimulating IL-10 production. Several derivatives of PBN have been developed as potential therapeutic agents, such as **CPI-1429** (Fig. 10.8). A promising one is **NXY-059**, 2,4-disulphophenyl-*N*-*tert*-butylnitrone, also called **Cerovive**® (Fig. 10.8). It has been shown to improve outcome in a primate stroke model even when therapy was begun as late as 4 h after ischaemia and is under test in humans. Again, it is only a weak antioxidant *in vitro*[216] and may be working by the other mechanisms mentioned above. Its hydrophilic structure suggests a poor ability to cross the blood–brain barrier (unlike PBN), and it may work only because the barrier is damaged by the stroke. An even more hydrophilic agent is LPBNAH (Fig. 10.8)[76] whereas a more hydrophobic agent that has been studied in some animal stroke models is **STAZN, stilbazulenyl nitrone** (Fig. 10.8).[218]

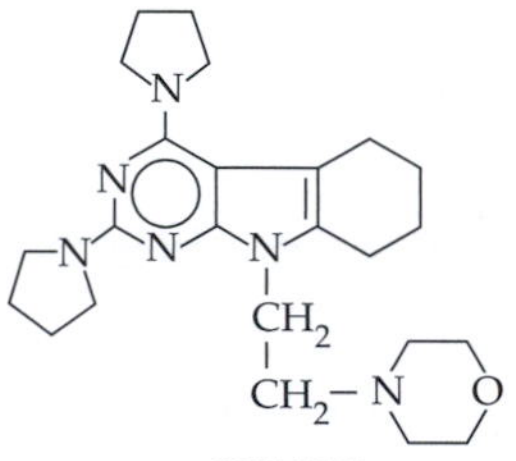

U101033

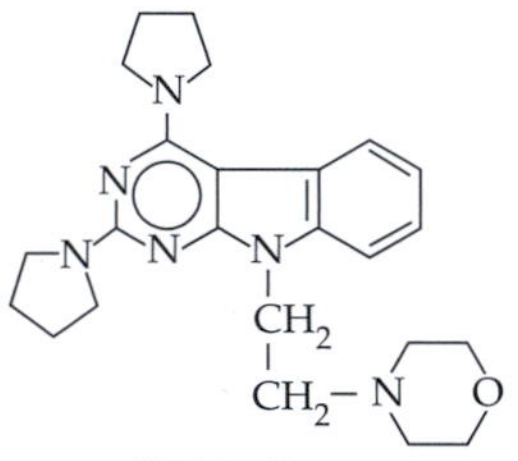

U104067

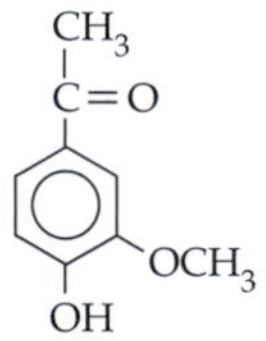

Apocynin

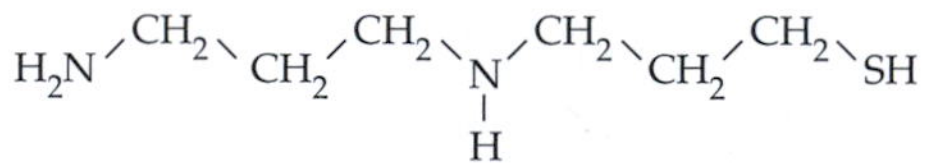

WR-1065
(-S-phosphate on pro-drug)

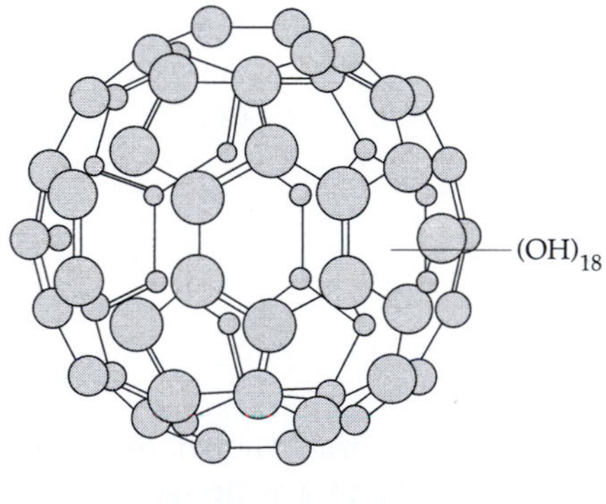

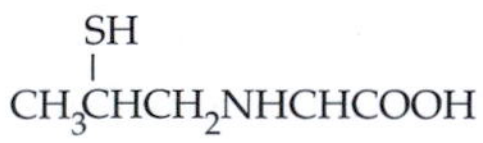

MPG

Polyhydroxylated C_{60}

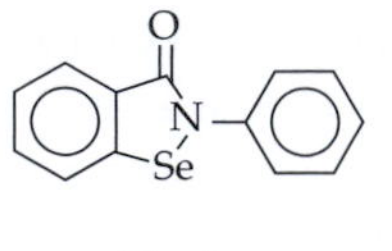

$(OH)_{18}$

Ebselen

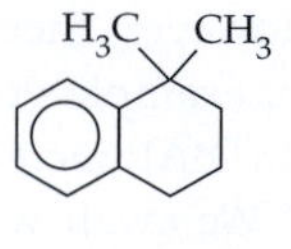

BXT-51072

Figure 10.8 (*Cont.*)

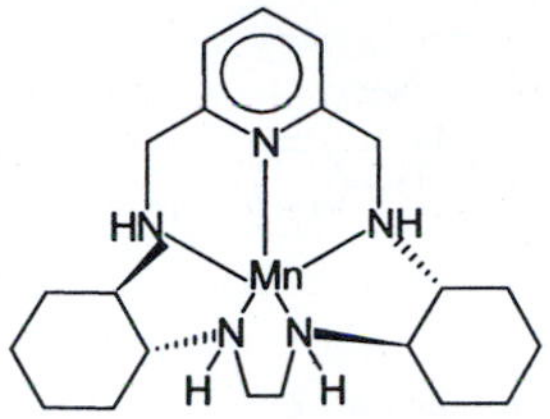

M40403

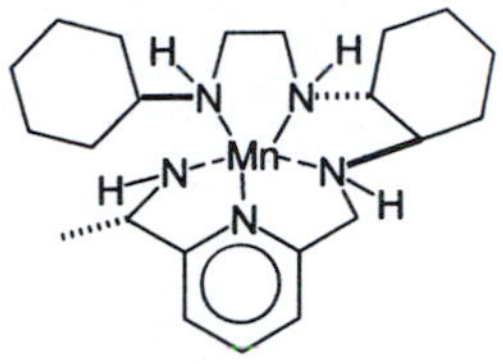

M40401

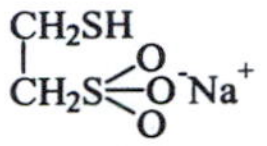

MESNA

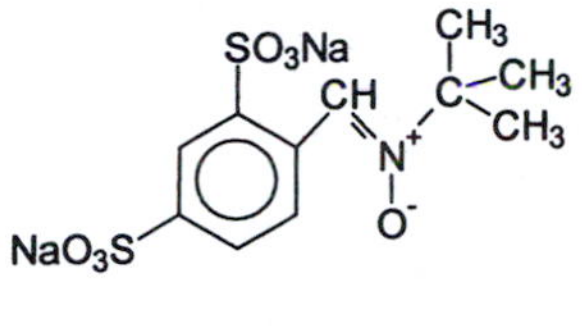

NXY-059

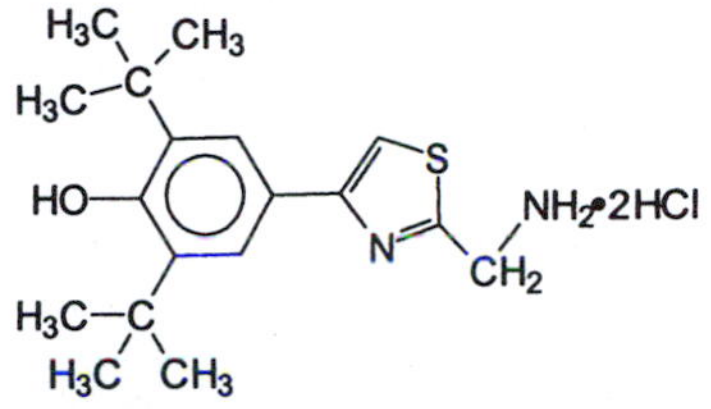

BN82451

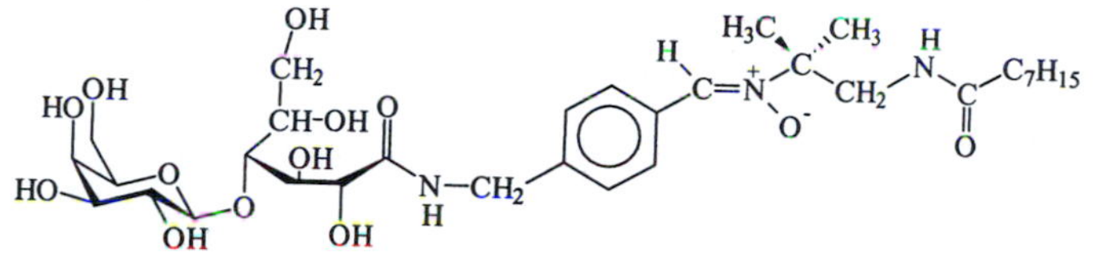

LPBNAH

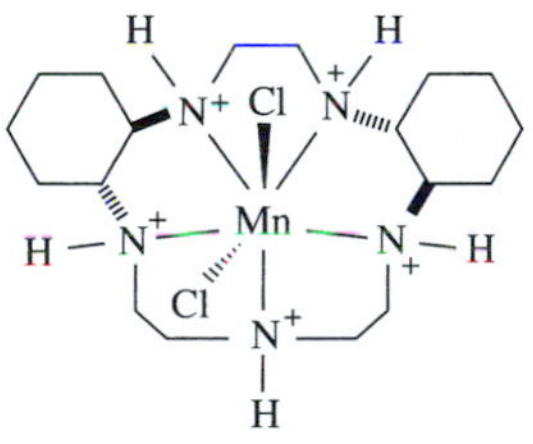

SC-55858

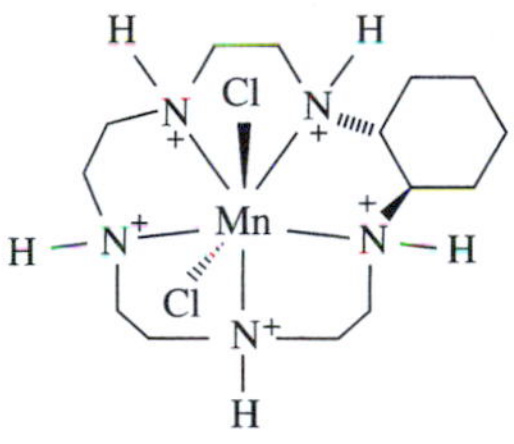

SC-54417

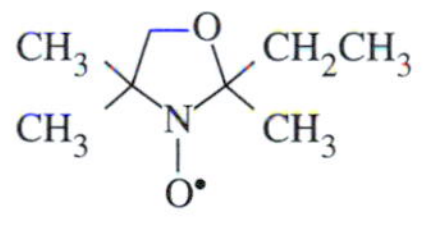

OXANO

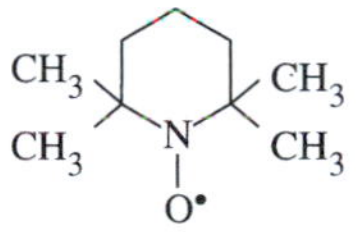

TEMPO

Figure 10.8 (*Cont.*)

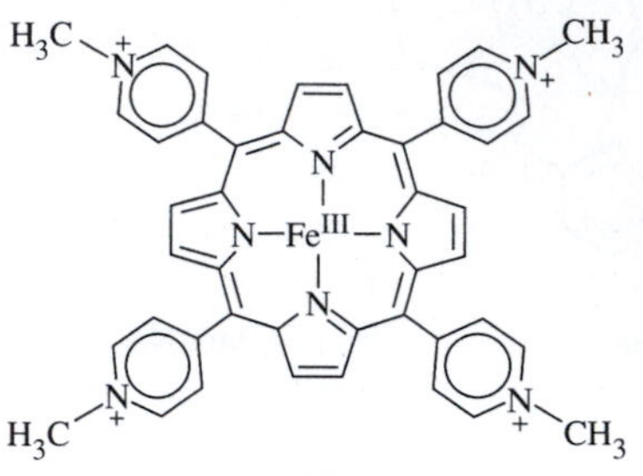

FeTMPyP
(In MnTMPyP, Mn replaces Fe)

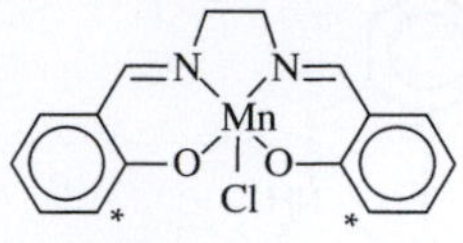

EUK-8

(in EUK134 there are 2
–OCH$_3$ group on the
carbons marked *, in
EUK189 2 –OCH$_2$CH$_3$
groups)

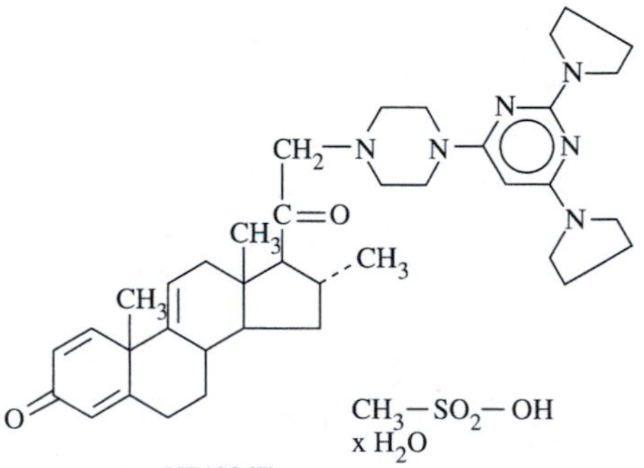

U74006F

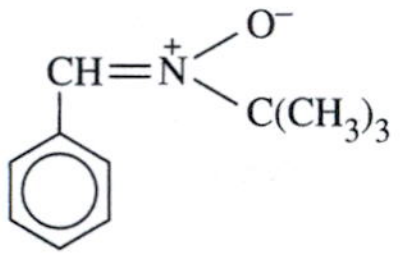

CH_3-SO_2-OH
x H$_2$O

PBN

U78517F

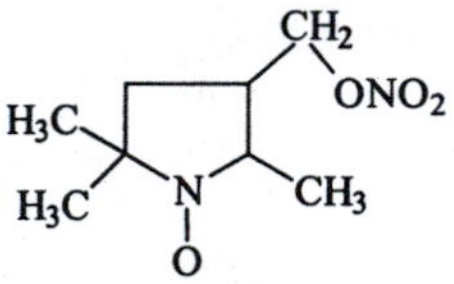

3-Nitratomethyl-PROXYL
(NMP)

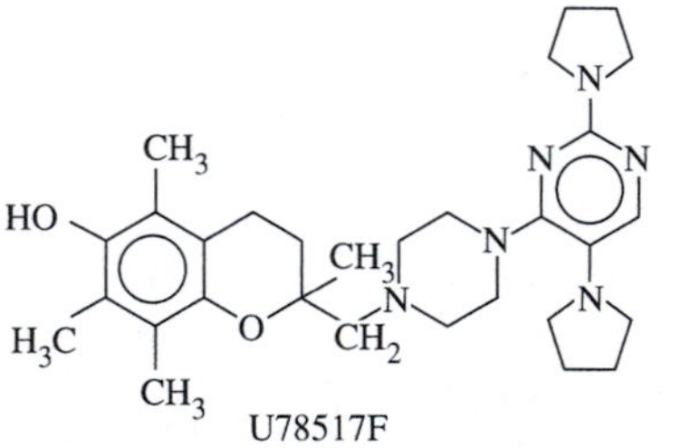

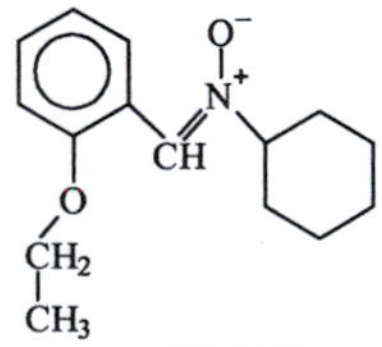

CPI-1429

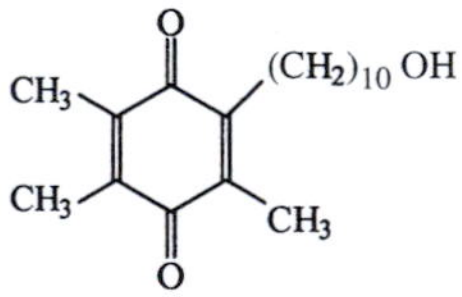

Idebenone

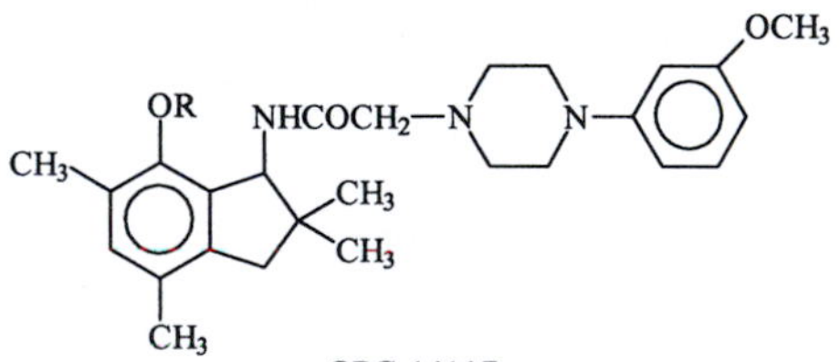

OPC-14117

Figure 10.8 (*Cont.*)

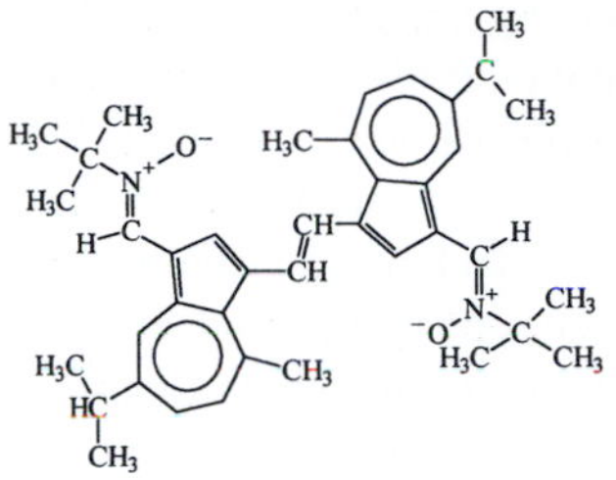

STAZN

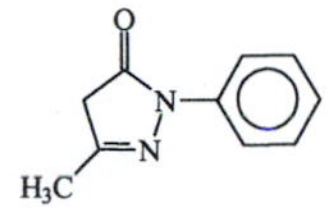

(MCI-186, sometimes called edaravone)

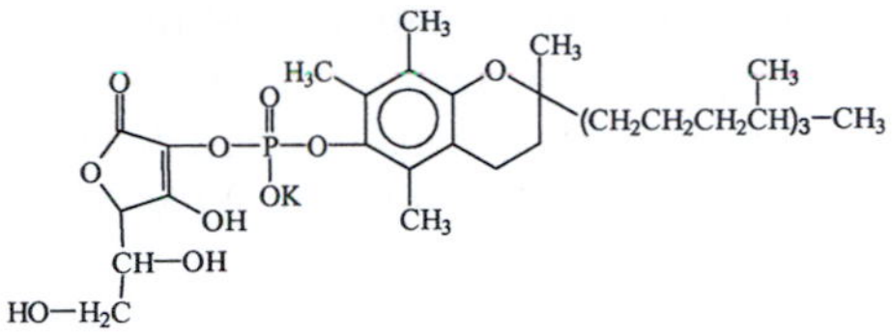

EPC-K1

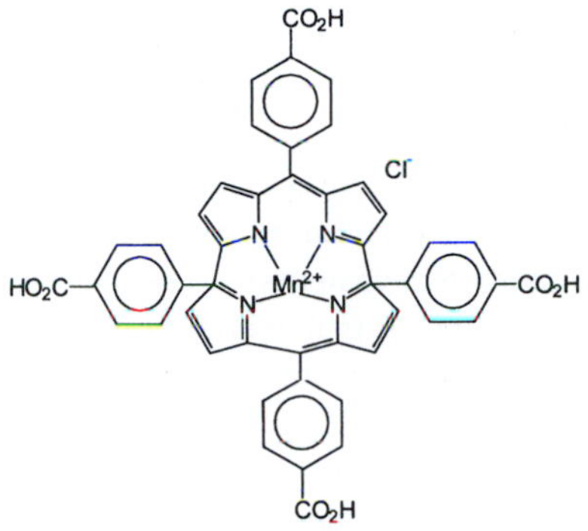

MnTBAP

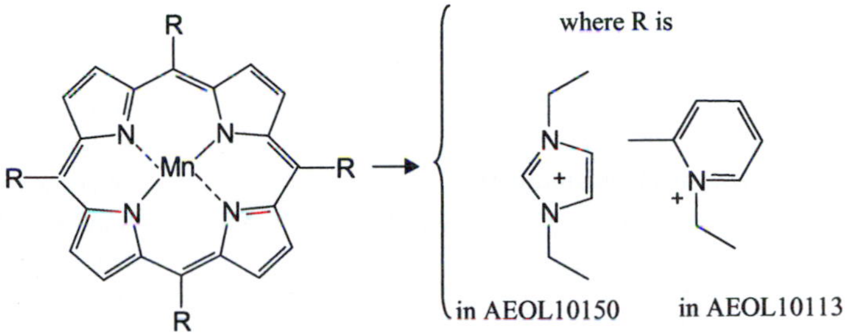

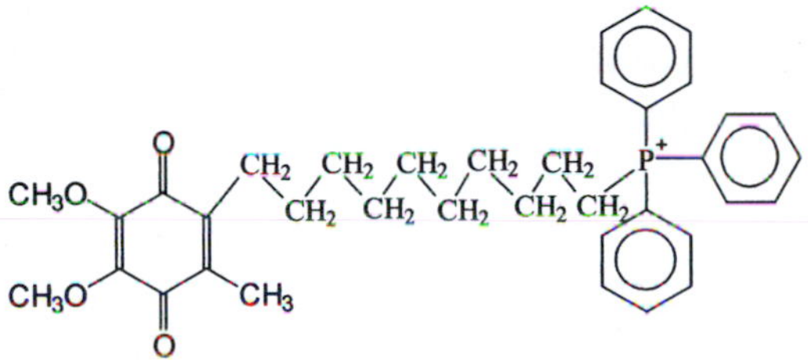

MITO-Q_{10}

Figure 10.8 Structures of some antioxidants mentioned in the text. Molecules such as **buckminsterfullerene** (made of 60 carbon atoms) show high reactivity towards radical addition ('radical sponges'), and polyhydroxylated (18–20 –OH groups) or carboxylated fullerenes have been synthesized as antioxidants (*J. Med. Chem.* **42**, 4614, 1999; *Parkinson Relat. Disord.* **7**, 243, 2001; *Free Rad. Biol. Med.* **37**, 1191, 2004; *Am. J. Physiol.* **287**, R21, 2004). But be careful; fullerene nanoparticles have been reported to *induce* oxidative stress in fish (*Environ. Health Perspect.* **112**, 1058, 2004) and can cause lipid peroxidation in cultured cells (*Biomaterials* **26**, 7587, 2005). MPG, mercaptopropionylglycine.

The PBN molecule is a nitrone and reacts withf radicals to give a nitroxide (Section 5.2). Indeed, some nitroxides have been proposed as antioxidants, such as **OXANO** and **TEMPO** (Fig. 10.8).[219] They react with $O_2^{\bullet-}$

$$R-N-O^{\bullet} + O_2^{\bullet-} + H^+ \rightleftharpoons O_2 + R-NOH$$

as can the resulting hydroxylamines

$$R-NOH + O_2^{\bullet-} + H^+ \rightleftharpoons R-N-O^{\bullet} + H_2O_2$$

One could also use hydroxylamines as antioxidants, of course. For example, *N-t-butyl hydroxylamine*, formed during the spontaneous decomposition of PBN, is a better antioxidant than PBN itself.[220] Several hydroxamates (such as *N-methylhexanoylhydroxamate*),

$$CH_3(CH_2)_4 - \overset{\overset{\displaystyle O}{\|}}{C} - \overset{\overset{\displaystyle OH}{|}}{N} - CH_3$$

have been developed as antioxidants, e.g. to prevent damage mediated by myoglobin/H_2O_2 systems.[221]

If both the above reactions occurred *in vivo*, then the nitroxide (or hydroxylamine) would catalyse $O_2^{\bullet-}$ dismutation. An alternative, apparently preferred,[219] catalytic cycle is between nitroxide and oxo-ammonium cation

$$R-N-O^{\bullet} + O_2^{\bullet-} + 2H^+ \rightleftharpoons R-N=O + H_2O_2$$

$$R-N=O + O_2^{\bullet-} \rightleftharpoons R-N-O^{\bullet} + O_2$$

In vivo, however, nitroxides undergo other redox reactions. For example, they can oxidize ascorbate, thiols, NAD(P)H, or Fe^{2+} ions and react with $ONOO^-$-derived nitrating species. Nitroxides have radioprotective effects (Section 8.19) and can decrease tissue damage in some animal model systems of shock, ischaemia–reperfusion and inflammation.[222] Some disposable plastic syringes can contaminate solutions with nitroxide.[223] A compound (**3-nitratomethylPROXYL**, Fig. 10.8) that is both a nitroxide and an NO$^{\bullet}$ donor (from its nitro group) has been developed.[224]

10.6.6 Vitamins C and E and their derivatives

Diseases causing prolonged deficiency of α-tocopherol produce neurological damage that can be ameliorated by giving supplements of this vitamin to the affected patients (Section 3.20.2). Administration of α-tocopherol to premature babies or patients suffering from haemolytic syndromes caused by an inborn lack of glutathione synthetase or G6PDH has been reported to confer some benefit (Sections 1.5.3 and 6.4). However, attempts to use α-tocopherol to treat diabetes, anthracycline-induced cardiotoxicity, cancer, Huntington's and Parkinson's diseases, have been disappointing, although there may be limited benefit in AD (Section 9.20). Remember that it takes a considerable time to raise the α-tocopherol content of tissues, especially brain, whereas oxidative damage can often be fast (e.g. within minutes in some reoxygenation injury experiments). A second reason for limited efficacy is that oxidative damage frequently occurs by mechanisms other than lipid peroxidation. Third, high-dose α-tocopherol does not, in any case, seem good at inhibiting lipid peroxidation in humans (Section 10.4.2).

Several structural analogues of α-tocopherol, some with improved antioxidant activity (as assayed *in vitro* and/or tested in animals), have been described. One is **BO-653** (Table 10.13), which has shown antiatherosclerotic effects in animals and, unlike probucol (Section 10.6.7 below), does not lower HDL levels. However, it might also decrease proteasome activity.[225] A water-soluble analogue of α-tocopherol, Trolox C, is widely used *in vitro* as an antioxidant (e.g. Section 5.17), a 'cardioselective' α-tocopherol analogue, **MDL 74 405** has been developed (Table 10.13), and various molecules in which Trolox or α-tocopherol are linked with NO$^{\bullet}$-donating groups have been described.[226] For most of these compounds, few (if any) human studies have been reported. **Troglitazone**, an antidiabetic agent with antioxidant properties is being used on patients, although not without problems (Table 10.13). **Raxofelast** has been reported to improve vascular endothelial dysfunction in diabetes; it is hydrolysed to the antioxidant IRF1005 *in vivo* (Table 10.13). Vitamin E succinate has been claimed to have anticancer properties (Section 3.20.2.9).

Various esters of ascorbic acid, for example **ascorbyl palmitate** and **2-octadecylascorbate**, have been synthesized as lipophilic versions of ascorbate.

Table 10.13 Some synthetic antioxidants

Compound	Structure	Comments
Synthetic chain-breaking antioxidants related to tocopherols		
Trolox		Water-soluble form of α-tocopherol; the hydrophobic side-chain is replaced by a hydrophilic –COOH group. Good scavenger of peroxyl and alkoxyl radicals, giving a Trolox radical that can be recycled by ascorbate. Often does not work well as an antioxidant in membranes—too hydrophilic to enter. Used as a standard in assays of total antioxidant capacity (Section 5.17).
TMG		Water-soluble forms of tocopherol (*Cardiovasc. Res.* **28**, 235, 1994; *Dig. Dis. Sci.* **48**, 54, 2003; *Free Rad. Biol. Med.* **26**, 858, 1999; *Br. J. Haematol.* **117**, 699, 2002). The compound IRFI016 is sometimes called **Raxofelast** and was reported to aid wound healing (Section 6.12.3); IRFI005 is its deacetylated (antioxidant) form. The compound PMC was reported to have antithrombotic effects in mice.
IRFI005/1006		

The –OH marked * on IRFI005 is acetylated in IRFI006.

Table 10.13 (*Cont.*)

Compound	Structure	Comments
PMC		
CS-045 (Troglitazone)		An analogue of α-tocopherol; acts as a hypoglycaemic agent by mimicking or enhancing the effect of insulin. Marketed as **Rezulin** in several countries for diabetic patients, but hepatotoxicity has caused problems. This may be due to its oxidation to peroxyl radicals, semiquinones, and quinones by CYPs and peroxidases (*Drug Metab. Disp.* **27**, 1260, 1999; *Chem. Res. Tox.* **16**, 679, 2003; and **18**, 1567, 2005).
MDL 74,405		Quaternary ammonium compound. Chain-breaking antioxidant that apparently concentrates in the heart when administered to animals but also enters other tissues. Protective in myocardial ischaemia–reperfusion models in several animals; also against models of inflammatory bowel disease in rodents. Related compounds containing a tertiary amine function have been tested in animals as neuroprotective agents (*J. Med. Chem.* **38**, 453, 1995; Cardiovasc. Res. 28, 235, 1994). Not much used recently.
CY-659S		Anti-inflammatory in animals (*Eur. J. Pharmacol.* **438**, 189, 2002), e.g. against contact hypersensitivity.

BO-563

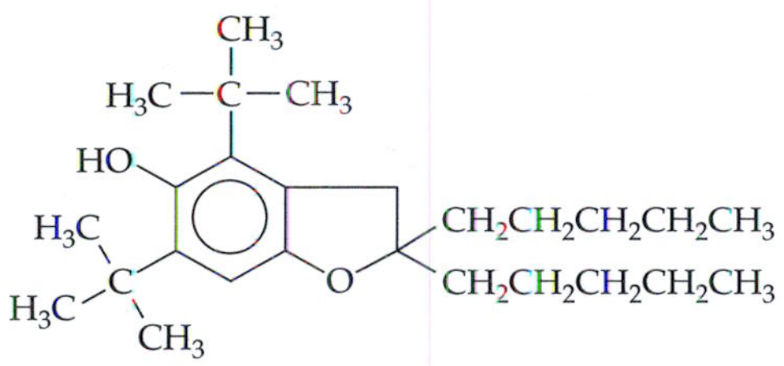

CH_3
$H_3C-C-CH_3$
HO
$H_3C-C-CH_3$
CH_3
O
$CH_2CH_2CH_2CH_2CH_3$
$CH_2CH_2CH_2CH_2CH_3$

Lipophilic α-tocopherol analogue (*J. Am. Chem. Soc.* **122**, 5438, 2000; *Proc. Natl. Acad. Sci.* **95**, 10123, 1998)

Sperm-directed antioxidant

α-Tocopherol attached to a polymer that contains a ligand to carbohydrate-binding proteins on the sperm surface.

Apparently able to efficiently deliver α-tocopherol to sperm (*Nature Chem. Biol.* **1**, 248, 2005).

Other synthetic chain breaking antioxidants

Butylated hydroxyanisole (BHA)

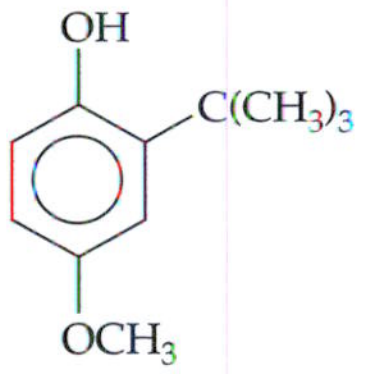

OH
$C(CH_3)_3$
OCH_3

The major (90%) constituent (3-*tert*-butyl-4-hydroxyanisole) of commercial BHA is shown. Acts by hydrogen donation, typical chain-breaking antioxidant. Generally recognized as safe but large doses ($\geq$ 1% of diet) deplete liver GSH and cause forestomach cancer in rats (*Toxicol. Lett.* **37**, 251, 1987; *Food Chem. Tox.* 24, 1167,1986). High doses can antagonize the action of other carcinogens in animals, by inducing phase II enzymes (*Crit. Rev. Toxicol.* **15**, 109, 1985). Metabolized in animals by O-demethylation to the diphenol ***tert*-butylhydroquinone** (TBHQ) followed by glucuronidation and sulphation. This compound also has antioxidant properties; can undergo oxidation to a semiquinone radical *in vitro*, and then on to a quinone (*tert*-butylquinone).

Propofol (2,6-diisopropylphenol)

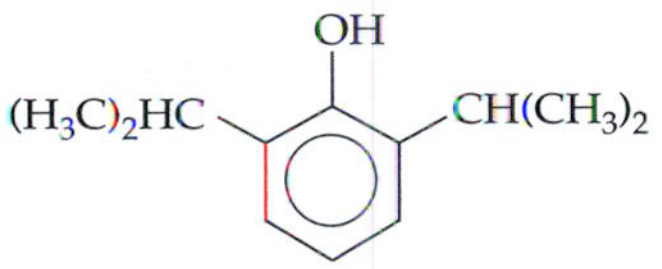

OH
$CH(CH_3)_2$
$(H_3C)_2HC$

Anaesthetic and sedative, used in humans. Has antioxidant properties *in vitro*, unclear if these contribute to its effects *in vivo* (*Anesthesiology* **5**, 1151, 2004).

Table 10.13 (*Cont.*)

Compound	Structure	Comments
Butylated hydroxytoluene (BHT)		Often added to foodstuffs; generally recognized as safe but very high doses can antagonize action of vitamin K and cause bleeding in animals.
Propyl gallate		Fairly water-soluble; good inhibitor of lipid peroxidation; lipoxygenase inhibitor. Binds iron ions and reduces Fe(III) to Fe^{2+}.
Nordihydroguaiaretic acid (NDGA)		Occurs naturally in resinous exudates of *Larrea divaricata* (American creosote bush) and in some other plants. Binds iron ions and reduces Fe(III) to Fe^{2+}, powerful lipoxygenase inhibitor. Some toxicity to animals (Section 3.22.4).
N,N'-Diphenyl-*p*-phenylene diamine (DPPD)		Sometimes used for animal studies of *in vivo* lipid peroxidation. Aromatic amines often used as antioxidants in the lubricant and polymer industries.

LY178002 (R=H), LY256548 (R=CH₃)

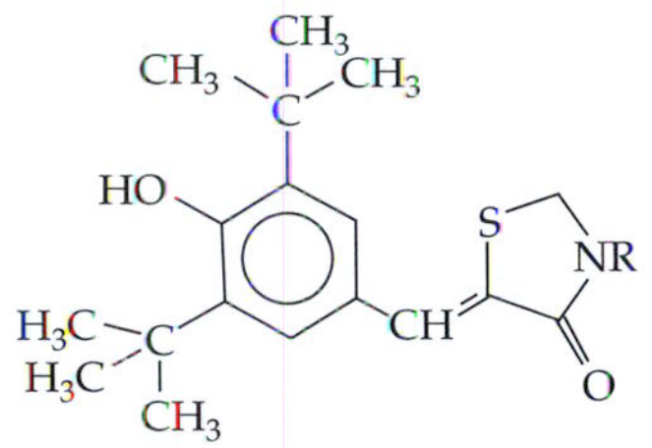

Inhibitors of lipid peroxidation, orally active in animal models of rheumatoid arthritis and cerebral ischaemia–reperfusion.

ONO-3144

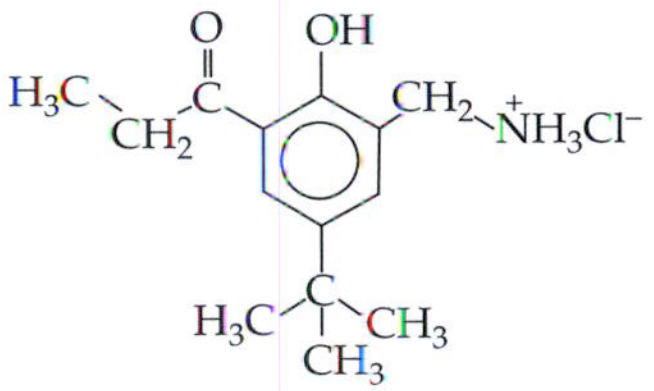

Chain-breaking antioxidant; anti-inflammatory in animal models.

MK-477

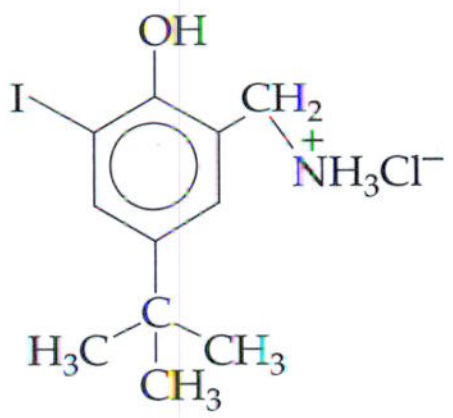

Chain-breaking antioxidant; anti-inflammatory in animal models.

Nitecapone

See Fig. 9.32

Section 9.19

Table 10.13 (*Cont.*)

Compound	Structure	Comments
6-Hydroxy-1,4-dimethylcarbazole (HDC)		Inhibitor of lipid peroxidation.
Promethazine		Inhibits lipid peroxidation in vitro; antihistamine and sedative.
Chlorpromazine		Used as a tranquillizer. Its antioxidant action in microsomes may partly depend on its enzymic conversion into hydroxylated products.
Ethoxyquin (Santoquin)		Powerful enzyme inducer *in vivo*. Used in longevity experiments (Section 10.4.2).
Carvedilol		Antihypertensive drug. Moderate inhibitor of lipid peroxidation *in vitro*, but its hydroxylated metabolite (–OH at point X) **SB211475** is more potent (*Eur. J. Pharm.* **251**, 237, 1996). It decreased levels of HNE in the hearts of patients with dilated cardiomyopathy (*Circulation* **105** 2867, 2002), but had no effect on urinary F$_2$-IPs in volunteers (*Eur. J. Clin. Pharmacol.* **60**, 83, 2004).

For more details see[228].

They have been used as food preservatives and tested as antioxidants in some animal models, but do not appear to have attracted much interest for therapeutic use. **EPC-K1** (Fig. 10.8) is a combined phosphate ester of vitamins E and C that has been reported as protective in a rat stroke model.[227]

10.6.7 Other chain-breaking antioxidants[228]

Probucol has antiatherosclerotic effects *in vivo* as well as antioxidant properties *in vitro*, although the latter may not explain the former (Section 9.3). Probucol also protects animals against adriamycin cardiotoxicity (Section 9.15.2). A succinate ester of probucol, **AGI-1067** (Fig. 9.6) is in clinical trials as an antiatherosclerotic agent, and other derivatives are being considered for use in treating transplant rejection and rheumatoid arthritis.[229] Probucol has one bad effect, in tending to decrease plasma HDL levels, but AGI-1067 appears not to (it is not clear why adding the succinate alters this property).

Coenzyme Q (CoQ) has antiatherosclerotic effects in some animals, and limited beneficial effects in human neurodegenerative diseases (Sections 9.3 and 9.16.6.6). These may or may not involve its antioxidant actions–the data are insufficient to decide. The modified CoQ **idebenone** (Fig. 10.8) has also been used, with indications of positive effects (Section 9.22.1). By contrast, the phenolic antioxidant **OPC-14117** (Fig. 10.8), although showing some benefit in animal models of neurodegenerative disease, did not help patients with Huntington's disease.[188] The compound **BN82451** (Fig. 10.8) increased survival in a transgenic mouse model of this disease, but does not appear to have been tested in humans.[230]

The chain-breaking antioxidants BHA and BHT (Table 10.13) are widely used in the food industry to prevent rancidity. Their toxicity is low; perhaps surprisingly, they have not been explored much as therapeutic agents, although comparable phenolic structures can be seen in probucol and in many other agents tested in humans (Table 10.13). Butylated hydroxytoluene can also increase transcription of c-*fos* and c-*jun*, and interact with the ARE to increase activities of defence enzymes (Sections 4.5.9 and 4.5.10). Because of alleged toxicity problems of BHA and BHT (at absurdly high doses;

Table 10.13), there are attempts to replace them as preservatives in certain foodstuffs by 'natural' phenolic compounds such as flavonoids, hydroxytyrosol, or rosemary antioxidants (which could turn out to be equally toxic at very high doses). Plastic often contain BHT, and traces can leach out from Parafilm and PVC tubing, sometimes affecting experiments.[231,232] **Propofol**, the active ingredient of the anaesthetic **Diprivan**, resembles BHT (Table 10.13) and has antioxidant activities *in vitro* at levels close to those that can be present *in vivo* during anaesthesia, although whether these are exerted *in vivo* is uncertain.

The therapeutic potential of plant phenols is also under investigation; much work has been done on mixtures such as *Ginkgo biloba* extract (Section 3.22.4 and 9.16.6.7) or **Daflon**,[233] a mixture of diosmin (90%) and hesperidin (10%). More data on their clinical efficacy are needed. Flavonoids and derivatives of them are under investigation as antiinflammatory and anticancer agents and for the treatment of vascular problems, for example in diabetes, since some may inhibit protein glycation[234] and aldose reductase activity as well as exerting antioxidant effects. When added to the diet of rats, the 'yellow curry spice' **curcumin** (Section 3.22.1) decreased IP levels and neuronal damage when the animals later had $A\beta$ infused into the brain.[235] Curcumin also slowed plaque development in AD transgenic mice.[236] Similarly, green tea extract or epigallocatechin gallate (EGCG) injected into mice diminished damage caused by later administration of MPP^+ (Section 9.19.3).[237] Of course, the safety of high doses of any plant phenol should never be assumed just because it is a natural product, nor must it be assumed that any benefit observed is due to antioxidant action. Indeed, these effects of curcumin and EGCG probably were not, or at least not completely.[236,237]

10.6.8 The lazaroids[238]

Attempts have been made to 'add on' antioxidant activities to drugs with other therapeutic properties, such as cholesterol-lowering agents, $NO^\bullet$ donors,[226] agonists of $PPAR\alpha$ or γ receptors, ion channel blockers, NSAIDs, antiarrhythmic agents such as lidocaine, and compounds that inhibit tyrosinase, elastase, calpains, thromboxane synthetase, iNOS or nNOS. Indeed, the original aim in developing the **lazaroids** as neuroprotective agents was to add antioxidant activity to a steroid nucleus, since high doses of methylprednisolone had been claimed as effective in diminishing brain lipid peroxidation after trauma and improving clinical outcome (it's doubtful that this is true, however).[239] The lazaroids inhibit iron-dependent lipid peroxidation in brain homogenates *in vitro* and exerted neuroprotective effects in various animal models of traumatic injury to the brain or spinal cord. The most studied was **U-74006F (Freedox)**, sometimes called **tirilazad mesylate**, which underwent several clinical trials for the treatment of stroke or traumatic injury to the nervous system. Sadly, there was no observable clinical benefit in the majority of cases and possible deleterious effects in stroke.[240] Nevertheless, studies suggested modest benefit in cases of subarachnoid haemorrhage in male but not female patients, apparently because females metabolize the drug faster. There is a lack of evidence that antioxidant action mediates any beneficial effects of the lazaroids *in vivo*, and the structure of U-74006F (Fig. 10.8) does not suggest that it will have much chain-breaking antioxidant activity.

Tirilazad seems to accumulate in the blood–brain barrier, perhaps protecting the microvascular endothelium, and its penetration into the brain is limited. An alternative is the **pyrrolopyrimidines** such as **U-101033E** and **U-104067F** (Fig. 10.8), antioxidants which appear to enter the brain more readily. Another drug being tested on stroke patients is **edaravone** (Fig. 10.8), with some suggestion of benefit.[240] Its structure does not suggest a high antioxidant activity, although keto-enol tautomerism may occur so that the structure shown in Fig. 10.8 is in equilibrium with a monophenol with some chain-breaking antioxidant activity.[241] Edaravone has also been suggested to be beneficial in animal models of cardiac and joint inflammation. Perhaps its actions are more anti-inflammatory than antioxidant.

10.6.9 Thiol compounds

Thiols scavenge numerous RS, but can also be cytotoxic, at least in part by generating oxygen- and sulphur-radicals (Section 2.5.5). Cysteine oxidizes much faster than either GSH or *N*-acetylcysteine and is correspondingly more cytotoxic, and homocysteine has been proposed to exert pro-oxidant effects *in vivo* (Section 10.5.9). Penicillamine and bucillamine[242] may exert side-effects in rheumatoid arthritis patients by forming sulphur radicals that bind to proteins and create new antigens (Section 9.10.6.2).

10.6.9.1 *Glutathione*
GSH is often suggested as potentially therapeutically useful. Areas of interest include the preservation of organs for transplantation (for example, GSH is added to University of Wisconsin solution; Section 9.6) and protection against tissue damage by cytotoxic drugs such as cyclophosphamide. Aerosolized GSH solutions have been suggested as a means of diminishing lung damage by RS (e.g. in cystic fibrosis; Table 9.6) although when tested in asthma patients they induced bronchoconstriction (not very beneficial!).[243] Remember that glutathione is a dicarboxylic acid (Fig. 3.13), so the free acid dissolved in insufficiently-buffered solution will have a low pH and could be irritant for that reason.

Glutathione is not easily taken up by cells. However, methyl, isopropyl and ethyl monoesters (esterified on the glycine carboxyl group) have been described, which can cross membranes and be hydrolysed to GSH within the cell (Fig. 10.9). Diethylesters (esterified on both the glycine carboxyl group and the side-chain carboxyl group of the glutamate) have also been tested, and may be more efficient delivery systems than monoesters. **L-2-oxathiazolidine-4-carboxylate (OTC)** can be hydrolysed to cysteine *in vivo*, which may lead to increased GSH synthesis. Hydrolysis requires the enzyme 5-oxoprolinase (Fig. 10.9). However, OTC has been tested in HIV-infected subjects, with no apparent benefit.[244] By contrast, it ameliorated allergen-induced airway injury in a mouse model of asthma, in part by decreasing VEGF production.[245]

10.6.9.2 N-*Acetylcysteine*[246]
N-Acetylcysteine is used as an antioxidant in many laboratory experiments and is effective in treating

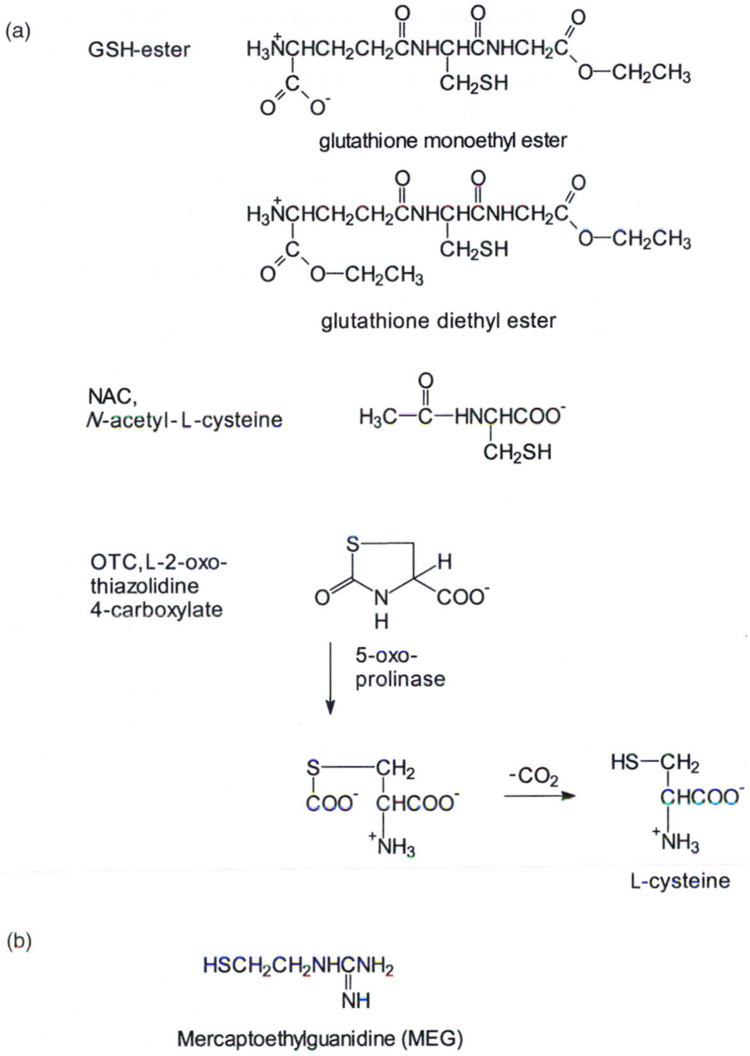

Figure 10.9 (a) Some agents that can increase GSH levels in cells. For more information see *Adv. Pharmacol.* **38**, 65, 1996. (b) Structure of mercaptoethylguanidine (MEG).

paracetamol overdosage (Section 8.10). It can protect by entering cells and being hydrolysed to cysteine, a precursor of GSH. Additionally, *N*-acetylcysteine itself can scavenge several RS (including $HOCl$, $ONOO^-$, $RO_2^\bullet$, $OH^\bullet$ and H_2O_2). It has been widely used in humans for treatment of several respiratory disorders (e.g. BPD in babies [Section 6.11.8] and ARDS [Section 9.7]), and in HIV [Section 9.23]); it has little toxicity but its therapeutic benefits are questionable.[247] More positive results (although not uniformly so) have been obtained in its use to prevent cardiovascular problems in patients with kidney failure, as well as kidney damage in patients with renal dysfunction who were administered radiocontrast media before radiography.[248] However, in one such study the protection occurred without effect on urinary F_2-IP levels—possibly indicative of a non-antioxidant protective mechanism.[249] *N*-Acetylcysteine slowed lung deterioration in patients with **idiopathic pulmonary fibrosis**, a progressive and usually fatal disorder characterized by fibrosis and remodelling of the lung. However, its mechanism of action is not clear.[250] **N-Acetylcysteine amide (AD4)** has been reported to cross the blood–brain barrier, unlike *N*-acetylcysteine itself, and showed protective effects against MOG-induced autoimmune encephalomyelitis (Section 9.17.2) and against MPTP toxicity in rats.[251]

10.6.9.3 *Other thiols*

Mercaptoethylguanidine (Fig. 10.9) is a powerful scavenger of $ONOO^-$ and HOCl and inhibits iNOS; it has beneficial effects in several animal models of inflammation.[252] Lipoic acid (Section 3.18.4) can act as an antioxidant *in vitro* and has been used in diabetes (Section 9.4). In rats, it prevented falls in GSH levels with age.[91] Several structurally modified forms of lipoic acid with improved antioxidant activity have been described, some of which can cross the blood–brain barrier.[253]

Many thiols have been tested for their ability to protect cells and animals against ionizing radiation (Section 8.19). They include GSH, cysteine, bucillamine, cysteamine, **dimercaprol (British anti-Lewisite**; Section 8.15.2), penicillamine, **mesna** (the sodium salt of **2-mercaptoethanesulphonic acid**; Fig. 10.8), and *S*-2-(3-aminopropylamino)ethyl phosphorothioic acid, a prodrug (**amifostine**) which is hydrolysed to the free thiol (**WR-1065**; Fig. 10.8) *in vivo* and has been used to protect normal tissues during radiotherapy. 'WR' signifies that this radioprotector (like many others) was developed at the Walter Reed Army Hospital in the USA.[254] The net charge on the thiol contributes to its radioprotective effect; if this is negative it can be repelled by the net negative change of DNA.

Mercaptopropionylglycine (MPG) (Fig. 10.8) decreases ROS production and protects against ischaemia–reperfusion injury in animal models of myocardial stunning and infarction (Section 9.5.4).

10.6.10 Glutathione peroxidase 'mimetics'[228]

Selenocysteine plays a key role at the active sites of GPx enzymes (Section 3.8), and attempts have thus been made to design low-molecular-mass selenium compounds with similar catalytic activity. The first was **ebselen (PZ51)**, 2-phenyl-1,2-benzisoselenazol-3 (2*H*)-one (Fig. 10.8). After reduction by GSH, ebselen decomposes peroxides in a catalytic manner. Other thiols, including *N*-acetylcysteine, reduced thioredoxin, and dihydrolipoate (DHLA) can replace GSH as cofactors, DHLA being especially effective. Thioredoxin reductase can use NADPH to reduce ebselen, and thus ebselen has also been described as a 'peroxiredoxin mimic'.[255] Reduction of ebselen opens the ring containing the Se, converting it to −SeH (**selenol**), which then reacts with the peroxide to re-form ebselen. The selenol can also react with another ebselen molecule to form a diselenide, which contributes to catalysis. Ebselen additionally has direct antioxidant activities *in vitro*, for example scavenging HOCl, singlet O_2, $ONOO^-$, and $RO_2^{\bullet}$. Ebselen binds to −SH groups on proteins, and much of it in plasma is probably attached to albumin −SH groups.

Ebselen has shown protective effects in several animal models of disease (e.g. metabolic syndrome [Section 9.4.6] and noise-induced hearing loss [Section 8.17]), and its toxicity appears low. As well as showing antioxidant activity, it can inhibit 5- and 15-lipoxygenases and NOS and may have direct inhibitory effects on phagocyte ROS production. Some clinical studies have suggested beneficial effects in patients with subarachnoid haemorrhage and stroke[188,240] but these remain to be confirmed. In any case, given its mixture of properties, it cannot be assumed that protection by ebselen is due only to antioxidant actions.

Other organoselenium compounds have been reported to possess GPx-like activity, including several diselenides (containing −Se−Se−groupings),[256] and **BXT−51075** (Fig. 10.8), one of a group of compounds which appear to exert greater protective effects than ebselen against oxidative stress in cell culture.

By analogy, several compounds containing the element **tellurium** (which, like sulphur and selenium, is in group VI of the periodic table) can scavenge peroxides and $ONOO^-$ and show other antioxidant effects *in vitro*.[257]

10.6.11 Mitochondrially-targeted antioxidants[258]

Since mitochondria are major sources of ROS *in vivo*, and damage to them contributes to ageing and disease, antioxidants selectively targeted to these organelles could be especially beneficial. One approach has been to link an antioxidant (such as a thiol, α-tocopherol, ebselen, CoQ or a spin trap) via hydrocarbon chains of variable length to the phosphorus of the lipophilic compound **triphenyl-phosphonium** (TPP), giving a **triphenylphospho-nium cation** $(Ph)_3P^+-R$, where R is the antioxidant. An example is **MitoQ$_{10}$** (Fig. 10.8). These compounds accumulate inside mitochondria in response to the inner membrane potential, and can protect cells in culture against the toxicity of added H_2O_2 or of hyperoxia. When fed to animals, they can enter all tissues, including the brain, and MitoQ$_{10}$ fed to rats protected subsequently-isolated hearts against ischaemia–reperfusion injury. Giving the rats CoQ$_{10}$ or TPP in the diet was not protective.[259] These compounds should prove useful in 'probing' the role of mitochondrial ROS in physiological and pathological processes, by scavenging such species and seeing what happens (e.g. Section 4.5.7). Triphenylphosphonium and similar compounds can also be used to target ROS-detecting molecules such as dihydroethidium to the mitochondria (Section 5.11.3).

10.7 Iron chelators[196]

Several chelating agents have been used in attempts to inhibit iron- or copper-dependent oxidative damage (Table 10.14). Examples already discussed include ICRF-187 (Section 9.15.2) and clioquinol (Section 9.20). Chelators can act by multiple mechanisms. Take a simple observation; adding a chelator (X) decreases the amount of OH$^\bullet$ observed from a metal ion–H_2O_2 mixture. How might X do this (for a detailed discussion see Section 2.4.5)?

1. X could chelate metal ions and alter their reduction potential and/or accessibility to stop them catalysing OH$^\bullet$ production. An example in the binding of iron ions to transferrin or lactoferrin.
2. Binding of metal ions to X does not stop OH$^\bullet$ formation, but the OH$^\bullet$ formed at the binding site reacts with X and does not escape into solution. For example, copper ions bound to albumin can still form OH$^\bullet$, but the protein absorbs it and is

damaged. Another example is OR10141 (Table 10.14).
3. X scavenges OH$^\bullet$ in free solution, competing for it with the 'detector molecule' being used to measure OH.

To help distinguish between these mechanisms, one can examine the fate of the chelator in the reaction mixture; it will be damaged if it is reacting with OH$^\bullet$. Similar principles apply to studies of effects of metal-chelating antioxidants on lipid peroxidation. Chelators that inhibit RS production are intrinsically preferable, since those that scavenge RS are destroyed as the reaction proceeds and may produce toxic chelator-derived radicals.

The first chelating agent reported to decrease the rate of $O_2^{\bullet-}$-dependent OH$^\bullet$ generation *in vitro* was DETAPAC. It decreases OH$^\bullet$ generation because Fe(III)–DETAPAC is reduced only slowly by $O_2^{\bullet-}$ (Table 2.6, legend). An Fe^{2+}–DETAPAC complex still reacts with H_2O_2 to form OH$^\bullet$, however, and more powerful reducing agents than $O_2^{\bullet-}$ (such as paraquat radical) *are* able to reduce Fe(III)–DETA-PAC. Hence DETAPAC is not a *general* inhibitor of iron-dependent OH$^\bullet$ generation. Phytic acid, *o*-phenanthroline, bathophenanthroline sulphonate and desferrioxamine are better inhibitors of iron-dependent formation of OH$^\bullet$ from $O_2^{\bullet-}$ and H_2O_2. Phytic acid, **inositol hexaphosphate**, has been used as an antioxidant in foodstuffs and could conceivably be protective in the colon, by binding iron in faeces (Section 6.2). Several plant phenolics can bind transition-metal ions (Section 3.22), and this may be the mechanism by which **7-mono-hydroxyethylrutoside** (Table 10.14) diminishes the cardiotoxicity of doxorubicin to mice.

10.7.1 Desferrioxamine

Desferrioxamine (DFO) is a powerful chelator of Fe (III). In the presence of physiological buffer systems, it inhibits iron-dependent lipid peroxidation and conversion of H_2O_2 to OH$^\bullet$ (Table 10.15). Desferrioxamine is produced by *Streptomyces pilosus* and is widely and effectively used for the prevention and treatment of iron overload in patients who have ingested toxic oral doses of iron salts, or who require multiple blood transfusions,

Table 10.14 Some chelating agents

Chelating agent	Comments
Penicillamine	Useful in promoting urinary excretion of copper ions in treatment of Wilson's disease. Also binds Fe^{2+}.
	$HS-C(CH_3)_2$
	$H_2N-CHCOOH$
EDTA	Chelates several metal ions. Manganese– and copper–EDTA chelates are usually less redox-active than the unchelated metal ions, whereas chelates of EDTA with Fe^{2+} or Fe(III) still react with H_2O_2 or $O_2^{\bullet-}$. Often EDTA promotes iron-dependent damage by keeping iron ions in solution in a redox-active form, but Fe^{2+}–EDTA rapidly oxidizes to Fe(III)–EDTA at pH 7.4, releasing $O_2^{\bullet-}$
	$Fe^{2+}-EDTA + O_2 \rightarrow Fe(III)-EDTA + O_2^{\bullet-}$
	EDTA can inhibit 'site-specific' damage by removing metal ions from a target (e.g. DNA). EDTA infusion into the blood has been used in some countries (**chelation therapy**) to treat patients with vascular problems, but its value is uncertain.
DETAPAC	Chelates iron, copper and other metal ions. Little used clinically because of side-effects, including zinc and magnesium depletion, but has been used *in vivo* to remove lead and plutonium, and to remove iron from thalassaemic patients who cannot tolerate desferrioxamine.
Rhodotorulic acid	Both this and desferrioxamine (below) are examples of **siderophores** (from the Greek words for 'iron' and 'carrier'). Siderophores are produced by microorganisms to chelate extracellular iron and bring it into the cell. Iron is usually bound as Fe(III). Siderophores are usually hydroxamates (such as desferrioxamine) or phenols. *M. tuberculosis* produces the **exochelins**, lipid-soluble siderophores.

Effective iron chelator in animals (*Blood* **91**, 1446, 1998).

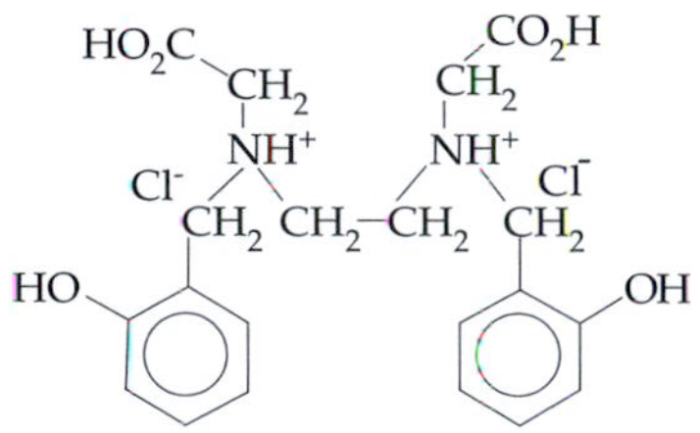

HBED

Can be given orally.

2–3-Dihydroxybenzoate

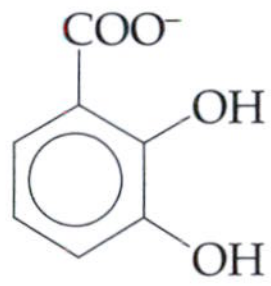

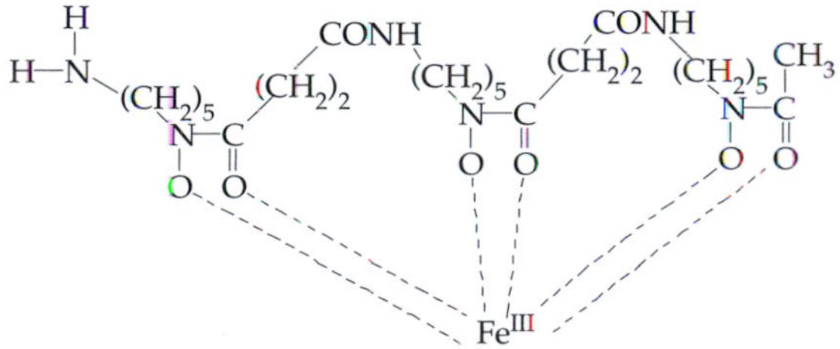

A linear molecule that 'bends round' to chelate Fe(III) with six ligands (i.e. it is a **hexadentate** chelator) forming a bright-red complex, **ferrioxamine**. Commercially available as **desferal** (desferrioxamine B methanesulphonate; relative molecular mass 657). Often called **deferoxamine** in the USA.

Desferrioxamine B

Effective iron chelator in animals. Can be given orally. An alternative is **salicylaldehyde isonicotinoylhydrazone**, SIH (*J. Mol. Cell. Cardiol.* **39**, 345, 2005; *Physiol. Res.* **53**, 683, 2004), which is used in the calcein assay for cellular iron pools (Fig. 3.21).

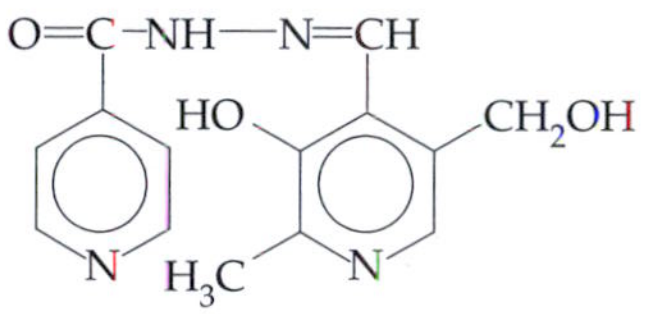

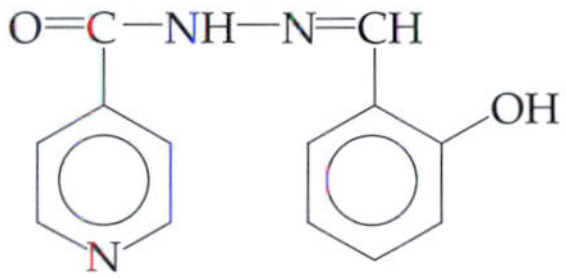

PIH

Table 10.14 (*Cont.*)

Chelating agent	Comments
o-Phenanthroline (1,10-phenanthroline)	Good chelator of Cu^{2+} ions (log stability constant = 6.3). Also binds Fe^{2+} (log stability constant = 5.8) and zinc. Can prevent H_2O_2-mediated damage to DNA in mammalian cells, probably by chelating iron. However, a Cu^{2+}-phenanthroline complex is able to promote DNA degradation (Section 4.3.4).
1,2-Dimethyl-3-hydroxy-pyridin-4-one[a]	One of a series of chelators, the **1-alkyl-3-hydroxy-2-methylpyrid-4-ones**, which can be given orally since they are absorbed through the gut. They enter tissues more readily than desferal and have shown promising results in the treatment of thalassaemia. They are bidentate; three molecules are needed to coordinate one iron completely.
OR10141	Reaction of Fe^{2+} chelated to this compound with H_2O_2 hydroxylates site-specifically on the aromatic ring to generate a better iron chelator (*J. Med. Chem.* **43**, 1418, 2000). X = co-ordinating solvent. * Site of hydroxylation

7-Monohydroxy-ethylrutoside

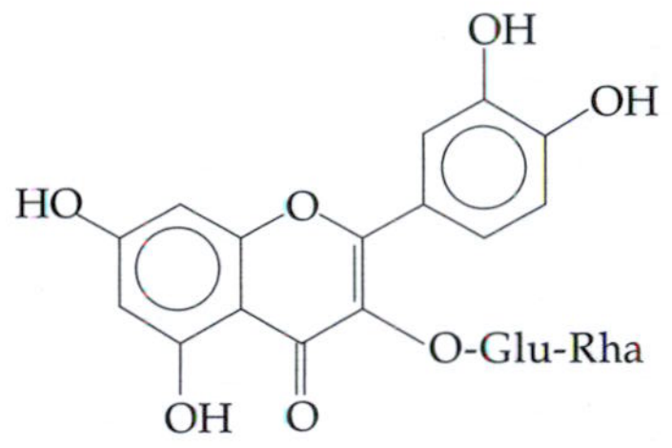

Effectiveness in protecting against cardiotoxicity in mice is comparable to that of ICRF-187 (*Br. J. Pharmacol.* **115**, 1260, 1995). Glu, glucose; Rha, rhamnose.

ICL670

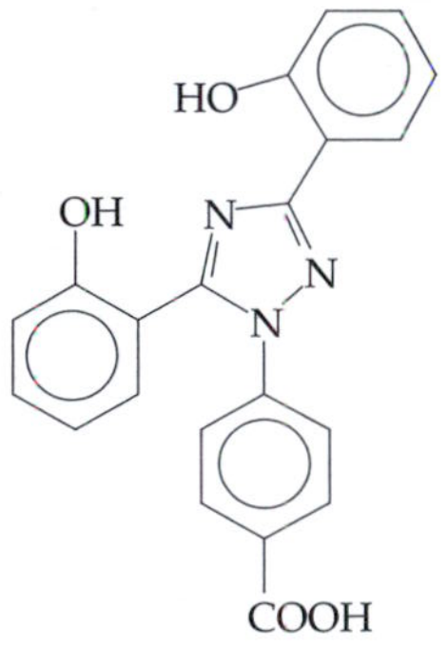

A tridentate ligand, under evaluation for treatment of thalassaemia (*Lancet* **361**, 1597, 2003).[270]

LAP oxidized

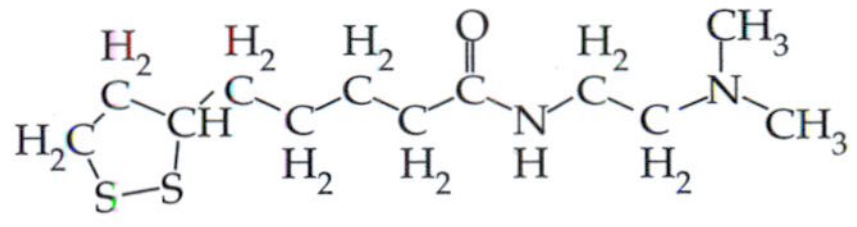

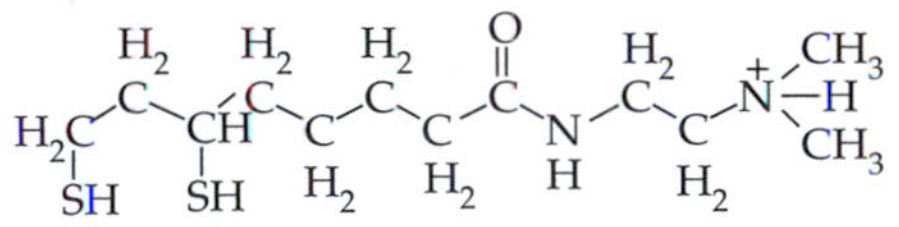

Derivative of lipoic acid (*Free Rad. Biol. Med.* **34**, 1295, 2003). Targets to lysosomes in cells.

LAP reduced, at acidic pH

Abbreviations: HBED, *N*, *N*-*bis*(2-hydroxybenzyl)ethylenediamine-*N*,*N*-diacetic acid; EDTA, ethylenediaminetetra-acetic acid; DETAPAC, diethylenetriaminepenta-acetic acid; PIH, pyridoxal isonicotinoyl hydrazone.

[a] Sometimes called **CP20**, **deferiprone** or **L1**. In **CP94** both –CH₃ groups are replaced by ethyl groups.

Table 10.15 Properties of desferrioxamine

Powerful chelator of Fe(III) (stability constant $\sim 10^{31}$)

Chelates several other metal ions with stability constants several orders of magnitude lower (e.g. Al(III), $\sim 10^{25}$; Cu^{2+}, $\sim 10^{14}$; Zn^{2+}, $\sim 10^{11}$); has been used to remove aluminium from dialysis patients (Section 8.15.11)

Reacts slowly with $O_2^{\bullet-}$ or $HO_2^{\bullet}$ ($k_2 \approx 10^3 \, M^{-1} s^{-1}$) to form nitroxide radicals that can inactivate yeast alcohol dehydrogenase and oxidize ascorbate, GSH and NAD(P)H

Moderately good scavenger of peroxyl ($RO_2^{\bullet}$) radicals in aqueous solution, again a nitroxide results

Reacts fast with $OH^{\bullet}$ ($k_2 \approx 10^{10} \, M^{-1} s^{-1}$); nitroxide radicals are again produced, so desferrioxamine is an excellent $OH^{\bullet}$ scavenger; ferrioxamine scavenges $OH^{\bullet}$ with the same rate constant

Reacts quickly with $CO_3^{\bullet-}$ ($k_2 \approx 1.7 \times 10^9 \, M^{-1} s^{-1}$) and $NO_2^{\bullet}$ radicals ($k_2 \approx 7.6 \times 10^6 \, M^{-1} s^{-1}$), nitroxide radicals yet again

Inhibits iron-dependent lipid peroxidation and $OH^{\bullet}$ generation from H_2O_2 in most systems; ferrioxamine does not inhibit, so a control with this substance can distinguish protection by iron binding from protection by direct scavenging of RS

Accelerates the oxidation of Fe^{2+} solutions, by binding the resulting Fe(III) more tightly than it does Fe^{2+}; this is the **ferroxidase** action of DFO, which produces $O_2^{\bullet-}$:

$$Fe^{2+} - DFO + O_2 \rightarrow Fe(III) - DFO + O_2^{\bullet-}$$

Penetrates only slowly into most animal cells; may enter by pinocytosis into lysosomes; poorly absorbed from gut but oral administration could conceivably be used to interfere with iron absorption

Can raise levels of HIF1α and promote a cell 'hypoxic response'

Most studies with desferrioxamine are carried out with the commercially available **desferal** (**desferrioxamine B methanesulphonate**).

Adapted from *Free Rad. Biol. Med.* **7**, 645, 1989; also see *Free Rad. Biol. Med.* **36**, 471, 2004 and[260,261].

for example to treat thalassaemia. Large doses of DFO can be injected into animals or humans; 50 mg/kg bodyweight per day appears fairly safe in thalassaemic patients provided that they do not become iron-deficient. Too much DFO can lead to auditory and visual problems, usually reversible when the excess is withdrawn, and an increased risk of serious infection with certain microorganisms, such as *Vibrio vulnificus* and *Yersinia enterocolitica*, and with fungi such as *Rhizopus*. Desferrioxamine is highly (but not absolutely; Table 10.15) specific for Fe(III). The Fe(III)–DFO complex (**ferrioxamine**) is difficult to reduce, not only by $O_2^{\bullet-}$, but also by more powerful reductants (Table 2.6). Despite its high stability constant for iron, DFO is inefficient at removing iron ions bound to transferrin or lactoferrin, which may be advantageous since iron left safely bound to these proteins does not stimulate free-radical reactions. Desferrioxamine is too hydrophilic to cross cell membranes, and seems to enter cells by pinocytosis, localizing in lysosomes.[262] Its limited toxicity allows it to be used *in vivo* to investigate the role of

iron ions in disease (Table 10.16), and it has sometimes been added to organ preservation fluids, for example for heart transplantation (Section 9.6).

Desferrioxamine can react directly with several RS, including $RO_2^{\bullet}$, $O_2^{\bullet-}$ (slowly), $OH^{\bullet}$, HOCl and oxo–haem species produced by mixing haem proteins with H_2O_2. It does not react with $ONOO^-$, but can be attacked by $ONOO^-$-derived species such as $CO_3^{\bullet-}$ and $NO_2^{\bullet}$ (Table 10.14). Hence it can inhibit damage caused by adding $ONOO^-$ to biological systems. Since it is a hydroxamate, DFO's oxidation by RS will generate nitroxide radicals, which could oxidize other biomolecules such GSH and ascorbate.[261] However, the toxicity of nitroxides is generally low (Section 10.6.5). Scavenging of RS by DFO may be of little significance *in vivo*, because the concentration achieved during normal therapeutic use (up to 20 μM plasma levels during infusion) is too low for scavenging to be feasible.

At therapeutically relevant concentrations, DFO can inhibit cell proliferation. It may act by depleting the cells of iron (so inhibiting iron-dependent

Table 10.16 Some animal models of oxidative stress in which desferrioxamine is protective

Effect reported	Comments
Decreases neutrophil-mediated acute lung injury in rats after complement activation.	A model for some forms of ARDS (Section 9.7).
Anti-inflammatory in several acute and acute-to-chronic models of inflammation, including an autoimmune disease model (experimental allergic encephalomyelitis) in rats (*J. Neuroimmunol.* **17**, 127, 1988).	Not necessarily acting by an antioxidant mechanism (Section 9.10).
Inhibits the toxic action of alloxan and paraquat.	Results variable (Sections 8.4 and 8.5).
Decreases liver damage by CCl_4.	Section 8.2.
Protective against reoxygenation injury after ischaemia in lung, heart, kidney, gut, brain and skin. Heart studies show protection against arrhythmias and stunning and perhaps decreased infarct size. Effects can be antioxidant, and/or by the induction of HIF1α, which can sometimes have a 'preconditioning' effect.[260]	Section 9.5; also see *J. Cereb. Blood Flow Metab.* **23**, 574, 2003.
Decreases antigen-antibody-induced kidney damage in rabbits	Damage may be due to $O_2^{\bullet-}$ and H_2O_2 produced by neutrophils, perhaps reacting with iron to form $OH^{\bullet}$.
Protective in rat and dog haemorrhagic shock models	*Shock* **17**, 339, 2002; *Free Radic. Res. Commun.* **6**, 29, 1989.

enzymes such as ribonucleoside diphosphate reductase; Section 7.2.2) and also by altering levels of the cyclins and cdk2.[263] Hence, if DFO is infused over several days, as has been done in some studies of its effects upon chronic inflammation or auto-immune disease in animals (Section 9.10), it is possible that any beneficial effects it exerts could involve inhibition of the proliferation of inflammatory cells such as lymphocytes. Desferrioxamine also increases levels of HIF-1 (Section 1.3.2) in many cell types, with subsequent increased transcription of genes under the control of this pathway (e.g. erythropoietin, glycolytic enzymes). Similar effects are seen with several other iron chelators and may involve removal of iron from prolyl hydroxylase, to inhibit its activity (Section 1.3.2).[260] Hence never assume that DFX is acting by antioxidant actions.

Because iron is essential for cell function, prolonged administration of any powerful iron-chelating agent to humans (others than patients suffering from iron overload) will probably cause side-effects. However, this should not preclude use of chelators in acute situations (Table 10.16). High-molecular-mass forms of DFO have been described, in which it is attached to such polymers as cellulose, dextran or hydroxyethyl starch. Conjugation of DFO to these polymers was reported not to diminish its

Fe(III)-binding activity, but to decrease the toxicity of high doses and to increase circulating plasma half-life in animals. They presumably enter cells by endocytosis and end up in the lysosomes—the hydroxyethyl starch remains there as it cannot be degraded by lysosomal enzymes.[262] These conjugates have been reported as protective in several animal models of disease, including septic shock, and to delay the onset of diabetes in spontaneously diabetic rats.[264] However, there have been few examples of the use of DFO or its conjugates to treat human disease, apart from iron overload of course. In one short-term study, intravenous infusion of DFO improved endothelial function (measured as forearm blood flow; Section 5.1.3.1) in patients with diseased coronary arteries.[265]

10.7.2 Other iron-chelating agents[266]

The gene encoding human lactoferrin has been cloned and expressed in plants, and in female mice and cows (both of which secrete the human protein in their milk). The human protein can be added to baby foods to decrease pro-oxidant effects of added iron, and was reported to decrease gastrointestinal damage by indomethacin in humans.[267] Bovine lactoferrin has been tested as a treatment, in combination with antibiotics, to aid eradication of *H. pylori* from the human stomach.[268]

The **hydroxypyridones** were introduced in an attempt to overcome a major drawback of DFO in treating thalassaemia; it is not absorbed through the gut and has to be administered by intravenous or subcutaneous infusion. Desferal is also expensive. There has therefore been a search for orally active chelating agents which, it is hoped, will be cheaper. Some work was carried out with HBED, PIH, desferrithiocin and 2,3-dihydroxybenzoate, but most attention has focused on the **3-hydroxypyrid-4-ones** (Table 10.14). For example, **1,2-dimethyl-3-hydroxypyridin-4-one (LI)** has undergone clinical trials in humans. Sadly, it appears more toxic than DFO, although still clinically useful. Other hydroxypyridones (such as the 1,2-diethyl compound) are under evaluation.[269]

The apparent increased toxicity of hydroxypyridones could be due to their chemistry. An iron ion can bind six ligands. Desferrioxamine is a **hexadentate** ligand, that is it occupies all six co-ordination sites. The DFO 'wraps around' the iron ion, encasing it in an envelope of organic material. By contrast, hydroxypyridones occupy only two co-ordination sites (i.e. they are **bidentate** ligands) and three hydroxypyridone molecules are needed to chelate one Fe(III) completely. Upon dilution, 3:1 hydroxypyridone: iron ion complexes might dissociate into 2:1 complexes, leaving available co-ordination sites on the iron that could allow catalysis of free-radical reactions. In addition, hydroxypyridones can mobilize iron ions from transferrin and lactoferrin, at least *in vitro*. Thus one could envisage a scenario in which 'safely' protein-bound iron (unable to stimulate free-radical reactions) could be mobilized and transferred to other sites in the body to cause oxidative damage. Whether this contributes to the side-effects of L1 is uncertain.

A few orally active tridentate ligands have been described. One is **ICL670** (Table 10.14) which has been tested in thalassaemia and its use has been approved by the USA FDA.[270] Some authors have described 'oxidative stress-activatable' iron chelators. For example, in the presence of H_2O_2 an Fe^{2+}-chelate of **OR10141** (Table 10.14) undergoes hydroxylation on the aromatic ring to generate a

better iron chelator. Hence these compounds putatively chelate iron at sites of oxidative stress, and not in the body generally. Another interesting compound is **LAP** (Table 10.14), a derivative of lipoamide designed to accumulate within lysosomes. It is more effective than DFO in protecting cells in culture against the toxic effects of H_2O_2.[262] An antioxidant derived from serine and vitamin B_6, **N-(4-pyridoxylmethylene)-L-serine**,

was found to protect mouse skin against damage by UV light, presumably by chelating iron.[271]

Iron-chelating ability can be 'added' to another drug, such as a MAO inhibitor. Examples are **M30**

and **M10**, structure as above but side-chain is

They have been suggested for use in PD, and M30 protects mice against MPTP neurotoxicity.[272]

10.8 Inhibitors of the generation of reactive species

Another approach to antioxidant protection is to inhibit RS formation.

10.8.1 Xanthine oxidase (XO) inhibitors

These were discussed in Fig. 1.16, so we make only brief comments here. Many animal experiments show that allopurinol protects against reoxygenation injury (Section 9.5). Since allopurinol is widely used to treat hyperuricaemia in humans, its toxicological profile is well-known and it is added to some organ preservation solutions (Section 9.6). Although XO makes only limited contributions to RS generation in most human tissues, it does occur in gut, atherosclerotic lesions (Section 9.3), the synovia of patients with rheumatoid arthritis (Section 9.10), the palmar fascia of patients with Dupuytren's contracture (Section 9.6.3) and the plasma of patients with thalassaemia (Section 6.4.4) and ARDS (Section 9.7). The therapeutic possibilities of treatment with allopurinol in these diseases have been discussed, but not fully evaluated clinically.

As well as inhibiting XO, oxypurinol (the major metabolite of allopurinol; Fig. 1.16) can scavenge HOCl *in vitro*, which might contribute to its protective effects under certain circumstances. *In vitro*, both allopurinol and oxypurinol react with $OH^•$, but the concentrations achieved *in vivo* are probably too low for this to be a significant mechanism of protection. An additional mechanism by which allopurinol, oxypurinol or other XO inhibitors could protect tissues is by preventing oxidation of hypoxanthine, so enhancing its salvage for reincorporation into adenine nucleotides when the tissue is reoxygenated (Section 9.5).

10.8.2 Inhibitors of phagocyte RS generation

Generation of RS by phagocytes sometimes contributes to tissue injury. Hence inhibitors of phagocyte recruitment can be useful, such as agents that inhibit the production, or antagonize the action of, 'proinflammatory' cytokines (e.g. infliximab, Section 9.10.2), compounds that decrease levels of adhesion molecules, antibodies directed against adhesion molecules, or synthetic 'decoy' adhesion molecules that compete with phagocytes for binding to endothelium. Compounds interfering with phagocyte RS production might also be useful—indeed, adenosine may act in this way (Section 9.5).

Several anti-inflammatory drugs have been hypothesized to decrease $O_2^{•-}$ formation by phagocytes (Section 9.10.6), and some of the beneficial effects of ebselen (Section 10.6.10) could be due to this. Diphenylene iodonium compounds inhibit the respiratory burst in isolated neutrophils, but are non-specific (Fig. 7.14). **Apocynin** (Fig. 10.8) is a plant phenol that is oxidized by MPO to a product that blocks assembly of the NADPH oxidase. Hence only activated phagocytes (producing the H_2O_2 necessary for peroxidase action) are affected. Apocynin has an anti-inflammatory effect in rats, but high levels are needed.[273] The compound **S17834** inhibits NADPH oxidase and was reported to be antiatherosclerotic in apoE-deficient mice, but seems to have attracted little attention.[274] **Tetomilast**[275] is under evaluation for the treatment of inflammatory bowel disease, although its benefits do not seems great (Section 9.11). **Tetrandrine**, an alkaloid from roots of the plant *Stephania tetrandra*, is used in China to treat silicosis in miners. It prevents NF-κB activation and hence may act by decreasing the levels of iNOS and COX-2.[276]

APPENDIX

Some basic chemistry

A1 Atomic structure

For the purposes of this book, it is sufficient to use a simple model of atomic structure in which atoms consist of a positively charged nucleus surrounded by one or more negatively charged electrons. The nucleus contains two types of particle of approximately equal mass, the positively charged **proton** and the uncharged **neutron**. By comparison with these particles, the mass of the electron is negligible, so that virtually all of the mass of the atom is contributed by its nucleus. The **atomic number** of an element is defined as the number of protons in its nucleus, the **mass number** as the number of protons plus neutrons. In the neutral atom, the atomic number also equals the number of electrons. The simplest atom is that of the element hydrogen, containing one proton (atomic number one, mass number one) and one electron. All other elements contain neutrons in the nucleus.

Some elements exist as **isotopes**, in which the atoms contain the same number of protons and electrons, but different numbers of neutrons. These isotopes can be stable or unstable, the unstable ones undergoing **radioactive decay** at various rates. In this process, the nucleus of the radioactive isotope changes, and a new element forms. For example, an isotope of the element uranium (atomic number 92) with a mass number of 238 undergoes nuclear disintegration to produce two fragments, one with two protons and two neutrons and the other with 90 protons and 144 neutrons, an isotope of the element thorium. The elements which largely concern us in this book, carbon, hydrogen, nitrogen and oxygen, exist almost exclusively as one isotopic form in nature (Table A1).

The electrons are negatively charged. Since they do not spiral into the positively-charged nucleus, they must possess energy to counteract the attractive force trying to pull them in. In 1900, Planck suggested that energy is quantized, i.e. energy changes only occur in small, definite amounts known as 'quanta'. Application of Planck's quantum theory to the atom, by Bohr, produced a model in which the electrons exist in specific orbits, or 'electron shells', each associated with a particular energy level. The 'K'-shell electrons, lying closest to the nucleus, have the lowest energy, and the energy successively increases as one proceeds outwards to the so-called L-, M- and N-shells. The K-shell can hold a maximum of two electrons, the L-shell, 8, M-shell, 18 and N-shell, 32. Table A2 shows the location of electrons in each of these shells for the elements up to atomic number 36.

Electrons have some of the properties of a particle, and some of the properties of a wave motion. The position of an electron at a given time cannot be precisely specified, but only the region of space where it is most likely to be. These regions are called **orbitals**. Each electron in an atom has its energy defined by four **quantum numbers**. The first, or **principal quantum number** (n), defines the main energy level the electron occupies. For the K-shell, $n = 1$; for L, $n = 2$; for M, $n = 3$; and for N, $n = 4$. The second, or **azimuthal quantum number** (l), governs the shape of the orbital and has values from zero up to $(n-1)$. When $l = 0$, the electrons are called 's' electrons; when $l = 1$, they are 'p' electrons; $l = 2$, 'd' electrons; and $l = 3$ gives 'f' electrons. The third quantum number is the **magnetic quantum number** (m) and, for each value of l, m has values

Table A1 Isotopes of some common elements

Element	Isotope	Number of protons in nucleus	Number of neutrons in nucleus	Comments
Chlorine	$^{35}_{17}Cl$	17	18	Both isotopes are stable and occur naturally, ^{35}Cl being more abundant
	$^{37}_{17}Cl$	17	20	
Carbon	$^{12}_{6}C$	6	6	Over 90% of naturally occurring carbon is $^{14}_{6}C$. Small amounts of the radioactive isotope $^{14}_{6}C$ are formed by the bombardment of atmospheric CO_2 with cosmic rays (streams of neutrons arising from outer space). This isotope undergoes slow radioactive decay (50% decay after 5600 years)
	$^{13}_{6}C$	6	7	
	$^{14}_{6}C$	6	8	
Nitrogen	$^{14}_{7}N$	7	7	^{15}N is a stable isotope of nitrogen often used as a 'tracer', e.g. $^{15}NO_3^-$ can be fed to humans to study its metabolism
	$^{15}_{7}N$	7	8	
Oxygen	$^{16}_{8}O$	8	8	Over 90% of naturally occurring oxygen is the isotope $^{16}_{8}O$
	$^{17}_{8}O$	8	9	
	$^{18}_{8}O$	8	10	
Hydrogen	$^{1}_{1}H$	1	0	Over 99% of hydrogen is $^{1}_{1}H$. Deuterium ($^{2}_{1}H$) is a stable isotope, whereas tritium ($^{3}_{1}H$) is radioactive. Deuterium oxide is known as 'heavy water', and is used in detecting singlet O_2 (Section 5.9).
	$^{2}_{1}H$	1	1	
	$^{3}_{1}H$	1	2	

The superscript number on the left of the symbol for the element is the mass number, and the subscript the atomic number. All atoms of a given element have the same number of protons, but sometimes have different numbers of neutrons, giving rise to isotopes.

of l, $(l–1)$, ..., 0, –1, ..., ..., $–l$. Finally, the fourth quantum number, or **spin quantum number**, can only have values of 1/2 or –1/2. Table A3 shows how electrons with these different quantum numbers fill the electron shells. **Pauli's principle** states that 'no two electrons can have the same four quantum numbers'. Since the spin quantum number has only two possible values ($\pm 1/2$), it follows that an orbital can hold a maximum of two electrons (Table A3).

In filling the available orbitals electrons enter the orbitals with the lowest energy first (**Aufbau principle**). The order is:

1s 2s 2p 3s 3p 4s 3d 4p 5s 4d 5p 6s 4f 5d 6p 7s 5f

Lowest energy   Increasing energy   Highest energy

Table A4 gives the electronic energy configurations of the elements with atomic numbers 1 to 32. When the elements are arranged in the **periodic table** (Figure A1), elements with similar electronic arrangements fall into similar **groups** (vertical rows), e.g. the group II elements all have two electrons in their outermost electron shell, and the group IV elements have four. Since the 4s-orbital is of lower energy than the 3d-orbitals, these latter orbitals remain empty until the 4s-orbital is filled (e.g. see potassium and calcium in Table A4). In subsequent elements the five 3d-orbitals receive electrons, creating the first row of the **d-block** in the periodic table (Figure A1). Some of these d-block elements are **transition elements**, meaning elements in which an inner shell of electrons is incomplete (in this case these are electrons in the fourth shell, but all the d-orbitals of the third shell are not yet full). The term transition element, as defined above, applies to scandium and subsequent elements as far as nickel, although it is often

Table A2 Location of electrons in shells for the elements with atomic numbers 1 to 36

Atomic number of element	Element	Symbol	Shell K	Shell L	Shell M	Shell N
1	Hydrogen	H	1			
2	Helium	He	2			
3	Lithium	Li	2	1		
4	Beryllium	Be	2	2		
5	Boron	B	2	3		
6	Carbon	C	2	4		
7	Nitrogen	N	2	5		
8	Oxygen	O	2	6		
9	Fluorine	F	2	7		
10	Neon	Ne	2	8		
11	Sodium	Na	2	8	1	
12	Magnesium	Mg	2	8	2	
13	Aluminium	Al	2	8	3	
14	Silicon	Si	2	8	4	
15	Phosphorus	P	2	8	5	
16	Sulphur	S	2	8	6	
17	Chlorine	Cl	2	8	7	
18	Argon	Ar	2	8	8	
19	Potassium	K	2	8	8	1
20	Calcium	Ca	2	8	8	2
21	Scandium	Sc	2	8	9	2
22	Titanium	Ti	2	8	10	2
23	Vanadium	V	2	8	11	2
24	Chromium	Cr	2	8	13	1
25	Manganese	Mn	2	8	13	2
26	Iron	Fe	2	8	14	2
27	Cobalt	Co	2	8	15	2
28	Nickel	Ni	2	8	16	2
29	Copper	Cu	2	8	18	1
30	Zinc	Zn	2	8	18	2
31	Gallium	Ga	2	8	18	3
32	Germanium	Ge	2	8	18	4
33	Arsenic	As	2	8	18	5
34	Selenium	Se	2	8	18	6
35	Bromine	Br	2	8	18	7
36	Krypton	Kr	2	8	18	8

extended to include the whole of the first row of the d-block.

If orbitals of equal energy are available, for example the three 2p-orbitals in the L-shell, or the five 3d-orbitals in the M-shell (Table A3), each is filled with one electron before any receives two (**Hund's rule**). Hence one can further analyse the electronic configurations in Table A4. For example, boron has two 1s, two 2s and one 2p electrons. Three 2p-orbitals of equal energy are available (Table A3), often written as $2p_x$, $2p_y$ and $2p_z$. If we represent each orbital as a box and an electron as an

Table A3 Orbitals available in the principal electron shells

Shell	Principal quantum number	Value of l (azimuthal quantum number)	Electron type	Value of m (magnetic quantum number)	Value of s (spin quantum number)	Maximum number of electrons in shell
K	1	0	s	0	±1/2	2 (1s–orbital)
L	2	0	s	0	±1/2	2 (2s–orbital) ⎫
		1	p	1, 0, −1	±1/2	3 × 2 (three 2p–orbitals) ⎬ 8
M	3	0	s	0	±1/2	2 (3s–orbital) ⎫
		1	p	1, 0, −1	±1/2	3 × 2 (three 2p–orbitals) ⎬ 18
		2	d	2, 1, 0, −1, −2	±1/2	5 × 2 (five 3d–orbitals) ⎭
N	4	0	s	0	±1/2	2 (4s–orbital) ⎫
		1	p	1, 0, −1	±1/2	3 × 2 (three 4p–orbitals) ⎪
		2	d	2, 1, 0, −1, −2	±1/2	5 × 2 (five 4d–orbitals) ⎬ 32
		3	f	3, 2, 1, 0, −1, −2, −3	±1/2	7 × 2 (seven 4f–orbitals) ⎭

arrow, boron can be represented as:

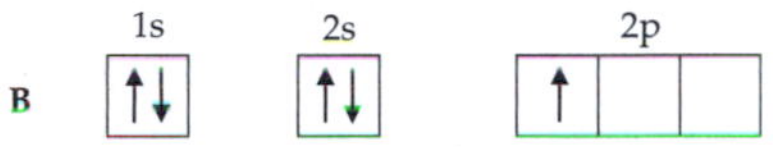

For the next element, carbon, the extra electron enters another 2p-orbital in obedience to Hund's rule:

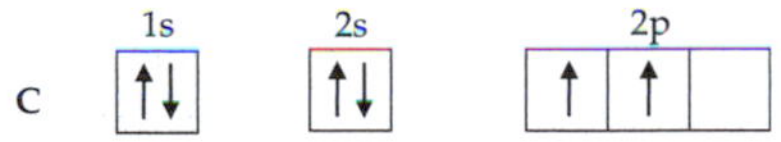

And for nitrogen:

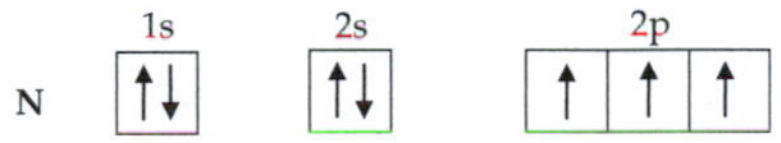

Further electrons will now begin to 'pair up' to fill the 2p-orbitals, for example the oxygen atom:

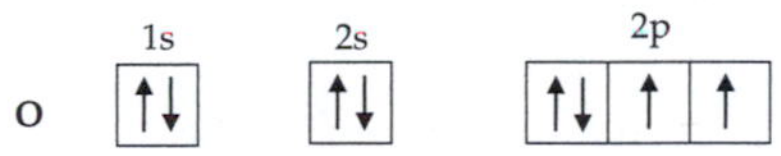

Table A5 uses the same 'electrons-in-boxes' notation for the elements in the first row of the d-block. Each of the five 3d-orbitals receives one electron, before any receives two.

A2 Bonding between atoms

The description of chemical bonding below is the simplest possible needed to understand this book.

A2.1 Ionic bonding

Essentially two types of chemical bond exist. The first is **ionic bonding**, and occurs when **electropositive** elements combine with **electronegative** ones. Electropositive elements, such as those in groups I and II of the periodic table (Figure A1), tend to lose their outermost electrons easily, whereas electronegative elements (group VII, and oxygen and sulphur in group VI) tend to accept extra electrons. By doing so, both gain the electronic configuration of the inert gases, which seems to be a particularly stable configuration in view of the lack of reactivity of these elements. Consider, for example, the combination of an atom of sodium with one of chlorine. Sodium, an electropositive group I element, has the electronic configuration $1s^2 2s^2 2p^6 3s^1$. If a sodium atom loses

Table A4 Electronic configuration of the elements

Element	Atomic number	Symbol	Configuration	Place in periodic table
Hydrogen	1	H	$1s^1$	Uncertain
Helium	2	He	$1s^2$	Group 0 (inert gases)
Lithium	3	Li	$1s^2 2s^1$	Group I (alkali metals)
Beryllium	4	Be	$1s^2 2s^2$	Group II (alkaline-earth metals)
Boron	5	B	$1s^2 2s^2 2p^1$	Group III
Carbon	6	C	$1s^2 2s^2 2p^2$	Group IV
Nitrogen	7	N	$1s^2 2s^2 2p^3$	Group V
Oxygen	8	O	$1s^2 2s^2 2p^4$	Group VI
Fluorine	9	F	$1s^2 2s^2 2p^5$	Group VII (halogen elements)
Neon	10	Ne	$1s^2 2s^2 2p^6$	Group 0
Sodium	11	Na	$1s^2 2s^2 2p^6 3s^1$	Group I
Magnesium	12	Mg	$1s^2 2s^2 2p^6 3s^2$	Group II
Aluminium	13	Al	$1s^2 2s^2 2p^6 3s^2 3p^1$	Group III
Silicon	14	Si	$1s^2 2s^2 2p^6 3s^2 3p^2$	Group IV
Phosphorus	15	P	$1s^2 2s^2 2p^6 3s^2 3p^3$	Group V
Sulphur	16	S	$1s^2 2s^2 2p^6 3s^2 3p^4$	Group VI
Chlorine	17	Cl	$1s^2 2s^2 2p^6 3s^2 3p^5$	Group VII
Argon	18	Ar	$1s^2 2s^2 2p^6 3s^2 3p^6$	Group 0
Potassium	19	K	$1s^2 2s^2 2p^6 3s^2 3p^6 4s^1$	Group I
Calcium	20	Ca	$1s^2 2s^2 2p^6 3s^2 3p^6 4s^2$	Group II
Scandium	21	Sc	$1s^2 2s^2 2p^6 3s^2 3p^6 4s^2 3d^1$	d-block
Titanium	22	Ti	$1s^2 2s^2 2p^6 3s^2 3p^6 4s^2 3d^2$	d-block
Vanadium	23	V	$1s^2 2s^2 2p^6 3s^2 3p^6 4s^2 3d^3$	d-block
Chromium	24	Cr	$1s^2 2s^2 2p^6 3s^2 3p^6 4s^1 3d^5$	d-block
Manganese	25	Mn	$1s^2 2s^2 2p^6 3s^2 3p^6 4s^2 3d^5$	d-block
Iron	26	Fe	$1s^2 2s^2 2p^6 3s^2 3p^6 4s^2 3d^6$	d-block
Cobalt	27	Co	$1s^2 2s^2 2p^6 3s^2 3p^6 4s^2 3d^7$	d-block
Nickel	28	Ni	$1s^2 2s^2 2p^6 3s^2 3p^6 4s^2 3d^8$	d-block
Copper	29	Cu	$1s^2 2s^2 2p^6 3s^2 3p^6 4s^1 3d^{10}$	d-block
Zinc	30	Zn	$1s^2 2s^2 2p^6 3s^2 3p^6 4s^2 3d^{10}$	d-block
Gallium	31	Ga	$1s^2 2s^2 2p^6 3s^2 3p^6 4s^2 3d^{10} 4p^1$	Group III
Germanium	32	Ge	$1s^1 2s^2 2p^6 3s^2 3p^6 4s^2 3d^{10} 4p^2$	Group IV

one electron, it now has the configuration $1s^2 2s^2 2p^6$, that of the inert gas neon. It is still sodium because its nucleus is unchanged, but the loss of an electron leaves the atom with a positive charge, forming an ion or, more specifically, a **cation** (positively charged ion). For chlorine, configuration $1s^2 2s^2 2p^6 3s^2 3p^5$, acceptance of one electron gives the argon electron configuration $1s^2 2s^2 2p^6 3s^2 3p^6$, and produces a negatively charged ion (**anion**) Cl^-.

In the case of a group II element such as magnesium, it must lose two electrons to gain an inert gas electron configuration. Thus one atom of magnesium can provide electrons for acceptance by two chlorine atoms, giving magnesium chloride a formula $MgCl_2$,

$$Mg \rightarrow Mg^{2+} + 2e^-$$
$$1s^2 2s^2 2p^6 3s^2 \quad 1s^2 2s^2 2p^6$$

(neon configuration)

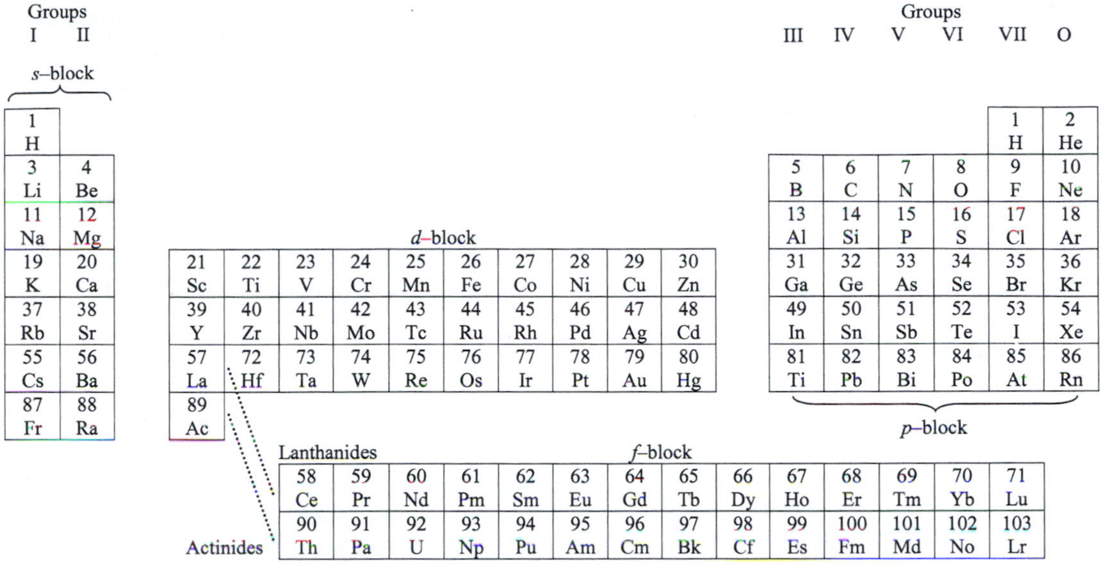

Figure A1 The periodic table.

Table A5 Electronic configuration of the elements scandium to zinc in the first row of the d-block of the periodic table

		3d					4s
Scandium	Ar	↑					↑ ↓
Titanium	Ar	↑	↑				↑ ↓
Vanadium	Ar	↑	↑	↑			↑ ↓
Chromium	Ar	↑	↑	↑	↑	↑	↑
Manganese	Ar	↑	↑	↑	↑	↑	↑ ↓
Iron	Ar	↑ ↓	↑	↑	↑	↑	↑ ↓
Cobalt	Ar	↑ ↓	↑ ↓	↑	↑	↑	↑ ↓
Nickel	Ar	↑ ↓	↑ ↓	↑ ↓	↑	↑	↑ ↓
Copper	Ar	↑ ↓	↑ ↓	↑ ↓	↑ ↓	↑ ↓	↑
Zinc	Ar	↑ ↓	↑ ↓	↑ ↓	↑ ↓	↑ ↓	↑ ↓

An atom of oxygen, however, can accept two electrons and combine with magnesium to form an oxide MgO:

$$O + 2e^- \rightarrow O^{2-}$$

$1s^2 2s^2 2p^4 \qquad 1s^2 2s^2 2p^6$

(neon configuration)

Once formed, anions and cations are held together by the attraction of their opposite charges. Each ion will exert an effect on each other ion in its vicinity, and these forces cause the ions to pack together into an **ionic crystal lattice**, as exemplified in Figure A2 for NaCl. Each Na^+ ion is surrounded by six Cl^- ions, and vice versa. Once the lattice has

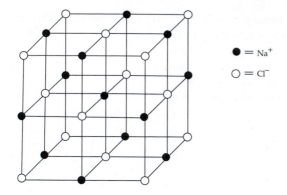

Figure A2 Crystal structure of sodium chloride. The exact type of lattice formed by an ionic compound depends on the relative sizes of the ions. NaCl forms a cubic lattice, as shown.

formed, it cannot be said that any one Na^+ ion 'belongs' to any one Cl^- ion, nor can 'molecules' of sodium chloride be said to exist. The formula of an ionic compound merely indicates the combining ratio of the elements involved. A lot of energy is needed to disrupt all the electrostatic forces between the many millions of ions in a crystal of an ionic compound, so such compounds are usually solids with high melting-points. Ionic compounds are mostly soluble in water, and the solutions conduct electricity because of the presence of ions to carry the current. The properties of an ionic compound are those of its constituent ions.

A2.2 Covalent bonding

This involves sharing a pair of electrons between the two bonded atoms. In 'normal' covalent bonding, each atom contributes one electron to the shared pair, but in **dative covalent bonding**, one atom contributes both. For example, hydrogen usually occurs as covalently-bonded **diatomic** molecules, H_2. If we represent the electron of each hydrogen atom by a cross (×) we can write:

$$H_\times + {}^\times H \rightarrow H_\times^\times H$$

where $\overset{\times}{\times}$ is the shared pair of electrons. Many other gaseous elements, including oxygen and chlorine, exist as covalently-bonded diatomic molecules.

When chlorine combines with hydrogen, the covalent compound hydrogen chloride is formed.

If we represent the outermost electrons of the chlorine atom as circles, we can write:

$$\overset{\text{OO}}{\underset{\text{OO}}{\text{OClO}}} + \text{H}_\times \rightarrow \text{H} {}_\times^{} \underset{\text{O OO}}{\overset{\text{OO}}{\text{Cl}}}$$

Hydrogen chloride

where $\overset{\times}{\text{O}}$ is the shared pair of electrons. Similarly for the covalent compound ammonia, NH_3:

$$\overset{\text{OO}}{\underset{\text{O}}{\text{O N}}} + 3H_\times \rightarrow \overset{\text{H}}{\underset{\text{H}}{\overset{\text{O×}}{\text{O N O}} \text{H}}}$$

In the above cases, each atom contributes one electron to the bond. Ammonia also undergoes dative covalent bonding using the spare pair (**lone pair**) of electrons on the nitrogen. For example, it forms a covalent bond with a proton (H^+). H^+ is formed by loss of one electron from a hydrogen atom, and so has no electrons.

$$\overset{\text{H}}{\underset{\text{H}}{\overset{\text{O×}}{\text{O N O}}\text{H}}} + \text{H}^+ \rightarrow \left[\overset{\text{H}}{\underset{\text{H}}{\text{H O}\overset{\text{O×}}{\text{N}}\text{O H}}} \right]^+$$

ammonia   ammonium ion, NH_4^+

Once formed, each of the four covalent bonds in NH_4^+ is indistinguishable from the others.

Covalent compounds do not conduct electricity and are usually gases, liquids or low-melting-point solids at room temperature, because the forces of interaction between the molecules are weak. By contrast, covalent bonds themselves are usually strong and hard to break. Covalent bonds, unlike ionic bonds, have definite directions in space, and so their length, and the angles between them, can be measured.

Orbital theory (Section A1) can also be applied to covalent compounds, the bonding electrons occupying **molecular orbitals** formed by interaction of the atomic orbitals in which they were originally located. Various possible interactions produce molecular orbitals of different energy levels, each of which can hold a maximum of two electrons with opposite values of the spin quantum number

(Pauli's principle). In the simplest case, H_2, two possible molecular orbitals can form by interaction of the 1s atomic orbitals of each H atom. The lowest energy orbital is the **bonding molecular orbital** (often written as $\sigma 1s$) in which the electron is most likely to be found between the two nuclei. There is also an **antibonding molecular orbital** (written as σ^*1s) of higher energy in which there is little chance of finding an electron between the two nuclei. A bonding molecular orbital is more stable than the atomic orbitals, whereas an antibonding molecular orbital is less stable. The two electrons in H_2 have opposite spin, and both occupy the bonding molecular orbital. Hence H_2 is much more stable than two H atoms. By contrast, helium atoms have the electron configuration $1s^2$, and if they combined to give He_2, both the bonding and antibonding molecular orbitals would contain two electrons, and there would be no effective gain in stability. Hence He_2 does not form.

P-type atomic orbitals can produce two types of molecular orbital (σ and π) by overlapping in different ways. Hence, for a 2p-orbital (say $2p_x$) combining with another one, there will be two bonding molecular orbitals, $\sigma 2p_x$ and $\pi 2p_x$, and two antibonding molecular orbitals, σ^*2p_x and π^*2p_x. Energy increases in the order:

$$\sigma 2p_x < \pi 2p_x < \pi^*2p_x < \sigma^*2p_x$$

With this in mind, we can consider bonding in three more complex cases: the gases nitrogen, oxygen and fluorine. The nitrogen atom has the configuration $1s^2 2s^2 2p^3$. If two atoms join to form N_2, the four 1s-electrons (two from each atom) fully occupy a $\sigma 1s$ bonding and a σ^*1s antibonding orbital, and so there is no net bonding. The four 2s-electrons similarly occupy $\sigma 2s$ and σ^*2s molecular orbitals, again no net bonding. Six electrons are left, located in two $2p_x$, two $2p_y$ and two $2p_z$ atomic orbitals. If the axis of the bond between the atoms is taken to be that of the $2p_x$ orbitals, they can overlap along this axis to produce a bonding $\sigma 2p_x$ molecular orbital that can hold both electrons. The $2p_y$ and $2p_z$ atomic orbitals cannot overlap along their axes, but they can overlap laterally to give bonding $\pi 2p_y$ and $\pi 2p_z$ molecular orbitals, each of which holds two electrons. The 2p antibonding orbitals are not occupied; and the net result is a triple covalent bond $N\equiv N$; one σ covalent bond and two π covalent bonds. The N_2 molecule is thus far more stable than individual N atoms.

The oxygen atom (configuration, $1s^2 2s^2 2p^4$) has one more electron, and so when O_2 forms there are two more electrons to consider. These must occupy the next highest molecular orbital in terms of energy. In fact, there are two such orbitals of equal energy, π^*2p_y and π^*2p_z. By Hund's rule, each receives one electron. Since the presence of two electrons in antibonding orbitals energetically cancels out one of the $\pi 2p$ bonding orbitals, the two oxygen atoms are effectively joined by a double bond, tha is $O=O$.

The fluorine molecule contains two more electrons than does O_2, and so the π^*2p_y and π^*2p_z orbitals are both full. Since three bonding and two antibonding molecular orbitals are occupied, the F_2 molecule effectively contains a single bond, $F-F$.

A2.3 Non-ideal character of bonds

The discussion so far has implied an equal sharing of the bonding electrons between two atoms joined by a covalent bond. However, this only occurs when both atoms have a similar attraction for the electrons, i.e. are equally electronegative. This is often not the case. Consider, for example, the water molecule, which contains two oxygen–hydrogen covalent bonds:

$$2H\times + \overset{\circ\circ}{\underset{\circ\circ}{O}} \rightarrow \overset{\times\circ}{\underset{\circ\circ}{O}}{}^{\circ}_{\times} H \quad {}^{H}$$

Oxygen is more electronegative than hydrogen, and so takes a slightly greater 'share' of the bonding electrons, giving it a slight negative charge (written as δ^-). The hydrogen thus has a slight positive charge, that is

$$\overset{\delta^+}{H}\diagdown\underset{O}{}\diagup\overset{\delta^+}{H}\quad\underset{\delta^-}{}$$

These charges give water many of its properties. They attract water molecules to each other, making it harder to separate them and so raising the boiling point of water to 100°C at normal atmospheric

pressure,

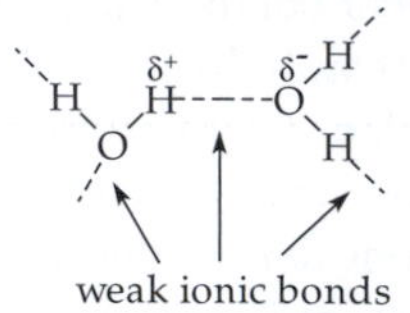

These weak ionic bonds are called **hydrogen bonds**. The δ^+ and δ^- charges also allow water to hydrate ions; water molecules cluster around ions and help to stabilize them, for example A^+ and B^- ions:

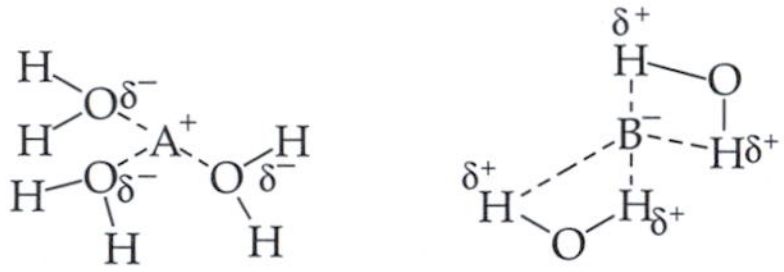

The energy released when ions become hydrated helps to provide the energy needed to disrupt the crystal lattice when ionic compounds dissolve in water. In some cases the energy of hydration is much smaller than the energy needed to disrupt the lattice, resulting in an ionic compound insoluble in water.

A2.4 Hydrocarbons and electron delocalization

Carbon has four electrons in its outermost shell (Table A4), and normally forms four covalent bonds. Carbon atoms can covalently bond to each other to form long chains. For example, butane has the structure

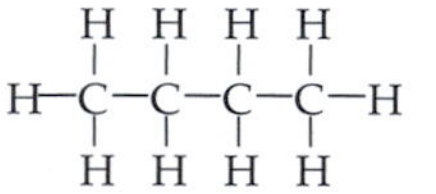

$$(C_4H_{10})$$

Butane is a **hydrocarbon**, that is it contains only carbon and hydrogen. Two other hydrocarbon gases, ethane and pentane, are released during lipid peroxidation (Section 4.12.5.1). They have the structures:

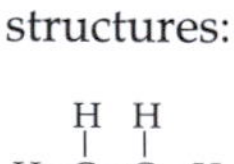

Carbon atoms can also form double covalent bonds (written as $\diagup C = C \diagdown$ and triple covalent bonds ($-C \equiv C-$) with each other. A double bond consists of four shared electrons (two pairs), and

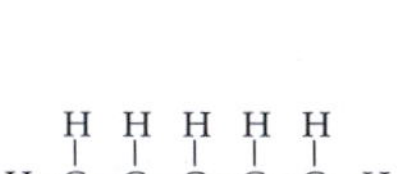

a triple bond has six shared electrons (three pairs). The simplest hydrocarbon containing a double bond is the gas **ethene**, sometimes called ethylene.

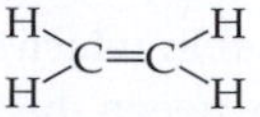

Ethene is produced in several assays for the detection of hydroxyl radicals (Section 5.3).

Ethyne, sometimes called acetylene, contains a triple bond and has the structure $H-C \equiv C-H$. Organic compounds containing carbon–carbon double or triple bonds are said to be **unsaturated**, for example PUFAs (Section 4.12).

The organic liquid **benzene** has the formula C_6H_6. Given that carbon forms four covalent bonds, the structure of benzene might be drawn as containing three carbon–carbon single bonds, and three double bonds, that is

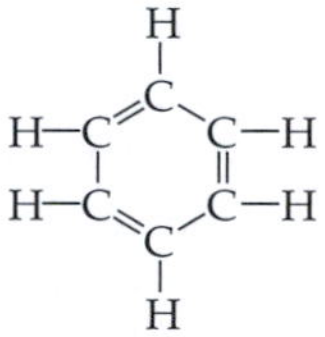

This structure cannot be correct, however, since benzene does not show the characteristic chemical reactions of compounds containing double bonds. A carbon–carbon single bond is normally 0.154 nm long (one nanometre, nm, is 10^{-9} metre), and a carbon–carbon double bond, 0.134 nm; yet all the bond lengths between the carbon atoms in benzene are equal at 0.139 nm, that is intermediate between the double and single bond lengths. The six electrons, which should have formed three double bonds, appear to be 'spread around' all six bonds. This is often drawn as:

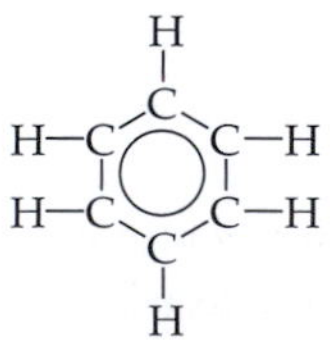

or, in abbreviated form,

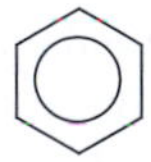

Compounds containing the benzene ring or similar ring structures are called **aromatic compounds**. Delocalization of electrons over several bonds greatly increases the stability of a molecule. Other examples can be seen in haem rings (Section 1.10.3) which show extensive delocalization of electrons, and in several ions such as nitrate (NO_3^-) and carbonate (CO_3^{2-}). In each case the negative charge is spread between each of the bonds,

(each O has, on average, one-third of the negative charge).

(each O has, on average, two-thirds of a negative charge).

A3 Moles and molarity

One **mole** of a substance is its relative molecular mass ('molecular weight') expressed in grams. Thus one mole of hydrogen (H_2) is 2 g, one mole of water 18 g and one mole of sodium hydroxide (NaOH) 40 g. One mole of any covalently-bonded substance contains the same number of molecules, 6.023×10^{23} to be precise (**Avogadro's number**). Thus $6.023 \times 10^{23} H_2$ molecules are found in 2 g of hydrogen, and 6.023×10^{23} water molecules in 18 g of water. One mole of the ionic solid NaOH will contain $6.023 \times 10^{23} Na^+$ ions and the same number of OH^- ions. For the ionic solid ZnF_2, one mole will contain $6.023 \times 10^{23} Zn^{2+}$ ions and twice that number of F^- ions.

Whereas moles are amounts, **molarity** is a concentration. Solution concentrations in biology are usually expressed in molar terms because this relates to the actual number of ions or molecules present in the solution. A **molar** solution has one mole of **solute** (the substance dissolved) present in $1 dm^3$ (or 1 litre) of solution.

One **millimole** (1 mmol) is 10^{-3} moles. Thus a **millimolar** (1 mM) solution has 1 mmol of solute per dm^3. One **micromole** (1 μmol) is 10^{-6} moles. Thus a **micromolar** (1 μM) solution has 1 μmole of solute per dm^3. A 1 mM solution has 1 μmol of solute per cm^3 (ml). One **nanomole** (1 nmol) is 10^{-9} moles. Thus a **nanomolar** (1 nM) solution has 1 nmol of solute per dm^3. A 1 μM solution has 1 nmol of solute per cm^3 (ml).

A4 pH and pK$_a$

The pH of a solution is a measure of its acidity; pH 7.0 is neutral, pH <7 acidic, and pH >7 alkaline. Most cells operate at pH values at or close to 7.4, but 'physiological pH' ranges from <2 in the stomach to >8 in the lumen of the small intestine and in the stroma of illuminated chloroplasts. The term pH is defined as

$$pH = -\log_{10}[H^+]$$

where the square brackets denote concentration. Thus pure water at 25°C contains 10^{-7} moles/dm^3 of H^+ ions and its pH is 7. As temperature rises, heterolytic fission of water is favoured, $[H^+]$ rises and pH falls, so pure water at 37°C is not neutral but slightly acidic.

An **acid** may be (somewhat simplistically) defined as a donor of hydrogen ions. **Strong acids** (HCl, HNO_3, H_2SO_4) are completely ionized when mixed with water to give dilute aqueous solutions (but not as the pure acids, which are covalently bonded). However, most acids in living systems are only partially ionized (so-called **weak acids**) and exist in an equilibrium:

$$HA \rightleftharpoons H^+ + A^-$$
$$\text{acid}$$

A^- is the **conjugate base** of the weak acid HA; a **base** is a hydrogen ion acceptor.

The **acid dissociation constant**, K_a, is the ratio of the concentrations

$$[H^+][A^-]/[HA]$$

at equilibrium. The bigger the value of K_a, the stronger the acid. Values of K_a are affected by temperature. Another term often used is pK_a

$$pK_a = -\log_{10} K_a$$

Thus the higher K_a, the smaller pK_a.

Mixtures of weak acids and their conjugate bases form **buffer solutions**; their pH changes only slightly when acid or alkali (in moderate amounts) are added.

The equation governing the behaviour of buffers is the **Henderson–Hasselbalch equation**:

$$pH = pK_a + \log_{10} [\text{base}]/[\text{acid}]$$

Thus if equal amounts of a weak acid and its conjugate base are mixed, the pH of the resulting solution equals the pK_a of the acid. If extra H^+ is added, it is buffered by movement of the equilibrium

$$HA \rightleftharpoons H^+ + A^-$$

towards the left; if alkali is added, $[H^+]$ falls and it is replaced by movement of the reaction towards the right. This is the essence of buffer action.

References

Chapter 1

1. Kasting, JF (1993) Earth's early atmosphere. *Science* **259**, 920.
2. Lane, N (2002) *Oxygen, the Molecule That Made the World*. Oxford University Press, Oxford, UK.
3. Olson, JM and Blankenship, RE (2004) Thinking about the evolution of photosynthesis. *Photosynth. Res.* **80**, 373.
4. Munns, SE and Arthur, PG (2002) Stability of O_2 deprivation in glass culture vessels facilitates fast reproducible cell death to cortical neurons under simulated ischemia. *Anal. Biochem.* **306**, 149.
5. Krieg, NR and Hoffman, PS (1986) Microaerophily and O_2 toxicity. *Ann. Rev. Microbiol.* **40**, 107.
6. Marquis, RE (1995) O_2-metabolism, oxidative stress and acid–base physiology of dental plaque biofilms. *J. Indust. Microbiol.* **15**, 198.
7. Morris, JG (1976) O_2 and the obligate anaerobe. *J. Appl. Bacteriol.* **40**, 229.
8. Baughn, AD and Malamy, MH (2004) The strict anaerobe *Bacteroides fragilis* grows in and benefits from nanomolar concentrations of O_2. *Nature* **427**, 441.
9. Imlay, JA (2002) How O_2 damages microbes: O_2 tolerance and obligate anaerobiosis. *Adv. Microbial Physiol.* **46**, 111.
10. Gallon, JR (1981) The O_2-sensitivity of nitrogenase: a problem for biochemists and micro-organisms. *TIBS* **6**, 19.
11. Oelze, J (2000) Respiratory protection of nitrogenase in *Azotobacter* species: is a widely held hypothesis unequivocally supported by experimental evidence? *FEMS Microbiol. Rev.* **24**, 321.
12. Ribbe, M *et al.* (1997) N_2 fixation by *Streptomyces thermoautotrophicus* involves a Mo-dinitrogenase and a Mn-superoxide oxidoreductase that couple N_2 reduction to the oxidation of $O_2^{\bullet-}$ produced from O_2 by a Mo–CO dehydrogenase. *J. Biol. Chem.* **272**, 26627.
13. Cleary, PP and Larkin, A (1979) Hyaluronic acid capsule: strategy for O_2 resistance in group A streptococci. *J. Bacteriol.* **140**, 1090.
14. Minning, DM *et al.* (1999) *Ascaris* haemoglobin is a $NO^{\bullet}$-activated 'deoxygenase'. *Nature* **401**, 497.

15. Merx, MW *et al.* (2005) O_2 supply and $NO^{\bullet}$ scavenging by myoglobin contribute to exercise endurance and cardiac function. *FASEB J.* **19**, 1015.
16. Bunn, HF and Poyton, RO (1996) O_2 sensing and molecular adaptation to hypoxia. *Physiol. Rev.* **76**, 839.
17. Smalley, JW *et al.* (2000) The periodontal pathogen *Porphyromonas gingivalis* harnesses the chemistry of the μ-oxo bishaem of iron protoporphyrin IX to protect against H_2O_2. *FEMS Microbiol. Lett.* **183**, 159.
18. Schofield, CJ and Ratcliffe, PJ (2004) O_2 sensing by HIF hydroxylases. *Nature Rev. Mol. Cell Biol.* **5**, 343.
19. Halliwell, B (1984) *Chloroplast Metabolism*. Oxford University Press, Oxford.
20. Halestrap, A (2005) A pore way to die. *Nature* **434**, 578.
21. Babcock, GT (1999) How O_2 is activated and reduced in respiration. *Proc. Natl. Acad. Sci. USA* **96**, 12971.
22. Kroemer, G and Reed, JC (2000) Mitochondrial control of cell death. *Nature Med.* **6**, 513.
23. Muller, F (2000) The nature and mechanism of $O_2^{\bullet-}$ production by the electron transport chain: its relevance to aging. *J. Amer. Aging Assoc.* **23**, 227.
24. Dyall, SD *et al.* (2004) Ancient invasions: from endosymbionts to organelles. *Science* **304**, 253.
25. Degroot, H and Littauer, A (1989) Hypoxia, reactive O_2 and cell injury. *Free Rad. Biol. Med.* **6**, 541.
26. Coon, MJ (2005) Cytochrome P450; Nature's most versatile biological catalyst. *Ann. Rev. Pharm. Tox.* **45**, 1.
27. Guengerich, FP (2001) Common and uncommon cytochrome P450 reactions related to metabolism and chemical toxicity. *Chem. Res. Toxicol.* **14**, 611.
28. Balentine, JD (1982) *Pathology of O_2 Toxicity*. Academic Press, New York.
29. Bruyninckx, WJ *et al.* (1978) Are physiological O_2 concentrations mutagenic? *Nature* **274**, 606.
30. Gray, JM *et al.* (2004) O_2 sensation and social feeding mediated by a *C. elegans* guanylate cyclase homologue. *Nature* **430**, 317.
31. Beerling, DJ *et al.* (1998) The influence of carboniferous palaeoatmospheres on plant function: an

experimental and modelling assessment. *Phil. Trans. R. Soc.* **353**, 131.

32. Gardner, PR and Fridovich, I (1991) Quinolinate synthetase: the O_2-sensitive site of *de novo* $NAD(P)^+$ biosynthesis. *Arch. Biochem. Biophys.* **284**, 106.

33. Gilbert, DL (ed) (1981) *O_2 and Living Processes: an Inter-disciplinary Approach.* Springer, New York.

34. Smerz, RW (2004) Incidence of O_2 toxicity during the treatment of dysbarism. *Undersea Hyperbaric Med.* **31**, 199.

35. Deneke, SM and Fanburg, BL (1980) Normobaric O_2 toxicity of the lung. *N. Engl. J. Med.* **303**, 76.

36. Speit, G *et al.* (2002) Genotoxicity of hyperbaric O_2. *Mut. Res.* **512**, 111.

37. Neriishi, K and Frank, L (1984) Castration prolongs tolerance of young male rats to pulmonary O_2 toxicity. *Am. J. Physiol.* **247**, R475.

38. Weinberger, B *et al.* (2002) O_2 toxicity in premature infants. *Toxicol. Appl. Pharmacol.* **181**, 60.

39. Hansmann, G (2004) Neonatal resuscitation on air: it is time to turn down the O_2 tanks? *Lancet* **364**, 1293.

40. Khaw, KS *et al.* (2002) Effects of high inspired O_2 fraction during elective Caesarean section under spinal anaesthesia on maternal and fetal oxygenation and lipid peroxidation. *Br. J. Anaesth.* **88**, 18.

41. Kehrer, JP and Autor, AP (1978) The effect of dietary fatty acids on the composition of adult rat lung lipids: relationship to oxygen toxicity. *Toxicol. Appl. Pharmacol.* **44**, 423.

42. Berenbrink, M *et al.* (2005) Evolution of O_2 secretion in fishes and the emergence of a complex physiological system. *Science* **307**, 1752.

43. Lehr, HA *et al.* (1999) Do vitamin E supplements in diets for laboratory animals jeopardize findings in animal models of disease? *Free Rad. Biol. Med.* **26**, 472.

44. Haugaard, N (1968) Cellular mechanisms of O_2 toxicity. *Physiol. Rev.* **48**, 311.

45. Liochev, SI and Fridovich, I (1993) Modulation of the fumarases of *E. coli* in response to oxidative stress. *Arch. Biochem. Biophys.* **301**, 379.

46. Morton, RL *et al.* (1998) Loss of lung mitochondrial aconitase activity due to hyperoxia in bronchopulmonary dysplasia in primates. *Am. J. Physiol.* **274**, L127.

47. Torbati, D *et al.* (1992) Free-radical generation in the brain precedes hyperbaric O_2-induced convulsions. *Free Rad. Biol. Med.* **13**, 101.

48. Chavko, M *et al.* (2003) Relationship between protein nitration and oxidation and development of hyperoxic seizures. *Nitric Oxide* **9**, 18.

49. Gu, XL *et al.* (2003) Hyperoxia induces retinal vascular endothelial cell apoptosis through formation of $ONOO^-$. *Am. J. Physiol.* **285**, C546.

50. Auten, RL *et al.* (2002) Blocking neutrophil influx reduces DNA damage in hyperoxia-exposed newborn rat lung. *Am. J. Respir. Cell Mol. Biol.* **26**, 391.

51. von Sonntag, C (1987) *The Chemical Basis of Radiation Biology.* Taylor & Francis, London.

52. Symons, MCR (1996) Radicals generated by bone cutting and fracture. *Free Rad. Biol. Med.* **20**, 831.

53. Shirkey, B *et al.* (2000) Active Fe-containing SOD and abundant *sodF* mRNA in *Nostoc commune* (Cyanobacteria) after years of desiccation. *J. Bacteriol.* **182**, 189.

54. Fridovich, I (1995) Superoxide radical and SODs. *Ann. Rev. Biochem.* **64**, 97.

55. Enroth, C *et al.* (2000) Crystal structures of bovine milk XDH and XO: structure-based mechanism of conversion. *Proc. Natl. Acad. Sci. USA* **97**, 10723.

56. Harrison, R (2004) Physiological roles of XOR. *Drug Metab. Rev.* **36**, 363.

57. Carlsson, J *et al.* (1978) H_2O_2 and $O_2^{\bullet-}$ formation in anaerobic broth media exposed to atmospheric O_2. *Appl. Env. Microbiol.* **36**, 223.

58. Kirsch, M *et al.* (2003) The autoxidation of THB revisited. *J. Biol. Chem.* **278**, 24481.

59. Saez, G *et al.* (1982) The production of free radicals during the autoxidation of cysteine and their effect on isolated rat hepatocytes. *Biochim. Biophys. Acta.* **719**, 24.

60. Rifkind, JM *et al.* (2004) Redox reactions of hemoglobin. *Antiox. Redox Signal.* **6**, 657.

61. Pietraforte, D *et al.* (2004) Scavenging of RNS by oxygenated hemoglobin: globin radicals and nitrotyrosines distinguish nitrite from $NO^{\bullet}$ reaction. *Free Rad. Biol. Med.* **37**, 1244.

62. Winterbourn, CC *et al.* (1976) Reactions involving $O_2^{\bullet-}$ and normal and unstable haemoglobins. *Biochem. J.* **155**, 493.

63. Bonaventura, C. *et al.* (1999) Internal electron transfer between hemes and Cu(II) bound at cysteine $\beta93$ promotes methemoglobin reduction by carbon monoxide. *J. Biol. Chem.* **274**, 5499.

64. Duncan, C *et al.* (1997) Protection against oral and gastrointestinal diseases: importance of dietary nitrate intake, oral nitrate reduction and enterosalivary nitrate circulation. *Comp. Biochem. Physiol.* **118A**, 939.

65. Wu, G *et al.* (2004) *E. coli* Hmp, an 'O_2-binding flavohaemoprotein', produces $O_2^{\bullet-}$ and self-destructs. *Arch. Microbiol.* **182**, 193.

66. Poole, RK and Hughes, MN (2000) New functions for the ancient globin family: bacterial responses to $NO^{\bullet}$ and nitrosative stress. *Mol. Microbiol.* **36**, 775.

67. Saborido, A *et al.* (2005) Isolated respiring heart mitochondria release ROS in states 4 and 3. *Free Radic. Res.* **39**, 921.

68. Freeman, BA and Crapo, JD (1981) Hyperoxia increases O_2 radical production in rat lungs and lung mitochondria. *J. Biol. Chem.* **256**, 10986.

69. St-Pierre, J *et al.* (2002) Topology of $O_2^{\bullet-}$ production from different sites in the mitochondrial electron transport chain. *J. Biol. Chem.* **277**, 44784.

70. Park, JI *et al.* (1998) The cytoplasmic CuZnSOD of *S. cerevisiae* is required for resistance to freeze–thaw stress. *J. Biol. Chem.* **273**, 22921.

71. Giulivi, C *et al.* (1999) The steady-state concentrations of O_2 radicals in mitochondria. In: *ROS in Biological Systems*. Kluwer Academic, Plenum Press Publishers, New York, USA.

72. Li, N *et al.* (2003) Mitochondrial complex I inhibitor rotenone induces apoptosis through enhancing mitochondrial ROS production. *J. Biol. Chem.* **278**, 8516.

73. Turrens, JF (2003) Mitochondrial formation of ROS. *J. Physiol.* **552**, 335.

74. Batandier, C *et al.* (2004) Opening of the MPT pore induces ROS production at the level of the respiratory chain complex I. *J. Biol. Chem.* **279**, 17197.

75. Barja, G (1999) Mitochondrial O_2 radical generation and leak: sites of production in state 4 and 3, organ specificity, and relation to aging and longevity. *J. Bioenerg. Biomembr.* **31**, 347.

76. Nohl, H *et al.* (2003) Cell respiration and formation of ROS: facts and artefacts. *Biochem. Soc. Trans.* **31**, 1308.

77. Anson, RM and Bohr, VA (2000) Mitochondria, oxidative DNA damage, and aging. *J. Amer. Aging Assoc.* **23**, 199.

78. Qi, X *et al.* (2004) SOD2 gene transfer protects against optic neuropathy induced by deficiency of complex I. *Ann. Neurol.* **56**, 182.

79. Canter, JA *et al.* (2005) Degree of heteroplasmy reflects oxidant damage in a large family with the mitochondrial DNA A8344G mutation. *Free Rad. Biol. Med.* **38**, 678.

80. Starkov, AA *et al.* (2004) Mitochondrial αKGDH complex generates ROS. *J. Neurosci.* **24**, 7779.

81. Brand, MD *et al.* (2004) Mitochondrial $O_2^{\bullet-}$: production, biological effects, and activation of uncoupling proteins. *Free Rad. Biol. Med.* **37**, 755.

82. Andrews, ZB *et al.* (2005) Mitochondrial uncoupling proteins in the CNS: in support of function and survival. *Neuroscience* **6**, 829.

83. Seaver, LC and Imlay, JA (2004) Are respiratory enzymes the primary sources of intracellular H_2O_2? *J. Biol. Chem.* **279**, 48742.

84. Goeptar, AR *et al.* (1995) O_2 and xenobiotic reductase activities of cytochrome P450. *Crit. Rev. Toxicol.* **25**, 25.

85. Peskin, AV *et al.* (1987) An unusual NAD(P)H-dependent $O_2^{\bullet-}$-generating redox system in hepatoma 22a nuclei. *Free Radic. Res. Commun.* **3**, 47.

86. Yusa, T *et al.* (1984) Hyperoxia enhances lung and liver nuclear $O_2^{\bullet-}$ generation. *Biochim. Biophys. Acta.* **798**, 2.

87. Macho, A *et al.* (2003) Involvement of ROS in capsaicinoid-induced apoptosis in transformed cells. *Free Radic. Res.* **37**, 611.

88. De Spiegeleer, P *et al.* (2004) Source of tryptone in growth medium affects oxidative stress in *E. coli*. *J. Appl. Microbiol.* **97**, 124.

89. Halliwell, B. (2003) Oxidative stress in cell culture: an under-appreciated problem? *FEBS Lett.* **540**, 3.

90. Kutala, VK *et al.* (2004) Simultaneous measurement of oxygenation in intracellular and extracellular compartments of lung microvascular endothelial cells. *Antiox. Redox Signal.* **6**, 597.

Chapter 2

1. Giles, GI and Jacob, C (2002) Reactive sulfur species: an emerging concept in oxidative stress. *Biol. Chem.* **383**, 375.

2. Beckman, JS and Koppenol, WH (1996) $NO^{\bullet}$, $O_2^{\bullet-}$ and $ONOO^{-}$: the good, the bad, and the ugly. *Am. J. Physiol.* **271**, C1424.

3. Buettner, GR (1993). The pecking order of free radicals and antioxidants: lipid peroxidation, α-tocopherol and ascorbate. *Arch. Biochem. Biophys.* **300**, 535.

4. Aruoma, OI and Halliwell, B (1987) $O_2^{\bullet-}$-dependent and ascorbate-dependent formation of $OH^{\bullet}$ from H_2O_2 in the presence of Fe. Are lactoferrin and transferrin promoters of $OH^{\bullet}$ generation? *Biochem. J.* **241**, 273.

5. Koppenol, WH and Butler, J (1985) Energetics of interconversion reactions of oxyradicals. *Adv. Free Rad. Biol. Med.* **1**, 91.

6. Butler, J and Land, E (1996) Pulse radiolysis. In: Punchard, NA and Kelly, F (eds) *Free Radicals. A Practical Approach*, p. 47. IRL Press, Oxford.

7. Folkes, LK *et al.* (1995) Kinetics and mechanisms of HOCl reactions. *Arch. Biochem. Biophys.* **323**, 120.

8. Rush, JD *et al.* (1996) Reaction of ferrate (VI) / ferrate (V) with H_2O_2 and $O_2^{\bullet-}$—a stopped-flow and premix pulse radiolysis study. *Free Radic. Res.* **24**, 187.

9. Halliwell, B (1978) $O_2^{\bullet-}$-dependent formation of $OH^{\bullet}$ in the presence of Fe salts. Its role in degradation of hyaluronic acid by a $O_2^{\bullet-}$-generating system. *FEBS Lett.* **96**, 238.

10. Bielski, BHJ and Cabelli, DE (1995) Chapter 3. In: Foote, CS et al. (eds) Active O_2 in Chemistry. Blackie, London.

11. Gutteridge, JM and Bannister, JV (1986) CuZn and MnSODs inhibit deoxyribose degradation by the $O_2^{\bullet-}$-driven Fenton reaction at two different stages. Biochem. J. **234**, 225.

12. Liochev, SI and Fridovich, I (2004) CO_2 mediates Mn(II)-catalyzed decomposition of H_2O_2 and peroxidation reactions. Proc. Natl. Acad. Sci. USA **101**, 12485.

13. Halliwell, B and Gutteridge, JMC (1992) Biologically-relevant metal ion-dependent $OH^{\bullet}$ generation. An update. FEBS Lett. **307**, 108.

14. Walling, C (1998) Intermediates in the reactions of Fenton type reagents. Acc. Chem. Res. **31**, 155.

15. Burkitt, MJ (2003) Chemical, biological, and medical controversies surrounding the Fenton reaction. Prog. React. Kinet. Mech. **28**, 75.

16. Symons, MCR and Gutteridge, JMC (1998) Free Radicals and Iron, Chemistry Biology and Medicine. Oxford University Press, UK.

17. Gutteridge, JMC (1990) $O_2^{\bullet-}$-dependent formation of $OH^{\bullet}$ from Fe(III) complexes and H_2O_2: an evaluation of 14 iron chelators. Free Radic. Res. Commun. **9**, 119.

18. Gutteridge, JMC et al. (1990) ADP-Fe as Fenton reactant: radical reactions detected by spin trapping, H abstraction and aromatic hydroxylation. Arch. Biochem. Biophys. **277**, 422.

19. Walling, C et al. (1975) Kinetics of the decomposition of H_2O_2 catalyzed by ferric EDTA complex. Proc. Natl. Acad. Sci. USA **72**, 140.

20. Shimon, MB et al. (1998) Specific Cu^{2+}-catalyzed oxidative cleavage of Na, K-ATPase at the extracellular surface. J. Biol. Chem. **273**, 51.

21. Frelon, S et al. (2003) $OH^{\bullet}$ is not the main RS involved in the degradation of DNA bases by Cu in the presence of H_2O_2. Chem. Res. Toxicol. **16**, 191.

22. Eberhardt, MK (1995) $OH^{\bullet}$. Formation and some reactions used in its identification. Trends Org. Chem. **5**, 115.

23. Mylonas, M et al. (2001) Stray Cu(II) may cause oxidative damage when coordinated to the -TESHHK-sequence derived from the C-terminal tail of histone H2A. Chem. Res. Toxicol. **14**, 1177.

24. Von Sonntag, C (1987) The Chemical Basis of Radiation Biology. Taylor and Francis, London.

25. Riesz, P et al. (1990) Sonochemistry of volatile and non-volatile solutes in aqueous solutions: epr and spin trapping studies. Ultrasonics **28**, 295.

26. Crum, LA et al. (1987) Free radical production in amniotic fluid and blood plasma by medical ultrasound. J. Ultrasound Med. **6**, 643.

27. Takahashi, H et al. (2002) Free radicals in pharmacoemulsification and aspiration procedures. Arch. Ophthalmol. **120**, 1348.

28. Munver, R et al. (2002) In vivo assessment of free radical activity during shock wave lithotripsy using a microdialysis system: the renoprotective action of allopurinol. J. Urol. **167**, 327.

29. Zhu, BZ et al. (2002) Metal-independent production of $OH^{\bullet}$ by halogenated quinones and H_2O_2: an esr spin trapping study. Free Rad. Biol. Med. **32**, 465.

30. Schäcker, M et al. (1991) Oxidation of Tris to 1-carbon compounds in a radical-producing model system, in microsomes, in hepatocytes and in rats. Free Radic. Res. Commun. **11**, 339.

31. Augusto, O et al. (2002) $NO_2^{\bullet}$ and $CO_3^{\bullet-}$: two emerging radicals in biology. Free Rad. Biol. Med. **32**, 841.

32. Andrekopoulos, C et al. (2004) HCO_3^- enhances α-synuclein oligomerization and nitration: intermediacy of $CO_3^{\bullet-}$ and $NO_2^{\bullet}$. Biochem. J. **378**, 435

33. Ramirez, DC et al. (2005) Cu-catalyzed protein oxidation and its modulation by CO_2. J. Biol. Chem. **280**, 27402.

34. Winterbourn, CC and Kettle, AJ (2003) Radical-radical reactions of $O_2^{\bullet-}$: a potential route to toxicity. Biochem. Biophys. Res. Commun. **305**, 729.

35. Konya, KG et al. (2000) Laser flash photolysis studies on the first $O_2^{\bullet-}$ thermal source. J. Am. Chem. Soc. **122**, 7518.

36. Dietzel, PDC et al. (2004) Tetraorganylammonium $O_2^{\bullet-}$ compounds: close to unperturbed $O_2^{\bullet-}$ in the solid state. J. Am. Chem. Soc. **126**, 4689.

37. Jones, CM et al. (2002) EPR spin trapping investigation into the kinetics of GSH oxidation by $O_2^{\bullet-}$: re-evaluation of the rate constant. Free Rad. Biol. Med. **32**, 982.

38. Voelker, BM and Sedlak, DL (1995) Iron reduction by photoproduced $O_2^{\bullet-}$ in seawater. Marine Chem. **50**, 93.

39. Sawyer, DT and Valentine, JS (1981) How super is $O_2^{\bullet-}$? Acc. Chem. Res. **14**, 393.

40. Sugimoto, H et al. (1987) Oxygenation of polychloro aromatic hydrocarbons by $O_2^{\bullet-}$ in aprotic media. J. Am. Chem. Soc. **109**, 8081.

41. Forni, LG and Willson, RL (1986) Thiyl and phenoxyl free radicals and NADH. Biochem. J. **240**, 897.

42. Yoshida, Y et al. (2004) Application of water-soluble radical initiator, AIPH, to a study of oxidative stress. Free Radic. Res. **38**, 375.

43. Soriani, M et al. (1994) Antioxidant potential of anaerobic human plasma: role of serum albumin and thiols as scavengers of $C^{\bullet}$. Arch. Biochem. Biophys. **312**, 180.

44. Paul, T *et al.* (2000) Strand cleavage of supercoiled DNA by water-soluble $RO_2^\bullet$. The overlooked importance of $RO_2^\bullet$ charge. *Biochemistry* **39**, 4129.

45. Paya, M *et al.* (1992) $RO_2^\bullet$ scavenging by a series of coumarins. *Free Radic. Res. Commun.* **17**, 293.

46. Aruoma, OI *et al.* (1995) Reaction of plant-derived and synthetic antioxidants with $CCl_3O_2^\bullet$. *Free Radic. Res.* **22**, 187.

47. Symons, MCR (1996) Radicals generated by bone cutting and fracture. *Free Rad. Biol. Med.* **20**, 831.

48. Wardman, P and von Sonntag, C (1995) Kinetic factors that control the fate of $RS^\bullet$ in cells. *Meth. Enzymol.* **251**, 31.

49. Schöneich, C *et al.* (1989) $RS^\bullet$ attack on PUFAs: a possible route to lipid peroxidation. *Biochem. Biophys. Res. Commun.* **101**, 113.

50. Saez, G *et al.* (1982) The production of free radicals during the autoxidation of cysteine and their effect on isolated rat hepatocytes. *Biochim. Biophys. Acta* **719**, 24.

51. Wang, R (2003) The gasotransmitter role of H_2S. *Antiox. Redox Signal.* **5**, 493.

52. Whiteman, M *et al.* (2004) The novel neuromodulator H_2S: an endogenous $ONOO^-$ 'scavenger'? *J. Neurochem.* **90**, 765.

53. Nauser, T and Schöneich, C (2003) Thiyl radical reaction with thymine: absolute rate constant for $H^\bullet$ abstraction and comparison to benzylic C–H bonds. *Chem. Res. Toxicol.* **16**, 1056.

54. Pogocki, D and Schöneich, C (2001) Thiyl radicals abstract $H^\bullet$ from carbohydrates: reactivity and selectivity. *Free Rad. Biol. Med.* **31**, 98.

55. Long, LH and Halliwell, B (2001) Oxidation and generation of H_2O_2 by thiol compounds in commonly used cell culture media. *Biochem. Biophys. Res. Commun.* **268**, 991.

56. Munday, R *et al.* (2004) Inhibition of Cu-catalyzed cysteine oxidation by nM concentrations of Fe salts. *Free Rad. Biol. Med.* **36**, 757.

57. Hu, VW *et al.* (2001) Metabolic radiolabeling: experimental tool or Trojan horse?[35] S-Methionine induces DNA fragmentation and p53-dependent ROS production. *FASEB J.* **15**, 1562.

58. Grisham, MB *et al.* (2001) $NO^\bullet$. I. Physiological chemistry of $NO^\bullet$ and its metabolites: implication in inflammation. *Am. J. Physiol.* **276**, G315.

59. Fukuto, JM *et al.* (2005) Nitroxyl (HNO): chemistry, biochemistry and pharmacology. *Ann. Rev. Pharm. Tox.* **45**, 335.

60. Möller, M *et al.* (2005) Direct measurement of $NO^\bullet$ and O_2 partitioning into liposomes and LDL. *J. Biol. Chem.* **280**, 8850.

61. Guittet, O *et al.* (1999) $NO^\bullet$: a radical molecule in quest of free radicals in proteins. *Cell. Mol. Life. Sci.* **55**, 1054.

62. Halliwell, B *et al.* (1999) $NO^\bullet$ and $ONOO^-$. The ugly, the uglier and the not so good. *Free Radic. Res.* **31**, 651.

63. Gorbunov, NV *et al.* (1995) Reduction of ferrylmyoglobin and ferrylhemoglobin by $NO^\bullet$: a protective mechanism against ferryl hemoprotein-induced oxidations. *Biochemistry* **34**, 6689.

64. Moncada, S and Higgs, EA (1995) Molecular mechanisms and therapeutic strategies related to $NO^\bullet$. *FASEB J.* **9**, 1319.

65. Bredt, DS (1999) Endogenous $NO^\bullet$ synthesis: biological functions and pathophysiology. *Free Radic. Res.* **31**, 577.

66. Brookes, PS *et al.* (1999) The assumption that $NO^\bullet$ inhibits mitochondrial ATP synthesis is correct. *FEBS Lett.* **445**, 261.

67. Huang, Z *et al.* (2005) Enzymatic function of hemoglobin as a NO_2^- reductase that produces $NO^\bullet$ under allosteric control. *J. Clin. Invest.* **115**, 2099.

68. Abu-Soud, HM and Hazen, SL (2000) $NO^\bullet$ is a physiological substrate for mammalian peroxidases. *J. Biol. Chem.* **275**, 37524.

69. Vernia, S *et al.* (2001) Differential sensitivity of rat hepatocyte CYP isoforms to self-generated $NO^\bullet$. *FEBS Lett.* **488**, 59.

70. Merx, MW *et al.* (2005) O_2 supply and $NO^\bullet$ scavenging by myoglobin contribute to exercise endurance and cardiac function. *FASEB J.* **19**, 1015.

71. Pearce, LL *et al.* (2002) The catabolic fate of $NO^\bullet$. The $NO^\bullet$ oxidase and $ONOO^-$ reductase activities of cytochrome oxidase. *J. Biol. Chem.* **277**, 13556.

72. Wennmalm, A *et al.* (1993) Metabolism and excretion of $NO^\bullet$ in humans. *Circ. Res.* **73**, 1121.

73. Kleinbongard, P *et al.* (2003) Plasma NO_2^- reflects constitutive $NO^\bullet$ synthase activity in mammals. *Free Rad. Biol. Med.* **35**, 790.

74. Cosby, K *et al.* (2003) Nitrite reduction to $NO^\bullet$ by deoxyhemoglobin vasodilates the human circulation. *Nature Med.* **9**, 1498.

75. Whiteman, M *et al.* (2003) Nitrite-mediated protection against HOCl–induced chondrocyte toxicity. A novel cytoprotective role of $NO^\bullet$ in the inflamed joint? *Arth. Rheum.* **48**, 3140.

76. Gladwin, MT (2004) Haldane, hot dogs, halitosis, and hypoxic vasodilation: the emerging biology of NO_2^-. *J. Clin. Invest.* **113**, 19.

77. Suzuki, H *et al.* (2003) Conditions for acid catalysed luminal nitrosation are maximal at the gastric cardia. *Gut* **52**, 1095.

78. Alderton, WK *et al.* (2001) NOS: structure, function and inhibition. *Biochem. J.* **357**, 593.

79. van Hinsbergh VWM (2001) NO$^\bullet$ or H$_2$O$_2$ for endothelium-dependent vasorelaxation. THB makes the difference. *Arterio. Thromb. Vasc. Biol.* **21**, 719.

80. Dweik, RA (2005) NO$^\bullet$, hypoxia and O$_2^{\bullet-}$; the good, the bad, and the ugly! *Thorax* **60**, 265.

81. Tsikas, D *et al.* (2000) Endogenous NOS inhibitors are responsible for the L-arginine paradox. *FEBS Lett.* **478**, 1.

82. Uematsu, M *et al.* (1995) Regulation of endothelial cell NOS mRNA expression by shear stress. *Am. J. Physiol.* **268**, C1371.

83. Pasto, M *et al.* (2001) Nasal polyp-derived O$_2^{\bullet-}$. *Am. J. Resp. Crit. Care Med.* **163**, 145.

84. Weinberg, JB (1998) NO$^\bullet$ production and NOS type 2 expression by human mononuclear phagocytes: a review. *Mol. Med.* **4**, 557.

85. Keynes, RG *et al.* (2003) O$_2^{\bullet-}$-dependent consumption of NO$^\bullet$ in biological media may confound *in vitro* experiments. *Biochem. J.* **369**, 399.

86. Alvarez, B and Radi, R (2003) ONOO$^-$ reactivity with amino acids and proteins. *Amino Acids* **25**, 295.

87. Eiserich, JP *et al.* (1996) Formation of nitrating and chlorinating species by reaction of NO$_2^-$ with HOCl. *J. Biol. Chem.* **271**, 19199.

88. Naseem, KM and Bruckdorfer, KR (1995) H$_2$O$_2$ at low concentrations strongly enhances the inhibitory effect of NO$^\bullet$ on platelets. *Biochem. J.* **310**, 149.

89. Wink, DA *et al.* (1996) The effect of various NO$^\bullet$-donor agents on H$_2$O$_2$- mediated toxicity. *Arch. Biochem. Biophys.* **331**, 241.

90. Kotamraju, S *et al.* (2003) NO$^\bullet$ inhibits H$_2$O$_2$-induced transferrin receptor-dependent apoptosis in endothelial cells: role of ubiquitin-proteasome pathway. *Proc. Natl. Acad. Sci. USA* **100**, 10653.

91. Greenacre, SAB and Ischiropoulos, H (2000) Tyrosine nitration: localization, quantification, consequences for protein function and signal transduction. *Free Radic. Res.* **34**, 541.

92. Macmillan-Crow, LA *et al.* (2001) Mitochondrial tyrosine nitration precedes chronic allograft nephropathy. *Free Rad. Biol. Med.* **31**, 1603.

93. Berlett, BS *et al.* (1996) ONOO$^-$ mediated nitration of tyrosine residues in E. coli glutamine synthetase mimics adenylation: relevance to signal transduction. *Proc. Natl. Acad. Sci. USA* **93**, 1776.

94. Zou, MH *et al.* (2002) Modulation by ONOO$^-$ of Akt- and AMP-activated kinase-dependent Ser^{1179} phosphorylation of endothelial NOS. *J. Biol. Chem.* **277**, 32552.

95. Balafanova, Z *et al.* (2002) NO$^\bullet$ induces nitration of PKC$_\varepsilon$, facilitating PKC$_\varepsilon$ translocation via enhanced PKC$_\varepsilon$-Rack2 interactions. *J. Biol. Chem.* **277**, 15021.

96. Dairou, J *et al.* (2005) Impairment of the activity of the xenobiotic-metabolizing enzymes NAT1/NAT2 by ONOO$^-$ in mouse skeletal muscle cells. *FEBS Lett.* **579**, 4719.

97. Lin, H *et al.* (2003) Mutation of tyrosine 190 to alanine eliminates the inactivation of CYP2B1 by ONOO$^-$. *Chem. Res. Toxicol.* **16**, 129.

98. Ji, Y *et al.* (2006) Nitration of tyrosine 92 mediates the activation of rat microsomal GST by ONOO$^-$. *J. Biol. Chem.* **281**, 1986.

99. Crow, JP *et al.* (1997) SOD catalyzes nitration of tyrosines by ONOO$^-$ in the rod and head domains of neurofilament-L. *J. Neurochem.* **69**, 1945.

100. Boulos, C *et al.* (2000) Diffusion of ONOO$^-$ into the human platelet inhibits COX via nitration of tyrosine residues. *J. Pharmacol. Exp. Ther.* **293**, 222.

101. Schmidt, P *et al.* (2003) Specific nitration at tyrosine 430 revealed by high resolution mass spectrometry as basis for redox regulation of bovine prostacyclin synthase. *J. Biol. Chem.* **278**, 12813.

102. Eaton, S *et al.* (2003) Myocardial carnitine palmitoyltransferase I as a target for oxidative modification in inflammation and sepsis. *Biochem. Soc. Trans.* **31**, 1133.

103. Schopfer, FJ *et al.* (2003) NO-dependent protein nitration: a cell signaling event or an oxidative inflammatory response? *TIBS* **28**, 646.

104. Swain, JA *et al.* (1994) ONOO$^-$ releases Cu from caeruloplasmin: implications for atherosclerosis. *FEBS Lett.* **342**, 49.

105. Vadseth *et al.* (2004) Pro-thrombotic state induced by post-translational modification of fibrinogen by RNS. *J. Biol. Chem.* **279**, 8820.

106. Kuhn, DM *et al.* (2002) ONOO$^-$-induced nitration of tyrosine hydroxylase. *J. Biol. Chem.* **277**, 14336.

107. Lee, JH *et al.* (2003) Inactivation of NADP$^+$-dependent isocitrate dehydrogenase by ONOO$^-$. Implications for cytotoxicity and alcohol-induced liver injury. *J. Biol. Chem.* **278**, 51360.

108. Goldstein, S and Czapski, G (2000) Reactivity of ONOO$^-$ versus simultaneous generation of $^\bullet$NO and O$_2^{\bullet-}$ toward NADH. *Chem. Res. Toxicol.* **13**, 736.

109. Kaur, H *et al.* (1997) ONOO$^-$-dependent aromatic hydroxylation and nitration of salicylate and phenylanine. Is OH$^\bullet$ involved? *Free Radic. Res.* **26**, 71.

110. Goldstein. S *et al.* (2001) Gibbs energy of formation of ONOO$^-$-order restored. *Chem. Res. Toxicol.* **14**, 657.

111. Yamakura, F *et al.* (2005) Nitrated and oxidized products of a single tryptophan residue in human

CuZnSOD treated with either $ONOO^- - CO_2$ or $MPO - H_2O_2 - NO_2^-$. *J. Biochem.* **138**, 57.

112. Eiserich, JP *et al.* (1999) Microtuble dysfunction by posttranslational nitrotyrosination of α-tubulin: A $NO^\bullet$-dependent mechanism of cellular injury. *Proc. Natl. Acad. Sci. USA* **96**, 6365.

113. Peluffo, H *et al.* (2004) Induction of motor neuron apoptosis by free 3-NT. *J. Neurochem.* **89**, 602.

114. Birnboim, HC *et al.* (2003) MHC class II-restricted peptides containing the inflammation-associated marker 3-NT evade central tolerance and elicit a robust cell-mediated immune response. *J. Immunol.* **171**, 528.

115. Aulak, KS *et al.* (2004) Dynamics of protein nitration in cells and mitochondria. *Am. J. Physiol.* **286**, H30.

116. Schopfer, FJ *et al.* (2005) Nitrolinoleic acid: an endogenous PPARγ ligand. *Proc. Natl. Acad. Sci. USA* **102**, 2340.

117. Lima, ES *et al.* (2005) Nitrated lipids decompose to $NO^\bullet$ and lipid radicals and cause vasorelaxation. *Free Rad. Biol. Med.* **39**, 532.

118. Skinner, KA *et al.* (1998) Nitrosation of uric acid by $ONOO^-$. Formation of a vasoactive $NO^\bullet$ donor. *J. Biol. Chem.* **273**, 24491.

119. Murray, J *et al.* (2003) Oxidative damage to mitochondrial complex I due to $ONOO^-$. *J. Biol. Chem.* **278**, 37223.

120. Stachowiak, O *et al.* (1998) Mitochondrial creatine kinase is a prime target of $ONOO^-$ induced modification and inactivation. *J. Biol. Chem.* **273**, 16694.

121. Whiteman, M and Halliwell, B (1997) Thiourea and DMTU inhibit $ONOO^-$-dependent damage: non-specificity as $OH^\bullet$ scavengers. *Free Rad. Biol. Med.* **22**, 1309.

122. Zhang, Y and Rosenberg, PA (2004) Caspase-1 and PARP inhibitors may protect against $ONOO^-$-induced neurotoxicity independent of their enzyme inhibitor activity. *Eur. J. Neurosci.* **20**, 1727.

123. Tempone, AG *et al.* (2001) *Bothrops moojeni* venom kills *Leishmania* spp. with H_2O_2 generated by its L-amino acid oxidase. *Biochem. Biophys. Res. Commun.* **280**, 620.

124. Ehara, T *et al.* (2002) Antimicrobial action of achacin is mediated by L-amino acid oxidase activity. *FEBS Lett.* **531**, 509.

125. Taormina, PJ *et al.* (2001) Inhibitory activity of honey against foodborne pathogens as influenced by the presence of H_2O_2 and level of antioxidant power. *Int. J. Food Microbiol.* **69**, 217.

126. Siess, M-H *et al.* (1996) Flavonoids and honey and propolis. *J. Agr. Food Chem.* **44**, 2297.

127. Henzler, T and Steudle, E (2000) Transport and metabolic degradation of H_2O_2 in *Chara corallina*: model calculations and measurements with the pressure probe suggest transport of H_2O_2 across water channels. *J. Exp. Bot.* **51**, 2053.

128. Branco, MR *et al.* (2004) Decrease of H_2O_2 plasma membrane permeability during adaptation to H_2O_2 in *S. cerevisiae*. *J. Biol. Chem.* **279**, 6501.

129. Long, LH *et al.* (2000) Artifacts in cell culture: rapid generation of H_2O_2 on addition of $(-)$-epigallocatechin, $(-)$-epigallocatechin gallate, $(+)$-catechin, and quercetin to commonly used cell culture media. *Biochem Biophys Res Commun*, **273**, 50.

130. Mahns, A *et al.* (2003) Irradiation of cells with UVA (320–400 nm) in the presence of cell culture medium elicits biological effects due to extracellular generation of H_2O_2. *Free Radic. Res.* **37**, 391.

131. Boveris, A and Cadenas, E (2000) Mitochondrial production of H_2O_2. Regulation by $NO^\bullet$ and the role of ubisemiquinone. *IUBMB Life* **50**, 245

132. Halliwell, B *et al.* (2004) Establishing biomarkers of oxidative stress. The measurement of H_2O_2 in human urine. *Curr. Med. Chem.* **11**, 1085.

133. Seaver LC and Imlay, JA (2001) H_2O_2 fluxes and compartmentalization inside growing *E. coli*. *J. Bacteriol.* **183**, 7182.

134. Brodie, AE and Reed, DJ (1987) Reversible oxidation of G3PDH thiols in human lung carcinoma cells by H_2O_2. *Biochem. Biophys. Res. Commun.* **148**, 120.

135. Jansen, WTM *et al.* (2002) H_2O_2-mediated killing of *C. elegans* by *Streptococcus pyogenes*. *Infect. Immun.* **70**, 5202.

136. Almagor, M *et al.* (1984) Role of $O_2^{\bullet-}$ in host cell injury induced by *Mycoplasma pneumoniae* infection. A study in normal and trisomy 21 cells. *J. Clin. Invest.* **73**, 842.

137. Chochola, J *et al.* (1995) Release of H_2O_2 from human T cell lines and normal lymphocytes co-infected with HIV-1 and mycoplasma. *Free Radic. Res.* **23**, 197.

138. Spencer, JPE *et al.* (1995) DNA damage in human respiratory tract epithelial cells. *FEBS Lett.* **375**, 179.

138A. Coyle, CH *et al.* (2006) Mechanisms of H_2O_2-induced oxidative stress in endothelial cells. *Free Rad. Biol. med.* **40**, 2206.

139. Daniels, V (1984) The Russell effect—a review of its possible uses in conservation and the scientific examination of materials. *Stud. Conserv.* **29**, 57.

140. Schraufstatter, IU *et al.* (1990) Mechanisms of OCl^- injury to target cells. *J. Clin. Invest.* **85**, 554.

141. Winterbourn CC and Kettle AJ. (2000) Biomarkers of MPO-derived HOCl. *Free Rad. Biol. Med.* **29**, 403.

142. Weiss, SJ (1989) Tissue destruction by neutrophils. *N. Engl. J Med.* **320**, 365.

143. Hannum, DM *et al.* (1995) Subunit sites of oxidative inactivation of E. coli F_1-ATPase by HOCl. *Biochem. Biophys. Res. Commun.* **212**, 868.

144. Dukan, S *et al.* (1999) ROS are partially involved in the bacteriocidal action of HOCl. *Arch. Biochem. Biophys.* **367**, 311.

145. Moreno, JJ and Pryor, WA (1992) Inactivation of $\alpha_1 P$ inhibitor by $ONOO^-$. *Chem. Res. Toxicol.* **5**, 425.

146. Glaser, CB *et al.* (1992) Oxidation of a specific methionine in thrombomodulin by activated neutrophil products blocks cofactor activity. *J. Clin. Invest.* **90**, 2565.

147. Spencer, JP *et al.* (2000) NO_2^--induced deamination and OCl^--induced oxidation of DNA in intact human respiratory tract epithelial cells. *Free Rad. Biol. Med.* **28**, 1039.

148. Hawkins, CL *et al.* (2002) $O_2^{\bullet -}$ can act synergistically with OCl^- to induce damage to proteins. *FEBS Lett.* **510**, 41.

149. Fliss, H and Menard, M (1991) HOCl-induced mobilization of Zn from metalloproteins. *Arch. Biochem. Biophys.* **287**, 175.

150. Ashby, MT *et al.* (2004) Redox buffering of HOCl by thiocyanate in physiologic fluids. *J. Am. Chem. Soc.* **126**, 15976.

151. Sundaramoorthy, M *et al.* (2005) Stereochemistry of the CPO active site: crystallographic and molecular-modelling studies. *Curr. Biol.* **5**, 461.

152. Peskin, AV and Winterbourn, CC (2003) Histamine chloramine reactivity with thiol compounds, ascorbate and methionine and with intracellular GSH. *Free Rad. Biol. Med.* **35**, 1252.

153. Foote, CS *et al.* (eds) (1995) *Active O_2 in Chemistry.* Blackie, London.

154. Martin, JP and Logsdon, N (1987) The role of O_2 radicals in dye-mediated photodynamic effects in *E. coli. B. J. Biol. Chem.* **262**, 7213.

155. Davies, MJ (2003) Singlet O_2-mediated damage to proteins and its consequences. *Biochem. Biophys. Res. Commun.* **305**, 761.

156. Cardoso, DR *et al.* (2005) Deactivation of triplet-excited riboflavin by purine derivatives: important role of uric acid in light-induced oxidation of milk sensitized by riboflavin. *J. Agric. Food. Chem.* **53**, 3679.

157. Cox, TM *et al.* (2005) King George III and porphyria: an elemental hypothesis and investigation. *Lancet* **366**, 332.

158. Morison, WL (2004) Photosensitivity. *N. Engl. J. Med.* **350**, 1111.

159. Clare, NJ (1955) Photosensitization in animals. *Adv. Vet. Sci. Comp. Med.* **2**, 182.

160. Ennever, JP *et al.* (1987) Rapid clearance of a structural isomer of bilirubin during phototherapy. *J. Clin. Invest.* **79**, 1674.

161. Detty, MR *et al.* (2004) Current clinical and preclinical photosensitizers for use in photodynamic therapy. *J. Med. Chem.* **47**, 3897.

162. Wagner, JR *et al.* (1993) The oxidation of blood plasma and LDL components by chemically generated $^1O_2$. *J. Biol. Chem.* **268**, 18502.

163. Cross, CE *et al.* (1997) General biological consequences of inhaled environmental toxicants. In: *The Lung: Scientific Foundations*, Crystal, RG *et al.* (eds) p. 2421. Raven Press, Philadelphia.

164. Zhou, JF *et al.* (2003) Oxidative stress and potential free radical damage associated with photocopying. A role for O_3? *Free Radic. Res.* **37**, 137.

165. Schmut, O *et al.* (1994) Destruction of human tear proteins by O_3. *Free Rad. Biol. Med.* **17**, 165.

166. Berlett, BS *et al.* (1996) Comparison of the effects of O_3 on the modification of amino acid residues in glutamine synthetase and bovine serum albumin. *J. Biol. Chem.* **271**, 4177.

167. Frischer, Th *et al.* (1997) Aromatic hydroxylation in nasal lavage fluid following ambient O_3 exposure. *Free Rad. Biol. Med.* **22**, 201.

168. Kanofsky, JR and Sima, PD (1993) $^1O_2$ generation at gas-liquid interfaces: a significant artifact in the measurements of $^1O_2$ yields from O_3–biomolecule interactions. *Photochem. Photobiol.* **58**, 335.

169. Nieva, J and Wentworth, P (2004) The antibody-catalyzed water oxidation pathway—a new chemical arm to immune defense? *TIBS* **29**, 274.

170. Smith, LL (2004) O_2, oxysterols, ouabain, and O_3: a cautionary tale. *Free Rad. Biol. Med.* **37**, 318.

Chapter 3

1. Armitage, JP (1999) Bacterial tactic responses. *Adv. Microb. Physiol.* **41**, 229.

2. Burmester, T (2005) A welcome shortage of breath. *Nature* **433**, 471.

3. Dernbach, E *et al.* (2004) Antioxidative stress-associated genes in circulating progenitor cells: evidence for enhanced resistance against oxidative stress. *Blood* **104**, 3591.

4. Finkel, T (2005) Radical medicine; treating ageing to cure disease. *Nature Rev. Mol. Cell. Biol.* **6**, 971.

5. Daniels, V (1989) Oxidative damage and the preservation of organic artefacts. *Free Radic. Res. Commun.* **5**, 213.

6. Scott, G (1993) *Atmospheric Oxidation and Antioxidants*, Vols I, II and III, Elsevier, Amsterdam.

7. Fridovich, I (1995) Superoxide radical and SODs. *Ann. Rev. BioChem.* **64**, 97.

8. Bertini, I *et al.* (1998) Structure and properties of CuZnSODs. *Adv. Inorg. Chem.* **45**, 127.

9. Liochev, SI and Fridovich, I (2001) CuZnSOD as a univalent NO^- oxidoreductase and as a DCF peroxidase. *J. Biol. Chem.* **276**, 35253.

10. Searcy, DG *et al.* (1995) Interaction of CuZnSOD with H_2S. *Arch. Biochem. Biophys.* **318**, 251.

11. Winterbourn, CC *et al.* (2002) Thiol oxidase activity of CuZnSOD. *J. Biol. Chem.* **277**, 1906.

12. Okado-Matsumoto, A and Fridovich I (2001) Subcellular distribution of SODs in rat liver. *J. Biol. Chem.* **276**, 38388.

13. Desideri, A and Falconi, M (2003) Prokaryotic CuZnSODs. *Biochem. Soc. Trans.* **31**, 1322.

14. Lynch, M and Kuramitsu, H (2000) Expression and role of SODs in pathogenic bacteria. *Microbes Infect.* **2**, 1245.

15. Spagnolo, L *et al.* (2004) Unique features of the *sodC*-encoded SOD from *M. tuberculosis*, a fully functional Cu-containing enzyme lacking Zn in the active site. *J. Biol. Chem.* **279**, 33447.

16. Furukawa, Y *et al.* (2004) O_2-induced maturation of SOD1: a key role for disulfide formation by the Cu chaperone CCS. *EMBO J.* **23**, 2872.

17. Carroll, MC *et al.* (2004) Mechanisms for activating CuZnSOD in the absence of the CCS Cu chaperone. *Proc. Natl. Acad. Sci. USA* **101**, 5964.

18. O'Neill, P *et al.* (1982) Evidence for catalytic dismutation of O_2^- by Co^{2+} derivatives of bovine SOD in aqueous solution as studied by pulse radiolysis. *Biochem. J.* **205**, 181.

19. Heikkila, RE *et al.* (1976) *In vivo* inhibition of SOD in mice by DDTC. *J. Biol. Chem.* **251**, 2182.

20. Kober, T *et al.* (2003) DDTC inhibits the catalytic activity of XO. *FEBS Lett.* **551**, 99.

21. Kachadourian, R *et al.* (2001) 2-Methoxyestradiol does not inhibit SOD. *Arch. Biochem. Biophys.* **392**, 349.

22. Schinina, ME *et al.* (1996) Amino acid sequence of chicken CuZnSOD and identification of GSH adducts at exposed cys residues. *Eur. J. Biochem.* **237**, 433.

23. Marklund, SL *et al.* (1976) A comparison between the common type and rare genetic variant of human CuZnSOD. *Eur. J. Biochem.* **65**, 415.

24. Fink, RC and Scandalios, JG (2002) Molecular evolution and structure-function relationships of the SOD gene families in angiosperms and their relationship to other eukaryotic and prokaryotic SODs. *Arch. Biochem. Biophys.* **399**, 19.

25. De Croo, S *et al.* (1988) Isoelectric focusing of SOD: report of the unique SOD A*2 allele in a US white population. *Human Hered.* **38**, 1.

26. Liochev, SI and Fridovich, I (2004) CO_2, not HCO_3^-, facilitates oxidations by CuZnSOD plus H_2O_2. *Proc. Natl. Acad. Sci. USA* **101**, 743.

27. Ramirez, DC *et al.* (2005) Mechanism of H_2O_2-induced CuZnSOD-centered radical formation as explored by immuno-spin trapping: the role of Cu- and $CO_3^{•-}$-mediated oxidations. *Free Rad. Biol. Med.* **38**, 201.

28. Karunakaran, C *et al.* (2005) Thiol oxidase activity of Cu, ZnSOD stimulates HCO_3^--dependent peroxidase activity via formation of $CO_3^{•-}$. *Chem. Res. Toxicol.* **18**, 494.

29. Davis, CA *et al.* (2004) Potent anti-tumor effects of an active site mutant of human MnSOD. *J. Biol. Chem.* **279**, 12769.

30. Lamarre, C *et al.* (2001) *C. albicans* expresses an unusual cytoplasmic MnSOD (SOD3 gene product) upon the entry and during the stationary phase. *J. Biol. Chem.* **276**, 43784.

31. Brouwer, M *et al.* (2003) Replacement of a cytosolic CuZnSOD by a novel cytosolic MnSOD in crustaceans that use Cu (haemocyanin) for O_2 transport. *Biochem. J.* **374**, 219.

32. Shatzman, AR and Kosman, DJ (1979) Biosynthesis and cellular distribution of the two SODs of *Dactylium dendroides*. *J. Bacteriol.* **137**, 313.

33. De Rosa, G *et al.* (1980) Regulation of SOD activity by dietary Mn. *J. Nutr.* **110**, 795.

34. Li, H *et al.* (2005) MnSOD polymorphism, pre-diagnostic antioxidant status, and risk of clinical significant prostate cancer. *Cancer Res.* **65**, 2498.

35. Gabbianelli, R *et al.* (1995) Metal uptake of recombinant cambialistic SOD from *Propionibacterium shermanii* is affected by growth conditions of host *E. coli.* cells. *Biochem. Biophys. Res. Commun.* **216**, 841.

36. Huang, JK *et al.* (2005) Biochemical characterization of a cambialistic SOD isoenzyme from diatom *Thallassiosira weissflogii*. *J. Agric. Food Chem.* **53**, 6319.

37. Chen, HY *et al.* (2002) Structural studies of an eukaryotic cambialistic SOD purified from the mature seeds of camphor tree. *Arch. Biochem. Biophys.* **404**, 218.

38. Kim, EJ *et al.* (1998) Expression and regulation of the sodF gene encoding Fe- and Zn-containing SOD in *Streptomyces coelicolor* Müller. *J. Bact.* **180**, 2014.

39. Wuerges, J *et al.* (2004) Crystal structure of NiSOD reveals another type of active site. *Proc. Natl. Acad. Sci. USA* **101**, 8569.

40. Bannister, JV and Calabrese, L (1987) Assays for SOD. *Meth. Biochem. Anal.* **32**, 279.

41. Beyer, WF, Jr and Fridovich, I (1987) Assaying for SOD: some large consequences of minor changes in conditions. *Anal. BioChem.* 161, 559.

42. Sutherland, MW and Learmonth, BA (1997) The tetra-zolium dyes MTS and XTT provide new quantitative assays for $O_2^{\bullet-}$ and SOD. *Free Radic. Res.* **27**, 283.

43. Hassan, HM *et al.* (1980) Inhibitors of SODs: a cautionary tale. *Arch. Biochem. Biophys.* **199**, 349.

44. Okado-Matsumoto, A and Fridovich, I (2001) Assay of SOD: cautions relevant to the use of cytochrome *c*, a sulfonated tetrazolium, and cyanide. *Anal. BioChem.* **298**, 337.

45. Halliwell, B (1977) Generation of H_2O_2, $O_2^{\bullet-}$ and $OH^{\bullet}$ during the oxidation of dihydroxyfumaric acid by peroxidase. *Biochem. J.* **163**, 441.

46. Nivière, V and Fontecave, M (2004) Discovery of $O_2^{\bullet-}$ reductase: an historical perspective. *J. Biol. Inorg. Chem.* **9**, 119.

47. Fournier, M *et al.* (2004) A new function of the *Desulfovibrio vulgaris* Hildenborough [Fe] hydro-genase in the protection against oxidative stress. *J. Biol. Chem.* **279**, 1787.

48. Liochev, SI and Fridovich, I (2000) CuZnSOD can act as a $O_2^{\bullet-}$ reductase and $O_2^{\bullet-}$ oxidase. *J. Biol. Chem.* **275**, 38482.

49. Farr, SB *et al.* (1986) O_2-dependent mutagenesis in *E. coli* lacking SOD. *Proc. Natl. Acad. Sci USA* **83**, 8268.

50. Benov, L and Fridovich, I (1996) Functional significance of the CuZnSOD in *E. coli. Arch. Biochem. Biophys.* **327**, 249.

51. González-Flecha, B and Demple, B (1995) Metabolic sources of H_2O_2 in aerobically growing *E. coli. J. Biol. Chem.* **270**, 13681.

52. Hassett, DJ *et al.* (1995) *Pseudomonas aeruginosa, sod*A and *sod*B mutants defective in Mn- and Fe- cofactored SOD activity demonstrate the importance of the Fe-cofactored form in aerobic metabolism. *J. Bacteriol.* **177**, 6330.

53. Outten, CE *et al.* (2005) Cellular factors required for protection from hyperoxia toxicity in *S. cerevisiae. Biochem. J.* **388**, 93.

54. Balzan, R *et al.* (1995) *E. coli* FeSOD targeted to the mitochondria of yeast cells protects the cells against oxidative stress. *Proc. Natl. Acad. Sci USA* **92**, 4219.

55. Guidot, DM *et al.* (1993) Absence of electron transport (Rh° state) restores growth of a MnSOD-deficient *S. cerevisiae* in hyperoxia. *J. Biol. Chem.* **268**, 26699.

56. Żyracka, E *et al.* (2005) Ascorbate abolishes auxotrophy caused by the lack of SOD in *S. cerevisiae*. Yeast can be a biosensor for antioxidants. *J. Biotechnol.* **115**, 271.

57. Peled-Kamar, M *et al.* (1997) Oxidative stress mediates impairment of muscle function in transgenic mice with elevated level of wild-type CuZnSOD. *Proc. Natl. Acad. Sci. USA* **94**, 3883.

58. Ho, YS *et al.* (1998) Transgenic models for the study of lung antioxidant defense: enhanced MnSOD activity gives partial protection to B6C3 hybrid mice exposed to hyperoxia. *Am. J. Respir. Cell Mol. Biol.* **18**, 538.

59. Reveillaud, I *et al.* (1992) Stress resistance of *Drosophila* transgenic for bovine CuZnSOD. *Free Radic. Res. Commun.* **17**, 73.

60. Lebovitz, RM *et al.* (1996) Neurodegeneration, myo-cardial injury and perinatal death in mitochondrial SOD-deficient mice. *Proc. Natl. Acad. Sci. USA* **93**, 9782.

61. Hinerfeld, D *et al.* (2004) Endogenous mitochondrial oxidative stress: neurodegeneration, proteomic analysis, specific respiratory chain defects, and efficacious antioxidant therapy in SOD2 null mice. *J. Neurochem.* **88**, 657.

62. Kokoszka, JE *et al.* (2001) Increased mitochondrial oxidative stress in the Sod2 (+/−) mouse results in the age-related decline of mitochondrial function culminating in increased apoptosis. *Proc. Natl. Acad. Sci USA* **98**, 2278.

63. Melov, S *et al.* (1998) A novel neurological phenotype in mice lacking mitochondrial MnSOD. *Nature Genet.* **18**, 159.

64. Asikainen, TM *et al.* (2002) Increased sensitivity of homozygous SOD 2 mutant mice to O_2 toxicity. *Free Rad. Biol. Med.* **32**, 175.

65. Ho, YS *et al.* (1998) The nature of antioxidant defense mechanisms: a lesson from transgenic studies. *Environ. Health Perspect.* **106** (Suppl 5), 1219.

66. Reaume, AG *et al.* (1996) Motor neurones in CuZnSOD-deficient mice develop normally but exhibit enhanced cell death after axonal injury. *Nature Genet.* **13**, 43.

67. Muller, FL *et al.* (2006) Absence of CuZnSOD leads to elevated oxidative stress and acceleration of age-dependent skeletal muscle atrophy. *Free Rad. Biol. Med.* **40**, 1993.

68. Didion, SP *et al.* (2002) Increased $O_2^{\bullet-}$ and vascular dysfunction in CuZnSOD-deficient mice. *Circ. Res.* **91**, 938.

69. Elchuri, S *et al.* (2005) CuZnSOD deficiency leads to persistent and widespread oxidative damage and hepatocarcinogenesis later in life. *Oncogene* **24**, 367.

70. Ghoshal, K *et al.* (1999) Transcriptional induction of metallothionein-I and -II genes in the livers of CuZnSOD knockout mice. *Biochem. Biophys. Res. Commun.* **264**, 735.

71. Sugino, N *et al.* (1999) Suppression of intracellular SOD activity by antisense oligonucleotides causes inhibition of progesterone production by rat luteal cells. *Biol. Reprod.* **61**, 1133.

72. Kirby, K, *et al.* (2002) RNA interference-mediated silencing of SOD2 in *Drosophila* leads to early

adult-onset mortality and elevated endogenous oxidative stress. *Proc. Natl. Acad. Sci. USA* **99**, 16162.

73. Dykens, JA and Shick, JM (1984) Photobiology of the symbiotic sea anemone, *Anthopleura elegantissima*: defences against photodynamic effects, and seasonal photoacclimatization. *Biol. Bull.* **167**, 683.

74. Tsan, MF *et al.* (2001) SOD and pulmonary O_2 toxicity: lessons from transgenic and knockout mice. *Int. J. Mol. Med.* **7**, 13.

75. Hass, MA and Massaro, D (1987) Differences in CuZnSOD induction in lungs of neonatal and adult rats. *Am. J. Physiol.* **253**, C66.

76. Asikainen, TM and White, CW (2005) Antioxidant defenses in the preterm lung: role for hypoxia-inducible factors in BPD? *Toxicol. Appl. Pharmacol.* **203**, 177.

77. Turrens, JF *et al.* (1984) Protection against O_2 toxicity by intravenous injection of liposome-entrapped catalase and SOD. *J. Clin. Invest.* **73**, 87.

78. Buzadzic, B *et al.* (1990) Antioxidant defenses in the ground squirrel *Citellus citellus*. 2. The effect of hibernation. *Free Rad. Biol. Med.* **9**, 407.

79. Hermes-Lima, M *et al.* (1998) Antioxidant defenses and metabolic depression. The hypothesis of preparation for oxidative stress in land snails. *Comp. Biochem. Physiol.* **120**, 437.

80. Almagor, M *et al.* (1984) Role of $O_2^{\bullet-}$ in host cell injury induced by *M. pneumoniae* infection. A study in normal and trisomy 21 cells. *J. Clin. Invest.* **73**, 842.

81. Austin, FE *et al.* (1981) Distribution of SOD, catalase, and peroxidase activities among *Treponema pallidum* and other spirochetes. *Infect. Immun.* **33**, 372.

82. Seib, KL *et al.* (2006) Defenses against oxidative stress in *N. gonorrhoeae*: a system tailored for a changing environment. *Microb. Molec. Biol. Rev.* **70**, 344.

83. Zheng, H *et al.* (1992) Regulation of catalase in *N. gonorrhoeae*. *J. Clin. Invest.* **90**, 1000.

84. Archibald, FS (1985) Mn: its acquisition by and function in the lactic acid bacteria. *CRC Crit. Rev. Microbiol.* **13**, 63.

85. Al-Maghrebi, M *et al.* (2002) Mn supplementation relieves the phenotypic deficits seen in SOD-null *E. coli*. *Arch. Biochem. Biophys.* **402**, 104.

86. Lapinskas, PJ *et al.* (1995) Mutations in PMR1 suppress oxidative damage in yeast cells lacking SOD. *Mol. Cell. Biol.* **15**, 1382.

87. Etherington, DJ *et al.* (1981) Collagen degradation in an experimental inflammatory lesion: studies on the role of the macrophage. *Acta Biol. Med. Germ.* **40**, 1625.

88. Imlay, JA *et al.* (2003) Pathways of oxidative damage. *Ann. Rev. Microbiol.* **57**, 395.

89. Kwon, ES *et al.* (2006) Inactivation of homocitrate synthase causes lysine auxotrophy in CuZn-containing SOD-deficient yeast *S. pombe*. *J. Biol. Chem.* **281**, 1345.

90. Vasquez-Vivar *et al.* (2000) Mitochondrial aconitase is a source of OH$^{\bullet}$. *J. Biol. Chem.* **275**, 14064.

91. Zhang, Y *et al.* (1990) The oxidative inactivation of mitochondrial electron transport chain components and ATPase. *J. Biol. Chem.* **265**, 16630.

92. Benov, L and Fridovich, I (1999) Why $O_2^{\bullet-}$ imposes an aromatic amino acid auxotrophy on *E. coli*. *J. Biol. Chem.* **274**, 4202.

93. Gaudu, P *et al.* (1996) The irreversible inactivation of RNR from *E. coli* by $O_2^{\bullet-}$. *FEBS Lett.* **387**, 137.

94. Wendt, S *et al.* (2003) Differential effects of ONOO$^-$ on human mitochondrial creatine kinase isoenzymes. Inactivation, octamer destabilization, and identification of involved residues. *J. Biol. Chem.* **278**, 1125.

95. Halliwell, B and Gutteridge, JMC (1990) Role of free radicals and catalytic metal ions in human disease. *Meth. Enzymol.* **186**, 1.

96. Halliwell, B and Gutteridge JMC (1984) O_2 toxicity, O_2 radicals, transition metals and disease. *Biochem. J.* **219**, 1.

97. Petrat, F *et al.* (2003) Reduction of Fe(III) ions complexed to physiological ligands by lipoyl dehydrogenase and other flavoenzymes *in vitro*. *J. Biol. Chem.* **278**, 46403.

98. Rowley, DA and Halliwell, B (1982) $O_2^{\bullet-}$-dependent formation of OH$^{\bullet}$ from NADH and NADPH in the presence of Fe salts. *FEBS Lett.* **142**, 39.

99. Park, S and Imlay JA (2003) High levels of intracellular cysteine promote oxidative DNA damage by driving the Fenton reaction. *J. Bacteriol.* **185**, 1942.

100. Woodmansee, AN and Imlay, JA (2002) Reduced flavins promote oxidative DNA damage in non-respiring *E. coli* by delivering electrons to intracellular free Fe. *J. Biol. Chem.* **277**, 34055.

101. Repine, JE *et al.* (1981) H_2O_2 kills *S. aureus* by reacting with staphylococcal Fe to form OH$^{\bullet}$. *J. Biol. Chem.* **256**, 7094.

102. Touati, D *et al.* (1995) Lethal oxidative damage and mutagenesis are generated by iron in Δfur mutants of *E. coli*: protective role of SOD. *J. Bacteriol.* **177**, 2305.

103. Nunoshiba, T *et al.* (1999) Role of Fe and $O_2^{\bullet-}$ for generation of OH$^{\bullet}$, oxidative DNA lesions, and mutagenesis in *E. coli*. *J. Biol. Chem.* **274**, 34832.

104. Benov, L and Fridovich, I (1998) Growth in Fe-enriched medium partially compensates *E. coli* for the lack of Mn- and Fe-SOD. *J. Biol. Chem.* **273**, 10313.

105. Kakhlon, O and Cabantchik, ZI (2002) The labile Fe pool: characterization, measurement, and participation in cellular processes. *Free Rad. Biol. Med.* **33**, 1037.

106. Oudit, GY *et al.* (2003) L-type Ca^{2+} channels provide a major pathway for Fe entry into cardiomyocytes in Fe-overload cardiomyopathy. *Nature Med.* **9**, 1187.

107. Kyle, ME *et al.* (1988) Endocytosis of SOD is required in order for the enzyme to protect hepatocytes from the cytotoxicity of H_2O_2. *J. Biol. Chem.* **263**, 3784.

108. Spencer, JP *et al.* (1995) DNA strand breakage and base modification induced by H_2O_2 treatment of human respiratory tract epithelial cells. *FEBS Lett.* **374**, 233.

109. MacManus-Spencer, LA and McNeill, K (2005) Quantification of $^1O_2$ production in the reaction of $O_2^{\bullet-}$ with H_2O_2 using a selective chemiluminescent probe. *J. Am. Chem. Soc.* **127**, 8954.

110. Kanofsky, JR (1986) Singlet O_2 production in $O_2^{\bullet-}$-halocarbon systems. *J. Am. Chem. Soc.* **108**, 2977.

111. Chance, B *et al.* (1979) Hydroperoxide metabolism in mammalian organs. *Physiol. Rev.* **59**, 527.

112. Winterbourn, CC and Stern, A (1987) Human red cells scavenge extracellular H_2O_2 and inhibit formation of HOCl and OH$^\bullet$. *J. Clin. Invest.* **80**, 1486.

113. Lledías, F *et al.* (1998) Oxidation of catalase by singlet O_2. *J. Biol. Chem.* **273**, 10630.

114. Reid, TJ III *et al.* (1981) Structure and heme environment of beef liver catalase at 2.5 Å resolution. *Proc. Natl. Acad. Sci. USA* **78**, 4767.

115. Sichak, SP and Dounce, AL (1987) A study of the catalase monomer produced by lyophilization. *Biochim. Biophys. Acta* **925**, 282.

116. Gordon, T (1986) Purity of catalase preparations: contamination by endotoxin and its role in the inhibition of airway inflammation. *Free Rad. Biol. Med.* **2**, 373.

117. Tian, Y *et al.* (2000) A commercial preparation of catalase inhibits NO$^\bullet$ production by activated murine macrophages: role of arginase. *Infect. Immun.* **68**, 3015.

118. Brava, J *et al.* (1999) Structure of catalase HPII from *E. coli* at 1.9 Å resolution. *Proteins* **34**, 155.

119. Lee, JS *et al.* (2005) KatA, the major catalase, is critical for osmoprotection and virulence in *P. aeruginosa* PA14. *Infect. Immun.* **73**, 4399.

120. Lardinois, OM (1995) Reactions of bovine liver catalase with $O_2^{\bullet-}$ and H_2O_2. *Free Radic. Res.* **22**, 251.

121. Kirkman, HN *et al.* (1999) Mechanisms of protection of catalase by NADPH. *J. Biol. Chem.* **274**, 13908.

122. Darr, D and Fridovich, I (1986) Irreversible inactivation of catalase by 3-amino-1,2,4-triazole. *Biochem. Pharmacol.* **35**, 3642.

123. Smith, T *et al.* (1998) Bacterial oxidation of mercury metal vapor, Hg(0). *Appl. Environ. Microbiol.* **64**, 1328.

124. DeMaster, EG *et al.* (1998) Mechanisms of inhibition of aldehyde dehydrogenase by NO$^-$, the active metabolite of the alcohol deterrent agent cyanamide. *Biochem. Pharmacol.* **55**, 2007.

125. Brunelli, L *et al.* (2001) Modulation of catalase peroxidatic and catalatic activity by NO$^\bullet$. *Free Rad. Biol. Med.* **30**, 709.

126. Heck, DE *et al.* (2003) UVB light stimulates production of ROS. Unexpected role for catalase. *J. Biol. Chem.* **278**, 22432.

127. Kawada, Y *et al.* (2004) Inhibitions of peroxisomal functions due to oxidative imbalance induced by mistargeting of catalase to cytoplasm is restored by vitamin E treatment in skin fibroblasts from Zellweger syndrome-like patients. *Mol. Genet. Metab.* **83**, 297.

128. Antunes, F *et al.* (2002) Relative contributions of heart mitochondria GPx and catalase to H_2O_2 detoxification in in vivo conditions. *Free Rad. Biol. Med.* **33**, 1260.

129. Bulitta, C *et al.* (1996) Cytoplasmic and peroxisomal catalases of the guinea pig liver: evidence for two distinct proteins. *Biochim. Biophys. Acta* **1293**, 55.

130. Barynin, VV *et al.* (2001) Crystal structure of Mn-catalase from *L. plantarum*. *Structure* **9**, 725.

131. Leopold, JA and Loscalzo, J (2005) Oxidative enzymopathies and vascular diseases. *Arterio. Thromb. Vasc. Biol.* **25**, 1332.

132. Ho, YS *et al.* (2004) Mice lacking catalase develop normally but show differential sensitivity to oxidant tissue injury. *J. Biol. Chem.* **279**, 32804.

133. Mackey, WJ and Bewley, GC (1989) The genetics of catalase in *Drosophila melanogaster*:isolation and characterization of acatalasemic mutants. *Genetics* **122**, 643.

134. Forsberg, L *et al.* (2001) A common functional C-T substitution polymorphism in the promoter region of the human catalase gene influences transcription factor binding, reporter gene transcription and is correlated to blood catalase levels. *Free Rad. Biol. Med.* **30**, 500.

135. Niederfuhr, A *et al.* (1998) A sequence-ready 3-Mb PAC contig covering 16 breakpoints of the Wilms tumor/anirida region of human chromosome 11p13. *Genomics* **53**, 155.

136. Brigelius-Flohé, R (1999) Tissue-specific functions of individual GPx. *Free Rad. Biol. Med.* **27**, 951.

137. Chaudiere, J *et al.* (1984) Mechanism of Se-GPx and its inhibition by mercaptocarboxylic acids and other mercaptans. *J. Biol. Chem.* **259**, 1043.

138. Bao, Y *et al.* (1997) Reduction of thymine hydroperoxide by PHGPx and GST. *FEBS Lett.* **410**, 210.

139. Maiorino, M *et al.* (2005) Functional interaction of PHGPx with sperm mitochondrion-associated cysteine-rich protein discloses the adjacent cysteine motif as a new substrate of the selenoperoxidase. *J. Biol. Chem.* **280**, 38395.

140. Hall, L *et al.* (1998) The majority of human GPx type 5 (GPX5) transcripts are incorrectly spliced: implications for the role of GPX5 in the male reproductive tract. *Biochem. J.* **333**, 5.

141. Burk, RF and Hill, KE (2005) Selenoprotein P: an extracellular protein with unique physical characteristics and a role in Se homeostasis. *Ann. Rev. Nutr.* **25**, 215.

142. Takebe, G. *et al.* (2002) A comparative study on the hydroperoxide and thiol specificity of the GPx family and selenoprotein P. *J. Biol. Chem.* **277**, 41254.

143. Jeong, D *et al.* (2002) Selenoprotein W is a glutathione-dependent antioxidant in vivo. *FEBS Lett.* **517**, 225.

144. Thienne, R *et al.* (1981) 3D-structure of glutathione reductase at 2Å resolution. *J. Mol. Biol.* **152**, 763.

145. Romero-Ramos, M *et al.* (2003) Semichronic inhibition of glutathione reductase promotes oxidative damage to proteins and induces both transcription and translation of tyrosine hydroxylase in the nigrostriatal system. *Free Radic. Res.* **37**, 1003.

146. Cheng, ML *et al.* (2004) G6PDH-deficient cells show an increased propensity for oxidant-induced senescence. *Free Rad. Biol. Med.* **36**, 580.

147. Salvemini, F *et al.* (1999) Enhanced GSH levels and oxidoresistance mediated by increased G6PDH expression. *J. Biol. Chem.* **274**, 2750.

148. Maeng, O *et al.* (2004) Cytosolic NADP$^+$-dependent isocitrate dehydrogenase protects macrophages from LPS-induced NO$^•$ and ROS. *Biochim. Biophys. Acta* **317**, 558.

149. Kosower, NW and Kosower, EM (1995) Diamide, an oxidant probe for thiols. *Meth. Enzymol.* **251**, 123.

150. Kaplowitz, N *et al.* (1996) GSH transporters: molecular characterization and role in GSH homeostasis. *Biol. Chem. Hoppe Seyler* **377**, 267.

151. Barhoumi, R *et al.* (1993) Concurrent analysis of intracellular GSH content and gap junctional intercellular communication. *Cytometry* **14**, 747.

152. Schafer, FQ and Buettner, GR (2001) Redox environment of the cell as viewed through the redox state of the GSSG/GSH couple. *Free Rad. Biol. Med.* **30**, 1191.

153. Abordo, EA *et al.* (1999) Accumulation of α-oxoaldehydes during oxidative stress: a role in cytotoxicity. *Biochem. Pharmacol.* **58**, 641.

154. Bellis, SL *et al.* (1994) Affinity purification of *Hydra* GSH binding proteins. *FEBS Lett.* **354**, 320.

155. Villa, LM *et al.* (1994) ONOO$^-$ induces both vasodilation and impaired vascular relaxation in the isolated perfused rat heart. *Proc. Natl. Acad. Sci. USA* **91**, 12383.

156. Hanna, PM and Mason, RP (1992) Direct evidence for inhibition of free radical formation from Cu(I) and H_2O_2 by GSH and other potential ligands using the EPR spin-trapping technique. *Arch. Biochem. Biophys.* **295**, 205.

157. Fernandez-Checa, JC and Kaplowitz, N (2005) Hepatic mitochondrial GSH: transport and role in disease and toxicity. *Toxicol. Appl. Pharmacol.* **204**, 263.

158. Wu, G *et al.* (2004) Glutathione metabolism and its implications for health. *J. Nutr.* **134**, 489.

159. Vaziri, ND *et al.* (2000) Induction of oxidative stress by GSH depletion causes severe hypertension in normal rats. *Hypertension* **36**, 142.

160. Meister, A (1995) Mitochondrial changes associated with GSH deficiency. *Biochim. Biophys. Acta* **1271**, 35.

161. Ballatori, N *et al.* (2005) Molecular mechanisms of reduced GSH transport: role of MRP/CFTR/ABCC and OATP/SLC21A families of membrane proteins. *Toxicol. Appl. Pharmacol.* **204**, 238.

162. Dalton, TP *et al.* (2004) Genetically altered mice to evaluate GSH homeostasis in health and disease. *Free Rad. Biol. Med.* **37**, 1511.

163. Lei, XG (2002) *In vivo* antioxidant role of GPx: evidence from knockout mice. *Meth. Enzymol.* **347**, 213.

164. Chu, FF *et al.* (2004) Bacteria-induced intestinal cancer in mice with disrupted Gpx1 and Gpx2 genes. *Cancer Res.* **64**, 962.

165. Yant, LJ *et al.* (2003) The selenoprotein GPX4 is essential for mouse development and protects from radiation and oxidative damage insults. *Free Rad. Biol. Med.* **34**, 496.

166. Suzuki, H *et al.* (2005) The *yliA, -B, -C,* and *-D* genes of *E. coli* K-12 encode a novel GSH importer with an ATP-binding cassette. *J. Bacteriol.* **187**, 5861.

167. Ferguson, GP and Booth, IR (1998) Importance of GSH for growth and survival of *E. coli* cells: detoxification of methylglyoxal and maintenance of intracellular K$^+$. *J. Bacteriol.* **180**, 4314.

168. Baek, YU *et al.* (2004) Disruption of γ-GCS results in absolute GSH auxotrophy and apoptosis in *C. albicans. FEBS Lett.* **556**, 47.

169. Hayes, JD *et al.* (2005) GSH transferases. *Ann. Rev. Pharmacol. Toxicol.* **45**, 51.

170. Edwards, R *et al.* (2000) Plant GSTs: enzymes with multiple functions in sickness and in health. *Trends Plant Sci.* **5**, 193.

171. Lu, WD and Atkins, WM (2004) A novel antioxidant role for ligandin behavior of GSTs: attenuation of the photodynamic effects of hypericin. *Biochemistry* **43**, 12761.

172. Jankowski, J *et al.* (2000) Isolation and characterization of coenzyme A glutathione disulfide as a parathyroid-derived vasoconstrictive factor. *Circulation* **102**, 2548.

173. Ram, JL *et al.* (1999) The spawning pheromone cysteine-glutathione disulfide ('nereithione') arouses a multicomponent nuptial behavior and electrophysiological activity in *N. succinea* males. *FASEB J.* **13**, 945.

174. Ghezzi, P *et al.* (2005) Thiol–disulfide balance: from the concept of oxidative stress to that of redox regulation. *Antiox. Redox Signal.* **7**, 964.

175. Shelton, MD *et al.* (2005) Glutaredoxin: role in reversible protein-S-glutathionylation and regulation of redox signal transduction and protein translocation. *Antiox. Redox Signal.* **7**, 348.

176. Beer, SM *et al.* (2004) Glutaredoxin 2 catalyzes the reversible oxidation and glutathionylation of mitochondrial membrane thiol proteins. *J. Biol. Chem.* **279**, 47939.

177. Dhindsa, RS (1987) Glutathione status and protein synthesis during drought and subsequent rehydration in *Tortula ruralis*. *Plant Physiol.* **83**, 816.

178. Ravichandran, V *et al.* (1994) *S*-Thiolation of G3PDH induced by the phagocytosis-associated respiratory burst in blood monocytes. *J. Biol. Chem.* **269**, 25010.

179. Wang, J *et al.* (2003) Stable and controllable RNA interference: investigating the physiological function of glutathionylated actin. *Proc. Natl. Acad. Sci USA* **100**, 5103.

180. Wells, WW *et al.* (1990) Mammalian thioltransferase (glutaredoxin) and protein disulfide isomerase have DHA reductase activity. *J. Biol. Chem.* **265**, 15361.

181. Björnstedt, M *et al.* (1995) Selenite and selenodiglutathione: reactions with thioredoxin systems. *Meth. Enzymol.* **252**, 209.

182. Gruber, CW *et al.* (2006) PDI: the structure of oxidative folding. *TIBS* **31**, 455.

183. Nordberg, J and Arnér, ESJ (2001) ROS, antioxidants, and the mammalian thioredoxin system. *Free Rad. Biol. Med.* **31**, 1287.

184. Rhee, SG *et al.* (2005) Controlled elimination of intracellular H_2O_2: regulation of peroxiredoxin, catalase, and GSH peroxidase via post-translational modification. *Antiox. Redox Signal.* **7**, 619.

185. Kanzok, SM *et al.* (2001) Substitution of the thioredoxin system for glutathione reductase in *D. melanogaster*. *Science* **291**, 643.

186. Cha, MK *et al.* (2004) *V. cholerae* thiol peroxidase-glutaredoxin fusion is a 2-cys TSA/AhpC subfamily acting as a lipid hydroperoxide reductase. *J. Biol. Chem.* **279**, 11035.

187. Zoccarato, F *et al.* (2004) Respiration-dependent removal of exogenous H_2O_2 in brain mitochondria. *J. Biol. Chem.* **279**, 4166.

188. Manevich, Y and Fisher, AB (2005) Peroxiredoxin 6, a 1-cys peroxiredoxin, functions in antioxidant defense and lung phospholipid metabolism. *Free Rad. Biol. Med.* **38**, 1422.

189. Wong, CM *et al.* (2004) Peroxiredoxin-null yeast cells are hypersensitive to oxidative stress and are genomically unstable. *J. Biol. Chem.* **279**, 23207.

190. Georgiou, G and Masip, L (2003) An overoxidation journey with a return ticket. *Science* **300**, 592.

191. Seaver, LC and Imlay, JA (2001) AHPR is the primary scavenger of endogenous H_2O_2 in *E. coli*. *J. Bacteriol.* **183**, 7173.

192. Cha, MK *et al.* (2004) *E. coli* periplasmic thiol peroxidase acts as lipid hydroperoxide peroxidase and the principal antioxidative function during anaerobic growth. *J. Biol. Chem.* **279**, 8769.

193. Wang, G *et al.* (2004) Role of a bacterial organic hydroperoxide detoxification system in preventing catalase inactivation. *J. Biol. Chem.* **279**, 51908.

194. Bryk, R *et al.* (2000) ONOO⁻ reductase activity of bacterial peroxiredoxins. *Nature* **407**, 211.

195. Dubuisson, M *et al.* (2004) Human peroxiredoxin 5 is a ONOO⁻ reductase. *FEBS Lett.* **571**, 161.

196. Diplock, AT (1985) *Fat-soluble Vitamins*. Heineman, London.

197. Awad, JA *et al.* (1994) Detection and localization of lipid peroxidation in Se- and vitamin E-deficient rats using F_2-IPs. *J. Nutr.* **124**, 810.

198. Beck, MA *et al.* (1998) GPx protects mice from viral-induced myocarditis *FASEB J.* **12**, 1143.

199. Moreno-Reyes, R *et al.* (1998) Kashin-Beck osteoarthropathy in rural Tibet in relation to Se and iodine status. *N. Engl. J. Med.* **339**, 1112.

200. Brown, TA and Shrift, A (1982) Se: toxicity and tolerance in higher plants. *Biol. Rev.* **57**, 59.

201. Bébien, M *et al.* (2002) Involvement of SOD in the response of *E. coli* to Se oxides. *J. Bacteriol.* **184**, 1556.

202. Kobayashi, Y *et al.* (2002) Selenosugars are key and urinary metabolites for Se excretion within the required to low-toxic range. *Proc. Natl. Acad. Sci. USA* **99**, 15932.

203. Sundquist, AR and Fahey RC (1989) The function of γ-glutamylcysteine and bis-γ-glutamylcystine reductase in *H. halobium*. *J. Biol. Chem.* **264**, 719.

204. Tausz, M *et al.* (2004) Root uptake, transport, and metabolism of externally applied GSH in *P. vulgaris* seedlings. *J. Plant Physiol.* **161**, 347.

205. Newton, GL *et al.* (2005) A mycothiol synthase mutant of *Mycobacterium smegmatis* produces novel thiols and has an altered thiol redox status. *J. Bacteriol.* **187**, 7309.

206. Ariyanayagam, MR and Fairlamb, AH (1999) *Entamoeba histolytica* lacks trypanothione metabolism. *Mol. Biochem. Parasitol.* **103**, 61.

207. Janowiak, BE and Griffith, OW (2005) GSH synthesis in *S. agalactiae*. *J. Biol. Chem.* **280**, 11829.

208. Krauth-Siegel, RL *et al.* (2005) Dithiol proteins as guardians of the intracellular redox milieu in parasites: old and new drug targets in trypanosomes and malaria-causing plasmodia. *Angew. Chem. Int. Ed.* **44**, 690.

209. McGonigle, S *et al.* (1998) Peroxidoxins: a new antioxidant family. *Parasitol. Today* **14**, 139.

210. Akanmu, D *et al.* (1991) The antioxidant action of ergothioneine. *Arch. Biochem. Biophys.* **288**, 10.

211. Gründemann, D *et al.* (2005) Discovery of the ergothioneine transporter. *Proc. Natl. Acad. Sci. USA* **102**, 5256.

212. Asmus, KD *et al.* (1996) One-electron oxidation of ergothioneine and analogues investigated by pulse radiolysis: redox reaction involving ergothioneine and vitamin C. *Biochem. J.* **315**, 625.

213. Erman, JE and Vitello, LB (2002) Yeast CCP: mechanistic studies via protein engineering. *Biochim. Biophys. Acta* **1597**, 193.

214. Moy, TI *et al.* (2004) Cytotoxicity of H_2O_2 produced by *E. faecium*. *Infect. Immun.* **72**, 4512.

215. Kawasaki, S *et al.* (1998) Effect of O_2 on the growth of *C. butyricum* (Type species of the genus *Clostridium*), and the distribution of enzymes for O_2 and for active O_2 species in Clostridia. *J. Ferment. Bioeng.* **86**, 368.

216. Nishiyama, Y *et al.* (2001) H_2O_2-forming NADH oxidase belonging to the peroxiredoxin oxidoreductase family: existence and physiological role in bacteria. *J. Bacteriol.* **183**, 2431.

217. Duffey, SS and Blum, MS (1977) Phenol and guaiacol: biosynthesis, detoxication and function in a polydesmid millipede, *Oxidus gracilis*. *Insect. Biochem.* **7**, 57.

218. Carlsson, J (1987) Salivary peroxidase: an important part of our defense against O_2 toxicity. *J. Oral Pathol.* **16**, 412.

219. Conner, GE *et al.* (2002) LPO and H_2O_2 metabolism in the airway. *Am. J. Respir. Crit. Care Med.* **166**, S57.

220. Passardi, F *et al.* (2005) Peroxidases have more functions than a Swiss army knife. *Plant Cell Rep.* **24**, 255.

221. Lardinois, OM *et al.* (1999) Spin trapping and protein cross-linking of the LPO protein radical. *J. Biol. Chem.* **274**, 35441.

222. Halliwell, B (1978) Lignin synthesis: generation of H_2O_2 and $O_2^{\bullet-}$ by HRP and its stimulation by Mn^{2+} and phenols. *Planta* **140**, 81.

223. Metodiewa, D and Dunford, HB (1989) The reactions of HRP, LPO and MPO with enzymatically generated $O_2^{\bullet-}$. *Arch. Biochem. Biophys.* **272**, 245.

224. Harman, LS *et al.* (1986) One- and two-electron oxidation of GSH by peroxidases. *J. Biol. Chem.* **261**, 1642.

225. Porter, DJT and Bright HJ (1983) The mechanism of oxidation of nitroalkanes by HRP. *J. Biol. Chem.* **258**, 9913.

226. Mader, M and Füssl, R (1982) Role of peroxidase in lignification of tobacco cells. *J. Biol. Chem.* **70**, 1132.

227. van Pée, KH and Unversucht, S (2003) Biological dehalogenation and halogenation reactions. *Chemosphere* **52**, 299.

228. Colin, C *et al.* (2005) V-dependent iodoperoxidases in *Laminaria digitata*, a novel biochemical function diverging from brown algal bromoperoxidases. *J. Biol. Inorg. Chem.* **10**, 156.

229. Sharp, KH *et al.* (2003) Crystal structure of the ascorbate peroxidase-ascorbate complex. *Nature Struct. Biol.* **10**, 303.

230. Hiner, ANP *et al.* (2000) Kinetic study of the inactivation of ascorbate peroxidase by H_2O_2. *Biochem. J.* **348**, 321.

231. Sieg, A *et al.* (1999) Detection of colorectal neoplasms by the highly sensitive hemoglobin–haptoglobin complex in feces. *Int. J. Colorect. Dis.* **14**, 267.

232. Yusa, T *et al.* (1984) Liposome-mediated augmentation of brain SOD and catalase inhibits CNS O_2 toxicity. *J. Appl. Phyisol.* **57**, 1674.

233. de Haan, JB *et al.* (1996) Elevation in the ratio of CuZnSOD to GPx activity induces features of cellular senescence and this effect is mediated by H_2O_2. *Hum. Mol. Genet.* **5**, 283.

234. Jovanovic, SV *et al.* (1998) Biomarkers of oxidative stress are significantly elevated in Down syndrome. *Free Rad. Biol. Med.* **25**, 1044.

235. Žitňanivá, I *et al.* (2004) Uric acid and allantoin levels in Down syndrome: antioxidant and oxidative stress mechanisms? *Clin. Chim. Acta* **341**, 139.

236. Praticò, D *et al.* (2000) Down's syndrome is associated with increased 8,12-*iso*-iPF$_{2\alpha}$-VI levels: evidence for enhanced lipid peroxidation *in vivo*. *Ann. Neurol.* **48**, 796.

237. Nunomura, A *et al.* (2000) Neuronal oxidative stress precedes Aβ deposition in Down syndrome. *J. Neuropathol. Exp. Neurol.* **59**, 1011.

238. Helguera, P *et al.* (2005) Ets-2 promotes the activation of a mitochondrial death pathway in DS neurons. *J. Neurosci.* **25**, 2295.

239. Wessling-Resnick, M (2006) Fe imports III. Transfer of Fe from the mucosa into circulation. *Am. J. Physiol.* **290**, G1.

240. Beard, JL and Connor, JR (2003) Iron status and neural functioning. *Ann. Rev. Nutr.* **23**, 41.

241. Maines, MD (1988) HO: function, multiplicity, regulatory mechanisms and clinical applications. *FASEB J.* **2**, 2557.

242. Cross, AJ *et al.* (2003) Haem, not protein or inorganic Fe, is responsible for endogeneous intestinal N-nitrosation arising from red meat. *Cancer Res.* **63**, 2358.

243. Atanasova, BD *et al.* (2005) Duodenal ascorbate and ferric reductase in human Fe deficiency. *Am. J. Clin. Nutr.* **81**, 130.

244. Hentze, MW *et al.* (2004) Balancing acts: molecular control of mammalian Fe metabolism. *Cell* **117**, 285.

245. Weinberg, ED (2003) The therapeutic potential of lactoferrin. *Expert Opin. Invest. Drugs* **12**, 841.

246. Halleen, JM *et al.* (1999) Intracellular fragmentation of bone resorption products by ROS generated by osteoclastic tartrate-resistant acid phosphatase. *J. Biol. Chem.* **274**, 22907.

247. Kruszewski, M (2003) Labile Fe pool: the main determinant of cellular response to oxidative stress. *Mutat. Res.* **531**, 81.

248. Petrat, F *et al.* (2001) Subcellular distribution of chelatable Fe: a laser scanning microscopic study in isolated hepatocytes and liver endothelial cells. *Biochem. J.* **356**, 61.

249. Kurz, T *et al.* (2004) Relocalized redox-active lysosomal Fe is an important mediator of oxidative-stress-induced DNA damage. *Biochem. J.* **378**, 1039.

250. Liu, X and Theil, EC (2005) Ferritins: dynamic management of biological Fe and O_2 chemistry. *Acc. Chem. Res.* **38**, 167.

251. Bolann, BJ and Ulvik, RJ (1993) Stimulated decay of $O_2^{\bullet-}$ caused by ferritin-bound copper. *FEBS Lett.* **328**, 263.

252. Wiedenheft, B *et al.* (2005) An archaeal antioxidant: characterization of a Dps-like protein from *Sulfolobus solfataricus. Proc. Natl. Acad. Sci. USA* **102**, 10551.

253. Girelli, D *et al.* (2001) Clinical, biochemical and molecular findings in a series of families with hereditary hyperferritinaemia-cataract syndrome. *Br J. Haematol.* **115**, 334.

254. Templeton, DM and Liu, Y (2003) Genetic regulation of cell function in response to Fe overload or chelation. *Biochim. Biophys. Acta* **1619**, 113.

255. Wang, J *et al.* (2004) Fe-mediated degradation of IRP2, an unexpected pathway involving a 2-oxoglutarate-dependent oxygenase activity. *Mol. Cell Biol.* **24**, 954.

256. Cooperman, SS *et al.* (2005) Microcytic anemia, erythropoietic protoporphyria, and neurodegeneration in mice with targeted deletion of Fe-regulatory protein 2. *Blood* **106**, 1084.

257. Núñez-Millacura, C *et al.* (2002) An oxidative stress-mediated positive-feedback Fe uptake loop in neuronal cells. *J. Neurochem.* **82**, 240.

258. Walter, PB *et al.* (2002) Fe deficiency and Fe excess damage mitochondria and mitochondrial DNA in rats. *Proc. Natl. Acad. Sci. USA* **99**, 2264.

259. Prohaska, JR and Gybina, AA (2004) Intracellular Cu transport in mammals. *J. Nutr.* **134**, 1003.

260. Brewer, GJ (2005) AntiCu therapy against cancer and diseases of inflammation and fibrosis. *Drug Disc. Today* **10**, 1103.

261. Johnson, WT and Thomas, AC (1999) Cu deprivation potentiates oxidative stress in HL-60 cell mitochondria. *Proc. Soc. Exp. Biol. Med.* **221**, 147.

262. Gutteridge, JMC *et al.* (1985) The behaviour of caeruloplasmin in stored human extracellular fluids in relation to ferroxidase II activity, lipid peroxidation and phenanthroline-detectable Cu. *Biochem. J.* **230**, 517.

263. Evans, PJ *et al.* (1989) Non-caeruloplasmin Cu and ferroxidase activity in mammalian serum. *Free Radic. Res. Commun.* **7**, 55.

264. Fox, PL *et al.* (2000) Ceruloplasmin and cardiovascular disease. *Free Rad. Biol. Med.* **28**, 1735.

265. Gutteridge, JMC and Stocks, J (1981) Caeruloplasmin: physiological and pathological perspectives. *CRC Crit. Rev. Clin. Lab. Sci.* **14**, 257.

266. Miyajima, H *et al.* (2003) Aceruloplasminemia, an inherited disorder of Fe metabolism. *Biometals* **16**, 205.

267. Park, YS *et al.* (1999) GPx-like activity of caeruloplasmin as an important lung antioxidant. *FEBS Lett.* **458**, 133.

268. Park, YS *et al.* (2000) Antioxidant binding of caeruloplasmin to MPO is inhibited, but oxidase, peroxidase and immunoreactive properties of caeruloplasmin remain intact. *Free Radic. Res.* **33**, 261.

269. Baron, CP and Andersen HJ (2002) Myoglobin-induced lipid oxidation. A review. *J. Agric. Food Chem.* **50**, 3887.

270. Herold, S *et al.* (2004) Reactivity studies of the Fe(III) and Fe(II) NO forms of human neuroglobin reveal a potential role against oxidative stress. *J. Biol. Chem.* **279**, 22841.

271. Gutteridge, JM (1986) Fe promoters of the Fenton reaction and lipid peroxidation can be released from haemoglobin by peroxides. *FEBS Lett.* **201**, 291.

272. Nagababu, E and Rifkind, JM (2000) Reaction of H_2O_2 with ferrylhemoglobin: $O_2^{\bullet-}$ production and heme degradation. *Biochemistry* **39**, 12503.

273. Lardinois, OM and Ortiz de Montellano, PR (2003) Intra- and intermolecular transfers of protein radicals in the reactions of sperm whale myoglobin with H_2O_2. *J. Biol. Chem.* **278**, 36214.

274. Hogg, N *et al.* (1994) The role of lipid hydroperoxides in the myoglobin-dependent oxidation of LDL. *Arch. Biochem. Biophys.* **314**, 39.

275. Romero, FJ *et al.* (1992) The reactivity of thiols and disulfides with different redox states of myoglobin, *J. Biol. Chem.* **267**, 1680.

276. Reeder, BJ and Wilson, MT (2005) DFX inhibits production of cytotoxic heme to protein cross-linked myoglobin: a mechanism to protect against oxidative stress with Fe chelation. *Chem. Res. Toxicol.* **18**, 1004.

277. Qian, SY *et al.* (2002) Identification of protein-derived tyrosyl radical in the reaction of cytochrome c and H_2O_2: characterization by ESR spin-trapping, HPLC and MS. *Biochem. J.* **363**, 281.

278. Evans, PJ *et al.* (1994) Promotion of oxidative damage to AA and α_1-AP by anti-inflammatory drugs in the presence of the haem proteins myoglobin and cytochrome c. *Biochem. Pharmacol.* **48**, 2173.

279. Baliga, R (1998) Role of CYP as a source of catalytic Fe in cisplatin-induced nephrotoxicity. *Kidney Int.* **54**, 1562.

280. Atamna, H *et al.* (2001) Heme deficiency selectively interrupts assembly of mitochondrial complex IV in human fibroblasts. *J. Biol. Chem.* **276**, 48410.

281. Kontoghiorghes, GJ and Weinberg, ED (1995) Fe: mammalian defense systems, mechanisms of disease, and chelation therapy approaches. *Blood Rev.* **9**, 33.

282. Posey, JE and Gherardini, FC (2000) Lack of a role for Fe in the Lyme disease pathogen. *Science* **288**, 1651.

283. Flo, TH *et al.* (2004) Lipocalin 2 mediates an innate immune response to bacterial infection by sequestering Fe. *Nature* **432**, 917.

284. Halliwell, B and Gutteridge, JMC (1990) The antioxidants of human extracellular fluids. *Arch. Biochem. Biophys.* **280**, 1.

285. Park, S *et al.* (2005) Substantial DNA damage from submicromolar intracellular H_2O_2 detected in Hpx$^-$ mutants of *E. coli*. *Proc. Natl. Acad. Sci. USA* **102**, 9317.

286. Toyokuni, S *et al.* (1995) Treatment of Wistar rats with a renal carcinogen, Fe(III)NTA, causes DNA protein cross-linking between thymine and tyrosine in their renal chromatin. *Int. J. Cancer* **62**, 309.

287. Paul, T (2000) Effects of a prolonged $O_2^{\bullet-}$ flux on transferrin and ferritin. *Arch. Biochem. Biophys.* **382**, 253.

288. O'Connell, MJ *et al.* (1986) Haemosiderin-like properties of free-radical-modified ferritin. *Biochem. J.* **240**, 297.

289. Simpson, RJ *et al.* (1992) Non-transferrin bound Fe species in the serum of hypotransferrinemic mice. *Biochim. Biophys. Acta.* **1156**, 19.

290. Beutler, E *et al.* (2000) Molecular characterization of a case of atransferrinemia. *Blood* **96**, 4071.

291. Cross, CE *et al.* (1984) Antioxidant protection: a function of tracheobronchial and gastrointestinal mucus. *Lancet* **1**, 1328.

292. Wood, C and Clauss, M (2004) Panda phlebotomies? The need for comparative screening for haemochromatosis. *Lancet* **364**, 1384.

293. Mete, A *et al.* (2005) Intestinal over-expression of Fe transporters induces Fe overload in birds in captivity. *Blood Cells Mol. Dis.* **34**, 151.

294. Gangaidzo, IT *et al.* (1999) Fe overload in urban Africans in the 1990s. *Gut* **45**, 278.

295. Vaulont, S *et al.* (2005) Of mice and men; the Fe age. *J. Clin. Invest.* **115**, 2079.

296. Ajioka, RS and Kushner, JP (2003) Clinical consequences of Fe overload in hemochromatosis homozygotes. *Blood* **101**, 3351.

297. Grootveld, M *et al.* (1989) NTBI in plasma or serum from patients with idiopathic hemochromatosis. *J. Biol. Chem.* **264**, 4417.

298. Phumala, N *et al.* (2003) Hemin: a possible cause of oxidative stress in blood circulation in beta-thalassemia/hemoglobin E disease. *Free Radic. Res.* **37**, 129.

299. Amer, J and Fibach, E (2005) Chronic oxidative stress reduces the respiratory burst response of neutrophils from β-thalassaemia patients. *Br. J. Haematol.* **129**, 435.

300. Bartsch, H and Nair, J (2005) Accumulation of lipid peroxidation-derived DNA lesions. *Mut. Res.* **591**, 34.

301. De Luca, C *et al.* (1999) Blood antioxidant status and urinary levels of catecholamine metabolites in β-thalassemia. *Free Radic. Res.* **30**, 453.

302. Hussain, SP *et al.* (2000) Increased p53 mutation load in nontumorous human liver of Wilson disease and hemochromatosis: oxyradical overload diseases. *Proc. Natl. Acad. Sci. USA* **97**, 12770.

303. Ogihara, H *et al.* (1995) Plasma Cu and antioxidant status in Wilson's disease. *Pediat. Res.* **37**, 219.

304. Von Herbay, A *et al.* (1994) Low vitamin E content in plasma of patients with alcoholic liver disease,

haemochromatosis and Wilson's disease. *J. Hepatol.* **20**, 41.

305. Nair, J *et al.* (2005) Apoptosis and age-dependent induction of nuclear and mitochondrial etheno-DNA adducts in LEC rats: enhanced DNA damage by dietary curcumin upon copper accumulation. *Carcinogenesis* **26**, 1307.

306. Yamamoto, H *et al.* (2001) In vivo evidence for accelerated generation of OH˙ in liver of LEC rats with acute heptatitis. *Free Rad. Biol. Med.* **30**, 547.

307. Tapia, L *et al.* (2004) MT is crucial for safe intracellular Cu storage and cell survival at normal and supraphysiological exposure levels. *Biochem. J.* **378**, 617.

308. Li, X *et al.* (2004) MT protects islets from hypoxia and extends islet graft survival by scavenging most kinds of ROS. *J. Biol. Chem.* **279**, 765.

309. Conrad, CC *et al.* (2000) Using MT$^{-/-}$ mice to study MT and oxidative stress. *Free Rad. Biol. Med.* **28**, 447.

310. Carrasco, J *et al.* (2003) Role of MT-III following CNS damage. *Neurobiol. Dis.* **13**, 22.

311. Cobbett, C and Goldsbrough, P (2002) Phytochelatins and MT: roles in heavy metal detoxification and homeostasis. *Annu. Rev. Plant Biol.* **53**, 159.

312. Lapointe, S *et al.* (1998) Binding of a bovine oviductal fluid catalase to mammalian spermatozoa. *Biol. Reprod.* **58**, 747.

313. El-Chemaly, S *et al.* (2003) H_2O_2-scavenging properties of normal human airway secretions. *Am. J. Resp. Crit. Care Med.* **167**, 425.

314. Fattman, CL *et al.* (2003) Extracellular SOD in biology and medicine. *Free Rad. Biol. Med.* **35**, 236.

315. Petersen, SV *et al.* (2004) EC-SOD binds to type I collagen and protects against oxidative fragmentation. *J. Biol. Chem.* **279**, 13705.

316. Nguyen, AD *et al.* (2004) Fibulin-5 is a novel binding protein for EC–SOD. *Circ. Res.* **95**, 1067.

317. Jung, O *et al.* (2003) EC-SOD is a major determinant of NO˙ bioavailability. In vivo and ex vivo evidence from ecSOD-deficient mice. *Circ. Res.* **93**, 622.

318. Carlsson, LM *et al.* (1995) Mice lacking ECSOD are more sensitive to hyperoxia. *Proc. Natl. Acad. Sci. USA* **92**, 6264.

319. Chu, Y *et al.* (2005) Vascular effects of the human ECSOD R213G variant. *Circulation* **112**, 1047.

320. Kelly, FJ and Mudway IS (2003) Protein oxidation at the air-lung interface. *Amino Acids* **25**, 375.

321. Wagener, F *et al.* (2001) Heme is a potent inducer of inflammation in mice and is counteracted by HO. *Blood* **98**, 1802.

322. Kristiansen, M *et al.* (2001) Identification of the haemoglobin scavenger receptor. *Nature* **409**, 198.

323. Lim SK *et al.* (2001) Role of haptoglobin in free hemoglobin metabolism. *Redox Rep.* **6**, 219.

324. Tolosano, E *et al.* (2002) Enhanced splenomegaly and severe liver inflammation in haptoglobin/ hemopexin double-null mice after acute hemolysis. *Blood* **100**, 4201.

325. Asleh, R *et al.* (2005) Haptoglobin genotype- and diabetes-dependent differences in Fe-mediated oxidative stress *in vitro* and *in vivo*. *Circ. Res.* **96**, 435.

326. Yamamoto, Y *et al.* (1992) Comparison of plasma levels of lipid hydroperoxides and antioxidants in hyperlipidemic Nagase analbuminemic rats, Sprague-Dawley rats and humans. *Biochem. Biophys. Res. Commun.* **189**, 518.

327. Mera, K *et al.* (2005) The structure and function of oxidized albumin in hemodialysis patients: its role in elevated oxidative stress via neutrophil burst. *Biochem. Biophys. Res. Commun.* **334**, 1322.

328. Quinlan, GJ *et al.* (1998) Administration of albumin to patients with sepsis syndrome: a possible beneficial role in plasma thiol repletion. *Clin. Sci.* **95**, 459.

329. Kaiser, VL *et al.* (2005) Trauma–hemorrhagic shock mesenteric lymph from rat contains a modified form of albumin that is implicated in endothelial cell toxicity. *Shock* **23**, 417.

330. Bito, R *et al.* (2005) Degradation of oxidative stress-induced denatured albumin in rat liver endothelial cells. *Am. J. Physiol.* **289**, C531.

331. Quinlan, GJ *et al.* (1992) Vanadium and Cu in clinical solutions of albumin and their potential to damage protein structure. *J. Pharmacol. Sci.* **81**, 611.

332. Gosriwatana, I *et al.* (1999) Quantification of non-transferrin-bound Fe in the presence of unsaturated transferrin. *Anal. Biochem.* **273**, 212.

333. Williams, SEJ *et al.* (2004) HO–2 is an O_2 sensor for a Ca-sensitive K^+ channel. *Science* **306**, 2093.

334. Kawashima, A *et al.* (2002) HO–1 deficiency: the first autopsy case. *Hum. Pathol.* **33**, 125.

335. Morse, D and Sethi, J (2002) CO and human disease. *Antiox. Redox Signal.* **4**, 331.

336. Dennery, PA *et al.* (2003) Resistance to hyperoxia with HO–1 disruption: role of Fe. *Free Rad. Biol. Med.* **34**, 124.

337. Otterbein, LE *et al.* (2003) CO suppresses arteriosclerotic lesions associated with chronic graft rejection and with balloon injury. *Nature Med.* **9**, 183.

338. Nakao, A *et al.* (2005) Biliverdin administration prevents the formation of intimal hyperplasia induced by vascular injury. *Circulation* **112**, 587.

339. Otterbein, L *et al.* (1995) Hemoglobin provides protection against lethal endotoxemia in rats: the role of HO-1. *Am. J. Resp. Cell. Mol. Biol.* **13**, 595.

340. Barañano, DE *et al.* (2002) Biliverdin reductase: a major physiologic cytoprotectant. *Proc. Natl. Acad. Sci. USA* **99**, 16093.

341. Liu, YR *et al.* (2003) Bilirubin as a potent antioxidant suppresses experimental autoimmune encephalomyelitis: implications for the role of oxidative stress in the development of multiple sclerosis. *J. Neuroimmunol.* **139**, 27.

342. Otani, K *et al.* (2001) Increased urinary excetion of bilirubin oxidative metabolites in septic patients: a new marker for oxidative stress *in vivo*. *J. Surg. Res.* **96**, 44.

343. Lin, S *et al.* (2005) Minocycline blocks bilirubin neurotoxicity and prevents hyperbilirubinemia-induced cerebellar hypoplasia in the Gunn rat. *Eur. J. Neurosci.* **22**, 21.

344. Pyne-Geithman, G *et al.* (2005) Bilirubin production and oxidation in CSF of patients with cerebral vasospasm after subarachnoid hemorrhage. *J. Cereb. Blood Flow Metab.* **25**, 1070.

345. Nath, KA *et al.* (1995) α-Ketoacids scavenge H_2O_2 *in vitro* and *in vivo* and reduce menadione-induced DNA injury and cytotoxicity. *Am. J. Physiol.* **268**, C227.

346. Knott, EM *et al.* (2005) Pyruvate-fortified cardioplegia suppresses oxidative stress and enhances phosphorylation potential of arrested myocardium. *Am. J. Physiol.* **289**, H1123.

347. Reiter, RJ and Tan DX (2003) Melatonin: a novel protective agent against oxidative injury of the ischemic/reperfused heart. *Cardiovasc. Res.* **58**, 10.

348. Marshall, KA *et al.* (1996) Evaluation of the antioxidant activity of melatonin *in vitro*. *Free Rad. Biol. Med.* **21**, 307.

349. Quinn, J *et al.* (2005) Chronic melatonin therapy fails to alter amyloid burden or oxidative damage in old Tg2576 mice: implications for clinical trials. *Brain Res.* **1037**, 209.

350. Antolín, I *et al.* (1997) Antioxidative protection in a high-melatonin organism: the dinoflagellate *Gonyaulax polyedra* is rescued from lethal oxidative stress by strongly elevated, but physiologically possible concentrations of melatonin. *J. Pineal Res.* **23**, 182.

351. Smith, AR *et al.* (2004) Lipoic acid as a potential therapy for chronic diseases associated with oxidative stress. *Curr. Med. Chem.* **11**, 1135.

352. Lee, WJ *et al.* (2005) α-Lipoic acid increases insulin sensitivity by activating AMPK in skeletal muscle. *Biochem. Biophys. Res. Commun.* **332**, 885.

353. Bryk, R *et al.* (2002) Metabolic enzymes of mycobacteria linked to antioxidant defense by a thioredoxin-like protein. *Science* **295**, 1073.

354. Ernster, L and Dallner, G (1995) Biochemical, physiological and medical aspects of ubiquinone function. *Biochim. Biophys. Acta* **1271**, 195.

355. Xia, L *et al.* (2003) The mammalian cytosolic selenoenyzme thioredoxin reductase reduces ubiquinone. *J. Biol. Chem.* **278**, 2141.

356. Do, TQ *et al.* (1996) Enhanced sensitivity of ubiquinone-deficient mutants of *S. cerevisiae* to products of autoxidized PUFAs. *Proc. Natl. Acad. Sci. USA* **93**, 7534.

357. Yamashita, S and Yamamoto, Y (1997) Simultaneous detection of ubiquinol and ubiquinone in human plasma as a marker of oxidative stress. *Anal. Biochem.* **250**, 66.

358. Watts, GF *et al.* (2002) Coenzyme Q_{10} improves endothelial dysfunction of the brachial artery in Type II diabetes mellitus. *Diabetologia* **45**, 420.

359. Papucci, L *et al.* (2003) Coenzyme Q_{10} prevents apoptosis by inhibiting mitochondrial depolarization independently of its free radical scavenging property. *J. Biol. Chem.* **278**, 28220.

360. Martinon, F *et al.* (2006) Gout-associated uric acid crystals activate the NALP3 inflammasome. *Nature* **440**, 237.

361. Simic, MG and Jovanovic, SV (1989) Antioxidation mechanisms of uric acid. *J. Am. Chem. Soc.* **111**, 5778.

362. Wu, X *et al.* (1994) Hyperuricaemia and urate nephropathy in urate oxidase-deficient mice. *Proc. Natl. Acad. Sci. USA* **91**, 742.

363. Ames, BN *et al.* (1981) Uric acid provides an antioxidant defense in humans against oxidant- and radical-caused aging and cancer. A hypothesis. *Proc. Natl. Acad. Sci. USA* **78**, 6858.

364. Robinson, KM *et al.* (2004) Triuret: a novel product of $ONOO^-$-mediated oxidation of urate. *Arch. Biochem. Biophys.* **423**, 213.

365. Whiteman, M and Halliwell, B (1996) Protection against $ONOO^-$-dependent tyrosine nitration and α_1-antiproteinase inactivation by ascorbic acid. A comparison with other biological antioxidants. *Free Radic. Res.* **25**, 275.

366. Santus, R *et al.* (2001) Redox reactions of the urate radical/ urate couple with $O_2^{\bullet-}$, the tryptophan neutral radical and selected flavonoids in neutral aqueous solutions. *Free Radic. Res.* **35**, 129.

367. Kanellis, J and Johnson, RJ (2003) Elevated uric acid and ischemic stroke: accumulating evidence that it is injurious and not neuroprotective. *Stroke* **34**, 1956.

368. Scott, GS *et al.* (2005) Uric acid protects against secondary damage after spinal cord injury. *Proc. Natl. Acad. Sci. USA* **102**, 3483.

369. Babizhayev, MA *et al.* (1994) L-Carnosine (β-alanyl-L-histidine) and carcinine (β-alanylhistamine) act as natural antioxidants with OH$^\bullet$ scavenging and lipid-peroxidase activities. *Biochem. J.* **304**, 509.

370. Park, YJ *et al.* (2005) Quantitation of carnosine in humans plasma after dietary consumption of beef. *J. Agric. Food Chem.* **53**, 4736.

371. Kohen, R *et al.* (1988) Antioxidant activity of carnosine, homocarnosine and anserine present in muscle and brain. *Proc. Natl. Acad. Sci. USA* **85**, 3175.

372. Aruoma, OI *et al.* (1989) Carnosine, homocarnosine and anserine: could they act as antioxidants *in vivo*? *Biochem. J.* **264**, 863.

373. Decker, EA *et al.* (2000) A re-evaluation of the antioxidant activity of purified carnosine. *Biochem. (Mosc.)* **65**, 766.

374. Winkler, P *et al.* (1984) Selective promotion of Fe^{2+} ion-dependent lipid peroxidation in Ehrlich ascites tumor cells by histidine as compared with other amino acids. *Biochim. Biophys. Acta.* **796**, 226.

375. Cantoni, O *et al.* (1994) The L-histidine mediated enhancement of H$_2$O$_2$-induced cytotoxicity is a general response in cultured mammalian cell lines and is always associated with the formation of DNA double strand breaks. *FEBS Lett.* **353**, 75.

376. Hipkiss, AR and Chana, H (1998) Carnosine protects proteins against methylglyoxal-mediated modifications. *Biochem. Biophys. Res. Commun.* **248**, 28.

377. Teufel, M *et al.* (2003) Sequence identification and characterization of human carnosinase and a closely-related non-specific dipeptidase. *J. Biol. Chem.* **278**, 6521.

378. Janssen, B *et al.* (2005) Carnosine as a protective factor in diabetic nephropathy. *Diabetes* **54**, 2320.

379. Benaroudj, N *et al.* (2001) Trehalose accumulation during cellular stress protects cells and cellular proteins from damage by oxygen radicals. *J. Biol. Chem.* **276**, 24261.

380. Różanowska, M *et al.* (1999) Free radical scavenging properties of melanin. Interaction of eu- and pheo-melanin models with reducing and oxidizing radicals. *Free Rad. Biol. Med.* **26**, 518.

381. Takeuchi, S *et al.* (2004) Melanin acts as a potent UVB photosensitizer to cause an atypical mode of cell death in murine skin. *Proc. Natl. Acad. Sci. USA* **101**, 15076.

382. Wang, Y and Casadevall, A (1994) Susceptibility of melanized and non-melanized *Cryptococcus neoformans* to nitrogen- and oxygen-derived oxidants. *Infect. Immun.* **62**, 3004.

383. Dunlap, WC *et al.* (1999) Sunscreens, oxidative stress and antioxidant functions in marine organisms and the Great Barrier Reef. *Redox Rep.* **4**, 301.

384. Ide, T *et al.* (2002) Greater oxidative stress in healthy young men compared with premenopausal women. *Arterio. Thromb. Vasc. Biol.* **22**, 438.

385. Nakano, M *et al.* (2003) Oxidative DNA damage (8OHdG) and body Fe status: a study of 2507 healthy people. *Free Rad. Biol. Med.* **35**, 826.

386. Bayir, H *et al.* (2004) Marked gender effect on lipid peroxidation after severe traumatic brain injury in adult patients. *J. Neurotrauma* **21**, 1.

387. Liehr, JG (1996) Antioxidant and pro-oxidant properties of estrogens. *J. Lab. Clin. Med.* **128**, 344.

388. Wiseman, H and Halliwell, B (1993) Carcinogenic antioxidants: diethylstilboestrol, hexoestrol and 17α-ethynyloestradiol. *FEBS Lett.* **322**, 159.

389. Vina, J *et al.* (2006) Role of ROS and (phyto)oestrogens in the modulation of adaptive response to stress. *Free Radic. Res.* **40**, 111.

390. Lean, JM *et al.* (2005) H$_2$O$_2$ is essential for estrogen-deficiency bone loss and osteoclast formation. *Endocrinol.* **146**, 728.

391. Ke, RW *et al.* (2003) Effect of short-term hormone therapy on oxidative stress and endothelial function in African American and Caucasian postmenopausal women. *Fertil. Steril.* **79**, 1118.

392. Padayatty, SJ *et al.* (2003) Vitamin C as an antioxidant: evaluation of its role in disease prevention. *J. Am. Coll. Nutr.* **22**, 18.

393. Nishikimi, M *et al.* (2003) Recent advances in biochemistry of L-ascorbic acid biosynthesis. *Recent Res. Devel. Biophys. Biochem.* **3**, 531.

394. Braun, L *et al.* (1999) Induction and peroxisomal appearance of gulonolactone oxidase upon clofibrate treatment in mouse liver. *FEBS Lett.* **458**, 359.

395. Halliwell, B (2001) Vitamin C and genomic stability. *Mutat. Res.* **475**, 29.

396. McCall, MR and Frei, B (1999) Can antioxidant vitamins materially reduce oxidative damage in humans? *Free Rad. Biol. Med.* **26**, 1034.

397. Duarte, TL and Lunec, J (2005) When is an antioxidant not an antioxidant? A review of novel actions and reactions of vitamin C. *Free Radic. Res.* **39**, 671.

398. Wilson, JY (2005) Regulation of vitamin C transport. *Ann. Rev. Nutr.* **25**, 105.

399. Sagun, K *et al.* (2005) Vitamin C enters mitochondria via facilitative glucose transporter (glut1) and confers mitochondrial protection against oxidative injury. *FASEB J.* **19**, 1657.

400. Clement, MV *et al.* (2001) The in vitro cytotoxicity of ascorbate depends on the culture medium used to perform the assay and involves H$_2$O$_2$. *Antiox. Redox Signal.* **3**, 157.

401. Long, CL *et al.* (2003) Ascorbic acid dynamics in the seriously ill and injured. *J. Surg. Res.* **109**, 144.

402. Chien, CT *et al.* (2004) Ascorbate supplement reduces oxidative stress in dyslipidemic patients undergoing apheresis. *Arterio. Thromb. Vasc. Biol.* **24**, 1111.

403. Kojo, S (2004) Vitamin C: basic metabolism and its function as an index of oxidative stress. *Curr. Med. Chem.* **11**, 1041.

404. Lenton, KJ *et al.* (2003) Vitamin C augments lymphocyte GSH in subjects with ascorbate deficiency. *Am. J. Clin. Nutr.* **77**, 189.

405. Kadiiska, MB *et al.* (1995) Fe supplementation generates OH$^•$ *in vivo*. *J. Clin. Invest.* **96**, **1653.**

406. Maskos, Z and Koppenol, WH (1991) Oxyradicals and multivitamin tablets. *Free Rad. Biol. Med.* **11**, 609.

407. Porter, WL (1995) Paradoxical behaviour of antioxidants in food and biological systems. *Tox. Ind. Health* **9**, 93.

408. Jansson, PJ *et al.* (2005) Fe prevents ascorbic acid (vitamin C) induced H_2O_2 accumulation in Cu contaminated drinking H_2O. *Free Radic. Res.* **39**, 1233.

409. Barton, JC MD *et al.* (1998) Management of hemochromatosis. *Ann. Intern. Med.* **129** (Suppl. 11S), 932.

410. Gastaldello, K *et al.* (1995) Resistance to erythropoietin in Fe-overloaded haemodialysis patients can be overcome by ascorbic acid administration. *Nephrol. Dial. Transplant.* **10** (Suppl. 6), 44.

411. Cook, JD and Reddy, MB (2001) Effect of ascorbic acid intake on nonheme-iron absorption from a complete diet. *Am. J. Clin. Nutr.* **73**, 93.

412. Cheng, R *et al.* (2002) Rate of formation of AGEs during ascorbate glycation and during aging in human lens tissue. *Biochim. Biophys. Acta* **1587**, 65.

413. Lee, SH *et al.* (2001) Vitamin C-induced decomposition of LOOH to endogenous genotoxins. *Science* **292**, 2083.

414. Sowell, J *et al.* (2004) Vitamin C conjugates of genotoxic lipid peroxidation products: structural charaterization and detection in human plasma. *Proc. Natl. Acad. Sci. USA* **101**, 17964.

415. Massey, LK *et al.* (2005) Ascorbate increases human oxaluria and kidney stone risk. *J. Nutr.* **135**, 1673.

416. Levine, M *et al.* (1996) Vitamin C pharmacokinetics in healthy volunteers: evidence for a recommended dietary allowance. *Proc. Natl. Acad. Sci. USA* **93**, 3704.

417. Hemilä, H *et al.* (2002) Vitamin C, vitamin E and beta-carotene in relation to common cold incidence in male smokers. *Epidemiol.* **13**, 32.

418. Zingg, JM and Azzi, A (2004) Non-antioxidant activities of vitamin E. *Curr. Med. Chem.* **11**, 1113.

419. Kaikkonen, J *et al.* (2001) Supplementation with vitamin E but not with vitamin C lowers lipid peroxidation *in vivo* in mildly hypercholesterolemic men. *Free Radic. Res.* **35**, 967.

420. Meagher, EA *et al.* (2001) Effects of vitamin E on lipid peroxidation in healthy persons. *JAMA* **285**, 1178.

421. Dierenfeld, ES (1989) Vitamin E deficiency in zoo reptiles, birds and ungulates. *J. Zoo Wildlife Med.* **20**, 3.

422. Muller, DPR and Goss-Sampson, MA (1990) Neurochemical, neurophysiological and neuropathological studies in vitamin E deficiency. *Crit. Rev. Neurobiol.* **5**, 239.

423. Maguire, LS *et al.* (2004) Fatty acid profile, tocopherol, squalene and phytosterol content of walnuts, almonds, peanuts, hazelnuts and the macadamia nut. *Int. J. Food Sci. Nutr.* **55**, 171.

424. Sundram, K *et al.* (2003) Palm fruit chemistry and nutrition. *Asia Pac. J. Clin. Nutr.* **12**, 355.

425. Mukai, K *et al.* (1993) Kinetic study of reactions between tocopheroxyl radical and fatty acids. *Lipids* **28**, 753.

426. Yoshida, Y *et al.* (2003) Comparative study on the action of tocopherols and tocotrienols as antioxidants: chemical and physical effects. *Chem. Phys. Lipids* **123**, 63.

427. Monroe, EB *et al.* (2005) Vitamin imaging and localization in the neuronal membrane. *J. Am. Chem. Soc.* **127**, 12152.

428. Lass, A and Sohal, RS (2000) Effect of coenzyme Q_{10} and α-tocopherol content of mitochondria on the production of $O_2^{•-}$. *FASEB J.* **14**, 87.

429. Yamamoto, Y *et al.* (2001) An unusual vitamin E constituent (α-tocomonoenol) provides enhanced antioxidant protection in marine organisms adapted to cold-water environments. *Proc. Natl. Acad. Sci. USA* **98**, 13144.

430. Burton, GW *et al.* (1990) Biokinetics of dietary *RRR*-α-tocopherol in the male guinea-pig at three dietary levels of vitamin C and two levels of vitamin E. *Lipids* **25**, 199.

431. Burk, RF *et al.* (2006) A combined deficiency of vitamins E and C causes severe CNS damage in guinea pigs. *J. Nutr.* **136**, 1576.

432. Sealey, WM and Gatlin III, DM. (2002) Dietary vitamin C and vitamin E interact to influence growth and tissue composition of juvenile hybrid striped bass (*Morone chrysops* ♀ *M.saxatilis* ♂) but have limited effects on immune responses. *J. Nutr.* **132**, 748.

433. Steger, PJK and Mühlebach, SF (1998) Lipid peroxidation of IV lipid emulsions in TPN bags: the influence of tocopherols. *Nutrition* **14**, 179.

434. Weinberg, RB *et al.* (2001) Pro-oxidant effect of vitamin E in cigarette smokers consuming a high

polyunsaturated fat diet. *Arterio. Thromb. Vasc. Biol.* **21**, 1029.

435. Nolan, B *et al.* (2005) High vitamin E and Se elevate, whereas DPPD plus caffeine lowers liver fat in alcohol-fed rats. *Nutr. Res.* **25**, 701.

436. Booth, SL *et al.* (2004) Effect of vitamin E supplementation on vitamin K status in adults with normal coagulation status. *Am. J. Clin. Nutr.* **80**, 143.

437. Stahl, W *et al.* (2002) Bioavailability and metabolism. *Mol. Aspects. Med.* **23**, 39.

438. Roxborough, HE *et al.* (2000) Inter- and intra-individual variation in plasma and red blood cell vitamin E after supplementation. *Free Radic. Res.* **33**, 437.

439. Roodenburg, AJC *et al.* (2000) Amount of fat in the diet affects bioavailability of lutein esters but not of α-carotene, β-carotene, and vitamin E in humans. *Am. J. Clin. Nutr.* **71**, 1187.

440. Traber, MG *et al.* (2005) α-Tocopherol modulates Cyp3a expression, increases γ-CEHC production, and limits tissue γ-tocopherol accumulation in mice fed high γ-tocopherol diets. *Free Rad. Biol. Med.* **38**, 773.

441. Wu, JHY *et al.* (2005) Nitration of γ-tocopherol prevents its oxidative metabolism by HepG2 cells. *Free Rad. Biol. Med.* **39**, 483.

442. Halliwell, B *et al.* (2005) Health promotion by flavonoids, tocopherols, tocotrienols and other phenols. Direct or indirect effects? Antioxidant or not? *Am. J. Clin. Nutr.* **81** (Suppl.), 268S.

443. Hensley, K *et al.* (2004) New perspectives on vitamin E: γ-tocopherol and CEHC metabolites in biology and medicine. *Free Rad. Biol. Med.* **36**, 1.

444. Schaefer, DM *et al.* (1995) Supranutritional administration of vitamins E and C improves oxidative stability of beef. *J. Nutr.* **125**, 1792S.

445. Navarro, F *et al.* (1998) Vitamin E and Se deficiency induces expression of the ubiquinone-dependent antioxidant system at the plasma membrane. *FASEB J.* **12**, 1665.

446. Kelley, EE *et al.* (1995) Relative α-tocopherol deficiency in cultured cells: free radical-mediated lipid peroxidation, lipid oxidizability, and cellular PUFA content. *Arch. Biochem. Biophys.* **319**, 102.

447. Singh, U *et al.* (2005) Vitamin E, oxidative stress, and inflammation. *Ann. Rev. Nutr.* **25**, 151.

448. Shiau, CW *et al.* (2006) α-Tocopheryl succinate induces apoptosis in prostate cancer cells through inhibition of Bcl-xL/Bcl-2 function. *J. Biol. Chem.* **281**, 11819.

449. Jiang, Q *et al.* (2004) γ-Tocopherol or combinations of vitamin E forms induce cell death in human prostate cancer cells by interrupting sphingolipid synthesis. *Proc. Natl. Acad. Sci. USA* **101**, 17825.

450. O'Byrne. D *et al.* (2000) Studies of LDL oxidation following α-, γ- or d-tocotrienyl acetate supplementation of hypercholesterolemic humans. *Free Rad. Biol. Med.* **29**, 834.

451. Krinsky, NI (1993) Actions of carotenoids in biological systems. *Ann. Rev. Nutr.* **13**, 561.

452. Britton, G *et al.* (eds) (2004) *Carotenoids Handbook.* Birkhauser Verlag, Basle, Switzerland.

453. Mortensen, A *et al.* (2001) The interaction of dietary carotenoids with radical species. *Arch. Biochem. Biophys.* **385**, 13.

454. Tebbe, B (2001) Relevance of oral supplementation with antioxidants for prevention and treatment of skin disorders. *Skin Pharmacol. Appl. Skin Physiol.* **14**, 296.

455. Alaluf, S *et al.* (2002) Dietary carotenoids contribute to normal human skin color and UV photosensitivity. *J. Nutr.* **132**, 399.

456. Hatta, A and Frei, B (1995) Oxidative modification and antioxidant protection of human LDL at high and low O_2 partial pressures. *J. Lipid Res.* **36**, 2383.

457. Różanowska, M *et al.* (2005) Pulse radiolysis study of the interaction of retinoids with peroxyl radicals. *Free Rad. Biol. Med.* **39**, 1399.

458. Dal-Pizzol, F *et al.* (2001) Mitogenic signaling mediated by oxidants in retinol treated Sertoli cells. *Free Radic. Res.* **35**, 749.

459. Aust, O *et al.* (2003) Lycopene oxidation product enhances gap junctional communication. *Food Chem. Toxicol.* **41**, 1399.

460. Bertram, JS (2004) Induction of connexin 43 by carotenoids: functional consequences. *Arch. Biochem. Biophys.* **430**, 120.

461. Yeh, SL and Hu, ML (2001) Induction of oxidative DNA damage in human foreskin fibroblast Hs68 cells by oxidized β-carotene and lycopene. *Free Radic. Res.* **35**, 203.

462. Hurst, JS *et al.* (2005) Toxicity of oxidized β-carotene to cultured human cells. *Exp. Eye Res.* **81**, 239.

463. Wertz, K *et al.* (2004) Lycopene: modes of action to promote prostate health. *Arch. Biochem. Biophys.* **430**, 127.

464. Rice-Evans, C *et al.* (1996) Structure-antioxidant activity relationships of flavonoids and phenolic acids. *Free Rad. Biol. Med.* **20**, 933.

465. Manach, C and Donovan, JL (2004) Pharmacokinetics and metabolism of dietary flavonoids in humans. *Free Radic. Res.* **38**, 771.

466. Taubert, D *et al.* (2003) Reaction rate constants of $O_2^{\bullet-}$ scavenging by plant antioxidants. *Free Rad. Biol. Med.* **35**, 1599.

467. Walle, T *et al.* (2001) CO_2 is the major metabolite of quercetin in humans. *J. Nutr.* **131**, 2648.

468. Song, J *et al.*(2002) Flavonoid inhibition of Na^+-dependent vitamin C transporter 1 (SVCT1) and glucose transporter isoform 2 (GLUT2), intestinal transporters for vitamin C and glucose. *J. Biol. Chem.* **277**, 15252.

469. Keli, SO *et al.* (1996) Dietary flavonoids, antioxidant vitamins and incidence of stroke. The Zutphen study. *Arch. Int. Med.* **154**, 637.

470. Manach, C *et al.* (2004) Polyphenols: food sources and bioavailability. *Am. J. Clin. Nutr.* **79**, 727.

471. Hodgson, JM and Puddey, IB (2005) Dietary flavonoids and cardiovascular disease: does the emperor have any clothes? *J. Hypertens.* **23**, 1461.

472. Landry, LG *et al.* (1995) *Arabidopsis* mutants lacking phenolic sunscreens exhibit enhanced UV-B injury and oxidative damage. *Plant Physiol.* **109**, 1159.

473. Grace, SC and Logan, BA (2000) Energy dissipation and radical scavenging by the plant phenylpropanoid pathway. *Phil. Trans. R. Soc. Lond.* **355**, 1499.

474. Frankel, EN *et al.* (1995) Principal phenolic phytochemicals in selected California wines and their antioxidant activity in inhibiting oxidation of human LDL. *J. Agric. Food Chem.* **43**, 890.

475. Lu, YP *et al.* (2001) Inhibitory effects of orally administered green tea, black tea, and caffeine on skin carcinogenesis in mice previously treated with UVB light (high-risk mice): relationship to decreased tissue fat. *Cancer Res.* **61**, 5002.

476. McAnulty, SR *et al.* (2005) Effect of daily fruit ingestion on ACE activity, blood pressure and oxidative stress in chronic smokers. *Free Radic. Res.* **39**, 1241.

477. Mukai, K *et al.* (2005) Structure–activity relationship of the tocopherol-regeneration reaction by catechins. *Free Rad. Biol. Med.* **38**, 1243.

478. Smith, DM *et al.* (2004) Docking studies and model development of tea polyphenol proteasome inhibitors: applications to rational drug design. *Proteins* **54**, 58.

479. Middleton E. Jr *et al.* (2000) The effects of plant flavonoids on mammalian cells: implications for inflammation, heart disease, and cancer. *Pharmacol. Rev.* **52**, 673.

480. August, DA *et al.* (1999) Ingestion of green tea rapidly decreases prostaglandin E_2 levels in rectal mucosa in humans. *Cancer Epidemiol. Biomark. Prev.* **8**, 709.

481. Wee, LM *et al.* (2003) Factors affecting the ascorbate- and phenolic-dependent generation of H_2O_2 in DMEM. *Free Radic. Res.* **37**, 1123.

482. Long, LH and Halliwell, B (2000) Coffee drinking increases levels of urinary H_2O_2 detected in healthy human volunteers. *Free Radic. Res.* **32**, 463.

483. Fang, J *et al.* (2005) Thioredoxin reductase is irreversibly modified by curcumin. *J. Biol. Chem.* **280**, 25284.

484. Okuda, T *et al.* (1993) Antioxidant phenolics in oriental medicine. In: *Active Oxygens, Lipid Peroxides and Antioxidants* (ed. Yagi, K). Japan Sci. Soc. Press, Tokyo, p.333.

485. Vaja, J *et al.* (1997) Antioxidant constituents from licorice roots: isolation, structure elucidation and antioxidative capacity towards LDL oxidation. *Free Rad. Biol. Med.* **23**, 302.

486. Tang, SY *et al.* (2004) Mechanism of cell death induced by an antioxidant extract of *Cratoxylum cochinchinense* (YCT) in Jurkat T cells: the role of ROS and Ca^{2+}. *Free Rad. Biol. Med.* **36**, 1588.

487. Verbeek, R *et al.* (2005) Oral flavonoids delay recovery from experimental autoimmune encephalomyelitis in mice. *Biochem. Pharmacol.* **70**, 220.

488. Altman, RD and Marcussen, KC (2001) Effects of a ginger extract on knee pain in patients with osteoarthritis. *Arthritis Rheum.* **44**, 2531.

489. Lim, GP *et al.* (2001) The curry spice curcumin reduces oxidative damage and amyloid pathology in an Alzheimer transgenic mouse. *J. Neurosci.* **21**, 8370.

Chapter 4

1. Halliwell, B and Whiteman, M (2004) Measuring RS and oxidative damage *in vivo* and in cell culture: how should you do it and what do the results mean? *Br. J. Pharmacol.* **142**, 231.

2. Sies, H (1991) *Oxidative Stress II. Oxidants and Antioxidants*. Acadamic Press, London.

3. Fuchs, GJ (2005) Antioxidants for children with kwashiorkor. *Br. Med. J.* **330**, 1095.

4. Pani, G *et al.* (2000) A redox signaling mechanism for density-dependent inhibition of cell growth. *J. Biol. Chem.* **275**, 38891.

5. Poli, G and Parola, M (1997) Oxidative damage and fibrogenesis. *Free Rad. Biol. Med.* **22**, 287.

6. Brown, MR *et al.* (1999) Overexpression of human catalase inhibits proliferation and promotes apoptosis in vascular smooth muscle cells. *Circ. Res.* **85**, 524.

7. Chen, X *et al.* (2004) Catalase transgenic mice: characterization and sensitivity to oxidative stress. *Arch. Biochem. Biophys.* **422**, 197.

8. Sun, JZ *et al.* (1996) Evidence for an essential role of ROS in the genesis of late preconditioning against myocardial stunning in conscious pigs. *J. Clin. Invest.* **97**, 562.

9. Gille, JJP and Joenje, H (1989) Chromosomal instability and progressive loss of chromosomes in

HeLa cells during adaptation to hyperoxic growth conditions. *Mutat. Res.* **219**, 225.

10. Li, JC *et al.* (2004) O_2 tolerance and coupling of mitochondrial electron transport. *J. Biol. Chem.* **279**, 46580.

11. Nicotera, P and Orrenius, S (1994) Molecular mechanisms of toxic cell death; an overview. *Meth. Toxicol.* 1B, 23 [and other articles in this volume].

12. Barouki, R and Morel, Y (2001) Repression of CYP1A1 gene expression by oxidative stress: mechanisms and biological implications. *Biochem. Pharmacol.* **61**, 511.

13. Mikalsen, SO and Sauner, T (1994) Increased gap junctional intracellular communication in Syrian hamster embryo cells treated with oxidative agents. *Carcinogenesis* **15**, 381.

14. Chen, QM *et al.* (1998) Molecular analysis of H_2O_2-induced senescent-like growth arrest in normal human fibroblasts: p53 and Rb control G_1 arrest but not cell replication. *Biochem. J.* **332**, 43.

15. Jagtap, P and Szabó, C (2005) PARP and the therapeutic effects of its inhibitors. *Nature Rev. Drug Disc.* 4, 421.

16. Masutani, M *et al.* (2000) The response of Parp knockout mice against DNA damaging agents. *Mutat. Res.* **462**, 159.

17. Matalon, S *et al.* (2003) Regulation of ion channel structure and function by reactive O_2-N_2 species. *Am. J. Physiol.* **285**, L1184.

18. Andreoli, SP *et al.* (1993) Oxidant-induced alterations in glucose and phosphate transport in LLC-PK1 cells: mechanisms of injury. *Am. J. Physiol.* **265**, F377.

19. Schliess, F and Häussinger, D (2002) The cellular hydration state: a critical determinant for cell death and survival. *Biol. Chem.* **383**, 577.

20. Gutterman, DD *et al.* (2005) Redox modulation of vascular tone. *Arterio. Thromb. Vasc. Biol.* **25**, 671.

21. Varela, D *et al.* (2004) NAD(P)H-oxidase-derived H_2O_2 signals Cl^- channel activation in cell volume regulation and cell proliferation. *J. Biol. Chem.* **279**, 13301.

22. McConkey, DJ and Orrenius, S (1997) The role of Ca in the regulation of apoptosis. *Biochem. Biophys. Res. Comm.* **239**, 357.

23. Squier, TC and Bigelow, DJ (2000) Protein oxidation and age-dependent alterations in Ca^{2+} homeostasis. *Front. Biosci.* **5**, 1.

24. Miller, BA (2006). The role of TRP channels in oxidative stress-induced cell death. *J. Membrane Biol.* **209**, 31.

25. Sandstrom, BE *et al.* (1994) New roles for quin 2: powerful transition-metal ion chelator that inhibits

Cu-, but potentiates Fe-driven, Fenton-type reactions. *Free Rad. Biol. Med.* **16**, 177.

26. Meinicke, AR *et al.* (1996) The Ca^{2+} sensor Ru red can act as a Fenton-type reagent. *Arch. Biochem. Biophys.* **328**, 239.

27. Mumby, S *et al.* (1998) Reactive Fe species in biological fluids activate the Fe–S cluster of aconitase. *Biochim. Biophys. Acta* **1380**, 102.

28. Gutteridge, JMC and Halliwell, B (1987) Radical-promoting loosely-bound Fe in biological fluids and the bleomycin assay. *Life Chem. Rep.* **4**, 113.

29. Esposito, BP *et al.* (2003) Labile plasma Fe in Fe overload: redox activity and susceptibility to chelation. *Blood* **102**, 2670.

30. Nilsson, UA *et al.* (2002) A simple and rapid method for the determination of 'free' iron in biological fluids. *Free Radic. Res.* **36**, 677.

31. Jacobs, EMG *et al.* (2005) Results of an international round robin for the quantification of serum NTBI: need for defining standardization and a clinically relevant isoform. *Anal. Biochem.* **341**, 241.

32. Healing, G *et al.* (1990) Intracellular Fe redistribution. An important determinant of reperfusion damage to rabbit kidneys. *Biochem. Pharmacol.* **39**, 1239.

33. Gutteridge, JM (1984) Cu-phenanthroline-induced site-specific O_2-radical damage to DNA. Detection of loosely bound trace Cu in biological fluids. *Biochem. J.* **218**, 983.

34. Scaffidi, P *et al.* (2002) Release of chromatin protein HMGB1 by necrotic cells triggers inflammation. *Nature* **418**, 191.

35. Reznikov, K *et al.* (2000) Clustering of apoptotic cells via bystander killing by peroxides. *FASEB J.* **14**, 1754.

36. Bratton, DL and Henson, PM (2005) Autoimmunity and apoptosis: refusing to go quietly. *Nature Med.* **11**, 26.

37. Züllig, S and Hengartner, MO (2004) Tickling macrophages, a serious business. *Science* **304**, 1123.

38. Chandra, J *et al.* (2000) Triggering and modulation of apoptosis by oxidative stress. *Free Rad. Biol. Med.* **29**, 323.

39. Villamor, N *et al.* (2004) Cytotoxic effects on B lymphocytes mediated by ROS. *Curr. Pharm. Design* **10**, 841.

40. Volbracht, C *et al.* (2005) The critical role of calpain versus caspase activation in excitotoxic injury induced by NO$^\bullet$ *J. Neurochem.* **93**, 1280.

41. Blumenthal, SB *et al.* (2005) Metalloporphyrins inactivate caspase-3 and -8. *FASEB J.* **19**, 1272.

42. Ricci, JE *et al.* (2004) Disruption of mitochondrial function during apoptosis is mediated by caspase cleavage of the p75 subunit of complex I of the electron transport chain. *Cell* **117**, 773.

43. Urbano, A *et al.* (2005) AIF suppresses chemical stress-induced apoptosis and maintains the transformed state of tumour cells. *EMBO J.* **24,**2815.

44. Orrenius, S (2004) Mitochondrial regulation of apoptotic cell death. *Toxicol. Lett.* **149**, 19.

45. Kagan, VE *et al.* (2005) Cytochrome c acts as a cardiolipin oxygenase required for release of proapoptotic factors. *Nature Chem. Biol.* **1**, 223.

46. Tyurina, YY *et al.* (2004) Lipid antioxidant, etoposide, inhibits phosphatidylserine externalization and macrophage clearance of apoptotic cells by preventing phosphatidylserine oxidation. *J. Biol. Chem.* **279**, 6056.

47. Singh, I *et al.* (1998) Cytokine-mediated induction of ceramide production is redox-sensitive. *J. Biol. Chem.* **273**, 20354.

48. Jacobson, MD (1996) ROS and programmed cell death. *TIBS* **21**, 83.

49. Akram, S *et al.* (2006) ROS-mediated regulation of Na^+–H^+ exchanger 1 gene expression connects intracellular redox status with cells' sensitivity to death triggers. *Cell Death Differ.* **13**, 628.

50. Vaquero, EC *et al.*(2004) ROS produced by NAD(P)H oxidase inhibit apoptosis in pancreatic cancer cells. *J. Biol. Chem.* **279**, 34643.

51. Teoh, M.LT *et al.* (2005) Tumorigenic poxviruses up-regulate intracellular $O_2^{\bullet-}$ to inhibit apoptosis and promote cell proliferation. *J. Virol.* **79**, 5799.

52. Hara, MR *et al.* (2005) *S*-nitrosylated GAPDH initiates cell death by nuclear translocation following Siah1 binding. *Nature Cell Biol.* **7**, 665.

53. Lillig, CH *et al.* (2005) Characterization of human glutaredoxin 2 as Fe-S protein: a possible role as redox sensor. *Proc. Natl. Acad. Sci. USA* **102**, 8168.

54. Pomposiello, PJ and Demple, B (2002) Global adjustment of microbial physiology during free radical stress. *Adv. Microb. Physiol.* **46**, 319.

54A. Lee, JW and Helmann, JD (2006). The PerR transcription factor senses H_2O_2 by metal-catalyzed histidine oxidation. *Nature* **440**, 363.

55. Hon, T *et al.* (2003) A mechanism of O_2 sensing in yeast. *J. Biol. Chem.* **278**, 50771.

56. Temple, MD *et al.* (2005) Complex cellular responses to ROS. *Trends Cell Biol.* **15**, 319.

57. Jang, HH *et al.* (2004) Two enzymes in one: two yeast peroxiredoxins display oxidative stress-dependent switching from a peroxidase to a molecular chaperone function. *Cell* **117**, 625.

58. Martindale, JL and Holbrook, NJ (2002) Cellular response to oxidative stress: signaling for suicide and survival. *J. Cell. Physiol.* **192**, 1.

59. Lee, K and Esselman, WJ (2002) Inhibition of PTPs by H_2O_2 regulates the activation of distinct MAPK pathways. *Free Rad. Biol. Med.* **33**, 1121.

60. Klotz, LO *et al.* (2002) $ONOO^-$ signaling: receptor tyrosine kinases and activation of stress-responsive pathways. *Free Rad. Biol. Med.* **33**, 737.

61. Sigaud, S *et al.* (2005) H_2O_2-induced proliferation of primary alveolar epithelial cells is mediated by MAP kinases. *Antiox. Redox Signal.* **7**, 6.

62. Houle, F *et al.* (2003) ERK mediates phosphorylation of tropomyosin-1 to promote cytoskeleton remodeling in response to oxidative stress: impact on membrane blebbing. *Mol. Biol. Cell* **14**, 1418.

63. Chu, CT *et al.* (2004) Oxidative neuronal injury. The dark side of ERK1/2. *Eur. J. Biochem.* **271**, 2060.

64. Essers, MAG *et al.* (2004) FOXO transcription factor activation by oxidative stress mediated by the small GTPase Ral and JNK. *EMBO J.* **23**, 4802.

65. Heo, J and Campbell, SL (2005) $O_2^{\bullet-}$ modulates the activity of Ras and Ras-related GTPases by a radical-based mechanism similar to that of $NO^{\bullet}$. *J. Biol. Chem.* **280**, 12438.

66. Kim, JH *et al.* (2003) H_2O_2 induces association between G3PDH and phospholipase D2 to facilitate phospholipase D2 activation in PC12 cells. *J. Neurochem.* **85**, 1228.

67. Gopalakrishna, R and Jaken, S (2000) PKC signaling and oxidative stress. *Free Rad. Biol. Med.* **28**, 1349.

68. Cao, C *et al.* (2003) GPx1 is regulated by the c-Abl and Arg tyrosine kinases. *J. Biol. Chem.* **278**, 39609.

69. Nathan, C (2003) Specificity of a third kind: ROS and N_2 intermediates in cell signaling. *J. Clin. Invest.* **111**, 769.

70. Rhee, SG *et al.* (2005) Intracellular messenger function of H_2O_2 and its regulation by peroxiredoxins. *Curr. Opin. Cell Biol.* **17**, 183.

71. Cho, SH *et al.* (2004) Redox regulation of PTEN and protein tyrosine phosphatases in H_2O_2-mediated cell signaling. *FEBS Lett.* **560**, 7.

72. Namgaladze, D *et al.* (2005) $O_2^{\bullet-}$ targets calcineurin signaling in vascular endothelium. *Biochem. Biophys. Res. Commun.* **334**, 1061.

73. Sumbayev, VV and Yasinska, IM (2005) Regulation of MAP kinase-dependent apoptotic pathway: implication of ROS and RNS. *Arch. Biochem. Biophys.* **436**, 406.

74. DeYulia, GJ *et al.* (2005) H_2O_2 generated extracellularly by receptor–ligand interaction facilitates cell signaling. *Proc. Natl. Acad. Sci. USA* **102**, 5044.

75. Nemoto, S *et al.* (2000) Role for mitochondrial oxidants as regulators of cellular metabolism. *Mol. Cell. Biol.* **20**, 7311.

76. Suzuki, H *et al.* (1998) Increase in intracellular H_2O_2 and upregulation of a nuclear respiratory gene evoked

by impairment of mitochondrial electron transfer in human cells. *Biochem. Biophys. Res. Commun.* **249**, 542.

77. Hoffmann, S *et al.* (2004) ROS derived from the mitochondrial respiratory chain are not responsible for the basal levels of oxidative base modifications observed in nuclear DNA of mammalian cells. *Free Rad. Biol. Med.* **36**, 765.

78. Scarpulla, RC (2002) Nuclear activators and coactivators in mammalian mitochondrial biogenesis. *Biochim. Biophys. Acta* 1576, 1.

79. Lawrence, T *et al.* (2005) IKKα limits macrophage NF-κB activation and contributes to the resolution of inflammation. *Nature* **434**, 1138.

80. Carlsen, H *et al.* (2002) *In vivo* imaging of NF-κB activity. *J. Immunol.* **168**, 1441.

81. Pahl, HL and Baeuerle, PA (1994) O_2 and the control of gene expression. *BioEssays* **16**, 497.

82. Natarajan, K *et al.* (1996) Caffeic acid phenethyl ester is a potent and specific inhibitor of activation of NF-κB. *Proc. Natl. Acad. Sci. USA* **93**, 9090.

83. Grilli, M *et al.* (1996) Neuroprotection by aspirin and sodium salicylate through blockade of NF-κB activation. *Science* **274**, 1383.

84. Hayakawa, M *et al.* (2003) Evidence that ROS do not mediate NF-κB activation. *EMBO J.* **22**, 3356.

85. Xiong, S *et al.* (2003) Signaling role of intracellular Fe in NF-κB activation. *J. Biol. Chem.* **278**, 17646.

86. Fries, DM *et al.* (2003) Expression of iNOS and intracellular protein tyrosine nitration in vascular smooth muscle cells. *J. Biol. Chem.* **278**, 22901.

87. Zhang, Y and Chen, F (2004) ROS, troublemakers between NF-κB and c-Jun NH_2-terminal kinase (JNK). *Cancer Res.* **64**, 1902.

88. Shaulian, E and Karin, M (2002) AP-1 as a regulator of cell life and death. *Nature Cell. Biol.* **4**, E131.

89. Itoh, K *et al.* (2004) Molecular mechanism activating Nrf2-Keap1 pathway in regulation of adaptive response to electrophiles. *Free Rad. Biol. Med.* **36**,1208.

90. Choi, S *et al.* (2003) Downregulation of p38 kinase pathway by cAMP response element-binding protein protects HL-60 cells from Fe chelator-induced apoptosis. *Free Rad. Biol. Med.* **35**, 1171.

91. Halliwell, B (2003) Oxidative stress in cell culture: an under-appreciated problem? *FEBS Lett.* **540**, 3.

92. Ishibashi, N *et al.* (1999) Modulation of chemokine expression during ischemia/reperfusion in transgenic mice overproducing human GPx. *J. Immunol.* **163**, 5666.

93. Mirochnitchenko, O *et al.* (2000) Endotoxemia in transgenic mice overexpressing human GPxs. *Circ. Res.* **87**, 289.

94. Marikovsky, M *et al.* (2003) CuZnSOD plays important role in immune response. *J. Immunol.* **170**, 2993.

95. McClung, JP *et al.* (2004) Development of insulin resistance and obesity in mice overexpressing cellular GPx. *Proc. Natl. Acad. Sci. USA.* **101**, 8852.

96. Shimokawa, H and Morikawa, K (2005) H_2O_2 is an endothelium-derived hyperpolarizing factor in animals and humans. *J. Mol. Cell. Cardiol.* **39**, 725.

97. Thiels, E and Klann, E (2002) Hippocampal memory and plasticity in SOD mutant mice. *Physiol. Behav.* **77**, 601.

98. Lauer, N *et al.* (2005) Critical involvement of H_2O_2 in exercise-induced up-regulation of endothelial NO synthase. *Cardiovasc. Res.* **65**, 254.

99. Gomez-Cabrera, MC *et al.* (2005) Decreasing XO-mediated oxidative stress prevents useful cellular adaptations to exercise in rats. *J. Physiol.* **567**, 113.

100. Bloomfield, G and Pears, C (2003) $O_2^{•-}$ signaling required for multicellular development of *Dictyostelium*. *J. Cell. Sci.* **116**, 3387.

101. Sohal, RS *et al.* (1988) Oxidative stress and cellular differentiation. *Ann. N. Y. Acad. Sci.* **551**, 59.

102. Toledo, I *et al.* (1994) Enzyme inactivation related to a hyperoxidant state during conidiation of *N. crassa*. *Microbiol.* **140**, 2391.

103. Luna, MC *et al.* (2000) Photodynamic therapy-mediated oxidative stress as a molecular switch for the temporal expression of genes ligated to the human Hsp. *Cancer Res.* **60**, 1637.

104. Rao, RV *et al.* (2004) Coupling ER stress to the cell death program. *Cell Death Differ.* **11**, 372.

105. Cabiscol, E *et al.* (2002) Mitochondrial Hsp60, resistance to oxidative stress, and the labile Fe pool are closely connected in *S. cerevisiae*. *J. Biol. Chem.* **277**, 44531.

106. Garrido, C *et al.* (2003) HSP27 and HSP70: potentially oncogenic apoptosis inhibitors. *Cell Cycle* **2**, 579.

107. Moon, JC *et al.* (2005) Oxidative stress-dependent structural and functional switching of a human 2-cys peroxiredoxin isotype II that enhances HeLa cell resistance to H_2O_2-induced cell death. *J. Biol. Chem.* **280**, 28775.

108. Mirochnitchenko, O *et al.* (1995) Thermosensitive phenotype of transgenic mice overproducing human GPx. *Proc. Natl. Acad. Sci. USA.* **92**, 8120.

109. Sancho, P *et al.* (2003) Differential effects of catalase on apoptosis induction in human promonocytic cells. Relationships with HSP expression. *Mol. Pharmacol.* **63**, 581.

110. Yerbury, JJ *et al.* (2005) The acute phase protein haptoglobin is a mammalian EC chaperone with an action similar to clusterin. *Biochemistry* **44**, 10914.

111. Haddad, JJ (2002) Pharmaco-redox regulation of cytokine-related pathways: from receptor signaling to pharmacogenomics. *Free Rad. Biol. Med.* **33**, 907.

112. Li, YP *et al.* (1998) Skeletal muscle myocytes undergo protein loss and ROS-mediated NF-κB activation in response to TNFα. *FASEB J.* **12**, 871.

113. Bruce, AJ *et al.* (1996) Altered neuronal and microglial responses to excitotoxic and ischemic brain injury in mice lacking TNF receptors. *Nature Med.* **2**, 788.

114. Hughes, G *et al.* (2005) Mitochondrial ROS regulate the temporal activation of NF-κB to modulate TNF-induced apoptosis: evidence from mitochondria-targeted antioxidants. *Biochem. J.* **389**, 83.

115. Alikhani, M *et al.* (2005) FOXO1 functions as a master switch that regulates gene expression necessary for TNF-induced fibroblast apoptosis. *J. Biol. Chem.* **280**, 12096.

116. Lee, TS and Chau, LY (2002) HO-1 mediates the anti-inflammatory effect of IL-10 in mice. *Nature Med.* **8**, 240.

117. von Sonntag, C (2006) *Free-Radical-Induced DNA Damage and its Repair.* Springer, Basle.

118. Barnes, DE and Lindahl, T (2004) Repair and genetic consequences of endogenous DNA base damage in mammalian cells. *Ann. Rev. Genet.* **38**, 445.

119. Mitchell, D *et al.* (2005) Damage and repair of ancient DNA. *Mutat. Res.* **571**, 265.

120. Evans, MD *et al.* (2004) Oxidative DNA damage and disease: induction, repair and significance. *Mutat. Res.* **567**, 1.

121. Rodriguez, M *et al.* (1995) Mapping of Cu/H_2O_2-induced DNA damage at nucleotide resolution in human genomic DNA by ligation-mediated PCR. *J. Biol. Chem.* **270**, 17633.

122. Altman, SA *et al.* (1995) Formation of DNA-protein cross-links in cultured mammalian cells upon treatment with Fe. *Free Rad. Biol. Med.* **19**, 897.

123. Toyokuni, S *et al.* (1995) Treatment of Wistar rats with a renal carcinogen, FeNTA, causes DNA-protein cross-linking between thymine and tyrosine in their renal chromatin. *Int. J. Cancer* **62**, 309.

124. Halliwell, B (1999) O_2 and N_2 are pro-carcinogens. Damage to DNA by reactive oxygen, chlorine and nitrogen species: measurement, mechanism and the effects of nutrition. *Mutat. Res.* **443**, 37.

125. Hofer, T *et al.* (2005) H_2O_2 causes greater oxidation in cellular RNA than in DNA. *Biol. Chem.* **386**, 333.

126. Gackowski, D *et al.* (2002) The level of 8OHdG is positively correlated with the size of the labile iron pool in human lymphocytes. *J. Biol. Inorg. Chem.* **7**, 548.

127. Zastawny, TH *et al.* (1995) DNA base modifications and membrane damage in cultured mammalian cells treated with Fe. *Free Rad. Biol. Med.* **18**, 1013.

128. Park, S and Imlay, JA (2003) High levels of intracellular cysteine promote oxidative DNA damage by driving the Fenton reaction. *J. Bact.* **185**, 1942.

129. Milligan, JR and Ward, JF (1994) Yield of single-strand breaks due to attack on DNA by scavenger-derived radicals. *Radiat. Res.* **137**, 295.

130. Li, Y and Trush, MA (1994) Reactive O_2-dependent DNA damage resulting from the oxidation of phenolic compounds by a Cu-redox cycle mechanism. *Cancer Res.* (Suppl.) **54**, 1895S.

131. Guan, JQ and Chance, MR (2005) Structural proteomics of macromolecular assemblies using oxidative footprinting and mass spectrometry. *TIBS* **30**, 583.

132. Cantoni, O and Giacomoni, P (1997) The role of DNA damage in the cytotoxic response to H_2O_2/histidine. *Gen. Pharmacol.* **29**, 513.

133. Duarte, V *et al.* (2001) Repair and mutagenic potential of oxaluric acid, a major product of singlet O_2-mediated oxidation of 8-oxodG. *Chem. Res. Toxicol.* **14**, 46.

134. Joffe, A *et al.* (2003) DNA lesions derived from the site selective oxidation of guanine by $CO_3^{\bullet-}$. *Chem. Res. Toxicol.* **16**, 1528.

135. Spencer, JPE *et al.* (2000) Nitrite-induced deamination and OCl$^-$-induced oxidation of DNA in intact human respiratory tract epithelial cells. *Free Rad. Biol. Med.* **28**, 1039.

136. Jiang, Q *et al.* (2003) 5-Chlorouracil, a marker of DNA damage from HOCl during inflammation. *J. Biol. Chem.* **278**, 32834.

137. Shen, Z *et al.* (2001) EPO catalyzes bromination of free nucleosides and double-stranded DNA. *Biochemistry* **40**, 2041.

138. Ito, K *et al.* (2005) Mechanism of site-specific DNA damage induced by O_3. *Mutat. Res.* **585**, 60.

139. Zhao, K *et al.* (2001) DNA damage by NO_2^- and ONOO$^{\bullet-}$: protection by dietary phenols. *Meth. Enzymol.* **335**, 296.

140. Nakano, T *et al.* (2003) DNA-protein cross-link formation mediated by oxanine. *J. Biol. Chem.* **278**, 25264.

141. Niles, JC *et al.* (2004) Spiroiminodihydantoin and guanidinohydantoin are the dominant products of 8-oxoguanosine oxidation at low fluxes of ONOO$^-$: mechanistic studies with ^{18}O. *Chem. Res. Toxicol.* **17**, 1510.

142. Graziewicz, MA *et al.* (2002) The mitochondrial DNA polymerase as a target of oxidative damage. *Nucl. Acids Res.* **30**, 2817.

143. Beckman, KB and Ames, BN (1999) Endogenous oxidative damage of mtDNA. *Mutat. Res.* **424**, 51.

144. Chen, JJ *et al.* (1996) Little or no repair of cyclobutyl pyrimidine dimers is observed in the organellar genomes of the young *Arabidopsis* seedling. *Plant Physiol.* **111**, 19.

145. Neeley, WL and Essigmann, JM (2006) Mechanisms of formation, genotoxicity and mutation of guanine oxidation products. *Chem. Res. Toxicol.* **19**, 491.

146. Hah, SS *et al.* (2005) Hydantoin derivative formation from oxidation of 8-oxodG and incorporation of ^{14}C-labeled 8-oxodG into the DNA of human breast cancer cells. *Bioorg. Med. Chem. Lett.* **15**, 3627.

147. Moraes, EC *et al.* (1990) Mutagenesis by H_2O_2 treatment of mammalian cells: a molecular analysis. *Carcinogenesis* **11**, 283.

148. Newcomb, TG *et al.* (1999) Detection of tandem CC → TT mutations induced by O_2 radicals using mutation-specific PCR. *Mutat. Res.* **427**, 21.

149. Henderson, JP *et al.* (2001) Bromination of deoxycytidine by EPO: a mechanism for mutagenesis by oxidative damage of nucleotide precursors. *Proc. Natl. Acad. Sci. USA* **98**, 1631.

150. Valinluck, V *et al.* (2004) Oxidative damage to methyl-CpG sequences inhibits the binding of the MBD of MeCP2. *Nucl. Acids Res.* **32**, 4100.

151. Nedelcu, AM *et al.* (2005) Sex as a response to oxidative stress: stress genes co-opted for sex. *Proc. R. Soc. Lond. B* **272**, 1935.

152. Bernstein, C (1998) Sex may be a significant factor in efficient repair of endogenous oxidative DNA damage in the germ line. In *DNA and Free Radicals; Technologies, Mechanisms and Applications.* (eds Aruoma, OI and Halliwell, B), OICA Press, p99.

153. Nakabeppu, Y *et al.* (2004) The defense mechanisms in mammalian cells against oxidative damage in nucleic acids and their involvement in the suppression of mutagenesis and cell death. *Free Radic. Res.* **38**, 423.

154. Khanna, KK and Jackson, SP (2001) DNA double-strand breaks: signaling, repair and the cancer connection. *Nature Genet.* **27**, 247.

155. Christmann, M *et al.* (2003) Mechanisms of human DNA repair: an update. *Toxicology* **193**, 3.

156. Kao, YT *et al.* (2005) Direct observation of thymine dimer repair in DNA by photolyase. *Proc. Natl. Acad. Sci. USA* **102**, 16128.

157. Fujikawa, K *et al.* (2002) 8-Chloro-dGTP, a HOCl-modified nucleotide, is hydrolyzed by hMTH1, the human MutT homolog. *FEBS Lett.* **512**,149.

158. Ishibashi, T *et al.* (2003) A novel mechanism of preventing mutations caused by oxidation of guanine nucleotides. *EMBO Rep.* **4**, 479.

159. Kuraoka, I *et al.* (2000) Removal of O_2 free-radical-induced 5′,8-purine cyclodeoxynucleosides from DNA by the NER pathway in human cells. *Proc. Natl. Acad. Sci. U.S.A.* **97**, 3832.

160. Dizdaroglu, M (2005) Base-excision repair of oxidative DNA damage by DNA glycosylases. *Mutat. Res.* **591**, 45.

161. Bohr, VA (2002) Repair of oxidative DNA damage in nuclear and mitochondrial DNA, and some changes with aging in mammalian cells. *Free Rad. Biol. Med.* **32**, 804.

162. Banerjee, A *et al.* (2006) Structure of a DNA glycosylase searching for lesions. *Science* **311**, 1153.

163. Friedman, N *et al.* (2005) Precise temporal modulation in the response of the SOS DNA repair network in individual bacteria. *PLoS Biol.* **3**, 1261.

164. Meira, LB *et al.* (2001) Heterozygosity for the mouse *apex* gene results in phenotypes associated with oxidative stress. *Cancer Res.* **61**, 5552.

165. Buchmeier, NA *et al.* (1995) DNA repair is more important than catalase for *Salmonella* virulence in mice. *J. Clin. Invest.* **95**, 1047.

166. Tuo, JS, *et al.* (2003) Primary fibroblasts of CS patients are defective in cellular repair of 8OHG and 8OHA resulting from oxidative stress. *FASEB J.* **17**, 668.

167. Reichenbach, J *et al.* (2002) Elevated oxidative stress in patients with AT. *Antiox. Redox Signal.* **4**, 465.

168. Browne, SE *et al.* (2004) Treatment with a catalytic antioxidant corrects the neurobehavioral defect in ataxia-telangiectasia mice. *Free Rad. Biol. Med.* **36**, 938.

169. Ito, K *et al.* (2004) Regulation of oxidative stress by ATM is required for self-renewal of haematopoietic stem cells. *Nature* **431**, 997.

170. Hung, RJ *et al.* (2005) Large-scale investigation of base excision repair genetic polymorphisms and lung cancer risk in a multicenter study. *J. Natl. Cancer Inst.* **97**, 567.

171. Monstrey, S *et al.* (2000) Biocompatibility and oxidative stability of radiolucent breast implants. *Plast. Reconstr. Surg.* **105**, 1429.

172. Paradies, G *et al.* (1997) Age-dependent decline in the cytochrome *c* oxidase activity in rat heart mitochondria: role of cardiolipin. *FEBS Lett.* **406**, 136.

173. Koppenol, WH (1990) Oxyradical reactions: from bond-dissociation energies to reduction potentials. *FEBS Lett.* **264**, 165.

174. Barden, AE *et al.* (2004) Fish oil supplementation in pregnancy lowers F_2-IPs in neonates at high risk of atopy. *Free Radic. Res.* **38**, 233.

175. Barber, DJW and Thomas, JK (1978) Reactions of radicals with lecithin bilayers. *Radiat. Res.* **74**, 51.

176. Aikens, J and Dix, JA (1991) Perhydroxyl radical (HOO•) initiated lipid peroxidation. *J. Biol. Chem.* **266**, 15091.

177. Frank, H *et al.*(1989) Mass spectrometric detection of cross-linked fatty acids formed during radical-induced lesion of lipid membranes. *Biochem. J.* **260**, 873.

178. Gardner, HW (1989) O_2 radical chemistry of PUFAs. *Free Rad. Biol. Med.* **7**, 65.

179. Fam, SS and Morrow, JD (2003) The isoprostanes: unique products of arachidonic acid oxidation-a review. *Curr. Med. Chem.* **10**, 1723.

180. Gutteridge, JMC (1982) The role of $O_2^{\bullet-}$ and $OH^\bullet$ in phospholipid peroxidation catalyzed by Fe salts. *FEBS Lett.* **150**, 454.

181. Halliwell, B and Gutteridge, JMC (1990) Role of free radicals and catalytic metal ions in human disease: an overview. *Meth. Enzymol.* **186**, 1.

182. Spiteller, G (1998) Linoleic acid peroxidation-the dominant lipid peroxidation process in LDL-and its relationship to chronic diseases. *Chem. Phys. Lipids* **95**, 105.

183. Tang, L (2000) The mechanism of Fe^{2+}-initiated lipid peroxidation in liposomes: the dual function of Fe^{2+}, the roles of the pre-existing lipid peroxides and the lipid peroxyl radical. *Biochem. J.* **352**, 27.

184. Sevanian, A *et al.* (1990) Microsomal lipid peroxidation: the role of NADPH-cytochrome P450 reductase and cytochrome P450. *Free Rad. Biol. Med.* **8**, 145.

185. Schacter, BA *et al.* (1972) Hemoprotein catabolism during stimulation of microsomal lipid peroxidation. *Biochim. Biophys. Acta* **279**, 221.

186. Girotti, AW and Kriska, T (2004) Role of lipid hydroperoxides in photo-oxidative stress signaling. *Antiox. Redox Signal.* **6**, 301.

187. Hix, S *et al.* (2000) *In vivo* metabolism of tert-butyl hydroperoxide to $CH_3^\bullet$ radicals. EPR spin-trapping and DNA methylation studies. *Chem. Res. Toxicol.* **13**,1056.

188. Coon, MJ *et al.* (1996) Peroxidative reactions of diversozymes. *FASEB J.* **10**, 428.

189. Richter, C (1987) Biophysical consequences of lipid peroxidation in membranes. *Chem. Phys. Lipids* **44**, 175.

190. Nigam, S and Schewe, T (2000) Phospholipase A_2s and lipid peroxidation. *Biochim. Biophys. Acta.* **1488**, 167.

191. Duprat, F *et al.* (1995) Susceptibility of cloned K^+ channels to ROS. *Proc. Natl. Acad. Sci. USA* **92**, 11796.

192. Bindoli, A (1988) Lipid peroxidation in mitochondria. *Free Rad. Biol. Med.* **5**, 247.

193. Saeed, S *et al.* (1999) ESR study on free radical transfer in fish lipid-protein interaction. *J. Sci. Food Agric.* **79**, 1809.

194. Hsieh, CC and Lin, BF (2005) The effects of vitamin E supplementation on autoimmune-prone New Zealand black x New Zealand white F_1 mice fed an oxidized oil diet. *Br. J. Nutr.* **93**, 655.

195. Kanazawa, K and Ashida, H (1998) Dietary hydroperoxides of linoleic acid decompose to aldehydes in stomach before being absorbed into the body. *Biochim. Biophys. Acta.* **1393**, 349.

196. Tsunada, S *et al.* (2003) Chronic exposure to subtoxic levels of peroxidized lipids suppresses mucosal cell turnover in rat small intestine and reversal by GSH. *Dig. Dis. Sci.* **48**, 210.

197. Dever, G *et al.* (2003) Phospholipid chlorohydrins cause ATP depletion and toxicity in human myeloid cells. *FEBS Lett.* **540**, 245.

198. Marathe, GK *et al.* (1999) Inflammatory PAF-like phospholipids in oxidized LDL are fragmented alkyl phosphatidylcholines. *J. Biol. Chem.* **274**, 28395.

199. Mackman, N (2003) How do oxidized phospholipids inhibit LPS signaling? *Arterio. Thromb. Vasc. Biol.* **23**, 1133.

200. Bochkov, VN *et al.* (2002) Protective role of phospholipid oxidation products in endotoxin-induced tissue damage. *Nature* **419**, 77.

201. Roberts, LJ *et al.* (2004) The biochemistry of the IP, neuroprostane, and isofuran pathways of lipid peroxidation. *Chem. Phys. Lipids* **128**, 173.

202. Musiek, ES *et al.* (2005) Cyclopentenone IPs inhibit the inflammatory response in macrophages. *J. Biol. Chem.* **280**, 35562.

203. Poliakov, E *et al.* (2004) Iso[7]LGD$_2$-protein adducts are abundant in vivo and free radical-induced oxidation of an arachidonyl phospholipid generates this D series isolevuglandin *in vitro*. *Chem. Res. Toxicol.* **17**, 613.

204. Wentzel, P and Eriksson, UJ (2002) 8-iso-PGF$_{2\alpha}$ administration generates dysmorphogenesis and increased lipid peroxidation in rat embryos *in vitro*. *Teratology* **66**, 164.

205. Moore, K (2004) IPs and the liver. *Chem. Phys. Lipids* **128**, 125.

206. Bochkov, VN and Leitinger, N (2003) Anti-inflammatory properties of lipid oxidation products. *J. Mol. Med.* **81**, 613.

207. Linseisen, J and Wolfram, G (1998) Absorption of COPs from ordinary foodstuff in humans. *Ann. Nutr. Metab.* **42**, 221.

208. Ryan, E *et al.* (2005) Qualitative and quantitative comparison of the cytotoxic and apoptotic potential of phytosterol oxidation products with their corresponding COPs. *Br. J. Nutr.* **94**, 443.

209. Esterbauer, H *et al.* (1991) Chemistry and biochemistry of 4-HNE, MDA and related aldehydes. *Free Rad. Biol. Med.* **11**, 81.

210. Chang, LW *et al.* (2005) *Trans, Trans*-2,4-Decadienal, a product found in cooking oil fumes, induces cell proliferation and cytokine production due to ROS in human bronchial epithelial cells. *Toxicol. Sci.* **87**, 337.

211. Marnett, LJ (2000) Oxyradicals and DNA damage. *Carcinogenesis* **21**, 361.

212. Niedernhofer, LJ *et al.* (2003) MDA, a product of lipid peroxidation, is mutagenic in human cells. *J. Biol. Chem.* **278**, 31426.

213. Schneider, C *et al.* (2001) Two distinct pathways of formation of 4-HNE. *J. Biol. Chem.* **276**, 20831.

214. Kristal, BS *et al.* (1996) 4-HHE is a potent inducer of the MPT. *J. Biol. Chem.* **271**, 6033.

215. Segall, HJ *et al.* (1985) *Trans*-4-HHE: a reactive metabolite from the macrocyclic pyrrolizidine alkaloid senecionine. *Science* **229**, 472.

216. Noël, S *et al.* (1999) Release of deuterated nonenal during beer aging from labeled precursors synthesized in the boiling kettle. *J. Agric. Food Chem.* **47**, 4323.

217. Feng, Z *et al.* (2004) *Trans*-4HNE inhibits NER in human cells: a possible mechanism for lipid peroxidation-induced carcinogenesis. *Proc. Natl Acad. Sci. USA.* **101**, 8598.

218. Parola, M *et al.* (1999) 4-HNE as a biological signal: molecular basis and pathophysiological implications *Antiox. Redox Signal.* **1**, 255.

219. Bennaars-Eiden, A *et al.* (2002) Covalent modification of epithelial fatty acid-binding protein by 4HNE *in vitro* and *in vivo*. *J. Biol. Chem.* **277**, 50693.

220. Bruns, CM *et al.* (1999) Human GST A4-4 crystal structures and mutagenesis reveal the basis of high catalytic efficiency with toxic lipid peroxidation products. *J. Mol. Biol.* **288**, 427.

221. Uchida, K *et al.* (1998) Acrolein is a product of lipid peroxidation reaction. *J. Biol. Chem.* **273**, 16058.

222. Fisher, D *et al.* (1972) Environmental effects on the autoxidation of retinol. *Biochem. J.* **130**, 259.

223. Itabe, H (1998) Oxidized phospholipids as a new landmark in atherosclerosis. *Prog. Lipid Res.* **37**, 181.

224. Engelmann, B (2004) Plasmalogens: targets for oxidants and major lipophilic antioxidants. *Biochem. Soc. Trans.* **32**, 147.

225. Albert, CJ *et al.* (2003) EPO-derived RBS target the vinyl ether bond of plasmalogens generating a novel chemoattractant, α-bromo fatty aldehyde. *J. Biol. Chem.* **278**, 8942.

226. Chattopadhyay, MK *et al.* (2003) Polyamines protect *E. coli* cells from the toxic effect of O_2. *Proc. Natl. Acad. Sci. USA* **100**, 2261.

227. Ivanova, S *et al.* (2002) Neuroprotection in cerebral ischemia by neutralization of 3-aminopropanal. *Proc. Natl. Acad. Sci. USA* **99**, 5579.

228. Peng, SL *et al.* (1997) Scleroderma: a disease related to damaged proteins? *Nature Med.* **3**, 276.

229. Li, S *et al.* (1995) Chemical instability of protein pharmaceuticals: mechanisms of oxidation and strategies for stabilization. *Biotechnol. Bioeng.* **48**, 490.

230. Tamarit J *et al.* (1998) Identification of the major oxidatively damaged proteins in *E. coli* exposed to oxidative stress. *J. Biol. Chem.* **273**, 3027.

231. Cabiscol, E *et al.* (2000) Oxidative stress promotes specific protein damage in *S. cerevisiae*. *J. Biol. Chem.* **275**, 27393.

232. Van der Vlies D *et al.* (2002) ER resident proteins of normal human dermal fibroblasts are the major targets for oxidative stress induced by H_2O_2. *Biochem. J.* **366**, 825.

233. Stadtman, ER (2004) Role of oxidant species in aging. *Curr. Med. Chem.* **11**, 1105.

234. Davies, MJ (2005) The oxidative environment and protein damage. *Biochim. Biophys. Acta* **1703**, 93.

235. Hampton, MB *et al.* (2002) Inactivation of cellular caspases by peptide-derived tryptophan and tyrosine peroxides. *FEBS Lett.* **527**, 289.

236. Taylor, SW *et al.* (2003) Oxidative post-translational modification of tryptophan residues in cardiac mitochondrial proteins. *J. Biol. Chem.* **278**, 19587.

237. Moskovitz, J and Stadtman, ER (2003) Se-deficient diet enhances protein oxidation and affects methionine sulfoxide reductase (MsrB) protein level in certain mouse tissues. *Proc. Natl. Acad. Sci. USA* **100**, 7486.

238. Bota, DA and Davies, KJA (2002) Lon protease preferentially degrades oxidized mitochondrial aconitase by an ATP-stimulated mechanism. *Nature Cell Biol.* **4**, 674.

239. Dunlop, RA *et al.* (2002) Recent developments in the intracellular degradation of oxidized proteins. *Free Rad. Biol. Med.* **33**, 894.

240. Adams, J (2004) The proteasome: a suitable antineoplastic target. *Nature Rev. Cancer* **4**, 349.

241. Lee, MH *et al.* (2001) Effect of proteasome inhibition on cellular oxidative damage, antioxidant defences and NO• production. *J. Neurochem.* **78**, 32.

242. Yew, EHJ *et al.* (2005) Proteasome inhibition by lactacystin in primary neuronal cells induces both potentially neuroprotective and pro-apoptotic transcriptional responses: a microarray analysis. *J. Neurochem.* **94**, 943.

243. Grune, T *et al.* (2003) Selective degradation of oxidatively modified protein substrates by the proteasome. *Biochem. Biophys. Res. Commun.* **305**, 709.

244. Whittier, JE *et al.* (2004) Hsp90 enhances degradation of oxidized calmodulin by the 20S proteasome. *J. Biol. Chem.* **279**, 46135.

245. Arnold, J and Grune, T (2002) PARP-mediated proteasome activation: a co-ordination of DNA repair and protein degradation? *Bioessays* **24**, 1060.

246. Yamanaka, K *et al.* (2003) Identification of the ubiquitin-protein ligase that recognizes oxidized IRP2. *Nature Cell Biol.* **5**, 336.

247. Dudek, EJ *et al.* (2005) Selectivity of the ubiquitin pathway for oxidatively modified proteins: relevance to protein precipitation diseases. *FASEB J.* **19**, 1707.

248. Friguet, B *et al.* (1994) Susceptibility of G6PDH modified by HNE and metal-catalyzed oxidation to proteolysis by the multicatalytic protease. *Arch. Biochem. Biophys.* **311**,168.

249. Davies, SS *et al.* (2004) Isoketals: highly reactive γ-ketoaldehydes formed from the H_2-isoprostane pathway. *Chem. Phys. Lipids* **128**, 85.

Chapter 5

1. Halliwell, B (1999) Establishing the significance and optimal intake of dietary antioxidants: the biomarker concept. *Nutr. Rev.* **57**, 104.

2. Carroll, MF and Schade, DS (2003) Timing of anti-oxidant vitamin ingestion alters postprandial proatherogenic serum markers. *Circulation* **108**, 24.

3. Jones, DP *et al.* (2000) Redox state of glutathione in human plasma. *Free Rad. Biol. Med.* **28**, 625.

4. Lee, DH *et al.* (2004) Is serum γGT a marker of oxidative stress? *Free Radic. Res.* **38**, 535.

5. Corti, A *et al.* (2005) The *S*-thiolating activity of membrane γ-GT: formation of cys–gly mixed disulfides with cellular proteins and in the cell microenvironment. *Antiox. Redox Signal.* **7**, 911.

6. Gonzalez-Flecha, B and Demple, B (1994) Intracellular generation of $O_2^{\bullet-}$ as a by-product of *Vibrio harveyi* luciferase expressed in *E. coli*. *J. Bacteriol.* **176**, 2293.

7. Mitchell, RJ and Gu, MB (2004) Construction and characterization of novel dual stress-responsive bacterial biosensors. *Biosens. Bioelectron.* **19**, 977.

8. Villamena, FA and Zweier, JL (2004) Detection of reactive O_2 and N_2 species by EPR spin trapping. *Antiox. Redox Signal.* **6**, 619.

9. Mason, RP (1996) *In vitro* and *in vivo* detection of free radical metabolites with ESR. In *Free Radicals: a Practical Approach* (Punchard, NA and Kelly, FJ, eds), p. 11. IRL Press, Oxford.

10. Knowles, PF *et al.* (1969) ESR evidence for enzymic reduction of O_2 to a free radical: the $O_2^{\bullet-}$ ion. *Biochem. J.* **111**, 53.

11. Takeshita, K and Ozawa, T (2004) Recent progress in *in vivo* ESR spectroscopy. *J. Radiat. Res.* **45**, 373.

12. Swartz, HM (2004) Using EPR to measure a critical but often unmeasured component of oxidative damage: O_2. *Antiox. Redox Signal.* **6**, 677.

13. Jackson, SK *et al.* (2002) Detection and removal of contaminating hydroxylamines from the spin trap DEPMPO, and re-evaluation of its use to indicate nitrone radical cation formation and S_N1 reactions. *Free Rad. Biol. Med.* **32**, 228.

14. Dikalov, S *et al.* (2005) Characterization of the high-resolution ESR spectra of $O_2^{\bullet-}$ adducts of DEPMPO and DMPO. Analysis of conformational exchange. *Free Radic. Res.* **39**, 825.

15. Takeshita, K *et al.* (2004) *In vivo* monitoring of $OH^{\bullet}$ generation caused by X-ray irradiation of rats using the spin trapping/EPR technique. *Free Rad. Biol. Med.* **36**, 1134.

16. Chen, G *et al.* (1990) Excretion, metabolism and tissue distribution of a spin trapping agent, PBN, in rats. *Free Radic. Res. Commun.* **9**, 317.

17. Connor, HD *et al.* (1994) New ROS causes formation of carbon-centered radical adducts in organic extracts of blood following liver transplantation. *Free Rad. Biol. Med.* **16**, 871.

18. Reinke, LA *et al.* (1998) Free radical formation during ketamine anaesthesia in rats: a cautionary note. *Free Rad. Biol. Med.* **24**, 1002.

19. Saito, K *et al.* (2004) Pharmacokinetic study of acyl-protected hydroxylamine probe, 1-acetoxy-3-carbamoyl-2,2,5,5-tetramethylpyrrolidine, for *in vivo* measurements of ROS. *Free Rad. Biol. Med.* **36**, 517.

20. Filosa, A *et al.* (2005) Quantitative evaluation of oxidative stress status on peripheral blood in β-thalassaemic patients by means of electron paramagnetic resonance spectroscopy. *Br. J. Haematol.* **131**, 135.

21. Mason, RP (2004) Using anti-DMPO to detect protein radicals in time and space with immuno-spin trapping. *Free Rad. Biol. Med.* **36**, 1214.

22. Nishizawa, C *et al.* (2004) $OH^{\bullet}$ generation caused by the reaction of singlet O_2 with a spin trap, DMPO, increases significantly in the presence of biological reductants. *Free Radic. Res.* **38**, 385.

23. Kalyanaraman, B (1995) Thiyl radicals in biological systems: significant or trivial? *Biochem. Soc. Symp.* **61**, 55.

24. Ramirez, DC *et al.* (2006) Immuno-spin trapping of DNA radicals. *Nature Meth.* **3**, 123.

25. Althaus, JS *et al.* (1998) Azulenyl nitrones: colorimetric detection of oxyradical end products and neuroprotection in the gerbil transient forebrain ischemia/reperfusion model. *Free Rad. Biol. Med.* **24**, 738.

26. Qian, SY *et al.* (2005) A novel protocol to identify and quantify all spin trapped free radicals from *in vitro*/in

vivo interaction of HO$^{\bullet}$ and DMSO: LC/ESR, LC/MS, and dual spin trapping combinations. *Free Rad. Biol. Med.* **38**, 125.

27. Halliwell, B and Kaur, H (1997) Hydroxylation of salicylate and phenylalanine as assays for OH$^{\bullet}$: a cautionary note visited for the third time. *Free Radic. Res.* **273**, 239.

28. Halliwell, B and Whiteman, M (2004) Measuring RS and oxidative damage *in vivo* and in cell culture: how should you do it and what do the results mean? *Br J. Pharmacol.* **142**, 231.

29. Eberhardt, MK (1995) OH$^{\bullet}$. Formation and some reactions used in its identification. *Trends Org. Chem.* **5**, 115.

30. Lamrini, R *et al.* (1998) Oxidative decarboxylation of benzoic acid by peroxyl radicals. *Free Rad. Biol. Med.* **24**, 280.

31. Powell, SR (1994) Salicylate trapping of OH$^{\bullet}$ as a tool for studying post-ischemic oxidative injury in the isolated rat heart. *Free Radic. Res.* **21**, 355.

32. Schapira, RM *et al.* (1995) OH$^{\bullet}$ production and lung injury in the rat following silica or TiO_2 instillation *in vivo. Am. J. Resp. Cell Mol. Biol.* **12**, 220.

33. Orhan, H *et al.* (2004) Simultaneous determination of tyrosine, phenylalanine and dG oxidation products by LC-MS as non-invasive biomarkers for oxidative damage. *J. Chromatog.* **799**, 245.

34. Huycke, MM and Moore, DR (2002) *In vivo* production of OH$^{\bullet}$ by *Enterococcus faecalis* colonizing the intestinal tract using aromatic hydroxylation. *Free Rad. Biol. Med.* **33**, 818.

35. Kalyanaraman, B *et al.* (1993) Formation of 2,5-DHB during the reaction between $^1O_2$ and salicylic acid. Analysis by ESR oximetry and HPLC with electrochemical detection. *J. Am. Chem. Soc.* **115**, 4007.

36. Whiteman, M and Halliwell, B (1997) Thiourea and DMTU inhibit ONOO$^-$-dependent damage: nonspecificity as OH$^{\bullet}$ scavengers. *Free Rad. Biol. Med.* **22**, 1309.

37. Halliwell, B (1995) Antioxidant characterization. Methodology and mechanism. *Biochem. Pharmacol.* **49**, 1341.

38. Kahn, V (1989) Tiron as a substrate for horseradish peroxidase. *Phytochemistry* **28**, 41.

39. Ghosh, M *et al.* (2002) Tiron exerts effects unrelated to its role as a scavenger of $O_2^{\bullet-}$: effects on Ca^{2+} binding and vascular responses. *Can. J. Physiol. Pharmacol.* **80**, 755.

40. Tian, Y *et al.* (2002) SOD-based third generation biosensor for $O_2^{\bullet-}$ anion. *Anal. Chem.* **74**, 2428.

41. Giulivi, C *et al.* (1999) The steady-state concentrations of O_2 radicals in mitochondria. In: *ROS in Biological*

Systems. Kluwer Academic, Plenum Press Publishers, New York, USA.

42. Kutala, VK *et al.* (2004) Reaction of $O_2^{\bullet-}$ with trityl radical: implications for the determination of $O_2^{\bullet-}$ by spectrophotometry. *Arch. Biochem. Biophys.* **424**, 81.

43. Freitas, I *et al.* (2002) In situ detection of ROS and NO$^{\bullet}$ production in normal and pathological tissues: improvement by differential interference contrast. *Exp. Gerontol.* **37**, 591.

44. Tarpey, MM *et al.* (2004) Methods for detection of reactive metabolites of O_2 and N_2: *in vitro* and *in vivo* considerations. *Am. J. Physiol.* **289**, R431.

45. Kleinbongard, P *et al.* (2003) Plasma NO_2^- reflects constitutive NO$^{\bullet}$ synthase activity in mammals. *Free Rad. Biol. Med.* **35**, 790.

46. Ischiropoulos, H (2003) Biological selectivity and functional aspects of protein tyrosine nitration. *Biochem. Biophys. Res. Commun.* **305**, 776.

47. Kaur, H *et al.* (1998) Artefacts in HPLC detection of 3-nitrotyrosine in human brain tissue. *J. Neurochem.* **70**, 2220.

48. Kanski, J *et al.* (2003) Proteomic identification of agedependent protein nitration in rat skeletal muscle. *Free Rad. Biol. Med.* **35**, 1229.

49. Halliwell, B (1997) What nitrates tyrosine? *FEBS Lett.* **411**, 157.

50. Whiteman, M *et al.* (2003) Lack of tyrosine nitration by HOCl in the presence of physiological concentrations of NO_2^-. Implications for the role of NO_2Cl in tyrosine nitration *in vivo. J. Biol. Chem.* **278**, 8380.

51. MacPherson, JC *et al.* (2001) Eosinophils are a major source of NO$^{\bullet}$-derived oxidants in severe asthma: characterization of pathways available to eosinophils for generating RNS. *J. Immunol.* **166**, 5763.

52. Eiserich, JP *et al.* (2002) MPO, a leukocyte-derived vascular NO$^{\bullet}$ oxidase. *Science* **296**, 2391.

53. Frost, MT *et al.* (2000) Analysis of free and proteinbound 3-NT in human plasma by a GC/MS method that avoids nitration artifacts. *Biochem. J.* **345**, 453.

54. Tsikas, D *et al.* (2005) Determination of 3-NT in human urine at the basal state by gas chromatography-tandem mass spectrometry and evaluation of the excretion after oral intake. *J. Chromatog.* **827**, 146.

55. Mani, AR *et al.* (2003) Nitration of endogenous *para*-hydroxyphenylacetic acid and the metabolism of 3-NT. *Biochem. J.* **374**, 521.

56. Shishehbor, MH *et al.* (2003) Statins promote potent systemic antioxidant effects through specific inflammatory pathways. *Circulation* **108**, 426.

57. Whiteman, M and Halliwell, B (1999) Loss of 3-NT on exposure to HOCl: implications for the use of 3-NT as

a biomarker *in vivo. Biochem. Biophys. Res. Commun.* **258**, 168.

58. Kettle, AJ (1996) Neutrophils convert tyrosyl residues in albumin to chlorotyrosine. *FEBS Lett.* **379**, 103.

59. Andersen, SO (2004) Chlorinated tyrosine derivatives in insect cuticle. *Insect Biochem. Mol. Biol.* **34**, 1079.

60. Kettle, AJ *et al.* (1994) Assays using HRP and phenolic substrates require SOD for accurate determination of H_2O_2 production by neutrophils. *Free Rad. Biol. Med.* **17**, 161.

61. Halliwell, B *et al.* (2004) Establishing biomarkers of oxidative stress: the management of H_2O_2 in human urine. *Curr. Med. Chem.* **11**, 1085.

62. Foote, CS and Clennan, EL (1995) Properties and reactions of singlet O_2. In: *Active Oxygen in Chemistry* (Foote, CS *et al.*, eds), p. 105. Blackie, London.

63. Miyamoto, S *et al.* (2003) Direct evidence of O_2 ($^1\Delta g$) production in the reaction of linoleic acid hydroperoxide with $ONOO^-$. *J. Am. Chem. Soc.* **125**, 4510.

64. Packer, JE *et al.* (1981) Free radicals and $^1O_2$ scavengers: reaction of a peroxy radical with β-carotene, diphenyl furan and DABCO. *Biochem. Biophys. Res. Commun.* **98**, 901.

65. Steinbeck, MJ *et al.* (1993) Extracellular production of $^1O_2$ by stimulated macrophages quantified using 9,10-diphenylanthracene and perylene in a polystyrene film. *J. Biol. Chem.* **268**, 15649.

66. Nye, AC *et al.* (1987) Diffusion of $^1O_2$ into human bronchial epithelial cells. *Biochim. Biophys. Acta* **928**, 1.

67. Vladimirov, YA (1996) Intrinsic (low-level) chemiluminescence. In: *Free Radicals: A Practical Approach* (Punchard, NA and Kelly, FJ, eds), p. 65. IRL Press, Oxford.

68. Williams, MD and Chance, B (1993) Spontaneous chemiluminescence of human breath. *J. Biol. Chem.* **258**, 3628.

69. Clement, MV *et al.* (2002) The cytotoxicity of dopamine may be an artifact of cell culture. *J. Neurochem.* **81**, 414.

70. Lawrence, A *et al.* (2003) Evidence for the role of a peroxidase compound I-type intermediate in the oxidation of GSH, NADH, ascorbate, and dichlorofluorescin by cytochrome c/H_2O_2. Implications for oxidative stress during apoptosis. *J. Biol. Chem.* **278**, 29410.

71. Zhao, H *et al.* (2005) Detection and characterization of the product of hydroethidine and intracellular $O_2^{\bullet-}$ by HPLC and limitations of fluorescence. *Proc. Natl. Acad. Sci. USA* **102**, 5727.

72. Shimomura, O *et al.* (1998) Evaluation of five imidazopyrazinone-type chemiluminescent $O_2^{\bullet-}$ probes and their application to the measurement of $O_2^{\bullet-}$ anion

generated by *Listeria monocytogenes. Anal. Biochem.* **259**, 230.

73. Collins, C *et al.* (2003) Analysis of 3'-phosphoglycolaldehyde residues in oxidized DNA by GC/negative chemical ionization/MS. *Chem. Res. Toxicol.* **16**, 1560.

74. Zhou, X *et al.* (2005) Quantification of DNA strand breaks and abasic sites by oxime derivatization and accelerator MS: application to γ-radiation and $ONOO^-$. *Anal. Biochem.* **343**, 84.

75. Kasai, H (1997) Analysis of a form of oxidative DNA damage, 80HdG, as a marker of cellular oxidative stress during carcinogenesis. *Mutat. Res.* **387**, 147.

76. Cooke, MS *et al.* (2005) DNA repair is responsible for the presence of oxidatively damaged DNA lesions in urine. *Mutat. Res.* **574**, 58.

77. Lin, HS *et al.* (2004) A high-throughput and sensitive methodology for the quantification of urinary 80HdG; measurement with GC–MS after single solid-phase extraction. *Biochem. J.* **380**, 541.

78. Rozalski, R *et al.* (2004) Diet is not responsible for the presence of several oxidatively damaged DNA lesions in mouse urine. *Free Radic. Res.* **38**, 1201.

79. Loft, S and Poulsen, HE (1996) Cancer risk and oxidative DNA damage in man. *J. Mol. Med.* **74**, 297.

80. Shi, M *et al.* (2005) Generation of 80HdG from DNA using rat liver homogenates. *Cancer Sci.* **96**, 13.

81. Pilger, A *et al.* (2002) Urinary excretion of 80HdG measured by HPLC with electrochemical detection. *J. Chromatog.* **778**, 393.

82. Sokhansanj, BA and Wilson III, DM (2004) Oxidative DNA damage background estimated by a system model of base excision repair. *Free Rad. Biol. Med.* **37**, 422.

83. Halliwell, B (2000) Why and how should we measure oxidative DNA damage in nutritional studies? How far have we come? *Am. J. Clin. Nutr.* **72**, 1082.

84. Cadet, J *et al.* (2003) Oxidative damage to DNA: formation, measurement and biochemical features. *Mutat. Res.* **531**, 5.

85. Collins, AR (2005) Assays for oxidative stress and antioxidant status: applications to research into the biological effectiveness of polyphenols. *Am. J. Clin. Nutr.* 81 (Suppl. 1), 261S.

86. Beckman, KB *et al.* (2000) A simpler, more robust method for the analysis of 8-oxoguanine in DNA. *Free Rad. Biol. Med.* **29**, 357.

87. Ravanat, JL *et al.* (2002) Cellular background level of 80HdG; an isotope based method to evaluate artefactual oxidation of DNA during its extraction and subsequent work-up. *Carcinogenesis* **23**, 1911.

88. Nakae, Y *et al.* (2005) A new technique for the quantitative assessment of 8-oxoG in nuclear DNA as a

marker of oxidative stress. Application to dystrophin-deficient DMD skeletal muscles. *Histochem. Cell Biol.* **124**, 335.

89. Loft, S *et al.* (1998) Experimental study of oxidative DNA damage. *Free Radic. Res.* **29**, 525.

90. Kamura, K *et al.* (1997) Effect of endurance exercise on the tissue 8OHdG content in dogs. *Free Radic. Res.* **26**, 523.

91. Halliwell, B (2002) Effect of diet on cancer development: is oxidative DNA damage a biomarker? *Free Rad. Biol. Med.* **32**, 968.

92. Ma, N *et al.* (2004) Accumulation of 8-NG in human gastric epithelium induced by *H. pylori* infection. *Biochem. Biophys. Res. Comm.* **319**, 506.

93. Sawa, T *et al.* (2006) Analysis of urinary 8NG, a marker of nitrative nucleic acid damage, by HPLC–ECD coupled with immunoaffinity purification: association with cigarette smoking. *Free Rad. Biol. Med.* **40**, 711.

94. Oikawa, S and Kawanishi, S (1999) Site-specific DNA damage at GGG sequence by oxidative stress may accelerate telomere shortening. *FEBS Lett.* **453**, 365.

95. Lu, T *et al.* (2004) Gene regulation and DNA damage in the ageing human brain. *Nature* **429**, 883.

96A. Otteneder, MB *et al.* (2006) *In vivo* oxidative metabolism of a major peroxidation-derived DNA adduct M_1dG. *Proc. Natl. Acad. Sci. USA* **103**, 6665.

96. Choi, J *et al.* (2002) Gene-specific oxidative DNA damage in *H. pylori*-infected human gastric mucosa. *Int. J. Cancer* **99**, 485.

97. Frank, A *et al.* (2004) Immunohistochemical detection of 1,N^6-ethenodeoxyadenosine in nuclei of human liver affected by diseases predisposing to hepato-carcinogenesis. *Carcinogenesis* **25**, 1027.

98. Leuratti, C *et al.* (2002) Detection of MDA–DNA adducts in human colorectal mucosa: relationship with diet and the presence of adenomas. *Cancer Epidemiol. Biomark. Prev.* **11**, 267.

99. Chen, HJC *et al.* (2004) Urinary excretion of 3, N^4-etheno-2′-deoxycytidine in humans as a biomarker of oxidative stress: association with cigarette smoking. *Chem. Res. Toxicol.* **17**, 896.

100. Morrow, JD (2005) Quantification of IPs as indices of oxidant stress and the risk of atherosclerosis in humans. *Arterio. Thromb. Vasc. Biol.* **25**, 279.

101. Cornelli, U *et al.* (2001) Bioavailability and antioxidant activity of some food supplements in men and women using the D-Roms test as a marker of oxidative stress. *J. Nutr.* **131**, 3208.

102. Venkataraman, S *et al.* (2004) Detection of lipid radicals using EPR. *Antiox. Redox Signal.* **6**, 631.

103. Hay, A *et al.* (2005) Development of a new EPR spin trap, DOD-8C for the trapping of lipid radicals at a predetermined depth within biological membranes. *Arch. Biochem. Biophys.* **435**, 336.

104. Qian, S *et al.* (2002) Characterization of the initial carbon-centered pentadienyl radical and subsequent radicals in lipid peroxidation: identification via on-line HPLC/ESR and MS. *Free Rad. Biol. Med.* **33**, 998.

105. Banni, S *et al.* (1996) No direct evidence of increased lipid peroxidation in hemodialysis patients. *Nephron.* **72**, 177.

106. Thompson, S and Smith, MT (1985) Measurement of the diene conjugated form of linoleic acid in plasma by HPLC: a questionable non-invasive assay of free radical activity? *Chem. Biol. Interac.* **55**, 357.

107. Park, Y and Pariza, MW (1998) Evidence that commercial calf and horse sera can contain substantial amounts of *trans*-10, *cis*-12 CLA. *Lipids* **33**, 817.

108. Larsen, TM *et al.* (2003) Efficacy and safety of dietary supplements containing CLA for the treatment of obesity: evidence from animal and human studies. *J. Lipid Res.* **44**, 2234.

109. Risérus, U *et al.* (2002) Supplementation with CLA causes isomer-dependent oxidative stress and elevated CRP. *Circulation* **106**, 1925.

110. Fessel, JP and Roberts, LJ (2005) Isofurans: novel products of lipid peroxidation that define the occurrence of oxidant injury in settings of elevated O_2 tension. *Antiox. Redox Signal.* **7**, 202.

111. Richelle, M *et al.* (1999) Urinary IP excretion is not confounded by the lipid content of the diet. *FEBS Lett.* **459**, 259.

112. Lee, CY *et al.* (2004) Rapid preparation of human urine and plasma samples for analysis of F_2–IPs by GC–MS. *Biochem. Biophys. Res. Comm.* **320**, 696.

113. Rahman, I and Kelly, F (2003) Biomarkers in breath condensate: a promising new non-invasive technique in free radical research. *Free Radic. Res.* **37**, 1253.

114. Poliakov, E *et al.* (2004) Iso[7]LGD$_2$-protein adducts are abundant *in vivo* and free radical-induced oxidation of an arachidonyl phospholipids generates this D series isolevuglandin *in vitro*. *Chem. Res. Toxicol.* **17**, 613.

115. Esterbauer, H *et al.* (1991) Chemistry and biochemistry of HNE, MDA and related aldehydes. *Free Rad. Biol. Med.* **11**, 81.

116. Frankel, EN *et al.* (1989) Rapid headspace GC of hexanal as a measure of lipid peroxidation in biological samples. *Lipids* **24**, 976.

117. Olsen, E *et al.* (2005) Analysis of early lipid oxidation in smoked, comminuted pork or poultry sausages with spices. *J. Agric. Food Chem.* **53**, 7448.

118. Phillips, M *et al.* (2003) Response: scientific basis of the breath methylated alkane contour. *Clin. Chim. Acta* **333**, 93.

119. Lärstad, M *et al.* (2005) Selective quantification of free 3-NT in exhaled breath condensate in asthma using GC/tandem MS. *Nitric Oxide* **13**, 134.

120. Weissmann, N *et al.* (2004) Measurement of exhaled H_2O_2 from rabbit lungs. *Biol. Chem.* **385**, 259.

121. Forteza, R *et al.* (2005) Regulated H_2O_2 production by Duox in human airway epithelial cells. *Am. J. Respir. Cell Mol. Biol.* **32**, 462.

122. Kanoh, S *et al.* (2005) Exhaled ethane. *Chest* **128**, 2387.

123. Gutteridge, JMC and Quinlan, GJ (1983) MDA formation from lipid peroxides in the TBA test: the role of lipid radicals, Fe salts, and metal chelators. *J. Appl. Biochem.* **5**, 293.

124. Cighetti, G *et al.* (1998) β-Ethoxyacrolein contamination increases MDA inhibition of milk XO activity. *Free Rad. Biol. Med.* **25**, 818.

125. Shimizu, T *et al.* (1981) Role of prostaglandin endoperoxides in the serum TBA reaction. *Arch. Biochem. Biophys.* **206**, 271.

126. Girón-Calle, J *et al.* (2002) Bound MDA in foods: bioavailability of the N-2-propenals of lysine. *J. Agric. Food Chem.* **50**, 6194.

127. Draper, HH *et al.* (2000) Urinary aldehydes as indicators of lipid peroxidation *in vivo*. *Free Rad. Biol. Med.* **29**, 1071.

128. Brown, ED *et al.* (1995) Urinary MDA-equivalents during ingestion of meat cooked at high or low temperatures. *Lipids* **30**, 1053.

129. Kosugi, H *et al.* (1993) Characteristics of the TBA reactivity of human urine as a possible consequence of lipid peroxidation. *Lipids* **28**, 337.

130. Korchazhkina, O *et al.* (2003) Measurement by reversed-phase HPLC of MDA in normal human urine following derivatisation with 2,4-DNPH. *J. Chromatog.* **794**, 353.

131. Kikugawa, K and Beppu, M (1987) Involvement of lipid oxidation products in the formation of fluorescent and cross-linked proteins. *Chem. Phys. Lipids* **44**, 277.

132. Drummen, GPC *et al.* (1999) Validation of the peroxidative indicators, *cis*-parinaric acid and parinaroyl-phospholipids, in a model system and cultured cardiac myocytes. *Biochim. Biophys. Acta* **1436**, 370.

133. Drummen, GPC *et al.* (2004) MS characterization of the oxidation of the fluorescent lipid peroxidation reporter molecule C11-BODIPY[581/591]. *Free Rad. Biol. Med.* **36**, 1635.

134. Davies, MJ *et al.* (1999) Stable markers of oxidant damage to proteins and their application in the study of human disease. *Free Rad. Biol. Med.* **27**, 1151.

135. Requena, JR *et al.* (2003) Recent advances in the analysis of oxidized proteins. *Amino Acids* **25**, 221.

136. Wells-Knecht, MC *et al.* (1993) Oxidized amino acids in lens proteins with age. *J. Biol. Chem.* **268**, 12348.

137. Lubec, G *et al.* (1994) Racemization and oxidation studies of hair protein in *Homo tirolensis*. *FASEB J.* **8**, 1166.

138. Malencik, DA and Anderson, SR (2003) Dityrosine as a product of oxidative stress and fluorescent probe. *Amino Acids* **25**, 233.

139. Kato, Y *et al.* (1998) Immunohistochemical detection of dityrosine in lipofuscin pigments in the aged human brain. *FEBS Lett.* **439**, 231.

140. Sakharov, DV *et al.* (2003) Photodynamic treatment and H_2O_2-induced oxidative stress result in different patterns of cellular protein oxidation. *Eur. J. Biochem.* **270**, 4859.

141. Pattison, DI and Davies, MJ (2004) Kinetic analysis of the reactions of HOBr with protein components: implications for cellular damage and use of 3-bromotyrosine as a marker of oxidative stress. *Biochemistry* **43**, 4799.

142. Dalle-Donne, I *et al.* (2003) Protein carbonylation in human diseases. *Trends Mol. Med.* **9**, 169.

143. Henrietta, AH and Davies, MJ (2004) Markers of protein oxidation: different oxidants give rise to variable yields of bound and released carbonyl products. *Free Rad. Biol. Med.* **36**, 1175.

144. Mirzaei, H and Regnier, F (2005) Affinity chromatographic selection of carbonylated proteins followed by identification of oxidation sites using tandem MS. *Anal. Chem.* **77**, 2386.

145. Lyras, L *et al.* (1996) Oxidative damage and motor neurone disease. Difficulties in the measurement of protein carbonyls in human brain tissue. *Free Radic. Res.* **24**, 397.

146. Shacter, E *et al.* (1994) Differential susceptibility of plasma proteins to oxidative modification: examination by western blot immunoassay. *Free Rad. Biol. Med.* **17**, 429.

147. Stagsted, J *et al.* (2004) Identification of specific oxidatively modified proteins in chicken muscles using a combined immunologic and proteomic approach. *J. Agric. Food Chem.* **52**, 3967.

148. Dragsted, LO (2003) Antioxidant actions of polyphenols in humans. *Int. J. Vitam. Nutr. Res.* **73**, 112.

149. Bartosz, G (2003) Total antioxidant capacity. *Adv. Clin. Chem.* **37**, 219.

150. Huang, D *et al.* (2005) The chemistry behind antioxidant capacity assays. *J. Agric. Food Chem.* **53**, 1841.

151. Wayner, DDM *et al.* (1987) The relative contributions of vitamin E, urate, ascorbate and proteins to the total peroxyl radical-trapping antioxidant activity of human blood plasma. *Biochim. Biophys. Acta* **924**, 408.

152. Lönnrot, K *et al.* (1996) The effect of ascorbate and ubiquinone supplementation on plasma and CSF total antioxidant capacity. *Free Rad. Biol. Med.* **21**, 211.

153. Ratty, AK *et al.* (1988) Interaction of flavonoids with 1,1-diphenyl-2-picrylhydrazyl free radical, liposomal membranes and soybean lipoxygenase-1. *Biochem. Pharmacol.* **37**, 989.

154. Kocherginsky, NM *et al.* (2005) Use of nitroxide spin probes and EPR for assessing reducing power of beer. *J. Agric. Food Chem.* **53**, 1052.

155. Cao, G and Prior, RL (2000) Postprandial increases in serum antioxidant capacity in older women. *J. Appl. Physiol.* **89**, 877.

156. Halliwell, B (2003) Health benefits of eating chocolate? *Nature* **426**, 787.

157. Long, LH *et al.* (2000) The antioxidant activities of seasonings used in Asian cooking. Powerful antioxidant activity of dark soy sauce revealed using the ABTS assay. *Free Radic. Res.* **32**, 181.

Chapter 6

1. Lemaire, P *et al.* (1993) Pro-oxidant and antioxidant processes in gas gland and other tissues of cod (*Gadus morhua*). *J. Comp. Physiol.* **163**, 477.

2. Halliwell, B *et al.* (2000) The gastrointestinal tract: a major site of antioxidant action? *Free Radic. Res.* **33**, 819.

3. Grootveld, M *et al.* (1998) *In vivo* absorption, metabolism, and urinary excretion of α, β-unsaturated aldehydes in experimental animals. *J. Clin. Invest.* **101**, 1210.

4. Aw, TY (2005) Intestinal GSH: determinant of mucosal peroxide transport, metabolism, and oxidative susceptibility. *Toxicol. Appl. Pharmacol.* **204**, 320.

5. Gorelik, S *et al.* (2005) Lipid peroxidation and coupled vitamin oxidation in simulated and human gastric fluid inhibited by dietary polyphenols: health implications. *J. Agric. Food Chem.* **53**, 3397.

6. Chamulitrat, W (1999) Activation of the $O_2^{\bullet-}$-generating NADPH oxidase of intestinal lymphocytes produces highly reactive free radicals from sulfite. *Free Radic. Biol. Med.* **27**, 411.

7. Hassani, RAE *et al.* (2005) Duox2 is expressed all along the digestive tract. *Am. J. Physiol.* **288**, G933.

8. Ha, EM *et al.* (2005) A direct role for duox in *Drosophila* gut immunity. *Science* **310**, 847.

9. Babbs, CF (1990) Free radicals and the etiology of colon cancer. *Free Rad. Biol. Med.* **8**, 191.

10. Huycke, MM and Moore, DR (2002) *In vivo* production of OH$^{\bullet}$ by *Enterococcus faecalis* colonizing the intestinal tract using aromatic hydroxylation. *Free Rad. Biol. Med.* **33**, 818.

11. Wark, PA *et al.* (2004) Habitual consumption of fruits and vegetables: associations with human rectal GST. *Carcinogenesis* **25**, 2135.

12. Katsuki, K *et al.* (2004) Feeding induces expression of HSPs that reduce oxidative stress. *FEBS Lett.* **571**, 187.

13. Nagler, RM *et al.* (2002) Characterization of the differentiated antioxidant profile of human saliva. *Free Rad. Biol. Med.* **32**, 268.

14. Halliwell, B *et al.* (2005) Health promotion by flavonoids, tocopherols, tocotrienols, and other phenols: direct or indirect effects? Antioxidant or not? *Am. J. Clin. Nutr.* **81**, 268S.

15. Zhao, K *et al.* (2001) DNA damage by NO_2^- and $ONOO^-$: protection by dietary phenols. *Meth. Enzymol.* **335**, 296.

16. Barbehenn, RV *et al.* (2001) Antioxidant defenses in caterpillars: role of the ascorbate-recycling system in the midgut lumen. *J. Insect Physiol.* **47**, 349.

17. Bjelakovic, G *et al.* (2005) Authors' reply to 'Antioxidant supplements for prevention of gastrointestinal cancers.' *Lancet* **365**, 471.

18. Wu, W *et al.* (2000) Eosinophils generate brominating oxidants in allergen-induced asthma. *J. Clin. Invest.* **105**, 1455.

19. Loukides, S *et al.* (2002) The relationships among H_2O_2 in expired breath condensate, airway inflammation, and asthma severity. *Chest* **121**, 338.

20. Wood, LG *et al.* (2005) Induced sputum 8-IP concentration in inflammatory airway diseases. *Am. J. Respir. Crit. Care Med.* **171**, 426.

21. Comhair, SAA *et al.* (2005) SOD inactivation in pathophysiology of asthmatic airway remodeling and reactivity. *Am. J. Pathol.* **166**, 663.

22. Butteroni, C *et al.* (2004) Cloning and expression of the *Olea europaea* allergen Ole e 5, the pollen CuZn-SOD. *Int. Arch. Allergy Immunol.* **137**, 9.

23. Hoidal, JR *et al.* (2003) The role of endogenous NADPH oxidases in airway and pulmonary vascular smooth muscle function. *Antiox. Redox Signal.* **5**, 751.

24. Que, LG *et al.* (2005) Protection from experimental asthma by an endogenous bronchodilator. *Science* **308**, 1618.

25. Merritt, TA *et al.* (1993) Reduction of the surface-tension-lowering ability of surfactant after exposure to HOCl. *Biochem. J.* **295**, 19.

26. Narasaraju, TA *et al.* (2003) Protein nitration in rat lungs during hyperoxia exposure: a possible role of MPO. *Am. J. Physiol.* **285**, L1037.

27. Quinlan, GJ *et al.* (2002) Fe and the redox status of the lungs. *Free Rad. Biol. Med.* **33**, 1306.

28. Zingg, JM and Azzi, A (2004) Non-antioxidant activities of vitamin E. *Curr. Med. Chem.* **11**, 1113.

29. Carpagnano, GE *et al.* (2004) Supplementary O_2 in healthy subjects and those with COPD increases oxidative stress and airway inflammation. *Thorax* **59**, 1016.

30. Cross, CE *et al.* (1994) Oxidants, antioxidants, and respiratory tract lining fluids. *Environ. Health Perspect.* **102** (Suppl. 10), 185.

31. van der Vliet, A *et al.* (1999) Determination of low-molecular-mass antioxidant concentrations in human respiratory tract lining fluids. *Am. J. Physiol.* **276**, L289.

32. Riccioni, G and D'Orazio, N (2005) The role of Se, Zn and antioxidant vitamin supplementation in the treatment of bronchial asthma: adjuvant therapy or not? *Expert Opin. Invest. Drugs* **14**, 1145.

33. Romieu, I *et al.* (2002) Antioxidant supplementation and lung functions among children with asthma exposed to high levels of air pollutants. *Am. J. Resp. Crit. Care Med.* **166**, 703.

34. Schock, BC *et al.* (2004) Ascorbic acid in nasal and tracheobronchial airway lining fluids. *Free Rad. Biol. Med.* **37**, 1393.

35. Winterbourn, CC (1985) Free-radical production and oxidative reactions of hemoglobin. *Environ. Health Perspect.* **64**, 321.

36. Johnson, RM *et al.* (2005) Hemoglobin autoxidation and regulation of endogenous H_2O_2 levels in erythrocytes. *Free Rad. Biol. Med.* **39**, 1407.

37. D'Agnillo, F and Chang, TM (1998) Absence of hemoprotein-associated free radical events following oxidant challenge of crosslinked hemoglobin-SOD catalase. *Free Rad. Biol. Med.* **24**, 906.

38. Ando, K *et al.* (2002) Increased release of free Fe ions in human erythrocytes during aging in the circulation. *Free Radic. Res.* **36**, 1079.

39. Ney, PA *et al.* (1990) Synergistic effects of oxidation and deformation on erythrocyte monovalent cation leak. *Blood* **75**, 1192.

40. Nozik-Grayck, E *et al.* (2003) HCO_3^--dependent $O_2^{\bullet-}$ release and pulmonary artery tone. *Am. J. Physiol.* **285**, H2327.

41. Romero, N *et al.* (2003) Reaction of human hemoglobin with $ONOO^-$. *J. Biol. Chem.* **278**, 44049.

42. Lee, TH *et al.* (2003) Peroxiredoxin II is essential for sustaining life span of erythrocytes in mice. *Blood* **101**, 5033.

43. Percy, MJ *et al.* (2005) Disorders of oxidized haemoglobin. *Blood Rev.* **19**, 61.

44. Clemens, MR and Waller, HD (1987) Lipid peroxidation in erythrocytes. *Chem. Phys. Lipids* **45**, 251.

45. Stagsted, J and Young, JF (2002) Large differences in erythrocyte stability between species reflect different antioxidative defense mechanisms. *Free Radic. Res.* **36**, 779.

46. Burton, GW *et al.* (1986) Vitamin E in young and old human red blood cells. *Biochim. Biophys. Acta* **860**, 84.

47. May, JM *et al.* (2004) Human erythrocyte recycling of ascorbic acid. *J. Biol. Chem.* **279**, 14975.

48. Mcmillan, DC *et al.* (2005) Lipids versus proteins as major targets of pro-oxidant, direct-acting hemolytic agents. *Toxicol. Sci.* **88**, 274.

49. Aslan, M and Freeman, BA (2004) Oxidant-mediated impairment of $NO^{\bullet}$ signaling in sickle disease–mechanisms and consequences. *Cell. Mol. Biol.* **50**, 95.

50. Shalev, O and Hebbel, RP (1996) Extremely high avidity association of Fe(III) with the sickle red cell membrane. *Blood* **88**, 349.

51. Winterbourn, CC *et al.* (1981) Unstable haemoglobin haemolytic crises: contributions of pyrexia and neutrophil oxidants. *Br. J. Haematol.* **49**, 111.

52. Feng, L *et al.* (2005) Structure of oxidized α-haemoglobin bound to AHSP reveals a protective mechanism for haem. *Nature* **435**, 697.

53. Dumaswala, UJ *et al.* (2001) GSH protects chemokine-scavenging and antioxidative defense functions in human RBCs. *Am. J. Physiol.* **280**, C867.

54. Notaro, R *et al.* (2000) Human mutations in G6PDH reflect evolutionary history. *FASEB J.* **14**, 485.

55. Paglialunga, F *et al.* (2004) G6PDH is indispensable for erythropoiesis after embryonic–adult hemoglobin switch. *Blood* **104**, 3148.

56. Tsai, KJ *et al.* (1998) Impaired production of $NO^{\bullet}$, $O_2^{\bullet-}$, and H_2O_2 in G6PDH-deficient granulocytes. *FEBS Lett.* **436**, 411.

57. Paglia, DE (1993) Acute episodic hemolysis in the African black rhinoceros as an analogue of human G6PDH deficiency. *Am. J. Hematol.* **42**, 36.

58. Chevion, M *et al.* (1982) The chemistry of favism-inducing compounds. *Eur. J. Biochem.* **127**, 405.

59. Spolarics, Z *et al.* (2001) Increased incidence of sepsis and altered monocyte functions in severely-injured type A-G6PDH-deficient African American trauma patients. *Crit. Care Med.* **29**, 728.

60. Salo, DC *et al.* (1990) SOD undergoes proteolysis and fragmentation following oxidative modification and inactivation. *J. Biol. Chem.* **265**, 11919.

61. Shimizu, K *et al.* (2004) Coordination of oxidized protein hydrolase and the proteasome in the clearance of cytotoxic denatured proteins. *Biochem. Biophys. Res. Comm.* **324**, 140.

62. Terpstra, V and van Berkel, TJ (2000) Scavengers receptors on liver Kupffer cells mediate the *in vivo*

uptake of oxidatively damaged red blood cells in mice. *Blood* **95**, 2157.

63. Comporti, M *et al.* (2002) Fe release, oxidative stress and erythrocyte ageing. *Free Rad. Biol. Med.* **32**, 568.

64. Timmins, GS *et al.* (2004) NO$^{\bullet}$ generated from isoniazid activation by KatG: source of NO$^{\bullet}$ and activity against *M. tuberculosis*. *Antimicrob. Ag. Chemother.* **48**, 3006.

65. Maples, KR *et al.* (1988) *In vivo* rat hemoglobin thiyl free radical formation following administration of phenylhydrazine and hydrazine-based drugs. *Drug Metab. Disp.* **16**, 799.

66. Evelo, CT *et al.* (1998) Two mechanisms for toxic effects of hydroxylamines in human erythrocytes: involvement of free radicals and risk of potentiation. *Blood Cells Mol. Dis.* **24**, 280.

67. Munday, R (1989) Toxicity of thiols and disulphides: involvement of free-radical species. *Free Rad. Biol. Med.* **7**, 659.

68. Oliveira, PL and Oliveira, MF (2002) Vampires, Pasteur and ROS. *FEBS Lett.* **525**, 3.

69. Oliveira, MF *et al.* (2002) On the pro-oxidant effects of haemozoin. *FEBS Lett.* **512**, 139.

70. Monti, D *et al.* (2002) Does chloroquine really act through oxidative stress? *FEBS Lett.* **522**, 3.

71. Greenwood, B and Mutabingwa, T (2002) Malaria in 2002. *Nature* **415**, 670.

72. Oliveira, MF *et al.* (2000) Haemozoin formation in the midgut of the blood-sucking insect *Rhodnius prolixus*. *FEBS Lett.* **477**, 95.

73. Graça-Souza, AV *et al.* (1999) Urate synthesis in the blood-sucking insect *Rhodnius prolixus*. *J. Biol. Chem.* **274**, 9673.

74. Kumar, S *et al.* (2003) The role of ROS on *Plasmodium* melanotic encapsulation in *Anopheles gambiae*. *Proc. Natl. Acad. Sci. USA* **100**, 14139.

75. Hood, AT *et al.* (1996) Protection from lethal malaria in transgenic mice expressing sickle hemoglobin. *Blood* **87**, 1600.

76. Pasvol, G (1996) Malaria and resistance genes–they work in wondrous ways. *Lancet* **348**, 1532.

77. Schwarzer, E *et al.* (2003) Malaria-parasitized erythrocytes and hemozoin nonenzymatically generate large amounts of hydroxy fatty acids that inhibit monocyte functions. *Blood* **101**, 722.

78. Lüersen, K *et al.* (2000) *P. falciparum*-infected red blood cells depend on a functional GSH *de novo* synthesis attributable to an enhanced loss of GSH. *Biochem. J.* **346**, 545.

79. Müller, S (2004) Redox and antioxidant systems of the malaria parasite *P. falciparum*. *Mol. Microbiol.* **53**, 1291.

80. Komaki-Yasuda, K *et al.* (2003) Disruption of the *P. falciparum* 2-Cys peroxiredoxin gene renders parasites hypersensitive to reactive O_2 and N_2 species. *FEBS Lett.* **547**, 140.

81. Clark, IA *et al.* (1984) Radical-mediated damage to parasites and erythrocytes in P. vinckei infected mice after injection of t-butyl hydroperoxide. *Clin. Exp. Immunol.* **56**, 524.

82. Eckstein-Ludwig, U *et al.* (2003) Artemisinins target the SERCA of *P.falciparum*. *Nature* **424**, 957.

83. Vippagunta, SR *et al.* (1999) Deferoxamine: stimulation of hematin polymerization and antagonism of its inhibition by chloroquine. *Biochem. Pharmacol.* **58**, 817.

84. Griffiths, G *et al.* (2000) Lipid hydroperoxide levels in plant tissues. *J. Exp. Bot.* **51**, 1363.

85. Neill, SJ *et al.* (2002) H_2O_2 and NO$^{\bullet}$ as signalling molecules in plants. *J. Exp. Bot.* **53**, 1237.

86. Vanin, AF *et al.* (2004) Endogenous $O_2^{\bullet-}$ production and the NO_2^-/NO_3^- ratio control the concentration of bioavailable free NO$^{\bullet}$ in leaves. *J. Biol. Chem.* **279**, 24100.

87. Lamotte, O *et al.* (2005) NO$^{\bullet}$ in plants: the biosynthesis and cell signalling properties of a fascinating molecule. *Planta* **221**, 1.

88. Veljovic-Jovanovic, S *et al.* (2002) Are leaf H_2O_2 concentrations commonly overestimated? The potential influence of artefactual interference by tissue phenolics and ascorbate. *Plant Physiol. Biochem.* **40**, 501.

89. Thoma, I *et al.* (2004) The isoprostanoid pathway in plants. *Chem. Phys. Lipids* **128**, 135.

90. Umbach, AL *et al.* (2005) Characterization of transformed *Arabidopsis* with altered alternative oxidase levels and analysis of effects of ROS in tissue. *Plant Physiol.* **139**, 1806.

91. Considine, MJ *et al.* (2003) $O_2^{\bullet-}$ stimulates a proton leak in potato mitochondria that is related to the activity of uncoupling protein. *J. Biol. Chem.* **278**, 22298.

92. Woo, EJ *et al.* (2000) Germin is a Mn containing homohexamer with oxalate oxidase and SOD activities. *Nature Struct. Biol.* **7**, 1036.

93. Ferreira, KN *et al.* (2004) Architecture of the photosynthetic O_2-evolving center. *Science* **303**, 1831.

94. Szabó, I *et al.* (2005) Light and oxygenic photosynthesis: energy dissipation as a protection mechanism against photo-oxidation. *EMBO Rep.* **6**, 629.

95. Iwata, S and Barber, J (2004) Structure of photosystem II and molecular architecture of the O_2-evolving centre. *Curr. Opin. Struct. Biol.* **14**, 447.

96. Halliwell, B (1987) Oxidative damage, lipid peroxidation and antioxidant protection in chloroplasts. *Chem. Phys. Lipids* **44**, 327.

97. Pospíšil, P *et al.* (2004) OH$^\bullet$ generation by photo-system II. *Biochemistry* **43**, 6783.

98. Johansson, E *et al.* (2004) Progression and specificity of protein oxidation in the life cycle of *Arabidopsis thaliana*. *J. Biol. Chem.* **279**, 22204.

99. Berenbaum, M (1995) Phototoxicity of plant secondary metabolites: insect and mammalian perspectives. *Arch. Insect. Biochem. Physiol.* **29**, 119.

100. Ehrenshaft, M *et al.* (1998) SOR1, a gene required for photosensitizer and singlet O_2 resistance in *Cercospora* fungi, is highly conserved in divergent organisms. *Mol. Cell* **1**, 603.

101. Bilski, P *et al.* (2000) Vitamin B$_6$ (pyridoxine) and its derivatives are efficient singlet O_2 quenchers and potential fungal antioxidants. *Photochem. Photobiol.* **71**, 129.

102. Van Wuytswinkel, O *et al.* (1999) Fe homeostasis alteration in transgenic tobacco overexpressing ferritin. *Plant J.* **17**, 93.

103. Kampfenkel, K *et al.* (1995) Effects of Fe excess on *N. plumbaginifolia* plants. *Plant Physiol.* **107**, 725.

104. Liu, Z *et al.* (2004) Crystal structure of spinach major light-harvesting complex at 2.72 Å resolution. *Nature* **428**, 287.

105. Baroli, I *et al.* (2004) Photo-oxidative stress in a xanthophyll-deficient mutant of *Chlamydomonas*. *J. Biol. Chem.* **279**, 6337.

106. Alscher, RG *et al.* (2002) Role of SODs in controlling oxidative stress in plants. *J. Exp. Bot.* **53**, 1331.

107. Chu, CC *et al.* (2005) A CCS that confers three types of CuZnSOD activity in Arabidopsis. *Plant Physiol.* **139**, 425.

108. Smith, IK *et al.* (1994) Increased levels of GSH in a catalase-deficient mutant of barley (*Hordeum vulgare L*). *Plant Sci. Lett.* **37**, 29.

109. Rodriguez Milla, MA *et al.* (2003) GSH peroxidase genes in *Arabidopsis* are ubiquitous and regulated by abiotic stresses through diverse signaling pathways. *Plant J.* **36**, 602.

110. Herbette, S *et al.* (2002) Two GPX-like proteins from *Lycopersicon esculentum* and *Helianthus annuus* are antioxidant enzymes with PHGPx and thioredoxin peroxidase activities. *Eur. J. Biochem.* **269**, 2414.

111. Edwards, R *et al.* (2000) Plant GSTs; enzymes with multiple functions in sickness and in health. *Trends Plant Sci.* **5**, 193.

112. Rouhier, N and Jacquot, JP (2005) The plant multigenic family of thiol peroxidases. *Free Rad. Biol. Med.* **38**, 1413.

113. Iigusa, H *et al.* (2005) O_2 and H_2O_2 enhance light-induced carotenoid synthesis in *Neurospora crassa*. *FEBS Lett.* **579**, 4012.

114. Foyer, CH and Noctor, G (2005) Oxidant and antioxidant signalling in plants: a re-evaluation of the concept of oxidative stress in a physiological context. *Plant Cell Envir.* **28**, 1056.

115. Miyake, C and Asada, K (1996) Inactivation mechanisms of ascorbate peroxidase at low concentrations of ascorbate; H_2O_2 decomposes compound I of ascorbate peroxidase. *Plant Cell Physiol.* **37**, 423.

116. Ogawa, K (2005) GSH-associated regulation of plant growth and stress responses. *Antiox. Redox Signal.* **7**, 973.

117. Hancock, RD and Viola, R (2005) Biosynthesis and catabolism of L-ascorbic acid in plants. *Crit. Rev. Plant Sci.* **24**, 167.

118. Yamamoto, A *et al.* (2005) Suppressed expression of the apoplastic ascorbate oxidase gene increases salt tolerance in tobacco and *Arabidopsis* plants. *J. Exp. Bot.* **56**, 1785.

119. Cahoon, EB *et al.* (2003) Metabolic redesign of vitamin E biosynthesis in plants for tocotrienol production and increased antioxidant content. *Nature Biotechnol.* **21**, 1082.

120. Kanwischer, M *et al.* (2005) Alterations in tocopherol cyclase activity in transgenic and mutant plants of *Arabidopsis* affect tocopherol content, tocopherol composition, and oxidative stress. *Plant Physiol.* **137**, 713.

121. Trebst, A *et al.* (2002) A specific role for tocopherol and of chemical $^1O_2$ quenchers in the maintenance of photosystem II structure and function in *Chlamydomonas reinhardtii*. *FEBS Lett.* **516**, 156.

122. Hundal, T *et al.* (1995) Antioxidant activity of reduced plastoquinone in chloroplast thylakoid membranes. *Arch. Biochem. Biophys.* **324**, 117.

123. Aro, EM *et al.* (1993) Photoinhibition of PSII. Inactivation, protein damage and turnover. *Biochim. Biophys. Acta* **1143**, 113.

124. Kimura, S *et al.* (2004) DNA repair in higher plants; photoreactivation is the major DNA repair pathway in non-proliferating cells while excision repair (nucleotide excision repair and base excision repair) is active in proliferating cells. *Nucleic Acids Res.* **32**, 2760.

125. Romero, HM *et al.* (2004) Investigations into the role of the plastidial peptide methionine sulfoxide reductase in response to oxidative stress in *Arabidopsis*. *Plant Physiol.* **136**, 3784.

126. Moreau, S *et al.* (1996) Leghemoglobin-derived radicals. Evidence for multiple protein-derived radicals and the initiation of peribacteroid membrane damage. *J. Biol. Chem.* **271**, 32557.

127. Groten, K *et al.* (2005) The roles of redox processes in pea nodule development and senescence. *Plant Cell Envir.* **28**, 1293.

128. Nakamura, A *et al.* (2000) Peroxidative formation of lipid hydroperoxides in etiolated leaves. *Pestic. Biochem. Physiol.* **66**, 206.

129. Calderbank, A (1968) The bipyridylium herbicides. *Adv. Pest Control Res.* **8**, 127.

130. Kingston-Smith, AH and Foyer, CH (2000) Bundle sheath proteins are more sensitive to oxidative damage than those of the mesophyll in maize leaves exposed to paraquat or low temperatures. *J. Exp. Bot.* **51**, 123.

131. Taylor, NL *et al.* (2002) Environmental stress causes oxidative damage to plant mitochondria leading to inhibition of glycine decarboxylase. *J. Biol. Chem.* **277**, 42663.

132. Harper, DB and Harvey, BMR (1978) Mechanisms of paraquat tolerance in perennial ryegrass. Role of SOD, catalase and peroxidase. *Plant Cell Envir.* **1**, 211.

133. Van Breusegem, F *et al.* (2001) The role of ROS in plant signal transduction. *Plant. Sci.* **161**, 405.

134. Murgia, I *et al.* (2004) *A. thaliana* plants over-expressing thylakoidal ascorbate peroxidase show increased resistance to paraquat-induced photo-oxidative stress and to NO$^\bullet$-induced cell death. *Plant J.* **38**, 940.

135. Miyagawa, Y *et al.* (2000) Evaluation of the defense system in chloroplasts to photooxidative stress caused by paraquat using transgenic tobacco plants expressing catalase from *E. coli*. *Plant Cell Physiol.* **41**, 311.

136. Allen, RD (1995) Dissection of oxidative stress tolerance using transgenic plants. *Plant Physiol.* **107**, 1049.

137. Shen, B *et al.* (1997) Increased resistance to oxidative stress in transgenic plants by targeting mannitol biosynthesis to chloroplasts. *Plant Physiol.* **113**, 1177.

138. Zer, H *et al.* (1994) The protective effect of desferrioxamine on paraquat-treated pea (*Pisum sativum*). *Physiol. Plant.* **92**, 437.

139. Babbs, CF *et al.* (1989) Lethal OH$^\bullet$ production in paraquat-treated plants. *Plant Physiol.* **90**, 1267.

140. Stancliffe, TC and Pirie, A (1971) The production of $O_2^{\bullet-}$ radicals in reactions of the herbicide diquat. *FEBS Lett.* **17**, 297.

141. Floyd, RA *et al.* (1989) Increased 8OHdG content of chloroplast DNA from O_3-treated plants. *Plant Physiol.* **91**, 644.

142. Bowler, C and Fluhr, R (2000) The role of Ca^{2+} and activated O_2 as signals for controlling cross-tolerance. *Trends Plant Sci.* **5**, 241.

143. Sanmartin, M *et al.* (2003) Over-expression of ascorbate oxidase in the apoplast of transgenic tobacco results in altered ascorbate and GSH redox states and increased sensitivity to O_3. *Planta* **216**, 918.

144. Conklin, PL (2001) Recent advances in the role and biosynthesis of ascorbic acid in plants. *Plant Cell Envir.* **24**, 383.

145. Loreto, F and Velikova, V (2001) Isoprene produced by leaves protects the photosynthetic apparatus against O_3 damage, quenches O_3 products, and reduces lipid peroxidation of cellular membranes. *Plant Physiol.* **127**, 1781.

146. Cooney, RV *et al.* (1993) γ-Tocopherol detoxification of NO_2: superiority to α-tocopherol. *Proc. Natl. Acad. Sci. USA* **90**, 1771.

147. Rabinowitch, HD and Fridovich, I (1995) Growth of *Chlorella sorokiniana* in the presence of sulfite elevates cell content of SOD and imparts resistance towards paraquat. *Planta* **164**, 524.

148. Smirnoff, N (2000) Ascorbic acid: metabolism and functions of a multi-facetted molecule. *Curr. Opin. Plant Biol.* **3**, 229.

149. Feierabend, J *et al.* (1992) Photoinactivation of catalase occurs under both high- and low-temperature stress conditions and accompanies photoinhibition of PSII. *Plant Physiol.* **100**, 1554.

150. Ma, F and Cheng, L (2003) The sun-exposed peel of apple fruit has higher xanthophyll cycle-dependent thermal dissipation and antioxidants of the ascorbate-GSH pathway than the shaded peel. *Plant Sci.* **165**, 819.

151. Im, YJ *et al.* (2005) Production of a thermostable archaeal SOR in plant cells. *FEBS Lett.* **579**, 5521.

152. Wise, RR (1995) Chilling-enhanced photooxidation: the production, action and study of ROS produced during chilling in the light. *Photosynth. Res.* **45**, 79.

153. Kerdnaimongkol, K and Woodson, WR (1999) Inhibition of catalase by antisense RNA increases susceptibility to oxidative stress and chilling injury in transgenic tomato plants. *J. Amer. Soc. Hort. Sci.* **124**, 330.

154. Kranner, I and Birtić, S (2005) A modulating role for antioxidants in desiccation tolerance. *Intergr. Comp. Biol.* **45**, 734.

155. Munné-Bosch, S *et al.* (1999) Enhanced formation of α-tocopherol and highly oxidized abietane diterpenes in water-stressed rosemary plants. *Plant Physiol.* **121**, 1047.

156. McKersie, BD *et al.* (1996) Water-deficit tolerance and field performance of transgenic alfalfa over-expressing SOD. *Plant Physiol.* **111**, 1177.

157. Leprince, O *et al.* (1993) The mechanisms of desiccation tolerance in developing seeds. *Seed Sci. Res.* **3**, 231.

158. Hendry, GAF (1993) Oxygen, free radical processes and seed longevity. *Seed Sci. Res.* **3**, 141.

159. Downs, CA *et al.* (2002) Oxidative stress and seasonal coral bleaching. *Free Rad. Biol. Med.* **33**, 533.

160. Yamasaki, Y *et al.* (2004) Production of $O_2^{\bullet-}$ and H_2O_2 by the red tide dinoflagellate *Karenia mikimotoi*. *J. Biosci. Bioeng.* **97**, 212.

161. Bloemendal, H *et al.* (2004) Ageing and vision: structure, stability and function of lens crystallins. *Prog. Biophys. Mol. Biol.* **86**, 407.

162. Parker, NR *et al.* (2004) Protein-bound kynurenine is a photosensitizer of oxidative damage. *Free Rad. Biol. Med.* **37**, 1479.

163. Molnár, GA *et al.* (2005) Accumulation of the OH$^{\bullet}$ markers *meta-*, *ortho*-tyrosine and DOPA in cataractous lenses is accompanied by a lower protein and phenylalanine content of the H_2O-soluble phase. *Free Radic. Res.* **39**, 1359.

164. Ma, W *et al.* (2004) The effect of stress withdrawal on gene expression and certain biochemical and cell biological properties of peroxide-conditioned cell lines. *FASEB J.* **18**, 480.

165. Hahn, P *et al.* (2004) Disruption of ceruloplasmin and hephaestin in mice causes retinal Fe overload and retinal degeneration with features of age-related macular degeneration. *Proc. Natl. Acad. Sci. USA* **101**, 13850.

166. Hahn, P *et al.* (2003) Maculas affected by age-related macular degeneration contain increased chelatable Fe in the retinal pigment epithelium and Bruch's membrane. *Arch. Ophthalmol.* **121**, 1099.

167. Garner, B *et al.* (2000) Formation of OH$^{\bullet}$ in the human lens is related to the severity of nuclear cataract. *Exp. Eye Res.* **70**, 81.

168. Spector, A (1995) Oxidative stress-induced cataract: mechanism of action. *FASEB J.* **9**, 1173.

169. Nourooz-Zadeh, J and Pereira, P (2000) F_2-IPs, potential specific markers of oxidative damage in human retina. *Ophthal. Res.* **32**, 133.

170. Koliakos, GG *et al.* (2003) 8-Isoprostaglandin F2α and ascorbic acid concentration in the aqueous humour of patients with exfoliation syndrome. *Br. J. Ophthalmol.* **87**, 353.

171. Mukherjee, PK *et al.* (2004) Neuroprotectin D1: a DHA-derived docosatriene protects human retinal pigment epithelial cells from oxidative stress. *Proc. Natl. Acad. Sci. USA* **101**, 8491.

172. Sun, H and Nathans, J (2001) ABCR, the ATP-binding cassette transporter responsible for Stargardt macular dystrophy, is an efficient target of all-*trans*-retinal-mediated photooxidative damage *in vitro*. *J. Biol. Chem.* **276**, 11766.

173. Tamai, K *et al.* (2002) Lipid hydroperoxide stimulates subretinal choroidal neovascularization in the rabbit. *Exp. Eye Res.* **74**, 301.

174. Newsome, DA *et al.* (1994) Antioxidants in the retinal pigment epithelium. *Prog. Ret. Eye Res.* **13**, 101.

175. Sparrow, JR *et al.* (2003) A2E-epoxides damage DNA in retinal pigment epithelial cells. *J. Biol. Chem.* **278**, 18207.

176. Choy, CK *et al.* (2000) Ascorbic acid concentration and total antioxidant activity of human tear fluid measured using the FRASC assay. *Invest. Ophthalmol. Vis. Sci.* **41**, 3293.

177. Boonstra, A and Kijlstra, A (1984) The identification of transferrin, an Fe-binding protein in rabbit tears. *Exp. Eye Res.* **38**, 561.

178. Kuizenga, A *et al.* (1987) Inhibition of OH$^{\bullet}$ formation by human tears. *Invest. Ophthalmol. Vis. Sci.* **28**, 305.

179. Breusted, DA *et al.* (2005) The 1.8-Å crystal structure of human tear lipocalin reveals an extended branched cavity with capacity for multiple ligands. *J. Biol. Chem.* **280**, 484.

180. Balasubramanian, D (2005) Photodynamics of cataract: an update on endogenous chromophores and antioxidants. *Photochem. Photobiol.* **81**, 498.

181. Linsenmayer, TF *et al.* (2005) Nuclear ferritin in corneal epithelial cells: tissue-specific nuclear transport and protection from UV-damage. *Prog. Retin. Eye Res.* **24**, 139.

182. Sastre, J *et al.* (2005) Age-associated oxidative damage leads to absence of γ-cystathionase in over 50% of rat lenses: relevance in cataractogenesis. *Free Rad. Biol. Med.* **38**, 575.

183. Wolf, N *et al.* (2005) Age-related cataract progression in five mouse models for antioxidant protection or hormonal influence. *Exp. Eye Res.* **81**, 276.

184. Lou, MF (2003) Redox regulation in the lens. *Prog. Retin. Eye Res.* **22**, 657.

185. Maeda, A *et al.* (2005) Microsomal GST1 in the RPE: protection against oxidative stress and a potential role in aging. *Biochemistry* **44**, 480.

186. Sandbach, JM *et al.* (2001) Ocular pathology in mitochondrial SOD (Sod2)-deficient mice. *Invest. Ophthalmol. Vis. Sci.* **42**, 2173.

187. Takata, I *et al.* (1996) Glycated CuZnSOD in rat lenses: evidence for the presence of fragmentation *in vivo*. *Biochem. Biophys. Res. Commun.* **219**, 243.

188. Bennaars-Eiden, A *et al.* (2002) Covalent modification of epithelial fatty acid-binding protein by 4-HNE *in vitro* and *in vivo*. *J. Biol. Chem.* **277**, 50693.

189. Taylor, A (1993) Cataract: relationship between nutrition and oxidation. *J. Am. Coll. Nutr.* **12**, 138.

190. Ringvold, A *et al.* (1998) Ascorbate in the corneal epithelium of diurnal and nocturnal species. *Invest. Ophthalmol. Vis. Sci.* **39**, 2774.

191. Ohta, Y *et al.* (2002) Prolonged marginal ascorbic acid deficiency induces oxidative stress in retina of guinea pigs. *Int. J. Vitam. Nutr. Res.* **72**, 63.

192. Cheng, R *et al.* (2001) Similarity of the yellow chromophores isolated from human cataracts with those from ascorbic acid-modified calf lens proteins: evidence for ascorbic acid glycation during cataract formation. *Biochim. Biophys. Acta* **1537**, 14.

193. Kutty, RK *et al.* (1995) Induction of HO-1 in the retina by intense visible light: suppression by the antioxidant DMTU. *Proc. Natl. Acad. Sci. USA* **92**, 1177.

194. McGahan, MC and Fleischer, LN (1986) A micromethod for the determination of Fe^{2+} and total Fe-binding capacity in intraocular fluids and plasma using electrothermal atomic absorption spectroscopy. *Anal. Biochem.* **156**, 397.

195. Chen, W *et al.* (1998) Expression of the protective proteins hemopexin and haptoglobin by cells of the neural retina. *Exp. Eye Res.* **67**, 83.

196. Marchetti, MA *et al.* (2005) Methionine sulfoxide reductases B1, B2 and B3 are present in the human lens and confer oxidative stress resistance to lens cells. *Invest. Ophthalmol.* **46**, 2107.

197. Caballero, M *et al.* (2004) Effects of donor age on proteasome activity and senescence in trabecular meshwork cells. *Biochem. Biophys. Res. Comm.* **323**, 1048.

198. Pittman, KM *et al.* (2002) Nitration of MnSOD during ocular inflammation. *Exp. Eye Res.* **74**, 463.

199. Kirschfeld, K (1982) Carotenoid pigments: their possible role in protecting against photo-oxidation in eyes and photoreceptor cells. *Proc. Roy. Soc. Lond.* **B216**, 71.

200. Schupp, C *et al.* (2004) Lutein, zeaxanthin, macular pigment, and visual function in adult cystic fibrosis patients. *Am. J. Clin. Nutr.* **79**, 1045.

201. Leung, I *et al.* (2001) Absorption and tissue distribution of zeaxanthin and lutein in rhesus monkeys after taking *Fructus lycii* (Gou Qi Zi) extract. *Invest. Ophthalmol. Vis. Sci.* **42**, 466.

202. Meyer, CH and Sekundo, W (2005) Nutritional supplementation to prevent cataract formation. *Dev. Ophthalmol.* **38**, 103.

203. Mares, JA (2004) High-dose antioxidant supplementation and cataract risk. *Nutr. Rev.* **62**, 28.

204. Bessler, NM (2004) Verteporfin therapy in age-related macular degeneration (VAM): an open-label multicenter photodynamic therapy study of 4435 patients. *Retina* **24**, 512.

205. Aitken, RJ and Baker, MA (2006) Oxidative stress, sperm survival and fertility control. *Mol. Cell Endocrinol.* **250**, 66.

206. Sikka, SC (2004) Role of oxidative stress and antioxidants in andrology and assisted reproductive technology. *J. Androl.* **25**, 5.

207. Brouwers, JF and Gadella, BM (2003) *In situ* detection and localization of lipid peroxidation in individual bovine sperm cells. *Free Rad. Biol. Med.* **35**, 1382.

208. Loft, S *et al.* (2003) Oxidative DNA damage in human sperm influences time to pregnancy. *Hum. Reprod.* **18**, 1265.

209. Ford, WCI (2004) Regulation of sperm function by ROS. *Hum. Reprod. Update* **10**, 387.

210. Herrero, MB *et al.* (2001) Tyrosine nitration in human spermatozoa: a physiological function of $ONOO^-$, the reaction product of $NO^•$ and $O_2^{•-}$. *Mol. Hum. Reprod.* **7**, 913.

211. Ishii, T *et al.* (2005) Accelerated impairment of spermatogenic cells in SOD1-knockout mice under heat stress. *Free Radic. Res.* **39**, 697.

212. Agarwal, A *et al.* (2005) Role of oxidative stress in female reproduction. *Reprod. Biol. Endocrinol.* **3**, 28.

213. Ho, YS *et al.* (1998) Reduced fertility in female mice lacking CuZnSOD. *J. Biol. Chem.* **273**, 7765.

214. Smith, WL and Langenbach, R (2001) Why there are two COX isozymes. *J. Clin. Invest.* **107**, 1491.

215. Wai-sum, O *et al.* (2006) Male genital tract antioxidant enzymes – their ability to preserve sperm DNA integrity. *Mol. Cell Endocrinol.* **250**, 80.

216. Raijmakers, MT *et al.* (2003) GSH and GSTs A1–1 and P1–1 in seminal plasma may play a role in protecting against oxidative damage to spermatozoa. *Fertil. Steril.* **79**, 169.

217. Kikuchi, M *et al.* (2003) Seminal plasma lactoferrin but not transferrin reflects gonadal function in dogs. *J. Vet. Med. Sci.* **65**, 679.

218. Sanocka, D *et al.* (2003) Male genital tract inflammation: The role of selected interleukins in regulation of pro-oxidant and antioxidant enzymatic substances in seminal plasma. *J. Androl.* **24**, 448.

219. Bender, HS *et al.* (1988) Effects of gossypol on the antioxidant defense system of the rat testis. *Arch. Androl.* **21**, 59.

220. Baumgrass, R *et al.* (2001) Reversible inhibition of calcineurin by the polyphenolic aldehyde gossypol. *J. Biol. Chem.* **276**, 47914.

221. Nakai, N *et al.* (2003) Oxidative DNA damage induced by toluene is involved in its male reproductive toxicity. *Free Radic. Res.* **37**, 69.

222. Guérin, P *et al.* (2001) Oxidative stress and protection against ROS in the pre-implantation embryo and its surroundings. *Hum. Reprod. Update* **7**, 175.

223. Hempstock, J *et al.* (2003) The contribution of placental oxidative stress to early pregnancy failure. *Hum. Pathol.* **34**, 1265.

224. Matsuoka, I *et al.* (1995) Impact of erythrocytes on mouse embryonal development *in vitro. FEBS Lett.* **371**, 297.

225. Nasr-Esfahani, M *et al.* (1991) The origin of ROS in mouse embryos cultured *in vitro. Development* **113**, 551.

226. Pierce, GB *et al.* (1991) H_2O_2 as a mediator of programmed cell death in the blastocyst. *Differentiation* **46**, 181.

227. Gazzolo, D *et al.* (2005) Non protein bound Fe concentrations in amniotic fluid. *Clin. Biochem.* **38**, 674.

228. Avissar, N *et al.* (1994) Human placenta makes extracellular GPx and secretes it into maternal circulation. *Am. J. Physiol.* **267**, E68

229. Hammer, A *et al.* (2001) MPO-dependent generation of OCl^--modified proteins in human placental tissues during normal pregnancy. *Lab. Invest.* **81**, 543.

230. Hnat, MD *et al.* (2005) Hsp-70 and 4HNE adducts in human placental villous tissue of normotensive, preeclamptic and intrauterine growth restricted pregnancies. *Am. J. Obst. Gynecol.* **193**, 836.

231. Poston, L *et al.* (2006) Vitamin C and Vitamin E in pregnant women at risk for pre-eclampsia (VIP trial): randomized placebo-controlled trial. *Lancet* **367**, 1145.

232. Poston, L and Raijmakers, MT (2004) Trophoblast oxidative stress, antioxidants and pregnancy outcome—a review. *Placenta* **25** (Suppl 1), S72.

233. Casanueva, E *et al.* (2005) Vitamin C supplementation to prevent premature rupture of the chorioamniotic membranes: a randomized trial. *Am. J. Clin. Nutr.* **81**, 859.

234. Regan, CL *et al.* (2001) No evidence for lipid peroxidation in severe preeclampsia. *Am. J. Obstet. Gynecol.* **185**, 572.

235. Moretti, M *et al.* (2004) Increased breath markers of oxidative stress in normal pregnancy and in pre-eclampsia. *Am. J. Obstet. Gynecol.* **190**, 1184.

236. Ishihara, O *et al.* (2004) IPs, prostaglandins and tocopherols in pre-eclampsia, normal pregnancy and non-pregnancy. *Free Radic. Res.* **38**, 913.

237. Shibata, E *et al.* (2003) Enhancement of mitochondrial oxidative stress and up-regulation of antioxidant protein peroxiredoxin III/SP-22 in the mitochondria of human pre-eclamptic placentae. *Placenta* **24**, 698.

238. Longini, M *et al.* (2005) IPs in amniotic fluid: a predictive marker for fetal growth restriction in pregnancy. *Free Rad. Biol. Med.* **38**, 1537.

239. Wells, PG and Winn, LM (1996) Biochemical toxicology of chemical teratogenesis. *Crit. Rev. Biochem. Mol. Biol.* **31**, 1.

240. Wentzel, P and Eriksson, UJ (2002) 8-Iso-$PGF_{2\alpha}$ administration generates dysmorphogenesis and increased lipid peroxidation in rat embryos *in vitro. Teratology* **66**, 164.

241. Hagay, ZJ *et al.* (1995) Prevention of diabetes-associated embryopathy by overexpression of the free radical scavenger CuZnSOD in transgenic mouse embryos. *Am. J. Obstet. Gynecol.* **173**, 1036.

242. Hansen, JM and Harris, C (2004) A novel hypothesis for thalidomide-induced limb teratogenesis: redox misregulation of the NF-κB pathway. *Antiox. Redox Signal.* **6**, 1.

243. Wan, H *et al.* (2004) *Foxa2* is required for transition to air breathing at birth. *Proc. Natl. Acad. Sci. USA* **101**, 14449.

244. Kaarteenaho-Wilk, R and Kinnula, VL (2004) Distribution of antioxidant enzymes in developing human lung, respiratory distress syndrome, and bronchopulmonary dysplasia. *J. Histochem. Cytochem.* **52**, 1231.

245. Archer, SL *et al.* (2004) O_2 sensing in the human ductus arteriosus: redox-sensitive K^+ channels are regulated by mitochondria-derived H_2O_2. *Biol. Chem.* **385**, 205.

246. Brennan, LA *et al.* (2003) Increased $O_2^{\bullet -}$ generation is associated with pulmonary hypertension in fetal lambs: a role for NADPH oxidase. *Circ. Res.* **92**, 683.

247. Comporti, M *et al.* (2004) Plasma F_2-IPs are elevated in newborns and inversely correlated to gestational age. *Free Rad. Biol. Med.* **37**, 724.

248. Brault, S *et al.* (2004) Cytotoxicity of the E_2-IP 15-E_{2T}-IsoP on oligodendrocyte progenitors. *Free Rad. Biol. Med.* **37**, 358.

249. Back, SA *et al.* (2005) Selective vulnerability of preterm white matter to oxidative damage defined by F_2-IPs. *Ann. Neurol.* **58**, 108.

250. Tsukahara, H *et al.* (2004) Oxidative stress in neonates: evaluation using specific biomarkers. *Life Sci.* **75**, 933

251. Sullivan, JL (1988) Fe, plasma antioxidants, and the 'O_2 radical disease of prematurity'. *Am. J. Dis. Child* **142**, 1341.

252. Quiles, JL *et al.* (2006) Coenzyme Q concentration and total antioxidant capacity of human milk at

different stages of lactation in mothers of preterm and full-term infants. *Free Radic. Res.* **40**, 199.

253. Karg, E *et al.* (2001) Ferroxidases and XO in plasma of healthy newborn infants. *Free Radic. Res.* **35**, 555.

254. Welty, SE (2003) Antioxidants and oxidations in bronchopulmonary dysplasia: there are no easy answers. *J. Pediatr.* **143**, 697.

255. Davis, JM *et al.* (2003) Pulmonary outcome at 1 year corrected age in premature infants treated at birth with recombinant human CuZnSOD. *Pediatrics* **111**, 469.

256. Moison, RMW *et al.* (1993) Induction of lipid peroxidation of pulmonary surfactant by plasma of preterm babies. *Lancet* **341**, 79.

257. Evans, PJ *et al.* (1992) Bleomycin-detectable Fe in the plasma of premature and full-term neonates. *FEBS Lett.* **303**, 210.

258. Hirano, K *et al.* (2001) Blood transfusion increases radical promoting non-transferrin bound Fe in preterm infants. *Arch. Dis. Child* **84**, F188.

259. Yu, T *et al.* (2003) Effect of asphyxia on non-protein-bound Fe and lipid peroxidation in newborn infants. *Dev. Med. Child Neurol.* **45**, 24.

260. Ogihara, T *et al.* (2003) Non-protein-bound transition metals and OH$^•$ generation in CSF of newborn infants with hypoxic ischemic encephalopathy. *Pediatr. Res.* **53**, 594.

261. Jain, SK (1989) The neonatal erythrocyte and its oxidative susceptibility. *Semin. Hematol.* **26**, 286.

262. Ciccoli, L *et al.* (2003) Fe release in erythrocytes and plasma non protein-bound Fe in hypoxic and non hypoxic newborns. *Free Radic. Res.* **37**, 51.

263. Picaud, JC *et al.* (2004) Lipid peroxidation assessment by MDA measurement in parenteral nutrition solutions for newborn infants: a pilot study. *Acta Paediatr.* **93**, 241.

264. Chessex, P *et al.* (2001) Photoprotection of solutions of parenteral nutrition decreases the infused load as well as the urinary excretion of peroxides in premature infants. *Semin. Perinatol.* **25**, 55.

265. Massarenti, P *et al.* (2004) 4-HNE is markedly higher in patients on a standard long-term home parenteral nutrition. *Free Radic. Res.* **38**, 73.

266. Tan, S *et al.* (1996) Maternal infusion of antioxidants (Trolox and ascorbic acid) protects the fetal heart in rabbit fetal hypoxia. *Pediatr. Res.* **39**, 499.

267. Shoji, H *et al.* (2003) Effect of human breast milk on urinary 8OHdG excretion in infants. *Pediatr. Res.* **53**, 850.

268. Chamulitrat, W *et al.* (2004) A constitutive NADPH oxidase-like system containing gp91*phox* homologs in human keratinocytes. *J. Invest. Dermatol.* **122**, 1000.

269. Schmid-Grendelmeier, P *et al.* (2005) IgE-mediated and T cell-mediated auto-immunity against MnSOD in atopic dermatitis. *J. Allerg. Clin. Immunol.* **115**, 1068.

270. Gutteridge, JMC *et al.* (1985) Cu and Fe complexes catalytic for O_2 radical reactions in sweat from human athletes. *Clin. Chim. Acta* **145**, 267.

271. Wondrak, GT *et al.* (2004) 3-Hydroxypyridine chromophores are endogenous sensitizers of photooxidative stress in human skin cells. *J. Biol. Chem.* **279**, 30009.

272. Anonymous (1996) Phototoxic celery. *Lancet* **348**, 742.

273. Anderson, RR (2004) Shedding some light on tattoos? *Photochem. Photobiol.* **80**, 155.

274. Nishigori, C *et al.* (2004) Role of ROS in skin carcinogenesis. *Antiox. Redox Signal.* **6**, 561.

275. Møller, P *et al.* (2002) Sunlight-induced DNA damage in human mononuclear cells. *FASEB J.* **16**, 45.

276. Berneburg, M *et al.* (2004) Induction of the photoaging-associated mitochondrial common deletion *in vivo* in normal human skin. *J. Invest. Dermatol.* **122**, 1277.

277. Yamazaki, S *et al.* (1999) Cholesterol 7-hydroperoxides in rat skin as a marker for lipid peroxidation. *Biochem. Pharmacol.* **58**, 1415.

278. Tanaka, N *et al.* (2001) Immunohistochemical detection of lipid peroxidation products, protein-bound acrolein and 4-HNE protein adducts, in actinic elastosis of photodamaged skin. *Arch. Dermatol. Res.* **293**, 363.

279. Kunisada, M *et al.* (2005) 8OHdG formation induced by chronic UVB exposure makes *ogg1* knockout mice susceptible to skin carcinogenesis. *Cancer Res.* **65**, 6006.

280. Luo, JL *et al.* (2001) UV-induced DNA damage and mutations in Hupki (human p53 knock-in) mice recapitulate p53 hotspot alterations in sun-exposed human skin. *Cancer Res.* **61**, 8158.

281. Tyrrell, RM (2004) Solar UVA radiation: an oxidizing skin carcinogen that activates HO-1. *Antiox. Redox Signal.* **6**, 835.

282. Reelfs, O *et al.* (2004) UVA radiation-induced immediate Fe release is a key modulator of the activation of NF-κB in human skin fibroblasts. *J. Invest. Dermatol.* **122**, 1440.

283. Bissett, DL *et al.* (1991) Chronic UV radiation-induced increase in skin Fe and the photoprotective effect of topically applied Fe chelators. *Photochem. Photobiol.* **54**, 215.

284. Trouba, KJ *et al.* (2002) Oxidative stress and its role in skin disease. *Antiox. Redox Signal.* **4**, 665.

285. Chaudhari, U *et al*. (2001) Efficacy and safety of infliximab monotherapy for plaque-type psoriasis: a randomized trial. *Lancet* **357**, 1842.

286. Vyas, PM *et al*. (2005) ROS generation and its role in the differential cytotoxicity of the arylhydroxylamine metabolites of sulfamethoxazole and dapsone in normal human epidermal keratinocytes. *Biochem. Pharmacol.* **70**, 275.

287. Valacchi, G *et al*. (2003) Induction of stress proteins and MMP-9 by 0.8 ppm of O_3 in murine skin. *Biochem. Biophys. Res. Commun.* **305**, 741.

288. Brezová, V *et al*. (2005) ROS produced upon photoexcitation of sunscreens containing TiO_2 (an EPR study). *J. Photochem. Photobiol. B* **79**, 121.

289. Kramer-Stickland, K *et al*. (1999) UV-B-Induced photooxidation of vitamin E in mouse skin. *Chem. Res. Toxicol.* **12**, 187.

290. Kammeyer, A *et al*. (1999) Urocanic acid isomers are good $OH^\bullet$ scavengers: a comparative study with structural analogues and with uric acid. *Biochim. Biophys. Acta* **1428**, 117.

291. Rijken, F *et al*. (2004) Responses of black and white skin to solar-simulating radiation: differences in DNA photodamage, infiltrating neutrophils, proteolytic enzymes induced, keratinocyte activation, and IL-10 expression. *J. Invest. Dermatol.* **122**, 1448.

292. Hasse, S *et al*. (2004) Perturbed 6-tetrahydrobiopterin recycling via decreased dihydropteridine reductase in vitiligo: more evidence for H_2O_2 stress. *J. Invest. Dermatol.* **122**, 307.

293. Biesalski, HK and Obermueller-Jevic, UC (2001) UV light, β-carotene and human skin-beneficial and potentially harmful effects. *Arch. Biochem. Biophys.* **389**, 1.

294. Hemminki, K *et al*. (2002) Demonstration of UV-dimers in human skin DNA *in situ* 3 weeks after exposure. *Carcinogenesis* **23**, 605.

295. Shindo, Y *et al*. (1993) Antioxidant defense mechanisms in murine epidermis and dermis and their responses to UV light. *J Invest. Dermatol.* **100**, 260.

296. Thiele, JJ *et al*. (1999) Sebaceous gland secretion is a major physiologic route of vitamin E delivery to skin. *J. Invest. Dermatol.* **113**, 1006.

297. Hanada, K *et al*. (1998) Novel function of metallothionein in photoprotection: metallothionein-null mouse exhibits reduced tolerance against UV-B injury in the skin. *J. Invest. Dermatol.* **111**, 582.

298. Bulteau, AL *et al*. (2002) Impairment of proteasome function upon UVA- and UVB-irradiation of human keratinocytes. *Free Rad. Biol. Med.* **32**, 1157.

299. Wagener, FA *et al*. (2003) The heme-HO system: a molecular switch in wound healing. *Blood* **102**, 521.

300. Roy, S *et al*. (2006) Dermal wound healing is subject to redox control. *Mol. Ther.* **13**, 211.

301. Li, W *et al*. (2000) H_2O_2-mediated, lysyl-oxidase-dependent chemotaxis of vascular smooth muscle cells. *J. Cell. Biochem.* **78**, 550.

302. Shukla, A *et al*. (1997) Depletion of GSH, ascorbic acid, vitamin E and antioxidant defence enzymes in a healing cutaneous wound. *Free Radic. Res.* **26**, 93.

303. Hanselmann, C *et al*. (2001) HO-1: a novel player in cutaneous wound repair and psoriasis? *Biochem. J.* **353**, 459.

304. Luo, JD *et al*. (2004) Gene therapy of eNOS and MnSOD restores delayed wound healing in type 1 diabetic mice. *Circulation* **110**, 2484.

305. Musalmah, M *et al*. (2005) Comparative effects of palm vitamin E and α-tocopherol on healing and wound tissue antioxidant enzyme levels in diabetic rats. *Lipids* **40**, 575.

306. Wlaschek, M and Scharffetter-Kochanek, K (2005) Oxidative stress in chronic venous leg ulcers. *Wound Rep. Reg.* **13**, 452.

307. Taylor, JE *et al*. (2005) Extent of Fe pick-up in deferoxamine-coupled polyurethane materials for therapy of chronic wounds. *Biomaterials* **26**, 6024.

308. Horton, JW (2003) Free radicals and lipid peroxidation mediated injury in burn trauma: the role of antioxidant therapy. *Toxicology* **189**, 75.

309. Ritter, C *et al*. (2003) Plasma oxidative parameters and mortality in patients with severe burn injury. *Intensive Care Med.* **29**, 1380.

310. Vorauer-Uhl, K *et al*. (2002) Reepithelialization of experimental scalds effected by topically applied SOD: controlled animal studies. *Wound Rep. Reg.* **10**, 366.

311. Altavilla, D *et al*. (2005) Lipid peroxidation inhibition by raxofelast improves angiogenesis and wound healing in experimental burn wounds. *Shock* **24**, 85.

312. Saez, JC *et al*. (1984) $O_2^{\bullet-}$ radical involvement in the pathogenesis of burn shock. *Circ. Shock* **12**, 229.

313. Laufs, U *et al*. (2005) Physical inactivity increases oxidative stress, endothelial dysfunction, and atherosclerosis. *Arterio. Thromb. Vasc. Biol.* **25**, 809.

314. Powers, SK *et al*. (2005) Mechanisms of disuse muscle atrophy: role of oxidative stress. *Am. J. Physiol.* **288**, R337.

315. Davies, KJA *et al*. (1982) Free radicals and tissue damage produced by exercise. *Biochem. Biophys. Res. Commun.* **107**, 1198.

316. Witt, EF *et al.* (1992) Exercise, oxidative damage and effects of antioxidant manipulation. *J. Nutr.* **122** (3 Suppl.), 766.

317. Smith, JA *et al.* (1990) Exercise, training and neutrophil microbicidal activity. *Int. J. Sports Med.* **11**, 179.

318. Sen, CK (1995) Oxidants and antioxidants in exercise. *J. Appl. Physiol.* **79**, 675.

319. Leeuwenburgh, C and Heinecke, JW (2001) Oxidative stress and antioxidants in exercise. *Curr. Med. Chem.* **8**, 829.

320. Bloomer, RJ and Goldfarb, AH (2004) Anaerobic exercise and oxidative stress: a review. *Can. J. Appl. Physiol.* **29**, 245.

321. Mastaloudis, A *et al.* (2004) Antioxidant supplementation prevents exercise-induced lipid peroxidation, but not inflammation, in ultramarathon runners. *Free Rad. Biol. Med.* **36**, 1329.

322. Okamura, K *et al.* (1997) Effect of endurance exercise on the tissue 8OHdG content in dogs. *Free Radic. Res.* **26**, 523.

323. Poulsen, HE *et al.* (1996) Extreme exercise and oxidative DNA modification. *J. Sports Sci.* **14**, 343.

324. Sato, Y *et al.* (2003) Increase of human MTH1 and decrease of 8OHdG in leukocyte DNA by acute and chronic exercise in healthy male subjects. *Biochem. Biophys. Res. Commun.* **305**, 333.

325. McAnulty, S *et al.* (2005) Effect of resistance exercise and carbohydrate ingestion on oxidative stress. *Free Radic. Res.* **39**, 1219.

326. Goto, C *et al.* (2003) Effect of different intensities of exercise on endothelium-dependent vasodilation in humans. *Circulation* **108**, 530.

327. Hellsten, Y *et al.* (1997) Oxidation of urate in human skeletal muscle during exercise. *Free Rad. Biol. Med.* **22**, 169.

328. Waring, WS *et al.* (2003) Uric acid reduces exercise-induced oxidative stress in healthy adults. *Clin. Sci.* **105**, 425.

329. Close, GL *et al.* (2005) Microdialysis studies of EC ROS in skeletal muscle: factors influencing the reduction of cytochrome *c* and hydroxylation of salicylate. *Free Rad. Biol. Med.* **39**, 1460.

330. Xia, R *et al.* (2003) Skeletal muscle sarcoplasmic reticulum contains a NADH-dependent oxidase that generates $O_2^{\bullet-}$. *Am. J. Physiol.* **285**, C215.

331. Gomez-Cabrera, MC *et al.* (2005) Decreasing XO-mediated oxidative stress prevents useful cellular adaptations to exercise in rats. *J. Physiol.* **567**, 113.

332. Kinugawa, S *et al.* (2005) Limited exercise capacity in heterozygous MnSOD gene-knockout mice. *Circulation* **111**, 1480.

333. Reid, MB *et al.* (1994) *N*-Acetylcysteine inhibits muscle fatigue in humans. *J. Clin. Invest.* **94**, 2468.

334. Aoi, W *et al.* (2004) Oxidative stress and delayed-onset muscle damage after exercise. *Free Rad. Biol. Med.* **37**, 480.

335. McAnulty, SR *et al.* (2005) Effect of α-tocopherol supplementation on plasma homocysteine and oxidative stress in highly trained athletes before and after exhaustive exercise. *J. Nutr. Biochem.* **16**, 530.

336. Childs, A *et al.* (2001) Supplementation with vitamin C and *N*-acetyl-cysteine increases oxidative stress in humans after an acute muscle injury induced by eccentric exercise. *Free Rad. Biol. Med.* **31**, 745.

337. van Praag, H *et al.* (2005) Exercise enhances learning and hippocampal neurogenesis in aged mice. *J. Neurosci.* **25**, 8680.

338. Yang, ZP *et al.* (1996) Diisopropylphosphorofluoridate-induced muscle hyperactivity associated with enhanced lipid peroxidation *in vivo*. *Biochem. Pharmacol.* **52**, 357.

Chapter 7

1. Marsh, ENG (1995) A radical approach to enzyme catalysis. *BioEssays* **17**, 431.

2. Eklund, H *et al.* (2001) Structure and function of the radical enzyme RNR. *Prog. Biophys. Mol. Biol.* **77**, 177.

3. Guittet, O *et al.* (2000) $ONOO^-$-mediated nitration of the stable free radical tyrosine residue of the RNR small subunit. *Biochemistry* **39**, 4640.

4. Högbom, M *et al.* (2004) The radical site in chlamydial RNR defines a new R2 subclass. *Science* **305**, 245.

5. Marsh, ENG *et al.* (2004) SAM radical enzymes. *Bioorg. Chem.* **32**, 326.

6. Reed, GH and Mansoorabadi, SO (2003) The positions of radical intermediates in the active sites of adenosylcobalamin-dependent radical enzymes. *Curr.Opin. Struct. Biol.* **13**, 716.

7. Knappe, J and Wagner, FV (2001) Stable glycyl radical from PFL and RNR(III). *Adv. Protein Chem.* **58**, 277.

8. Echave, P *et al.* (2003) Novel antioxidant role of ADH E from *E. coli*. *J. Biol. Chem.* **278**, 30193.

9. Ragsdale, SW (2003) PFOR and its radical intermediate. *Chem. Rev.* **103**, 2333.

10. Tittmann, K *et al.* (2005) Radical phosphate transfer mechanism for the thiamin diphosphate- and FAD-dependent pyruvate oxidase from *Lactobacillus plantarum*. *Biochemistry* **44**, 13291.

11. Whittaker, JW (2005) The radical chemistry of galactose oxidase. *Arch. Biochem. Biophys.* **433**, 227.

12. Takikawa, O (2005) Biochemical and medical aspects of the indoleamine 2,3-dioxygenase-initiated L-tryptophan metabolism. *Biochem. Biophys. Res. Comm.* **338**, 12.

13. Dunford, HB (1995) One-electron oxidations by peroxidases. *Xenobiotica* **25**, 725.

14. Moreno, JC *et al.* (2002) Inactivating mutations in the gene for thyroid oxidase 2 (*Thox2*) and congenital hypothyroidism. *N. Engl. J. Med.* **347**, 95.

15. Kim, H *et al.* (2000) Role of peroxiredoxins in regulating intracellular H_2O_2 and H_2O_2-induced apoptosis in thyroid cells. *J. Biol. Chem.* **275**, 18266.

16. Hand, CE and Honek, JF (2005) Biological chemistry of naturally occurring thiols of microbial and marine origin. *J. Nat. Prod.* **68**, 293.

17. Goodell, B *et al.* (2003) *Wood Deterioration and Preservation*. ACS Symposium Series **845**, American Chemical Society, Washington DC, USA.

18. Davin, LB and Lewis, NG (2005) Lignin primary structures and dirigent sites. *Curr. Opin. Biotech.* **16**, 407.

19. Barceló, AR (2005) Xylem parenchyma cells deliver the H_2O_2 necessary for lignification in differentiating xylem vessels. *Planta* **220**, 747.

20. Mayer, AM and Staples, RC (2002) Laccase: new functions for an old enzyme. *Phytochemistry* **60**, 551.

21. Choinowski, T *et al.* (1999) The crystal structure of lignin peroxidase at 1.70Å resolution reveals a −OH group on the C^{β} of tryptophan 171: a novel radical site formed during the redox cycle. *J. Mol. Biol.* **286**, 809.

22. Kapich, AN *et al.* (2005) Involvement of lipid peroxidation in the degradation of a non-phenolic lignin model compound by Mn peroxidase of the litter-decomposing fungus *Stropharia coronilla*. *Biochem. Biophys. Res. Comm.* **330**, 371.

23. Pogni, R *et al.* (2005) Tryptophan-based radical in the catalytic mechanism of versatile peroxidase from *Bjerkandera adusta*. *Biochemistry* **44**, 4267.

24. Kirk, TK *et al.* (1985) Free $OH^{\bullet}$ is not involved in an important reaction of lignin degradation by *Phanerochaete chrysosporium* Burds. *Biochem. J.* **226**, 455.

25. Campbell, AK (1989) Living light: biochemistry, function and biomedical applications. *Essays Biochem.* **24**, 41.

26. Janssens, BJ *et al.* (2002) Protection of peroxide-treated fish erythrocytes by coelenterazine and coelenteramine. *Free Radic. Res.* **36**, 967.

27. Hanson, GT *et al.* (2004) Investigating mitochondrial redox potential with redox-sensitive GFP indicators. *J. Biol. Chem.* **279**, 13044.

28. Shapiro, SD (2003) Mobilizing the army. *Nature* **421**, 223.

29. Babior, BM *et al.* (2002) The neutrophil NADPH oxidase. *Arch. Biochem. Biophys.* **397**, 342.

30. Bernhagen, J (2005) Macrophage migration and function: from recruitment in vascular disease to redox regulation in the immune and neuroendocrine networks. *Antiox. Redox Signal.* **7**, 1182.

31. Loegering, DJ *et al.* (1996) Macrophage dysfunction following the phagocytosis of IgG-coated erythrocytes: production of lipid peroxidation products. *J. Leuk. Biol.* **59**, 357.

32. Panés, J *et al.* (1999) Leukocyte–endothelial cell adhesion: avenues for therapeutic intervention. *Br. J. Pharmacol.* **126**, 537.

33. Ley, K and Deem, TL (2005) Oxidative modification of leukocyte adhesion. *Immunity* **22**, 5.

34. Nathan, C (2003) O_2 and the inflammatory cell. *Nature* **422**, 675.

35. Zhao, T and Bokoch, GM (2005) Critical role of proline-rich tyrosine kinase 2 in reversion of the adhesion-mediated suppression of ROS generation by human neutrophils. *J. Immunol.* **174**, 8049.

36. Westendorp, RGJ *et al.* (1997) Genetic influence on cytokine production and fatal meningococcal disease. *Lancet* **349**, 170.

37. Levy, O (2004) Antimicrobial proteins and peptides: anti-infective molecules of mammalian leukocytes. *J. Leuk. Biol.* **76**, 909.

38. Hampton, MB *et al.* (1998) Inside the neutrophil phagosome: oxidants, MPO, and bacterial killing. *Blood* **92**, 3007.

39. Segal, AW (2005) How neutrophils kill microbes. *Ann. Rev. Immunol.* **23**, 197.

40. Fletcher, MP and Seligmann, BE (1986) PMN heterogeneity: long-term stability of fluorescent membrane potential responses to the chemoattractant fmetleuphe in healthy adults and correlation with respiratory burst activity. *Blood* **68**, 611.

41. Swain, SD *et al.* (2002) Neutrophil priming in host defense: role of oxidants as priming agents. *Antiox. Redox Signal.* **4**, 69.

42. Edwards, SW and Lloyd, D (1988) The relationship between $O_2^{\bullet-}$ generation, cytochrome b and O_2 in activated neutrophils. *FEBS Lett.* **227**, 39.

43. Coakley, RJ *et al.* (2002) Ambient pCO_2 modulates intracellular pH, intracellular oxidant generation, and IL-8 secretion. *J. Leuk. Biol.* **71**, 603.

44. Brinkmann, V *et al.* (2004) Neutrophil extracellular traps kill bacteria. *Science* **303**, 1532.

45. Wang, Q *et al.* (1999) Infection-associated decline of cape buffalo blood catalase augments serum trypanocidal activity. *Infect. Immun.* **67**, 2797.

46. Segal, BH *et al.* (2000) XO contributes to host defense against *Burkholderia cepacia* in the p47$^{phox-/-}$ mouse model of CGD. *Infect. Immun.* **68**, 2374.

47. Helmerhorst, EJ *et al.* (2001) The human salivary peptide histatin 5 exerts its antifungal activity through the formation of ROS. *Proc. Natl. Acad. Sci. USA* **98**, 14637.

48. Repine, JE *et al.* (1981) H_2O_2 kills *S. aureus* by reacting with staphylococcal Fe to form OH$^•$. *J. Biol. Chem.* **256**, 7094.

49. Babior, BM *et al.* (2003) Investigating antibody-catalyzed O_3 generation by human neutrophils. *Proc. Natl. Acad. Sci. USA* **100**, 3031.

50. Nathan, C and Shiloh, MU (2000) Reactive O_2 and N_2 intermediates in the relationship between mammalian hosts and microbial pathogens. *Proc. Natl. Acad. Sci. USA* **97**, 8841.

51. Albina, JE (1995) On the expression of NOS by human macrophages. Why no NO? *J. Leuk. Biol.* **58**, 643.

52. Wheeler, MA *et al.* (1997) Bacterial infection induces NOS in human neutrophils. *J. Clin. Invest.* **99**, 110.

53. Rosen, H *et al.* (2002) Human neutrophils use the MPO-H_2O_2-Cl$^-$ system to chlorinate but not nitrate bacterial proteins during phagocytosis. *J. Biol. Chem.* **277**, 30463.

54. Rothfork, JM *et al.* (2004) Inactivation of a bacterial virulence pheromone by phagocyte-derived oxidants: new role for the NADPH oxidase in host defense. *Proc. Natl. Acad. Sci. USA* **101**, 13867.

55. Staudinger, BJ *et al.* (2002) mRNA expression profiles for *E. coli* ingested by normal and phagocyte oxidase-deficient human neutrophils. *J. Clin. Invest.* **110**, 1151.

56. O'Rourke, EJ *et al.* (2003) Pathogen DNA as a target for host-generated oxidative stress: role for repair of bacterial DNA damage in *H. pylori* colonization. *Proc. Natl. Acad. Sci. USA* **100**, 2789.

57. De Groote, MA *et al.* (1997) Periplasmic SOD protects *Salmonella* from products of phagocyte NADPH-oxidase and NOS. *Proc. Natl. Acad. Sci. USA* **94**, 13997.

58. Liu, GY *et al.* (2005) *S. aureus* golden pigment impairs neutrophil killing and promotes virulence through its antioxidant activity. *J. Exp. Med.* **202**, 209.

59. Wagner, BA *et al.* (2004) Role of thiocyanate, Br$^-$ and HOBr in H_2O_2-induced apoptosis. *Free Radic. Res.* **38**, 167.

60. Burner, U *et al.* (1999) Transient and steady-state kinetics of the oxidation of substituted benzoic acid hydrazides by MPO. *J. Biol. Chem.* **274**, 9494.

61. Learn, DB *et al.* (1990) Taurine and hypotaurine content of human leukocytes. *J. Leuk. Biol.* **48**, 174.

62. Aruoma, OI *et al.* (1988) The antioxidant action of taurine, hypotaurine and their metabolic precursors. *Biochem. J.* **256**, 251.

63. Palazzolo, AM *et al.* (2005) GFP-expressing *E. coli* as a selective probe for HOCl generation within neutrophils. *Biochemistry* **44**, 6910.

64. Marchetti, C *et al.* (2004) Genetic characterization of MPO deficiency in Italy. *Hum. Mutat.* **23**, 496.

65. Hamers, MN *et al.* (1984) Kinetics and mechanism of the bactericidal action of human neutrophils against *E. coli. Blood* **64**, 635.

66. Ghibaudi, E and Laurenti, E (2003) Unraveling the catalytic mechanism of LPO and MPO. *Eur. J. Biochem.* **270**, 4403.

67. Abu-Soud, HM and Hazen, SL (2000) NO$^•$ modulates the catalytic activity of MPO. *J. Biol. Chem.* **275**, 5425.

68. Kumar, S *et al.* (2004) Inducible peroxidases mediate nitration of *Anopheles* midgut cells undergoing apoptosis in response to *Plasmodium* invasion. *J. Biol. Chem.* **279**, 53475.

69. Small, AL and McFall-Ngai, MJ (1999) Halide peroxidase in tissues that interact with bacteria in the host squid *Euprymna scolopes. J. Cell. Biochem.* **72**, 445.

70. Wang, JG and Slungaard, A (2006) Role of EPO in host defense and disease pathology. *Arch. Biochem. Biophys.* **445**, 256.

71. Albert, CJ *et al.* (2003) EPO-derived RBS target the vinyl ether bond of plasmalogens generating a novel chemoattractant, α-bromo fatty aldehyde. *J. Biol. Chem.* **278**, 8942.

72. Kanofsky, JR *et al.* (1988) Singlet O_2 production by human eosinophils. *J. Biol. Chem.* **263**, 9692.

73. Tarr, M and Valenzeno, DP (2003) Singlet O_2: the relevance of extracellular production mechanisms to oxidative stress *in vivo. Photochem. Photobiol. Sci.* **2**, 355.

74. Wu, W *et al.* (1999) EPO nitrates protein tyrosyl residues. *J. Biol. Chem.* **274**, 25933.

75. Kutter, D *et al.* (2000) Screening for total and partial EPO deficiency by flow cytometry: prevalence in a general population, pathology and genetic implications. *Redox Rep.* **5**, 225.

76. Heneberg, P and Dráber, P (2005) Regulation of cys-based protein tyrosine phosphatases *via* ROS/RNS in mast cells and basophils. *Curr. Med. Chem.* **12**, 1859.

77. Drabikova, K *et al.* (2002) Reactive O_2 metabolite production is inhibited by histamine and H1-antagonist dithiaden in human PMN leukocytes. *Free Radic. Res.* **36**, 975.

78. Cregar, L *et al.* (1999) Neutrophil MPO is a potent and selective inhibitor of mast cell tryptase. *Arch. Biochem. Biophys.* **366**, 125.

79. Elsen, S *et al.* (2004) Cryptic $O_2^{\bullet-}$-generating NADPH oxidase in dendritic cells. *J. Cell Sci.* **117**, 2215.

80. Vandivier, RW *et al.* (2002) Elastase-mediated phosphatidylserine receptor cleavage impairs apoptotic cell clearance in cystic fibrosis and bronchiectasis. *J. Clin. Invest.* **109**, 661.

81. Wasil, M *et al.* (1987) The antioxidant action of human EC fluids. Effect of human serum and its protein components on the inactivation of α_1-antiproteinase by HOCl and by H_2O_2. *Biochem. J.* **243**, 219.

82. Wu, SM and Pizzo, SV (2001) α2-Macroglobulin from RA synovial fluid: functional analysis defines a role for oxidation in inflammation. *Arch. Biochem. Biophys.* **391**, 119.

83. Whiteman, M and Halliwell, B (1996) Protection against $ONOO^-$-dependent tyrosine nitration and α_1-antiproteinase inactivation by ascorbic acid. *Free Radic. Res.* **25**, 275.

84. Marquez, LA *et al.* (1990) Kinetic studies on the reaction of compound II of MPO with ascorbic acid. Role of ascorbic acid in MPO function. *J. Biol. Chem.* **265**, 5666.

85. Del Maestro, RF *et al.* (1981) Increase in macrovascular permeability induced by enzymatically generated free radicals. II. Role of $O_2^{\bullet-}$, H_2O_2 and $OH^{\bullet}$. *Microvasc. Res.* **5**, 423.

86. Rojkind, M *et al.* (2002) Role of H_2O_2 and oxidative stress in healing responses. *Cell. Mol. Life Sci.* **59**, 1872.

87. Steinhauser, ML *et al.* (1998) Macrophage/fibroblast coculture induces MIP1α production mediated by ICAM-1 and oxygen radicals. *J. Leuk. Biol.* **64**, 636.

88. DeForge, LE *et al.* (1993) Regulation of IL-8 gene expression by oxidant stress. *J. Biol. Chem.* **268**, 25568.

89. Lekstrom-Himes, JA *et al.* (2005) Inhibition of human neutrophil IL-8 production by H_2O_2 and dysregulation in chronic granulomatous disease. *J. Immunol.* **174**, 411.

90. Kanayama, A *et al.* (2002) Oxidation of IκBα at met 45 is one cause of taurine chloramines-induced inhibition of NF-κB activation. *J. Biol. Chem.* **277**, 24049.

91. Matata, BM and Galiñanes, M (2002) $ONOO^-$ is an essential component of cytokines production mechanism in human monocytes through modulation of NF-κB DNA binding activity. *J. Biol. Chem.* **277**, 2330.

92. Curzio, M (1988) Interaction between neutrophils and 4-hydroxyalkenals and consequences on neutrophil motility. *Free Radic. Res. Commun.* **5**, 55.

93. Hazen, SL *et al.* (1998) Human neutrophils employ the MPO-H_2O_2-Cl^- system to oxidize α-amino acids to a family of reactive aldehydes. *J. Biol. Chem.* **273**, 4997.

94. Park, YS *et al.* (2000) Antioxidant binding of caeruloplasmin to MPO: MPO is inhibited, but oxidase, peroxidase and immunoreactive properties of caeruloplasmin remain intact. *Free Radic. Res.* **33**, 261.

95. Vinten-Johansen, J *et al.* (2003) Adenosine in myocardial protection in on-pump and off-pump cardiac surgery. *Ann. Thorac. Surg.* **75**, S691.

96. Fliss, H *et al.* (1983) Oxidation of methionine residues in proteins of activated human neutrophils. *Proc. Natl. Acad. Sci. USA* **80**, 7160.

97. deRojas-Walker, T *et al.* (1995) $NO^{\bullet}$ induces oxidative damage in addition to deamination in macrophage DNA. *Chem. Res. Toxicol.* **8**, 473.

98. Chapman, ALP *et al.* (2002) Chlorination of bacterial and neutrophil proteins during phagocytosis and killing of *S. aureus*. *J. Biol. Chem.* **277**, 9757.

99. Hannah, S *et al.* (1995) Hypoxia prolongs neutrophil survival *in vitro*. *FEBS Lett.* **372**, 233.

100. Scheel-Toellner, D *et al.* (2004) ROS limit neutrophil life span by activating death receptor signaling. *Blood* **104**, 2557.

101. Pietarinen-Runtti, P *et al.* (2000) Expression of antioxidant enzymes in human inflammatory cells. *Am. J. Physiol.* **278**, C118.

102. Higgins, CP *et al.* (1978) Polymorphonuclear leukocyte species differences in the disposal of H_2O_2. *Proc. Soc. Exp. Biol. Med.* **158**, 478.

103. Lee, C *et al.* (2000) Biphasic regulation of leukocyte $O_2^{\bullet-}$ generation by $NO^{\bullet}$ and $ONOO^-$. *J. Biol. Chem.* **275**, 38965.

104. van der Veen, RC *et al.* (2000) $O_2^{\bullet-}$ prevents $NO^{\bullet}$-mediated suppression of helper T lymphocytes: decreased autoimmune encephalomyelitis in NADPH oxidase knockout mice. *J. Immunol.* **164**, 5177.

105. Bogdan, C *et al.* (2000) Reactive O_2 and N_2 intermediates in innate and specific immunity. *Curr. Opin. Immunol.* **12**, 64.

106. Chatterjee, S and Fisher, AB (2004) ROS to the rescue. *Am. J. Physiol.* **287**, L704.

107. Blüml, S *et al.* (2005) Oxidized phospholipids negatively regulate dendritic cell maturation induced by TLRs and CD40. *J. Immunol.* **175**, 501.

108. Pepys, MB and Hirschfield, GM (2003) C-reactive protein: a critical update. *J. Clin. Invest.* **111**, 1805.

109. Baldus, S *et al.* (2003) MPO serum levels predict risk in patients with acute coronary syndromes. *Circulation* **108**, 1440.

110. Zhang, R *et al.* (2002) Defects in leukocyte-mediated initiation of lipid peroxidation in plasma as studied in MPO-deficient subjects: systematic identification of multiple endogenous diffusible substrates for MPO in plasma. *Blood* **99**, 1802.

111. Woods, AA and Davies, MJ (2003) Fragmentation of extracellular matrix by HOCl. *Biochem. J.* **376**, 219.

112. Baldus, S *et al.* (2001) Endothelial transcytosis of MPO confers specificity to vascular ECM proteins as targets of tyrosine nitration. *J. Clin. Invest.* **108**, 1759.

113. Zhang, R *et al.* (2002) MPO functions as a major enzymatic catalyst for initiation of lipid peroxidation at sites of inflammation. *J. Biol. Chem.* **277**, 46116.

114. Baldus, S *et al.* (2004) MPO enhances $NO^\bullet$ catabolism during myocardial ischemia and reperfusion. *Free Rad. Biol. Med.* **37**, 902.

115. Takizawa, S *et al.* (2002) Deficiency of MPO increases infarct volume and nitrotyrosine formation in mouse brain. *J. Cereb. Blood Flow Metab.* **22**, 50.

116. Foucher, P *et al.* (1999) Anti-MPO-associated lung disease. *Am. J. Respir. Crit. Care Med.* **160**, 987.

117. Tarng, DC *et al.* (2002) Increased oxidative damage to peripheral blood leukocyte DNA in chronic peritoneal dialysis patients. *J. Am. Soc. Nephrol.* **13**, 1321.

118. Satoh, M *et al.* (2001) Oxidative stress is reduced by the long-term use of vitamin E-coated dialysis filters. *Kidney Int.* **59**, 1943.

119. Udipi, K *et al.* (2000) Modification of inflammatory response to implanted biomedical materials *in vivo* by surface bound SOD mimics. *J. Biomed. Mater. Res.* **51**, 549.

120. Halliwell, B (2004) Ageing and disease: from Darwinian medicine to antioxidants? *Innovation* **4**, 12.

121. Van de Loo, FAJ *et al.* (2003) Deficiency of NADPH oxidase components p47phox and gp91phox caused granulomatous synovitis and increased connective tissue destruction in experimental arthritis model. *Am. J. Pathol.* **163**, 1525.

122. Balish, E *et al.* (2005) Susceptibility of germfree phagocyte oxidase- and NOS2-deficient mice, defective in the production of reactive metabolites of both O_2 and N_2, to mucosal and systemic candidiasis of endogenous origin. *Infect. Immun.* **73**, 1313.

123. Gao, XP *et al.* (2002) Role of NADPH oxidase in the mechanism of lung neutrophil sequestration and microvessel injury induced by gram-negative sepsis: studies in $p47^{phox-/-}$ and $gp91^{phox-/-}$ mice. *J. Immunol.* **168**, 3974.

124. Ross, AD *et al.* (2004) Enhancement of collagen-induced arthritis in mice genetically deficient in ECSOD. *Arth. Rheum.* **50**, 3702.

125. Benov, L and Fridovich, I (1996) *E. coli* exhibits negative chemotaxis in gradients of H_2O_2, OCl^- and N-chlorotaurine: products of the respiratory burst of phagocytic cells. *Proc. Natl. Acad. Sci. USA* **93**, 4999.

126. Haas, A. and Goebel, W (1992) Microbial strategies to prevent O_2-dependent killing by phagocytes. *Free Radic. Res. Commun.* **16**, 137.

127. Roos, D *et al.* (2003) Oxidative killing of microbes by neutrophils. *Microbes Infect.* **5**, 1307.

128. Nishida, S *et al.* (2005) Fungal metabolite gliotoxin targets flavocytochrome b_{558} in the activation of the human neutrophil NADPH oxidase. *Infect. Immun.* **73**, 235.

129. Chaturvedi, V *et al.* (1996) Oxidative killing of *C. neoformans* by human neutrophils. *J. Immunol.* **156**, 3836.

130. Allen, LAH *et al.* (2005) *H. pylori* disrupts NADPH oxidase targeting in human neutrophils to induce extracellular $O_2^{\bullet-}$ release. *J. Immunol.* **174**, 3658.

131. Raynaud, C *et al.* (1998) Extracellular enzyme activities potentially involved in the pathogenicity of *M. tuberculosis*. *Microbiol.* **144**, 577.

132. Sumimoto, H *et al.* (2005) Molecular composition and regulation of the Nox family NAD(P)H oxidases. *Biochem. Biophys. Res. Comm.* **338**, 677.

133. Lardy, B *et al.* (2005) NADPH oxidase homologs are required for normal cell differentiation and morphogenesis in *Dictyostelium discoideum*. *Biochim. Biophys. Acta* **1744**, 199.

134. Bergin, D *et al.* (2005) $O_2^{\bullet-}$ production in *Galleria mellonella* hemocytes: identification of proteins homologous to the NADPH oxidase complex of human neutrophils. *Infect. Immun.* **73**, 4161.

135. Tam, NNC *et al.* (2003) Androgenic regulation of oxidative stress in the rat prostate. *Am. J. Pathol.* **163**, 2513.

136. Tammariello, SP *et al.* (2000) NADPH oxidase contributes directly to oxidative stress and apoptosis in NGF-deprived sympathetic neurons. *J. Neurosci.* **20**, RC53.

137. Thabut, G *et al.* (2002) TNFα increases airway smooth muscle oxidants production through a NADPH oxidase-like system to enhance myosin light chain phosphorylation and contractility. *J. Biol. Chem.* **277**, 22814.

138. Al-Shabrawey, M *et al.* (2005) Inhibition of NAD(P)H oxidase activity blocks VEGF overexpression and neovascularization during ischemic retinopathy. *Am. J. Pathol.* **167**, 599.

139. Geiszt, M *et al.* (2003) Dual oxidases represent novel H_2O_2 sources supporting mucosal surface host defense. *FASEB J.* **17**, 1502.

140. Hordijk, P (2006) Regulation of NADPH oxidases. *Circ. Res.* **98**, 453.

141. Geiszt, M *et al.* (2003) Proteins homologous to $p47^{phox}$ and $p67^{phox}$ support $O_2^{\bullet-}$ production by NOX1 in colon epithelial cells. *J. Biol. Chem.* **278**, 20006.

142. Mitsushita, J *et al.* (2004) The $O_2^{\bullet-}$-generating oxidase Nox1 is functionally required for Ras oncogene transformation. *Cancer Res.* **64**, 3580.

143. Edens, WA *et al.* (2001) Tyrosine cross-linking of extracellular matrix is catalyzed by Duox, a multi-domain oxidase/peroxidase with homology to the phagocyte oxidase subunit gp91^{phox}. *J. Cell Biol.* **154**, 879.

144. Brandes, RP and Kreuzer, J (2005) Vascular NADPH oxidases: molecular mechanisms of activation. *Cardiovasc. Res.* **65**, 16.

145. Kelley, EE *et al.* (2004) Binding of XO to glycosaminoglycans limits inhibition by oxypurinol. *J. Biol. Chem.* **279**, 43362.

146. Gavazzi, G *et al.* (2006) Decreased blood pressure in NOX1-deficient mice. *FEBS Lett.* **580**, 497.

147. Hilenski, LL *et al.* (2004) Distinct subcellular localizations of Nox1 and Nox4 in vascular smooth muscle cells. *Arterio. Thromb. Vasc. Biol.* **24**, 677.

148. Patterson, C *et al.* (1999) Stimulation of a vascular smooth muscle cell NADPH oxidase by thrombin. *J. Biol. Chem.* **274**, 19814.

149. Ormezzano, O *et al.* (2005) F_2-isoprostane level is associated with the angiotensin II type 1 receptor-153A/G gene polymorphism. *Free Rad. Biol. Med.* **38**, 583.

150. Zhan, CD *et al.* (2004) Up-regulation of kidney NAD(P)H oxidase and calcineurin in SHR: reversal by lifelong antioxidant supplementation. *Kidney Int.* **65**, 219.

151. Cuzzocrea, S *et al.* (2004) $O_2^{\bullet-}$: a key player in hypertension. *FASEB J.* **18**, 94.

152. Tai, MH *et al.* (2005) Increased $O_2^{\bullet-}$ in rostral ventrolateral medulla contributes to hypertension in spontaneously hypertensive rats via interactions with $NO^{\bullet}$. *Free Rad. Biol. Med.* **38**, 450.

153. Ushio-Fukai, M and Alexander, RW (2004) ROS as mediators of angiogenesis signaling. *Mol. Cell. Biochem.* **264**, 85.

154. Kase, H *et al.* (2005) Supplementation with THB prevents the cardiovascular effects of Ang II-induced oxidative and nitrosative stress. *J. Hypertens.* **23**, 1375.

155. Kobayashi, S *et al.* (1995) Characterization of the $O_2^{\bullet-}$-generating system in human peripheral lymphocytes and lymphoid cell lines. *J. Biochem.* **117**, 758.

156. Kwon, J *et al.* (2005) Receptor-stimulated oxidation of SHP-2 promotes T-cell adhesion through SLP-76-ADAP. *EMBO J.* **24**, 2331.

157. Badr, KF and Abi-Antoun, TE (2005) Isoprostanes and the kidney. *Antiox. Redox Signal.* **7**, 236.

158. Malle, E *et al.* (2003) MPO in kidney disease. *Kidney Int.* **64**, 1956.

159. Shah, SV (2004) Oxidants and Fe in chronic kidney disease. *Kidney Int.* **66**, S50.

160. Kitiyakara, C *et al.* (2003) Salt intake, oxidative stress, and renal expression of NOX. *J. Am. Soc. Nephrol.* **14**, 2775.

161. Garvin, JL and Ortiz, PA (2003) The role of ROS in the regulation of tubular function. *Acta Physiol. Scand.* **179**, 225.

162. Haque, MZ and Majid, DSA (2004) Assessment of renal functional phenotype in mice lacking gp91^{phox} subunit of NADPH oxidase. *Hypertension* **43**, 335.

163. Guo, W *et al.* (2003) Quantitative assessment of tyrosine nitration of MnSOD in angiotensin II-infused rat kidney. *Am. J. Physiol.* **285**, H1396.

164. Kazemian, P *et al.* (2001) Respiratory control in neonatal mice with NOX deficiency. *Respir. Physiol.* **126**, 89.

165. Suliman, HB *et al.* (2004) SOD3 promotes full expression of the *EPO* response to hypoxia. *Blood* **104**, 43.

166. Sabetkar, M *et al.* (2002) The nitration of proteins in platelets: significance in platelet function. *Free Rad. Biol. Med.* **33**, 728.

167. Görlach, A (2005) Redox regulation of the coagulation cascade. *Antiox. Redox Signal.* **7**, 1398.

168. Nardi, M *et al.* (2004) Complement-independent Ab-induced peroxide lysis of platelets requires 12-lipoxygenase and a platelet NOX pathway. *J. Clin. Invest.* **113**, 973.

169. Yang, S *et al.* (2004) Expression of NOX4 in osteoclasts. *J. Cell. Biochem.* **92**, 238.

170. Ly, JD and Lawen, A (2003) Transplasma membrane electron transport: enzymes involved and biological function. *Redox Rep.* **8**, 3.

171. Baker, MA *et al.* (2004) VDAC1 is a transplasma membrane NADH-ferricyanide reductase. *J. Biol. Chem.* **279**, 4811.

172. Apel, K and Hirt, H (2004) ROS: metabolism, oxidative stress, and signal transduction. *Ann. Rev. Plant Biol.* **55**, 373.

173. Carol, RJ *et al.* (2005) A RhoGDP dissociation inhibitor spatially regulates growth in root hair cells. *Nature* **438**, 1013.

174. Kwak, JM *et al.* (2003) NADPH oxidase *AtrbohD* and *AtrbohF* genes function in ROS-dependent ABA signaling in *Arabidopsis*. *EMBO J.* **22**, 2623.

175. Boldogh, I *et al.* (2005) ROS generated by pollen NOX provide a signal that augments antigen-induced allergic airway inflammation. *J. Clin. Invest.* **115**, 2169.

176. Gechev, TS and Hille, J (2005) H_2O_2 as a signal controlling plant programmed cell death. *J. Cell. Biochem.* **168**, 17.

177. Gapper, G and Dolan, L (2006) Control of plant development by ROS. *Plant Physiol.* **141**, 341.

178. Loeffler, C *et al.* (2005) B$_1$-Phytoprostanes trigger plant defense and detoxification responses. *Plant Physiol.* **137**, 328.

179. Jennings, DB *et al.* (1998) Roles of mannitol and mannitol dehydrogenase in active oxygen-mediated plant defense. *Proc. Natl. Acad. Sci. USA* **95**, 15129.

180. Crawford, NM and Guo, FQ (2005) New insights into NO$^\bullet$ metabolism and regulatory functions. *Trends Plant Sci.* **10**, 195.

181. Job, C *et al.* (2005) Patterns of protein oxidation in *Arabidopsis* seeds and during germination. *Plant Physiol.* **138**, 790.

182. Schopfer, P *et al.* (2001) Release of reactive O$_2$ intermediates (O$_2^{\bullet-}$, H$_2$O$_2$, and OH$^\bullet$) and peroxidase in germinating radish seeds controlled by light, gibberellin, and abscisic acid. *Plant Physiol.* **125**, 1591.

183. Marx, C *et al.* (2003) Thioredoxin and germinating barley: targets and protein redox changes. *Planta* **216**, 454.

184. Passardi, E *et al.* (2005) Peroxidases have more functions than a Swiss army knife. *Plant Cell Rep.* **24**, 255.

185. Fry, SC *et al.* (2001) Fingerprinting of polysaccharides attacked by OH$^\bullet$ *in vitro* and in the cell walls of ripening pear fruit. *Biochem. J.* **357**, 729.

186. Berger, S *et al.* (2001) Enzymatic and non-enzymatic lipid peroxidation in leaf development. *Biochim. Biophys. Acta* **1533**, 266.

187. Matsui, K (2006) Green leaf volatiles: hydroperoxide lyase pathway of oxylipin metabolism. *Curr. Opin. Pl. Biol.* **9**, 274.

188. Hörnsten, L *et al.* (2002) Cloning of the Mn LOX gene reveals homology with the LOX gene family. *Eur. J. Biochem.* **269**, 2690.

189. Kemal, C *et al.* (1987) Reductive inactivation of soybean LOX-1 by catechols: a possible mechanism for regulation of LOX activity. *Biochemistry* **26**, 7064.

190. O'Donnell, VB *et al.* (1999) 15-LOX catalytically consumes NO$^\bullet$ and impairs activation of guanylate cyclase. *J. Biol. Chem.* **274**, 20083.

191. Hatanaka, A (1993) The biogeneration of green odour by green leaves. *Phytochemistry* **34**, 1201.

192. Thoma, I *et al.* (2003) Cyclopentenone isoprostanes induced by ROS trigger defense gene activation and phytoalexin accumulation in plants. *Plant J.* **34**, 363.

193. Soberman, RJ and Christmas, P (2003) The organization and consequences of eicosanoid signaling. *J. Clin. Invest.* **111**, 1107.

194. Schewe, T (2002) 15-LOX-1: a prooxidant enzyme. *Biol. Chem.* **383**, 365.

195. Smith, WL (2005) COX, peroxide tone and the allure of fish oil. *Curr. Opin. Cell Biol.* **17**, 174.

196. Morse, DE *et al.* (1977) H$_2$O$_2$ induces spawning in mollusks, with activation of prostaglandin endoperoxide synthetase. *Science* **196**, 298.

197. Gao, L *et al.* (2003) Formation of prostaglandins E$_2$ and D$_2$ via the IP pathway. *J. Biol. Chem.* **278**, 28479.

198. Salomon, RG (2005) Distinguishing levuglandins produced through the COX and IP pathways. *Chem. Phys. Lipids* **134**, 1.

199. Moos, PJ *et al.* (2003) Electrophilic prostaglandins and lipid aldehydes repress redox-sensitive transcription factors p53 and hypoxia-inducible factor by impairing the selenoprotein thioredoxin reductase. *J. Biol. Chem.* **278**, 745.

200. Mullally, JE *et al.* (2001) Cyclopentenone prostaglandins of the J series inhibit the ubiquitin isopeptidase activity of the proteasome pathway. *J. Biol. Chem.* **276**, 30366.

201. Maccarrone, M *et al.* (1997) NO donors activate the COX and peroxidase activities of prostaglandin H synthase. *FEBS Lett.* **410**, 470.

202. Williams, PC *et al.* (2005) *In vivo* aspirin supplementation inhibits NO$^\bullet$ consumption by human platelets. *Blood* **106**, 2737.

203. Laughton, MJ *et al.* (1991) Inhibition of mammalian 5-LOX and COX by flavonoids and phenolic dietary additives. Relationship to antioxidant activity and to Fe ion-reducing ability. *Biochem. Pharmacol.* **42**, 1673.

Chapter 8

1. Maiti, S *et al.* (2005) *In vivo* and *in vitro* oxidative regulation of rat AST IV. *J. Biochem. Mol. Toxicol.* **19**, 109.

2. Mills, EM *et al.* (1996) CN$^-$-induced apoptosis and oxidative stress in differentiated PC12 cells. *J. Neurochem.* **67**, 1039.

3. Chellman, GJ *et al.* (1986) Role of epididymal inflammation in the induction of dominant lethal mutations in Fischer 344 rat sperm by CH$_3$Cl. *Proc. Natl. Acad. Sci. USA* **83**, 8087.

4. Saez, JC *et al.* (1987) CCl$_4$ at hepatotoxic levels blocks reversibly gap junctions between rat hepatocytes. *Science* **236**, 967.

5. Plaa, GL (2000) Chlorinated methanes and liver injury: highlights of the past 50 years. *Ann. Rev. Pharmacol. Toxicol.* **40**, 43.

6. McGregor, D and Lang, M (1996) CCl$_4$: genetic effects and other modes of action. *Mutat. Res.* **366**, 181.

7. Basu, S (2003) CCl$_4$-induced lipid peroxidation: eicosanoid formation and their regulation by antioxidant nutrients. *Toxicology* **189**, 113.

8. Casini, AF *et al.* (1987) Lipid peroxidation, protein thiols and Ca^{2+} homeostasis in bromobenzene-induced liver damage. *Biochem. Pharmacol.* **36**, 3689.

9. Kharasch, ED *et al.* (2000) Human halothane metabolism, lipid peroxidation, and cytochrome P(450)2A6 and P(450)3A4. *Eur. J. Clin. Pharmacol.* **55**, 853.

10. Pohl, LR (1993) An immunochemical approach of identifying and characterizing protein targets of toxic reactive metabolites. *Chem. Res. Toxicol.* **6**, 786.

11. Toraason, M *et al.* (2003) Effect of perchloroethylene, smoking, and race on oxidative DNA damage in female dry cleaners. *Mutat. Res.* **539**, 9.

12. Pohl, LR (1979) Biochemical toxicology of CHCl$_3$. *Rev. Biochem. Toxicol.* **1**, 79.

13. Lungarella, G *et al.* (1987) BrCCl$_3$-induced damage to bronchiolar Clara cells. *Res. Comm. Chem. Pathol. Pharmacol.* **57**, 213.

14. Umemura, T *et al.* (1996) Oxidative DNA damage and cell proliferation in the livers of B6C3F1 mice exposed to pentachlorophenol in their diet. *Fund. Appl. Toxicol.* **30**, 285.

15. Shen, D *et al.* (2005) GSH redox state regulates mitochondrial ROS production. *J. Biol. Chem.* **280**, 25305.

16. Wyde, ME *et al.* (2001) Induction of hepatic 8OHdG adducts by 2,3,7,8-tetrachlorodibenzo-*p*-dioxin in Sprague–Dawley rats is female-specific and estrogen-dependent. *Chem. Res. Toxicol.* **14**, 849.

17. Horvath, ME *et al.* (2001) Vitamin E protects against Fe-hexachlorobenzene induced porphyria and formation of 8OHdG in the liver of C57BL/10ScSn mice. *Toxicol. Lett.* **122**, 97.

18. Kitzler, J and Fridovich, I (1986) The effects of paraquat on *E. coli*: distinction between bacteriostasis and lethality. *J. Free Rad. Biol. Med.* **2**, 245.

19. Liochev, SI *et al.* (1994) NADPH: ferredoxin oxidoreductase acts as a paraquat diaphorase and is a member of the *sox*RS regulon. *Proc. Natl. Acad. Sci. USA* **91**, 1328.

20. Korbashi, P *et al.* (1986) Fe mediates paraquat toxicity in *E. coli*. *J. Biol. Chem.* **261**, 12472.

21. Hassan, HM and Fridovich, I (1979) Paraquat and *E. coli*. Mechanism of production of extracellular O$_2^{\bullet-}$. *J. Biol. Chem.* **254**, 10846.

22. Smith, LL and Wyatt, I (1981) The accumulation of putrescine into slices of rat lung and brain and its relationship to the accumulation of paraquat. *Biochem. Pharmacol.* **30**, 1053.

23. Landrigan, PJ *et al.* (1983) Paraquat and marijuana: epidemiologic risk assessment. *Am. J. Public Health* **73**, 784.

24. Keeling, PL and Smith, LL (1982) Relevance of NADPH depletion and mixed disulphide formation in rat lung to the mechanism of cell damage following paraquat administration. *Biochem. Pharmacol.* **31**, 3243.

25. Thomas, CE and Aust, SD (1986) Reductive release of Fe from ferritin by cation free radicals of paraquat and other bipyridyls. *J. Biol. Chem.* **261**, 13064.

26. Burkitt, MJ *et al.* (1993) ESR spin-trapping investigation into the effects of paraquat and desferrioxamine on OH$^{\bullet}$ generation during acute iron poisoning. *Mol. Pharmacol.* **43**, 257.

27. Waintrub, ML *et al.* (1990) XO is increased and contributes to paraquat-induced acute lung injury. *J. Appl. Physiol.* **68**, 1755.

28. Denicola, A and Radi, R (2005) ONOO$^-$ and drug-dependent toxicity. *Toxicology* **208**, 273.

29. Frank, L (1981) Prolonged survival after paraquat. *Biochem. Pharmacol.* **30**, 2319.

29A. Wang, Y *et al.* (2006) Pr6 gene-targeted mice show increased lung injury with paraquat-induced oxidative stress. *Antiox. Redox. Signal.* **8**, 229.

30. Burk, RF (1995) Pathogenesis of diquat-induced liver necrosis in Se-deficient rats: assessment of the roles of lipid peroxidation and selenoprotein P. *Hepatology* **21**, 561.

31. Winterbourn, CC and Munday, R (1989) GSH-mediated redox cycling of alloxan. *Biochem. Pharmacol.* **38**, 271.

32. Ho, E *et al.* (2000) PBN inhibits NFκB activation offering protection against chemically induced diabetes. *Free Rad. Biol. Med.* **28**, 604.

33. Malaisse, WJ *et al.* (1982) Determinants of the selective toxicity of alloxan to the pancreatic B cell. *Proc. Natl. Acad. Sci. USA* **79**, 927.

34. Grankvist, K *et al.* (1981) CuZnSOD, MnSOD, catalase and GPx in pancreatic islets and other tissues in the mouse. *Biochem. J.* **199**, 393.

35. Holmgren, A and Lyckeborg, C (1980) Enzymatic reduction of alloxan by thioredoxin and NADPH-thioredoxin reductase. *Proc. Natl. Acad. Sci. USA* **77**, 5149.

36. Herson, PM and Ashford, MLJ (1999) GSH inhibits β-NAD$^+$-activated non-selective cation currents in the rat insulin-secreting cell line CRI–GI. *J. Physiol.* **514**, 47.

37. Hadjivassiliou, V *et al.* (1998) Insulin secretion, DNA damage, and apoptosis in human and rat islets of Langerhans following exposure to NO$^{\bullet}$, ONOO$^-$ and cytokines. *Nitric Oxide* **2**, 429.

38. Grankvist, K and Marklund, SL (1983) Opposite effects of two metal-chelators on alloxan-induced diabetes in mice. *Life Sci.* **33**, 2535.

39. el-Hage, A *et al.* (1986) Mechanism of the protective activity of ICRF-187 against alloxan-induced diabetes in mice. *Res. Commun. Chem. Pathol. Pharmacol.* **52**, 341.

40. Eizirik, DL *et al.* (1986) 1,10 phenanthroline, a metal chelator, protects against alloxan- but not streptozotocin-induced diabetes. *Free Rad. Biol. Med.* **2**, 189.

41. Kubisch, HM *et al.* (1994) Transgenic CuZnSOD modulates susceptibility to type I diabetes. *Proc. Natl. Acad. Sci. USA* **91**, 9956.

42. Chen, H *et al.* (2005) MnSOD and catalase transgenes demonstrate that protection of islets from oxidative stress does not alter cytokine toxicity. *Diabetes* **54**, 1437.

43. Li, Y *et al.* (1996) Role of CuZnSOD in xenobiotic activation. 1. Chemical reactions involved in the CuZnSOD-accelerated oxidation of the benzene metabolite, 1,4-hydroquinone. *J. Pharmacol. Exp. Ther.* **49**, 404.

44. Bolten, JL *et al.* (2000) Role of quinones in toxicology. *Chem. Res. Toxicol.* **13**, 135.

45. Winterbourn, CC *et al.* (1979) The reaction of menadione with haemoglobin. *Biochem. J.* **179**, 665.

46. Fischer-Nielsen, A *et al.* (1995) Menadione-induced DNA fragmentation without 8OHdG formation in isolated rat hepatocytes. *Biochem. Pharmacol.* **49**, 1469.

47. Cenas, N *et al.* (2004) Interactions of quinones with thioredoxin reductase. *J. Biol. Chem.* **279**, 2583.

48. Beyer, RE *et al.* (1996) The role of DT-diaphorase in the maintenance of the reduced antioxidant form of coenzyme Q in membrane systems. *Proc. Natl. Acad. Sci. USA* **93**, 2528.

49. Siegel, D and Ross, D (2000) Immunodetection of NAD(P)H: quinone oxidoreductase 1 (NQO1) in human tissues. *Free Rad. Biol. Med.* **29**, 246.

50. Zhou, GD *et al.* (2004) Effects of NQO1 deficiency on levels of cyclopurines and other oxidative DNA lesions in liver and kidney of young mice. *Int. J. Cancer* **112**, 877.

51. Bindoli, A *et al.* (1992) Biochemical and toxicological properties of the oxidation products of catecholamines. *Free Rad. Biol. Med.* **13**, 391.

52. Serra, PA *et al.* (2000) Mn increases L-DOPA autoxidation in the striatum of the freely moving rat: potential implications to L-DOPA long-term therapy of PD. *Br. J. Pharmacol.* **130**, 937.

53. Xu, R *et al.* (1996) Characterization of products from the reactions of *N*-acetyldopamine quinone with *N*-acetylhistidine. *Arch. Biochem. Biophys.* **329**, 56.

54. Cohen. G and Heikkila, RE (1984) Alloxan and 6-hydroxydopamine: cellular toxins. *Meth. Enzymol.* **105**, 510.

55. Barkats, M *et al.* (2002) Neuronal transfer of the human CuZnSOD gene increases the resistance of dopaminergic neurons to 6-hydroxydopamine. *J. Neurochem.* **82**, 101.

56. Callio, J *et al.* (2005) MnSOD protects against 6-hydroxydopamine injury in mouse brains. *J. Biol. Chem.* **280**, 18536.

57. Liu, L *et al.* (1996) The study of DNA oxidative damage in benzene-exposed workers. *Mutat. Res.* **370**, 145.

58. Chen, KM *et al.* (2004) Detection of nitrated benzene metabolites in bone marrow of B6C3F$_1$ mice treated with benzene. *Chem. Res. Toxicol.* **17**, 370.

59. de la Paz, MP *et al.* (2003) Neurologic outcomes of toxic oil syndrome patients 18 years after the epidemic. *Environ. Health Perspect.* **111**, 1326.

60. Khan, ME *et al.* (1999) Fe exacerbates aniline-associated splenic toxicity. *J. Toxicol. Environ. Health* **57**, 173.

61. Lau, GW *et al.* (2004) The role of pyocyanin in *P. aeruginosa* infection. *Trends Mol. Med.* **10**, 599.

62. Britigan, BE *et al.* (1997) Augmentation of oxidant injury to human pulmonary epithelial by the *Pseudomonas aeruginosa* siderophore pyochelin. *Infect. Immun.* **65**, 1071.

63. Heikkila, RE *et al.* (1974) Prevention of alloxan-induced diabetes by ethanol administration. *J. Pharmacol. Exp. Ther.* **190**, 501.

64. Navasumrit, P *et al.* (2000) Ethanol-induced free radicals and hepatic DNA strand breaks are prevented *in vivo* by antioxidants: effects of acute and chronic ethanol exposure. *Carcinogenesis* **21**, 93.

65. Tsukamoto, H and Lu, SC (2001) Current concepts in the pathogenesis of alcoholic liver injury. *FASEB J.* **15**, 1335.

66. Caro, AA and Cederbaum, AI (2004) Oxidative stress, toxicology, and pharmacology of CYP2E1. *Ann. Rev. Pharmacol. Toxicol.* **44**, 27.

67. Montoliu, C *et al.* (1995) Ethanol increases CYP2E1 and induces oxidative stress in astrocytes. *J. Neurochem.* **65**, 2561.

68. Fuchs, FD (2005) Vascular effects of alcoholic beverages. *Hypertension* **45**, 851.

69. Ikonomidou, C *et al.* (2000) Ethanol-induced apoptotic neurodegeneration and fetal alcohol syndrome. *Science* **287**, 1056.

70. Ji, C *et al.* (2004) Role of TNFα in ethanol-induced hyperhomocysteinemia and murine alcoholic liver injury. *Hepatology* **40**, 442.

71. Fletcher, LM *et al.* (2002) Excess alcohol greatly increases the prevalence of cirrhosis in hereditary hemochromatosis. *Gastroenterol.* **122**, 281.

72. Herrera, DG *et al.* (2003) Selective impairment of hippocampal neurogenesis by chronic alcoholism: protective effects of an antioxidant. *Proc. Natl. Acad. Sci. USA* **100**, 7919.

73. Ledig, M *et al.* (1981) SOD activity in rat brain during acute and chronic alcohol intoxication. *Neurochem. Res.* **6**, 385.

74. Aleynik, SI *et al.* (1998) Increased circulating products of lipid peroxidation in patients with alcoholic liver disease. *Alcohol. Clin. Exp. Res.* **22**, 192.

75. Adachi, J *et al.* (2004) Plasma PC–OOH as a new marker of oxidative stress in alcoholic patients. *J. Lipid Res.* **45**, 967.

76. Moss, M *et al.* (2000) The effects of chronic alcohol abuse on pulmonary GSH homeostasis. *Am. J. Respir. Crit. Care Med.* **161**, 414.

77. Ramachandran, V *et al.* (2001) *In utero* ethanol exposure causes mitochondrial dysfunction, which can result in apoptotic cell death in fetal brain: a potential role for 4HNE. *Alcohol. Clin. Exp. Res.* **25**, 862.

78. Ren, JC *et al.* (2005) Exposure to ethanol induces oxidative damage in the pituitary gland. *Alcohol* **35**, 91.

79. Puntarulo, S *et al.* (1999) Interaction of 1-hydroxyethyl radical with antioxidant enzymes. *Arch. Biochem. Biophys.* **372**, 355.

80. Shaw, S and Jayatilleke, E (1990) The role of aldehyde oxidase in ethanol-induced hepatic lipid peroxidation in the rat. *Biochem. J.* **268**, 579.

81. Tuma, DJ *et al.* (2001) Elucidation of reaction scheme describing MDA-acetaldehyde-protein adduct formation. *Chem. Res. Toxicol.* **14**, 822.

82. Han, QP and Dryhurst, G (1996) Influence of GSH on the oxidation of 1-methyl-6-hydroxyl-1,2,3,4-tetrahydro-β-carboline: chemistry of potential relevance to the addictive and neurodegenerative consequences of ethanol abuse. *J. Med. Chem.* **39**, 1494.

83. Tillonen, J *et al.* (1998) Role of catalase in *in vitro* acetaldehyde formation by human colonic contents. *Alcohol. Clin. Exp. Res.* **22**, 1113.

84. Vallett, M *et al.* (1997) Free radical production during ethanol intoxication, dependence, and withdrawal. *Alcohol. Clin. Exp. Res.* **21**, 275.

85. Kessova, IG *et al.* (2003) Alcohol-induced liver injury in mice lacking CuZnSOD. *Hepatology* **38**, 1136.

86. Apte, M (2002) Oxidative stress: does it 'initiate' hepatic stellate cell activation or only 'perpetuate' the process? *J. Gastroenterol. Hepatol.* **17**, 1045.

87. Comporti, M *et al.* (2005) F_2-IPs stimulate collagen synthesis in activated hepatic stellate cells: a link with liver fibrosis? *Lab. Invest.* **85**, 1381.

88. Laurent, A *et al.* (2004) Pivotal role of $O_2^{\bullet-}$ and beneficial effect of antioxidant molecules in murine steatohepatitis. *Hepatology* **39**, 1277.

89. Banan, A *et al.* (1999) Ethanol-induced barrier dysfunction and its prevention by growth factors in human intestinal monolayers: evidence for oxidative and cytoskeletal mechanisms. *J. Pharmacol. Exp. Ther.* **291**, 1075.

90. Mezey, E *et al.* (2004) A randomized placebo controlled trial of vitamin E for alcoholic hepatitis. *J. Hepatol.* **40**, 40.

91. Lucena, MI *et al.* (2002) Effects of silymarin MZ-80 on oxidative stress in patients with alcoholic cirrhosis. *Int. J. Clin. Pharmacol. Ther.* **40**, 2.

92. Silva, JM and O'Brien, PJ (1989) Allyl alcohol and acrolein-induced toxicity in isolated rat hepatocytes. *Arch. Biochem. Biophys.* **275**, 551.

93. Ferrali, M *et al.* (1990) Fe release and erythrocyte damage in allyl alcohol intoxication in mice. *Biochem. Pharmacol.* **40**, 1485.

94. Boelsterli, UA and Goldlin, C (1991) Biomechanisms of cocaine-induced hepatocyte injury mediated by the formation of reactive metabolites. *Arch. Toxicol.* **65**, 351.

95. Zimmerman, EF *et al.* (1994) Role of O_2 free radicals in cocaine-induced vascular disruption in mice. *Teratology* **49**, 192.

96. Cadet, JL *et al.* (1995) $O_2^{\bullet-}$ radicals mediate the biochemical effects of MDMD: evidence from using CuZnSOD transgenic mice. *Synapse* **21**, 169.

97. Camarero, J *et al.* (2002) Studies, using *in vivo* microdialysis, on the effect of the dopamine uptake inhibitor GBR 12909 on 3,4-MDMA ('ecstasy')-induced dopamine release and free radical formation in the mouse striatum. *J. Neurochem.* **81**, 961.

98. Itzhak, Y and Achat-Mendes, C (2004) Methamphetamine and MDMA (Ecstasy) neurotoxicity: 'of mice and men'. *IUBMB Life* **56**, 249.

99. Jeng, W *et al.* (2005) Methamphetamine-enhanced embryonic oxidative DNA damage and neurodevelopmental deficits. *Free Rad. Biol. Med.* **39**, 317.

100. Hamelink, C *et al.* (2005) Comparison of cannabidiol, antioxidants, and diuretics in reversing binge ethanol-induced neurotoxicity. *J. Pharmacol. Exp. Ther.* **314**, 780.

101. Lastres-Becker, I *et al.* (2005) Cannabinoids provide neuroprotection against 6-hydroxydopamine toxicity *in vivo* and *in vitro*: relevance to PD. *Neurobiol. Dis.* **19**, 96.

102. Jaeschke, H *et al.* (2003) The role of oxidant stress and RNS in acetaminophen hepatotoxicity. *Toxicol. Lett.* **144**, 279.

103. Lee, SST *et al.* (1996) Role of CYP2E1 in the hepatotoxicity of acetaminophen. *J. Biol. Chem.* **271**, 12063.

104. Stern, ST *et al.* (2005) Contribution of acetaminophen-cysteine to acetaminophen nephrotoxicity II. Possible involvement of the γ-glutamyl cycle. *Toxicol. Appl. Pharmacol.* **202**, 160.

105. Cribb, AE *et al.* (2005) The ER in xenobiotic toxicity. *Drug Metab. Rev.* **37**, 405.

106. Awad, JA and Morrow, JD (1995) Excretion of F_2-isoprostanes in bile; a novel index of hepatic lipid peroxidation. *Hepatology* **22**, 962.

107. Mehendale, HM and Limaye, PB (2005) Calpain: a death protein that mediates progression of liver injury. *Trends Pharmacol. Sci.* **26**, 232.

108. Evans, PJ *et al.* (1994) Metal ions catalytic for free radical reactions in the plasma of patients with fulminant hepatic failure. *Free Radic. Res.* **20**, 139.

109. Phimister, AJ *et al.* (2005) Consequences of abrupt GSH depletion in murine Clara cells: ultrastructural and biochemical investigations into the role of GSH loss in naphthalene cytotoxicity. *J. Pharmacol. Exp. Ther.* **314**, 506.

110. Cross, CE *et al.* (2006) Combating oxidative stress at respiratory tract biosurfaces. *Free Rad. Biol. Med.* **40**, 1693.

111. Romieu, I *et al.* (2004) Genetic polymorphism of GSTM1 and antioxidant supplementation influence lung function in relation to O_3 exposure in asthmatic children in Mexico city. *Thorax* **59**, 8.

112. Samet, JM *et al.* (2001) Effect of antioxidant supplementation on O_3-induced lung injury in human subjects. *Am. J. Resp. Crit. Care Med.* **164**, 819.

113. Grievink, L *et al.* (2000) Anti-oxidants and air pollution in relation to indicators of asthma and COPD: a review of the current evidence. *Clin. Exp. Allergy* **30**, 1344.

114. Long, NC *et al.* (2001) O_3 causes lipid peroxidation but little antioxidant depletion in exercising and nonexercising hamsters. *J. Appl. Physiol.* **91**, 1694.

115. Montuschi, P *et al.* (2002) O_3-induced increase in exhaled 8-IP in healthy subjects is resistant to inhaled budesonide. *Free Rad. Biol. Med.* **33**, 1403.

116. Ballinger, CA *et al.* (2005) Antioxidant-mediated augmentation of O_3-induced membrane oxidation. *Free Rad. Biol. Med.* **38**, 515.

117. Wiester, MJ *et al.* (2000) O_3 adaptation in mice and its association with ascorbic acid in the lung. *Inhal. Toxicol.* **12**, 577.

118. Jackson, RM and Frank, L (1984) O_3-induced tolerance to hyperoxia in rats. *Am. Rev. Resp. Dis.* **129**, 425.

119. Augusto, O *et al.* (2002) $NO_2^{\bullet}$ and $CO_3^{\bullet-}$: two emerging radicals in biology. *Free Rad. Biol. Med.* **32**, 841.

120. Finlayson-Pitts, BJ and Pitts Jr, JN (1997) Tropospheric air pollution: O_3, airborne toxics, polycyclic aromatic hydrocarbons, and particles. *Science* **276**, 1045.

121. Franze, T *et al.* (2005) Protein nitration by polluted air. *Env. Sci. Technol.* **39**, 1673.

122. Greis, KD *et al.* (1996) Identification of nitration sites on surfactant protein A by tandem electrospray MS. *Arch. Biochem. Biophys.* **335**, 396.

123. Huie, RE (1994) The reaction kinetics of $NO_2^{\bullet}$. *Toxicology* **89**, 193.

124. Kirsch, M *et al.* (2002) The pathobiochemistry of $NO_2^{\bullet}$. *Biol. Chem.* **383**, 389.

125. Pryor, WA and Lightsey, JW (1981) Mechanisms of $NO_2^{\bullet}$ reactions: initiation of lipid peroxidation and the production of HNO_2. *Science* **214**, 435.

126. Ford, E *et al.* (2002) Kinetics of the reactions of $NO_2^{\bullet}$ with GSH, cysteine, and uric acid at physiological pH. *Free Rad. Biol. Med.* **32**, 1314.

127. Kelly, FJ *et al.* (1996) Antioxidant kinetics in lung lavage fluid following exposure of humans to $NO_2^{\bullet}$. *Am. J. Resp. Crit. Care Med.* **154**, 1700.

128. Mitsuhashi, H *et al.* (2001) Is sulfite an antiatherogenic compound in wine? *Clin. Chem.* **47**, 1872.

129. Zhang, X *et al.* (2004) A mechanism of sulfite neurotoxicity: direct inhibition of glutamate dehydrogenase. *J. Biol. Chem.* **279**, 43035.

130. McCord, JM and Fridovich, I (1969) The utility of SOD in studying free radical reactions. *J. Biol. Chem.* **244**, 6056.

131. Chamulitrat, W (1999) Activation of the $O_2^{\bullet-}$-generating NADPH oxidase of intestinal lymphocytes produces highly reactive free radicals from sulfite. *Free Rad. Biol. Med.* **27**, 411.

132. Liu, KJ *et al.* (1999) Evaluation of DEPMPO as a spin trapping agent in biological systems. *Free Rad. Biol. Med.* **26**, 714.

133. Mottley, C and Mason, RP (1988) Sulfate free radical formation by the peroxidation of (bi)sulfite and its reaction with $OH^{\bullet}$ scavengers. *Arch. Biochem. Biophys.* **267**, 681.

134. Halliwell, B and Poulsen, HE (eds) (2006) *Cigarette Smoke and Oxidative Stress.* Springer Verlag, Basle, Switzerland.

135. O'Reilly, EJ *et al.* (2005) Smokeless tobacco use and the risk of PD mortality. *Mov. Disord.* **20**, 1383.

136. Flicker, TM and Green, SA (1998) Detection and separation of gas-phase carbon-centered radicals

from cigarette smoke and diesel exhaust. *Anal. Chem.* **70**, 2008.

137. Klein, I *et al.* (2003) Effect of cigarette smoke on oral peroxidase activity in human saliva: role of HCN. *Free Rad. Biol. Med.* **35**, 1448.

138. van der Vaart, H *et al.* (2004) Acute effects of cigarette smoke on inflammation and oxidative stress: a review. *Thorax* **59**, 713.

139. Chen, HJ and Chiu, WL (2005) Association between cigarette smoking and urinary excretion of 1, N^2-ethenoguanine measured by isotope dilution liquid chromatography-electrospray ionization/tandem MS. *Chem. Res. Toxicol.* **18**, 1593.

140. Göen, T *et al.* (2005) Sensitive and accurate analyses of free 3-NT in exhaled breath condensate by LC-MS/MS. *J. Chromatogr.* **826**, 261.

141. Jaimes, EA *et al.* (2004) Stable compounds of cigarette smoke induce endothelial $O_2^{\cdot-}$ production via NADPH oxidase activation. *Arterio. Thromb. Vasc. Biol.* **24**, 1031.

142. Nowak, D *et al.* (1990) Nicotine increases human polymorphonuclear leukocytes chemotactic response–a possible additional mechanism of lung injury in cigarette smokers. *Exp. Pathol.* **39**, 37.

143. Petrache, I *et al.* (2005) Ceramide upregulation causes pulmonary cell apoptosis and emphysema-like disease in mice. *Nature Med.* **11**, 491.

144. Bruno, RS *et al.* (2006) Faster plasma vitamin E disappearance in smokers is normalized by vitamin C supplementation. *Free Rad. Biol. Med.* **40**, 689.

145. Dietrich, M *et al.* (2002) Antioxidant supplementation decreases lipid peroxidation biomarker F_2-IPs in plasma of smokers. *Cancer Epidemiol. Biomark. Prevent.* **11**, 7.

146. Patrignani, P *et al.* (2000) Effects of vitamin E supplementation on F_2-IP and thromboxane biosynthesis in healthy cigarette smokers. *Circulation* **102**, 539.

147. Bruno, RS and Traber, MG (2005) Cigarette smoke alters human vitamin E requirements. *J. Nutr.* **135**, 671.

148. Bielicki, JK *et al.* (1995) Cu and gas-phase cigarette smoke inhibit plasma LCAT activity by different mechanisms. *J. Lipid Res.* **36**, 322.

149. Prieme, H *et al.* (1997) No effect of supplementation with vitamin E, ascorbic acid, or coenzyme Q10 on oxidative DNA damage estimated by 8OHdG excretion in smokers. *Am. J. Clin. Nutr.* **65**, 503.

150. Fiala, ES *et al.* (2005) Induction of preneoplastic lung lesions in guinea pigs by cigarette smoke inhalation and their exacerbation by high dietary levels of vitamins C and E. *Carcinogenesis* **26**, 605.

151. Kinnula, VL (2005) Focus on antioxidant enzymes and antioxidant strategies in smoking related airway diseases. *Thorax* **60**, 693.

152. Gensch, E *et al.* (2004) Tobacco smoke control of mucin production in lung cells requires O_2 radicals AP-1 and JNK. *J. Biol. Chem.* **279**, 39085.

153. Rahman, I and MacNee, W (1999) Lung GSH and oxidative stress: implications in cigarette smoke-induced airway disease. *Am. J. Physiol.* **277**, L1067.

154. Asami, S *et al.* (1996) Increase of a type of oxidative DNA damage, 8OHG and its repair activity in human leukocytes by cigarette smoking. *Cancer Res.* **56**, 2546.

155. Collier, AC and Pritsos, CA (2003) ETS in the workplace: markers of exposure, polymorphic enzymes and implications for disease state. *Chem. Biol. Interact.* **146**, 211.

156. Dietrich, M *et al.* (2003) Vitamin C supplementation decreases oxidative stress biomarker F_2-IPs in plasma of nonsmokers exposed to ETS. *Nutr. Cancer* **45**, 176.

157. Chen, CL *et al.* (2002) $OH^{\bullet}$ formation and oxidative DNA damage induced by areca quid *in vivo*. *J. Tox. Environ. Health A.* **65**, 327.

158. Pryor, WA (1992) Biological effects of cigarette smoke, wood smoke and the smoke from plastics: the use of ESR. *Free Rad. Biol. Med.* **13**, 659.

159. La Londe, C *et al.* (1994) Aerosolized deferoxamine prevents lung and systemic injury caused by smoke inhalation. *J. Appl. Physiol.* **77**, 2057.

160. Wang, S *et al.* (1999) Early alterations of lung injury following acute smoke exposure by 21-aminosteroid treatment. *Toxicol. Pathol.* **27**, 334.

161. Nel, A (2005) Air pollution-related illness: effects of particles. *Science* **308**, 804.

162. Li, N *et al.* (2003) Particulate air pollutants and asthma. A paradigm for the role of oxidative stress in PM-induced adverse health effects. *Clin. Immunol.* **109**, 250.

163. Risom, L *et al.* (2003) Oxidative DNA damage and defence gene expression in the mouse lung after short-term exposure to diesel exhaust particles by inhalation. *Carcinogenesis* **24**, 1847.

164. Mudway, IS *et al.* (2004) An *in vitro* and *in vivo* investigation of the effects of diesel exhaust on human airway lining fluid antioxidants. *Arch. Biochem. Biophys.* **423**, 200.

165. Castranova, V (2004) Signaling pathways controlling the production of inflammatory mediators in response to crystalline silica exposure: role of RO/N species. *Free Rad. Biol. Med.* **37**, 916.

166. Fubini, B and Hubbard, A (2003) ROS and RNS generation by silica in inflammation and fibrosis. *Free Rad. Biol. Med.* **34**, 1507.

167. Shukla, A *et al.* (2003) Multiple roles of oxidants in the pathogenesis of asbestos-induced diseases. *Free Rad. Biol. Med.* **34**, 1117.

168. Fattman, CL *et al.* (2006) Increased sensitivity to asbestos-induced lung injury in mice lacking EC-SOD. *Free Rad. Biol. Med.* **40**, 601.

169. Marczynski, B *et al.* (2000) Association between 8OHdG levels in DNA of workers highly exposed to asbestos and their clinical data, occupational and non-occupational confounding factors, and cancer. *Mutat. Res.* **468**, 203.

170. McNeilly, JD *et al.* (2005) Soluble transition metals in welding fumes cause inflammation via activation of NF-κB and AP-1. *Toxicol. Lett.* **158**, 152.

171. Zhang, Q *et al.* (2002) Roles of bioavailable Fe and Ca in coal dust-induced oxidative stress: possible implications in coal workers' lung disease. *Free Radic. Res.* **36**, 285.

172. Karlsson, HL *et al.* (2005) Subway particles are more genotoxic than street particles and induce oxidative stress in cultured human lung cells. *Chem. Res. Toxicol.* **18**, 19.

173. Valko, M *et al.* (2005) Metals, toxicity and oxidative stress. *Curr. Med. Chem.* **12**, 1161.

174. Hei, TK and Filipic, M (2004) Role of oxidative damage in the genotoxicity of As. *Free Rad. Biol. Med.* **37**, 574.

175. Chou, WC *et al.* (2004) Role of NADPH oxidase in As-induced ROS formation and cytotoxicity in myeloid leukemia cells. *Proc. Natl. Acad. Sci. USA* **101**, 4578.

176. An, Y *et al.* (2004) Immunohistochemical analysis of oxidative DNA damage in As-related human skin samples from As-contaminated area of China. *Cancer Lett.* **214**, 11.

177. Diaz, Z *et al.* (2005) Trolox selectively enhances As-mediated oxidative stress and apoptosis in APL and other malignant cell lines. *Blood* **105**,1237.

178. Kasprzak, KS (2002) Oxidative DNA and protein damage in metal-induced toxicity and carcinogenesis. *Free Rad. Biol. Med.* **32**, 958.

179. Bal, W *et al.* (2003) Mechanism of Ni assault on the zinc finger of DNA repair protein XPA. *Chem. Res. Toxicol.* **16**, 242.

180. Gunton, JE *et al.* (2005) Cr supplementation does not improve glucose tolerance, insulin sensitivity, or lipid profile. *Diabetes Care* **28**, 712.

181. Slade, PG *et al.* (2005) Guanine-specific oxidation of double-stranded DNA by Cr(VI) and ascorbic acid forms spiroiminodihydantoin and 8OHdG. *Chem. Res. Toxicol.* **18**, 1140.

182. Sørensen, M *et al.* (2005) Transition metals in personal samples of $PM_{2.5}$ and oxidative stress in human volunteers. *Cancer Epidemiol. Biomark. Prev.* **14**, 1340.

183. Eberhardt, MK (1995) The OH$^\bullet$. Formation and some reactions used in its identification. *Trends Org. Chem.* **5**, 115.

184. Liochev, SI and Fridovich, I (2005) The roles of CO_2 in cobalt-catalyzed peroxidations. *Arch. Biochem. Biophys.* **439**, 99.

185. Contrino, J *et al.* (1988) Effect of mercury on human polymorphonuclear leukocyte function *in vitro. Am. J. Pathol.* **132**, 110.

186. Chen, C *et al.* (2005) Increased oxidative DNA damage, as assessed by urinary 8OHdG concentrations, and serum redox status in persons exposed to mercury. *Clin. Chem.* **51**, 759.

187. Gurer, H and Ercal, N (2000) Can antioxidants be beneficial in the treatment of lead poisoning? *Free Rad. Biol. Med.* **29**, 927.

188. Liochev, SI and Fridovich, I (1991) The roles of $O_2^{\bullet-}$, HO$^\bullet$, and secondarily derived radicals in oxidation reactions catalyzed by vanadium salts. *Arch. Biochem. Biophys.* **291**, 379.

189. Quinlan GJ *et al.* (1992) Vanadium and Cu in clinical albumin solutions and their potential to damage protein structure. *J. Pharm. Sci.* **81**, 611.

190. Krejsa, CM *et al.* (1997) Role of oxidative stress in the action of vanadium phosphotyrosine phosphatase inhibitors. *J. Biol. Chem.* **272**, 11541.

191. Kumazawa, R *et al.* (2002) Effects of Ti ions and particles on neutrophil function and morphology. *Biomaterials* **23**, 3757.

192. Exley, C (2004) The pro-oxidant activity of Al. *Free Rad. Biol. Med.* **36**, 380.

193. Quinlan, GJ *et al.* (1988) Action of Pb(II) and Al(III) ions on Fe-stimulated lipid peroxidation in liposomes, erythrocytes and rat liver microsomal fractions. *Biochim. Biophys. Acta* **962**, 196.

194. Kapiotis, S *et al.* (2005) Al^{3+} stimulate the oxidizability of LDL by Fe^{2+}: implication in hemodialysis mediated atherogenic LDL modification. *Free Radic. Res.* **39**, 1225.

195. Pratico, D *et al.* (2002) Al modulates brain amyloidosis through oxidative stress in APP transgenic mice. *FASEB J.* **16**, 1138.

196. Zhang, Y *et al.* (2004) ONOO⁻-induced neuronal apoptosis is mediated by intracellular Zn release and 12-LOX activation. *J. Neurosci.* **24**, 10616.

197. Noh, KM and Koh, JY (2000) Induction and activation by Zn of NADPH oxidase in cultured cortical neurons and astrocytes. *J. Neurosci.* **20**, 111.

198. Gutteridge, JMC *et al.* (1983) Free radical damage to polyene antifungal antibiotics: changes in biological activity and TBA reactivity. *J. Appl. Biochem.* **5**, 53.

199. Cuquerella, MC *et al.* (2003) Photochemical properties of ofloxacin involved in oxidative DNA damage: a comparison with rufloxacin. *Chem. Res. Toxicol.* **16**, 562.

200. Angrave, FE and Avery, SV (2001) Antioxidant functions required for insusceptibility of *S cerevisiae* to tetracycline antibiotics. *Antimicrob. Ag. Chemother.* **45**, 2939.

201. Koistinaho, M *et al.* (2005) Minocycline protects against permanent cerebral ischemia in wild type but not in MMP-9-deficient mice. *J. Cereb. Blood Flow Metab.* **25**, 460.

202. Gutteridge, JM *et al.* (1998) Phagomimetic action of antimicrobial agents. *Free Radic. Res.* **28**, 1.

203. Dong, C *et al.* (2005) Tryptophan 7-halogenase (PrnA) structure suggests a mechanism for regioselective chlorination. *Science* **309**, 2216.

204. Yeowell, HN and White, JR (1982) Fe requirement in the bactericidal mechanism of streptonigrin. *Antimicrob. Ag. Chemother.* **22**, 961.

205. Hassett, DJ *et al.* (1987) Bacteria form intracellular free radicals in response to paraquat and streptonigrin: demonstration of the potency of OH$^\bullet$. *J. Biol. Chem.* **262**, 13404.

206. Kono, Y (1982) O_2 enhancement of bactericidal activity of rifamycin SV on *E. coli* and aerobic oxidation of rifamycin SV to rifamycin S catalyzed by Mn^{2+}: the role of $O_2^{\bullet-}$. *J. Biochem.* **91**, 381.

207. Lesniak, W *et al.* (2005) Ternary complexes of gentamicin with Fe and lipid catalyze formation of ROS. *Chem. Res. Toxicol.* **18**, 357.

208. Ramasammy, LS *et al.* (1987) Failure of inhibition of lipid peroxidation by vitamin E to protect against gentamicin nephrotoxicity in the rat. *Biochem. Pharmacol.* **36**, 2125.

209. Sergi, B *et al.* (2004) The role of antioxidants in protection from ototoxic drugs. *Acta Otolaryngol.* **552** (Suppl.), 42.

210. Miller, JM *et al.* (2002) 8-Iso-prostaglandin $F_{2\alpha}$, a product of noise exposure, reduces inner ear blood flow. *Audiol. Neurootol.* **8**, 207.

211. Lynch, ED and Kil, J (2005) Compounds for the prevention and treatment of noise-inducing hearing loss. *Drug Disc. Today* **10**, 1291.

212. Endo, T *et al.* (2005) Elevation of SOD increases acoustic trauma from noise exposure. *Free Rad. Biol. Med.* **38**, 492.

213. Klein, K *et al.* (2003) Meningitis-associated hearing loss: protection by adjunctive antioxidant therapy. *Ann. Neurol.* **54**, 451.

214. Bánfi, B *et al.* (2004) NOX3, $O_2^{\bullet-}$-generating NADPH oxidase of the inner ear. *J. Biol. Chem.* **279**, 46065.

215. Liu, J *et al.* (1996) Immobilization stress causes oxidative damage to lipid, protein, and DNA in the brain of rats. *FASEB J.* **10**, 1532.

216. Kim, ST *et al.* (2005) Immobilization stress causes increases in THB, dopamine, and neuromelanin and oxidative damage in the nigrostriatal system. *J. Neurochem.* **95**, 89.

217. Silva, RH *et al.* (2004) Role of hippocampal oxidative stress in memory deficits induced by sleep deprivation in mice. *Neuropharmacol.* **46**, 895.

218. Irie, M *et al.* (2005) Depression and possible cancer risk due to oxidative DNA damage. *J. Psychiatr. Res.* **39**, 553.

219. Epel, ES *et al.* (2004) Accelerated telomere shortening in response to life stress. *Proc. Natl. Acad. Sci. USA* **101**, 17312.

220. Oh, TY *et al.* (2005) Synergism of *H. pylori* infection and stress on the augmentation of gastric mucosal damage and its prevention with α-tocopherol. *Free Rad. Biol. Med.* **38**, 1447.

221. Biaglow, JE *et al.* (1986) Biochemistry of reduction of nitroheterocycles. *Biochem. Pharmacol.* **35**, 77.

222. Kumagai, Y *et al.* (2000) ζ-Crystallin catalyzes the reductive activation of 2,4,6-trinitrotoluene to generate ROS: a proposed mechanism for the induction of cataracts. *FEBS Lett.* **478**, 295.

223. Hetherington, LH *et al.* (1996) Two- and one-electron dependent *in vitro* reductive metabolism of nitroaromatics by *Mytilus edulis*, *Carcinus maenas* and *Asterias rubens*. *Comp. Biochem. Physiol.* **113C**, 231.

224. Krainev, AG *et al.* (1998) Enzymatic reduction of 3-nitrotyrosine generates $O_2^{\bullet-}$. *Chem. Res. Toxicol.* **11**, 495.

225. Moreno, SNJ *et al.* (1985) Reduction of the metallochromic indicators arsenoazo III and antipyrylazo III to their free radical metabolites by cytoplasmic enzymes. *FEBS Lett.* **180**, 229.

226. Carugo, O and Carugo, KD (2005) When X-rays modify the protein structure: radiation damage at work. *TIBS* **30**, 213.

227. Pearson, CG *et al.* (2004) Enhanced mutagenic potential of 8OHdG when present within a clustered DNA damage site. *Nucl. Acids Res.* **32**, 263.

228. Tondel, M *et al.* (2005) Urinary 8OHdG in Belarussian children relates to urban living rather than radiation dose after the Chernobyl accident: a pilot study. *Arch. Environ. Contam. Toxicol.* **48**, 515.

229. Stone, R (2005) Russian cancer study adds to the indictment of low-dose radiation. *Science* **310**, 959.

230. Brown, JM (2000) Exploiting the hypoxic cancer cell: mechanism and therapeutic strategies. *Mol. Med. Today* **6**, 157.

231. Dürken, M *et al.* (2000) Impaired plasma antioxidative defense and increased nontransferrinbound Fe during high-dose chemotherapy and radiochemotherapy preceding bone marrow transplantation. *Free Rad. Biol. Med.* **28**, 887.

232. Ghosal, D *et al.* (2005) How radiation kills cells: survival of *Deinococcus radiodurans* and *Shewanella oneidensis* under oxidative stress. *FEMS Microbiol. Rev.* **29**, 361.

233. Persson, HL *et al.* (2005) Radiation-induced cell death: importance of lysosomal destabilization. *Biochem. J.* **389**, 877.

234. Carpenter, M *et al.* (2005) Inhalation delivery of MnSOD-plasmid/liposomes protects the murine lung from irradiation damage. *Gene Ther.* **12**, 2005.

235. Epperly, MW *et al.* (1999) MnSOD plasmid/liposome pulmonary radioprotective gene therapy: modulation of irradiation-induced mRNA for IL-1, TNF-α and TGF-β correlates with delay of organizing alveolitis/fibrosis. *Biol. Blood Marrow Transplant.* **5**, 204.

236. Kolesnick, R and Fuks, Z (2003) Radiation and ceramide-induced apoptosis. *Oncogene* **22**, 5897.

237. Misra, H and Fridovich, I (1976) SOD and the O_2 enhancement of radiation lethality. *Arch. Biochem. Biophys.* **176**, 577.

238. Bairati, I *et al.* (2005) Randomized trial of antioxidant vitamins to prevent acute adverse effects of radiation therapy in head and neck cancer patients. *J. Clin. Oncol.* **23**, 5805.

239. Schreiber, GA *et al.* (1993) Detection of irradiated food—methods and routine applications. *Int. J. Rad. Biol.* **63**, 105.

Chapter 9

1. Halliwell, B *et al.* (1992) Free radicals, antioxidants and human disease. Where are we now? *J. Lab. Clin. Med.* **119**, 598.

2. Southorn, PA (1988) Free radicals in medicine. II: involvement in human disease. *Mayo Clin. Proc.* **63**, 390.

3. Giralt, M *et al.* (1996) GSH, GST and ROS in human scalp sebaceous glands in male pattern baldness. *J. Invest. Dermatol.* **107**, 154.

4. Halliwell, B and Gutteridge, JMC (1984) Lipid peroxidation, O_2 radicals, cell damage and antioxidant therapy. *Lancet* **1**, 1396.

5. Solaini, G and Harris, DA (2005) Biochemical dysfunction in heart mitochondria exposed to ischaemia and reperfusion. *Biochem. J.* **390**, 377.

6. Gutteridge, JMC and Mitchell, J (1999) Redox imbalance in the critically ill. *Br. Med. Bull.* **55**, 49.

7. Sepulveda, RT and Watson, RR (2002) Treatment of antioxidant deficiencies in AIDS patients. *Nutr. Res.* **22**, 27.

8. Scorah, CJ *et al.* (1996) Total vitamin C, ascorbic acid, and DHA concentrations in plasma of critically ill patients. *Am. J. Clin. Nutr.* **63**, 760.

9. Crimi, E *et al.* (2004) The beneficial effects of antioxidant supplementation in enteral feeding in critically ill patients: a prospective, randomized, double-blind, placebo-controlled trial. *Anesth. Analg.* **99**, 857.

10. Jackson, MJ and Edwards, RHT (1998) Therapeutic trials of antioxidants in muscle diseases. In: *Oxidative Stress in Skeletal Muscle* (Reznick, AZ *et al.* eds), p. 327. Birkhäuser Verlag, Basel, Switzerland.

11. Ross, R (1993) The pathogenesis of atherosclerosis: a perspective for the 1990s. *Nature* **362**, 801.

12. Steinberg, D (2002) Atherogenesis in perspective: hypercholesterolemia and inflammation as partners in crime. *Nature Med.* **8**, 1211.

13. Nicholls, SJ and Hazen, SL (2005) MPO and cardiovascular disease. *Arterio. Thromb. Vasc. Biol.* **25**, 1102.

14. Kobayashi, S *et al.* (2003) Interaction of oxidative stress and inflammatory response in coronary plaque instability. *Arterio. Thromb. Vasc. Biol.* **23**, 1398.

15. Palinski, W and Napoli, C (2002) The fetal origins of atherosclerosis: maternal hypercholesterolemia, and cholesterol-lowering or antioxidant treatment during pregnancy influence in utero programming and postnatal susceptibility to atherogenesis. *FASEB J.* **16**, 1348.

16. Walzem, RL *et al.* (1995) Older plasma lipoproteins are more susceptible to oxidation: a linking mechanism for the lipid and oxidation theories of atherosclerotic cardiovascular disease. *Proc. Natl. Acad. Sci. USA* **92**, 7460.

17. Cines, DB *et al.* (1998) Endothelial cells in physiology and in the pathophysiology of vascular disorders. *Blood* **91**, 3527.

18. Topper, JN *et al.* (1996) Identification of vascular endothelial genes differentially responsive to fluid mechanical stimuli: COX-2, MnSOD and endothelial cell NOS are selectively up-regulated by steady laminar shear stress. *Proc. Natl. Acad. Sci. USA* **93**, 10417.

19. Murphy, JE *et al.* (2005) Biochemistry and cell biology of mammalian scavenger receptors. *Atherosclerosis* **182**, 1.

20. Darley-Usmar, V and Halliwell, B (1996) Blood radicals. *Pharm. Res.* **13**, 649.

21. Robbesyn, F *et al.* (2004) Dual role of oxidized LDL on the NF-κB signaling pathway. *Free Radic. Res.* **38**, 541.

22. Brand, K *et al.* (1997) Role of NF-κB in atherogenesis. *Exp. Physiol.* **82**, 297.

23. Szmitko, PE *et al.* (2003) Biomarkers of vascular disease linking inflammation to endothelial activation. *Circulation* **108**, 2041.

24. Cipollone, F *et al.* (2004) Balance between PGD synthase and PGE synthase is a major determinant of atherosclerotic plaque instability in humans. *Arterio. Thromb. Vasc. Biol.* **24**, 1259.

25. Praticò, D *et al.* (1997) Localization of distinct F_2-isoprostanes in human atherosclerotic lesions. *J. Clin. Invest.* **100**, 2028.

26. Devchand, PR *et al.* (2004) Oxidative stress and PPARs. *Circ. Res.* **95**, 1137.

27. Davies, SS *et al.* (2001) Oxidized alkyl phospholipids are specific, high affinity PPARγ ligands and agonists. *J. Biol. Chem.* **276**, 16015.

28. Swain, J and Gutteridge, JMC (1995) Prooxidant Fe and Cu, with ferroxidase and XO activities in human atherosclerotic lesions. *FEBS Lett.* **368**, 513.

29. Denicola, A *et al.* (2002) Diffusion of NO• into LDL. *J. Biol. Chem.* **277**, 932.

30. Thomas, SR *et al.* (2003) Oxidative stress and endothelial NO• bioactivity. *Antioxid. Redox Signal.* **5**, 181.

31. Kuhlencordt, PJ *et al.* (2001) Genetic deficiency of iNOS reduces atherosclerosis and lowers plasma lipid peroxides in apoE-knockout mice. *Circulation* **103**, 3099.

32. Boger, RH (2004) ADMA, an endogenous inhibitor of NOS, explains the 'L-arginine paradox' and acts as a novel cardiovascular risk factor. *J. Nutr.* **134**, 2842S.

33. Evans, PJ *et al.* (1995) Metal ion release from mechanically-disrupted human arterial wall. Implications for the development of atherosclerosis. *Free Radic. Res.* **23**, 465.

34. Völker, W *et al.* (1997) Cu-induced inflammatory reactions of rat carotid arteries mimic restenosis/arteriosclerosis-like neointima formation. *Atherosclerosis* **130**, 29.

35. Pentikäinen, MO *et al.* (2001) MPO and OCl^-, but not Cu ions, oxidize heparin-bound LDL particles and release them from heparin. *Arterio. Thromb. Vasc. Biol.* **21**, 1902.

36. Wang, LJ *et al.* (1998) Expression of HO-1 in atherosclerotic lesions. *Am. J. Pathol.* **152**, 711.

37. Jeney,V *et al.* (2002) Pro-oxidant and cytotoxic effects of circulating heme. *Blood* **100**, 879.

38. Ishikawa, K *et al.* (2001) HO-1 inhibits atherogenesis in Watanabe heritable hyperlipidemic rabbits. *Circulation* **104**, 1831.

39. Ren, M *et al.* (2005) Fe chelation inhibits atherosclerosis lesion development and reduces lesion Fe concentrations in the cholesterol-fed rabbit. *Free Rad. Biol. Med.* **38**, 1206.

40. You, SA and Wang, Q (2005) Ferritin in atherosclerosis. *Clin. Chim. Acta* **357**, 1.

41. Pannala, AS *et al.* (1998) Interaction of $ONOO^-$ with carotenoids and tocopherols within LDL. *FEBS Lett.* **423**, 297.

42. Thukkani, AK *et al.* (2003) MPO-derived RCS from human monocytes target plasmalogens in LDL. *J. Biol. Chem.* **278**, 36365.

43. Coleman, LG *et al.* (2004) LDL oxidized by HOCl causes irreversible platelet aggregation when combined with low levels of ADP, thrombin, epinephrine, or macrophage-derived chemokine (CCL22). *Blood* **104**, 380.

44. Brennan, ML *et al.* (2001) Increased atherosclerosis in MPO-deficient mice. *J. Clin. Invest.* **107**, 419.

45. Sentman, ML *et al.* (2001) EC-SOD deficiency and atherosclerosis in mice. *Arterio. Thromb. Vasc. Biol.* **21**, 1477.

46. Thukkani, AK *et al.* (2003) Identification of α-chloro fatty aldehydes and unsaturated lysophosphatidylcholine molecular species in human atherosclerotic lesions. *Circulation* **108**, 3128.

47. Fu, S *et al.* (1998) Evidence for roles of radicals in protein oxidation in advanced human atherosclerotic plaque. *Biochem. J.* **333**, 519.

48. Navab, M *et al.* (2004) The oxidative hypothesis of atherogenesis: the role of oxidized phospholipids and HDL. *J. Lipid Res.* **45**, 993.

49. Sendobry, SM *et al.* (1997) Attenuation of diet-induced atherosclerosis in rabbits with a highly selective 15-LOX inhibitor lacking significant antioxidant properties. *Br. J. Pharmacol.* **120**, 1199.

50. Waddington, EI *et al.* (2003) Fatty acid oxidation productions in human atherosclerotic plaque: an analysis of clinical and histopathological correlates. *Atherosclerosis* **167**, 111.

51. Shishehbor, MH *et al.* (2003) Association of nitrotyrosine levels with cardiovascular disease and modulation by statin therapy. *JAMA* **289**, 1675.

52. Rota, S *et al.* (1998) Atherogenic lipoproteins support assembly of the prothrombinase complex and thrombin generation: modulation by oxidation and vitamin E. *Blood* **91**, 508.

53. Parhami, F *et al.* (1997) Lipid oxidation products have opposite effects on calcifying vascular cell and bone cell differentiation. *Arterio. Thromb. Vasc. Biol.* **17**, 680.

54. Upston, JM *et al.* (2002) Disease stage-dependent accumulation of lipid and protein oxidation products in human atherosclerosis. *Am. J. Pathol.* **160**, 701.

55. Rimner, A *et al.* (2005) Relevance and mechanism of oxysterol stereospecificity in coronary artery disease. *Free Rad. Biol. Med.* **38**, 535.

56. Biasi, F *et al.* (2004) Oxysterol mixtures prevent proapoptotic effects of 7-ketocholesterol in macrophages: implications for proatherogenic gene modulation. *FASEB J.* **18**, 693.

57. Meisinger, C *et al.* (2005) Plasma oxidized LDL, a strong predictor for acute coronary heart disease events in apparently healthy, middle-aged men from the general population. *Circulation* **112**, 651.

58. Horiuchi, S *et al.* (2003) Scavenger receptors for oxidized and glycated proteins. *Amino Acids* **25**, 283.

59. Upston, JM *et al.* (2002) Oxidized lipid accumulates in the presence of α-tocopherol in atherosclerosis. *Biochem. J.* **363**, 753.

60. Martinet, W *et al.* (2002) Elevated levels of oxidative DNA damage and DNA repair enzymes in human atherosclerotic plaques. *Circulation* **106**, 927.

61. Hazen, SL and Chisolm, GM (2002) Oxidized phosphatidylcholines: pattern recognition ligands for multiple pathways of the innate immune response. *Proc. Natl. Acad. Sci. USA* **99**, 12515.

62. Shoenfeld, Y *et al.* (2004) Are anti-oxidized LDL antibodies pathogenic or protective? *Circ. Res.* **110**, 2552.

63. Nilsson, J *et al.* (2003) Immunomodulation of atherosclerosis. *Arterio. Thromb. Vasc. Biol.* **25**, 18.

64. Freyschuss, A *et al.* (2001) On the anti-atherogenic effect of the antioxidant BHT in cholesterol-fed rabbits: inverse relation between serum triglycerides and atheromatous lesions. *Biochim. Biophys. Acta* **1534**, 129.

65. Witting, P *et al.* (1999) Dissociation of atherogenesis from aortic accumulation of lipid hydro(pero)xides in WHHL rabbits. *J. Clin. Invest.* **104**, 213.

66. Wågberg, M *et al.* (2001) DiNAC, the disulfide dimer of NAc, inhibits atherosclerosis in WHHL rabbits: evidence for immunomodulatory agents as a new approach to prevent atherosclerosis. *J. Pharmacol. Exp. Ther.* **299**, 76.

67. Waddington, E *et al.* (2004) Red wine polyphenolic compounds inhibit atherosclerosis in apolipoprotein E-deficient mice independently of effects on lipid peroxidation. *Am. J. Clin. Nutr.* **79**, 54.

68. Wagner, AH *et al.* (2000) Improvement of NO•-dependent vasodilatation by HMG-CoA reductase inhibitors through attenuation of endothelial $O_2^{•-}$ formation. *Arterio. Thromb. Vasc. Biol.* **20**, 61.

69. Yang, H *et al.* (2004) Retardation of atherosclerosis by overexpression of catalase or both CuZnSOD and catalase in mice lacking apoplipoprotein E. *Circ. Res.* **95**, 1075.

70. Praticò, D *et al.* (2001) Lipid peroxidation in mouse models of atherosclerosis. *Trends Cardiovasc. Med.* **11**, 112.

71. Esterbauer, H *et al.* (1992) The role of lipid peroxidation and antioxidants in oxidative modification of LDL. *Free Rad. Biol. Med.* **13**, 341.

72. Ziouzenkova, O *et al.* (1998) Cu can promote oxidation of LDL by markedly different mechanisms. *Free Rad. Biol. Med.* **24**, 607.

73. Reaven, P (1996) The role of dietary fat in LDL oxidation and atherosclerosis. *Nutr. Metab. Cardiovasc. Dis.* **6**, 57.

74. Retsky, KL *et al.* (1999) Inhibition of Cu-induced LDL oxidation by vitamin C is associated with decreased Cu-binding to LDL and 2-oxo-histidine formation. *Free Rad. Biol. Med.* **26**, 90.

75. Hatta, A and Frei, B (1995) Oxidative modification and antioxidant protection of human LDL at high and low O_2 partial pressures. *J. Lipid Res.* **36**, 2383.

76. Raveh, O *et al.* (2002) O_2 availability as a possible limiting factor in LDL oxidation. *Free Radic. Res.* **36**, 1109.

77. Burkitt, MJ (2001) A critical overview of the chemistry of Cu-dependent LDL oxidation: roles of lipid hydroperoxides, α-tocopherol, thiols, and ceruloplasmin. *Arch. Biochem. Biophys.* **394**, 117.

78. Staprans, I *et al.* (1994) Oxidized lipids in the diet are a source of oxidized lipid in chylomicrons of human serum. *Arterio. Thromb. Vasc. Biol.* **14**, 1900.

79. Vila, A *et al.* (2002) Spontaneous transfer of phospholipid and cholesterol hydroperoxides between cell membranes and LDL: assessment of reaction kinetics and prooxidant effects. *Biochemistry* **41**, 13705.

80. Kalyanaraman, B *et al.* (1992) Synergistic interaction between the probucol phenoxyl radical and ascorbic acid in inhibiting the oxidation of LDL. *J. Biol. Chem.* **267**, 6789.

81. Bräsen, JH *et al.* (2002) Comparison of the effects of α-tocopherol, ubiquinone-10 and probucol at therapeutic doses on atherosclerosis in WHHL rabbits. *Atherosclerosis* **163**, 249.

82. Laughton, MJ *et al.* (1991) Inhibition of mammalian 5-LOX and COX by flavonoids and phenolic dietary additives. Relationship to antioxidant activity and to iron ion-reducing ability. *Biochem. Pharmacol.* **42**, 1673.

83. Sadik, CD *et al.* (2003) Inhibition of 15-LOX by flavonoids: structure-activity relations and mode of action. *Biochem. Pharmacol.* **65**, 773.

84. Bowry, VW *et al.* (1995) Prevention of tocopherol-mediated peroxidation in ubiquinol-10-free human LDL. *J. Biol. Chem.* **270**, 5756.

85. Patterson, RA *et al.* (2003) Prooxidant and antioxidant properties of human serum ultrafiltrates toward LDL: important role of uric acid. *J. Lipid Res.* **44**, 512

86. Otero, P *et al.* (1997) Antioxidant and prooxidant effects of ascorbic acid, dehydroascorbic acid and flavonoids on LDL submitted to different degrees of oxidation. *Free Radic. Res.* **27**, 619.

87. Carr, AC *et al.* (2000) Vitamin C protects against and reverses specific HOCl- and chloramine-dependent modifications of LDL. *Biochem. J.* **346**, 491.

88. Vissers, MN *et al.* (2001) Effect of consumption of phenols from olives and extra virgin olive oil on LDL oxidizability in healthy humans. *Free Radic. Res.* **35**, 619.

89. Riemersma, RA *et al.* (2003) Seasonal variation in Cu-mediated LDL oxidation *in vitro* is related to varying plasma concentration of oxidized lipids in summer and winter. *Free Radic. Res.* **37**, 341.

90. Hoeg, JM *et al.* (1996) Overexpression of LCAT in transgenic rabbits prevents diet-induced atherosclerosis. *Proc. Natl. Acad. Sci. USA* **93**, 11448.

91. Fogelman, AM (2004) When good cholesterol goes bad. *Nature Med.* **10**, 902.

92. Mackness, M and Mackness, B (2004) Paraoxonase 1 and atherosclerosis: is the gene or the protein more important? *Free Rad. Biol. Med.* **37**, 1317.

93. Francis, GA (2000) HDL oxidation: *in vitro* susceptibility and potential *in vivo* consequences. *Biochim. Biophys. Acta* **1483**, 217.

94. Zheng, L *et al.* (2004) ApoA-I is a selective target for MPO-catalysed oxidation and functional impairment in subjects with cardiovascular disease. *J. Clin. Invest.* **114**, 529.

95. Pennathur, S *et al.* (2004) Human atherosclerotic intima and blood of patients with established coronary artery disease contain HDL damaged by RNS. *J. Biol. Chem.* **279**, 42977.

96. Berglund, L and Ramakrishnan, R (2004) Lipoprotein (a). *Arterio. Thromb. Vasc. Biol.* **24**, 2219.

97. Aviram, M and Rosenblat, M (2005) Paraoxonases and cardiovascular diseases: pharmacological and nutritional influences. *Curr. Opin. Lipidol.* **16**, 393.

98. Chen, H *et al.* (2005) MnSOD and catalase transgenes demonstrate that protection of islets from oxidative stress does not alter cytokine toxicity. *Diabetes* **54**, 1437.

99. Kulkarni, RN and Kahn, CR (2004) HNFs-linking the liver and pancreatic islets in diabetes. *Science* **303**, 1311.

100. Piganelli, JD *et al.* (2002) A metalloporphyrin-based SOD mimic inhibits adoptive transfer of autoimmune diabetes by a diabetogenic T-cell clone. *Diabetes* **51**, 347.

101. Bowman, MA *et al.* (1994) Prevention of diabetes in the NOD mouse: implications for therapeutic intervention in human disease. *Immunol. Today* **15**, 115.

102. Olcott, AP *et al.* (2004) A salen-manganese catalytic free radical scavenger inhibits Type 1 diabetes and islet allograft rejection. *Diabetes* **53**, 2574.

103. Betera, S *et al.* (2003) Gene transfer of MnSOD extends islet graft function in a mouse model of autoimmune diabetes. *Diabetes* **52**, 387.

104. Bottino, R *et al.* (2004) Response of human islets to isolation stress and the effect of antioxidant treatment. *Diabetes* **53**, 2559.

105. Davi, G *et al.* (2004) Determinants of F_2-IP biosynthesis and inhibition in man. *Chem. Phys. Lipids* **128**, 149.

106. Rehman, A *et al.* (1999) Increased oxidative damage to all DNA bases in patients with type 2 diabetes mellitus. *FEBS Lett.* **448**, 120.

107. Vincent, AM *et al.* (2004) Oxidative stress in the pathogenesis of diabetic neuropathy. *Endocr. Rev.* **25**, 612.

108. Thornalley, PJ *et al.* (1996) Negative association between erythrocyte GSH concentration and diabetic complications. *Clin. Sci.* **91**, 575.

109. Cowell, RM and Russell, JW (2004) Nitrosative injury and antioxidant therapy in the management of diabetic neuropathy. *J. Invest. Med.* **52**, 33.

110. Chang, TI *et al.* (2003) Oxidant regulation of gene expression and neural tube development: insights gained from diabetic pregnancy on molecular causes of neural tube defects. *Diabetologia* **46**, 538.

111. Brownlee, M (2005) The pathobiology of diabetic complications. *Diabetes* **54**, 1615.

112. Khan, ZA *et al.* (2005) Glucose-induced regulation of novel iron transporters in vascular endothelial cell dysfunction. *Free Radic. Res.* **39**, 1203.

113. Schulze, PC *et al.* (2004) Hyperglycemia promotes oxidative stress through inhibition of thioredoxin function by thioredoxin-interacting protein. *J. Biol. Chem.* **279**, 30369.

114. Sampson, MJ *et al.* (2002) Plasma F_2-IPs direct evidence of increased free radical damage during acute hyperglycemia in type 2 diabetes. *Diabetes Care* **25**, 537.

115. Creager, MA *et al.* (2003) Diabetes and vascular disease. *Circulation* **108**, 1527.

116. Robertson, RP (2004) Chronic oxidative stress as a central mechanism for glucose toxicity in pancreatic islet β-cells in diabetes. *J. Biol. Chem.* **279**, 42351.

117. Sakuraba, H *et al.* (2002) Reduced β-cell mass and expression of oxidative stress-related DNA damage in the islet of Japanese Type II diabetic patients. *Diabetologia* **45**, 85.

118. Hudson, BI *et al.* (2005) Diabetic vascular disease: it's all the RAGE. *Antiox. Redox Signal.* **7**, 1588.

119. Cai, W *et al.* (2004) High levels of dietary advanced glycation end products transform LDL into a potent redox-sensitive MAP kinase stimulant in diabetic patients. *Circulation* **110**, 285.

120. Suleiman, M *et al.* (2005) Haptoglobin polymorphism predicts 30-day mortality and heart failure in patients with diabetes and acute myocardial infarction. *Diabetes* **54**, 2802.

121. Islam, KN *et al.* (1995) Fragmentation of ceruloplasmin following non-enzymatic glycation reaction. *J. Biochem.* **118**, 1054.

122. Burke, AP *et al.* (2004) Morphologic findings of coronary atherosclerotic plaques in diabetics. *Arterio. Thromb. Vasc. Biol.* **24**, 1266.

123. Vasan, S *et al.* (2003) Therapeutic potential of breakers of advanced glycation end product-protein crosslinks. *Arch. Biochem. Biophys.* **419**, 89.

124. Voziyan, PA and Hudson, BG (2005) Pyridoxamine as a multifunctional pharmaceutical: targeting pathogenic glycation and oxidative damage. *Cell. Mol. Life Sci.* **62**, 1671.

125. Davi, G *et al.* (2005) Lipid peroxidation in diabetes mellitus. *Antiox. Redox Signal.* **7**, 256.

126. Hinokio, Y *et al.* (2002) Urinary excretion of 8OHdG as a predictor of the development of diabetic nephropathy. *Diabetologia* **45**, 877.

127. Gopaul, NK *et al.* (2001) Oxidative stress could precede endothelial dysfunction and insulin resistance in Indian Mauritians with impaired glucose metabolism. *Diabetologia* **44**, 706.

128. Hansel, B *et al.* (2004) Metabolic syndrome is associated with elevated oxidative stress and dysfunctional dense HDL particles displaying impaired antioxidative activity. *J. Clin. Endocrinol. Metab.* **89**, 4963.

128A. Houstis, N *et al.* (2006) ROS have a causal role in multiple forms of insulin resistance. *Nature* **440**, 944.

129. Chander, PN *et al.* (2004) Nephropathy in ZDF rat is associated with oxidative and nitrosative stress: prevention by chronic therapy with a $ONOO^-$ scavenger ebselen. *J. Am. Soc. Nephrol.* **15**, 2391.

130. Monnier, VM (2001) Transition metals redox: reviving an old plot for diabetic vascular disease. *J. Clin. Invest.* **107**, 799.

131. McClung, JP *et al.* (2004) Development of insulin resistance and obesity in mice overexpressing cellular GPx. *Proc. Natl. Acad. Sci. USA* **101**, 8852.

132. Sacco, M *et al.* (2003) Primary prevention of cardiovascular events with low-dose aspirin and vitamin E in type 2 diabetic patients. *Diabetes Care* **26**, 3264.

133. Sola, S *et al.* (2005) Irbesartan and lipoic acid improve endothelial function and reduce markers of inflammation in the metabolic syndrome. *Circulation* **111**, 343.

134. Lee, DH *et al.* (2004) Does supplemental vitamin C increase cardiovascular disease risk in women with diabetes? *Am. J. Clin. Nutr.* **80**, 1194.

135. Carden, DL and Granger, DN (2000) Pathophysiology of ischaemia-reperfusion injury. *J. Pathol.* **190**, 255.

136. Harrison, R (2002) Structure and function of XOR: where are we now? *Free Rad. Biol. Med.* **33**, 774.

137. Szakmany, T *et al.* (2003) Lack of effect of prophylactic *N*-acetylcysteine on postoperative organ dysfunction following major abdominal tumour surgery: randomized, placebo-controlled, double-blinded clinical trial. *Anaesth. Intes. Care* **31**, 267.

138. Nathens, AB *et al.* (2002) Randomized, prospective trial of antioxidant supplementation in critically ill surgical patients. *Ann. Surg.* **236**, 814.

139. Mallick, IH *et al.* (2004) Ischemia-reperfusion injury of the intestine and protective strategies against injury. *Dig. Dis. Sci.* **49**, 1359.

140. Powell, CS and Jackson, RM (2003) Mitochondrial complex I, aconitase, and succinate dehydrogenase during hypoxia-reoxygenation: modulation of enzyme activities by MnSOD. *Am. J. Physiol.* **285**, L189.

141. Nielsen, VG *et al.* (1997) XO mediates myocardial injury after hepatoenteric ischemia-reperfusion. *Crit. Care Med.* **25**, 1044.

142. Bianciardi, P *et al.* (2004) XOR activity in ischemic human and rat intestine. *Free Radic. Res.* **38**, 919.

143. Stahl, GL *et al.* (1992) H_2O_2-induced cardiovascular reflexes. *Circ. Res.* **71**, 295.

144. Li, G *et al.* (1997) Catalase-overexpressing transgenic mouse heart is resistant to ischemia-reperfusion injury. *Am. J. Physiol.* **273**, H1090.

145. Jain, M *et al.* (2004) Increased myocardial dysfunction after ischemia-reperfusion in mice lacking G6PDH. *Circulation* **109**, 898.

146. Forgione, MA *et al.* (2002) Heterozygous cellular GPx deficiency in the mouse. *Circulation* **106**, 1154.

147. Bernier, M *et al.* (1989) Reperfusion arrhythmias: dose-related protection by anti-free-radical interventions. *Am. J. Physiol.* **256**, H1344.

148. Bolli, R and Marbán (1999) Molecular and cellular mechanisms of myocardial stunning. *Physiol. Rev.* **79**, 609.

149. Li, Q *et al.* (2001) Gene therapy with EC-SOD protects conscious rabbits against myocardial infarction. *Circulation* **103**, 1893.

150. Xia, Y *et al.* (1996) Adenosine deaminase inhibition prevents free radical-mediated injury in the post-ischemic heart. *J. Biol. Chem.* **271**, 10096.

151. Lasley, RD *et al.* (1988) Allopurinol enhanced adenine nucleotide repletion after myocardial ischemia in the isolated rat heart. *J. Clin. Invest.* **81**, 16.

152. Sadek, HA *et al.* (2003) Cardiac ischemia/reperfusion, aging, and redox-dependent alterations in mitochondrial function. *Arch. Biochem. Biophys.* **420**, 201.

153. Granville, DJ *et al.* (2004) Reduction of ischemia and reperfusion-induced myocardial damage by cytochrome P450 inhibitors. *Proc. Natl. Acad. Sci. USA* **101**, 1321.

154. Kakkar, AK and Lefer, DJ (2004) Leukocyte and endothelial adhesion molecule studies in knockout mice. *Curr. Opin. Pharmacol.* **4**, 154.

155. Jordan, JE *et al.* (1999) The role of neutrophils in myocardial ischemia-reperfusion injury. *Cardiovasc. Res.* **43**, 860.

156. Hart, ML *et al.* (2004) Initiation of complement activation following oxidative stress. *Mol. Immunol.* **41**, 165.

157. Xia, Z *et al.* (2005) 15F$_{2t}$-IP exacerbates myocardial ischemia-reperfusion injury of isolated rat hearts. *Am. J. Physiol.* **289**, H1366.

158. Turoczi, T *et al.* (2003) HFE mutation and dietary Fe content interact to increase ischemia/reperfusion injury of the heart in mice. *Circ. Res.* **92**, 1240.

159. Chevion, M *et al.* (1993) Cu and Fe are mobilized following myocardial ischemia: possible predictive criteria for tissue injury. *Proc. Natl. Acad. Sci. USA* **90**, 1102.

160. Puppo, A and Halliwell, B (1988) Formation of $OH^{\bullet}$ in biological systems. Does myoglobin stimulate $OH^{\bullet}$ formation from H_2O_2? *Free Radic. Res. Commun.* **4**, 415.

161. Bolli, R (2001) Cardioprotective function of iNOS and role of $NO^{\bullet}$ in myocardial ischemia and preconditioning: an overview of a decade of research. *J. Mol. Cell. Cardiol.* **33**, 1897.

162. Lokuta, AJ *et al.* (2005) Increased nitration of sarcoplasmic reticulum Ca^{2+}-ATPase in human heart failure. *Circulation* **111**, 988.

163. Maack, C *et al.* (2003) Oxygen free radical release in human failing myocardium is associated with increased activity of Rac1-GTPase and represents a target for statin treatment. *Circulation* **108**, 1567.

164. Takimoto, E *et al.* (2005) Oxidant stress from NOS3 uncoupling stimulates cardiac pathologic remodeling from chronic pressure load. *J. Clin. Invest.* **115**, 1221.

165. Schwedhelm, E *et al.* (2004) Urinary 8-iso-prostaglandin $F_{2\alpha}$ as a risk marker in patients with coronary heart disease. *Circulation* **109**, 843.

166. Cracowski, JL (2004) IPs: an emerging role in vascular physiology and disease? *Chem. Phys. Lipids* **128**, 75.

167. Flaherty, JT *et al.* (1994) Recombinant human SOD (h-SOD) fails to improve recovery of ventricular function in patients undergoing coronary angioplasty for acute myocardial infarction. *Circulation* **89**, 1982.

168. Mumby, S *et al.* (2001) Risk of Fe overload is decreased in beating heart coronary artery surgery compared to conventional bypass. *Biochim. Biophys. Acta* **1537**, 204.

169. Mumby, S *et al.* (2000) Fe overload in paediatrics undergoing cardiopulmonary bypass. *Biochim. Biophys. Acta* **1500**, 342.

170. Matata, BM *et al.* (2000) Off-pump bypass graft operation significantly reduces oxidative stress and inflammation. *Ann. Thorac. Surg.* **69**, 785.

171. Guan, W *et al.* (2003) Effect of allopurinol pretreatment on free radical generation after primary coronary angioplasty for acute myocardial infarction. *J. Cardiovasc. Pharmacol.* **41**, 699.

172. Laurindo, FRM *et al.* (1991) Evidence for $O_2^{\bullet-}$-dependent coronary artery vasospasm after angioplasty in intact dogs. *Circulation* **83**, 1705.

173. Tsimikas, S *et al.* (2004) Percutaneous coronary intervention results in acute increases in oxidized phospholipids and lipoprotein(a). *Circulation* **109**, 3164.

174. Szöcs, K *et al.* (2002) Upregulation of Nox-based NAD(P)H oxidases in restenosis after carotid injury. *Arterio. Thromb. Vasc. Biol.* **22**, 21.

175. Tardif, JC *et al.* (1997) Probucol and multivitamins in the prevention of restenosis after coronary angioplasty. *N. Engl. J. Med.* **337**, 365.

176. Jacobson, GM *et al.* (2003) Novel NAD(P)H oxidase inhibitor suppresses angioplasty-induced $O_2^{\bullet-}$ and neointimal hyperplasia of rat carotid artery. *Circ. Res.* **92**, 637.

177. Laukkanen, MO *et al.* (2002) Adenovirus-mediated EC-SOD gene therapy reduces neointima formation in balloon-denuded rabbit aorta. *Circulation* **106**, 1999.

178. Choy, KJ *et al.* (2003) Coenzyme Q_{10} supplementation inhibits aortic lipid oxidation but fails to attenuate intimal thickening in balloon-injured New Zealand white rabbits. *Free Rad. Biol. Med.* **35**, 300.

179. West, NEJ *et al.* (2001) Enhanced $O_2^{\bullet-}$ production in experimental venous bypass graft intimal hyperplasia. *Arterio. Thromb. Vasc. Biol.* **21**, 189.

180. Coghlan, JG *et al.* (1994) Allopurinol pretreatment improves postoperative recovery and reduces lipid peroxidation in patients undergoing coronary artery bypass grafting. *J. Thorac. Cardiovasc. Surg.* **107**, 248.

181. Davies, MG *et al.* (1996) Lazaroid therapy (methylaminochroman: U83836E) reduces vein graft intimal hyperplasia. *J. Surg. Res.* **63**, 128.

182. Godfried, SL and Deckelbaum, LI (1995) Natural antioxidants and restenosis after percutaneous transluminal coronary angioplasty. *Am. Heart J.* **129**, 203.

183. Hanley, PJ and Daut, J (2005) K_{ATP} channels and preconditioning: A re-examination of the role of mitochondrial K_{ATP} channels and an overview of alternative mechanisms. *J. Mol. Cell. Cardiol.* **39**, 17.

184. Facundo, HTF *et al.* (2006) Ischemic preconditioning requires increases in RO release independent of mitochondrial K^+ channel activity. *Free Rad. Biol. Med.* **40**, 469.

185. Tang, XL *et al.* (2002) Oxidant species trigger late preconditioning against myocardial stunning in conscious rabbits. *Am. J. Physiol.* **282**, H281.

186. Powell, SR *et al.* (2005) Oxidized and ubiquitinated proteins may predict recovery of postischemic cardiac function: essential role of the proteasome. *Antiox. Redox Signal.* **7**, 538.

187. Yamaguchi, T *et al.* (2003) Late preconditioning by ethanol is initiated via an oxidant-dependent signaling pathway. *Free Rad. Biol. Med.* **34**, 365.

188. Shi, Y *et al.* (2005) Delayed cardioprotection with isoflurane: role of ROS and RNS. *Am. J. Physiol.* **288**, H175.

189. Akgür, FM *et al.* (2000) Role of $O_2^{\bullet-}$ in hemorrhagic shock-induced P-selectin expression. *Am. J. Physiol.* **279**, H791.

190. Sanan, S and Sharma, G (1986) Effect of desferrioxamine mesylate (Desferal) in anesthetized dogs with clinical hemorrhagic shock. *Ind. J. Med. Res.* **83**, 655.

191. Salvemini, D and Cuzzocrea, S (2002) Oxidative stress in septic shock and disseminated intravascular coagulation. *Free Rad. Biol. Med.* **33**, 1173.

192. Victor, VM *et al.* (2005) Role of free radicals in sepsis: antioxidant therapy. *Curr. Pharm. Des.* **11**, 3141.

193. Cui, X *et al.* (2004) Severity of sepsis alters the effects of $O_2^{\bullet-}$ inhibition in a rat sepsis model. *J. Appl. Physiol.* **97**, 1349.

194. Ophir, A *et al.* (1993) $OH^{\bullet}$ generation in the cat retina during reperfusion following ischemia. *Exp. Eye Res.* **57**, 351.

195. Crawford, RMM and Braendle, R (1996) O_2 deprivation stress in a changing environment. *J. Exp. Bot.* **47**, 145.

196. Piantadosi, CA (2002) Biological chemistry of CO. *Antiox. Redox Signal.* **4**, 259.

197. Thom, SR *et al.* (2004) Delayed neuropathology after CO poisoning is immune-mediated. *Proc. Natl. Acad. Sci. USA* **101**, 13660.

198. Bailey, SR *et al.* (2005) ROS from smooth muscle mitochondria initiate cold-induced constriction of cutaneous arteries. *Am. J. Physiol.* **289**, H243.

199. Muelleman, RL *et al.* (1997) The use of pegorgotein in the treatment of frostbite. *Wilderness Environ. Med.* **8**, 17.

200. Hermes-Lima, M and Storey, KB (1993) Antioxidant defenses in the tolerance of freezing and anoxia by garter snakes. *Am. J. Physiol.* **265**, R646.

201. Buzadzic, B *et al.* (1990) Antioxidant defenses in the ground squirrel, *Citellus citellus*. 2. The effect of hibernation. *Free Rad. Biol. Med.* **9**, 407.

202. Phillips, CL and Grunstein, RR (2006) Obstructive sleep apnoea: time for a radical change ? *Eur. Resp. J.* **27**, 671.

203. Møller, P *et al.* (2001) Acute hypoxia and hypoxic exercise induce DNA strand breaks and oxidative DNA damage in humans. *FASEB J.* **15**, 1181.

204. Phillips, M *et al.* (2004) Heart allograft rejection: detection with breath alkanes in low levels (the HARDBALL study). *J. Heart Lung Transplant.* **23**, 701.

205. Fang, JC *et al.* (2002) Effect of vitamins C and E on progression of transplant-associated arteriosclerosis: a randomized trial. *Lancet* **359**, 1108.

206. Ollinger, R *et al.* (2005) Bilirubin. *Circulation* **112**, 1030.

207. Pollak, R *et al.* (1993) A randomized double-blind trial of the use of human recombinant SOD in renal transplantation. *Transplantation* **55**, 57.

208. Elsner, R *et al.* (1998) Diving seals, ischemia-reperfusion and O_2 radicals. *Comp. Biochem. Physiol., Part A* **119**, 975.

209. MacMillan-Crow, LA *et al.* (2001) Mitochondrial tyrosine nitration precedes chronic allograft nephropathy. *Free Rad. Biol. Med.* **31**, 1603.

210. Rauen, U *et al.* (2000) Hypothermia injury/cold-induced apoptosis-evidence of an increase in

chelatable Fe causing oxidative injury in spite of low $O_2^{\bullet-}/H_2O_2$ formation. *FASEB J.* **14**, 1953.

211. Risby, TH *et al.* (1994) Evidence for free radical-mediated lipid peroxidation at reperfusion of human orthotopic liver transplants. *Surgery* **115**, 94.

212. Grezzana, TJM *et al.* (2004) Oxidative stress, hepatocellular integrity, and hepatic function after initial reperfusion in human hepatic transplantation. *Transplant. Proc.* **36**, 843.

213. Burke, A *et al.* (2002) A prospective analysis of oxidative stress and liver transplantation. *Tranplantation* **74**, 217.

214. Martin, HM *et al.* (2004) XOR is present in bile ducts of normal and cirrhotic liver. *Free Rad. Biol. Med.* **37**, 1214.

215. Schemmer, P *et al.* (1999) Reperfusion injury in livers due to gentle *in situ* organ manipulation during harvest involves hypoxia and free radicals. *J. Pharmacol. Exp. Ther.* **290**, 235.

216. Zwacka, RM *et al.* (1998) Redox gene therapy for ischemia/reperfusion injury of the liver reduces AP1 and NFκB activation. *Nature Med.* **4**, 698.

217. Ward, PH *et al.* (1992) O_2-derived free radicals mediate liver damage in rats subjected to tourniquet shock. *Free Radic. Res. Commun.* **17**, 313.

218. Park, JW *et al.* (2005) Skeletal muscle reperfusion injury is enhanced in ECSOD knockout mouse. *Am. J. Physiol.* **289**, H181.

219. Pattwell, D *et al.* (2003) Ischemia and reperfusion of skeletal muscle lead to the appearance of a stable lipid free radical in the circulation. *Am. J. Physiol.* **284**, H2400.

220. Dorion, D *et al.* (1993) Role of XO in reperfusion injury of ischemic skeletal muscles in the pig and human. *J. Appl. Physiol.* **75**, 246.

221. Soong, CV *et al.* (1994) Reduction of free radical generation minimizes lower limb swelling following femoropopliteal bypass surgery. *Eur. J. Vasc. Surg.* **8**, 435.

222. Wijnen, MHWA *et al.* (2001) Antioxidants reduce oxidative stress in claudicants. *J. Surg. Res.* **96**, 183.

223. Rossi, P *et al.* (2004) Revascularization decreases 8-isoprostaglandin $F_{2\alpha}$ excretion in chronic lower limb ischemia. *Prostagland. Leuk. Essent. Fatty Acids* **71**, 97.

224. Chiao, JJC *et al.* (1994) Fe delocalization occurs during ischemia and persists on reoxygenation of skeletal muscle. *J. Lab. Clin. Med.* **124**, 432.

225. Murrell, GAC *et al.* (1987) Free radicals and Dupuytren's contracture. *Br. Med. J.* **295**, 1373.

226. Southard, JH and Belzer, FO (1995) Organ preservation. *Ann. Rev. Med.* **46**, 235.

227. Evans, PJ *et al.* (1996) Catalytic metal ions and the loss of GSH from University of Wisconsin preservation solution. *Transplantation* **62**, 1046.

228. Nelson, SK *et al.* (2005) Oxidative stress in organ preservation; a multi-faceted role to cardioplegia. *Biomed. Pharmacother.* **59**, 149.

229. Li, X *et al.* (2004) Metallothionein protects islets from hypoxia and extends islet graft survival by scavenging most kinds of ROS. *J. Biol. Chem.* **279**, 765.

230. Suzuki, K *et al.* (2004) Dynamics and mediators of acute graft attrition after myoblast transplantation to the heart. *FASEB J.* **18**, 1153.

231. Diaz, DD *et al.* (1992) Hematoma-induced flap necrosis and free radical scavengers. *Acta Otolaryngol. Head Neck Surg.* **118**, 516.

232. Kinnula, VL *et al.* (1997) Assessment of XO in human lung and lung transplantation. *Eur. Respir. J.* **10**, 676.

233. Zhang, Q *et al.* (2005) Activation of endothelial NADPH oxidase during normoxic lung ischemia is K_{ATP} channel dependent. *Am. J. Physiol.* **289**, L954.

234. Kozower, BD *et al.* (2003) Immunotargeting of catalase to the pulmonary endothelium alleviates oxidative stress and reduces acute lung transplantation injury. *Nature Biotechnol.* **221**, 392.

235. Thiemermann, C *et al.* (2001) Inhaled CO: deadly gas or novel therapeutic? *Nature Med.* **7**, 534.

236. Reid, D *et al.* (2001) Fe overload and NO$^{\bullet}$-derived oxidative stress following lung transplantation. *J. Heart Lung Transplant.* **20**, 840.

237. Williams, A *et al.* (1999) Compromised antioxidant status and persistent oxidative stress in lung transplant recipients. *Free Radic. Res.* **30**, 383.

238. Gray, KD *et al.* (2004) Pulmonary MnSOD is nitrated following hepatic ischemia-reperfusion. *Surg. Infect.* **5**, 166.

239. Ward, PA (1996) Role of complement in lung inflammatory injury. *Am. J. Pathol.* **149**, 1081.

240. Thiel, M *et al.* (2005) Oxygenation inhibits the physiological tissue-protecting mechanism and thereby exacerbates acute inflammatory lung injury. *PLoS Biol.* **3**, e174.

241. Zergeroglu, MA *et al.* (2003) Mechanical ventilation-induced oxidative stress in the diaphragm. *J. Appl. Physiol.* **95**, 1116.

242. Kassim, SY *et al.* (2005) NADPH oxidase restrains the MMP activity of macrophages. *J. Biol. Chem.* **280**, 30201.

243. van der Vliet, A *et al.* (1996) Oxidative stress in cystic fibrosis: does it occur and does it matter? *Adv. Pharmacol.* **38**, 491.

244. Ballatori, N *et al.* (2005) Molecular mechanisms of GSH transport: role of the MRP/CFTR/ABCC and

OATP/SLC21A families of membrane proteins. *Toxicol. Appl. Pharmacol.* **204**, 238.

245. Shao, MXG and Nadel, JA (2005) Neutrophil elastase induces MUC5AC mucin production in human airway epithelial cells via a cascade involving protein kinase C, ROS, and TNF-α-converting enzyme. *J. Immunol.* **175**, 4009.

246. Wood, LG *et al.* (2003) Improved antioxidant and fatty acid status of patients with CF after antioxidant supplementation is linked to improved lung function. *Am. J. Clin. Nutr.* **77**, 150.

247. Ciofu, O *et al.* (2005) Occurrence of hypermutable *P. aeruginosa* in CF patients is associated with the oxidative stress caused by chronic lung inflammation. *Antimicrob. Ag. Chemother.* **37**, 311.

248. Lepage, G *et al.* (1996) Supplementation with carotenoids corrects increased lipid peroxidation in children with CF. *Am. J. Clin. Nutr.* **64**, 87.

249. Scofield, RH *et al.* (2005) Modification of lupus-associated 60-kDa Ro protein with the lipid oxidation product 4HNE increases antigenicity and facilitates epitope spreading. *Free Rad. Biol. Med.* **38**, 719.

250. Dixit, K *et al.* (2005) Immunological studies on ONOO⁻ modified human DNA. *Life Sci.* **77**, 2626.

251. Heeringa, P *et al.* (1997) Systemic injection of products of activated neutrophils and H_2O_2 in MPO-immunized rats leads to necrotizing vasculitis. *Am. J. Pathol.* **151**, 131.

252. Kurien, BT and Scofield, RH (2003) Free radical mediated peroxidative damage in SLE. *Life Sci.* **73**, 1655.

253. Collins, LV *et al.* (2004) Endogenously oxidized mitochondrial DNA induces *in vivo* and *in vitro* inflammatory responses. *J. Leuk. Biol.* **75**, 995.

254. Buttari, B *et al.* (2005) Oxidized β_2-glycoprotein I induces human dendritic cell maturation and promotes a T helper type 1 response. *Blood* **106**, 3880.

255. Martinuzzo, ME *et al.* (2001) Increased lipid peroxidation correlates with platelet activation but not with markers of endothelial cell and blood coagulation. *Br. J. Haematol.* **114**, 845.

256. Emerit, I *et al.* (1996) $O_2^{\bullet-}$-mediated clastogenesis and anticlastogenic effects of exogenous SOD. *Proc. Natl. Acad. Sci. USA* **93**, 12799.

257. Tafazoli, S *et al.* (2005) Oxidative stress mediated idiosyncratic drug toxicity. *Drug Metab. Rev.* **37**, 311.

258. Cracowski, JL *et al.* (2006) Postocclusive reactive hyperemia inversely correlates with urinary 15-F_{2t}-1P levels in systemic sclerosis. *Free Rad. Biol. Med.* **40**, 1732.

259. Morgan, PE *et al.* (2005) Increased levels of serum protein oxidation and correlation with disease activity in SLE. *Arth. Rheum.* **52**, 2069.

260. Sambo, P *et al.* (2001) Oxidative stress in scleroderma. *Arth. Rheum.* **44**, 2653.

261. Evans, MD *et al.* (2000) Aberrant processing of oxidative DNA damage in SLE. *Biochem. Biophys. Res. Commun.* **273**, 894.

262. Greenwald, RA (1991) Therapeutic usages of oxygen radical scavengers in human diseases: myths and realities. *Free Radic. Res. Commun.* **12–13**, 531.

263. Wang, ZQ *et al.* (2004) A newly identified role for $O_2^{\bullet-}$ in inflammatory pain. *J. Pharmacol. Exp. Ther.* **309**, 869.

264. Iida, M and Saito, K (1999) Failure of endotoxin-free SOD to reduce some paw edemas and adjuvant arthritis in rats. *Inflamm. Res.* **48**, 63.

265. Gutteridge, JMC *et al.* (1995) The behaviour of caeruloplasmin in stored human extracellular fluids in relation to ferroxidase II activity, lipid peroxidation and phenanthroline-detectable Cu. *Biochem. J.* **230**, 517.

266. Halliwell, B (2000) Oral inflammation and RS: a missed opportunity? *Oral Dis.* **6**, 136.

267. Waddington, RJ *et al.* (2000) ROS: a potential role in the pathogenesis of periodontal diseases. *Oral Dis.* **6**, 138.

268. Goulet, V *et al.* (2004) Cleavage of human transferrin by *Porphyromonas gingivalis* gingipains promotes growth and formation of OH•. *Infect. Immun.* **72**, 4351.

269. Sweeney, SE and Firestein, GS (2004) Rheumatoid arthritis: regulation of synovial inflammation. *Int. J. Biochem. Cell Biol.* **36**, 372.

270. Jasin, HE (1993) Oxidative modification of inflammatory synovial fluid IgG. *Inflammation* **17**, 167.

271. McNulty, AL *et al.* (2005) DHA transport in human chondrocytes is regulated by hypoxia and is a physiologically relevant source of ascorbic acid in the joint. *Arth. Rheum.* **52**, 2676.

272. Regan, E *et al.* (2005) EC-SOD and oxidant damage in osteoarthritis. *Arth. Rheum.* **52**, 3479.

273. Darden, AG *et al.* (1996) Osteoclastic $O_2^{\bullet-}$ production and bone resorption: stimulation and inhibition by modulators of NADPH oxidase. *J. Bone Min. Res.* **11**, 671.

274. Parhami, F (2003) Possible role of oxidized lipids in osteoporosis: could hyperlipidemia be a risk factor? *Prostagland. Leuk. Essent. Fatty Acids* **68**, 373.

275. Yang, S *et al.* (2004) Expression of Nox4 in osteoclasts. *J. Cell Biochem.* **92**, 238.

276. Wang, X *et al.* (2004) Overexpression of human MMP-12 enhances the development of inflammatory arthritis in transgenic rabbits. *Am. J. Pathol.* **165**, 1375.

277. Whiteman, M *et al.* (2004) ONOO⁻ mediates Ca-dependent mitochondrial dysfunction and cell death via activation of calpains. *FASEB J.* **18**, 1395.

278. Bates, EJ *et al.* (1985) Inhibition of proteoglycan synthesis by H_2O_2 in cultured bovine articular cartilage. *Biochim. Biophys. Acta* **838**, 221.

279. Schalkwijk, J *et al.* (1986) An experimental model for H_2O_2-induced tissue damage. *Arth. Rheum.* **29**, 532.

280. Maini, SR (2004) Infliximab treatment of rheumatoid arthritis. *Rheum. Dis. Clin. North Am.* **30**, 329.

281. Liew, FY and McInnes, IB (2005) A fork in the pathway to inflammation and arthritis. *Nature Med.* **11**, 601.

282. Grootveld, M *et al.* (1991) Oxidative damage to hyaluronate and glucose in synovial fluid during exercise of the inflamed rheumatoid joint. Detection of abnormal low-molecular-mass metabolites by proton-n.m.r. spectroscopy. *Biochem. J.* **273**, 459.

283. Kaur, H *et al.* (1996) OH$^{•}$ generation by rheumatoid blood and knee joint synovial fluid. *Ann. Rheum. Dis.* **55**, 915.

284. Gutteridge, JM (1987) Bleomycin-detectable Fe in knee-joint synovial fluid from arthritic patients and its relationship to the extracellular antioxidant activities of caeruloplasmin, transferrin and lactoferrin. *Biochem. J.* **245**, 415.

285. Kawasaki, N *et al.* (1994) Determination of non-protein-bound Fe in human synovial fluid by high-performance liquid chromatography with electrochemical detection. *J. Chromatogr. B* **656**, 436.

285A. Kobayashi, H *et al.* (2006) Regulatory role of HO-1 in inflammation of RA. *Arth. Rheum.* **54**, 1132.

286. Grinnell, S *et al.* (2005) Responses of lymphocytes of patients with rheumatoid arthritis to IgG modified by O_2 radicals or $ONOO^-$. *Arth. Rheum.* **52**, 80.

287. Jiang, D *et al.* (2005) Regulation of lung injury and repair by Toll-like receptors and hyaluronan. *Nature Med.* **11**, 1173.

288. Frears, ER *et al.* (1996) Inactivation of TIMP-1 by $ONOO^-$. *FEBS Lett.* **381**, 21.

289. Edwards, SW *et al.* (1983) Decrease in apparent K_m for O_2 after stimulation of respiration of rat polymorphonuclear leukocytes. *FEBS Lett.* **161**, 60.

290. Edmonds, SE *et al.* (1993) An imaginative approach to synovitis-the role of hypoxic reperfusion damage in arthritis. *J. Rheumatol.* **20** (Suppl. 37), 26.

291. Martin, JP Jr and Batkoff, B (1987) Homogentisic acid autoxidation and O_2 radical generation: implications for the etiology of alkaptonuric arthritis. *Free Rad. Biol. Med.* **3**, 241.

292. van de Loo, FAJ *et al.* (2003) Deficiency of NADPH oxidase components p47phox and gp91phox caused granulomatous synovitis and increased connective tissue destruction in experimental arthritis models. *Am. J. Pathol.* **163**, 1525.

293. Hultqvist, M and Holmdahl, R (2005) *Ncf1* (*p47phox*) polymorphism determines oxidative burst and the severity of arthritis in rats and mice. *Cell. Immunol.* **233**, 97.

294. Birukov, KG *et al.* (2004) Epoxycyclopentenone-containing oxidized phospholipids restore endothelial barrier function via Cdc42 and Rac. *Circ. Res.* **95**, 892.

295. Halliwell, B (1995) O_2 radicals, NO$^{•}$ and human inflammatory joint disease. *Ann. Rheum. Dis.* **54**, 505.

296. Yin, MJ *et al.* (1998) The anti-inflammatory agents aspirin and salicylate inhibit the activity of $I\kappa B$ kinase-β. *Nature* **396**, 77.

297. Rigobello, MR *et al.* (2005) Effect of auranofin on the mitochondrial generation of H_2O_2. Role of thioredoxin reductase. *Free Radic. Res.* **39**, 687.

298. Ganz, T (2003) Hepcidin, a key regulator of Fe metabolism and mediator of anemia of inflammation. *Blood* **102**, 783.

299. Winyard, PG *et al.* (1987) Mechanism of exacerbation of rheumatoid synovitis by total-dose-Fe-dextran infusion: *in vivo* demonstration of Fe-promoted oxidant stress. *Lancet* **1**, 69.

300. Roosendaal, G *et al.* (1999) Blood-induced joint damage. *Arth. Rheum.* **42**, 1033.

301. Blake, DR *et al.* (1985) Cerebral and ocular toxicity induced by desferrioxamine. *Q. J. Med.* **219**, 345.

302. Pavlick, KP *et al.* (2002) Role of reactive metabolites of O_2 and N_2 in inflammatory bowel disease. *Free Rad. Biol. Med.* **33**, 311.

303. Keshavarzian, A *et al.* (2003) Increases in free radicals and cytoskeletal protein oxidation and nitration in the colon of patients with inflammatory bowel disease. *Gut* **52**, 720.

304. Seril, DN *et al.* (2003) Oxidative stress and ulcerative colitis-associated carcinogenesis: studies in humans and animal models. *Carcinogenesis* **24**, 353.

305. Drew, JE *et al.* (2005) Novel sites of cytosolic GSH peroxidase expression in colon. *FEBS Lett.* **579**, 6135.

306. Chu, FF *et al.* (2004) Bacteria-induced intestinal cancer in mice with disrupted *Gpx1* and *Gpx2* genes. *Cancer Res.* **64**, 962.

307. Aghdassi, E *et al.* (2003) Antioxidant vitamin supplementation in Crohn's disease decreases oxidative stress: a randomized controlled trial. *Am. J. Gastroenterol.* **98**, 348.

308. D'Inca, R *et al.* (2004) Oxidative DNA damage in the mucosa of ulcerative colitis increases with disease duration and dysplasia. *Inflamm. Bowel Dis.* **10**, 23.

309. Kruidenier, L *et al.* (2003) Attenuated mild colonic inflammation and improved survival from severe Dss-colitis of transgenic CuZnSOD mice. *Free Rad. Biol. Med.* **34**, 753.

310. Aruoma, OI *et al.* (1987) The scavenging of oxidants by sulphasalazine and its metabolites. *Biochem. Pharmacol.* **36**, 3739.

311. Ahnfelt-Ronne, I *et al.* (1990) Clinical evidence supporting the radical scavenger mechanism of 5-aminosalicylic acid. *Gastroenterol.* **98**, 1162.

312. Liu, ZC *et al.* (1995) Oxidation of 5-aminosalicylic acid by HOCl to a reactive iminoquinone. *Drug Metab. Disp.* **23**, 246.

313. Schoenberg, MH *et al.* (1991) The involvement of O_2 radicals in acute pancreatitis. *Klin. Wochenschr.* **69**, 1025.

314. Poch, B *et al.* (1999) The role of polymorphonuclear leukocytes and O_2-derived free radicals in experimental acute pancreatitis: mediators of local destruction and activators of inflammation. *FEBS Lett.* **461**, 268.

315. Altavilla, D *et al.* (2003) Lipid peroxidation inhibition reduces NF-κB activation and attenuates cerulein-induced pancreatitis. *Free Radic. Res.* **37**, 425.

316. Bartsch, H and Nair, J (2005) Accumulation of lipid peroxidation-derived DNA lesions: potential lead markers for chemoprevention of inflammation-driven malignancies. *Mut. Res.* **591**, 34.

317. Uden, S *et al.* (1990) Antioxidant therapy for recurrent pancreatitis: placebo-controlled trial. *Aliment. Pharm. Ther.* **4**, 357.

318. Park, S *et al.* (2004) Amelioration of oxidative stress with ensuing inflammation contributes to chemoprevention of *H. pylori*-associated gastric carcinogenesis. *Antiox. Redox Signal.* **6**, 549.

319. Wang, G *et al.* (2005) Oxidative stress defense mechanisms to counter Fe-promoted DNA damage in *H. pylori. Free Radic. Res.* **39**, 1183.

320. Alamuri, P and Maier, RJ (2004) Methionine sulphoxide reductase is an important antioxidant enzyme in the gastric pathogen *H. pylori. Mol. Microbiol.* **53**, 1397.

321. Kuwahara, H *et al.* (2000) *H. pylori* urease suppresses bactericidal activity of $ONOO^-$ via CO_2 production. *Infect. Immun.* **68**, 4378.

322. Everett, SM *et al.* (2002) Antioxidant vitamin supplements do not reduce ROS activity in *H. pylori* gastritis in the short term. *Br. J. Nutr.* **87**, 3.

323. Keenan, JI *et al.* (2005) NADPH oxidase involvement in the pathology of *H. pylori* infection. *Free Rad. Biol. Med.* **38**, 1188.

324. Gehrke, SG *et al.* (2003) Hemochromatosis and transferrin receptor gene polymorphisms in chronic hepatitis C: impact on Fe status, liver injury and HCV genotype. *J. Mol. Med.* **81**, 780.

325. Horiike, S *et al.* (2005) Accumulation of 8-nitroguanine in the liver of patients with chronic hepatitis C. *J. Hepatol.* **43**, 403.

326. Elchuri, S *et al.* (2005) CuZnSOD deficiency leads to persistent and widespread oxidative damage and hepatocarcinogenesis later in life. *Oncogene* **24**, 367.

327. Jain, SK *et al.* (2002) Oxidative stress in chronic hepatitis C: not just a feature of late stage disease. *J. Hepatol.* **36**, 805.

328. Mezey, E *et al.* (2004) A randomized placebo controlled trial of vitamin E for alcoholic hepatitis. *J. Hepatol.* **40**, 40.

329. Aboutwerat, A *et al.* (2003) Oxidant stress is a significant feature of primary biliary cirrhosis. *Biochim. Biophys. Acta* **1637**, 142.

330. Seki, S *et al.* (2002) Immunohistochemical detection of 8OHdG, a marker of oxidative DNA damage, in human chronic cholecystitis. *Histopathol.* **40**, 531.

331. Massagué, J (2004) G1 cell-cycle control and cancer. *Nature* **432**, 298.

332. Vogelstein, B and Kinzler, KW (2004) Cancer genes and the pathways they control. *Nature Med.* **10**, 789.

333. Bensaad, K and Vousden, KH (2005) Saviour and slayer: the two faces of p53. *Nature Med.* **11**, 1278.

334. Sufan, RI *et al.* (2004) The role of VHL tumor suppressor protein and hypoxia in renal clear cell carcinoma. *Am. J. Physiol.* **287**, F1.

335. Totter, TR (1980) Spontaneous cancer and its possible relationship to O_2 metabolism. *Proc. Natl. Acad. Sci. USA* **77**, 1763.

336. Halliwell, B (2002) Effect of diet on cancer development: is oxidative DNA damage a biomarker? *Free Rad. Biol. Med.* **32**, 968.

337. Zimmerman, R and Cerutti, P (1984) Active O_2 acts as a promoter of transformation in mouse embryo C3H/10T1/2C18 fibroblasts. *Proc. Natl. Acad. Sci. USA* **81**, 2085.

338. Weitzman, SA *et al.* (1985) Phagocytes as carcinogens: malignant transformation produced by human neutrophils. *Science* **227**, 1231.

339. Jackson, JH (1994) Potential molecular mechanisms of oxidant-induced carcinogenesis. *Environ. Health Prespect.* **102** (Suppl. 10), 155.

340. Kensler, TW and Taffe, BG (1986) Free radicals in tumor promotion. *Adv. Free Rad. Biol. Med.* **2**, 347.

341. Cooke, MS *et al.* (2003) Oxidative DNA damage: mechanisms, mutation and disease. *FASEB J.* **17**, 1195.

342. Arbiser, JL *et al.* (2002) Reactive O_2 generated by Nox1 triggers the angiogenic switch. *Proc. Natl. Acad. Sci. USA* **99**, 715.

343. Lim, SD *et al.* (2005) Increased Nox1 and H_2O_2 in prostate cancer. *Prostate* **62**, 200.

344. Rivera, A and Maxwell, SA (2005) The p53-induced gene-6 (proline oxidase) mediates apoptosis through a calcineurin-dependent pathway. *J. Biol. Chem.* **280**, 29346.

345. Nakabeppu, Y *et al.* (2004) The defense mechanisms in mammalian cells against oxidative damage in nucleic acids and their involvement in the suppression of mutagenesis and cell death. *Free Radic. Res.* **38**, 423.

346. Irani, K *et al.* (1997) Mitogen signalling mediated by oxidants in Ras-transformed fibroblasts. *Science* **275**, 1649.

347. Cobbs, CS *et al.* (2001) Evidence for ONOO⁻-mediated modifications to p53 in human gliomas: possible functional consequences. *Arch. Biochem. Biophys.* **394**, 167.

348. Wu, HH *et al.* (1999) Direct redox modulation of p53 protein: potential sources of redox control and potential outcomes. *Gene Ther. Mol. Biol.* **4**, 119.

349. Klaunig, JE and Kamendulis, LM (2004) The role of oxidative stress in carcinogenesis. *Ann. Rev. Pharmacol. Toxicol.* **44**, 239.

350. Pervaiz, S and Clément, MV (2004) Tumor intracellular redox status and drug resistance-serendipity or a casual relationship? *Curr. Pharm. Des.* **10**, 1969.

351. Storz, P (2005) ROS in tumor progression. *Front. Biosci.* **10**, 1881.

352. Oberley, TD (2002) Oxidative damage and cancer. *Am. J. Pathol.* **160**, 403.

353. Radisky, DC *et al.* (2005) Rac1b and ROS mediate MMP-3-induced EMT and genomic instability. *Nature Med.* **436**, 123.

354. Barreiro, E *et al.* (2005) Both oxidative and nitrosative stress are associated with muscle wasting in tumour-bearing rats. *FEBS Lett.* **579**, 1646.

355. Fukuyama, M *et al.* (2005) Overexpression of a novel $O_2^{\bullet-}$-producing enzyme, NOX1, in adenoma and well-differentiated adenocarcinoma of the human colon. *Cancer Lett.* **221**, 97.

356. Petros, JA (2005) mtDNA mutations increase tumorigenicity in prostate cancer. *Proc. Natl. Acad. Sci. USA* **102**, 719.

357. Van Remmen, H *et al.* (2003) Life-long reduction in MnSOD activity results in increased DNA damage and higher incidence of cancer but does not accelerate aging. *Physiol. Genomics* **16**, 29.

358. Hagen, TM *et al.* (1994) Extensive oxidative DNA damage in hepatocytes of transgenic mice with chronic active hepatitis destined to develop hepatocellular carcinoma. *Proc. Natl. Acad. Sci. USA* **91**, 12808.

359. Li, Q *et al.* (2005) Inflammation-associated cancer: NF-κB is the lynchpin. *Trends Immunol.* **26**, 318.

360. Watanabe, N *et al.* (2002) Gene expression profile analysis of rheumatoid synovial fibroblast cultures revealing the overexpression of genes responsible for tumor-like growth of rheumatoid synovium. *Biochem. Biophys. Res. Commun.* **294**, 1121.

361. Swerdlow, AJ *et al.* (2005) Cancer incidence and mortality in patients with insulin-treated diabetes: a UK cohort study. *Br. J. Cancer* **92**, 2070.

362. Olinski, R *et al.* (1995) DNA base modifications and antioxidant enzyme activities in human benign prostatic hyperplasia. *Free Rad. Biol. Med.* **18**, 807.

363. Kondo, S *et al.* (1999) Persistent oxidative stress in human colorectal carcinoma, but not in adenoma. *Free Rad. Biol. Med.* **27**, 401.

364. Hofseth, LJ *et al.* (2003) NO•-induced cellular stress and p53 activation in chronic inflammation. *Proc. Natl. Acad. Sci. USA* **100**, 143.

365. Sawa, T and Ohshima, H (2005) Nitrative DNA damage in inflammation and its possible role in carcinogenesis. *Nitric Oxide* **14**, 91.

366. Kinnula, V and Crapo, JD (2004) SOD in malignant cells and human tumors. *Free Rad. Biol. Med.* **36**, 718.

367. Sander, CS *et al.* (2003) Oxidative stress in malignant melanoma and non-melanoma skin cancer. *Br. J. Dermatol.* **148**, 913.

368. Petkau, A *et al.* (1977) Modification of SOD in rat mammary carcinoma. *Res. Comm. Chem. Pathol. Pharmacol.* **17**, 125.

369. Kamsler, A *et al.* (2001) Increased oxidative stress in ataxia telangiectasia evidenced by alterations in redox state of brains from atm-deficient mice. *Cancer Res.* **61**, 1849.

370. Pagano, G *et al.* (2004) Gender- and age-related distinctions for the *in vivo* prooxidant state in Fanconi anaemia patients. *Carcinogenesis* **25**, 1899.

371. Biasi, F *et al.* (2002) Associated change of lipid peroxidation and TGFβ1 levels in human colon cancer during tumor progression. *Gut* **50**, 361.

372. Weinberg, ED (1996) The role of Fe in cancer. *Eur. J. Cancer Prevent.* **5**, 19.

373. Elliott, RL *et al.* (1993) Breast carcinoma and the role of Fe metabolism. A cytochemical, tissue culture, and ultrastructural study. *Ann. NY Acad. Sci.* **698**, 159.

374. Britten, KJ *et al.* (1986) The distribution of Fe and Fe binding proteins in spleen with reference to Hodgkin's disease. *Br. J. Cancer* **54**, 277.

375. Carmine, T *et al.* (1995) Presence of Fe catalytic for free radical reactions in patients undergoing chemotherapy: implications for therapeutic management. *Cancer Lett.* **94**, 219.

376. Hussain, SP *et al.* (2000) Increased p53 mutation load in nontumorous human liver of Wilson disease and

hemochromatosis: oxyradical overload diseases. *Proc. Natl. Acad. Sci. USA* **97**, 12770.

377. Toyokuni, S (1996) Fe-induced carcinogenesis: the role of redox regulation. *Free Rad. Biol. Med.* **20**, 553.

378. Choudhury, S *et al.* (2003) Evidence of alterations in base excision repair of oxidative DNA damage during spontaneous hepatocarcinogenesis in LEC rats. *Cancer Res.* **63**, 7704.

379. Hecht, SS and Hoffmann, D (1988) Tobacco-specific nitrosamines, an important group of carcinogens in tobacco and tobacco smoke. *Carcinogenesis* **9**, 875.

380. Morgan, RW and Hoffmann, GR (1983) Cycasin and its mutagenic metabolites. *Mut. Res.* **114**, 19.

381. Manderville, RA (2005) A case for the genotoxicity of ochratoxin A by bioactivation and covalent DNA adduction. *Chem. Res. Toxicol.* **18**, 1091.

382. Bolten, JL *et al.* (2000) Role of quinones in toxicology. *Chem. Res. Toxicol.* **13**, 135.

383. Felty, Q *et al.* (2005) Estrogen-induced mitochondrial ROS as signal-transducing messengers. *Biochemistry* **44**, 6900.

384. Burdick, AD *et al.* (2003) Benzo(a)pyrene quinones increase cell proliferation, generate ROS, and transactivate the EGF receptor in breast epithelial cells. *Cancer Res.* **63**, 7825.

385. Gower, JD (1988) A role for dietary lipids and antioxidants in the activation of carcinogens. *Free Rad. Biol. Med.* **5**, 95.

386. Reed, GA *et al.* (1986) Epoxidation of (±)-7,8-dihydroxy-7,8-dihydrobenzo[α]pyrene during (bi) sulfite autoxidation: activation of a procarcinogen by a cocarcinogen. *Proc. Natl. Acad. Sci. USA* **83**, 7499.

387. Van Schooten, FJ *et al.* (2004) MPO-463G → A reduces MPO activity and DNA adduct levels in bronchoalveolar lavages of smokers. *Cancer Epidemiol. Biomark. Prevent.* **13**, 828.

388. O'Brien, ML *et al.* (2005) Role of oxidative stress in peroxisome proliferator-mediated carcinogenesis. *Crit. Rev. Toxicol.* **35**, 61.

389. Qu, B *et al.* (2001) Mechanism of clofibrate hepatotoxicity: mitochondrial damage and oxidative stress in hepatocytes. *Free Rad. Biol. Med.* **31**, 659.

390. Bingham, SA *et al.* (1996) Does increased endogenous formation of *N*-nitroso compounds in the human colon explain the association between red meat and colon cancer? *Carcinogenesis* **17**, 515.

391. Wagner, DA *et al.* (1985) Effects of vitamins C and E on endogenous synthesis of *N*-nitrosoamino acids in humans: precursor-product studies with [^{15}N] nitrate. *Cancer Res.* **45**, 6519.

392. Zhao, K *et al.* (2001) DNA damage by nitrite and ONOO$^-$: protection by dietary phenols. *Meth. Enzymol.* **335**, 296.

393. Appenroth, D *et al.* (1997) Protective effects of vitamin E and C on cisplatin nephrotoxicity in developing rats. *Arch. Toxicol.* **71**, 677.

394. Geller, HM *et al.* (2001) Oxidative stress mediates neuronal DNA damage and apoptosis in response to cytosine arabinoside. *J. Neurochem.* **78**, 265.

395. Ramanathan, B *et al.* (2005) Resistance to paclitaxel is proportional to cellular TAC. *Cancer Res.* **65**, 8455.

396. Fang, J *et al.* (2002) Tumor-targeted delivery of PEG-conjugated D-amino acid oxidase for antitumor therapy via enzymatic generation of H$_2$O$_2$. *Cancer Res.* **62**, 3138.

397. Pelicano, H *et al.* (2004) ROS stress in cancer cells and therapeutic implications. *Drug Resist. Updates* **7**, 97.

398. Kachadourian, R *et al.* (2001) 2-Methoxyestradiol does not inhibit SOD. *Arch. Biochem. Biophys.* **392**, 349.

399. Minotti, G *et al.* (2004) Anthracyclines: molecular advances and pharmacologic developments in antitumor activity and cardiotoxicity. *Pharmacol. Rev.* **56**, 185.

400. Mihm, MJ *et al.* (2002) Intracellular distribution of ONOO$^-$ during doxorubicin cardiomyopathy: evidence for selective impairment of myofibrillar creatine kinase. *Br. J. Pharmacol.* **135**, 581.

401. Cvetković, RS and Scott, LJ (2005) Dexrazoxane. *Drugs* **65**, 1005.

402. Doroshow, JH *et al.* (2001) Oxidative DNA base modifications in peripheral blood mononuclear cells of patients treated with high-dose infusional doxorubicin. *Blood* **97**, 2839.

403. Kotamraju, S *et al.* (2002) Transferrin receptor-dependent Fe uptake is responsible for doxorubicin-mediated apoptosis in endothelial cells. *J. Biol. Chem.* **277**, 17179.

404. Cartoni, A *et al.* (2004) Oxidative degradation of cardiotoxic anticancer anthracyclines to phthalic acids. *J. Biol. Chem.* **279**, 5088.

405. Reszka, KJ *et al.* (2005) Inactivation of anthracyclines by cellular peroxidase. *Cancer Res.* **65**, 6346.

406. Chen, J and Stubbe, J (2005) Bleomycins: towards better therapeutics. *Nature Rev. Cancer* **5**, 102.

407. Gutteridge, JMC and Fu, XC (1981) Enhancement of bleomycin-Fe free radical damage to DNA by antioxidants and their inhibition of lipid peroxidation. *FEBS Lett.* **123**, 71.

408. Nagase, T *et al.* (2002) A pivotal role of cytosolic PLA$_2$ in bleomycin-induced pulmonary fibrosis. *Nature Med.* **8**, 480.

409. Fattman, CL *et al.* (2003) Enhanced bleomycin-induced pulmonary damage in mice lacking EC-SOD. *Free Rad. Biol. Med.* **35**, 763.

410. O'Farrell, PA *et al.* (1999) Crystal structure of human bleomycin hydrolase, a self-compartmentalizing cysteine protease. *Structure* **7**, 619.

411. Hay, JG *et al.* (1987) The effects of Fe and desferrioxamine on the lung injury produced by intravenous bleomycin and hyperoxia. *Free Radic. Res. Commun.* **4**, 109.

412. Wang, Q *et al.* (1991) Amelioration of bleomycin-indced pulmonary fibrosis in hamsters by combined treatment with taurine and niacin. *Biochem. Pharmacol.* **42**, 1115.

413. Zhou, Z *et al.* (2005) CO suppresses bleomycin-induced lung fibrosis. *Am. J. Pathol.* **166**, 27.

414. Matsuda, Y *et al.* (1982) Correlation between level of defense against active O_2 in *E. coli* K12 and resistance to bleomycin. *J. Antibiot.* **35**, 931.

415. Factor, VM *et al.* (2000) Vitamin E reduces chromosomal damage and inhibits hepatic tumor formation in a transgenic mouse model. *Proc. Natl. Acad. Sci. USA* **97**, 2196.

416. Venkateswaran, V *et al.* (2004) Antioxidants block prostate cancer in *lady* transgenic mice. *Cancer Res.* **64**, 5891.

417. Pathak, AK *et al.* (2005) Chemotherapy alone vs. chemotherapy plus high dose multiple antioxidants in patients with advanced non small cell lung cancer. *J. Am. Coll. Nutr.* **24**, 16.

418. Lesperance, ML *et al.* (2002) Mega-dose vitamins and minerals in the treatment of non-metastatic breast cancer: an historical cohort study. *Breast Cancer Res. Treat.* **76**, 137.

419. Ladas, EJ *et al.* (2004) Antioxidants and cancer therapy: a systematic review. *J. Clin. Oncol.* **22**, 517.

420. Benner, SE *et al.* (1993) Regression of oral leukoplakia with α-tocopherol: a community clinical oncology program chemoprevention study. *J. Natl. Cancer Inst.* **85**, 44.

421. Carey, J, ed. (2002) *Brain Facts; a Primer on the Brain and Nervous System*. The Society for Neuroscience, Washington DC.

422. Halliwell, B (2006) Oxidative stress and neurodegeneration: where are we now? *J. Neurochem.* **97**, 1634.

423. Fields, RD and Stevens-Graham, B (2002) New insights into neuron-glia communication. *Science* **298**, 556.

424. Ballabh, P *et al.* (2004) The blood-brain barrier: an overview. Structure, regulation, and clinical implications. *Neurobiol. Dis.* **16**, 1.

425. Smith, D *et al.* (2003) Lactate: a preferred fuel for human brain metabolism *in vivo*. *J. Cereb. Blood Flow Metab.* **23**, 658.

426. Zeevalk, GD *et al.* (2005) Mitochondrial inhibition and oxidative stress; reciprocating players in neurodegeneration. *Antiox. Redox Signal.* **7**, 1117.

427. Brouillet, E *et al.* (2005) 3-NPA: a mitochondrial toxin to uncover physiological mechanisms underlying striatal degeneration in Huntington's disease. *J. Neurochem.* **95**, 1521.

428. Egan, MF *et al.* (2003) The BDNF va166met polymorphism affects activity-dependent secretion of BDNF and human memory and hippocampal function. *Cell* **112**, 257.

429. Bredt, DS (1999) Endogenous $NO^{\bullet}$ synthesis: biological functions and pathophysiology. *Free Radic. Res.* **31**, 577.

430. Desvignes, C *et al.* (1999) Evidence that the nNOS inhibitor 7-nitroindazole inhibits MAO in the rat: *in vivo* effects on extracellular striatal dopamine and 3,4-dihydroxyphenylacetic acid. *Neurosci. Lett.* **264**, 5.

431. Muscoli, C *et al.* (2004) $O_2^{\bullet-}$-mediated nitration of spinal MnSOD: a novel pathway in NMDA-mediated hyperalgesia. *Pain* **111**, 96.

432. Phillis, JW and O'Regan, MH (2004) A potentially critical role of phospholipases in central nervous system ischemic, traumatic, and neurodegenerative disorders. *Brain Res. Rev.* **44**, 13.

433. Gonzalez-Zulueta, M *et al.* (1998) MnSOD protects nNOS neurons from NMDA and $NO^{\bullet}$-mediated neurotoxicity. *J. Neurosci.* **18**, 2040.

434. Fonfria, E *et al.* (2005) Amyloid β-peptide$_{1-42}$ and H_2O_2-induced toxicity are mediated by TRPM2 in rat primary striatal cultures. *J. Neurochem.* **95**, 715.

435. Wrona, MZ and Dryhurst, G (1998) Oxidation of serotonin by $O_2^{\bullet-}$ radical: implications to neurodegenerative brain disorders. *Chem. Res. Toxicol.* **11**, 639.

436. Burdo, JR and Connor, JR (2003) Brain Fe uptake and homeostatic mechanisms: an overview. *BioMetals* **16**, 63.

437. Schenck, JF and Zimmerman, EA (2004) High-field MRI of brain Fe: birth of a biomarker? *NMR Biomed.* **17**, 433.

438. Lin, D *et al.* (2005) 4-Oxo-2-nonenal is both more neurotoxic and more protein reactive than 4HNE. *Chem. Res. Toxicol.* **18**, 1219.

439. Mark, RJ *et al.* (1997) A role for 4-HNE, an aldehyde product of lipid peroxidation, in disruption of ion homeostasis and neuronal death induced by Aβ. *J. Neurochem.* **68**, 225.

440. Sheu, KF and Blass, JP (1999) The α-KGDH complex. *Ann. NY Acad. Sci.* **893**, 61.

441. Hou, X *et al.* (2004) Isomer-specific contractile effects of a series of synthetic F_2-IPs on retinal and cerebral microvasculature. *Free Rad. Biol. Med.* **36**, 163.

442. Kondo, M *et al.* (2002) 15-Deoxy-$\Delta^{12,14}$-prostaglandin J_2: the endogenous electrophile that induces neuronal apoptosis. *Proc. Natl. Acad. Sci. USA* **99**, 7367.

443. Sinet, PM *et al.* (1980) H_2O_2 production by rat brain *in vivo. J. Neurochem.* **34**, 1421.

444. Nimmerjahn, A *et al.* (2005) Resting microglial cells are highly dynamic surveillants of brain parenchyma *in vivo. Science* **308**, 1314.

445. Miksys, S and Tyndale, RF (2004) The unique regulation of brain cytochrome P450 2 (CYP2) family enzymes by drugs and genetics. *Drug Metab. Rev.* **36**, 313.

446. Howard, LA *et al.* (2003) Brain CYP2E1 is induced by nicotine and ethanol in rat and is higher in smokers and alcoholics. *Br. J. Pharmacol.* **138**, 1376.

447. Krizbai, IA *et al.* (2005) Effect of oxidative stress on the junctional proteins of cultured cerebral endothelial cells. *Cell. Mol. Neurobiol.* **25**, 129.

448. Kim, GW *et al.* (2003) Neurodegeneration in striatum induced by the mitochondrial toxin 3-nitropropionic acid: role of MMP-9 in early blood-brain barrier disruption? *J. Neurosci.* **23**, 8733.

449. Anekonda, TS and Reddy, PH (2006) Neuronal protection by sirtuins in AD. *J. Neurochem.* **96**, 305.

450. Puntambekar, P *et al.* (2005) Essential role of Rac1/NADPH oxidase in NGF induction of TRPV1 expression. *J. Neurochem.* **95**, 1689.

451. Sánchez-Carbente, MR *et al.* (2005) Motoneuronal death during spinal cord development is mediated by oxidative stress. *Cell Death Differ.* **12**, 279.

452. Burmester, T and Hankeln, T (2004) Neuroglobin: a respiratory protein of the nervous system. *News Physiol. Sci.* **19**, 110.

453. Patenaude, A *et al.* (2005) Emerging roles of thioredoxin cycle enzymes in the CNS. *Cell Mol. Life Sci.* **62**, 1063.

454. Melov, S *et al.* (1998) A novel neurological phenotype in mice lacking mitochondrial MnSOD. *Nature Genet.* **18**, 159.

455. Thiels, E *et al.* (2000) Impairment of long-term potentiation and associative memory in mice that overexpress EC-SOD. *J. Neurosci.* **20**, 7631.

456. Demchenko, IT *et al.* (2002) Regulation of the brain's vascular responses to O_2. *Circ. Res.* **91**, 1031.

457. Klivenyi, P *et al.* (2000) Mice deficient in cellular GPx show increased vulnerability to malonate, 3-nitropropionic acid, and MPTP. *J. Neurosci.* **20**, 1.

458. Valentine, WM *et al.* (2005) Brainstem axonal degeneration in mice with deletion of selenoprotein P. *Toxicol. Pathol.* **33**, 570.

459. Dringen, R *et al.* (2005) Peroxide detoxification by brain cells. *J. Neurosci. Res.* **79**, 157.

460. Ong, WY *et al.* (2000) Changes in GSH in the hippocampus of rats injected with kainate: depletion in neurons and upregulation in glia. *Exp. Brain Res.* **132**, 510.

461. Wong, PTH *et al.* (2006) High plasma cyst(e)ine level may indicate poor clinical outcome in acute stroke patients: possible involvement of H_2S. *J. Neuropath. Exp. Neurol.* **65**, 109.

462. Hovatta, I *et al.* (2005) Glyoxalase 1 and glutathione reductase 1 regulate anxiety in mice. *Nature* **438**, 662.

463. Passage, E *et al.* (2004) Ascorbic acid treatment corrects the phenotype of a mouse model of Charcot-Marie-Tooth disease. *Nature Med.* **10**, 396.

464. Astuya, A *et al.* (2005) Vitamin C uptake and recycling among normal and tumour cells from the CNS. *J. Neurosci. Res.* **79**, 146.

465. Bornstein, SR *et al.* (2003) Impaired adrenal catecholamine system function in mice with deficiency of the ascorbic acid transporter (SVCT2). *FASEB J.* **17**, 1928.

466. Huang, J *et al.* (2001) DHA, a blood-brain barrier transportable form of vitamin C, mediates potent cerebroprotection in experimental stroke. *Proc. Natl. Acad. Sci. USA* **98**, 11720.

467. Roy, S *et al.* (2002) Vitamin E sensitive genes in the developing rat fetal brain: a high-density oligonucleotide microarray analysis. *FEBS Lett.* **530**, 17.

468. Muller, DP and Goss-Sampson, MA (1990) Neurochemical, neurophysiological and neuropathological studies in vitamin E deficiency. *Crit. Rev. Neurobiol.* **5**, 239.

469. Pillai, SR *et al.* (1993) α-Tocopherol concentrations of the nervous system and selected tissues of adult dogs fed three levels of vitamin E. *Lipids* **28**, 1101.

470. Martin, A *et al.* (2002) Roles of vitamins E and C on neurodegenerative diseases and cognitive performance. *Nutr. Rev.* **60**, 308.

471. Mcdonald, SR *et al.* (2005) Concurrent administration of coenzyme Q_{10} and α-tocopherol improves learning in aged mice. *Free Rad. Biol. Med.* **38**, 729.

472. Spencer, JPE *et al.* (2004) Cellular uptake and metabolism of flavonoids and their metabolites: implications for their bioactivity. *Arch. Biochem. Biophys.* **423**, 148.

473. Englander, EW *et al.* (2002) Rat MYH, a glycosylase for repair of oxidatively damaged DNA, has brain-specific isoforms that localize to neuronal mitochondria. *J. Neurochem.* **83**, 1471.

474. Kruman, II *et al.* (2004) Suppression of uracil-DNA glycosylase induces neuronal apoptosis. *J. Biol. Chem.* **279**, 43952.

475. Narasimhaiah, R *et al.* (2005) Oxidative damage and defective DNA repair is linked to apoptosis of migrating neurons and progenitors during cerebral cortex development in Ku70-deficient mice. *Cereb. Cortex* **15**, 696.

476. El-Khamisy, SF *et al.* (2005) Defective DNA single-strand break repair in spinocerebellar ataxia with axonal neuropathy-1. *Nature* **434**, 108.

477. Agarwal, R and Shukla, GS (1999) Potential role of cerebral GSH in the maintenance of blood-brain barrier integrity in rat. *Neurochem. Res.* **24**, 1507.

478. Berry, KAZ and Murphy, RC (2005) Free radical oxidation of plasmalogen glycerophosphocoline containing esterified DHA: structure determination by MS. *Antiox. Redox Signal.* **7**, 157.

479. Montine, TJ *et al.* (2002) Neuronal oxidative damage from activated innate immunity is EP$_2$ receptor-dependent. *J. Neurochem.* **83**, 463.

480. Schaper, M *et al.* (2002) Cerebral vasculature is the major target of oxidative protein alterations in bacteria meningitis. *J. Neuropathol. Exp. Neurol.* **61**, 605.

481. Kastenbauer, S *et al.* (2002) Oxidative stress in bacterial meningitis in humans. *Neurology* **58**, 186.

482. Gilgun-Sherki, Y *et al.* (2005) Analysis of gene expression in MOG-induced EAE after treatment with a novel brain-penetrating antioxidant. *J. Mol. Neurosci.* **27**, 125.

483. Spitsin, SV *et al.* (2002) Comparison of uric acid and ascorbic acid in protection against EAE. *Free Rad. Biol. Med.* **33**, 1363.

484. Verbeek, R *et al.* (2005) Oral flavonoids delay recovery from experimental autoimmune encephalomyelitis in SJL mice. *Biochem. Pharmacol.* **70**, 220.

485. Tang, J *et al.* (2005) Role of NADPH oxidase in the brain injury of intracerebral hemorrhage. *J. Neurochem.* **94**, 1342.

486. Taylor, JM and Crack, PJ (2004) Impact of oxidative stress on neuronal survival. *Clin. Exp. Pharmacol. Physiol.* **31**, 397.

487. Wagener, KR *et al.* (2003) Heme and Fe metabolism: role in cerebral hemorrhage. *J. Cereb. Blood Flow Metab.* **23**, 629.

488. Pong, K (2004) Ischaemic preconditioning: therapeutic implications for stroke? *Exp. Opin. Ther. Targets* **8**, 1.

489. Choi, DW (2005) Cellular defences destroyed. *Nature* **433**, 696.

490. Liu, PK *et al.* (1996) Damage, repair and mutagenesis in nuclear genes after mouse forebrain ischemia-reperfusion. *J. Neurosci.* **16**, 6795.

491. Endres, M *et al.* (2004) Increased postischemic brain injury in mice deficient in uracil-DNA glycosylase. *J. Clin. Invest.* **113**, 1711.

492. Hurtado, O *et al.* (2003) Inhibition of glutamate release by delaying ATP fall accounts for neuroprotective effects of antioxidants in experimental stroke. *FASEB J.* **17**, 2082.

493. Linder, N *et al.* (1999) Cellular expression of XOR protein in normal human tissues. *Lab. Invest.* **79**, 967.

494. de Bilbao, F *et al.* (2004) Resistance to cerebral ischemic injury in UCP2 knockout mice: evidence for a role of UCP2 as a regulator of mitochondrial GSH levels. *J. Neurochem.* **89**, 1283.

495. Cho, S *et al.* (2005) The class B scavenger receptor CD36 mediates free radical production and tissue injury in cerebral ischemia. *J. Neurosci.* **25**, 2504.

496. Miura, T *et al.* (1998) Temperature-dependent lipid peroxidation of rat brain homogenate. *Res. Commun. Mol. Pathol. Pharmacol.* **100**, 117.

497. Jian, S *et al.* (2003) Feasibility and safety of moderate hypothermia after acute ischemic stroke. *Int. J. Dev. Neurosci.* **21**, 353.

498. Williams, AJ *et al.* (2004) Delayed treatment of ischemia/reperfusion brain injury. *Stroke* **35**, 1186.

499. Van der Worp, HB *et al.* (1998) Dietary vitamin E levels affect outcome of permanent focal cerebral ischemia in rats. *Stroke* **29**, 1002.

500. Asai, A *et al.* (2002) Selective proteasomal dysfunction in the hippocampal CA1 region after transient forebrain ischemia. *J. Cereb. Blood Flow Metab.* **22**, 705.

501. Bayir, H *et al.* (2004) Marked gender effect on lipid peroxidation after severe brain injury in adult patients. *J. Neurotrauma* **21**, 1.

502. Bao, F *et al.* (2004) An anti-CD11d integrin antibody reduces COX expression and protein and DNA oxidation after spinal cord injury in rats. *J. Neurochem.* **90**, 1194.

503. Yu, L *et al.* (2004) Selective inactivation or reconstitution of adenosine A$_{2A}$ receptors in bone marrow cells reveals their significant contribution to the development of ischemic brain injury. *Nature Med.* **10**, 1081.

504. Bruce, AJ *et al.* (1996) Altered neuronal and microglial responses to excitotoxic and ischemic brain injury in mice lacking TNF receptors. *Nature Med.* **2**, 788.

505. Liu, D *et al.* (2003) Spinal cord injury increases Fe levels: catalytic production of OH$^{•}$. *Free Rad. Biol. Med.* **34**, 64.

506. Macdonald, RL *et al.* (2004) Time course of production of OH$^{\bullet}$ after subarachnoid hemorrhage in dogs. *Life Sci.* **75**, 979.

507. Asaeda, M *et al.* (2005) A non-enzymatic derived arachidonyl peroxide, 8-IP $F_{2\alpha}$, in CSF of patients with aneurysmal subarachnoid hemorrhage participates in the pathogenesis of delayed cerebral vasospasm. *Neurosci. Lett.* **373**, 222.

508. Chang, EF *et al.* (2003) HO-2 protects against lipid peroxidation-mediated cell loss and impaired motor recovery after traumatic brain injury. *J. Neurosci.* **23**, 3689.

509. Qu, Y *et al.* (2005) Effect of targeted deletion of the HO-2 gene on hemoglobin toxicity in the striatum. *J. Cereb. Blood Flow Metab.* **25**, 1466.

510. Watanabe, Y *et al.* (2003) Gene transfer of EC-SOD reduces cerebral vasospasm after subarachnoid hemorrhage. *Stroke* **34**, 434.

511. Halliwell, B (2006) The proteasome: a source and a target of oxidative stress. In: *Ubiquitin and the Proteasome in Neurodegeneration* (Stefanis, L and Keller, JN, eds.), Kluwer, Germany.

512. Ischiropoulos, H and Beckman, JS (2003) Oxidative stress and nitration in neurodegeneration: cause, effect, or association? *J. Clin. Invest.* **111**, 163.

513. Bence, NF *et al.* (2001) Impairment of the ubiquitin-proteasome system by protein aggregation. *Science* **292**, 1552.

514. von Bohlen und Halbach, O *et al.* (2004) Genes, proteins, and neurotoxins involved in PD. *Prog. Neurobiol.* **73**, 151.

515. Andreoletti, O *et al.* (2002) Astrocytes accumulate 4-HNE adducts in murine scrapie and human CJD. *Neurobiol. Dis.* **11**, 386.

516. Sullivan, PG *et al.* (2004) Proteasome inhibition alters neural mitochondrial homeostasis and mitochondria turnover. *J. Biol. Chem.* **279**, 20699.

517. Zhou, B *et al.* (2001) A novel pantothenate kinase gene (*PANK2*) is defective in Hallervorden-Spatz syndrome. *Nature Genet.* **28**, 345.

518. Kruman, II *et al.* (2004) Cell cycle activation linked to neuronal cell death initiated by DNA damage. *Neuron* **41**, 549.

519. Orr, HT (2004) Neuron protection agency. *Nature* **431**, 747.

520. Moore, DJ *et al.* (2005) Molecular pathophysiology of PD. *Ann. Rev. Neurosci.* **28**, 57.

521. Zecca, L *et al.* (2003) Neuromelanin of the substantia nigra: a neuronal black hole with protective and toxic characteristics. *Trends Neurosci.* **26**, 578.

522. Fedorow, H *et al.* (2005) Dolichol is the major lipid component of human substantia nigra neuromelanin. *J. Neurochem.* **92**, 990.

523. Choi, J *et al.* (2004) Oxidative modifications and down-regulation of UCHL1 associated with idiopathic PD and AD. *J. Biol. Chem.* **279**, 13256.

524. Jenner, P (2003) Oxidative stress in PD. *Ann. Neurol.* **53**, S26.

525. The Parkinson Study Group (2004) Levodopa and the progression of PD. *N. Engl. J. Med.* **351**, 2498.

526. Clement, MV *et al.* (2002) The cytotoxicity of dopamine may be an artifact of cell culture. *J. Neurochem.* **81**, 414.

527. Olanow, CW (2004) The scientific basis for the current treatment of PD. *Ann. Rev. Med.* **55**, 41.

528. Glover, V *et al.* (1993) Effect of dopaminergic drugs on SOD: implications for senescence. *J. Neural Trans.* (Suppl.) **40**, 37.

529. Iida, M *et al.* (1999) Dopamine D2 receptor-mediated antioxidant and neuroprotective effects of ropinirole, a dopamine agonist. *Brain Res.* **838**, 51.

530. Przedborski, S *et al.* (2001) The parkinsonian toxin MPTP: a technical review of its utility and safety. *J. Neurochem.* **76**, 1265.

531. Pennathur, S *et al.* (1999) Mass spectrometric quantification of 3-NT, *ortho*-tyrosine, and *o,o'*-dityrosine in brain tissue of MPTP-treated mice, a model of oxidative stress in PD. *J. Biol. Chem.* **274**, 34621.

532. Shang, T *et al.* (2004) MPP^{+}-induced apoptosis in cerebellar granule neurons is mediated by transferrin receptor Fe-dependent depletion of THB and nNOS-derived $O_2^{\bullet-}$. *J. Biol. Chem.* **279**, 19099.

533. Brown, RC *et al.* (2005) Neurodegenerative diseases: an overview of environmental risk factors. *Environ. Health Perspect.* **113**, 1250.

534. McCormack, AL *et al.* (2005) Role of oxidative stress in paraquat-induced dopaminergic cell degeneration. *J. Neurochem.* **93**, 1030.

535. McCormack, AL and Di Monte, DA (2003) Effects of L-dopa and other amino acids against paraquat-induced nigrostriatal degeneration. *J. Neurochem.* **85**, 82.

536. Thiruchelvam, M *et al.* (2005) Overexpresion of SOD or GPx protects against the paraquat + maneb-induced PD phenotype. *J. Biol. Chem.* **280**, 22530.

537. Pezzoli, G *et al.* (1995) *n*-Hexane-induced parkinsonism: pathogenetic hypotheses. *Movement Dis.* **10**, 279.

538. Sanders, SG *et al.* (2001) MRI features of equine nigropallidal encephalomalacia. *Vet. Radiol. Ultrasound.* **42**, 291.

539. Champy, P *et al.* (2004) Annonacin, a lipophilic inhibitor of mitochondrial complex I, induces nigral and striatal neurodegeneration in rats: possible relevance for atypical parkinsonism in Guadeloupe. *J. Neurochem.* **88**, 63.

540. Caboni, P *et al.* (2004) Rotenone, deguelin, their metabolites, and the rat model of PD. *Chem. Res. Toxicol.* **17**, 1540.

541. Zhang, X *et al.* (2005) Neuroprotection by Fe chelator against proteasome inhibitor-induced nigral degeneration. *Biochem. Biophys. Res. Commun.* **333**, 554.

542. McNaught, KSP *et al.* (1998) Isoquinoline derivatives as endogenous neurotoxins in the aetiology of PD. *Biochem. Pharmacol.* **56**, 921.

543. Soto-Otero, R *et al.* (1998) Studies on the interaction between 1,2,3,4-tetrahydro-β-carboline and cigarette smoke: a potential mechanism of neuroprotection for PD. *Brain Res.* **802**, 155.

544. Castagnoli, KP *et al.* (2001) Neuroprotection in the MPTP parkinsonian C57BL/6 mouse model by a compound isolated from tobacco. *Chem. Res. Toxicol.* **14**, 523.

545. Beal, MF (2004) Mitochondrial dysfunction and oxidative damage in AD and PD and coenzyme Q_{10} as a potential treatment. *J. Bioenerg. Biomembr.* **36**, 381.

546. Liu, B and Hong, JS (2003) Role of microglia in inflammation-mediated neurodegenerative diseases: mechanisms and strategies for therapeutic intervention. *J. Pharmacol. Exp. Ther.* **304**, 1.

547. Burke, WJ *et al.* (2003) 3,4-Dihydroxyphenyl-acetaldehyde is the toxic dopamine metabolite *in vivo*: implications for PD pathogenesis. *Brain Res.* **989**, 205.

548. Aoyama, K *et al.* (2006) Neuronal GSH deficiency and age-dependent neurodegeneration in the EAAC1 deficient mouse. *Nature Neurosci.* **9**, 119.

549. Kirik, D *et al.* (2003) Nigrostriatal α-synucleinopathy induced by viral vector-mediated overexpression of human α-synuclein: a new primate model of PD. *Proc. Natl. Acad. Sci. USA* **100**, 2884.

550. Li, W and Lee, MK (2005) Antiapoptotic property of human α-synuclein in neuronal cell lines is associated with the inhibition of caspase-3 but not caspase-9 activity. *J. Neurochem.* **93**, 1542.

551. Kaur, D *et al.* (2003) Genetic or pharmacological Fe chelation prevents MPTP-induced neurotoxicity *in vivo*: a novel therapy for PD. *Neuron* **37**, 899.

552. Betarbet, R *et al.* (2006) Interacting pathways to neurodegeneration in PD. *Neurobiol. Dis.* **22**, 404.

553. Caparros-Lefebvre, D and Steele, J (2005) Atypical parkinsonism on Guadeloupe, comparison with the parkinsonism-dementia complex of Guam, and environmental toxic hypotheses. *Env. Tox. Pharmacol.* **19**, 407.

554. Castegna, A *et al.* (2004) Proteomic analysis of brain proteins in the gracile axonal dystrophy (*gad*) mouse, a syndrome that emanates from dysfunctional UCHL1, reveals oxidation of key proteins. *J. Neurochem.* **88**, 1540.

555. Li, HM *et al.* (2005) Association of DJ-1 with chaperones and enhanced association and colocalization with mitochondrial Hsp70 by oxidative stress. *Free Radic. Res.* **39**, 1091.

556. Mattson, MP (2004) Pathways toward and away from AD. *Nature* **430**, 631.

557. Casserly, I and Topol, E (2004) Convergence of atherosclerosis and AD: inflammation, cholesterol, and misfolded proteins. *Lancet* **363**, 1139.

558. Ravaglia, G *et al.* (2005) Homocysteine and folate as risk factors for dementia and AD. *Am. J. Clin. Nutr.* **82**, 636.

559. Lim, GP *et al.* (2005) A diet enriched with the omega-3 fatty acid DHA reduces amyloid burden in an aged AD mouse model. *J. Neurosci.* **25**, 3032.

560. Piccini, A *et al.* (2005) β-Amyloid is different in normal aging and in AD. *J. Biol. Chem.* **280**, 34186.

561. Dodart, JC *et al.* (2002) Immunization reverses memory deficits without reducing brain Aβ burden in AD model. *Nature Neurosci.* **5**, 452.

562. Park, L *et al.* (2005) NADPH oxidase-derived ROS mediate the cerebrovascular dysfunction induced by the amyloid β peptide. *J. Neurosci.* **25**, 1769.

563. Barnham, KJ *et al.* (2004) Neurodegenerative diseases and oxidative stress. *Nature Rev. Drug Disc.* **3**, 205.

564. Puglielli, L *et al.* (2005) AD β-amyloid activity mimics cholesterol oxidase. *J. Clin. Invest.* **115**, 2556.

565. Abramov, AY *et al.* (2004) β-Amyloid peptides induce mitochondrial dysfunction and oxidative stress in astrocytes and death of neurons through activation of NADPH oxidase. *J. Neurosci.* **24**, 565.

566. Yan, SD and Stern, DM (2005) Mitochondrial dysfunction and AD: role of ABAD. *Int. J. Exp. Path.* **86**, 161.

567. Wang, J *et al.* (2005) Increased oxidative damage in nuclear and mitochondrial DNA in AD. *J. Neurochem.* **93**, 953.

568. Ahmed, N *et al.* (2005) Protein glycation, oxidation and nitration adduct residues and free adducts of CSF in AD and link to cognitive impairment. *J. Neurochem.* **92**, 255.

569. Choi, J *et al.* (2005) Oxidative modifications and aggregation of CuZnSOD associated with AD and PD. *J. Biol. Chem.* **280**, 11648.

570. Makjanic, J *et al.* (1998) Absence of aluminium in neurofibrillary tangles in AD. *Neurosci. Lett.* **240**, 123.

571. Benvenisti-Zarom, L *et al.* (2005) The oxidative neurotoxicity of clioquinol. *Neuropharmacol.* **49**, 687.

572. Zagol-Ikapitte, I *et al.* (2005) PGH$_2$-derived adducts of protein correlate with AD severity. *J. Neurochem.* **94**, 1140.

573. Taubes, G (2003) Insulin insults may spur AD. *Science* **301**, 40.

574. Ong, WY and Halliwell, B (2004) Fe, atherosclerosis, and neurodegeneration: a key role for cholesterol in promoting Fe-dependent oxidative damage? *Ann. NY Acad. Sci.* **1012**, 51.

575. Green, PS *et al.* (2004) Neuronal expression of MPO is increased in AD. *J. Neurochem.* **90**, 724.

576. Markesbery, WR *et al.* (2005) Lipid peroxidation is an early event in the brain in amnestic MCI. *Ann. Neurol.* **58**, 730.

577. Wang, J *et al.* (2006) Increased oxidative damage in nuclear and mtDNA in MCI. *J. Neurochem.* **96**, 825.

578. Blacker, D (2005) Mild cognitive impairment–no benefit from vitamin E, little from donepezil. *N. Engl. J. Med.* **352**, 2439.

579. Montine, TJ *et al.* (2005) F$_2$-IPs in AD and other neurodegenerative diseases. *Antiox. Redox Signal.* **7**, 269.

580. Sultana, R *et al.* (2006) Redox proteomics identification of oxidized proteins in AD hippocampus and cerebellum: an approach to understand pathological and biochemical alterations in AD. *Neurobiol. Aging* In press

581. Shan, X *et al.* (2003) The identification and characterization of oxidized RNAs in AD. *J. Neurosci.* **23**, 4913.

582. Praticò, D *et al.* (2001) Increased lipid peroxidation precedes amyloid plaque formation in an animal model of Alzheimer amyloidosis. *J. Neurosci.* **21**, 4183.

583. Conte, V *et al.* (2004) Vitamin E reduces amyloidosis and improves cognitive function in Tg2576 mice following repetitive concussive brain injury. *J. Neurochem.* **90**, 758.

584. Yao, J *et al.* (2004) Aging, gender and *APOE* isotype modulate metabolism of Alzheimer's Aβ peptides and F$_2$-IPs in the absence of detectable amyloid deposits. *J. Neurochem.* **90**, 1011.

585. Drake, J *et al.* (2003) Oxidative stress precedes fibrillar deposition of AD amyloid β-peptide (1–42) in a transgenic *C. elegans* model. *Neurobiol. Aging* **24**, 415.

586. Li, F *et al.* (2004) Increased plaque burden in brains of APP mutant MnSOD heterozygous knockout mice. *J. Neurochem.* **89**, 1308.

587. Ciechanover, A and Brundin, P (2003) The ubiquitin proteasome system in neurodegenerative diseases: sometimes the chicken, sometimes the egg. *Neuron* **40**, 427.

588. Keck, S *et al.* (2003) Proteasome inhibition by paired helical filament-τ in brains of patients with AD. *J. Neurochem.* **85**, 115.

589. Pratico, D *et al.* (2002) Aluminium modulates brain amyloidosis through oxidative stress in APP transgenic mice. *FASEB J.* **16**, 1138.

589A. Pepys, MB (2006) Amyloidosis. *Ann. Rev. Med* **57**, 223.

590. Yoshida, T *et al.* (2005) The potential role of Aβ in the pathogenesis of age-related macular degeneration. *J. Clin. Invest.* **115**, 2793.

591. Fratta, P *et al.* (2005) Proteasome inhibition and aggresome formation in sporadic inclusion-body myositis and in Aβ-precursor protein-overexpressing cultured human muscle fibers. *Am. J. Pathol.* **167**, 517.

592. Stewart, CR *et al.* (2005) Oxidation of LDL induces amyloid-like structures that are recognized by macrophages. *Biochemistry* **44**, 9108.

593. Fowler, DM *et al.* (2006) Functional amyloid formation within mammalian tissue. *PLOS Biol.* **4**, e6.

594. Suhr, OB *et al.* (2001) Scavenger treatment of free radical injury in familial amyloidotic polyneuropathy: a study on Swedish transplanted and nontransplanted patients. *Scand. J. Clin. Lab. Invest.* **61**, 11.

595. Ando, Y *et al.* (1997) Oxidative stress is found in amyloid deposits in systemic amyloidosis. *Biochem. Biophys. Res. Commun.* **232**, 497.

596. Ando, Y (2003) New therapeutic approaches for familial amyloidotic polyneuropathy (FAP). *Amyloid* **10** (Suppl. 1), 55.

597. Dib, M (2003) Amyotrophic lateral sclerosis. *Drugs* **63**, 289.

598. Valentine, JS *et al.* (2005) CuZnSOD and ALS. *Ann. Rev. Biochem.* **74**, 563.

599. Lee, M *et al.* (2001) Effect of overexpression of wild-type and mutant CuZnSOD on oxidative stress and cell death induced by H$_2$O$_2$, 4-HNE or serum deprivation: potentiation of injury by ALS-related mutant SOD and protection by Bcl-2. *J. Neurochem.* **78**, 209.

600. Williamson, TL and Cleveland, DW (1999) Slowing of axonal transport is a very early event in the toxicity of ALS-linked SOD1 mutants to motor neurons. *Nature Neurosci.* **2**, 50.

601. Pasinelli, P *et al.* (2004) ALS-associated SOD1 mutant proteins bind and aggregate with Bcl-2 in spinal cord mitochondria. *Neuron* **43**, 19.

602. Boillé, S *et al.* (2006) Onset and progression in inherited ALS determined by motor neurons and microglia. *Science* **312**, 1389.

603. Lino, MM *et al.* (2002) Accumulation of SOD1 mutants in postnatal motoneurons does not cause motoneuron pathology or motoneuron disease. *J. Neurosci.* **22**, 4825.

604. von Lewinski, F and Keller, BU (2005) Ca^{2+}, mitochondria and selective motoneuron vulnerability: implications for ALS. *Trends Neurosci.* **28**, 494.

605. Ryberg, H *et al.* (2004) CSF levels of free 3-NT are not elevated in the majority of patients with ALS or AD. *Neurochem. Int.* **45**, 57.

606. Casoni, F *et al.* (2005) Protein nitration in a mouse model of familial ALS. *J. Biol. Chem.* **280**, 16295.

607. Poon, HF *et al.* (2005) Redox proteomics analysis of oxidatively modified proteins in G93A-SOD1 transgenic mice--A model of FALS. *Free Rad. Biol. Med.* **39**, 453.

608. Bogdanov, M *et al.* (2000) Increased oxidative damage to DNA in ALS patients. *Free Rad. Biol. Med.* **29**, 652.

609. Ralph, GS *et al.* (2005) Silencing mutant SOD1 using RNAi protects against neurodegeneration and extends survival in an ALS model. *Nature Med.* **11**, 429.

610. Brown, RH Jr (2005) ALS- a new role for old drugs. *N. Engl. J. Med.* **352**, 1376.

611. Graf, M *et al.* (2005) High dose vitamin E therapy in ALS as add-on therapy to riluzole: results of a placebo-controlled double-blind study. *J. Neural Trans.* **112**, 649.

612. Schulz, JB *et al.* (2000) Oxidative stress in patients with Friedreich ataxia. *Neurology* **55**, 1719.

613. Lodi, R *et al.* (2006) Friedreich's ataxia: from disease mechanisms to therapeutic interventions. *Antiox. Redox. Signal* **8**, 438.

614. Marx, J (2005) Huntington's research points to possible new therapies. *Science* **310**, 43.

615. Klivenyi, P *et al.* (2003) Increased survival and neuroprotective effects of BN82451 in a transgenic mouse model of HD. *J. Neurochem.* **86**, 267.

616. Nguyen, T *et al.* (2005) Clioquinol down-regulates mutant huntingtin expression *in vitro* and mitigates pathology in a HD mouse model. *Proc. Natl. Acad. Sci. USA* **102**, 11840.

617. Dedeoglu, A *et al.* (2003) Creatine therapy provides neuroprotection after onset of clinical symptoms in HD transgenic mice. *J. Neurochem.* **85**, 1359.

618. Collins, SJ *et al.* (2004) Transmissible spongiform encephalopathies. *Lancet* **363**, 51.

619. Wong, BS *et al.* (2001) Increased levels of oxidative stress markers detected in the brains of mice devoid of prion protein. *J. Neurochem.* **76**, 565.

620. McLennan, NF *et al.* (2004) Prion protein accumulation and neuroprotection in hypoxic brain damage. *Am. J. Pathol.* **165**, 227.

621. Klamt, F *et al.* (2001) Imbalance of antioxidant defense in mice lacking cellular prion protein. *Free Rad. Biol. Med.* **30**, 1137.

622. Turnbull, S *et al.* (2003) Generation of H_2O_2 from mutant forms of the prion protein fragment PrP121–131. *Biochemistry* **42**, 7675.

623. Guentchev, M *et al.* (2000) Evidence for oxidative stress in experimental prion disease. *Neurobiol. Dis.* **7**, 270.

624. Minghetti, L *et al.* (2000) Increased brain synthesis of prostaglandin E_2 and F_2-IP in human and experimental transmissible spongiform encephalopathies. *J. Neuropathol. Exp. Neurol.* **59**, 866.

625. Sigurdsson, EM *et al.* (2003) Cu chelation delays the onset of prion disease. *J. Biol. Chem.* **278**, 46199.

626. Mitchison, HM *et al.* (2004) Selectivity and types of cell death in the NCLs. *Brain Pathol.* **14**, 86.

626A. Klionsky DJ (2006) Good riddance to bad rubbish. *Nature* **441**, 819.

627. Lohr, JB *et al.* (2003) Oxidative mechanisms and tardive dyskinesia. *CNS Drugs* **17**, 47.

628. Steele, JC (2005) Parkinsonism-dementia complex of guam. *Mov. Disord.* **20**, S99.

629. Cox, PA *et al.* (2005) Diverse taxa of cyanobacteria produce β-N-methylamino-L-alanine, a neurotoxic amino acid. *Proc. Natl. Acad. Sci. USA* **102**, 5074.

630. Getahun, H *et al.* (2003) Food-aid cereals to reduce neurolathyrism related to grass-pea preparation during famine. *Lancet* **362**, 1808.

631. Hiscott, J *et al.* (2001) Hostile takeovers: viral appropriation of the NF-κB pathway. *J. Clin. Invest.* **107**, 143.

632. Akaike, T (2001) Role of free radicals in viral pathogenesis and mutation. *Rev. Med. Virol.* **11**, 87.

633. Valyi-Nagy, T *et al.* (2000) Herpes simplex virus type 1 latency in the murine nervous system is associated with oxidative damage to neurons. *Virology* **278**, 309.

634. Valyi-Nagy, T and Dermody, TS (2005) Role of oxidative damage in the pathogenesis of viral infections of the nervous system. *Histol. Histopathol.* **20**, 957.

635. Nicolini, A *et al.* (2001) HIV-1 Tat protein induces NF-κB activation and oxidative stress in microglial cultures by independent mechanisms. *J. Neurochem.* **79**, 713.

636. van der Ven, AJAM *et al.* (1998) GSH homeostasis is disturbed in CD4-positive lymphocytes of HIV-seropositive individuals. *Eur. J. Clin. Invest.* **28**, 187.

637. Gross, A *et al.* (1996) Elevated hepatic γ-GCS activity and abnormal sulfate levels in liver and muscle tissue may explain abnormal cysteine and GSH levels in SIV-infected rhesus macaques. *AIDS Res. Hum. Retrovir.* **12**, 1639.

638. Müller, F *et al.* (2000) Virological and immunological effects of antioxidant treatment in patients with HIV infection. *Eur. J. Clin. Invest.* **30**, 905.

639. Batterham, M *et al.* (2001) A preliminary open label dose comparison using an antioxidant regimen to determine the effect on viral load and oxidative stress in men with HIV/AIDS. *Eur. J. Clin. Nutr.* **55**, 107.

640. Stephensen, CB *et al.* (2005) Plasma cytokines and oxidative damage in HIV-positive and HIV-negative adolescents and young adults: a protective role for IL-10? *Free Radic. Res.* **39**, 859.

641. Kondo, N *et al.* (2004) Redox-sensing release of human thioredoxin from T lymphocyte with negative feedback loops. *J. Immunol.* **172**, 442.

642. Gülow, K *et al.* (2005) HIV-1 Tat substitutes for oxidative signaling in activation-induced T cell death. *J. Immunol.* **174**, 5249.

643. Liu, T *et al.* (2004) ROS mediate virus-induced STAT activation. *J. Biol. Chem.* **279**, 2461.

644. Dalpke, AH *et al.* (2003) Oxidative injury to endothelial cells due to EBV-induced autoantibodies against MnSOD. *J. Med. Virol.* **71**, 408.

645. de la Asunción, JG *et al.* (1998) AZT treatment induces molecular and ultrastructural oxidative damage to muscle mitochondria. *J. Clin. Invest.* **102**, 4.

646. Hulgan, T *et al.* (2003) Oxidant stress is increased during treatment of HIV infection. *Clin. Infect. Dis.* **37**, 1711.

647. McComsey, GA and Morrow, JD (2003) Lipid oxidative markers are significantly increased in lipoatrophy but not in sustained asymptomatic hyperlactatemia. *J. Acquir. Immune Defic. Syndr.* **34**, 45.

Chapter 10

1. Ames, BN *et al.* (1993) Oxidants, antioxidants and the degenerative diseases of ageing. *Proc. Natl. Acad. Sci. USA* **90**, 7915.

2. Yan, LJ and Sohal, RS (2000) Prevention of flight activity prolongs the life span of the housefly, *Musca domestica*, and attenuates the age-associated oxidative damage to specific mitochondrial proteins. *Free Rad. Biol. Med.* **29**, 1143.

3. Guarente, L and Picard, F (2005) CR–the *SIR2* connection. *Cell* **120**, 473.

4. Purdom, S and Chen, QM (2003) p66[Shc]: at the crossroad of oxidative stress and the genetics of aging. *Trends Mol. Med.* **9**, 206.

5. Hursting, SD *et al.* (2003) CR, aging and cancer prevention: mechanisms of action and applicability to humans. *Ann. Rev. Med.* **54**, 131.

6. Piper, MD *et al.* (2005) Counting the calories: the role of specific nutrients in extension of life span by food restriction. *J. Gerontol.* **60A**, 549.

7. Halliwell, B (2004) Ageing and disease: from Darwinian medicine to antioxidants. *Innovation* **4**, 13.

8. Keaney, JF *et al.* (2003) Obesity and systemic oxidative stress. *Arterio. Thromb. Vasc. Biol.* **23**, 434.

9. Lau, DC *et al.* (2005) Adipokines: molecular links between obesity and atherosclerosis. *Am. J. Physiol.* **288**, H2031.

10. Furukawa, S *et al.* (2004) Increased oxidative stress in obesity and its impact on metabolic syndrome. *J. Clin. Invest.* **114**, 1752.

11. Willcox, BJ *et al.* (2004) How much should we eat? The association between energy intake and mortality in a 36-year follow-up study of Japanese-American men. *J. Gerontol.* **59A**, 789.

12. Mattison, JA *et al.* (2003) CR in rhesus monkeys. *Exp. Gerontol.* **38**, 35.

13. Hadley, EC *et al.* (2005) The future of aging therapies. *Cell* **120**, 557.

14. Melliou, E and Chinou, I (2005) Chemistry and bioactivity of royal jelly from Greece. *J. Agric. Food Chem.* **53**, 8987.

15. Weinert, BT and Timiras, PS (2003) Theories of aging. *J. Appl. Physiol.* **95**, 1706.

16. Kirkwood, TBL (2005) Understanding the odd science of aging. *Cell* **120**, 437.

17. Finkel, T and Holbrook, NJ (2000) Oxidants, oxidative stress and the biology of ageing. *Nature* **408**, 239.

18. Kenyon, C (2005) The plasticity of aging: insights from long-lived mutants. *Cell* **120**, 449.

19. Murphy, CT *et al.* (2003) Genes that act downstream of DAF-16 to influence the lifespan of *C. elegans*. *Nature* **424**, 277.

20. Herndon, LA *et al.* (2002) Stochastic and genetic factors influence tissue-specific decline in ageing *C. elegans*. *Nature* **419**, 808.

21. Walker, DW *et al.* (2000) Evolution of lifespan in *C. elegans*. *Nature* **405**, 296.

22. Kayser, EB *et al.* (2004) Mitochondrial oxidative phosphorylation is defective in the long-lived mutant *clk-1*. *J. Biol. Chem.* **279**, 54479.

23. Petriv, OI and Rachubinski, RA (2004) Lack of peroxisomal catalase causes a progeric phenotype in *C. elegans*. *J. Biol. Chem.* **279**, 19996.

24. Tatar, M *et al.* (2003) The endocrine regulation of aging by insulin-like signals. *Science* **299**, 1346.

25. Holzenberger, M *et al.* (2003) IGF-1 receptor regulates lifespan and resistance to oxidative stress in mice. *Nature* **421**, 182.

26. Brown-Borg, HM and Rakoczy, SG (2005) GSH metabolism in long-living Ames dwarf mice. *Exp. Gerontol.* **40**, 115.

27. Kurosu, H *et al.* (2005) Suppression of aging in mice by the hormone klotho. *Science* **309**, 1829.

28. van der Horst, A *et al.* (2004) FOXO4 is acetylated upon peroxide stress and deacetylated by the longevity protein hSir2^{SIRT1}. *J. Biol. Chem.* **279**, 28873.

29. Tyner, SD *et al.* (2002) p53 mutant mice that display early ageing-associated phenotypes. *Nature* **415**, 45.

30. Lee, CK *et al.* (2004) The impact of α-lipoic acid, coenzyme Q_{10}, and CR on life span and gene expression patterns in mice. *Free Rad. Biol. Med.* **36**, 1043.

31. Jiang, CH *et al.* (2001) The effects of aging on gene expression in the hypothalamus and cortex of mice. *Proc. Natl. Acad. Sci. USA* **98**, 1930.

32. Blalock, EM *et al.* (2003) Gene microarrays in hippocampal aging: statistical profiling identifies novel processes correlated with cognitive impairment. *J. Neurosci.* **23**, 3807.

33. Lu, T *et al.* (2004) Gene regulation and DNA damage in the ageing human brain. *Nature* **429**, 883.

34. Kayo, T *et al.* (2001) Influences of aging and CR on the transcriptional profile of skeletal muscle from rhesus monkeys. *Proc. Natl. Acad. Sci. USA* **98**, 5093.

35. Pridmore, SA and Adams, GC (1991) The fertility of HD-affected individuals in Tasmania. *Aust. NZ J. Psychiatry* **25**, 262.

36. Martin, GM (2005) Genetic modulation of senescent phenotypes in *Homo sapiens*. *Cell* **120**, 523.

37. Varela, I *et al.* (2005) Accelerated ageing in mice deficient in Zmpste24 protease is linked to p53 signalling activation. *Nature* **437**, 564.

37A. Scaffidi, P and Misteli, T (2006) Lamin-A dependent nuclear defects in human ageing. *Science* **312**, 1059.

38. Campisi, J (2005) Senescent cells, tumor suppression, and organismal aging: good citizens, bad neighbours. *Cell* **120**, 513.

39. Nyström, T (2005) Role of oxidative carbonylation in protein quality control and senescence. *EMBO J.* **24**, 1311.

40. Wood, JG *et al.* (2004) Sirtuin activators mimic CR and delay ageing in metazoans. *Nature* **430**, 686.

41. Walle, T *et al.* (2004) High absorption but very low bioavailability of oral resveratrol in humans. *Drug Metab. Dis.* **32**, 1377.

42. Nemoto, S *et al.* (2004) Nutrient availability regulates SIRT1 through a forkhead-dependent pathway. *Science* **306**, 2105.

43. Massagué, J (2004) G1 cell-cycle control and cancer. *Nature* **432**, 298.

44. Anderson, RM *et al.* (2003) Nicotinamide and *PNC1* govern lifespan extension by CR in *S. cerevisiae*. *Nature* **423**, 181.

45. Nisoli, E *et al.* (2005) CR promotes mitochondrial biogenesis by inducing the expression of eNOS. *Science* **310**, 314.

46. Picard, F *et al.* (2004) Sirt1 promotes fat mobilization in white adipocytes by repressing PPAR-γ. *Nature* **429**, 771.

47. Corton, JC *et al.* (2004) Mimetics of CR include agonists of lipid-activated nuclear receptors. *J. Biol. Chem.* **279**, 46204.

48. Rogina, B and Helfand, SL (2004) Sir2 mediates longevity in the fly through a pathway related to CR. *Proc. Natl. Acad. Sci. USA* **101**, 15998.

49. Sharpless, NE and DePinho, RA (2005) Crime and punishment. *Nature* **436**, 636.

50. Chondrogianni, N *et al.* (2005) Overexpression of proteasome β_5 subunit increases the amount of assembled proteasome and confers ameliorated response to oxidative stress and higher survival rates. *J. Biol. Chem.* **280**, 11840.

51. Ben-Porath, I and Weinberg, RA (2004) When cells gets stressed: an integrative view of cellular senescence. *J. Clin. Invest.* **113**, 8.

52. Itahana, K *et al.* (2004) Mechanisms of cellular senescence in human and mouse cells. *Biogerontol.* **5**, 1.

53. Blander, G *et al.* (2003) SOD1 knock-down induces senescence in human fibroblasts. *J. Biol. Chem.* **278**, 38966.

54. Serra, V *et al.* (2003) EC-SOD is a major antioxidant in human fibroblasts and slows telomere shortening. *J. Biol. Chem.* **278**, 6824.

55. Tchirkov, A and Lansdorp, PM (2003) Role of oxidative stress in telomere shortening in cultured fibroblasts from normal individuals and patients with ataxia-telangiectasia. *Hum. Mol. Genet.* **12**, 227.

56. Opresko, PL *et al.* (2005) Oxidative damage in telomeric DNA disrupts recognition by TRF and TRF2. *Nucl. Acids Res.* **33**, 1230.

57. Foksinski, M *et al.* (2004) Urinary excretion of DNA repair products correlates with metabolic rates as well as with maximum life spans of different mammalian species. *Free Rad. Biol. Med.* **37**, 1449.

58. Barja, G (2004) Aging in vertebrates, and the effect of caloric restriction: a mitochondrial free radical production-DNA damage mechanism? *Biol. Rev.* **79**, 235.

59. Speakman, JR *et al.* (2004) Uncoupled and surviving: individual mice with high metabolism have greater mitochondrial uncoupling and live longer. *Aging Cell* **3**, 87.

60. Moghaddas, S *et al.* (2003) Aging defect at the Q_o site of complex III augments oxyradical production in rat heart interfibrillar mitochondria. *Arch. Biochem. Biophys.* **414**, 59.

61. Knoll, J (1988) The striatal dopamine dependency of life span in male rats. *Mech. Age. Dev.* **46**, 237.

62. Navarro, A and Boveris, A (2004) Rat brain and liver mitochondria develop oxidative stress and lose enzymatic activities on aging. *Am. J. Physiol.* **287**, R1244.

63. Hagen, TM *et al.* (1997) Mitochondrial decay in hepatocytes from old rats: membrane potential declines, heterogeneity and oxidants increase. *Proc. Natl. Acad. Sci. USA* **94**, 3064.

64. Szibor, M and Holtz, J (2003) Mitochondrial ageing. *Basic Res. Cardiol.* **98**, 210.

65. Schubert, C (2005) Deity of disease. *Nature Med.* **11**, 814.

66. Gredilla, R and Barja, G (2005) Minireview: the role of oxidative stress in relation to CR and longevity. *Endocrinol.* **146**, 3713.

67. Rojas, C *et al.* (1993) Relationship between lipid per-oxidation, fatty acid composition, and ascorbic acid in the liver during carbohydrate and CR in mice. *Arch. Biochem. Biophys.* **306**, 59.

68. Lambert, AJ and Merry, BJ (2004) Effect of CR on mitochondrial ROS production and bioenergetics: reversal by insulin. *Am. J. Physiol.* **286**, R71.

69. Hagopian, K *et al.* (2005) Long-term CR reduces proton leak and H_2O_2 production in liver mitochondria. *Am. J. Physiol.* **288**, E674.

70. Barros, MH *et al.* (2004) Higher respiratory activity decreases mitochondrial ROS release and increases life span in *S. cerevisiae*. *J. Biol. Chem.* **279**, 49883.

71. Giorgio, M *et al.* (2005) Electron transfer between cytochrome c and p66^{shc} generates ROS that trigger mitochondrial apoptosis. *Cell* **122**, 221.

72. Cutler, RG (2003) Genetic stability, dysdifferentiation, and longevity determinant genes. In: *Critical Reviews of Oxidative Stress and Ageing* (Cutler, RG and Rodriguez, H eds), p. 1146. World Scientific Press, Singapore.

73. Sampayo, JN *et al.* (2003) Oxidative stress in *C. elegans*: protective effects of SOD/catalase mimetics. *Aging Cell* **2**, 319.

74. Keaney, M *et al.* (2004) SOD mimetics elevate SOD activity *in vivo* but do not retard aging in the nematode *C. elegans*. *Free Rad. Biol. Med.* **37**, 239.

75. Orr, WC *et al.* (2003) Effects of overexpression of CuZn and MnSODs, catalase, and thioredoxin reductase genes on longevity in *D. melanogaster*. *J. Biol. Chem.* **278**, 26418.

76. Poeggeler, B *et al.* (2005) Mitochondrial medicine: neuroprotection and life extension by the new amphiphilic nitrone LPBNAH acting as a highly potent antioxidant agent. *J. Neurochem.* **95**, 962.

77. Ishii, N *et al.* (2004) CoQ_{10} can prolong *C. elegans* lifespan by lowering oxidative stress. *Mech. Ageing Dev.* **125**, 41.

78. Lipman, RD *et al.* (1998) Disease incidence and longevity are unaltered by dietary antioxidant supplementation initiated during middle age in C57BL/6 mice. *Mech. Age. Dev.* **103**, 269.

79. Enioutina, EY *et al.* (2000) Enhancement of common mucosal immunity in aged mice following their supplementation with various antioxidants. *Vaccine* **18**, 2381.

80. Simán, CM and Eriksson, UJ (1996) Effect of BHT on α-tocopherol content in liver and adipose tissue of rats. *Toxicol. Lett.* **87**, 103.

81. Sohal, RS *et al.* (1985) Fe induces oxidative stress and may alter the rate of aging in the housefly, *Musca domestica*. *Mech. Ageing Dev.* **32**, 33.

82. Liu, J *et al.* (2002) Memory loss in old rats is associated with brain mitochondrial decay and RNA/DNA oxidation: partial reversal by feeding acetyl-L-carnitine and/or R-α-LA. *Proc. Natl. Acad. Sci. USA* **99**, 2356.

83. Sun, J *et al.* (2004) Effects of simultaneous over-expression of Cu/ZnSOD and MnSOD on *Drosophila melanogaster* life span. *Mech. Age. Dev.* **125**, 341.

84. van Remmen, H *et al.* (2003) Life-long reduction in MnSOD activity results in increased DNA damage and higher incidence of cancer but does not accelerate aging. *Physiol. Genom.* **16**, 29.

85. Bayne, AV *et al.* (2005) Enhanced catabolism of mitochondrial $O_2^{\bullet-}$/H_2O_2 and aging in transgenic *Drosophila*. *Biochem. J.* **391**, 277.

86. Orr, W *et al.* (2005) Overexpression of γGCS extends life span in *D. melanogaster*. *J. Biol. Chem.* **280**, 37331.

87. Salganik, R *et al.* (2001) Antioxidants selectively protecting neurochemical functions in rats overproducing ROS. *J. Anti Aging Med.* **4**, 49.

88. Poon, HF *et al.* (2005) Proteomic analysis of specific brain proteins in aged SAMP8 mice treated with α-LA: implications for aging and age-related neurodegenerative disorders. *Neurochem. Int.* **46**, 159.

89. van der Loo, B *et al.* (2002) Cardiovascular aging is associated with vitamin E increase. *Circulation* **105**, 1635.

90. Carrillo, MC *et al.* (1992) Age-related changes in antioxidant enzyme activities are region and organ, as well as sex, selective in the rat. *Mech. Ageing Dev.* **65**, 187.

91. Suh, JH *et al.* (2004) Decline in transcriptional activity of Nrf2 causes age-related loss of GSH synthesis, which is reversible with LA. *Proc. Natl. Acad. Sci. USA* **101**, 3381.

92. Kim, HJ and Nel, AE (2005) The role of phase II antioxidant enzymes in protecting memory T cells from spontaneous apoptosis in young and old mice. *J. Immunol.* **175**, 2948.

93. Chung, HY *et al.* (1993) Modulation of renal XOR in aging: gene expression and ROS generation. *J Nutr. Health Aging* **3**, 19.

94. Beier, K *et al.* (1993) The impact of aging on enzyme proteins of rat liver peroxisomes: quantitative analysis by immunoblotting and immunoelectron microscopy. *Virchows Arch., B, Cell Pathol.* **63**, 139.

95. Son, TG *et al.* (2005) Aging effect on MPO in rat kidney and its modulation by calorie restriction. *Free Radic. Res.* **39**, 283.

96. Rebrin, I *et al.* (2003) Effects of age and caloric restriction on GSH redox state in mice. *Free Rad. Biol. Med.* **35**, 626.

97. Calabrese, V *et al.* (2004) Increased expression of Hsp in rat brain during aging: relationship with mitochondrial function and GSH redox state. *Mech. Age. Dev.* **125**, 325.

98. Jones, DP *et al.* (2002) Redox analysis of human plasma allows separation of pro-oxidant events of aging from decline in antioxidant defenses. *Free Rad. Biol. Med.* **33**, 1290.

99. Stuerenburg, HJ and Kunze, K (1999) Concentrations of free carnosine (a putative membrane-protective antioxidant) in human muscle biopsies and rat muscles. *Arch. Gerontol. Geriatr.* **29**, 107.

100. Wilson, JX (2005) Regulation of vitamin C transport. *Ann. Rev. Nutr.* **25**, 105.

101. Zainal, TA *et al.* (2000) CR of rhesus monkeys lowers oxidative damage in skeletal muscle. *FASEB J.* **14**, 1825.

102. Dremina, ES *et al.* (2005) Protein tyrosine nitration in rat brain is associated with raft proteins, flotillin-1 and α-tublulin: effect of biological aging. *J. Neurochem.* **93**, 1262.

103. Kanski, J *et al.* (2005) Proteomic identification of 3-nitrotyrosine-containing rat cardiac proteins: effects of biological aging. *Am. J. Physiol.* **288**, H371.

104. Knyushko, TV *et al.* (2005) 3-Nitrotyrosine modification of SERCA2a in the aging heart: a distinct signature of the cellular redox environment. *Biochemistry* **44**, 13071.

105. Ishii, N *et al.* (2002) Protein oxidation during aging of the nematode *C. elegans*. *Free Rad. Biol. Med.* **33**, 1021.

106. Ward, WF *et al.* (2005) Effects of age and CR on lipid peroxidation: measurement of oxidative stress by F$_2$-IP levels. *J. Gerontol.* **60A**, 847.

107. Youssef, JA *et al.* (2003) Age-dependent, gray matter-localized, brain-enhanced oxidative stress in male Fischer 344 rats: brain levels of F$_2$-IPs and F$_4$-neuroprostanes. *Free Rad. Biol. Med.* **34**, 1631.

108. Stadtman, ER and Berlett, BS (1998) Reactive O$_2$-mediated protein oxidation in aging and disease. *Drug Metab. Rev.* **30**, 225.

109. Cabiscol, E and Levine, RL (1995) Carbonic anhydrase III. Oxidative modification *in vivo* and loss of phosphatase activity during aging. *J. Biol. Chem.* **270**, 14742.

110. Friguet, B (2006) Oxidative protein degradation and repair in ageing and oxidative stress. *FBBS Lett* **580**, 2910.

111. Zeng, BY *et al.* (2005) Proteasomal activity in brain differs between species and brain regions and changes with age. *Mech. Ageing Dev.* **126**, 760.

112. Delaval, E *et al.* (2004) Age-related impairment of mitochondrial matrix aconitase and ATP-stimulated protease in rat liver and heart. *Eur. J. Biochem.* **271**, 4559.

113. Kirkwood, TBL (2005) Time of our lives. *EMBO Rep.* **6**, S4.

114. Stadtman, ER and Levine, RL (2003) Free radical-mediated oxidation of free amino acids and amino acid residues in proteins. *Amino Acids* **25**, 207.

115. Seehafer, SS and Pearce, DA (2006) You say lipofuscin, we say ceroid: defining autofluorescent storage material. *Neuorobiol. Aging* **27**, 576.

116. Chowdhury, PK *et al.* (2004) Generation of fluorescent adducts of MDA and amino acids: toward an understanding of lipofuscin. *Photochem. Photobiol.* **79**, 21.

117. Li, J and Holbrook, NJ (2003) Common mechanisms for declines in oxidative stress tolerance and proliferation with ageing. *Free Rad. Biol. Med.* **35**, 292.

118. Franceschi, C *et al.* (2005) Genes involved in immune response/inflammation, IGF1/insulin pathway and response to oxidative stress play a major role in the genetics of human longevity: the lesson of centenarians. *Mech. Ageing Dev.* **126**, 351.

119. Berzlanovich, AM *et al.* (2005) Do centenarians die healthy? An autopsy study. *J. Gerontol.* **60A**, 862.

120. Riley, SJ and Stouffer, GA (2002) The antioxidant vitamins and coronary heart disease. *Am. J. Med. Sci.* **324**, 314.

121. Morens, DM *et al.* (1996) Case–control study of idiopathic PD and dietary vitamin E intake. *Neurology* **46**, 1270.

122. Gaziano, JM (1994) Antioxidant vitamins and coronary artery disease risk. *Am. J. Med.* **97**, 18S.

123. Christen, WG *et al.* (2000) Design of Physicians' Health Study II–a randomized trial of β-carotene, vitamins E and C, and multivitamins, in prevention of cancer, cardiovascular disease, and eye disease, and review of results of completed trials. *Ann. Epidemiol.* **10**, 125.

124. Gey, KF (1995) Ten-year retrospective on the antioxidant hypothesis of arteriosclerosis: threshold plasma level of antioxidant micronutrients related to minimum cardiovascular risk. *J. Nutr. Biochem.* **6**, 206.

125. Hertog, MGL *et al.* (1993) Dietary antioxidant flavonoids and risk of coronary heart disease; the Zutphen elderly study. *Lancet* **342**, 1007.

126. Neuhouser, ML (2004) Dietary flavonoids and cancer risk: evidence from human population studies. *Nutr. Cancer* **50**, 1.

127. Kardinaal, AF *et al.* (1993) Antioxidants in adipose tissue and risk of myocardial infarctions: the EURAMIC study. *Lancet* **342**, 1379.

128. Su, LCJ *et al.* (1998) Differences between plasma and adipose tissue biomarkers of carotenoids and tocopherols. *Cancer Epidemiol. Biomark. Prev.* **7**, 1043.

129. Halliwell, B (1999) Establishing the significance and optimal intake of dietary antioxidants: the biomarker concept. *Nutr. Rev.* **57**, 104.

130. Velayutham, M *et al.* (2005) GSH-mediated formation of O_2 free radicals by the major metabolite of oltipraz. *Chem. Res. Toxicol.* **18**, 970.

131. Lawlor, DA *et al.* (2004) Those confounded vitamins: what can we learn from the differences between observational versus randomized trial evidence? *Lancet* **363**, 1724.

132. Halliwell, B (2000) The antioxidant paradox. *Lancet* **355**, 1179.

133. Verhagen, H *et al.* (1997) Effect of Brussels sprouts on oxidative DNA-damage in man. *Cancer Lett.* **114**, 127.

134. Priemé, H *et al.* (1997) No effect of supplementation with vitamin E, ascorbic acid or CoQ_{10} on oxidative DNA damage estimated by 8OHdG excretion in smokers. *Am. J. Clin. Nutr.* **65**, 503.

135. Møller, P (2005) Genotoxicity of environmental agents assessed by the alkaline comet assay. *Basic Clin. Pharmacol. Toxicol.* **96** (Suppl. 1), 3.

136. McAnulty, SR *et al.* (2005) Effect of daily fruit ingestion on angiotensin converting enzyme activity, blood pressure, and oxidative stress in chronic smokers. *Free Radic. Res.* **39**, 1241.

137. Stephens, NG *et al.* (1996) Randomised controlled trial of vitamin E in patients with coronary disease: Cambridge Heart Antioxidant Study (CHAOS) *Lancet* **347**, 781.

138. Brown, BG and Crowley, J (2005) Is there any hope for vitamin E? *JAMA* **293**, 1387.

139. Heart Protection Study Collaborative Group (2002). MRC/BHF heart protection study of antioxidant vitamin supplementation in 20,536 high-risk individuals: a randomized placebo-controlled trial. *Lancet* **360**, 23.

140. Miller III , ER *et al.* (2005) Meta-analysis: high-dosage vitamin E supplementation may increase all-cause mortality. *Ann. Intern. Med.* **142**, 37.

141. Kris-Etherton, PM *et al.* (2004) Antioxidant vitamin supplements and cardiovascular disease. *Circulation* **110**, 637.

142. Knekt, P *et al.* (2004) Antioxidant vitamins and coronary heart disease risk: a pooled analysis of 9 cohorts. *Am. J. Clin. Nutr.* **80**, 1508.

143. Kelemen, M *et al.* (2005) Hormone therapy and antioxidant vitamins do not improve endothelial vasodilator function in postmenopausal woman with established coronary artery disease: a substudy of the WAVE trial. *Atherosclerosis* **179**, 193.

144. Lee, IM *et al.* (2005) Vitamin E in the primary prevention of cardiovascular disease and cancer. *JAMA* **294**, 56.

145. Brown, BG *et al.* (2001) Simvastatin and niacin, antioxidant vitamins, or the combination for the prevention of coronary disease. *N. Engl. J. Med.* **345**, 1583.

146. Yang, CS (2000) Vitamin nutrition and gastro-esophageal cancer. *J. Nutr.* **130**, 338S.

147. Bjelakovic, G *et al.* (2004) Antioxidant supplements for prevention of gastrointestinal cancers: a systemic review and meta-analysis. *Lancet* **364**, 1219.

148. Taylor, PR *et al.* (2004) Science peels the onion of Se effects on prostate carcinogenesis. *J. Natl. Cancer. Inst.* **96**, 645.

149. ATBC Study Group (2003) Incidence of cancer and mortality following α-tocopherol and β-carotene supplementation. *JAMA* **290**, 476.

150. Hercberg, S (2005) The history of β-carotene and cancers: from observational to intervention studies. What lessons can be drawn for future research on polyphenols? *Am. J. Clin. Nutr.* **81** (Suppl.), 218S.

151. Wright, ME *et al.* (2004) Development of a comprehensive dietary antioxidant index and application to lung cancer risk in a cohort of male smokers. *Am. J. Epidemiol.* **160**, 68.

152. Hak, AE *et al.* (2003) Plasma carotenoids and tocopherols and risk of myocardial infarction in a low-risk population of US male physicians. *Circulation* **108**, 802.

153. Duffield-Lillico, AJ and Begg, CB (2004) Reflections on the landmark studies of β-carotene supplementation. *J. Natl. Cancer. Inst.* **96**, 1729.

154. Neuhouser, ML *et al.* (2003) Fruits and vegetables are associated with lower lung cancer risk only in the placebo arm of the β-carotene and retinol efficacy trial (CARET). *Cancer Epidemiol. Biomark. Prevent.* **12**, 350.

155. Paolini, M *et al.* (2001) Induction of CYP enzymes and over-generation of O_2 radicals in β-carotene supplemented rats. *Carcinogenesis* **22**, 1483.

156. Wolf, G (2002) The effect of low and high doses of β-carotene and exposure to cigarette smoke on the lungs of ferrets. *Nutr. Rev.* **60**, 88.

157. Galan, P *et al.* (2005) Antioxidant status and risk of cancer in the SU.VI.MAX study: is the effect of supplementation dependent on baseline levels? *Br. J. Nutr.* **94**, 125.

158. Fletcher, AE *et al.* (2003) Antioxidant vitamins and mortality in older persons: findings from the nutrition add-on study to the MRC trial of assessment and management of older people in the community. *Am. J. Clin. Nutr.* **78**, 999.

159. Holmquist, C *et al.* (2003) Multivitamin supplements are inversely associated with risk of myocardial infarction in men and women–Stockholm heart epidemiology program (SHEEP). *J. Nutr.* **133**, 2650.

160. Mitchell, BL *et al.* (2003) Supplementation with vitamins or minerals and immune function: can the elderly benefit? *Nutr. Res.* **23**, 1117.

161. Hemilä, H and Kaprio, J (2004) Vitamin E and respiratory tract infections in elderly persons. *JAMA* **292**, 2834.

162. Giovannucci, E (2005) Tomato products, lycopene, and prostate cancer: a review of the epidemiological literature. *J. Nutr.* **135**, 2030S.

163. Raitt, MH *et al.* (2005) Fish oil supplementation and risk of ventricular tachycardia and ventricular fibrillation in patients with implantable defibrillators. *JAMA* **293**, 2884.

164. Akbar, M *et al.* (2005) DHA: a positive modulator of Akt signaling in neuronal survival. *Proc. Natl. Acad. Sci. USA* **102**, 10858.

165. Shoji, H *et al.* (2006) Effect of DHA and EPA acid supplementation on oxidative stress levels during pregnancy. *Free Radic. Res.* **40**, 379.

166. Zou, CG and Banerjee, R (2005) Homocysteine and redox signaling. *Antiox. Redox Signal.* **7**, 547.

167. Fairfield, KM and Fletcher, RH (2002) Vitamins for chronic disease prevention in adults. *JAMA* **287**, 3116.

168. Reverter-Branchat, G *et al.* (2004) Oxidative damage to specific proteins in replicative and chronological-aged *S. cerevisiae*. *J. Biol. Chem.* **279**, 31983.

169. Heath, ALM *et al.* (2003) Health implication of Fe overload: the role of diet and genotype. *Nutr. Rev.* **61**, 45.

170. Mainous III, AG *et al.* (2005) Fe, lipids, and risk of cancer in the Framingham offspring cohort. *Am. J. Epidemiol.* **161**, 1115.

171. Ren, M *et al.* (2005) The Fe chelator desferrioxamine inhibits atherosclerotic lesion development and decreases lesion Fe concentrations in the cholesterol-fed rabbit. *Free Rad. Biol. Med.* **38**, 1206.

172. Sinha, R *et al.* (2005) Meat, meat cooking methods and preservation, and risk for colorectal adenoma. *Cancer Res.* **65**, 8034.

173. Tanguy, S *et al.* (2003) Ageing exacerbates the cardiotoxicity of H_2O_2 through the Fenton reaction in rats. *Mech. Age. Dev.* **124**, 229.

174. Yokoyama, T *et al.* (2000) Serum vitamin C concentration was inversely associated with subsequent 20-year incidence of stroke in a Japanese rural community. *Stroke* **31**, 2287.

175. Voko, Z *et al.* (2003) Dietary antioxidants and the risk of ischemic stroke: the Rotterdam study. *Neurology* **61**, 1273.

176. Hak, AE *et al.* (2004) Prospective study of plasma carotenoids and tocopherols in relation to risk of ischemic stroke. *Stroke* **35**, 1584.

177. Suter, PM (2000) Effect of vitamin E, vitamin C and β-carotene on stroke risk. *Nutr. Rev.* **58**, 184.

178. Törnwall, ME *et al.* (2004) Postintervention effect of α-tocopherol and β-carotene on different strokes. *Stroke* **35**, 1908.

179. Forster, MJ *et al.* (2000) Reversible effects of long-term CR on protein oxidative damage. *J. Gerontol.* **55**, B522.

180. Radak, Z *et al.* (2001) Regular exercise improves cognitive function and decreases oxidative damage in rat brain. *Neurochem. Int.* **38**, 17.

181. Podewils, LJ *et al.* (2005) Physical activity, *APOE* genotype, and dementia risk: findings from the cardiovascular healthy cognition study. *Am. J. Epidemiol.* **161**, 639.

182. Martin, A *et al.* (2002) Roles of vitamins E and C on neurodegenerative diseases and cognitive performance. *Nutr. Rev.* **60**, 308.

183. Reich, EE *et al.* (2001) Interactions between apoE gene and dietary α-tocopherol influence cerebral oxidative damage in aged mice. *J. Neurosci.* **21**, 5993.

184. Ikeda-Douglas, CJ *et al.* (2004) Prior experience, antioxidants, and mitochondrial cofactors improve cognitive function in aged beagles. *Vet. Ther.* **5**, 5.

185. Andres-Lacueva, C *et al.* (2005) Anthocyanins in aged blueberry-fed rats are found centrally and may enhance memory. *Nutr. Neurosci.* **8**, 111.

186. Youdim, KA *et al.* (2004) Flavonoids and the brain: interactions at the blood–brain barrier and their physiological effects on the central nervous system. *Free Rad. Biol. Med.* **37**, 1683.

187. Carlsen, H *et al.* (2003) Berry intake increases the activity of the γ-glutamylcysteine synthetase promoter in transgenic reporter mice. *J. Nutr.* **133**, 2137.

188. Moosmann, B and Behl, C (2002) Antioxidants as treatment for neurodegenerative disorders. *Expert Opin. Investig. Drugs* **11**, 1407.

189. De Caterina, R *et al.* (2002) LDL level reduction by the HMGCoA inhibitor simvastatin is accompanied by a related reduction of F_2-IP formation in hypercholesterolemic subjects. *Circulation* **106**, 2543.

190. Weinberg, RB *et al.* (2001) Pro-oxidant effect of vitamin E in cigarette smokers consuming high polyunsaturated fat diet. *Arterio. Thromb. Vasc. Biol.* **21**, 1029.

191. Williams, A *et al.* (1999) Compromised antioxidant status and persistent oxidative stress in lung transplant recipients. *Free Radic. Res.* **30**, 383.

192. Rabl, H *et al.* (1993) A multivitamin infusion prevents lipid peroxidation and improves transplantation performance. *Kidney Int.* **43**, 912.

193. Loong, CC *et al.* (2004) Antioxidant supplementation may improve renal transplant function: a preliminary report. *Transplant. Proc.* **36**, 2438.

194. Sanders, SK *et al.* (1997) Vitamin E supplementation of cattle and shelf-life of beef for the Japanese market. *J. Anim. Sci.* **75**, 2634.

195. Halliwell, B (1991) Drug antioxidant effects. A basis for drug selection? *Drugs* **42**, 569.

196. Halliwell, B (1999) Food-derived antioxidants, evaluating their importance in food and *in vivo*. *Food Sci. Agric. Chem.* **1**, 67.

197. Whiteman, M and Halliwell, B (1996) Protection against $ONOO^-$-dependent tyrosine nitration and α_1-antiproteinase inactivation by ascorbic acid. *Free Radic. Res.* **55**, 383.

198. Metz, TO *et al.* (2003) Pyridoxamine traps intermediates in lipid peroxidation reactions *in vivo*. *J. Biol. Chem.* **278**, 42012.

199. Hansson, L *et al.* (1994) Expression and characterization of biologically active human EC-SOD in milk of transgenic mice. *J. Biol. Chem.* **269**, 5358.

200. Somack, R *et al.* (1991) Preparation of long-acting SOD using high molecular weight PEG (41,000–72,000 daltons). *Free Radic. Res. Commun.* **12–13**, 553.

201. Eum, WS *et al.* (2004) *In vivo* protein transduction: biologically active intact PEP-1-SOD fusion protein efficiently protects against ischemic insult. *Free Rad. Biol. Med.* **37**, 1656.

202. Kozower, BD *et al.* (2003) Immunotargeting of catalase to the pulmonary endothelium alleviates oxidative stress and reduces lung transplantation injury. *Nature Biotech.* **21**, 392.

203. Nishikawa, M *et al.* (2005) Inhibition of metastatic tumor growth by targeted delivery of antioxidant enzymes. *J. Control. Release* **109**, 101.

204. Maksimenko, AV *et al.* (2004) The combination of modified antioxidant enzymes for anti-thrombotic protection of the vascular wall: the significance of covalent connection of SOD and catalase activities. *J. Pharm. Pharmacol.* **56**, 1463.

205. Luo, J *et al.* (2002) PEG immediately repairs neuronal membranes and inhibits free radical production after acute spinal cord injury. *J. Neurochem.* **83**, 471.

206. Hernandez-Saavedra, D *et al.* (2005) Anti-inflammatory properties of a chimeric recombinant SOD: SOD2/3. *Biomed. Pharmacother.* **59**, 204.

207. Kubota, Y *et al.* (2004) Significant contamination of SODs and catalases with LPS-like substances. *Toxicol. In Vitro* **18**, 711.

208. Li, Y and Davis, JM (2003) Delivering antioxidants by zip code. *Am. J. Physiol.* **285**, L281.

209. Im, YJ *et al.* (2005) Production of a thermostable archaeal SOR in plant cells. *FEBS Lett.* **579**, 5521.

210. Zhong, Z *et al.* (2002) Viral gene delivery of SOD attenuates experimental cholestasis-induced liver fibrosis in the rat. *Gene Ther.* **9**, 183.

211. Wang, Y *et al.* (2004) Adenovirus-mediated transfer of the 1-cys peroxiredoxin gene to mouse lung protects against hyperoxic injury. *Am. J. Physiol.* **286**, L1188.

212. Day, BJ (2004) Catalytic antioxidants: a radical approach to new therapeutics. *Drug Disc. Today* **9**, 558.

213. Ferrer-Sueta, G *et al.* (2003) Reactions of Mn porphyrins with $ONOO^-$ and carbonate radical anion. *J. Biol. Chem.* **278**, 27432.

214. Konorev, EA *et al.* (2002) Paradoxical effects of metalloporphyrins on doxorubicin-induced apoptosis: scavenging of ROS versus induction of HO-1 *Free Rad. Biol. Med.* **33**, 988.

215. Maples, KR *et al.* (2004) Nitrone-related therapeutics. *CNS Drugs* **18**, 1071.

216. Maples, KR *et al.* (2001) Comparison of the radical trapping ability of PBN, S-PBN and NXY-059. *Free Radic. Res.* **34**, 417.

217. Knecht, KT and Mason, RP (1993) *In vivo* spin trapping of xenobiotic free radical metabolites. *Arch. Biochem. Biophys.* **303**, 185.

218. Ley, JJ *et al.* (2005) Stilbazulenyl nitrone, a second-generation azulenyl nitrone antioxidant, confers enduring neuroprotection in experimental focal cerebral ischemia in the rat: neurobehavior, histopathology, and pharmacokinetics. *J. Pharmacol. Exp. Ther.* **313**, 1090.

219. Goldstein, S *et al.* (2003) The role of oxoammonium cation in the SOD-mimic activity of cyclic nitroxides. *J. Am. Chem. Soc.* **125**, 789.

220. Atamna, H *et al.* (2001) N-*t*-Butyl hydroxylamine is an antioxidant that reverses age-related changes in mitochondria *in vivo* and *in vitro. FASEB J.* **15**, 2196.

221. Collis, CS *et al.* (1993) Comparison of N-methyl hexanoyl hydroxamic acid, a novel antioxidant, with DFO and N-acetylcysteine against reperfusion-induced dysfunctions in isolated rat heart. *J. Cardiovasc. Pharmacol.* **2**, 336.

222. Cuzzocrea, S *et al.* (2004) Potential therapeutic effect of antioxidant therapy in shock and inflammation. *Curr. Med. Chem.* **11**, 1147.

223. Buettner, GR and Sharma, MK (1993) The syringe nitroxide radical-part II. *Free Radic. Res. Commun.* **19**, S227.

224. Haj-Yehia, A *et al.* (2000) Development of 3-nitratomethyl-proxyl (NMP): a novel, bifunctional SOD mimic-NO•-donor. *Drug Dev. Res.* **50**, 528.

225. Takabe, W *et al.* (2006) Chemical structure-dependent gene expression of proteasome subunits via regulation of the ARE. *Free Radic. Res.* **40**, 21.

226. López, GV *et al.* (2005) Design, synthesis, and biological characterization of potential antiatherogenic NO• releasing tocopherol analogs. *Bioorg. Med. Chem.* **13**, 5787.

227. Zhang, WR *et al.* (2001) Attenuation of oxidative DNA damage with a novel antioxidant EPC-K1 in rat brain neuronal cells after transient middle cerebral artery occlusion. *Neurol. Res.* **23**, 676.

228. Andersson, CM *et al.* (1996) Advances in the development of pharmaceutical antioxidants. *Adv. Drug Res.* **28**, 67.

229. Meng, CQ *et al.* (2004) Discovery of novel phenolic antioxidants as inhibitors of VCAM-1 expression for use in chronic inflammatory diseases. *J. Med. Chem.* **47**, 6420.

230. Klivenyi, P *et al.* (2003) Increased survival and neuroprotective effects of BN82451 in a transgenic mouse model of HD. *J. Neurochem.* **86**, 267.

231. Selby, C *et al.* (1996) Inhibition of somatic embryo maturation in Sitka spruce [*Picea sitchensis* (Bong) Carr] by BHT, a volatile antioxidant released by parafilm. *Plant Cell Rep.* **16**, 192.

232. Hill, SS *et al.* (2003) Plasticizers, antioxidants, and other contaminants found in air delivered by PVC tubing used in respiratory therapy. *Biomed. Chromatogr.* **17**, 250.

233. Lyseng-Williamson, KA and Perry, CM (2003) Micronised purified flavonoid fraction. *Drugs* **63**, 71.

234. Wu, CH and Yen, GC (2005) Inhibitory effect of naturally occurring flavonoids on the formation of advanced glycation endproducts. *J. Agric. Food Chem.* **53**, 3167.

235. Frautschy, SA *et al.* (2001) Phenolic anti-inflammatory antioxidant reversal of Aβ-induced cognitive deficits and neuropathology. *Neurobiol. Aging* **22**, 993.

236. Yang, F *et al.* (2005) Curcumin inhibits formation of Aβ oligomers and fibrils, binds plaques, and reduces amyloid *in vivo. J. Biol. Chem.* **280**, 5892.

237. Mandel, S *et al.* (2004) Cell signaling pathways in the neuroprotective actions of the green tea polyphenol (-)-epigallocatechin-3-gallate: implications for neurodegenerative diseases. *J. Neurochem.* **88**, 1555.

238. Hall, ED *et al.* (1997) Pyrrolopyrimidines: novel brain-penetrating antioxidants with neuroprotective activity in brain injury and ischaemia models. *J. Pharmacol. Exp. Ther.* **281**, 895.

239. CRASH trial collaborators (2005) Final results of MRC CRASH, a randomized placebo-controlled trial of intravenous corticosteroid in adults with head injury-outcomes at 6 months. *Lancet* **365**, 1957.

240. Margaill, I *et al.* (2005) Antioxidant strategies in the treatment of stroke. *Free Rad. Biol. Med.* **39**, 429.

241. Watanabe, K *et al.* (2003) Structure-activity relationship of 3-methyl-1-phenyl-2-pyrazolin-5-one (edaravone). *Redox Rep.* **8**, 151.

242. Horwitz, LD (2003) Bucillamine: a potent thiol donor with multiple clinical applications. *Cardiovasc. Drug Rev.* **21**, 77.

243. Marrades, RM *et al.* (1997) Nebulized GSH induces bronchoconstriction in patients with mild asthma. *Am. J. Respir. Crit. Care Med.* **156**, 425.

244. Raju, PA *et al.* (1994) GSH precursor and antioxidant activities of NAc and OTC compared in *in vitro* studies of HIV replication. *AIDS Res. Hum. Retrovir.* **10**, 961.

245. Lee, KS *et al.* (2005) A prodrug of cysteine, OTC, regulates vascular permeability by reducing VEGF expression in asthma. *Mol. Pharmacol.* **68**, 1281.

246. Cotgreave, I (1996) N-Acetylcysteine: pharmacological considerations and experimental and clinical applications. *Adv. Pharmacol.* **38**, 205.

247. Decramer, M *et al.* (2005) Effects of *N*-acetylcysteine on outcomes in COPD (BRONCUS): a randomized placebo-controlled trial. *Lancet* **365**, 1552.

248. Shalansky, SJ *et al.* (2005) NAC for prevention of radiocontrast induced nephrotoxicity: the importance of dose and route of administration. *Heart* **91**, 997.

249. Efrati, S *et al.* (2003) The effect of *N*-acetylcysteine on renal function, NO•, and oxidative stress after angiography. *Kidney Int.* **64**, 2182.

250. Hunninghake, GW (2005) Antioxidant therapy for idiopathic pulmonary fibrosis. *N. Engl. J. Med.* **353**, 2285.

251. Bahat-Stroomza, M *et al.* (2005) A novel antioxidant that crosses the blood brain barrier protects dopaminergic neurons in experimental models of PD. *Eur. J. Neurosci.* **21**, 637.

252. Wilmott, RW *et al.* (2000) MEG inhibits the inflammatory response in a murine model of chronic infection with *Pseudomonas aeruginosa. J. Pharmacol. Exp. Ther.* **292**, 88.

253. Guillonneau, C *et al.* (2003) Synthesis and pharmacological evaluation of new 1,2-dithiolane based antioxidants. *Eur. J. Med. Chem.* **38**, 1.

254. Nair, CKK *et al.* (2001) Radioprotectors in radiotherapy. *J. Radiat. Res.* **42**, 21.

255. Zhao, R and Holmgren, A (2004) Ebselen is a dehydroascorbate reductase mimic, facilitating the recycling of ascorbate via mammalian thioredoxin systems. *Antiox. Redox Signal.* **6**, 99.

256. Sun, Y *et al.* (2004) Se-containing 15-mer peptides with high GPx-like activity. *J. Biol. Chem.* **279**, 37235.

257. Pariagh, S *et al.* (2005) Asymmetric organotellurides as potent antioxidants and building blocks of protein conjugates. *Org. Biomol. Chem.* **3**, 975.

258. Smith, RAJ *et al.* (2003) Using mitochondria-targeted molecules to study mitochondrial radical production and its consequences. *Biochem. Soc. Trans.* **31**, 1295.

259. Adlam, VJ *et al.* (2005) Targeting an antioxidant to mitochondria decreases cardiac ischemia–reperfusion injury. *FASEB J.* **19**, 1088.

260. Prass, K *et al.* (2002) DFO induces delayed tolerance against cerebral ischemia *in vivo* and *in vitro. J. Cereb. Blood Flow Metab.* **22**, 520.

261. Davies, MJ *et al.* (1987) DFO (Desferal) and $O_2^{\bullet-}$. *Biochem. J.* **246**, 725.

262. Persson, HL and Richardson, DR (2005) Fe-binding drugs targeted to lysosomes: a potential strategy for the treatment of inflammatory lung disorders. *Expert Opin. Invest. Drugs* **14**, 997.

263. Le, NTV and Richardson, DR (2003) Potent Fe chelators increase the mRNA levels of the universal cyclin-dependent kinase inhibitor p21$^{CIP1/WAF1}$, but paradoxically inhibit its translation: a potential mechanism of cell cycle dysregulation. *Carcinogenesis* **24**, 1045.

264. Moch, D *et al.* (1995) Protective effects of hydroxyethyl starch-DFO in early sepsis. *Shock* **4**, 425.

265. Duffy, SJ *et al.* (2001) Fe chelation improves endothelial function in patients with coronary artery disease. *Circulation* **103**, 2799.

266. Kalinowski, JS and Richardson, DR (2005) The evolution of Fe chelators for the treatment of Fe overload disease and cancer. *Pharm. Rev.* **57**, 547.

267. Troost, FJ *et al.* (2003) Recombinant human lactoferrin ingestion attenuates indomethacin-induced enteropathy *in vivo* in healthy volunteers. *Eur. J. Clin. Nutr.* **57**, 1579.

268. Di Mario, F *et al.* (2003) Use of bovine lactoferrin for *H. pylori* eradication. *Dig. Liver Dis.* **35**, 706.

269. Hoffbrand, AV *et al.* (2003) Role of deferiprone in chelation therapy for transfusional iron overload. *Blood* **102**, 17.

270. Cappellini, MD (2005) Fe-chelating therapy with the new oral agent ICL670 (Exjade). *Best Pract. Res. Clin. Haematol.* **18**, 289.

271. Kitazawa, M *et al.* (2005) Protective effects of an antioxidant derived from serine and vitamin B_6 on skin photoaging in hairless mice. *Photochem. Photobiol.* **81**, 970.

272. Gal, S *et al.* (2005) Novel multifunctional neuroprotective Fe chelators-MAO inhibitor drugs for neurodegenerative diseases. *In vivo* selective brain MAO inhibition and prevention of MPTP-induced striatal dopamine depletion. *J. Neurochem.* **95**, 79.

273. Simons, JM *et al.* (1990) Metabolic activation of natural phenols into selective oxidative burst agonists by activated human neutrophils. *Free Rad. Biol. Med.* **8**, 251.

274. Cayatte, AJ *et al.* (2001) S17834, a new inhibitor of cell adhesion and atherosclerosis that targets NADPH oxidase. *Arterio. Thromb. Vasc. Biol.* **21**, 1577.

275. O'Mahony, S (2005) Tetomilast. *IDrugs* **8**, 502.

276. Ho, LJ *et al.* (2004) Plant alkaloid tetrandrine downregulates IκBα kinases IκBα-NF-κB signaling pathway in human peripheral blood T cell. *Br. J. Pharmacol.* **143**, 919.

INDEX

The most extensive discussion of any indexed topic is indicated in **bold type** The word 'structure' in parentheses indicates the place in the text where the structure of the compound is shown. The abbreviation 'def.' in parentheses indicates where a term is defined in the text.

A23187 195
Aβ, *see* β-amyloid peptides
Aβ_{1-40} 600–601
Aβ_{1-42} **600–601**, 602
Aβ25–35 600
Aβ-HNE 602
AAPH 51, 52(*structure*), 162, 304, 317, 337, 484, 507, 649
ABAD, *see* Aβ-binding alcohol dehydrogenase
abalone 434
abasic sites 309
ABCR 375–376
abdominal obesity 514
Abelson family 210
abetalipoproteinaemia 171, 173, 631
Aβ-binding alcohol dehydrogenase 601
abl oncogene 547
C-abl tyrosine kinase 124, 210
abscess 429
abscisic acid 429
ABTS 86, 290, 337–339, 340(*structure*), 649
ABTS$^{\bullet+}$ 290, 338, 340(*structure*)
ABTS method 338
acaeruloplasminaemia 139, 581
Acanthamoeba castellanii 90
acanthocytes 173
acatalasaemia 109
  in erythrocytes 348, 349
ACE inhibitors 647
acetaldehyde 108, 255, 457–459, 469
acetaminophen, *see* paracetamol
acetate 255
acetone 14, 82, 114, 457–458, 468, 578
acetonitrile 46
1-acetoxy-3-carbamoyl-2, 2, 5, 5-
      tetramethylpyrrolidine 276(*structure*)
O-acetyl-ADP-ribose 622
2-acetylaminofluorene 558(*structure*), 559
acetylation 440, 548, 627
N-acetylcarnitine 628
acetylcholine 56, 394, 530, 574
  in AD 598

acetylcholinesterase 394, 599
acetyl coenzyme A 10, 397
N-acetylcysteine 386, 393, 481, 516, 527, 567, 582, 585, 647, 667(*structure*)
  against paracetamol 463
  as therapeutic antioxidant 666
  in ALS 605
  in HIV 611
  protection against doxorubicin toxicity 567
N-acetylcysteine amide 582, 668
N-acetyldopamine 454
acetylene 465, 686
N-acetylglucosamine 533(*structure*)
acetyl-LDL receptors 497
N-acetylmethionine 417
N-acetyl-p-benzoquinoneimine 463(*structure*)
acetylphenylhydrazine 351, 352(*structure*)
N$^{\alpha}$-acetyl-N$^{\epsilon}$-(2-propenal)lysine 328(*structure*)
acetylsalicylic acid, *see* aspirin
acetylSCoA, *see* acetyl coenzyme A
N-acetyltransferases 62–63, 440
acetyltyramine-fluorescein probe 333
Achatina Fulica Ferussac 66
Acholeplasma laidlawii 88
achromatic zone 86
acid 687(*def.*)
acid dissociation constant 687(*def.*)
Acidianus ambivalens 90
acidosis 10(*def.*), 116, 583
acid rain 371, 465
acid reflex 542
acivicin 116(*structure*)
aclacinomycin A 266
acne 388, 390, 532
aconitase 10, 19, 39, 97–99, 101, 137, 141, 265, 517, 568, 576, 584, 587, 593, 600, 606
  in ageing 630
aconitase A 208
aconitase assay
  for iron 196
  for superoxide 285, 345